Computed Tomography and Magnetic Resonance Tomography of Intracranial Tumors

A Clinical Perspective

Second, Fully Revised and Expanded Edition

Edited by
E. Kazner · S. Wende · T. Grumme
O. Stochdorph · R. Felix · C. Claussen

Authors
C. Claussen · R. Fahlbusch · R. Felix · T. Grumme · J. Heinzerling
J.R. Iglesias-Rozas · E. Kazner · K. Kretzschmar · M. Laniado
W. Lanksch · W. Müller-Forell · T.H. Newton · W. Schörner
G. Schroth · B. Schulz · O. Stochdorph · G. Sze · S. Wende

With 738 Figures in 2993 Separate Illustrations

Springer-Verlag Berlin Heidelberg NewYork
London Paris Tokyo Hong Kong

Translator: Terry C. Telger, Fort Worth, Texas (USA)

Title of the German Edition: Computer- und Kernspin-Tomographie intrakranieller Tumoren aus klinischer Sicht. Zweite, völlig neubearbeitete und erweiterte Auflage

ISBN-13: 978-3-642-74313-9 e-ISBN-13: 978-3-642-74311-5
DOI: 10.1007/978-3-642-74311-5

Library of Congress Cataloging-in-Publication Data. Computer- und Kernspin-Tomographie intrakranieller Tumoren aus klinischer Sicht. English. Computed tomography and magnetic resonance tomography of intracranial tumors : a clinical perspective / edited by E. Kazner . . . [et al.] ; authors, C. Claussen ... [et al.] ; translator, T.C. Telger. – 2nd, fully rev. and expanded ed. p. cm. Translation of: Computer- und Kernspin-Tomographie intrakranieller Tumoren aus klinischer Sicht. Bibliography : p. Includes index. 1. Brain – Tumors – Diagnosis. 2. Brain – Tomography. 3. Brain – Tumors. I. Kazner, E. (Ekkehard) II. Claussen, Claus, 1945. III. Title. [DNLM : 1. Brain – radiography. 2. Brain Neoplasms – radiography. 3. Magnetic Resonance, Imaging. 4. Orbital Neoplasms – radiography. 5. Tomography, X-Ray Computed. WL 358 C7385] RC280.B7C5713 1989 616.99'2810757 – dc20 DNLM/DLC for Library of Congress. 89-10116 CIP.

Softcover reprint of the hardcover 2nd edition 1989

2122/3130-543210 – Printed on acid-free paper

List of Authors

Prof. Dr. med. Claus Claussen
Oberarzt der Strahlenklinik und Poliklinik der Universitätskliniken Rudolf Virchow der Freien Universität Berlin, Standort Charlottenburg, Spandauer Damm 130, D-1000 Berlin 19

Prof. Dr. med. Rudolf Fahlbusch
Direktor der Neurochirurgischen Klinik der Universität Erlangen-Nürnberg, Schwabachanlage 6, D-8520 Erlangen

Prof. Dr. med. Roland Felix
Direktor der Strahlenklinik und Poliklinik der Universitätskliniken Rudolf Virchow der Freien Universität Berlin, Standort Charlottenburg, Spandauer Damm 130, D-1000 Berlin 19

Prof. Dr. med. Thomas Grumme
Chefarzt der Neurochirurgischen Klinik, Zentralklinikum Augsburg, Stenglinstraße, D-8900 Augsburg

Dr. rer. nat. Jürgen Heinzerling
C.H.F. Müller, UB der Philips GmbH, Röntgenstraße 24, D-2000 Hamburg 63

Priv.-Doz. Dr. med. José R. Iglesias-Rozas
Abteilung für Neurochirurgie der Universitätskliniken Rudolf Virchow der Freien Universität Berlin, Standort Charlottenburg und Standort Wedding, Augustenburger Platz 1, D-1000 Berlin 65

Prof. Dr. med. Ekkehard Kazner †
Leiter der Abteilung für Neurochirurgie der Universitätskliniken Rudolf Virchow der Freien Universität Berlin, Standort Charlottenburg, Spandauer Damm 130, D-1000 Berlin 19

Prof. Dr. med. Konrad Kretzschmar
Oberarzt der Abteilung für Neuroradiologie, Johannes Gutenberg-Universität, Langenbeckstraße 1, D-6500 Mainz

Dr. med. Michael Laniado
Strahlenklinik und Poliklinik der Universitätskliniken Rudolf Virchow der Freien Universität Berlin, Standort Charlottenburg, Spandauer Damm 130, D-1000 Berlin 19

Prof. Dr. med. Wolfgang Lanksch
Oberarzt der Neurochirurgischen Klinik im Klinikum Großhadern der Ludwig-Maximilians-Universität, Marchioninistraße 15, D-8000 München 70

Dr. med. Wibke Müller-Forell
Abteilung für Neuroradiologie, Johannes Gutenberg-Universität, Langenbeckstraße 1, D-6500 Mainz

Thomas Hans Newton, MD
Department of Radiology, University of California Medical Center, San Francisco, CA 94143, USA

Dr. med. Wolfgang Schörner
Strahlenklinik und Poliklinik der Universitätskliniken Rudolf Virchow der Freien Universität Berlin, Standort Charlottenburg, Spandauer Damm 130, D-1000 Berlin 19

Dr. med. Gerhard Schroth
Abteilung für Neuroradiologie, Universität Tübingen, Osianderstraße 22, D-7400 Tübingen

Dr. med. Barbara Schulz
Oberärztin der Abteilung für Neurochirurgie der Universitätskliniken Rudolf Virchow der Freien Universität Berlin, Standort Wedding, Augustenburger Platz 1, D-1000 Berlin 65

Prof. Dr. med. Otto Stochdorph
Emer. Vorstand des Instituts für Neuropathologie der Ludwig-Maximilians-Universität München, Untertaxetweg 79, D-8035 Gauting

Gordon Sze, MD
Memorial Sloan Kettering Cancer Center (Cornell University Medical College), New York City, NY 10021, USA

Prof. Dr. med. Sigurd Wende
Leiter der Abteilung für Neuroradiologie, Johannes Gutenberg-Universität, Langenbeckstraße 1, D-6500 Mainz

Preface to the Second Edition

This book represents the second, fully revised edition of the original volume published in 1982. Experience in neuroradiology has confirmed the outstanding value of computed tomography (CT) for the diagnosis of space-occupying lesions within the skull and orbit. It might be assumed, then, that the second edition of this book would simply represent a numerically expanded continuation of the popular first edition.

That is not the case, however. Advances in imaging techniques have prompted the creation of a new book whose expanded title reflects its more comprehensive nature. The added illustrations, the revised text, and the expanded circle of editors and contributors document this.

Since publication of the first edition, a new modality, magnetic resonance imaging (MRI), has become an established neuroradiologic study. We felt it was essential to include this new modality in our book and explore its capabilities as an adjunct or alternative to CT scanning. Because of the high acquisition costs of MRI and the still small number of MR units currently in operation, we have relied in part on images furnished by other institutions and private practitioners, to whom we are indebted. Many problems relating to MR, both in terms of equipment and image interpretation, have yet to be resolved. There is no denying that we still have much to learn.

Additional experience with CT diagnosis has been gained since publication of the first edition. Most of the original material remains valid, but we can now draw on a total of 8516 brain tumors and 1043 orbital lesions evaluated by CT and MRI in Berlin, Mainz, Munich, and Augsburg.

Recognizing the topical importance of acquired immune deficiency syndrome, we have included a new chapter on the diagnostic imaging of brain diseases in AIDS patients. We extend our thanks to Dr. Newton and Dr. Sze of the United States for furnishing this chapter. We also thank Dr. Heinzerling for contributing the section on magnetic resonance spectroscopy.

The first and principal author of this book, Prof. Dr. E. Kazner, was the guiding spirit for the first edition. With great dedication that served as an inspiration to his coworkers, he took the second edition in hand and greatly advanced it through his efforts. Sadly, his all too early death kept him from seeing this new book to its completion. We have tried to remain true to his intentions by providing a reference that is truly state-of-the-art in its scientific content.

We also are indebted for this second edition to the many private practitioners and participating institutions who referred their patients to us for evaluation and provided us with necessary clinical data. Below we cite in alphabetic order the department heads who, with their colleagues, lent valuable support to our efforts:

Free University, Berlin: Prof. Dr. J. Cervós-Navarro, Neuropathology; Prof. Dr. D. Janz, Neurology; Prof. Dr. J. Wollensak, Ophthalmology. Rudolf Virchow Hospital: Prof. Dr. H. Witt, Radiology.

Johannes Gutenberg University Mainz: Prof. Dr. H.H. Goebel, Neuropathology; Prof. Dr. J. Helms, Otorhinolaryngology; Prof. Dr. H.-C. Hopf, Neurology; Prof. Dr. A. Nover, Ophthalmology; Prof. Dr. K. Schürmann, Neurosurgery; Prof. Dr. J. Spranger, Pediatrics.

Ludwig Maximilian University, Munich: Prof. Dr. T. Brandt, Neurology; Prof. Dr. R. Enzenbach, Neuroanesthesia; Prof. Dr. H.-B. Hadorn, Pediatrics; Prof. Dr. E.-R. Kastenbauer, Otorhinolaryngology; Prof. Dr. J. Lissner, Radiology; Prof. Dr. O. Lund, Ophthalmology; Prof. Dr. F. Marguth, Neurosurgery.

Central Hospital, Augsburg: Dr. E. Klotz, Diagnostic Radiology.

We express special thanks to all participating physicians and technicians, who performed most of the CT and MR examinations presented here.

We thank Mrs. Hanne Hofmann for her secretarial work in preparing the manuscript, and are grateful to Mrs. Christa Penseroth and Mr. Roland Bittner for the graphics and photographic work. We extend special thanks to Mrs. Christine Kazner for her great help in the general preparation of the book.

Once again, we are indebted to Dr. Dr. h.c. mult. H. Götze, Mr. W. Bergstedt, Mrs. T. Deigmöller, and Mrs. M. Gründler of Springer-Verlag for their unfailing cooperation and their excellent work in the production of this volume.

Mainz, Augsburg,
Munich, Berlin

S. Wende, T. Grumme,
O. Stochdorph, R. Felix, C. Claussen

Preface to the First Edition

The current book represents a distillation of the experience gained in diagnosis of intracranial tumors with computed X-ray tomography at the University Hospitals of Berlin, Mainz, and München. To what purpose? Standard radiological techniques such as pneumoencephalography with lumbar puncture and cerebral arteriography with puncture of the common carotid artery are invasive procedures which entail a certain amount of risk as well as discomfort for the patient. Furthermore, diagnoses made with these procedures rely primarily on indirect signs of an intracranial space-occupying lesion – such as displacement of the air-filled ventricles or of normal cerebral vessels. Only a few types of tumor are demonstrated directly with these techniques.

In contrast, computed tomography demonstrates the pathology directly in almost all cases, and this with a minimum of risk and discomfort. In addition, normal intracranial structures are demonstrated, so that the tumor's effect on its surroundings can be evaluated.

Today, almost a decade after Hounsfield's revolutionary invention, diagnosis of brain tumors without computed tomography is almost unthinkable, if not in fact irresponsible.

Computed tomography is an integral part of preoperative diagnostics. The tumor is clearly demonstrated, accurately located, and often defined as to histological type. In addition, it is usually possible to decide whether the tumor is operable or not. As a result, unnecessary and risky operations can be avoided – in cases where the tumor proves to be larger than expected and in which vital centers are involved, for example. Computed tomography is also ideally suited for postoperative follow-up, for planning adjunctive radiation therapy, and for determining the success of irradiation or other conservative treatment. The enormous cost of computed tomography is justified only by improved diagnostic accuracy and, concurrently, elimination of costs for other diagnostic procedures. Computed tomography is capable of detecting up to 98% of brain tumors and is far more accurate than any other single diagnostic technique. Even histological diagnoses can be predicted with an accuracy approaching 90% in certain types of tumor.

Cost-benefit analysis has shown conclusively that computed tomography has resulted in a considerable reduction in overall cost, since diagnosis may be performed on an outpatient basis in many cases, since average time in hospital is reduced, and since other expensive procedures may be eliminated. The three CT study groups at the University Hospitals of Berlin, Mainz, and München examined over 40000 patients in the period from 1975 to the middle of 1980. This includes 3750 patients with brain tumors and over 600 patients with orbital lesions. Extensive experience in the use of computed tomography as well as the opportunity to compare CT findings with surgical results and neuropathological studies are summarized in this book. It is intended to help clinicians and general practitioners in determining the location and type of tumor, using CT findings together with the clinical data and the results of supplementary diagnostic techniques.

The editors conceived the project in 1975 with the intention of developing the most comprehensive experience possible in the appearance of brain tumors in computed tomography. Regular meetings allowed a continuous interchange of experience as well as analysis of problem cases. As a result all three study groups developed a comparable level of knowledge, which provided a common standard for evaluation of CT findings. This allowed the presentation of the collected experience in a genuine cooperative study by neuroradiologists, neurosurgeons, and neuropathologists.

The study was initiated with the help of the Volkswagenwerk Foundation, the Ludwig-Maximilians-Universität München, the Senat of Berlin, the Freie Universität Berlin, the Deutsche Forschungsgemeinschaft, and the Johannes-Gutenberg-Universität Mainz. The generous financial support from these institutions made possible the purchase of computed tomography systems with which fundamental knowledge in CT diagnosis of intracranial lesions could be developed.

We should like to thank the many general practitioners and participating institutions who referred their patients to us for diagnostic procedures and provided us with the clinical data in these cases. The following listing presents in alphabetical order the department heads at various institutions who, with their colleagues, lent valuable support to our efforts:

Freie Universität Berlin: Prof. Dr. J. Cervós-Navarro, Dept. of Neuropathology; Prof. Dr. H.J. Eberlein, Dept. of Anesthesiology; Prof. Dr. R. Felix, Radiology Dept.; Prof. Dr. W. Girke, Neurology Dept.; Prof. Dr. F. Hanefeld, Dept. of Pediatrics; Prof. Dr. D. Janz, Neurology Dept.; Prof Dr. E. Kastenbauer, Dept. of Otorhinolaryngology; Prof. Dr. W. Schwab, formerly Dept. of Otorhinolaryngology; Prof. Dr. J. Wollensak, Dept. of Ophthalmology; Prof. Dr. R. Wüllenweber, formerly Dept. of Neurosurgery.

Johannes-Gutenberg-Universität Mainz: Prof. Dr. R. Frey †, Dept. of Anesthesiology; Prof. Dr. J. Helms, Dept. of Otorhinolaryngology; Prof. Dr. H.-Ch. Hopf, Neurology Dept.; Prof. Dr. A. Nover, Dept. of Ophthalmology; Prof. Dr. J.M. Schröder, Dept. of Neuropathology; Prof. Dr. K. Schürmann, Dept. of Neurosurgery; Prof. Dr. J. Spranger, Dept. of Pediatrics.

Ludwig-Maximilians-Universität München: Prof. Dr. K. Betke, Dept. of Pediatrics; Prof. Dr. R. Enzenbach, Dept. of Neuroanesthesiology; Prof. Dr. J. Lissner, Dept. of Radiology; Prof. Dr. O. Lund, Dept. of Ophthalmology; Prof. Dr. F. Marguth, Dept. of Neurosurgery; Prof. Dr. H. Naumann, Dept. of Otorhinolaryngology; Prof. Dr. A.Schrader, Neurology Dept.

We should like to express our particular thanks to all participating physicians and technicians who performed the great majority of CT studies presented here.

Mrs. Ilka Förster and Mrs. Brigitte Graef were of invaluable help in preparing the manuscript. Graphics and photography were provided by Mr. M. Tidnam.

We are grateful to Dr. h.c. H. Götze, Mr. W. Bergstedt, and the employees of Springer-Verlag for their cooperation and effort in the excellent layout and production of the book.

Finally, the editors E. Kazner and W. Lanksch would like to express their appreciation and special thanks to Prof. Dr. F. Marguth. Director of the Neurosurgical Dept. Klinikum Großhadern, Ludwig-Maximilians-Universität München, for his unflagging support of their efforts over the years.

Berlin, Mainz, München

E. Kazner, S. Wende, Th. Grumme,
W. Lanksch, O. Stochdorph

Contents

A. Introduction

Until well into the twentieth century, neurologic signs and symptoms were the only means available for the detection and localization of intracranial tumors. Diagnostic neuroradiology traces its origin to Dandy, who in 1918 *injected air into the cerebral ventricles* by the direct puncture of a fontanelle or through a bur hole as a means of outlining the ventricles on X-ray films. In 1919 he additionally described lumbar puncture as a means of introducing air into the ventricular system.

Cerebral angiography was developed by Moniz in 1927. This was the first procedure that permitted brain tumors to be directly visualized on the basis of their pathologic blood supply. In 1929 Berger introduced *electroencephalography* for the diagnosis of intracranial lesions. This method continues to play a major role, especially in evaluating functional disorders of the brain. The *radionuclide imaging* of brain tumors was first performed in the late 1940s (Moore 1948; Selverstone and Solomon 1948).

In 1955 Leksell introduced *echoencephalography*, which permits the accurate measurement of midline shifts and ventricular distension with relatively simple apparatus.

A new era in the diagnosis of intracranial space-occupying lesions began in 1972, when Godfrey N. Hounsfield announced at a London press conference his initial results with *computed tomography*, which he had developed for the firm EMI. In 1979 Hounsfield and Allan M. Cormack received the Nobel Prize for Medicine for their revolutionary advance of the roentgenographic technique.

In the past 15 years computed tomography (CT) has become *the* standard imaging modality for intracranial tumors. Its essential features have changed little during that period, and the study still relies on differences in the relative densities of tumor and normal brain tissue before and after the intravenous injection of contrast medium. However, significant improvements in spatial resolution and more modest improvements in density resolution have further enhanced the ability of CT to delineate and identify lesions of the brain, orbit, and skull base. Today CT permits a direct or indirect examination of the skull on multiple planes, and modern scanners can construct images from available data in a matter of seconds. In many cases, however, the image quality is inadequate for a definitive diagnosis. Dynamic CT has proved advantageous only in certain types of investigation.

The physicists Bloch, Purcell and colleagues described the phenomenon of "nuclear magnetic resonance" in 1946 (Bloch et al. 1946; Purcell et al. 1946) and 6 years later received the Nobel Prize for Physics. In 1973 Lauterbur utilized this phenomenon to make an image. Magnetic resonance (MR) scanners have been undergoing clinical trials since 1981/82, and the results have been most encouraging. The technical investment involved with this imaging modality is high, and a single examination is correspondingly cost-intensive, but the quality of the MR image has surpassed all expectations. Major advantages of magnetic resonance imaging (MRI) are the lack of ionizing radiation, the ability to acquire images in three planes, and the ability to define normal intracranial structures and their relations to pathologic processes with no artifacts emanating from bone.

B. Classification of Brain Tumors

1. History and Problems of Tumor Classification

In 1914, L. Bruns stated in Krause's *General Surgery of Brain Disorders* that brain tumors include all neoplasias growing within the cranium and that they comprise three groups: (1) true tumors, (2) infectious granulomas, and (3) parasites. Current usage is more precise and is limited to the first of Bruns' categories. Even so, brain tumors constitute a large and very heterogeneous group. A taxonomic approach to classification is necessary if we are to make sense of an initially disorganized set of observations, compare the findings of different observers, and attempt a prognostic evaluation.

In principle, we might apply any number of criteria to the classification of intracranial tumors, such as the age and sex of the patient, tumor location, clinical presentation, macroscopic appearance, and histologic features. Histologic findings offer a practical basis for classifying tumors of all the body tissues. This histogenetic classification by *tissue* of origin is not the same as a cytogenetic classification. It is true that the form and structure of individual tumor cells are related to the parent tissue. However, the statement "*Omnis cellula e cellula eiusdem generis* (every cell is derived from a cell of the same general type)" does not mean "*...e cellula eiusdem speciei* (from a cell of the same specific type)." Thus, a tumor cell which closely resembles a cell of normal tissue is not necessarily derived from a fully differentiated cell of that type, but in many cases results from the differentiation of the daughter cell of an uncommitted, pluripotent stem cell.

Thus, the classification of intracranial tumors by parent tissue would seem to offer a rational solution (see Stochdorph 1981). It is unnecessary to invoke the germ-layer theory ("neuroectodermal" tumors), which in any case has become obsolete in human embryology. Because the parent tissues are assignable to specific anatomic structures, the histogenetic approach to classification very often tells us something about the topographic anatomy of the tumor in question. However, we must be careful not to confuse site with structure: a tumor is not necessarily a meningioma just because it is located within the meninges.

By far the largest group of brain tumors in the broad sense are those that arise from tissue components of the brain itself, i.e., the part of the CNS contained within the skull. (Division of the CNS into brain and spinal cord is a linguistic convention resulting from the simplified conception of the body as consisting of head, trunk, and limbs, and has no structural basis.) Brain tumors in the stricter sense are all those that arise from tissues inside the space enclosed by the meninges.

Like any other organ, the brain is made up of parenchyma and stroma (the vascularized mesenchyma). The chief functional components of the brain parenchyma are the nerve cells or neurons. The nerve cell consists of a perikaryon (cell body with nucleus), dendrites (afferent processes), and an axon (efferent process). The gray matter of the brain is composed chiefly of nerve cell bodies and the "neuropil," a dense network of interwoven dendrites and axons. The white matter consists chiefly of bundled axons. The neuronal population of the CNS interacts functionally with the nerve cells of the afferent ganglion system (spinal ganglia and their intracranial counterparts) and the olfactory sensory neurons and also with two effector systems – the muscle fibers with end plates and the neurons of the efferent ganglion system (the autonomic nervous system).

The nerve cells of the CNS are supported by astrocytic and oligodendrocytic glia. The astrocytes serve as "all-purpose" cells, while the oligodendrocytes form the myelin sheaths. The astrocyte population includes protoplasmic and fibrillary cell types which Wolff (1980) describes as "adaptive differentiation and reaction forms." In terms of cellular kinetics, the nerve cells of the CNS have entered an irreversible postmitotic phase in which they retain at most a limited capacity for DNA synthesis, occasionally leading to the presence of two or more nuclei. The glial cells, therefore, constitute the principal substrate for tumor formation in the gray matter and white matter of the brain.

The glial cells were first described as a tissue component by Virchow (1862), who gave them the name neuroglia, meaning "nerve glue." He also introduced the term "glioma" for tumors arising from the neuroglia, regarding them as "partial hyperplasias." He classified these tumors by their secondary characteristics as "soft and hard or, more accurately, as cellular or medullary, fibrous and telangiectatic" gliomas. Virchow (1864/65) believed that tumors with areas resembling mucous tissue were transitional types between the soft glioma and the myxoglioma, characterized by a looser tissue meshwork. "If the cellularity of the tumor increases significantly, the meshwork becomes more dense, and the tumor becomes a true medullary glioma, which may undergo transformation to medullary sarcoma... Such transitions between myxoma, glioma, and sarcoma may occur in the same tumor, and this mixed pattern was apparent in the largest, fist-size tumors which I observed in the occipital lobe of the cerebrum." Virchow (1864/65) goes on to state that tumors such as fibromas, lipomas, chondromas, myxomas, osteoid chondromas, and gliomas can and should be differentiated from the sarcomas, but that a special name should be reserved for tumors of connective tissue that show a general histologic type rather than a strict analogy to normal tissue.

Besides characterizing gliomas by their gross characteristics as hard, soft, telangiectatic, etc., Virchow also noted that gliomas tend to be poorly demarcated with respect to surrounding brain. Rindfleisch (1878) later wrote that "one of the most striking characteristics of gliomas leads me to prefer the term 'gliomatous degeneration of brain structures' over the name glioma. When inspecting a glioma in situ, one can usually say with some certainty which part of the brain – the thalamus, the striate body, the anterior part of Vieussens' center, a larger area of the cortex – has undergone gliomatous transformation. The shapes of these structures are still recognizable, yet nothing remains of their normal histology, which has been replaced by gliomatous tissue. Simple round, nodular gliomas do not occur, and often it is difficult to appreciate the shape of the glioma, so closely does it resemble the replaced structure in color and consistency, and so smoothly does it blend with healthy surrounding brain."

The ill-defined margins of gliomas result from the fact that these tumors do not originate from a small, circumscribed group of cells, as metastases do. "Observations of early stages of (malignant) tumor growth in man indicate that the tumors arise either from a field of transformed cells or from several closely adjacent fields of cells which coalesce with further development" (Eder 1977). Of particular importance for gliomas is the hypothesis, advanced by Willis (1948), that tumors undergo an initial phase of "spreading neoplastic change" followed by a secondary phase of cellular proliferation. Often a reciprocal relationship exists between the extent of the initial "field of origin" and the proliferation kinetics of the secondary phase. The more intense the proliferation in the secondary phase, the greater the tendency for the glioma to acquire well-defined borders. At the other end of the scale is "gliomatosis," in which the field of origin involves large areas of brain but the cellular density of the tumor is only slightly greater than that of normal tissue. When the field of origin is extensive, proliferation may begin more or less concurrently at multiple sites, creating the impression of multifocal tumor growth since the areas between the proliferative centers still appear normal.

Tumor growth occurring in adjacent areas at different points in time should not be misconstrued as infiltrative growth. The tumor cells do not advance more deeply into the feltwork of dendrites and axons; rather, the sites of tumor growth simply spread to involve ever greater areas of tissue. The inherent proliferative tendency of the local tissues is a major factor in this process and explains, for example, why the subpial cortical layer overlying cortex seemingly uninvolved by a subjacent white matter tumor may show considerable cellular proliferation with ingrowth into the leptomeninges. Even when a preexisting tumor has been excised in toto at operation, delayed proliferation in surrounding areas can simulate a recurrence.

After Virchow (1862) introduced the concept of neuroglia, attention soon turned toward the finer structure of this tissue, leading in turn to the recognition of different glial cell types. Weigert's histologic stain made it possible to identify the fibrous glia as a kind of supporting tissue, while the silver incrustation method of Golgi (1894) demonstrated the existence of "long-branched" and "short-branched" cell forms (Koelliker 1896), to which Stroebe (1895) gave the collective name "astrocytes." Del Río Hortega (1921) identified oligodendroglial cells or oligodendrocytes as being part of the "third element" of brain tissue (besides nerve cells and astrocytes) recognized by Ramón y Cajal (1913).

In the parts of the brain which derive their structure largely from nerve cells and their processes (the *neuronal* areas of the gray and white matter), the glial cells consist basically of astrocytes and oligodendrocytes. This is not true of *paraneuronal* structures, however, which are composed of elements other than nerve cells and their fibers. They include the ependyma lining the ventricles of the brain, the tissue of the choroid plexus, and other circumventricular organs (Hofer 1965) such as the neurohypophysis, the organum vasculosum of the lamina terminalis, the subfornical organ, the subcommissural organ, the pineal body, and the area postrema. The subpial layer of the cortex is transitional between the neuronal and paraneuronal structures. Our understanding of the circumventricular brain structures is still far from complete. The older classification schemes and the more recent systems derived from them take little note of these special cell types, and virtually no attention has been given to their tissue patterns in tumors (Stochdorph 1955).

Gliomas of the cerebral and cerebellar hemispheres develop chiefly in the gray and white matter, although involvement of the ependymal "organ" (Leonhardt 1980) and other paraneuronal structures is occasionally seen. In 1894, Golgi stated that gliomas are composed of "branched, radiating cells similar to those found in large numbers in all parts of the central nervous system." Kaufmann noted in 1922 that some gliomas contain large numbers of cells with processes, called "spider cells" or astrocytes, and that tumors with a very large proportion of these cells should be classified as astromas or astrocytomas (the term astrocytoma had been proposed by von Lenhossék in 1895). Bailey and Hiller identified oligodendrogliomas in 1924. Ependymomas had been previously described.

Advances in neurosurgery directed interest toward the clinical relevance of histologic findings in gliomas. It became apparent that classifying tumors by their cellularity alone did not provide a sound basis for making a postoperative prognosis. Thus, gliomas of the oligodendrocytic type which have a long preoperative history and offer an excellent prospect for extended postoperative survival may demonstrate a much greater cellularity than an anaplastic glioma of the astrocytic type which carries a more gloomy prognosis.

In an effort to solve this problem, Bailey and Cushing (1926) proposed an embryogenetic classification in which the lack of differentiation of rapidly proliferating tumor cells was interpreted not as anaplasia (dedifferentiation), but as a failure of maturation (incomplete differentiation). Their first classification was a hierarchical one envisioning a gradual progression and maturation from primitive – and strongly proliferating – progenitor cells. Because of contradictions inherent in this interpretation (such as naming a cerebellar tumor of adolescence with excellent prognosis after the very immature spongioblasts) and an unwieldy number of differentiation stages, the principle of the embryogenetic classification was largely abandoned. But this also involved discarding a tenet of the embryogenetic theory that pertained to the composition of gliomas, namely that the incompletely differentiated cells in a glioma might continue to differentiate by epigenesis, thus accounting for the presence of different cell types in the tumor. Instead, it became necessary to assume a strict preformation of each cell type. The premise of glioma cells descending in orderly fashion from a particular glial cell type led to a simplification of the initially complicated scheme of Bailey and Cushing, and only a few types of glioma, presumably quite distinct from one another, came to be recognized: astrocytoma, oligodendroglioma, ependymoma, and glioblastoma multiforme. The latter was considered to be a separate entity and "the true cancer of the brain" (Zülch 1956).

However, it appears unlikely that fully differentiated astrocytes in a glioma, for example, could regain the capacity for unchecked proliferation. The rather slow cell turnover in the glial cell population as well as any reactive (and presumably neoplastic) proliferation are probably mediated primarily by a type of stem cell that resembles oligodendroglia or "resting" microglia and tends to occur mainly about the ventricles, as [^{3}H]thymidine labeling studies suggest (Bunge et al. 1962; Kleihues and Schultze 1968). Once differentiation toward a particular cell type has commenced, apparently it is still possible for bivalent cell divisions to occur, causing one daughter cell to mature into an astrocyte, for example, and another into an oligodendrocyte (Niessing 1980).

Even in normal tissue, conditions must be ideal before the glial cell types can be clearly differentiated from one another. Experience shows that gliomas with a completely uniform cell type are rarely if ever observed. As a rule, the tumor cells cannot be uniformly assigned to a particular differentiated cell type, and considerable heterogeneity exists within the cell population as a whole. Several histologic patterns may be observed: (1) The individual tumor cell may differ markedly from the "model" of a particular, fully differentiated glial cell type and may have the appearance of an undifferentiated cell form like that in "myelinating glia." (2) Some tumors may present an exotic, "salt-and-pepper" cell mix reminiscent of differentiated glial cell types. (3) Examination of different fields may disclose fields with predominantly astrocytic differentiation alternating with fields showing predominantly oligodendrocytic differentiation. The first of these patterns may be interpreted as incomplete differentiation, the second may result from unequal bivalent divisions, and the third may reflect the proliferation of individual tumor cell clones.

Thus, even reasonably well differentiated gliomas can rarely be assigned to one specific glial cell type and are best classified according to the principle of "*a potiori fit denominatio*" (naming the whole for its predominant part). But classifying a tumor in this way introduces a subjective element that is inconsistent with an accurate, quantitative approach to tumor diagnosis. What is more, gliomas are like many other tumors in that a specimen may show a degree of anaplasia out of proportion to the average proliferative tendency of the lesion. Lack of differentiation is a characteristic feature of tumor cells. The sum of these deficits determines the overall degree of tissue anaplasia, which may increase as the deficit of subsequent tumor cell generations becomes compounded. Thus, anaplasia or dedifferentiation is always a property of the tissue and does not apply to individual cells.

Even Bailey and Cushing recognized that glioblastoma multiforme may be derived from protoplasmatic astrocytes. Kernohan et al. (1949) concluded from their observations at the Mayo Clinic that many cases of glioblastoma multiforme represent maximal dedifferentiation of an astrocytoma (or ependymoma) and advised that the term glioblastoma be discarded. Willis made the same recommendation in 1948. In 1950, Ringertz developed a scheme similar to that proposed by Henschen in 1934, in which glioblastomas are not recognized as a separate, primary entity but as atypical variants of different types of glioma. For practical reasons, Ackerman and Rosai (1974) suggested an even simpler classification into astrocytomas, malignant astrocytomas, oligodendrogliomas, ependymomas, and undifferentiated gliomas. They argued against the continued use of the term glioblastoma on the grounds that it implies an embryogenetic derivation and conveys the impression of a specific tumor type, when in fact the lesion is simply the undifferentiated form of any type of glioma.

Taking carcinoma of the lip as an example, Broders (1926) showed that a correlation exists between the degree of anaplasia and the clinical course of some tumors. Thus, the severity of cellular and tissue changes can be helpful in establishing a prognosis and, as suggested by Broders, can be incorporated into a numerical grading scheme. Usually a system comprising grades 1–4, representing the presence of a quantifiable trait in up to 25%, 50%, 75% or 100% of the cells, cell groups, high-power fields, etc., is used to facilitate statistical evaluation.

Kernohan et al. (1949) applied this principle by subdividing the continuous spectrum of tumors in the astrocytoma-glioblastoma group and the ependymomas into four grades of malignancy. In common practical application (conscious or otherwise) of this four-grade

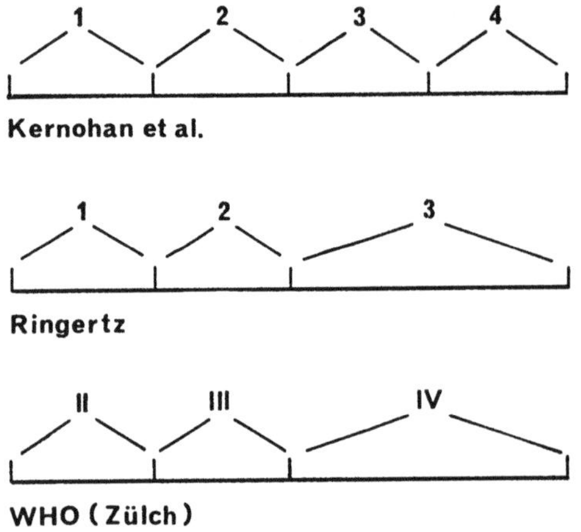

Fig. B1. Classification of anaplasia and prognosis of gliomas by grades or stages

principle, the pathologist first attempts to determine whether the histologic findings imply a long or short postoperative course and then states whether this assessment can be made with a high or low degree of confidence. Choosing twice between two alternatives results in a four-grade type of classification. Ringertz (1950), on the other hand, stressed the advantages of a three-grade system, which Henschen (1955) claims is less complicated but is still adequate for clinical and histologic purposes. Our own experience strongly supports Henschen's view. Grade 3 in the latter classification corresponds to grades 3 *and* 4 in the four-grade scheme (see Fig. B1).

If we arrange the principal groups of gliomas according to (1) the prevalence of normally differentiated glial cell forms and (2) the degree to which anaplastic phenomena define the histologic picture, we obtain a two-dimensional system with glial cell types on one axis and degree of anaplasia on the other. This permits us to represent the various proposed classification schemes in graphic form (see Fig. B2a–d). In the scheme of Henschen and Ringertz (Fig. B2c), for example, we find that the correlation with normal glial cell types is high in well-differentiated tumors but becomes less precise as the degree of anaplasia increases.

Classification by grades of malignancy is reasonable and useful only within a single tumor type or within a group of closely related tumor types, such as the glial tumors. Unfortunately, the staging system employed in the

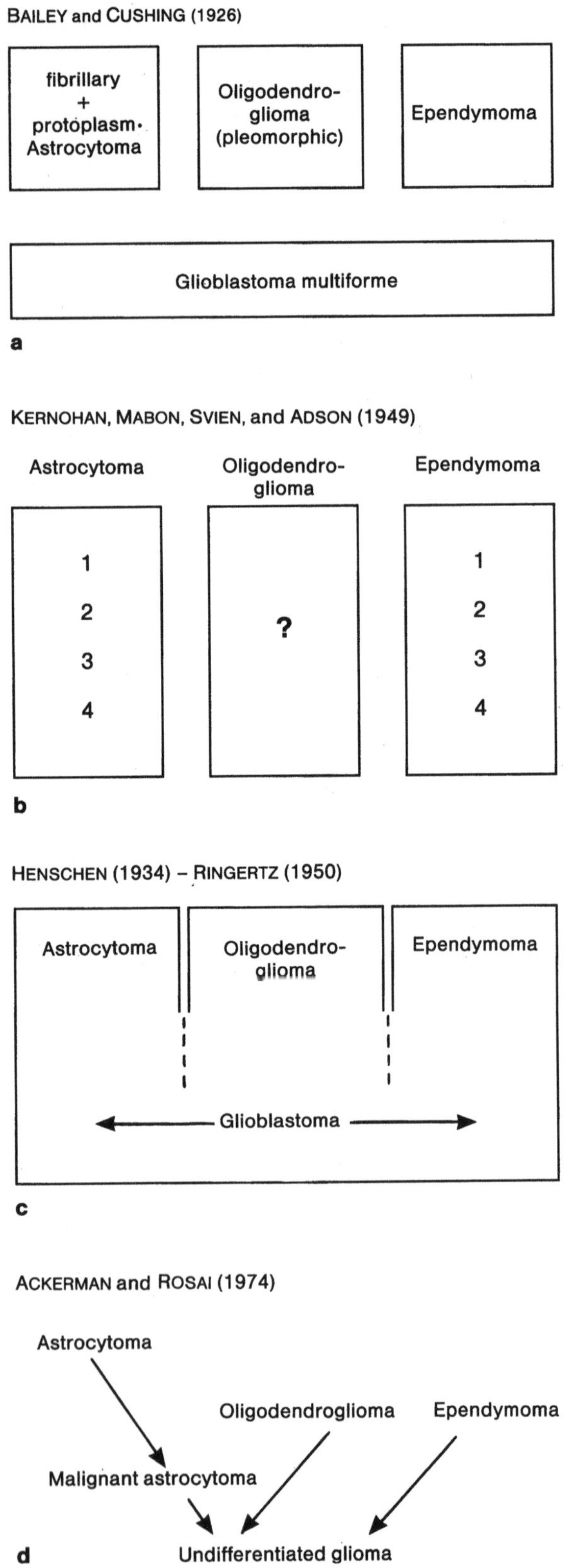

Fig. B2. Classification of gliomas according to Bailey and Cushing (**a**), Kernohan et al. (**b**), Henschen and Ringertz (**c**), and Ackerman and Rosai (**d**)

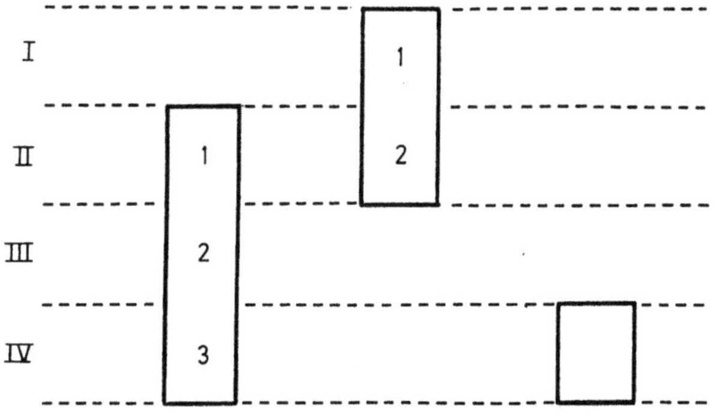

Fig. B3. Degrees of anaplasia (Arabic numerals) and prognostic classification (Roman numerals). *Left*: astrocytoma and glioblastoma group; *center*: pilocytic astrocytomas; *right*: medulloblastomas

WHO classification edited by Zülch (1979) has an entirely different meaning, although the term "grading" is used. This system disregards histologic anaplasia within a given tumor group as an index for clinical prognosis, relying instead on clinical experience for the comparison of totally unrelated tumors without regard for the range of anaplasia within a given tumor type (see Fig. B3). For example, medulloblastomas are assigned to "grade" IV even though it is generally agreed that there are hardly any prognostically significant differences in degree of anaplasia among medulloblastomas, making it impossible to assign these tumors to grades 1–3. Other tumors are placed in "grades" I and III while lacking a "grade" II form. Fully differentiated astrocytomas and oligodendrocytomas are assigned to "grade" II. Since there are a total of four grades, this means that there are only two higher categories, effectively resulting in only three "grades" for the astrocytoma-glioblastoma group and the oligodendroglioma-glioblastoma group – the same as in Ringertz' classification, except that the designations are one number higher (see Fig. B1).

There is a danger that the "grading" system of the WHO classification will lead to much confusion. If reference is made in the literature to the CT appearance of a grade 2 glioma, for example, it will be unclear whether the tumor is a moderately anaplastic glioma (under the previous system) or a "grade" II lesion showing no clear evidence of anaplasia and thus lacking a strong proliferative tendency.

Yet another criticism may be leveled against the WHO classification. Glioblastomas and medulloblastomas are listed jointly in a section following astrocytic and oligodendrocytic gliomas, even though they are two completely different entities that affect different age groups and are unrelated histologically. This approach also separates the astrocytoma-glioblastoma group, whose internal consistency has already been noted.

For statistical purposes, we recommend the ICD-O (*I*nternational *C*lassification of *D*iseases for *O*ncology), which includes a large number of alternative terms, many of which are not simply synonyms but reflect different schools of thought. The fourth place in the ICD-O code number, preceding the slash, is usually available for further subclassifications for internal use.

The CT appearance of tumors results both from the increase in tissue density caused by proliferation and from the decrease in tissue density caused by edema. Hematoxylin-eosin (H&E) preparations clearly demonstrate the proliferation-induced changes in nuclear configuration and cell density and in that respect correlate with CT findings. Magnetic resonance (MR) signals, on the other hand, are more strongly influenced by cytoplasmic changes, which are not well depicted in H&E preparations due to breakup and expansion of the cytoplasmic body. When MR findings are used to guide a stereotactic biopsy, the area of interest may be affected by cytoplasmic changes that precede the onset of proliferation and lead to a *false negative* histologic report. In cases of this kind, inflammatory infiltration stimulated by the patient's immune system may be the only apparent, albeit tentative, sign of incipient neoplastic change.

In some circumstances cellular morphologies and tissue patterns are inadequate for a definitive histologic diagnosis. Histochemical methods of analysis can provide an excellent resource in these cases. With these methods, most notably the peroxidase-antiperoxidase technique, it is possible to detect and label proteins of potential diagnostic importance. The detection of gliofibrillary acid protein (GFAP) is of major value in tumors of the CNS and is especially useful in the demonstration of astrocytes (Rubinstein 1982; Gullotta et al. 1985). Also valuable is the detection of neuron-specific enolase and the S-100 protein, a substance whose origin and significance are not yet fully understood but which is useful for labeling cells derived from the neural plate and neural crests.

2. Specific Tumors

In a classification of intracranial tumors based on tissue of origin, autochthonous brain tumors are listed first, with tumors of the brain matter itself preceding tumors of structures that can be grossly delineated from brain: the choroid plexus, pineal body, and neurohypophysis. Foremost among brain tumors in the strict sense are tumors of the glial series, followed by tumors of the ependymal "organ," whose cells represent modified glial cells; neuronal tumors; medulloblastomas, derived from a pluripotent matrix; and autochthonous mesenchymal tumors derived from the vascularized mesenchyma of the brain.

The differentiation of tumor cells along astrocytic lines yields the typical **astrocytoma**. As in normal histology, we can distinguish *protoplasmic* short-branched types and *fibrillary* long-branched types. The latter may be found in both the gray and the white matter, as opposed to normal fibrillary astrocytes which occur almost exclusively in the white matter. They probably represent a reactive phenomenon analogous to reactive gliosis (Wolff 1980). *Gemistocytic* astrocytes (gemistocytes) have a cell body resembling that of a protoplasmatic astrocyte but contain fibers like a fibrillary astrocyte, again most likely due to a reactive process. Astrocytomas of low malignancy (grade 1 of Kernohan and of Ringertz, WHO "grade" II) are characterized by a low cell density, an absence of mitotic figures, and a quiescent tissue pattern. **Anaplastic astrocytomas** (grade 2 of Kernohan and of Ringertz, WHO "grade" III) show a greater cell density, more abundant mitoses, a chaotic vascular structure, and alteration of the blood-brain barrier making the vessel walls permeable to contrast media.

Oligodendrogliomas are characterized by the presence of hypercellular areas with a typical honeycomb structure – round nuclei suspended in clear cytoplasm with well-defined cell boundaries – the result of regressive cytoplasmic changes. Calcium-encrusted protein droplets lie freely in the tissue and on capillary walls. Outside the hypercellular areas it is common to find a *"croissance périneuronale"* (Scherer 1936), meaning an increased number of satellite cells around the nerve cells. Enhanced proliferation in the superficial layer of the cortex is also frequently seen. As early as 1929, Bailey and Bucy noted variations in cell size and transitions to astrocytic forms. It is difficult or impossible to establish a diagnosis of **anaplastic oligodendroglioma** from cytologic features alone, especially in cases of low-grade malignancy (Kernohan). When areas closely resembling a Ringertz grade 3 or a Kernohan grade 3–4 oligodendroglioma (WHO "grade" IV), and thus an oligodendrocytic glioblastoma, are noted in a tumor which otherwise presents a relatively quiescent tissue pattern, a diagnosis of anaplastic oligodendroglioma may be made with reasonable confidence.

Differentiation between astrocytoma and oligodendroglioma is problematic in glial cell tumors that do not yet display an obviously malignant histologic pattern and either present indifferent cell forms that cannot be positively identified as astrocytic or oligodendrocytic or else contain a mixture of differentiated astrocytic and oligodendrocytic forms or adjacent nests of both cell types. For purposes of statistical evaluation, the first pattern may be classified under either heading. Cooper (1935) suggested the term **oligoastrocytoma** for the second, mixed type of pattern. Some authors apply this designation to the third pattern as well, which is also termed a **mixed glioma**. It bears repeating that gliomas almost never represent a pure culture of a particular line of differentiation. There is diversity of opinion concerning the point at which a tumor should be called a mixed glioma. The condition known as **gliomatosis** usually involves the growth of indifferent glial cell forms in extensive, primary "fields of origin" with a very low degree of associated neoplastic proliferation.

Just as Virchow (1864/65) wished to retain the term "sarcoma" for the group of undifferentiated connective tissue tumors despite the separate recognition of fibromas, lipomas, etc., there may be justification for retaining the term **glioblastoma** for certain glial cell tumors, despite the well-founded objections of Ackerman and Rosai (1974) against the term. If used, it should be applied only to the most anaplastic forms of glial cell tumors; it should not be used to designate a separate tumor entity. Glioblastomas combine a marked "ataxia" of differentiation with a profound loss of differentiation in their histologic picture. As dedifferentiation increases, tumors showing a predominance of astrocytic, oligodendrocytic, or ependymal cell forms increasingly come to resemble one another in their histologic features and clinical course, and subtle diagnostic distinctions become pointless. Apparently, some glial cell tumors progress in a way that causes them to change their appearance from one phase of their existence to the next. Thus, the histologic features of a recurrent tumor may recapitulate those of the primary growth in every detail, or a progressive loss of differentiation may be apparent from one recurrence to the next. If the intraoperative appearance of a tumor is consistent with glioblastoma but the preoperative history is exceptionally long, histologic evaluation may explain the situation by identifying the lesion as an oligodendrocytic glioblastoma (Ringertz grade 3 oligodendroglioma, Kernohan grade 3–4, WHO "grade" IV) that has undergone protracted growth before reaching its final grade of dedifferentiation. It is not always possible to assign an extremely anaplastic tumor to a particular glial cell type or line of differentiation (astrocytic, etc.), since even a glioma with indifferent cells or a mixed glioma may, with increasing dedifferentiation, ultimately present as a glioblastoma.

The close relationship between glial cells (especially astrocytes) and vascular structures is reflected in the brisk vascular proliferation that occurs in glioblastomas. The vessels are especially abundant around sites of necrosis. In some cases the accompanying mesenchymal proliferation exceeds the neoplastic glial cell proliferation, giving rise to a "mixed glioblastoma and fibrosarcoma" (Rubinstein 1972), also called a **gliosarcoma**. Proliferation of connective tissue fibers among the tumor cells is most commonly seen in tumors with large numbers of astrocytic giant cells and occasionally in well-differentiated glial tumors with little cellularity (Friede 1978). The term monstrocellular sarcoma (Zülch) is applied to a seemingly heterogeneous group of tumors that includes **giant cell glioblastomas** in addition to other types.

Recently an additional glial cell type has been identified within the ependymal "organ." These cells, called tanycytes, have a variety of forms ranging from typical cuboidal ependymal cells to "unipolar," "bipolar," and astrocytic forms. They are a component of the ependymal plate and especially of the circumventricular organs that form on or near the median plane of the embryonic brain (Leonhardt). They appear to be far less differentiated than ordinary astrocytes. Tumors composed of cells of this line of differentiation present a spectrum of cell morphologies ranging from ependymal cells to tanycytic forms and "piloidal" astrocytes (Friede and Pollak 1978), so named by Penfield (1932) due to the presence of bundles of delicate glial fibers like those seen in isomorphic gliosis. Bailey and Cushing (1926, 1930) referred to tumors with the latter cell forms as spongioblastomas and fibrillary astrocytomas. Bergstrand (1932) called them embryonic gliocytomas. The WHO classification identifies them as **pilocytic astrocytomas**, after Penfield's term. Kuhlendahl and Stochdorph (1968) suggested the term Bergstrand's tumor, while Jellinger (1977) spoke of tanycytomas, referring to their origin, as did Weindl et al. (1975). These tumors account for some 90% of cerebellar tumors in adolescents, and they comprise 10% of low-grade astrocytomas of the cerebral hemispheres in larger patient series (Ringertz and Nordenstam 1951). Other sites of occurrence are the walls of the third ventricle including the lamina terminalis, the infundibulum, the optic chiasm, and the proximal segment of the optic nerve.

The ependyma lining the ventricles (Fleischhauer 1972) is unique in that its glial elements predominate over its neuronal elements even though it is an intrinsic part of the cerebral hemispheres. While nerve cells are present in the form of "CSF-contact neurons," they do not determine the structure of the tissue. The CSF space, which is partitioned off from the amniotic cavity in embryonic life by fusion of the neural folds, is bounded by surface epithelium with a basement membrane only in the area of the choroid plexus. At all other sites the superficial layer lacks an epithelium and simply blends with the adjacent tissue like the crust on a piece of bread. True ependymal cells are

GFAP-negative. The ventricle wall forms the primary matrix for tumor growth. The principal embryonic tumors arising from this matrix in children and adolescents are **cerebral ependymomas**, which Zülch (1956) characterized by their location and age of occurrence. They are very cellular, contain abundant mitoses, show varying degrees of differentiation, and display the cytologic features of ependymoblastomas. Adult forms present as ependymal glioblastomas. In contrast to ordinary glial cell tumors, **ependymomas of the fourth ventricle** display exophytic growth, and their histologic pattern suggests a hyperplasia of the ependymal cell layer. The **subependymomas** (subependymal glomerate astrocytomas) first described by Ribbert (1909) also demonstrate exophytic growth and represent a hyperplasia of the glial layer rather than of the ependymal cells. They are clinically important only when they occur at sites of anatomic narrowing such as the foramen of Monro. **Subependymal giant cell astrocytomas**, which mostly occur in association with tuberous sclerosis, also originate in the glial layer of the ependyma. Despite their name they do not express GFAP in all cases (Rubinstein 1982) and thus may be related to the "parenchymal cells" of the circumventricular organs. Like ependymomas of the foramen of Monro, they are clinically important only when they cause obstruction to CSF flow.

The astrocytic glial cells of the ependymal layer often establish contact with vessel walls through a foot-like expansion similar to that of astrocytes in the gray and white matter. Perivascular extensions of this kind resemble the processes seen in astrocytomas undergoing early dedifferentiation (astroblastomas) and in ependymomas. Russell and Rubinstein (1977) state that these processes are finer in ependymomas than in astroblastomas, and the tissue background is more dense. Bailey (1932) described bodies resembling diplosomes or basal corpuscles ("blepharoplasts") occurring in astroblastomas. Russell and Rubinstein suggest that the astroblastomas described by them may be a separate tumor type rather than a dedifferentiated form of astrocytoma (cf. Weiser 1985).

Because the nerve cells of the mature brain remain in a postmitotic state, **neuronal tumors** of the brain imply some degree of dysontogenesis. The term "ganglioglioma" might also be appropriate for these tumors, since most do not arise from an isolated proliferation of nerve cells. Using terms analogous to those used for ganglioneuromas of the peripheral nervous tissue, we may refer to less differentiated neuronal tumors of the brain as partially differentiated gangliogliomas, ganglioneuroblastomas, and neuroblastomas. Connective tissue proliferation can be very marked, especially around blood vessels, and can create the nidus for a recurrence having the character of a fibrous histiocytoma (see below). Nodular lesions composed of dysontogenetic nerve cells and occurring in the hypothalamic region are called hamartomas, though they are in fact ectopias and are more aptly referred to as choristomas. There is a curious lesion of the cerebellum, variously called dysplastic gangliocytoma, purkinjeoma, or Lhermitte-Duclos disease, in which the granular layer of the cerebellar cortex is occupied by monstrous neurons as large as Purkinje cells, and the folia appear expanded as by a space-occupying lesion.

Medulloblastomas of the cerebellum have a pronounced embryonic character. Their matrix is pluripotent and apparently is related to the tissues of the circumventricular organs. Accordingly, the degree of differentiation encountered ranges from neuronal tumors at the neuroblastoma stage to occasional well-differentiated nerve cells. Differentiation along astrocytic, oligodendrocytic, or tanycytic lines may also occur, and there may even be elements of ependymal differentiation ("ependymal medulloblastoma"). The occasional presence of striated muscle fibers ("myomedulloblastoma") and rosette formation suggest a relation to the matrix of the pineal body, also a site where medulloblastoma-like tumors occur. The tissue of the area postrema, consisting of both a neuronal and a mesenchymal component, is repeated in the architecture of "desmoplastic medulloblastomas," which may be an anaplastic version of hemangioblastoma. These tumors affect both children and adults and possess rather characteristic clinical and histologic features. Some authors remove them from the medulloblastoma group and classify them as circumscribed arachnoid sarcomas or cerebellar sarcomas.

The rare **medulloepitheliomas** and **cerebral neuroblastomas** are also embryonic tumors and are included with cerebellar medulloblastomas in the group of "primitive neuroectodermal tumors" (PNET) (Rorke 1983).

Lymphoproliferative and myeloproliferative processes probably affect the brain more frequently than is generally assumed. Most primary **malignant** (Hodgkin's and non-Hodgkin's) **lymphomas** are immunocytic and lymphoblastic varieties (Jellinger and Radaszkiewicz 1976). But all other forms may also occur in the setting of generalized disease, including Hodgkin's lymphoma. **Leukemic** neoplasias can also involve the brain through secondary spread, whether by intracerebral seeding or by extension from a meningeal focus.

Intracranial **fibrous histiocytomas** are comparatively rare. Controversy still surrounds the place of pleomorphic fibrous xanthomas, which are positive for GFAP in immunohistochemical studies (xanthomatous transformation of astrocytes or GFAP uptake by stromal cells?) (Kepes et al. 1979). Some giant cell tumors (**"monstrocellular sarcomas"**), especially those with lipid storage, may be "xanthoastrocytomas" (Kepes 1979), if not pleomorphic malignant fibrous histiocytomas.

In **histiocytosis X**, the collective term for Hand-Schüller-Christian disease, eosinophilic granuloma, and Abt-Letterer-Siwe disease, it is not uncommon for lesions to involve the hypothalamus. It is unclear whether the process is truly neoplastic.

Another area of uncertainty concerns tumors descended from microglia. Isolation of the oligodendroglia by Del Río Hortega (1921) from the "third element" of Cajal left behind cell forms in the "microglia" group consisting of glial stem cells ("resting microglia") as well as macrophages adapted to the CNS milieu ("progressive microglia") and closely related to the mononuclear phagocytic system (MPS). Because cells of malignant lymphomas can sometimes be demonstrated by the impregnation method described by Del Río Hortega for microglia, Rubinstein (1972) suggested the term **reticulum cell sarcoma/microglioma** for these tumors. The question of cerebral MPS tumors is still unresolved.

Choroid plexus, the only tissue that can truly be called neuroepithelial, develops in areas where the neural tube differentiates into a single layer of epithelium. Tumor-like hypertrophy of this tissue leads to the development of **plexus papillomas**, which may be associated with hydrocephalus (hypersecretory?) in children. The rare mucus-forming plexus adenomas (Rubinstein 1972) may represent a metaplastic transition to the tissue of the subcommissural organ. Malignant plexus papillomas and plexus carcinomas are extremely rare. Dissemination via the CSF is not equivalent to metastasis in the accepted sense.

Tumors arising in the pineal body may differentiate along the line of pine(al)ocytes, the degree of differentiation being expressed by the terms **"pine(al)ocytoma"** or **"pine(al)-oblastoma"** (for the much less differentiated forms). Since nests of glia are consistently found in the pineal body of adults, the pineal tumors properly include astrocytomas, occasionally with giant cell forms (Schmincke 1930) or even neuronal components. (Germ cell tumors of the pineal body were also called "anisomorphic" pinealomas in the older literature.)

As noted earlier, "pilocytic" astrocytomas are found in the wall of the third ventricle (including the neurohypophysis). These lesions, known also as "infundibulomas," may coexist with collections of storage cells in the pituitary stalk that resemble the granular cell tumors composed of modified Schwann cells of peripheral nerve fibers. These cell collections are usually found incidentally and rarely cause a mass effect. Sternberg (1921) and Priesel (1922) considered them to be ectopias and referred to them as **choristomas**. Although this name gives no information as to histology, it is still in use. The occurrence of these lesions is considered evidence of a metabolic relationship between the sheath cells of peripheral nerve fibers and the glial cells of the circumventricular organs.

Suprasellar germinomas are germ cell tumors which differ from their pineal counterparts (see below) only in their location. They were called ectopic pinealomas in the older literature.

The most important tumors that develop in the region of the meninges, i.e., in the subarachnoid space and also in the choroid plexus stroma, are those that arise from the tissues of the leptomeninges and whose cells tend to differentiate along the lines of arachnothelial forms. The basic shape of the arachnothelial cell is a flat disc. Time-lapse studies in tissue cultures reveal peculiar spinning movements of individual cells which are imparted to surrounding cells and lead to the formation of onion-like laminated structures, often with central hyaline degeneration of cells and with calcium salt deposition forming a psammomatous body from the laminated structure. On sections, the stacked arrangement of the cells has commonly been interpreted in the literature as representing a spindle cell shape similar to fibroblasts, even though cross-sections through cell bundles are not seen, and the shapes of individual cells are observable among the stacks. **Meningiomas** rarely demonstrate mitotic activity. Loss of the laminated and stacked structures coupled with the presence of mitotic figures should raise suspicion of a heightened growth tendency (grade 2), a fact of clinical importance only if the tumor resection is incomplete. Further loss of differentiation creates the histologic picture of **meningeal sarcoma** (grade 3). Some meningiomas are highly vascular, and some present well-defined cell boundaries as a result of lipid deposition.

Vascular meningiomas require differentiation from **hemangiopericytomas**, which occur in the meninges as in other parts of the body. These tumors are rarely benign and are associated with high rates of recurrence and metastasis. Designation of these tumors and of supratentorial hemangioblastomas (see below) as "angioblastic meningiomas" merely substitutes a topographic classification for a histogenetic one.

Scheithauer and Rubinstein (1976) redefined "chondroblastic meningiomas" as meningeal mesenchymal chondrosarcomas, separating them from the class of meningiomas.

The melanocytes of the pia mater form yet another component of the meningeal tissue. They can proliferate and produce a leptomeningeal melanosis with no mass effect, or they may form circumscribed **meningeal melanomas** or even malignant melanomas that can metastasize to other organs.

A rare tumor of dural origin is the **fibroma**. Another rare tumor developing in the pia mater bears a histologic resemblance to "soft fibromas." A new cell population occurring between the arachnothelium and the innermost layer of the dura, the neurothelium, was discovered by Andres in 1967. These cells are fragile and prone to autolysis, and their disappearance can simulate the presence of a subdural space. In response to hemorrhage they proliferate to form the granulation tissue of "pachymeningitis interna haemorrhagica." These cells also form the nidus for endothelioma- or histiocytoma-like tumors.

The processes of nerve cells outside the central nervous system are invested by a population of sheath cells which differ from the neuroglia. The sheath cells of the nerve fibers (the Schwann cells of uniaxonal fibers and Remak cells of multiaxonal fibers) are closely related to the perineural sheath cells that envelop the fascicles. The descendants of these sheath cells give rise to two types of tumor: **neurofibromas** and **neurinomas**, the latter known also as schwannomas, neurilemomas, and neurolemmomas. Neurofibromas are characterized both by an accumulation of mucoid (basement membrane?) material, which begins subperineurally, and by a proliferation of sheath cells. The histologic picture of neurinomas is characterized by proliferation only. Nerve roots are similar to peripheral nerves in their fascicular makeup, except that the root fascicles are covered by leptomeninx rather than perineurium. This prevents the accumulation of mucoid material, which is quickly removed via the CSF, and explains why even in generalized neurofibromatosis (von Recklinghausen's disease) the tumors of cranial nerve roots always take the form of neurinomas rather than neurofibromas. In the initial phase of neurinoma development, the proliferation of sheath cells stimulates the outgrowth of axon collaterals, causing the neurinoma temporarily to acquire the character of a true neuroma as defined by Virchow (1864/65).

Adenomas of the anterior lobe of the pituitary are known to produce mass effects in some instances. The simplified classification into chromophobic, eosinophilic, and basophilic types is being gradually discarded in favor of a classification based on the hormone produced (e.g., ACTH, prolactin, somatotropin) and the storage phase.

Angiomas are not included among the tumors described in this book, and the only tumorlike lesion of vascular structures that will be considered is the **hemangioblastoma**. This tumor most commonly occurs infratentorially at various sites in the cerebellum. Supratentorial sites are much less frequent, the most common being the area of the planum sphenoidale (Earle 1980). Confusion regarding the best designation for these tumors can be avoided by using the eponym "Lindau's tumor." Recently the detection of GFAP in the stroma cells (Kepes 1979) has rekindled debate as to the origin of these cells and their lipid inclusions. Multifocal growth is possible and can mimic a recurrence. Desmoplastic medulloblastomas may show unmistakable similarities to hemangioblastoma. Mesenchymal tumors that are included under the heading of "monstrocellular sarcomas" are derived from the vascularized mesenchyma rather than from vascular structures and should not be classified among the angiomas.

Given the complex development of the CNS, it is not unusual to find tumorlike masses of **dysontogenetic** origin in central nervous tissues. Some of these lesions are ectopias while others are hamartomas with anomalous overgrowth of a tissue component.

The temporal lobe is the most favored site for the occurrence of circumscribed gliomalike foci which, while often epileptogenic, show no discernible proliferative tendency or mass effect. The histologic picture of these **hamartomas** is highly variable and may resemble any intrinsic brain tumor of very low malignancy, including gangliogliomas, or may simulate reactive gliosis. A mosaic pattern composed of astrocytic, oligodendrocytic, and other areas is not uncommon. It remains unclear whether these hamartomas represent "arrested" gliomas or a hyperplastic, keloidlike regenerative process secondary to an encephalitic or ischemic tissue injury sustained in very early life. True neoplastic transformation is possible.

Among the vascular malformations or hemangiomas, the capillary hemangiomas (telangiectasias) have no clinical or neurosurgical importance, while the arteriovenous angiomas (formerly termed arteriovenous aneurysms) rarely produce a significant mass effect. **Cavernous hemangiomas** (cavernomas) consist of blood spaces which are crowded together as a result of (pressure?) atrophy of brain tissue. Their walls have the structure of giant capillaries, and the spaces communicate with the normal circulation sufficiently to enhance after intravenous contrast injection.

Small nests of keratinizing or nonkeratinizing squamous epithelium or small epithelial cysts are consistently found in the intermediate zone between the anterior and posterior lobes of the pituitary in adults. The potential at that site for ectopic differentiation along the lines of the stomodeal epithelium defines the histologic picture of **craniopharyngioma** (Erdheim's tumor) and the histologic variants of epidermoids and epithelium-lined **Rathke's pouch cysts**.

Cysts lined by mucus-forming epithelium with yellow pigment granules may be found in the tela choroidea near the foramen of Monro, where the choroid plexus is reflected from the lateral ventricles onto the roof of the third ventricle. These cysts contain a colloid material of very high radiopacity. The epithelium of these **colloid cysts** most closely resembles the non-neuronal elements of the olfactory mucosa. (The term "neuroepithelial cyst" is inappropriate, as there is no evidence that the cysts arise from the neural tube.)

The intrameningeal ectopias include **endodermal cysts**, whose epithelial lining resembles that of the alimentary tract.

Meningeal **lipomas** are another dysontogenetic ectopia and result from the differentiation of fat lobules in the leptomeninx, most likely reflecting the pluripotent nature of the primitive mesenchyma.

The ectopic differentiation of cutaneous structures in the meninges can produce an **epidermoid** or **dermoid cyst**, the latter distinguished by the presence of skin appendages such as sebaceous glands. These cysts grow at an extremely slow rate by the accumulation of exfoliated keratinous material and may attain huge size before producing a mass effect.

The dysontogenetic nature of intracranial **germ cell tumors** is even more striking than in the tumors cited above. **Teratomas** occur chiefly in the area of the pineal body (extremely asymmetrical cephalopagus?); suprasellar sites are far less common. **Embryonic carcinomas** present a less varied histologic picture that includes endodermal structures of the yolk sac. **Choriocarcinoma** is differentiated along the lines of trophoblastic structures. **Germinomas** are germ cell tumors that lack embryogenetic potential. They are the counterpart to seminomas of the testis and to dysgerminomas of the ovary. They tend to have a uniform cell population (occasionally with giant cells), which incites a lymphocytic tissue reaction or sometimes a granulomatous reaction with tuberculoid structures and Langhans giant cells. Like teratomas, germinomas chiefly affect the pineal body and are less frequent in the suprasellar region, where they were formerly called "ectopic pinealomas" in the belief that pineal germinomas were anisomorphic pinealomas.

The dysontogenetic disorders include **tuberous sclerosis**, whose lesions may affect the brain, heart, kidneys, lung, and skin without regard for germ-layer associations. Lesions of the cerebral cortex conform to the pattern of resting hyperplasia, while lesions of the ependyma present as characteristic **subependymal giant cell "astrocytomas"**.

Tumors arising in the skeletal elements of the cranium include **osteomas, osteogenic sarcomas, chondromas, chondromyxoid fibromas,** and in the broader sense **fibrous dysplasia. Chordomas** are reasonably common tumors that reproduce the histologic pattern of the notochord. The form known as **chondroid chordoma** can present problems in terms of differential diagnosis.

Intracranial extension is a secondary attribute of various tumors that arise outside the cranial cavity and spread to the cranial interior through locally invasive growth. Foremost among these are **adenoid cystic carcinomas**, formerly called cylindromas, which arise from the mucosae of the paranasal sinuses. The cranial cavity also may be invaded by **esthesioneuroblastomas** (olfactory neuroblastomas), which develop from the neuronal population of the olfactory area and thus from a population independent of the neural tube and crests. These tumors can invade the anterior cranial fossa from the upper part of the nasal cavity. **Rhabdomyosarcoma**, a fairly common tumor of the orbit or ear in children, may exhibit similar behavior.

Tumors of the glomus jugulare also can spread by extension into the cranial cavity from a primary extracranial focus. They arise from peripheral nervous structures which relate to peripheral ganglia in much the same way as the circumventricular organs of the brain relate to its neuronal structures. These peripheral structures, called paraganglia, are either active in the production of neurohormones, like the adrenal medulla, or perform sensory functions. Tumors arising from these sensory elements, as they occur in the carotid body and in the glomus jugulare, are called **paragangliomas** or **chemodectomas**.

Besides primary intracranial growths and tumors that spread to the cranial cavity by local invasion, the brain may be affected by secondary tumors or **metastases**. The tumors that most commonly involve the brain by direct hematogenous spread are bronchogenic carcinoma, breast carcinoma, malignant melanoma, and hypernephroid renal carcinoma. Some metastases produce a mass effect through the development of perifocal edema. In the absence of edema, the space-occupying effect does not occur and only a volume-replacing effect (Merrem 1962) is seen as the lesion makes room for itself through local tissue destruction. Metastatic sarcomas of the brain are far less common than metastases from carcinoma or malignant melanoma. Some carcinomas involve the brain through tertiary spread. An example is gastric carcinoma, which metastasizes first to the cranial vault, where it incites a local pachymeningitic reaction, infiltrates the meninges, and produces a meningeal carcinomatosis which ultimately gives rise to intracerebral foci.

C. Technique of CT and MR Examinations

1. Technique of CT Examination

a) CT Scanners

The three original groups participating in our study used the EMI Mark I scanner from 1975 to the middle of 1977 and the EMI CT 1010 scanner after mid-1977. The Siemens Somatom DR has been used in Augsburg and Berlin since 1983, and the Philips Tomoscan CT 350 in Mainz since mid-1986.

b) Preparation for CT and Conduct of the Examination

The CT scans for *standard examinations* were performed parallel to the orbitomeatal line. The head was flexed 15° for examination of the cerebellar region and was extended 20° for scanning the basal temporal lobes and the orbit.

The large gantry aperture and tilt were utilized to obtain *coronal scans*, for which the patient was positioned prone with the head extended.

Image artifacts were minimized by close attention to correct examination technique and by optimum positioning of the patient, which in some cases required general anesthesia. Even so, method-related artifacts could not be entirely eliminated. This applies especially to the area between the petrous bones and to the basal skull region. Artifacts emanating from dental fillings cannot always be avoided in the coronal projection.

We have eliminated *metal clips* as a source of artifacts by modifying our neurosurgical techniques and, since 1975, restricting the use of such clips to aneurysms and large arteriovenous angiomas.

We routinely begin CT examinations with a *noncontrast* sequence extending from the base to the vertex of the skull. In our experience it is advantageous to obtain a complete sequence of slices, even after *contrast injection* (if required), so that multiple lesions will not go undetected. When an intracranial mass lesion was recognized, intermediate slices were often imaged in the region of the abnormality. The postcontrast scan was always performed immediately after the injection of contrast material.

We employed *image reconstruction* where needed to resolve certain questions. It proved especially useful for evaluating lesions close to the midline and lesions of the sellar region (Unsöld et al. 1982).

c) Intravenous Contrast Injection

In our view it is often futile to attempt to interpret CT images accurately or make a diagnosis of tissue type unless both pre- and postcontrast scans are obtained. Without contrast enhancement a large proportion of primarily isodense tumors, which accounted for almost 15% of brain tumors in our population, will not be visualized by CT. This was the case in 40% of isodense brain tumors in our series, or 6% of all patients with intracranial neoplasms. Contrast enhancement also provides better delineation of tumors in relation to perifocal edema and surrounding brain, especially in the case of metastases and glioblastomas. Moreover, the differences in tumor density before and after contrast injection yield important differential diagnostic information that cannot be obtained by any other means. The postcontrast scan is especially helpful in differentiating a vascular lesion from a tumor. On the other hand, using contrast-enhanced CT initially, without the benefit of a precontrast study, would needlessly increase the risk and the cost of the examination, since the indication for contrast medium primarily rests on the result of the noncontrast scan (see below). In addition, there are lesions that become isodense to surrounding tissue *after* contrast administration and are not visualized. This is illustrated by a cerebral infarction scanned in the early phase, when the blood-brain barrier still shows minimal breakdown, or in the late phase, when the blood-brain barrier is being restored. In some cases it would not be possible to distinguish a massive intracerebral hemorrhage from an intensely enhancing tumor.

The contrast dose for most adult examinations was between 20 and 30 g of iodine, depending on body weight, administered by bolus injection in a solution of approximately 300 mg iodine/ml. Recently we have adopted the practice of administering 30 g of iodine by infusion. Children were given much smaller doses, the usual amount being 1 ml of a solution of 300 mg iodine/ml per kg body weight. The preferred contrast media are nonionic preparations such as Omnipaque 300, Solutrast 300, or Ultravist 300. Meglumine salts of ionic contrast media, such as Angiografin, Rayvist 300, and Telebrix 300, are also satisfactory if still available.

Risks of Contrast Injection

The injection of contrast medium always carries a certain risk, even when a nonionic agent is used. Adverse reactions are always a possibility and cannot be excluded by preexposure testing (Lalli 1980; Wende and Speck 1981). Therefore:

- The patient must be questioned about any allergies he may have or any previous adverse reactions to contrast media that he may have experienced.
- The risks of the examination should be carefully weighed against the benefits, and alternative modalities considered, especially in patients with known risk factors (see below).
- The patient should be informed about the risks and benefits of the procedure.
- The examiner should be prepared to deal immediately with any adverse reactions that occur.

Given the very low frequency of contrast reactions that require treatment (Schrott et al. 1986), especially when nonionic media are used, special attention should be given to all appropriate prophylactic measures.

The examining physician should be present during the postcontrast study. "Every physician who routinely employs radiographic contrast media must be prepared to institute appropriate treatment without delay in the event of a significant adverse response" (Elke and Ferstl 1974).

The specific risks associated with contrast injection are discussed below.

Systemic Reactions

We shall not describe in detail the mild to severe systemic contrast reactions involving the skin and mucosae, the cardiovascular system, the respiratory system, and the autonomic and central nervous systems. These reactions most likely relate to a sudden release of biogenetic amines, such as histamine, and to activation of the complement and coagulation system. In 80% of cases they occur within 5 min following the contrast injection, and most can be adequately managed by trained medical personnel.

When nonionic contrast media are used, the incidence of these reactions falls to one-half to one-tenth the observed incidence of reactions to ionic contrast media (Dahlstrom et al. 1982; Tschakert 1983). The nature of the reactions and the measures taken to control them, however, are similar.

In recent years some treatment protocols, such as the oral administration of 32 mg methylprednisolone 12 and 2 h before the examination or the combined administration of H_1 and H_2 blockers, have proved effective in preventing adverse systemic reactions to conventional ionic contrast media (Lasser et al. 1984; Reimann et al. 1986). The value of this prophylaxis for nonionic contrast media has yet to be established. In any case, nonionic media should be used in patients with a history of allergy. There are many reports in the literature of patients who repeatedly manifested allergic reactions to ionic contrast agents, some severe, but who showed no adverse response to subsequent examination with nonionic media (Rapoport et al. 1982; Holtas 1984).

Even with the most conscientious technique, it is impossible to eliminate an occasional **death following i.v. contrast injection**. Shehadi and Tonilo (1980) reported a total of 18 deaths in 302083 patients (=0.006%) who received contrast medium by i.v. or i.a. injection. Ansell et al. (1980) reported 1 death in 7650 patients examined by contrast-enhanced CT (=0.01%), and Hobbs (1981) reported 4 deaths in 26712 patients (=0.01%).

Observations from 140048 CT examinations were reported in a 1986 collective study involving four major centers (Wende, Mainz; Voigt, Tübingen; Hammer, Linz; DuBoulay, London). Contrast medium was administered in 37% of the cases (=52124 patients). No deaths were recorded. However, the study contained a report of a patient with bronchial asthma who underwent contrast-enhanced CT (CECT). Following the injection of 5–10 ml of meglumine ioglicinate the patient experienced cyanosis, pulmonary spasms, and cardiac arrest that could not be reversed despite immediate intervention and anesthesia. Postmortem findings were consistent with the assumption of a fatal anaphylactic reaction induced by the contrast injection.

It will be appreciated, then, that the number of fatal contrast reactions in CECT is extremely small. Allowing for the fact that some of these incidents go unreported in the literature, it is reasonable to assume that the mortality rate is approximately the same as that associated with contrast injections for intravenous urography.

Given the growing frequency of reports of contrast-induced **renal dysfunction** in CT examinations, it is appropriate to consider these effects in some detail.

We know from radiology and from urologists who perform radiographic studies that i.v. pyelography is ordered in hospitalized patients and in outpatients even when renal disease is known to be present. Elevated creatinine levels are unlikely to be noticed, especially in outpatients, and in fact higher contrast doses are given to patients with renal disease so that an optimum excretory urogram will be obtained.

Renal dysfunction in response to contrast injection was first reported by Bergman et al. (1968) in their paper "Acute renal failure after drip infusion pyelography." In subsequent years other authors described similar phenomena, first in pyelography and angiography and later in connection with CECT. Most authors described reversible changes, although some deaths from irreversible renal failure were reported (Pillay et al. 1970; Dudzinski et al. 1971; Myers and Witten 1971; Barshay et al. 1973; Elke and Ferstl 1974; Kleinknecht et al. 1974; Port et al. 1974; Diaz-Buxo et al. 1975; Ansari and Baldwin 1976; Berezin 1977; Hanaway and Black 1977; Kamdar et al. 1977; Alexander et al. 1978; Baltzer 1978; Carvallo et al. 1978; Shafi et al. 1978; Swartz et al. 1978; Wagoner 1978; Warren et al. 1978; Weinrauch et al. 1978; Van Zee et al. 1978; Pierach 1979; Maurer 1980).

- Which patients are at increased risk for contrast-induced renal dysfunction?
- How is this condition manifested?
- What are its causes?
- How can it be prevented?

Patients undergoing CECT are considered to be at significant risk for renal failure when any of the following risk factors are present: renal insufficiency, insulin-dependent diabetes, hypertension and/or vascular disease, and dehydration. If two or more of these factors coexist, the risk of renal failure is potentiated.

High contrast doses in a kidney with minimal preexisting disease as well as repeated contrast doses over a period of several days can led to severe reversible or irreversible renal dysfunction.

Common manifestations of contrast-induced renal dysfunction are oliguria and an elevated serum creatinine. Oliguria develops an average of 12–24 h following the administration of contrast medium and usually clears within 8–10 days.

A transient impairment of renal function often goes unnoticed by both patient and physician. Close observation of the patient is necessary to identify the signs of renal dysfunction so that they can be reported to the attending physician.

The serum creatinine may rise to 6–8 mg/dl or even higher, signifying a severe renal dysfunction that may necessitate dialysis. Diaz-Buxo (1975) and Weinrauch et al. (1978) cited cases in which patients suffering contrast-induced renal failure required dialysis or even renal transplantation. Meeker (1978) described one death after CECT occurring in a 67-year-old man with age-related diabetes.

The cause of contrast-induced renal dysfunction is still poorly understood. Possible explanations include a change in intrarenal blood flow, increased blood viscosity with a decrease in renal blood flow, protein precipitation in the renal tubules, and an antibody response. The most likely cause is a direct nephrotoxic effect of the contrast medium on the kidneys, evidenced histologically by interstitial inflammation, edema, and acute necrosis in the proximal and distal portions of the tubule (Ansari and Baldwin 1976).

How can contrast-induced nephrotoxicity be avoided? The physician ordering a CT scan must provide the physician performing the examination with more than a simple request and a presumptive diagnosis. Relevant data on the patient's history, clinical findings, laboratory data, and the specific purpose of the study must be communicated. The examining physician is obliged to familiarize himself with the patient and should never assume that an adequate preliminary workup has been performed. By studying the data himself, he will be in a position to weigh the putative value of the CECT examination against the potential risk. CECT should never be the initial study in a routine diagnostic workup. Rather, the decision whether to perform CECT should be based on the history, the clinical examination report, the results of lower-risk studies, and the noncontrast CT scan.

The fluid and electrolyte balance should be evaluated before contrast medium is administered, and fluids given as required. Adequate fluid intake should be maintained for at least 12 h following the contrast injection.

The physician performing the CT examination is further obligated to inform the attending physician of possible renal dysfunction caused by the contrast medium and to recommend appropriate evaluation, i.e., measurement of urine output and serum creatinine for several days after CECT in patients at risk.

If CECT is deemed necessary on clinical grounds in a patient with severe renal insufficiency combined with diabetes and/or a vascular disorder, provision must be made for possible dialysis therapy for a period of 3 days following the contrast injection. CECT should be withheld from patients whose preexamination creatinine levels exceed 4.5 mg/dl.

Recently it has been suggested that the renal toxicity of contrast media as reflected in case reports or noncomparative studies may be overstated. A controlled study has shown that patients undergoing CT without contrast medium showed signs of renal dysfunction just as frequently as patients who received contrast medium during the examination (Cramer et al. 1985).

Based on evidence to date, it is reasonable to conclude that available intravenous contrast media will produce no clinically significant nephrotoxic effects when administered in doses up to 50 g iodine in adults who have no specific risk factors.

Effects on the Central Nervous System

Many tumors of the CNS cause a breakdown of the blood-brain barrier, allowing intravenous contrast medium to come in direct contact with otherwise inaccessible brain areas and their immediate surroundings. Indeed, Scott (1980) reported an increased rate of seizures in patients with intracranial metastases evaluated by CECT, although the contrast media consisted of highly concentrated preparations containing sodium salt. It is unlikely that the current nonionic contrast media would produce similar effects, since these preparations are already considered safe for subarachnoidal use.

A similar potential for injury exists in cerebral infarcts, although this has not been demonstrated even for ionic contrast media (Pullicino and Kendall 1980). Hammer (1984) published a risk-benefit analysis for the use of contrast medium in a presumed cerebral infarct and concluded that CECT is unnecessary in patients whose history, clinical presentation, and noncontrast CT findings are unremarkable.

Iodinated Contrast Media in Hyperthyroidism

Another problem concerns iodine-induced hyperthyroidism. We know that the administration of iodine can produce overt hyperthyroidism in patients with latent thyroid disease. This applies not just to contrast media but to any iodine-containing medication or antiseptic. History taking should therefore include questions about possible thyroid disease.

Iodine is not given to patients with manifest hyperthyroidism.

Plasmocytoma

Based on current knowledge, plasmocytoma is not an absolute contraindication to the use of contrast media. It is essential, however, that the patient be adequately hydrated. One to two liters of fluid should be given prior to the contrast examination.

Contrast Dose for CT

Various dose recommendations for contrast medium are stated in the literature. We have found 30 g of iodine to be sufficient for CT examinations (see above). American examiners use an average of 40 g, while some authors state that doses up to 80 g may be given with no side effects (Paling 1978; Davis et al. 1979; Hayman et al. 1979). The use of large contrast doses was first reported by Ethier et al. (1975) and Kramer et al. (1975), who claimed that large doses of iodine provided better definition of cerebral lesions and could, for example, demonstrate a larger number of metastatic foci than a smaller dose.

Davis et al. (1979) cautioned that 80 g of iodine should not be used in patients with a serum creatinine higher than 1.5 mg/dl or in patients who are dehydrated. These authors claim that there are no differences in the frequency, severity, and duration of renal dysfunction between patients receiving 80 g of iodine and those receiving 40 g. Hayman et al. (1980) recommend high doses of iodine (80 g) for scans taken with a 1-h delay as a means of demonstrating lesions that would otherwise go undetected.

Our experience has been that higher doses of iodine do not significantly improve the diagnosis of cerebral lesions. It is true that some tumors and especially metastases are more clearly defined when 80 g of iodine is administered. However, these lesions are also demonstrated with 30 g of iodine, and we feel there is little advantage to be gained by demonstrating, say, ten intracerebral metastases instead of just five. A high contrast dose is justified only in borderline cases where, for example, a CT correlate cannot be found for a given set of clinical symptoms using ordinary techniques.

High doses of iodine may increase the side effects of CT examinations, and the costs increase steeply. What is more, very high doses of contrast media, especially the ionic types, can completely disrupt the water and electrolyte balance in older patients and in infants.

The risk of high iodine doses, then, appears to outweigh the potential gain and therefore is not acceptable as a general rule.

The increased risk of high contrast doses is further demonstrated by an observation of Slasky and Lenkey (1981). These authors described the death of a 67-year-old woman who received 100 ml of sodium diatrizate for a urogram. The patient had received an injection of 150 ml of meglumine iothalamate for a CT study performed the same day, resulting in a total dose of 72 g of iodine. Within 24 h the patient became oliguric, her serum creatinine rose from 0.9 mg/dl to 4.1 mg/dl, and she developed pulmonary edema. She expired 5 days later.

Informing the Patient About the Procedure

We do not feel it is necessary to have the candidate for a CECT examination give explicit oral or written consent to the procedure. Nevertheless, the physician has an obligation to question the patient about any allergies he has and any previous adverse reactions to radiographic contrast media. At that time the patient should also be apprised of the risks of the procedure, whereupon his submission to the examination is considered to imply tacit consent.

The general policy in the U.S. is summarized in a 1975 publication of the American College of Radiology (Spring et al. 1984; Brown 1985):

> In performance of radiologic procedures carrying a relatively low risk and usually done at the request of the attending physician who is familiar with the clinical problems of the patient, it is not necessary, and at times may be unwise, to discuss with the patient the remote possibility of complications of the procedure. The radiolo-

gist should use his best judgment regarding consultation with the physician concerning the indication for the procedure and management of the examination. Radiologists should be reasonably prepared to deal with any emergency that might develop.

The importance of the examining physician being present at the examination is again emphasized.

d) Intrathecal Contrast Injection

In rare cases the intralumbar administration of nonionic myelographic contrast media (Amipaque, Solutrast M) for CT examination may be necessary:

a) To confirm or exclude communication between a cystic lesion and the CSF spaces, e.g., for cysts in the suprasellar region or for differential diagnosis (arachnoidal cyst/large cisterna magna)
b) To demonstrate an intracisternal mass lesion of CSF density, e.g., for an epidermoid cyst

Today we rarely use water-soluble contrast media to demonstrate tumors extending into the basal cisterns (sellar region, cerebellopontine angle region), as described by Greitz and Hindmarsh (1974), because of the side effects (see below) and the availability of better imaging modalities (MRI).

In our experience the contrast dose necessary for good CT visualization of the cisterns is 5–8 ml (150–200 mg iodine/ml) of an isotonic myelographic dye. Positioning the patient with the pelvis slightly elevated and the head flexed provides good filling of all cisterns 3–6 h after intrathecal administration of the contrast medium (Sprung and Grumme 1979).

Intrathecal injection of metrizamide may precipitate headache, vomiting, and dizziness. Confusional states have occasionally been reported in older patients (Schmidt 1980). Such responses are virtually unknown when the newer, water-soluble contrast media for myelography are used (Hammer and Deisenhammer 1985).

e) Interpretation of CT Images

CT interpretation relied partly on the analog image and partly on the digital values in regions of interest, which can be rapidly analyzed using special evaluative programs. We used a program that performs statistical calculations of density values in the region of interest and plots histograms of the same region. The accuracy of CT numbers was assured by using phantoms to periodically check the machine calibration.

The *X-ray absorption of suspected tumor tissue* was evaluated on the noncontrast analog image using the gray level of normal brain tissue as a reference standard. Each lesion was placed in one of four categories:

1. *Lesions that appear brighter than normal brain tissue on the analog image* as a result of **increased** X-ray absorption. These lesions are described as **hyperdense**.
2. *Lesions that appear darker than normal brain tissue* as a result of **decreased** X-ray absorption. These lesions are described as **hypodense**.
3. *Lesions that display the same gray level as normal brain tissue* because of equivalent X-ray absorption. These lesions are said to be **isodense**.
4. *Lesions containing areas that vary in their X-ray absorption.* These lesions do not display a uniform gray level and are said to be of **mixed density**.

The analog image was also used in determining *whether the density of a tumor increased after intravenous contrast injection.* The criterion for tumor enhancement was a visible increase in the brightness of the tumor on the CT image. A tumor whose X-ray absorption changed by only 1 – 4 HU was considered to be nonenhancing, since this change is comparable to that occurring in normal brain tissue when i.v. contrast is given, and no appreciable gray-level difference is apparent between tumor and brain. The second CT examination (postcontrast scan) was always performed immediately after injection of the contrast medium. In selected cases we repeated the scan of the tumor-bearing tissue slice after 10, 20, or 30 min.

CT was the first modality capable of demonstrating *perifocal edema.* With its relatively high water content, the edema appears as a hypodense area usually confined to the white matter.

Cerebellar edema likewise appears hypodense, its frequency and extent varying with the tumor type. A finger-shaped area of edema signifies extension of the tumor to the white matter and explains why even large meningiomas may be unassociated with major edema.

In an earlier work we proposed the following scheme for grading the extent of perifocal edema (Kazner et al. 1975):

Grade I edema	Rim of edema up to 2 cm in diameter around the tumor
Grade II edema	Peritumoral edema more than 2 cm in diameter and involving up to half of a cerebral hemisphere
Grade III edema	Peritumoral edema involving more than half of a cerebral hemisphere

f) Differential Diagnosis of Tissue Type

Opinions vary widely regarding the ability of CT to discriminate tissue type. Indeed, even common tumors that have a characteristic CT appearance, such as meningioma, glioblastoma, and pituitary adenoma, can pose major problems of differential diagnosis in any given case. Nevertheless, the correct tissue type can be established in more than 80% of cases when the CT presentation is evaluated in conjunction with the history and clinical findings. The accuracy rates in our own patients are 84% for meningioma, 83% for glioblastoma, and better than 90% for pituitary adenoma. Metastases were identified as such in about 80% of cases, owing largely to clues derived from the patient's history. Even less common brain tumors having a prevalence of less than 2% could be correctly identified in 56% of cases (Kazner and Steinhoff 1979). Given the experience gained in the past few years, we would expect that retrospective analysis of the earlier CT scans would yield an even better result.

Establishing the tissue type of an intracranial tumor relies not only on the CT presentation but also on the following clinical data:

1. Typical site of occurrence
2. Typical age of occurrence
3. Gender predilection
4. X-ray absorption or tissue density before and after contrast injection
5. Structural pattern
6. Tumor configuration
7. Perifocal edema

Zülch (1956), among others, directed attention to the first three factors long before the advent of computed tomography. These features are invaluable in the analysis and interpretation of CT images. Later we shall discuss these points in some detail with reference to specific tumor types, and they are reflected in our selection of illustrative scans.

The *analysis of CT scans* is based both on the *analog image*, or actual computed tomogram, and on the *digital values* (CT numbers), which convey a more accurate impression of true X-ray absorption than viewing the gray scales on an analog image. The analysis of dig-

Table 1. X-ray absorption (Hounsfield units) of normal and pathologic tissues and fluids in the cranial cavity and orbit (noncontrast CT)

Medium	Mean HU number in digital readout
Bone	to +1000
Calcifications	from + 60
Gray matter	+ 32 to + 40
White matter	+ 28 to + 32
CSF	+ 3 to + 14[a]
Flowing blood	+ 32 to + 44
Clotted blood, fresh	+ 64 to + 86
Clotted blood, old	+ 30 to + 60
Gliomas (uncalcified)	+ 18 to + 40
Glioblastomas (viable tumor parts)	+ 29 to + 38
Ependymomas	+ 28 to + 50
Medulloblastomas	+ 36 to + 58
Meningiomas (uncalcified)	+ 36 to + 56
Neurinomas	+ 28 to + 40
Pituitary adenomas	+ 35 to + 50
Lipomas	−120 to − 40
Dysontogenetic tumors (epidermoid, dermoid, teratoma)	−120 to + 10
Metastases	+ 22 to + 50
Tumor cysts	+ 6 to + 22
Necrotic areas in brain tumors	+ 19 to + 23
Peritumoral edema	+ 18 to + 26
Fresh brain infarct	+ 22 to + 26
Old brain infarct	+ 10 to + 16
Brain abscess, capsule	+ 28 to + 34
Contents of abscess	+ 19 to + 23
Intraorbital fat	− 90 to − 70

[a] High values due to partial volume effect in narrow ventricles.

ital readings is most useful in the differential diagnosis of hypodense lesions – from brain edema to intracranial lipoma – and of hyperdense lesions – from a recent hemorrhage to foci of calcification (see Table 1). The degree to which the density of a lesion increases after contrast injection, i.e., its degree of enhancement, can contribute greatly to differential diagnosis. Very intense enhancement should always raise suspicion of a vascular or highly vascularized lesion.

Our experience over the years has shown that there are a great many *characteristic CT presentations associated with specific tumor types*, and that these patterns are very useful in identifying the tissue type of the lesion. We have included as many of these scans as possible among the illustrations in this volume, because *specific CT patterns tend to recur in specific tumors*. The *sites of predilection* of the various tumor types are also illustrated. At the same time, *atypical findings* are presented to demonstrate the *limits of CT as a method of diagnosing tissue type.*

We have placed considerable emphasis on *differential diagnosis with CT*, which is discussed in some detail following the descriptions of specific tumors and tumor sites. The differential diagnosis of intracranial masses necessarily includes non-neoplastic space-occupying lesions, and these are discussed and illustrated fully in a separate chapter (Chap. F). The book is organized in a way that obviates the need for tables with prevalence data on individual tumor types and their locations, as Zülch (1958) has already done so well in his neuropathologic analysis of intracranial tumors. The CT appearance of a tumor is often so characteristic that differential diagnosis is limited to a few possibilities from the outset, making statistical data of minor importance compared with the actual CT criteria used in a given case to identify the disease.

Most tumor types in this book are graded according to their *biologic behavior* and *prognosis*. Our grading system broadly resembles that proposed by Zülch (1979), which has been included in the new WHO classification:

Table 2. CT evaluation according to density criteria, contrast enhancement, and frequency and extent of perifocal edema in

Histologic diagnosis	Number of patients	X-ray absorption of tumor tissue relative to brain tissue on noncontrast scan				Tumor not demonstrated by noncontrast scan	Tumor not directly demonstrated by CT
		Hypodense	Isodense	Hyperdense	Mixed density		
Astrocytoma	153	150	1	–	2	–	–
Anaplastic astrocytoma	157	52	20	30	55	5	–
Oligodendroglioma	174	45	8	24	97	–	–
Glioblastoma	711	65	80	61	505	16	2
Pilocytic astrocytoma	112	35	22	17	38	5	–
Ependymoma	54	7	5	22	20	1	–
Medulloblastoma	67	3	7	43	14	3	1
Malignant lymphoma or sarcoma	62	9	9	27	17	1	–
Choroid plexus papilloma	14	–	3	9	2	1	–
Meningioma	602	5	85	441	59	40	12*
Neurinoma	196	16	111	33	18	79	18*
Pituitary adenoma	377	16	66	248	47	20	1
Hemangioblastoma	41	27	3	5	6	2	–
Craniopharyngioma	81	11	5	30	35	4	1
Epidermoid, dermoid, teratoma	36	25	1	1	9	1	–
Other brain tumors	192	48	21	93	30	11	4
Brain metastases	575	97	99	194	184	17	5*
Brain tumors of unknown histology	146	33	25	53	35	17	5*
Total	3750	644	571	1331	1173	223	49**
Percent	100	17.2	15.2	35.5	31.3	6.0	1.3

Grade I **benign**: cure or at least 5 years' survival after extirpation
Grade II **semibenign**: postoperative survival 3–5 years
Grade III **moderately malignant**: postoperative survival 2–3 years
Grade IV **highly malignant**: postoperative survival 6–15 months

Our own experience with CT in the first edition of this book (1982) was based on a series of 3750 patients with intracranial tumors and metastases who were evaluated from December 1974 to March 1980 (see Table 2). The diagnostic criteria derived from these cases have remained generally valid since that time and have not been significantly altered by more recent experience with larger case numbers. In 3589 of the patients (95.7%), the intracranial tumor or tumors were detected by the initial CT examination. In 112 patients (3.0%) serial CT examinations were needed to detect the brain tumor, and in 49 (1.3%) CT missed a tumor that was subsequently detected by other methods. The great majority of these tumors were small and located close to the skull base (acoustic neurinomas less than 15 mm in diameter, meningiomas), and almost all had been examined with the old EMI Mark I scanner. Our earliest cases also included patients with small, high-sited parietal tumors that were missed because the CT scans did not extend to the apex of the skull. The CT diagnosis was later confirmed histologically in 3604 patients. Confirmation could not be obtained in 146 patients due to inoperability or other reasons.

Table 5 shows the distribution of histologic tumor types among the patients examined at all four participating centers. The large number of brain tumor patients is explained by the fact that the four groups of CT workers are largely oriented toward neurosurgery. The overrepresentation of some tumor groups, such as pituitary adenomas, is a result of the special interests of the staff at the participating neurosurgical departments. Close cooperation with the local tumor centers led to an unexpectedly high percentage of patients with brain metastases.

3750 patients with intracranial tumors

Postcontrast studies	Tumor enhancement		Demonstration of perifocal edema				Comments
	Positive	Negative	Total	Grade I	Grade II	Grade III	
140	2*	138	3	2	1	–	* Gemistocytic astrocytoma
143	117	26	106	51	47	8	
163	75	88	66	38	25	3	
695	671	24	652	160	376	116	
106	87	19	28	26	2	–	
49	41	8	23	14	6	3	
60	56	4	31	28	3	–	
56	54	2	45	20	22	3	
13	13	–	6	4	1	1	
546	531	15	369	147	181	41	* Tumors near skull base, too small, or wrong CT slice
194	173	21	53	47	5	1	* Tumors less than 15 mm in diameter
358	343	15	5	5	–	–	
40	21	19	10	9	1	–	
66	45	21	1	1	–	–	
28	4	24	2	2	–	–	
158	102	56	38	15	17	6	
540	510	30	500	172	253	75	* 1 × wrong CT slice
128	94	34	32	18	13	1	* Including 3 isodense pontine tumors
483	2939	544	1970	759	953	258	** Grade total equals only 99.2% due to failures of detection
100	84.4	15.6	52.5	20.2	25.4	6.9	

2. Technique of MR Examination

The technique of magnetic resonance imaging (MRI) has been discussed extensively in numerous publications (e.g., Loeffler and Oppelt 1981; Pykett et al. 1982; Ramm et al. 1986). Here we shall give a brief introduction to the essential clinical aspects of MRI to aid the reader in interpreting the MR scans given in the clinical portion of this book.

a) Basic Physical Principles of MRI

Hydrogen nuclei possess a property called *spin.* Because the nuclei carry an electric charge, the motion of the nuclei results in the creation of a magnetic field (magnetic moment). When the hydrogen nuclei are exposed to an external static magnetic field, as in MRI, the nuclei will interact with the external field by virtue of their magnetic moment. The magnetic moments, which are randomly arranged in the absence of an external magnetic field, become oriented either parallel or antiparallel to the applied field. The nuclei in the two orientations differ in their energy, so two different energy states are created. At body temperature a slightly larger number of hydrogen nuclei occupy the lower energy state than the higher energy state. The distribution of nuclei between the two energy states can be altered only by adding energy to the system or withdrawing energy from it. In MRI this is done by exciting the hydrogen nuclei with a radiofrequency pulse whose frequency, and thus energy, precisely equals the energy difference between the parallel and antiparallel states. Hydrogen nuclei absorbing this energy can then "rise" from the lower to the higher energy state. When the radiofrequency pulse is switched off, the system returns to its ground state by releasing energy to surrounding matter. During this process the excited hydrogen nuclei emit a radiofrequency signal that can be detected electronically. This "MR signal" is utilized to construct an image.

Relaxation at the molecular level is based on an interaction of excited hydrogen nuclei with surrounding atoms and molecules. The time course of this interaction is described by the T1 and T2 relaxation times.

This quantum mechanical description of magnetic resonance characterizes MRI as a technique of tissue analysis in which the density of hydrogen nuclei (spin density) and the relaxation times T1 and T2 determine the MR signal of the sample in a homogeneous magnetic field. However, the use of MR for imaging requires that the MR signal be encoded with spatial information so that the point of origin of the signal can be defined. This can be done by superimposing a second, spatially varying magnetic field of low strength onto the main static field. This "gradient field" is induced by means of special coils placed in the inner lining of the magnet. The effect of the gradients is to cause the main field strength to vary along one axis, providing spatial encoding of the MR signal. A detailed discussion of the various spatial encoding techniques may be found in Ramm et al. (1986).

b) Pulse Sequences

Two principal MR scanning methods have emerged for routine clinical imaging: spin echo (SE) and inversion recovery (IR) (Brant-Zawadzki et al. 1984; Bydder and Young 1985). Both methods employ a sequence of two pulses (a 90° and a 180° pulse) to excite the hydrogen nuclei and detect a signal. The pulse sequence is repeated several times to obtain sufficient data for image reconstruction. Thus, for an MR image matrix consisting of 256×256 points, it is necessary to repeat the pulse sequence 256 times. The choice of the scanning method (SE or IR) and the interval between pulses characterize the sequence and determine the signal level and thus the degree of contrast in the MR image.

The SE sequence consists of an initial 90° pulse followed by a 180° pulse. The interval between two 90° pulses is the pulse repetition time TR. The interval between the 90° and 180° pulses is the echo delay time TE. For routine clinical imaging TR ranges from 200 to 3000 ms, TE from 30 to 240 ms.

Today frequent use is made of SE sequences in which two (double-echo technique) or more successive 180° pulses (multi-echo technique) are applied, each pair of successive pulses separated by an interval equal to TE. A signal or image of the same tissue slice can be acquired after each 180° pulse. The advantage of this sequence is that two or more images of the same slice with different image contrasts (depending on the interval between the 90° pulse and the 180° pulse) can be obtained without increasing the scan time. Typically this sequence employs long TR of about 1200–3000 ms and TE of 30–120 ms (double-echo technique) or 30–240 ms (multi-echo technique).

The IR sequence employs an initial 180° pulse followed by a 90° pulse. The interval between two 180° pulses is the pulse repetition time TR; the interval between the 180° and 90° pulse is the inversion time TI. Most IR images are acquired using a long TR of 1000–2000 ms and a moderately long TI of 200–800 ms. A common method of improving image quality is to add a third, 180° pulse to the basic two pulses. The interval between the second and third pulses is again referred to as the echo delay time TE. Generally the TE for IR sequences is approximately 30 ms.

In an effort to shorten examination times in MRI, various fast imaging techniques have been suggested (FLASH, FISP, RARE). The FLASH (*f*ast *l*ow *a*ngle *sh*ot) technique, typical of the fast gradient-echo pulse sequences, has been available for routine clinical use since 1986. The FLASH technique differs from the conventional sequences in several respects (Haase et al. 1986):

1. A shorter pulse repetition time (TR≪T1)
2. Refocusing of spins by gradient reversal (gradient echo)
3. Radiofrequency pulses applied at flip angles < 90° (low-angle excitation)

Typical sequence parameters for FLASH imaging are a TR of about 40 ms and a TE between 10 and 15 ms. Image contrast is determined by the excitation pulse angle (alpha) of the radiofrequency pulse. Excitation angles of 40° to 60° have proved favorable for cerebral imaging, yielding predominantly T1- and proton-density-weighted images (Weiss et al. 1987).

The FISP (*f*ast *i*maging with *s*teady state *p*recession) technique is a pulse sequence related to the FLASH technique. Because the radiofrequency pulses in the FISP sequence alternately reverse their sign, the highest signals are elicited from tissues that have similar T1 and T2 relaxation times (Oppelt et al. 1986), most notably tissues that contain fluid. This sequence provides high signal intensity of cystic, necrotic, or CSF-containing lesions.

Another fast imaging principle is the RARE (*r*apid *a*cquisition *r*elaxation *e*nhanced) technique (Henning et al. 1984). In this sequence multiple 180° pulses are applied following an initial 90° excitation pulse. Multiple echoes are generated per excitation and can be used to reconstruct a sectional image. This reduces the number of excitations and shortens the scan time. Because "late" echoes contribute most data in the RARE technique, heavy T2 weighting is provided. For example, CSF yields a particularly bright signal resulting in myelographic RARE images.

While the fast MR imaging techniques result in shorter examination times, their value is limited by various artifacts that degrade image quality. Consequently, fast imaging has been unable to replace the established scanning protocols, especially T2-weighted SE sequences, which have become the mainstay for noncontrast cerebral imaging. Nevertheless, it has been found that special combinations of FLASH parameters (relatively long TR, short TE, 90° excitation angle, e.g., FLASH 315/14, 90°) can visualize the entire brain on T1-weighted scans in a short period of time (e.g., 15 slices in 83 s) with diagnostic image quality (Sander 1987). Whether fast MRI techniques will challenge conventional sequences for cerebral imaging depends on the further development of these techniques, and this is currently a topic of scientific discussion.

c) Image Contrast

In MRI, signal intensity (brightness) is determined by the sequence parameters TR, TE, and TI and also by the tissue parameters T1, T2, and proton density. Linear motion of the protons (e.g., in blood vessels) is another tissue parameter of importance in some circumstances. Regardless of the pulse sequence that is used, the first three tissue parameters always influence the contrast of the MR image. However, it is possible to enhance the effect of one of the three tissue parameters on image contrast by appropriate selection of the scanning method (SE or IR) and by manipulating the sequence parameters TR, TE, and TI (Semmler and Felix 1984). This is referred to as T1 weighting,

Table 3. Comparison of the signal intensities of various structures in relation to the signal intensity of normal brain tissue for various MR imaging sequences

	T1 weighting (SE 400/30)	Proton-density weighting (SE 1600/35)	T2 weighting (SE 1600-70)	Heavy T2 weighting (SE 1600/180)
CSF	↓↓↓	↓↓↓	↑	↑↑↑↑
Fatty tissue	↑↑↑	↑↑↑	↑↑↑	↑↑↑
Hemorrhage (chronic)	↑↑↑	↑↑↑	↑↑↑	↑↑↑
Vessel (with flowing blood)	↓↓↓	↓↓↓	↓↓↓	↓↓
Bone (cortex)[a]	↓↓↓	↓↓↓	↓↓↓	↓↓↓
Tumor (e.g., malignant glioma)	↓	↑ – ↑↑	↑↑↑	↑ – ↑↑
Necrosis	↓ – ↓↓	↓ – ↑	↑↑ – ↑↑↑	↑↑↑↑
Edema	↓	↑ – ↑↑	↑↑↑	↑↑↑↑

[a] Cancellous bone is made hyperintense by the presence of fat marrow. Calcifications produce areas of low signal, like bone.

The arrows indicate the signal intensity of the structures compared with that of healthy brain tissue. Down arrows: low, moderate, or marked hypointensity relative to brain; up arrows: low, moderate, marked, or very marked hyperintensity relative to brain.

T2 weighting, or proton-density weighting, depending on the tissue parameter that is being enhanced (Table 3).

SE images with a short TR (200–600 ms) and short TE (14–40 ms) are T1 weighted (e.g., SE 400/30). This means that the image contrast mainly reflects the differences in the T1 relaxation times of the structures in question. Tissues with a short T1 give a high signal (appear bright), while tissues with a long T1 give a low signal (appear dark). On SE 400/30 images, CSF (with a long T1) yields a very low signal intensity, and normal brain tissue (with intermediate T1 values) gives a moderately intense signal. The scalp and diploe appear very bright (hyperintense) by virtue of their high fat content (Fig. C1a). Pathologic processes usually appear hypointense to surrounding brain because of their prolonged T1 relaxation time. T1-weighted SE sequences provide images with good spatial resolution within relatively short scan times. These sequences are of value in the differential diagnosis of pathologic tissues with short T1 relaxation times, including chronic hematomas, fat-containing lesions, and contrast-enhancing tumors.

Proton-density weighting is achieved in an SE image by selecting a relatively long TR (1500–3000 ms) and a short TE (14–40 ms) (e.g., SE 1600/35). Proton-density-weighted images can be obtained along with T2-weighted images in almost all MR scanners without increasing the scan time by means of the double-echo technique. The advantage of SE 1600/35 images is their generally high signal-to-noise ratio with excellent anatomic resolution (Fig. C1b). Normal brain parenchyma on SE 1600/35 images displays a moderate to high signal intensity, the gray matter appearing brighter than the white matter. CSF appears hypointense despite its high spin density, since its very long T1 decreases the signal intensity even when a long TR is used. Pathologic tissues that have a high proton density because of their increased water content appear hyperintense to normal brain in this sequence.

On T2-weighted images, characterized by a long TR (1500–3000 ms) and long TE (60–240 ms) (e.g., SE 1600/70), tissues with a short T2 relaxation time give a low signal, while tissues with a long T2 give a bright signal. Normal brain tissue produces a signal of moderate intensity. The cortex appears hyperintense to the white matter, giving a contrast greater than that seen on proton-density-weighted images. CSF is nearly isointense to the white matter when the TE is about 90 ms or less. Pathologic processes, whose T2 values are generally prolonged, appear hyperintense to normal brain tissue (Fig. C1c). T2-weighted images are very sensitive in detecting lesions with prolonged T2 relaxation times (Brant-Zawadzki et al. 1984), and these sequences are generally preferred for screening examinations.

Increasing TE further enhances the effect of T2 differences and highlights contrast between healthy and diseased tissues. This principle is applied clinically in the multi-echo sequence. In the technique used in the institutions participating in this study (SE 1600/30–240, eight echoes), eight images of the same section are acquired with progressive T2 weighting of the successive images (Fig. C2). The heavily T2-weighted images are useful for differentiating various pathologic processes (tumor tissue, necrotic tissue, perifocal edema). Typically, heavily T2-weighted images (late echoes) present the following order of tissue intensities, from lowest to highest: healthy brain tissue, viable tumor, central necrosis, perifocal edema, CSF-containing structures. This can be very helpful in differentiating areas that show varying degrees of high signal intensity (Heindel et al. 1986; Rinck et al. 1985). Disadvantages of multi-echo sequences are prolonged imaging times and confinement to a few image sections.

The T1-weighted IR sequence with a long TR and moderately long TI (e.g., IR 1500/400) provides high gray matter–white matter contrast. The white matter (short T1) has a significantly higher signal intensity than the cortex and subcortical nuclei (longer T1). CSF appears virtually as an area of signal void (black). Pathologic processes (tumor, necrosis, edema) appear hypointense because of their long T1 values relative to the white matter (Fig. C1d). The advantage of IR sequences lies in the accurate anatomic definition of normal brain structures (Bydder and Young 1985). This in turn permits an accurate topographic definition of white matter lesions, which in the IR sequence contrast sharply with surrounding brain. Disadvantages of the IR technique are the relatively long acquisition times and the confinement to a few sections per measurement.

d) Practical Approach to MR Examination of the Brain

Before performing an MR scan, the investigator must define the following: scanning method and sequence parameters (TR, TE, TI), slice orientation, slice thickness, number of signal averages, and image matrix.

Pulse Sequence

Generally the entire brain is scanned using an SE sequence with a long TR applying a double-echo technique (e.g., SE 1600/35+70). As many as 16 contiguous slices (1 slice/100 ms TR) can be imaged in one measurement (multislice technique). However, experience has shown that image quality is improved when two measurements are performed. Noncontiguous slices are imaged in the first measurement, whereas the interleaved slices (gaps) are imaged in the second measurement. When an abnormality is noted, it is common practice to image the lesion with a T1-weighted sequence (e.g., SE 400/30 or IR 1500/400) or a heavily T2-weighted sequence (e.g., multi-echo technique). Imaging in different planes visualizes the topographic relationship of the lesion to surrounding structures.

Slice Orientation

The orthogonal planes (axial, sagittal, coronal) are imaged in routine examinations. Oblique projections, now available in most MR units, are not required for the diagnosis of most cerebral diseases.

To facilitate comparison with CT, the MR examination usually begins with axial scans. Midsagittal projections are acquired first for lesions of the sella, pineal body, or brainstem. Coronal images are the preferred initial view for lesions in the superior portion of the parietal lobe or lesions near the skull base, since coronal projections are less likely to produce partial volume effects in these areas.

Slice Thickness

The usual slice thickness for MR studies at intermediate field strength (0.5 T) is 10 mm. This may be reduced to 5 mm or 3 mm for the delineation of smaller anatomic structures and lesions (e.g., the sella or pituitary gland). Because a linear relationship exists between slice thickness and signal intensity, the reduction of signal-to-noise (S/N) ratio must be compensated by increasing the acquisition time (see Signal Averaging).

Signal Averaging

When imaging is performed with a short TR, signals of relatively low intensity are acquired. This results in a low S/N ratio with a corresponding degradation of image quality. The S/N ratio can be increased, and image quality improved, by performing two acquisitions in succession and then averaging the signals that are detected. Because the number of averages relates linearly to scan time while the S/N ratio varies with the square root of the number of averages, there are limits to how much image quality can be improved without greatly increasing the scan time. Sequences with a longer TR (> 1000 ms) yield adequate signal intensities, at least in units with field strengths of 0.5 T or more, and multiple acquisitions are not required. By contrast, a large number of averages are required for thin-section scanning.

Image Matrix
Acceptable spatial resolution generally requires projection onto a matrix of 256×256 pixels. The acquisition time T per sequence is calculated from TR, the number of data acquisitions n, and the number of lines N in the matrix: $T = TR \times N \times n$.

e) Image Interpretation

As in CT, the interpretation of MR images is based largely on morphologic criteria: the location and extent of a lesion, the structure and contour of a lesion, solitary occurrence or multiplicity. To date there is no good evidence that the level of signal intensity or the underlying relaxation times can provide tissue-specific information (Higer and Bielke 1986). Most lesions demonstrate decreased signal intensity on T1-weighted images and increased signal intensity on T2-weighted images because of their prolonged T1 and T2 relaxation times. This general rule does not apply to fat-containing or hemorrhagic lesions, which have relatively short T1 values (and relatively long T2 values) and tend to give high signals in T1-weighted images (Figs. C3, 4).

Calcifications, which are sensitively demonstrated by CT, often are not depicted by MRI and may be identified only in retrospect by comparison with the CT scan. However, larger calcifications may be detectable as regions of decreased signal on all MR imaging sequences. The low signal intensity of calcifications results from a paucity of mobile protons and extremely short T2 values. Cortical bone appears hypointense for the same reason (Fig. C5).

Blood vessels present a characteristic MR pattern. Because the hydrogen nuclei move out of the image volume between pulses, flowing blood may produce little or no MR signal in standard pulse sequences. Thus, in MRI blood vessels are identified without contrast agents by virtue of their characteristically low signal intensity (Fig. C6).

f) Contrast-Enhanced MRI

For a given pulse sequence, the contrast in MRI is determined by the tissue parameters of proton density and relaxation times (T1, T2). Substances that alter these tissue parameters can serve as contrast agents. Relaxation times are markedly influenced by paramagnetic substances, which are assuming increasing importance as MR contrast agents (Brash 1983; Felix et al. 1985; Semmler et al. 1985).

Principle of Paramagnetic MR Contrast Agents

Paramagnetic substances are characterized by their property of having unpaired electron spins. Electrons, much like the proton of the hydrogen nucleus, have an inherent angular momentum which gives them a magnetic moment. In most atoms the magnetic property of the electron shell is outwardly neutralized by the fact that electrons spinning in one direction cancel out with those spinning in the opposite direction (paired electron spins). Paramagnetic elements have electron spins that are unpaired, i.e., do not cancel out, resulting in a net magnetic moment. A single unpaired electron produces a local magnetic field that is approximately 1000 times greater than the local magnetic field of a hydrogen nucleus. The presence of paramagnetic metal ions and their strong local magnetic field amplifies the interaction of hydrogen nuclei with their environment, and the relaxation times are shortened. This shortening of relaxation times by paramagnetic agents is concentration dependent, and at low concentrations the effect on T1 predominates. A shortening of T1 increases the signal intensity of tissues, resulting in contrast enhancement on T1-weighted images. At higher concentrations T2 shortening becomes predominant, and signal intensity is diminished.

Among the paramagnetic ions tested to date, the trivalent gadolinium ion (Gd^{3+}) is of prime importance. This ion has seven unpaired electron spins, giving a strong magnetic moment. Like other metallic ions, Gd^{3+} is relatively toxic in the free state. It is stored in the liver and can cause parenchymal damage. Chelation of gadolinium with DTPA (diethylenetriaminepentaacetic acid) greatly reduces its toxicity while preserving its paramagnetic properties. Gd-DTPA (Magnevist, Schering, Berlin) is the first intravenous contrast agent for MRI to become available (Carr et al. 1984; Schörner et al. 1984; Claussen et al. 1985; Felix et al. 1985).

Characteristics of the Contrast Agent Gd-DTPA

The contrast agent consists of a stable aqueous solution of the Di-N-methylglucamine salt of the DTPA complex of gadolinium. This complex is extremely stable (dissociation constant 10^{-23}), so there are virtually no free gadolinium ions in aqueous solution. The high stability of the complex is a major reason for the extremely low toxicity of Gd-DTPA (Weinmann et al. 1984).

The pharmacokinetic behavior of Gd-DTPA is determined by the physicochemical properties of DTPA. The extreme hydrophilia and relatively high molecular weight of the Gd-DTPA molecule (molecular weight 590) account for the exclusively extracellular distribution of the contrast agent (Weinmann et al. 1984). Lipophilic membranes (e.g., cell membranes, blood-brain barrier) are impermeable to Gd-DTPA.

Following intravenous injection in man, the contrast agent is distributed rapidly in the intravascular and interstitial spaces of the body (distribution phase) and undergoes a gradual excretion of immediate onset (elimination half-life 1.6 h, Weinmann et al. 1984). Gd-DTPA is excreted unchanged, almost entirely through glomerular filtration. On average 83% of the administered dose is excreted within 6 h after i.v. injection, and 92% within 24 h.

Animal studies (Weinmann et al. 1984) indicate a very high acute, subacute, and neural tolerance of Gd-DTPA. The LD_{50} (dose at which 50% of animals die after slow intravenous injection) is approximately 100 times higher than the diagnostic dosage of 0.1 mmol Gd-DTPA/kg body weight, resulting in an excellent margin of safety – wider than that with conventional iodinated contrast media.

Animal studies have shown no evidence that Gd-DTPA can initiate an anaphylactic or allergic reaction like that occasionally seen with radiographic contrast media.

Technique of Contrast-Enhanced MRI

A dosage of 0.1 mmol Gd-DTPA/kg body weight is recommended for clinical examinations, corresponding to an injection volume of 0.2 ml/kg body weight (Niendorf et al. 1987). Strong enhancement of intracerebral lesions has been demonstrated between 5 min and 45 min following the injection (Schörner et al. 1986). A single injection of Gd-DTPA is sufficient for the visualization of an enhancing lesion; repeat injections are unnecessary.

T1-weighted pulse sequences are recommended for contrast-enhanced MRI (Laniado et al. 1986; Price and Runge 1986). It has been mentioned that the T1 and T2 relaxation times are shortened in the distribution space of Gd-DTPA. The shortening of T1 leads to the desired increase in signal intensity, whereas T2 shortening decreases the signal. At the clinical dosage of 0.1 mmol Gd-DTPA/kg body weight, the predominant effect on T1-weighted images is the shortening of T1.

SE sequences with a TR of 400–800 ms and a short TE of 16–40 ms have proved effective for contrast-enhanced MRI (Fig. C7a, b). IR sequences with a long TR and moderately long TI (e.g., IR 1500/400) are also satisfactory (Fig. C7c, d). IR images taken after the injection of Gd-DTPA show even greater enhancement of tumor tissue than on T1-weighted SE images. However, IR images have the disadvantage of a relatively long scan time.

Gd-DTPA does not cause significant enhancement of normal brain tissue. When the blood-brain barrier (BBB) is intact, the contrast material remains within the vascular structures of the brain and does not cause any visible change in the signal intensity of healthy brain tissue. However, breakdown of the BBB allows contrast agent to pass from the vessels into the interstitium (Runge et al. 1985), producing a circumscribed enhancement of the lesion in the area where the BBB is disrupted. Thus, MR enhancement by Gd-DTPA occurs via the same mechanism as enhancement using X-ray contrast material in CT.

As in contrast-enhanced CT, gadolinium enhancement in MR aids in differentiating lesions with an intact BBB from lesions that disrupt the integrity of the BBB. Breakdown of the BBB is a feature of brain tumors, infarcts, inflammatory lesions, and other processes. But enhancement can also occur in extra-axial tumors (e.g., meningiomas) which primarily lack a BBB (Bydder et al. 1985). As in CT, the degree and extent of the contrast enhancement can provide information to differentiate tumor types.

Gd-DTPA can improve the morphologic evaluation of intracranial tumors. The circumscribed enhancement produced by the contrast agent is helpful in delineating the boundaries of the lesion. This can improve the evaluation of very small lesions and lesions having a complex structure (Maravilla et al. 1986). Complex lesions include intraaxial brain tumors having heterogeneous signal intensities because of perifocal edema, necrosis, and cystic components as well as recurrent tumors with adjacent scar tissue. It can be quite difficult in these cases to distinguish tumor from surrounding tissues on nonenhanced MR images (Schörner et al. 1986). Lesions that show minimal or equivocal enhancement on CT scans may display a higher degree of contrast enhancement on MR images following the injection of Gd-DTPA.

Following the format of the first edition of this book, we shall present the CT characteristics of each tumor group and then compare them with the MR features of that group. Due to methodologic problems, the statements made about MR in the "boxes" that head each section should be viewed as generalizations rather than definitive guides.

1. In contrast to CT, experience to date with MR is based on a relatively small number of examinations.
2. So far, descriptions of MR features detailed enough to permit a specific histologic diagnosis have been published for only a few tumor types.
3. In contrast to CT, we cannot correlate the gray scale on MR images with absolute measured values. The myriad pulse sequences and the different field strengths are associated with a wide variety of gray levels and image contrasts.
4. In theory, relaxation times and proton-density measurements provide a means of achieving tissue discrimination. However, the results that have been published in this area are still too contradictory. It is possible that more accurate relaxation-time measurements will be forthcoming, but it remains to be seen whether this will provide data that are truly specific for individual tumor groups.

a 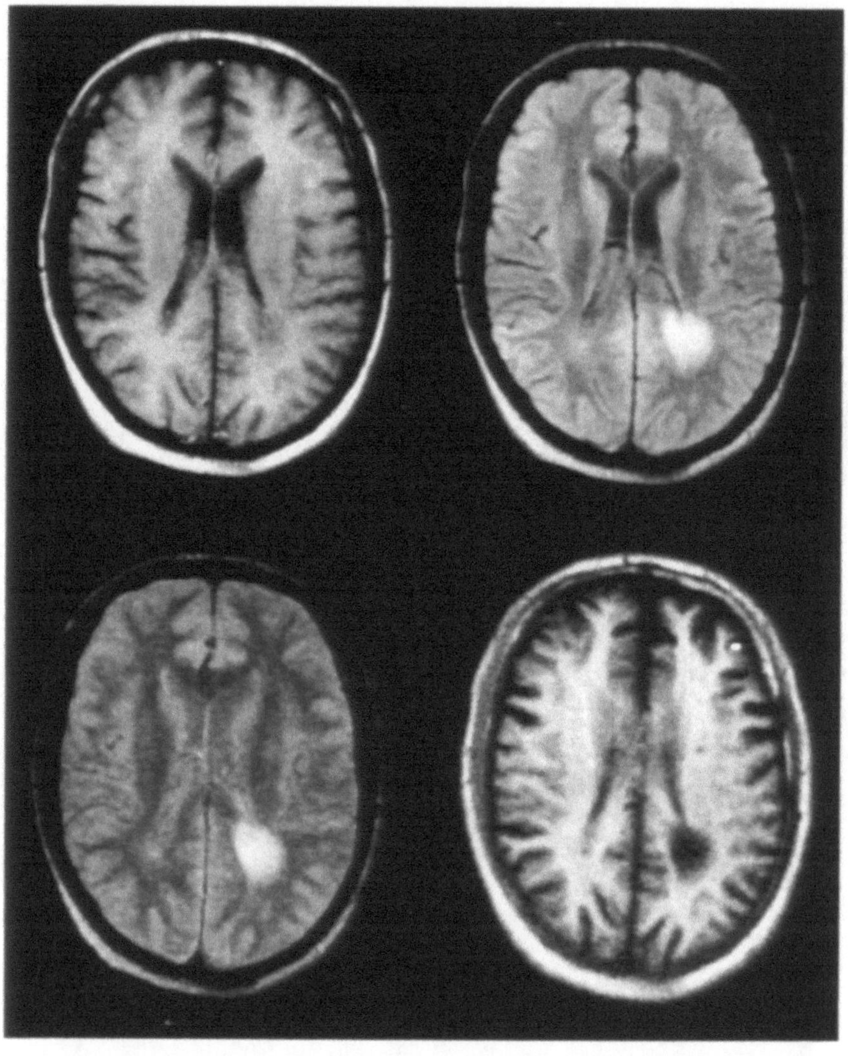 b

c d

Fig. C1a–d. Image contrast. Appearance of a lesion on pulse sequences commonly used for clinical MRI. (Patient A.G., acquired immune deficiency syndrome, lesion of unknown origin.) **a** SE 400/35: A subtle hypointensity is seen adjacent to the right occipital horn. **b** SE 1600/35: An area of markedly increased signal is demonstrated in the same location. **c** SE 1600/70: The hyperintense lesion contrasts sharply with adjacent structures. (Healthy brain structures can be differentiated with relatively high contrast; the ventricles and brain substance are almost identical in signal intensity.) **d** IR 1500/400: The lesion is markedly hypointense to the adjacent white matter (normal brain anatomy is displayed in high contrast)

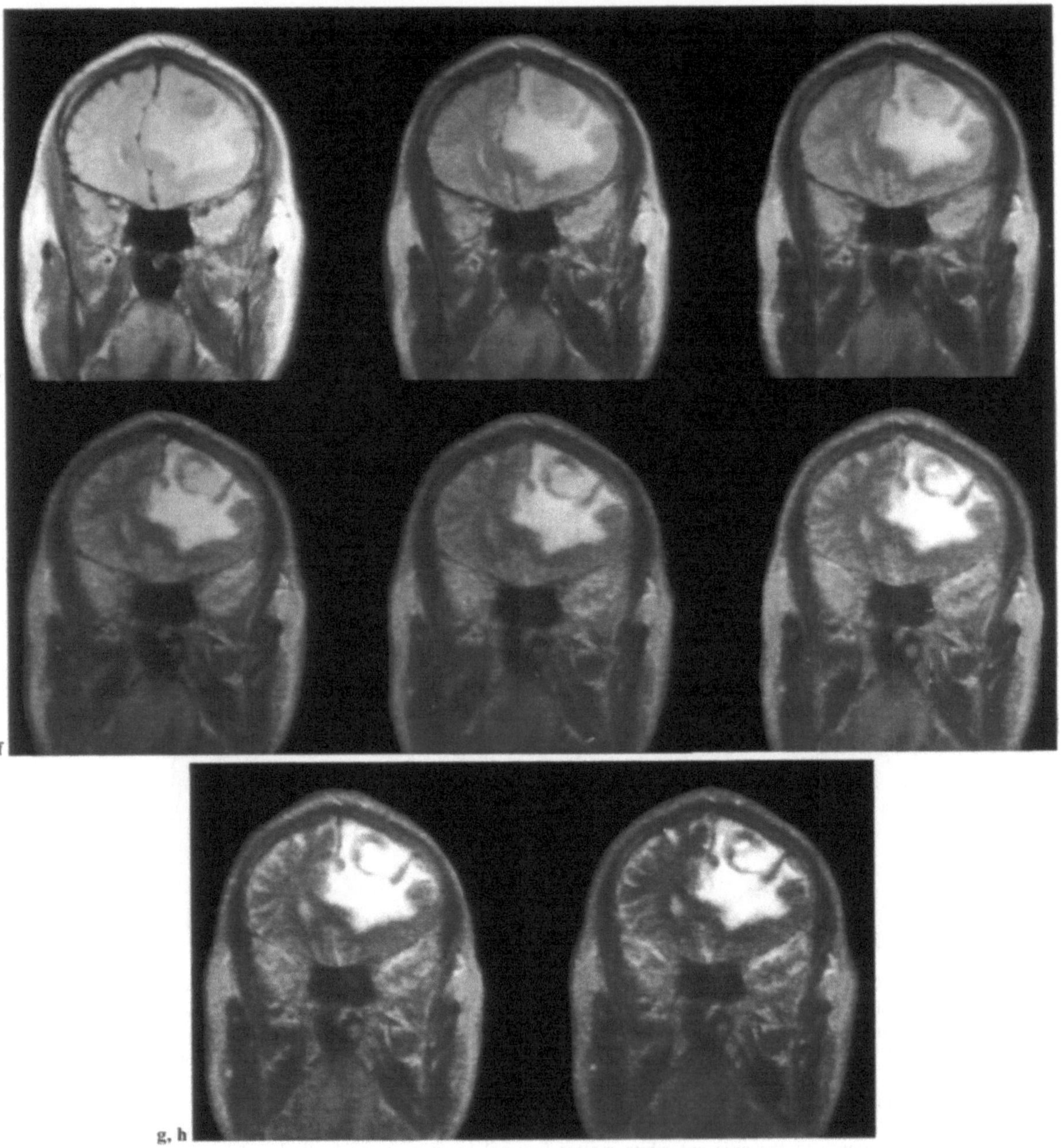

a–c d–f g, h

Fig. C2a–h. Multi-echo technique. The heterogeneous mass is a metastasis with central necrosis and perifocal edema. In the first echo [SE 1600/30, (**a**)] we can distinguish only the slightly hypointense necrosis from the slightly hyperintense edema. As the echo time is lengthened [SE 1600/60 (**b**), SE 1600/90 (**c**), SE 1600/120 (**d**), SE 1600/150 (**e**), SE 1600/180 (**f**), SE 1600/210 (**g**), SE 1600/240 (**h**)], the relative signal intensities of the edema and necrosis increase, and these structures are defined with increasing contrast. A hypointense ring representing the ring-like portion of the metastasis is also demonstrated

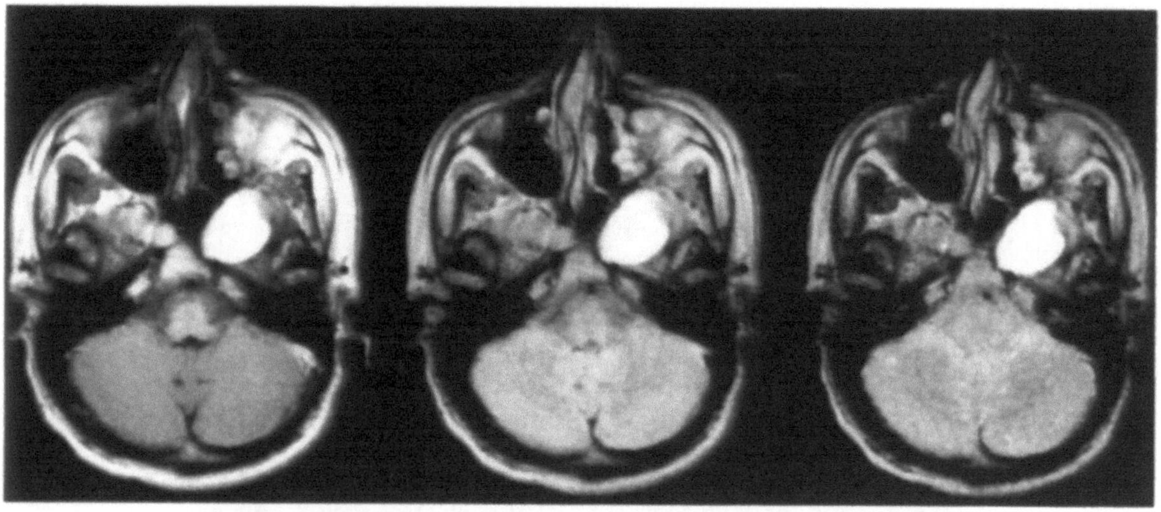

Fig. C3. Fat-containing lesion. The fatty contents of this saponified dermoid cyst give a bright signal in the SE 400/35 sequence (*left*). SE 1600/35+70 (*center* and *right*) shows a signal pattern characteristic of tissue with a short T1 relaxation time (here: fat)

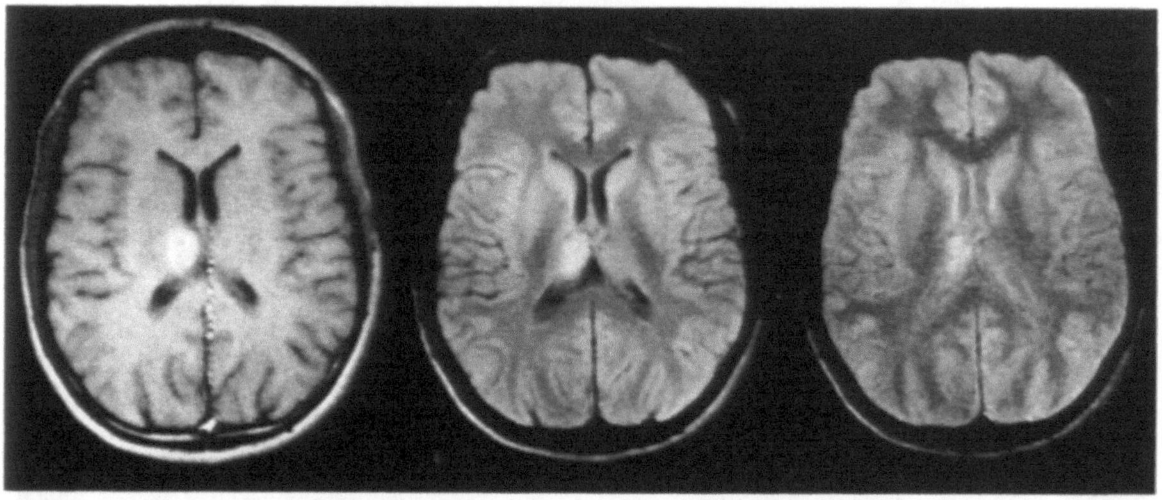

Fig. C4. Old intracerebral hemorrhage. The periventricular lesion appears hyperintense on all three sequences: SE 400/30 (*left*) and SE 1600/35+70 (*center* and *right*). The signal pattern is typical for tissue with a short T1 relaxation time (here: old hemorrhage)

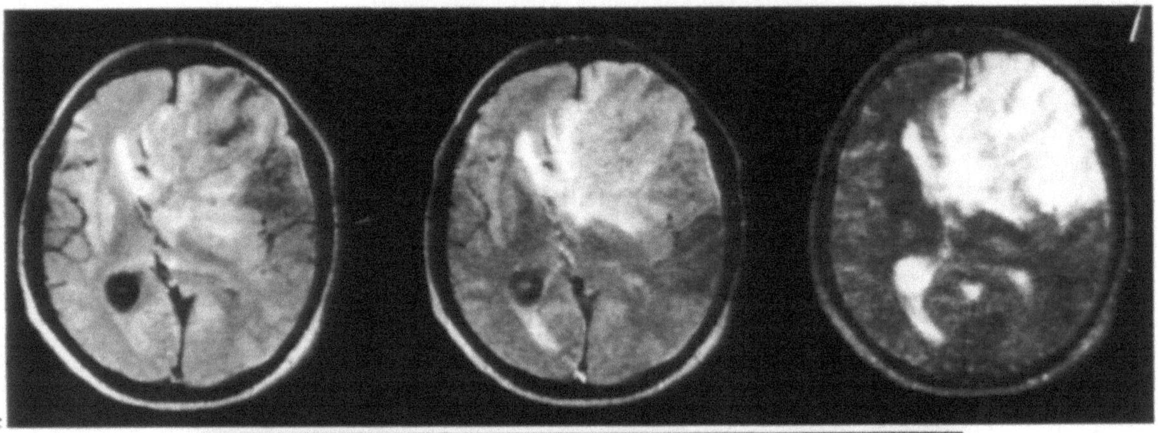

a–c

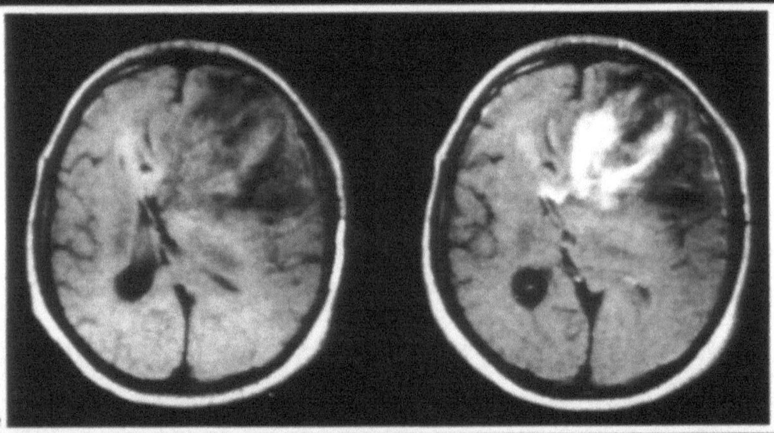

d, e

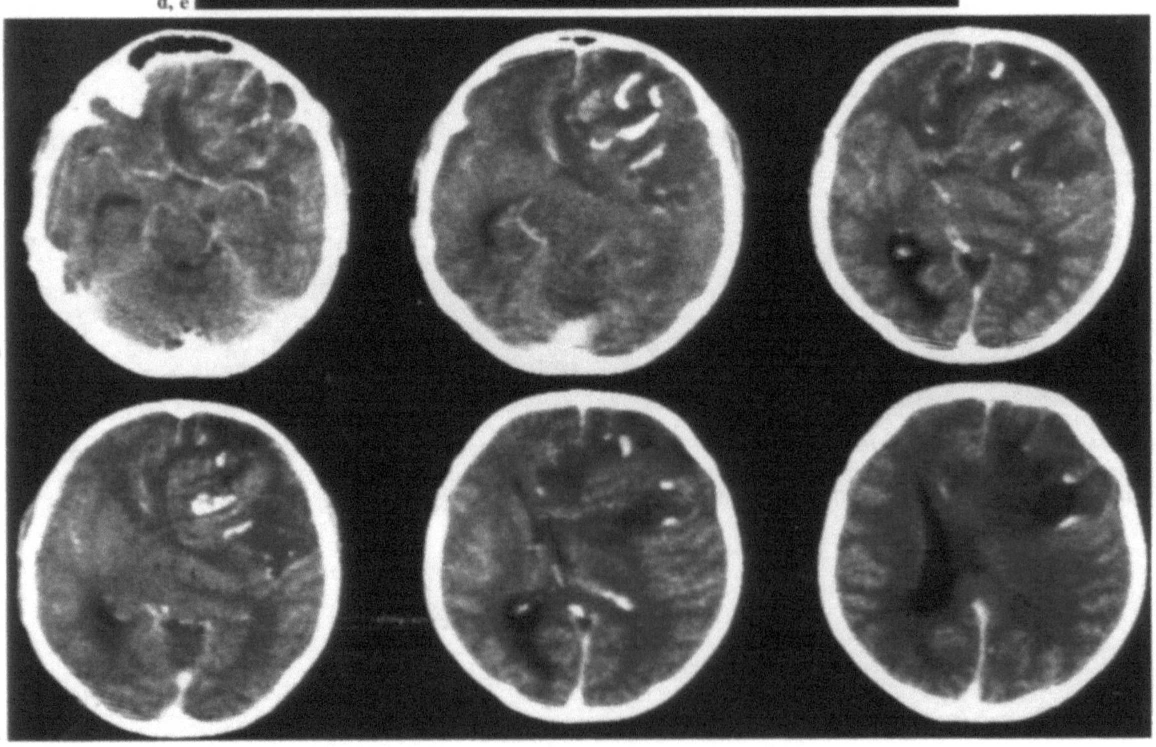

f–h

i–k

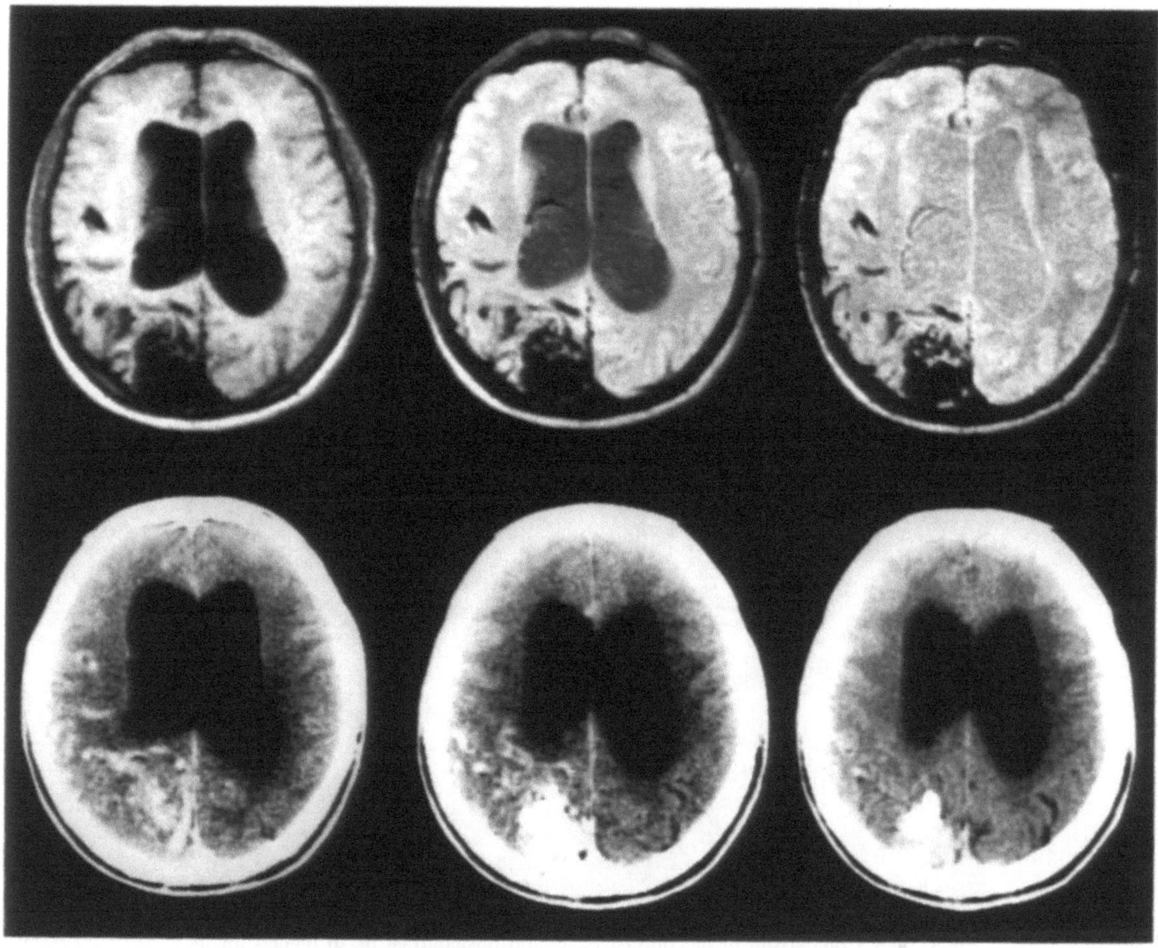

a–c

d–f

Fig. C6a–f. Appearance of vascular structures on MR images. Arteriovenous angioma. The vascular structures give a low signal on all sequences [SE 400/35 (**a**), SE 1600/35+70 (**b, c**)]. This, together with their morphology, identifies them as vessels. Corresponding contrast-enhanced CT scans (**d–f**)

◄

Fig. C5a–k. Calcifications. The CT scans (**f–k**) clearly demonstrate multiple plaque-like calcifications in an extensive frontal oligoastrocytoma. The MR images [SE 1600/30, 60, 210 (**a, b, c**), pre- and postcontrast SE 800/35 (**d, e**)] demonstrate a heterogeneous mass containing low-signal areas that represent calcifications. (These could be identified only in retrospect based on knowledge of the CT findings)

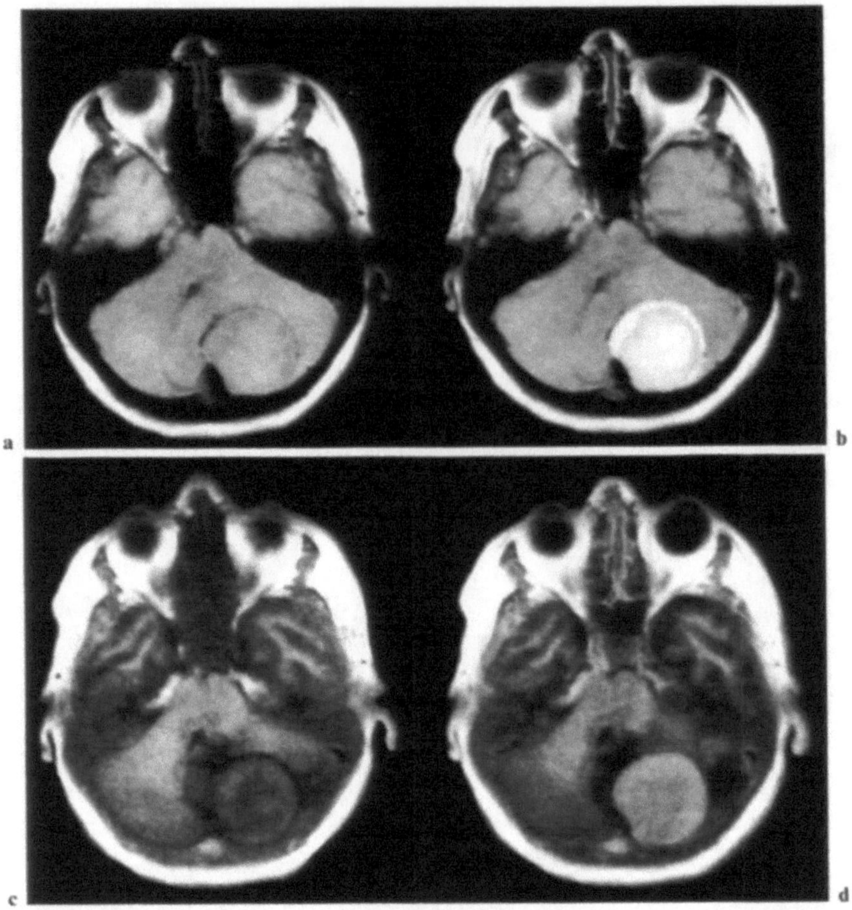

Fig. C7a–d. Comparison of precontrast (**a, c**) and postcontrast (**b, d**) images for the sequences SE 800/35 (**a, b**) and IR 1500/40 (**c, d**). The postcontrast images demonstrate uniform enhancement of the tumor (meningioma, histologically confirmed) in the posterior cranial fossa. The two sequences are of equal clinical value

3. MR Spectroscopy

While clinical MR imaging has been vastly improved since its beginnings in the early 1980s, classic MR spectroscopy has rarely been used clinically until recently. Though it has been a routine tool in physical chemistry for decades, progress toward its clinical implementation has been slow. Advances in localized MR spectroscopy have no doubt been stimulated by the perception that MR imaging has displayed "overwhelming sensitivity accompanied by disappointing specificity" (A. Margulis).

Hope for improved specificity now focuses more on spectroscopy than on imaging, even though the eventual role of MR spectroscopy may have to do more with elucidating the biochemistry of diseases than diagnosing disease and directing treatment in the individual patient.

a) Basic Principles of MR Spectroscopy

As explained in the previous section, the Larmor precession frequency of a nuclear spin is proportional to the product of the gyromagnetic ratio of the nucleus and the strength of the magnetic field at its location.[1] The gyromagnetic ratio is a fundamental constant belonging to all nuclei (see Table 4). The magnetic field experienced by a nuclear spin represents the sum of the externally applied static magnetic field B (often with gradient fields added for localization purposes) and the molecular magnetic fields originating from the magnetized sample. These fields arise from the neighboring atoms or, more precisely, from their electron clouds (Fig. C8). It follows that different partners chemically bonded to an atom, or even different bonding structures, should yield slightly different resonance frequencies for a given atom and a given external field strength. In fact, resonance shifts up to 100 ppm of the basic frequency can occur depending on the nucleus and bonding structure (Fig. C9). In proton imaging where strong field gradients are applied for frequency encoding, this is observed only as a fat-water shift. The roughly 3 ppm shift between water and fat protons produces double contouring at fat-water interfaces that are perpendicular to the read gradient.

The chemical shift enables us to assign a unique type of chemical bond to any resonance line of a specific nucleus when the distance from a reference line in the spectrum is known. The relative height of the line is a measure of the number of atoms from the sample contributing to the line. The width of the line determines the minimal shift of different bonds that can be resolved in the spectrum. Besides factors relating to the physical and chemical properties of the sample, the line width is determined to a large extent by inhomogeneities in the external magnetic field, which lead to a distribution of resonance frequencies and thus to a widening of any spectral line across the sample. MR spectroscopy, then, requires a considerably greater field homogeneity across the sample volume than does MR imaging. It should be noted, however, that in localized spectroscopy this applies only to the volume element from which the spectrum is acquired.

Only a few nuclei are sufficiently sensitive and abundant for measurement by in vivo MR spectroscopy. Among these nuclei are hydrogen-1 (^{1}H), phosphorus-31 (^{31}P), carbon-13 (^{13}C), and fluorine-19 (^{19}F).

Table 4. Biologically important MR nuclei

Nucleus	Spin	MR frequency at 1.5 T (MHz)	Relative sensitivity (constant field)	Natural abundance (%)
^{1}H	1/2	63.86	100.00	99.98
^{13}C	1/2	16.06	1.59	1.11
^{19}F	1/2	60.08	83.00	100.00
^{23}Na	3/2	16.89	9.25	100.00
^{31}P	1/2	25.85	6.63	100.00

[1] Actually it is more correct to speak of magnetic flux density than field strength, but because the latter term is so common among nonphysicists, and the field strength normally is proportional to the flux density in biologic media, field strength is used here as a synonym for flux density.

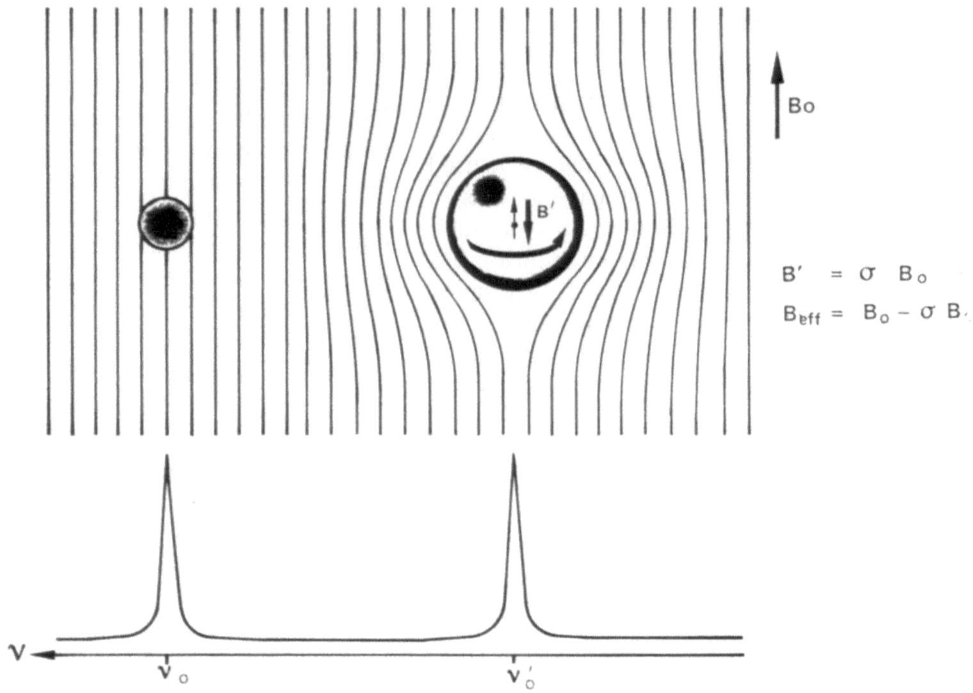

Fig. C8. Physical origin of the chemical shift. The externally applied magnetic field B_0 induces a precession of the electron cloud surrounding the nucleus, generating an opposite field B′. The nucleus experiences a net field B_{eff}, which is reduced by B′

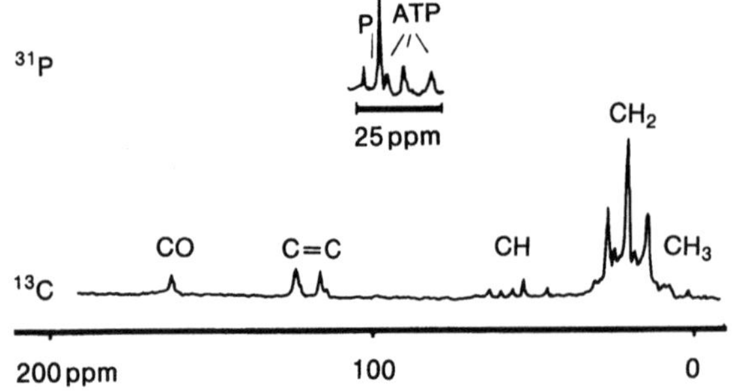

Fig. C9. Comparison of typical ^1H, ^{31}P, and ^{13}C spectra. ^1H offers the highest sensitivity but the smallest spectral separation. ^{13}C offers low sensitivity with a high spectral separation. *PCr*, phosphocreatine; *P*, inorganic phosphate. (After Roth 1984)

b) Experimental Considerations

Because nuclei far less sensitive than ^1H, such as ^{31}P, are used for spectroscopic studies, a relatively high magnetic field strength is necessary for in vivo experiments in order to limit the examination time. In addition, high field strengths yield better spectral resolution if the field is sufficiently homogeneous. This is because the line-widening relaxation effects (T1/T2) do not increase in proportion to the field strength, so the relative degree of line widening by relaxation is less in higher fields. Today a field strength of 1.5 T is generally considered to be the practical lower limit for clinical in vivo MR spectroscopy. This is also an acceptable compromise for high-quality proton imaging with the same instrument.

Classic in vivo MR spectroscopy employs sampling volumes only a few cubic centimeters in size. Because in vivo spectroscopy involves the examination of small volumes in a much larger heterogeneous sample, techniques must be used to achieve spatial localization, i.e., to restrict the origin of the MR signal to a particular volume of interest (VOI). The simplest way of accomplishing this in spectroscopy as well as imaging is to adapt the size and shape of the radiofrequency (RF) receiving coil to the VOI in the sample, as by the use of surface coils. This technique defines an approximate volume from which MR signals are collected. Surface coils were used for the first clinical trials of in vivo MR spectroscopy (Fig. C10), yielding good results in examinations of the limb muscles in patients with muscular disease such as McArdle's syndrome. While this technique is satisfactory for the analysis of superficial tissues, more precise localization of the signal origin is necessary for studies of deeper structures, and improved selection strategies are required. In the clinical spectroscopy of brain tumors, for example, the VOI is deeply placed and only a few cubic centimeters in size. This type of localization is best accomplished by using spatially resolved spectroscopic techniques. Various approaches have been devised, all incorporating special pulse sequences in combination with gradients applied for encoding and reading of the spectroscopic signal. The optimum strategy in a given situation depends on the sensitivities of the nuclei as well as on the RF power and gradient strengths that are to be delivered during the examination.

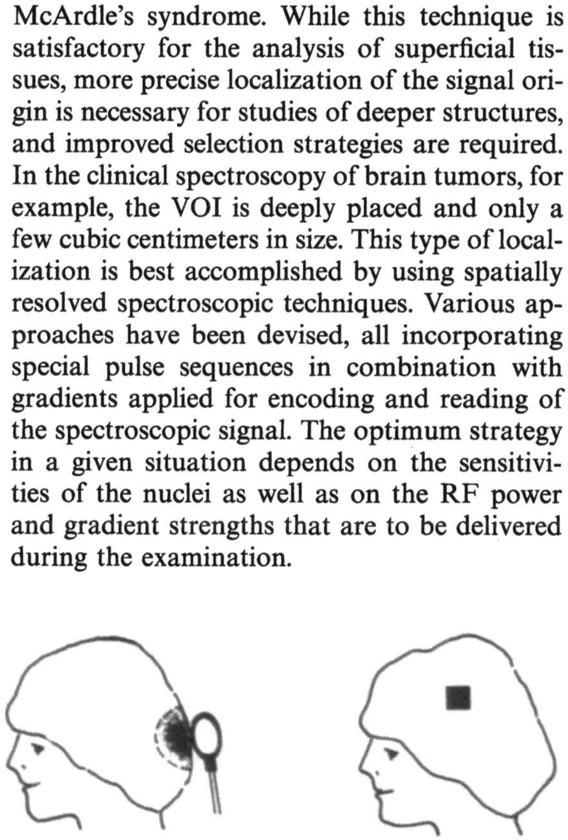

Fig. C10. Comparison of the VOI defined by localized spectroscopy (*right*) with the volume defined by a surface coil (*left*). Surface coils do not provide a sharply defined VOI and are best suited for the examination of superficial structures

c) Metabolic Studies

Because the metabolism of the living cell is mediated chiefly by hydrocarbons and phosphorus compounds (the latter being essential for energy metabolism), hydrogen, carbon, and phosphorus nuclei are natural candidates for metabolic investigations. Hydrogen is the most abundant element in biologic matter and the most sensitive of the nuclei. However, compounds such as amino acids, lactic acid, creatine, and other metabolites occur in very low concentrations and are difficult to measure spectroscopically in the presence of strong water and fat signals. Those compounds can be detected only by the use of special water-suppression techniques and in areas that have inherently low lipid signals, such as the brain.

Phosphorus spectra are easier to interpret. The concentrations of the phosphorus metabolites adenosine triphosphate (ATP), phosphocreatine (PCr), and inorganic phosphates (P_i) determine the energy state of the cell. The shift of the P_i signal provides a means of determining the cellular pH. The split in the spectral shifts of the phosphorus lines is much greater than with hydrogen (about 30 ppm versus 4 ppm), so a less homogeneous magnetic field is required. Numerous results from ^{31}P studies in animals are available, most dealing with muscle spectra.

So far few clinical results have been reported on carbon spectroscopy. While the most abundant isotope, ^{12}C (99%), is unsuited for MR because it has no magnetic moment, ^{13}C produces sharply defined resonance peaks covering a wide range of chemical shifts. Its low inherent sensitivity can be overcome by artificial enrichment, but at present the high cost of ^{13}C compounds makes this prohibitive. Another difficulty is that ^{13}C spectroscopy requires a two-RF-channel spectrometer for the simultaneous excitation of ^{1}H and ^{13}C nuclei.

d) Clinical MR Spectroscopy

Both ^{1}H and ^{31}P spectroscopy have found clinical application in metabolic studies of intracranial tumors. Most of these studies have been performed with 1.5-T or 2-T whole-body systems originally designed for proton imaging and adapted for MR spectroscopy.

Despite the limited homogeneity of imaging magnets (approximately 10 ppm over the field of view), satisfactory results are achieved, since only a small sampling volume of several cubic centimeters is selected for spectroscopic examination. Homogeneities on the order of 0.1 ppm are routinely obtained near the center of the magnet, and this is close to the inherent line width.

It is evident that the RF system must be matched to the nuclei of interest in terms of frequency range and resolution. Broad-band systems that can be tuned across the entire bandwidth spectrum are widely available. Nuclei other than hydrogen, sometimes called heteronuclei, require a much higher RF power output. This is especially true for ^{13}C measurements, where RF energy absorption in the patient with tissue heating is a significant concern and may ultimately limit the application of ^{13}C spectroscopy.

The Philips Gyroscan system permits almost instantaneous switching from the proton imaging frequency to, say, the phosphorus resonance frequency. However, the homogeneity of the magnetic field is insufficient to obtain well-resolved spectra, so it is still necessary to tune or "shim" the magnetic field in the VOI. Even with a superb inherent field homogeneity, shimming is made necessary by the magnetic susceptibility of the body (magnetization), which varies locally by several tenths of a ppm and introduces local inhomogeneities into the field. Shimming can be time consuming when done manually by the operator, but computer-assisted shimming has recently become available. The examination starts with standard ^{1}H MR imaging, and from these images the tumor is located and a VOI for localized spectroscopy is defined. Frequently two VOIs are established: a volume from the lesion itself and an equal volume of healthy tissue for comparison.

It takes approximately 15–20 min to acquire the phosphorus spectrum for a given brain area, comparable to the time required for imaging. At present the total time for a spatially resolved ^{31}P spectroscopic examination of the brain is approximately 45–60 min.

We shall now discuss some results of clinical MR spectroscopy. Unless stated otherwise, all spectra were measured at a field strength of 1.5 T.

e) ^{1}H Spectroscopy

Successful experiments with spatially resolved ^{1}H spectroscopy were performed using the SPARS technique of Luyten and Den Hollander (1985). Similar sequences were published earlier by Aue et al. (1984) and Ordidge (1985). SPARS (*spa*tially *r*esolved *s*pectroscopy) combines successive excitations of the sample in the x, y, and z directions, with suitable refocusing and dephasing pulses applied to select perpendicular slices from the sample. The combination of three slices yields a cube-shaped VOI from which signals are collected. The linear dimensions of this volume are determined by the slice thicknesses during excitation (Fig. C11a, b).

With the gradient strengths currently in use (approximately 10 mT/m), volumes smaller than 1 cm^3 can be achieved. However, the technique is suitable only for metabolites with relatively long T2 relaxation times (> 15 ms) and so is not appropriate for ^{31}P spectroscopy (Luyten et al. 1986). When applied in the presence of strong water signals like those occurring in brain tissue, the technique must be combined with water-suppression sequences. A ^{1}H spectrum of the normal human brain is illustrated in Fig. C12. The ^{1}H signals of the metabolites phosphocreatine, creatine, and N-acetyl aspartate (NAA) are displayed following water suppression. Signals from lactate, a sensitive indicator of oxygen supply, also have been identified in animal brain studies (Luyten and Den Hollander 1986) and subsequently in the clinical setting (Luyten et al. 1987) (Fig. C13). Elevated lactate levels were detected in patients with cerebral infarction, coinciding with areas of ischemia rather than with the infarcted tissue itself. Spectroscopy in these cases can detect changes at an earlier stage than conventional proton imaging.

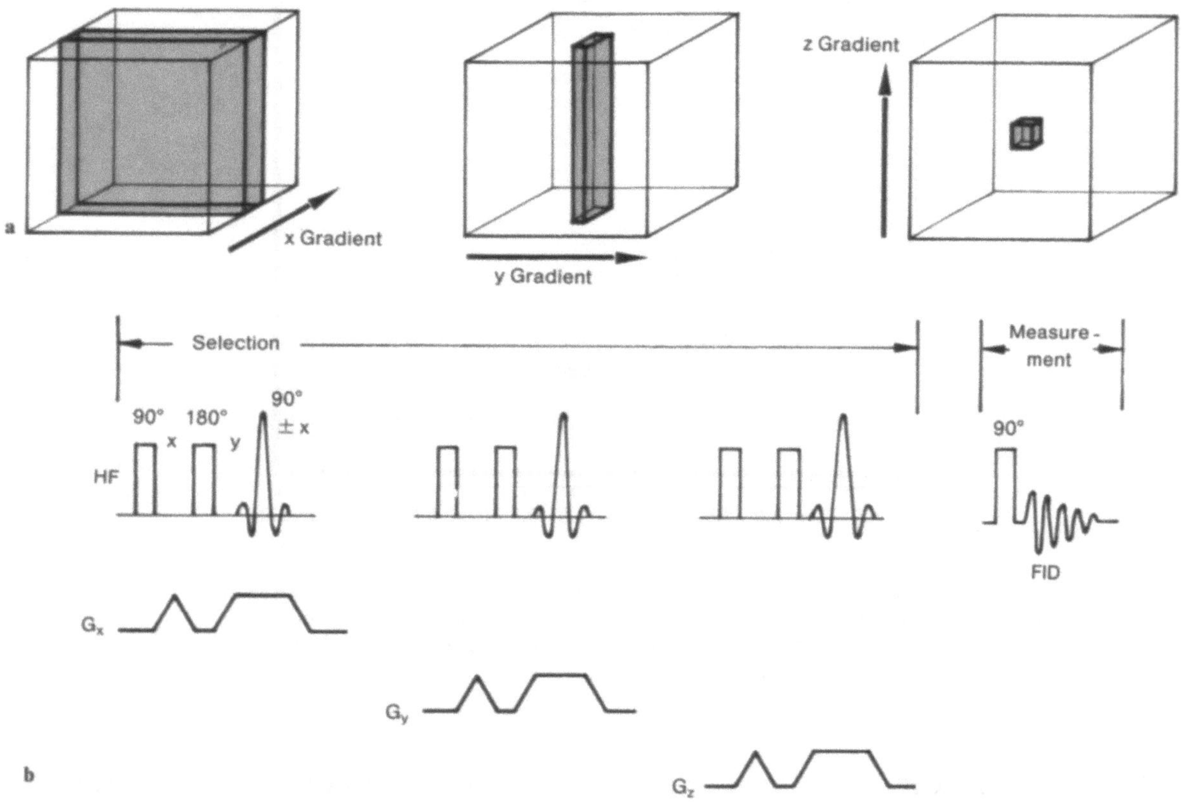

Fig. C11a, b. The SPARS principle of localized spectroscopy. **a** Basic principle. The magnetization of a slice in the x, y, and z directions is prepared by successive selective excitation and dephasing. This process defines a cube-shaped volume from which MR signals are collected. **b** Pulse sequence for SPARS

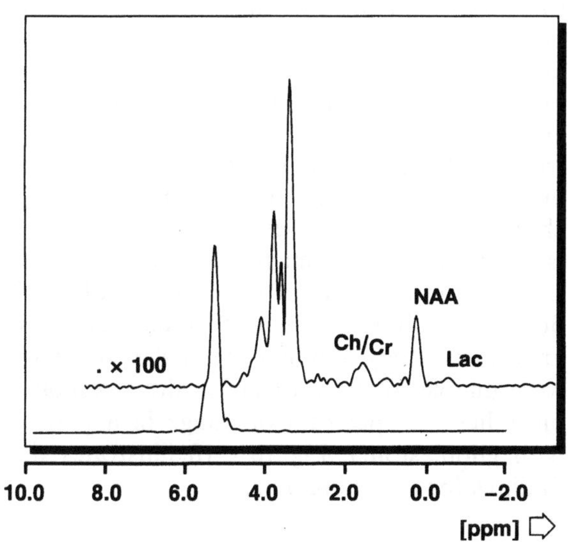

Fig. C12. Typical ^{1}H spectrum of a human brain. The water signal has been strongly suppressed. *NAA*, N-acetyl aspartate; *Cr*, creatine; *Ch*, choline; *Lac*, lactic acid. *Below*: The same spectrum without water suppression

Marien et al. (1987) observed a marked reduction of NAA (by 40%–60%) in the ^{1}H spectra of patients with astrocytoma in addition to a characteristic resonance at 1 ppm with a long T2 of approximately 380 ms. They found no increase in lactic acid levels. It remains to be determined whether different pathologic states can be discriminated on ^{1}H spectra. Nevertheless, as the examples at the end of this chapter will show, ^{1}H spectroscopy has stimulated greater interest among researchers who have had clinical experience with phosphorus, despite some technical difficulties that remain. New pulse sequences incorporating stimulated echo signals have improved the feasibility of clinical ^{1}H spectroscopy. A recent study (Bruhn et al. 1988) demonstrates marked differences between normal spectra and various tumor spectra when the selected VOI is sufficiently small.

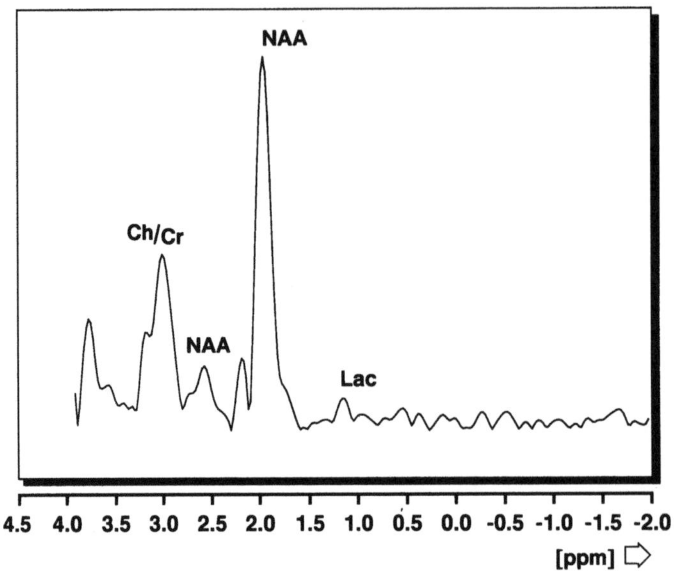

Fig. C13. A 1.5 T proton spectrum of a healthy volunteer: SPARS sequence with water suppression. The spectrum was acquired from 128 measurements with a TR of 2 s. The sampling volume was 25 cm^3. (After den Hollander and Luyten 1987)

f) ^{31}P Spectroscopy

The short T2 relaxation times of phosphorus metabolites necessitate a different approach to spatial localization than is used in SPARS. A modified ISIS technique (Ordidge 1985) is currently applied in the Philips Gyroscan system. A special close-fitting "headphone" coil is used for head examinations to obtain optimum signal sensitivity.

A typical ^{31}P spectrum of the brain is shown in Fig. C14. The normal spectrum is dominated by a PCr peak along with three peaks from ATP. The ATP peaks obscure the signals from ADP. Additional peaks represent P_i, phosphorus monoesters (PME), and phosphorus diesters (PDE).

Examinations in healthy subjects and in patients with gliomas, meningiomas, and metastases of other tumors showed generally increased levels of PME and decreased levels of P_i relative to the controls (Heindel et al. 1987). Alteration of pH was found only in one large glioma, whose ^{31}P spectrum indicated a shift toward alkaline values. This tumor, which displayed central necrosis on the MR image, also showed a marked reduction of ATP. Low ATP levels were also characteristic of tumors with large cystic components.

Although the specificity of ^{31}P spectroscopy seems doubtful in terms of identifying specific tumor types (except meningioma), this modality has definite value in monitoring therapeutic response and can detect such response at an earlier stage than is possible with MR imaging.

Figure C15 shows the MR image of an astrocytoma and the corresponding ^{31}P spectra of the tumor and of uninvolved tissue. Figure C16 shows the spectrum of a malignant prolactinoma. Positive therapeutic response is evidenced by a normalization of the ^{31}P spectrum (Baleriaux et al. 1986) with an increase in PCr and a decrease in PME and P_i. These changes are apparent even before regression is detected on MR images. Figure C17 illustrates the marked fall of PCr and rise of PME documented in response to the radiotherapy of an intracranial lymphoma. Heindel et al. (1987) were unable to demonstrate positive response on either the spectrum or image in a patient with glioblastoma. Figure C18 illustrates the findings for a meningioma.

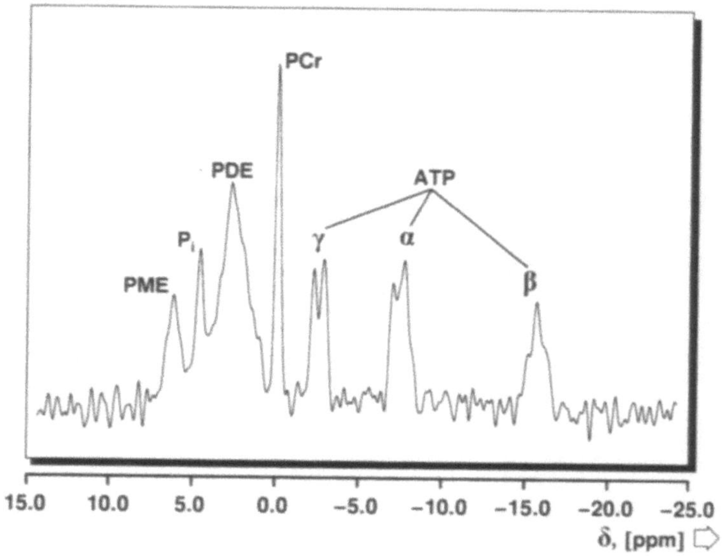

Fig. C14. ^{31}P brain spectrum. *PME, PDE,* phosphorus monoester and diester; P_i, inorganic phosphate; *PCr,* phosphocreatine. Modified ISIS technique, VOI $8 \times 7 \times 7$ cm^3. Field homogeneity was optimized by ^{1}H resonance (1.5 T field). The high-resolution ^{31}P spectrum even shows the J coupling between the adenosine triphosphate *(ATP)* signals

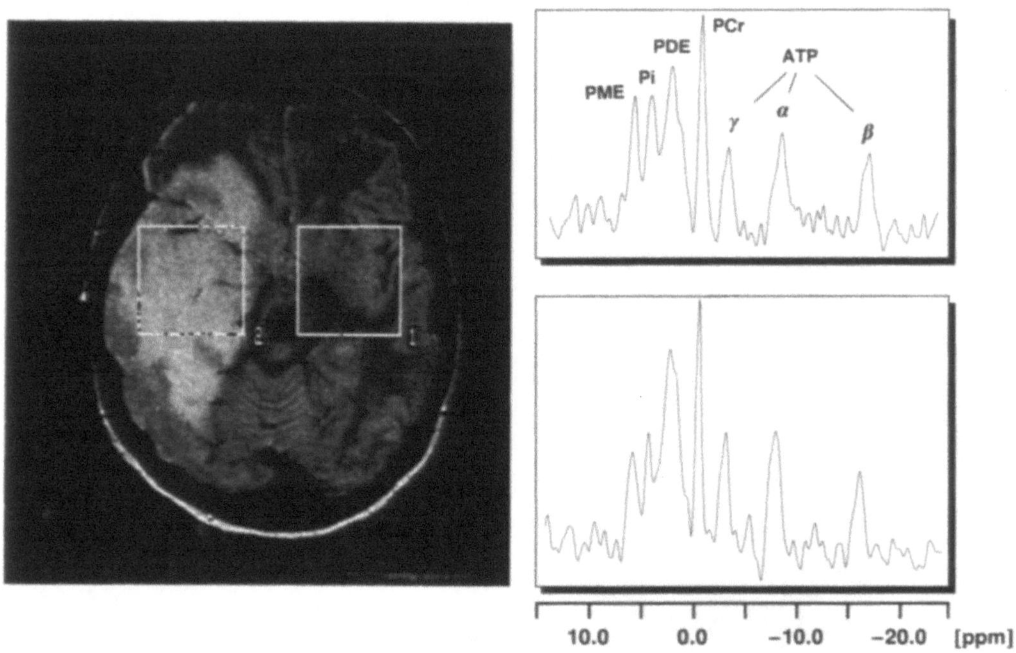

Fig. C15. Spatially resolved spectroscopy (modified ISIS technique). *Left*: axial MR image of astrocytoma (VOI 2). *Top right*: tumor spectrum showing increased PME. *Bottom right*: spectrum from uninvolved tissue (VOI 1). PCr is increased, PME reduced. The smaller separation of the PCr and P_i lines in the tumor spectrum signifies a lower pH

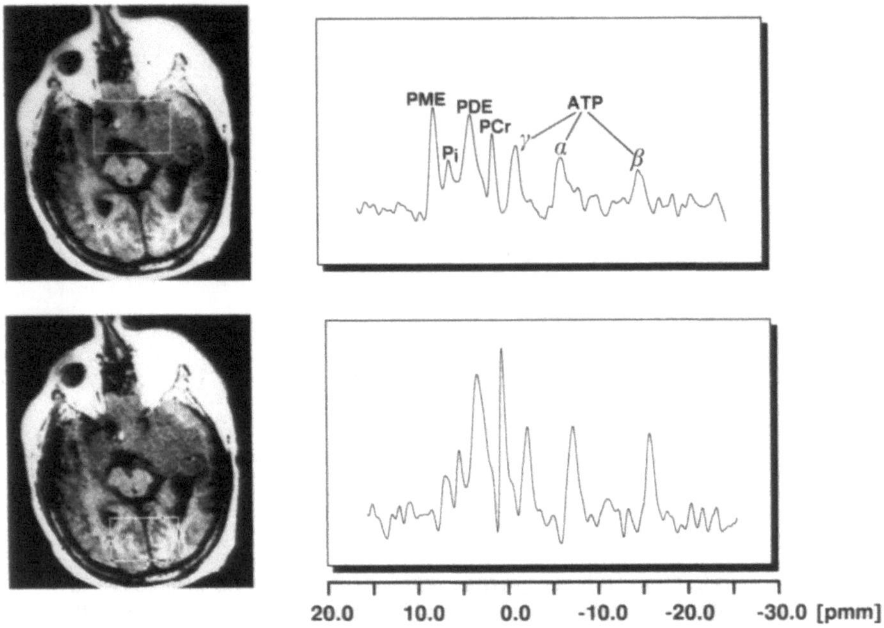

Fig. C16. ^{31}P brain spectrum in a patient with malignant prolactinoma. *Top*: MR scan showing the location of the VOI for spectroscopy. The tumor spectrum (1.5 T) shows a decrease in PCr and an increase in PME. *Bottom*: Normal spectrum from uninvolved tissue. (After Segebarth et al. 1987)

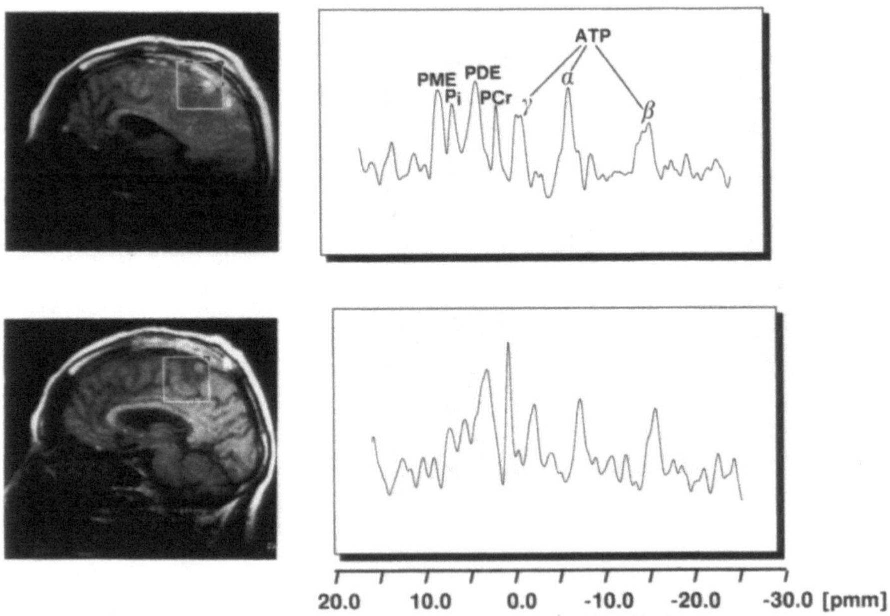

Fig. C17. Intracranial lymphoma before and after radiotherapy (2400 rad in 2 weeks). The increased PME levels and decreased PCr levels change toward values typical of normal brain in response to radiotherapy. (After Segebarth et al. 1987)

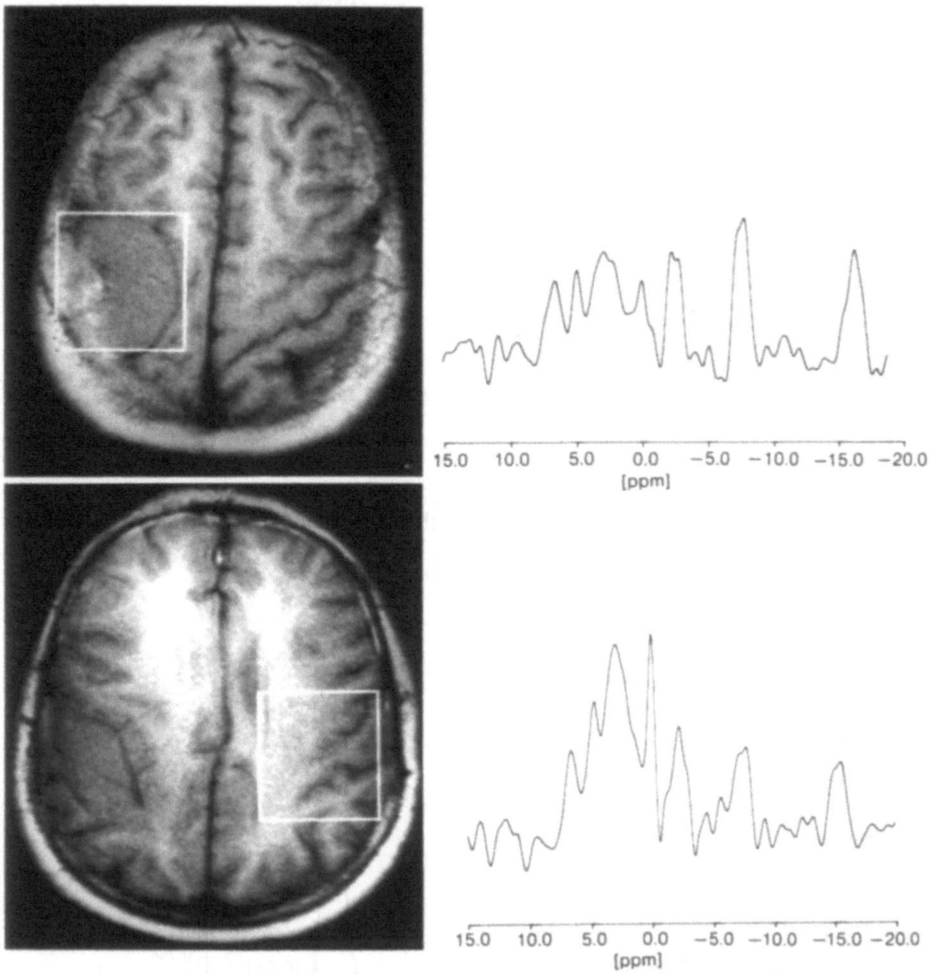

Fig. C18. a MR image and ^{31}P spectrum of a meningioma (1.5 T), VOI 4.5 × 4.5 × 5 cm^3. **b** MR image and spectrum from normal tissue in the contralateral hemisphere. (Courtesy of W. Heindel, Department of Radiology, University of Cologne)

g) Relaxation Time Measurements

Spatially resolved spectroscopy, like MR imaging, can be used to determine the T1 and T2 relaxation times. This can even be done for individual spectral lines, yielding more precise information on tissue characteristics than the integral values supplied by imaging. It also provides a way to measure the concentrations of different compounds that are resolved in the spectral trace.

h) Outlook

Spatially resolved ^{1}H and ^{31}P MR spectroscopy are currently undergoing limited clinical trials for the evaluation of brain tumors and brain metabolism. Although case numbers to date are small, available results suggest that ^{31}P spectroscopy in particular may become a valuable tool for monitoring therapeutic response in tumor patients, and that ischemic areas in the brain can be identified on the ^{1}H spectrum by the increase in lactic acid levels.

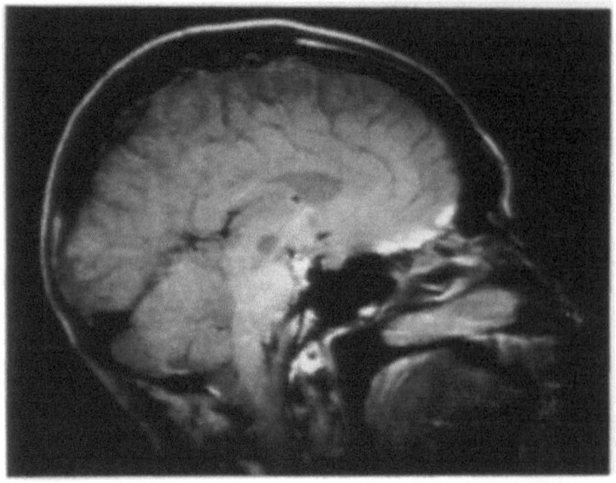

Fig. C19. Sagittal ^1H image (4 T) of a healthy subject

Figures C19–C21 are reproduced courtesy of H. Bomsdorf and colleagues, Philips Research Laboratories, Hamburg.

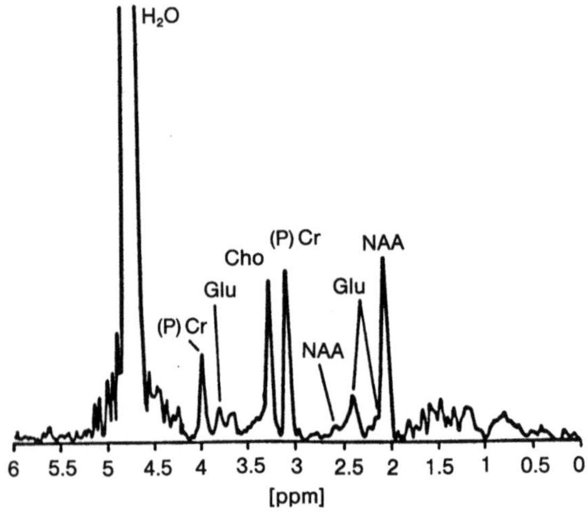

Fig. C20. 4-T ^1H spectrum of a healthy cerebellum acquired with a stimulated echo (STE) sequence. *Glu*, glutamic acid. NEX 128, TR 2500 ms, TE 272 ms, TSTE 48 ms. Sampling volume 15 cm^3

The question of specificity in tumor diagnosis remains unclear. Until recently it was thought that there was too much of an overlap, similar to the relaxation times in imaging, to allow for a specific diagnosis. But with improved techniques in ^1H spectroscopy such as stimulated echoes and with proton decoupling in ^{31}P spectroscopy, this situation may change. Recently (1987), a few research laboratories began using 4-T total-body magnets. To the surprise even of physicists, proton imaging of the human head and trunk proved to be feasible with an image quality acceptable at least for localizing lesions to be examined by spectroscopy. While the potential physiological hazards of applying high static fields, stronger gradients, and high levels of RF power are still discussed, 4-T systems offer increased sensitivity and spectral resolution which have yet to be exploited. Some early results are presented in Fig. C19, which shows a sagittal proton image acquired at 4 T, and in Figs. C20 and C 21, which show 4-T stimulated-echo ^1H spectra acquired from a subject with a normal cerebellum and from a patient with medulloblastoma. The tumor spectrum shows a reduction of NAA and a marked elevation of choline. The respective sampling volumes were 15 cm^3 and 20 cm^3, the examination time 4–8 min.

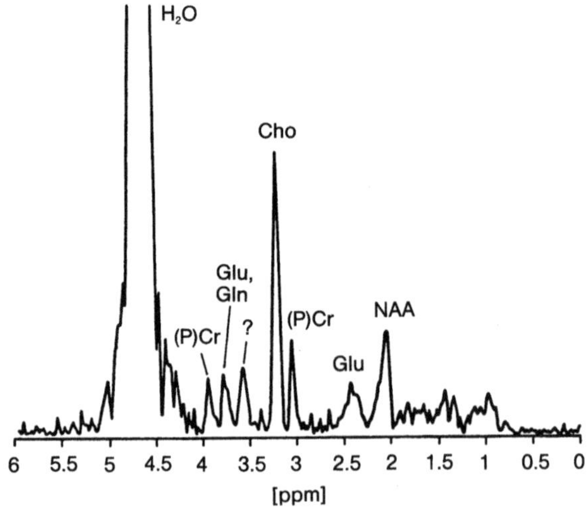

Fig. C21. 4-T ^1H spectrum of medulloblastoma. *Gln*, glutamine. NEX 256, TR 2000 ms, TE 272 ms, TSTE 48 ms, surface coil. Sampling volume 20 cm^3

The MR spectra shown in this section were supplied by Dr. D. Baleriaux and Dr. C. Segebarth, Erasmus Hospital of the Free University of Brussels; Dr. D. Arnold, Department of Neurology, McGill University, Montreal; Dr. W. Heindel, Department of Radiology, University of Cologne; Dr. J. den Hollander and Dr. P.R. Luyten, Philips Medical Systems, Eindhoven; and Dr. H. Bomsdorf, Philips Research Laboratories, Hamburg.

D. CT and MR Imaging of Brain Tumors

Patient Population

Our clinical population numbered 8516 patients with primary and metastatic brain tumors who underwent evaluation by **computed tomography** at the neurosurgical and neuroradiologic departments of the Berlin, Mainz, and Munich centers from 1975 to 1986 and at the Neurosurgical Department of Augsburg Central Hospital from 1983 to 1986. Table 5 lists all the tumors having an incidence greater than 1% in the total population; 98% of the lesions were confirmed histologically (open surgery, stereotactic biopsy, autopsy). "Rare" intracranial tumors having an incidence no greater than 1% are listed in Table 6. The frequencies of the individual tumor types correlate well with the statistical data reported by Cushing (1932), Olivecrona (1967), and Zülch (1986) for large clinical series. The disproportionate representation of some tumor groups is a result of the special interests of the staff at the participating centers or of the intrinsic differences that exist between the statistical outcomes of surgical and necropsy series. An example is pituitary adenoma, which has an incidence of 12.4% in our population compared with 17.8% stated by Cushing (1932) and 6.6% stated by Zülch (1986). The close cooperation with local tumor centers accounts for the high percentage of detected brain metastases in our series.

Magnetic resonance imaging was introduced at the Charlottenburg Clinic of the Free University of Berlin in late 1983. Initial results were so encouraging that research on MR contrast enhancement was extended to include a comparative study of the MR and CT features of a great many types of intracranial tumor. Close cooperation between the Neurosurgical Department of Augsburg Central Hospital and the independent radiologist Dr. Lewetz, as well as between the Neuroradiology Department of the Mainz University Clinic and the joint practice of Dr. Kühnert and his colleagues (Dietzenbach, Frankfurt) provided a major source of up-to-date, relevant MR data. Additional data were furnished by Prof. Fahlbusch and his group at the University of Erlangen-Nuremberg, and important illustrative materials were supplied by the MR research groups under the direction of Prof. Voigt in Tübingen and Prof. Lissner in Munich.

The field strengths of the MR units at the above research laboratories are indicated below (in tesla):

Augsburg	1.0 T
Berlin	0.35–0.5 T
Erlangen (Siemens Center)	0.35–1.0 T
Dr. Kühnert joint practice	0.35–0.5 T
Munich	1.0 T
Tübingen	1.5 T

Table 5. Patients with primary or metastatic brain tumors (n=8516) examined at the neurosurgical and neuroradiologic departments of the Berlin, Mainz, and Munich centers from 1975 to 1986 and at the Neurosurgical Clinic of Augsburg Medical Center from 1983 to 1986. All patients were examined by CT, and most were examined by MR from 1984/85

Histologic diagnosis	n	%
Astrocytoma	476	5.6
Anaplastic astrocytoma	337	4.0
Oligodendroglioma	388	4.6
Glioblastoma	1281	15.0
Pilocytic astrocytoma	230	2.7
Ependymoma	163	1.9
Medulloblastoma	131	1.5
Malignant lymphoma or sarcoma	144	1.7
Meningioma	1575	18.5
Neurinoma	565	6.6
Pituitary adenoma	1057	12.4
Hemangioblastoma	111	1.3
Craniopharyngioma	165	1.9
Epidermoid, dermoid, teratoma[a]	130	1.5
Other tumors[b]	420	5.0
Cerebral metastases	1175	13.8
Brain tumors of unknown histology	168	2.0
Total	8516	100.0

[a] Including one endodermal cyst
[b] Incidence < 1%; see Table 6

Table 6. Rare intracranial tumors and space-occupying lesions (*n*=420), each comprising < 1% of all such processes

Histologic diagnosis	*n*	%
Adenoid cystic carcinoma	2	0.02
Aneurysmatic bone cyst	2	0.02
Angiofibroma, angiosarcoma	8	0.10
Astroblastoma	12	0.14
Cavernoma	18	0.21
Chondroma	4	0.05
Chordoma	32	0.38
Choroid plexus papilloma	32	0.38
Colloid cyst	41	0.48
Embryonal carcinoma	1	0.01
Esthesioneuroblastoma	5	0.06
Fibroma, fibrosarcoma	4	0.05
Gangliocytoma	8	0.10
Ganglioglioma	6	0.07
Ganglioneuroblastoma, anaplastic ganglioglioma	3	0.04
Germinoma	13	0.15
Gliosarcoma	3	0.04
Granular cell tumor (choristoma)	2	0.02
Hamartoma	27	0.32
Hemangiopericytoma	20	0.24
Histiocytoma	15	0.18
Histiocytosis X	5	0.06
Hodgkin's lymphoma, leukemic infiltrate, myeloma	8	0.10
Lipoma	34	0.40
Monstrocellular sarcoma	2	0.02
Neuroblastoma	7	0.08
Osteochondrosarcoma	1	0.01
Osteoma	17	0.20
Paget's disease	2	0.02
Paraganglioma (glomus tumor)	4	0.05
Paranasal sinus carcinoma	4	0.05
Pinealoma, pinealoblastoma	25	0.30
Pituitary carcinoma	1	0.01
Plasmocytoma	5	0.06
Rhabdomyosarcoma	6	0.07
Subependymal giant cell astrocytoma	27	0.32
Undifferentiated neuroectodermal tumor (PNET)	14	0.17
Total	420	4.98

The total number of MR scans available for interpretation, including those from patients with non-neoplastic space-occupying lesions, was just over 1000, underscoring the high degree of selection. Only patients with an abnormal or highly suspicious CT scan were referred for MR evaluation.

Based on the data and findings from an earlier study of CT scans from 3750 patients with brain tumors (see Tables 1 and 2), we shall present numerous case reports which illustrate in systematic fashion the relative capabilities of both imaging modalities in the diagnosis of intracranial tumors. A comprehensive assessment of the value of both modalities for specific disease entities is presented in Table 14 (pp. 628–629).

1. Autochthonous Brain Tumors

a) Astrocytomas

Incidence	Approximately 5% of all brain tumors
Age predilection	25–45 years
Sex predilection	Slight preponderance in males
Typical sites	Frontal, frontotemporal, frontoprecentral, temporal, temporoparietal, pons
Main clinical features	Focal and generalized seizures, often existing for years
Angiography	Often negative in early stages; later evidence of mass lesion lacking vascular supply
CT	
Noncontrast scan	Circumscribed, homogeneous, relatively well delineated hypodensity near cortex or diffusely involving frontotemporal white matter
Contrast enhancement	Not significant
Postcontrast appearance	No significant change relative to unenhanced study
MR	
Noncontrast scan	Usually gives low signal on T1-weighted sequences; appears as conspicuous hyperintensity on T2-weighted images, often greater in extent than on CT scan
Gadolinium enhancement	Not appreciable

Differential diagnosis

Anaplastic astrocytoma
Oligodendroglioma without calcifications
Solitary nonenhancing metastasis
Recent brain infarct
Localized brain edema associated with basal or high parietal tumor
Intracerebral hematoma in course of resorption
Superficial cerebral venous thrombosis
Localized posttraumatic brain edema ("type I" contusion)
Phlegmonous encephalitis
Multiple sclerosis
Surface artifacts (especially in frontal region behind frontal sinus and in temporopolar region)

Slow-growing astrocytomas (fibrillary, protoplasmic, gemistocytic) are defined as grade II tumors in the WHO classification, although they display all the microscopic features of a benign tumor (see Chap. B). We referred to these lesions as grade I astrocytomas in earlier publications (Kazner et al. 1975; Wende et al. 1977).

Astrocytomas account for 5.6% of the intracranial tumors in our population. They have a peak incidence from 25 to 45 years but may also affect children and adolescents. There is a slight preponderance in males.

Typical Sites

Most cerebral astrocytomas occur in the frontal, frontotemporal, temporal, and temporoparietal regions. Other forms grow diffusely in the frontotemporal white matter. Astrocytomas also occur in the thalamus, midbrain, and pons (see Figs. D 1.1–17, 111, 112, 116, 117, 125–130).

Main Clinical Features

The major clinical manifestations of astrocytoma are focal and generalized seizures, which may have been present for many years. Neurologic deficits and signs of raised intracranial pressure tend to appear much later.

Additional Diagnostic Procedures

Additional clinical examinations do not provide specific diagnostic clues. Cerebral angiography shows no abnormalities in early stages. As tumor growth proceeds, signs of an intracranial space-occupying lesion become apparent, although angiograms still do not demonstrate an intrinsic tumor vascular supply.

Computed Tomography
(Figs. D 1.1–8, 12, 15, 16)

Noncontrast Scan
Slow-growing astrocytomas appear on plain CT scans as variably well-defined, homogeneous hypodensities, which very often are in contact with the brain surface (see Figs. D 1.1–3, 5–7, 15). Diffuse growths usually involve the frontotemporal white matter and present ill-defined borders (see Figs. D 1.2–4, 7). Astrocytomas of the lower brainstem appear as an expansion of the pons, usually with an associated decrease in radiographic density (see Figs. D 1.125–127).

The absorption values of astrocytomas are markedly decreased relative to normal brain tissue (18–24 HU) and approximate those of brain edema. It is likely that the high water content of grade II astrocytomas – 81%–82%, the same as edematous white matter – accounts for their low density on CT scans (Lanksch et al. 1976).

These findings are characteristic of fibrillary and protoplasmic astrocytomas but not of gemistocytic astrocytomas, which we found to present a heterogeneous density pattern that can include extensive isodense areas (Fig. D 1.7).

Postcontrast Scan
Slow-growing fibrillary and protoplasmic astrocytomas show *no apparent enhancement* on postcontrast CT scans. However, digital analysis shows an increase of absorption values by 2–3 HU in the tumor area, corresponding roughly to the increase seen in normal brain tissue after contrast injection.

Enhancement is occasionally seen in cortical areas adjacent to tumors located near the cortex, and this may be misinterpreted as contrast uptake by the tumor itself. Again, the gemistocytic astrocytomas are exceptional in this regard, and we observed marked contrast enhancement in two lesions of this type (Fig. D 1.7). These are the only astrocytomas with positive contrast enhancement (Table 2, pp. 22–23). Slight perifocal edema was also present around both tumors.

Magnetic Resonance Imaging
(Figs. D 1.9–17)

Noncontrast Scan
T1-weighted images give relatively little information on the tumor, which appears isointense or slightly hypointense to normal brain. No specific tumor structures are delineated. On the other hand, T2-weighted images clearly demonstrate an area of increased signal intensity. MR offers definite advantages over CT. The tumors consistently appear larger on MR images than on CT scans. Some grade II astrocytomas may not be detected by CT scanning, yet are easily identified with MR. The margins of astrocytomas are defined with much greater clarity by MR; they tend to be more diffuse than circumscribed when compared with earlier CT findings.

The slight perifocal brain edema that may be present in some cases cannot be demarcated by MR. However, samples of tissue taken from the margin of the tumor as defined by MR always show astrocytoma. MR is therefore clearly superior to CT regarding demonstration of the extent of the pathological process.

Postcontrast Appearance

As on CT scans, astrocytomas show no clinically significant contrast enhancement with Gd-DTPA.

Differential Diagnosis

The main condition requiring differentiation from astrocytoma is *circumscribed brain edema.* The edema associated with a fresh cerebral infarction is characterized by its occurrence in specific vascular distribution areas, although multiple small embolic infarctions may deviate from this pattern. In some cases a hypodense tumor can be distinguished from a brain infarct only by performing examinations at intervals, unless the clinical course is sufficient to establish the diagnosis.

Confusion with *circumscribed posttraumatic edema* (type I contusion according to Lanksch et al. 1978) is possible if the tumor patient is examined following a head injury (e.g., sustained during a seizure). Examinations repeated at intervals should establish the diagnosis.

Intracerebral hematomas in the course of resorption may appear as areas of decreased density in certain phases, simulating an astrocytoma (see Figs. F68, 69). Perifocal edema of the white matter does not support a diagnosis of astrocytoma. On the other hand, there are *metastases which do not enhance* with contrast medium and thus present only as areas of localized edema. These lesions may be mistaken for astrocytoma in a patient whose history is not suspicious for metastatic disease.

Uncalcified oligodendrogliomas are indistinguishable from astrocytomas on CT scans (see Fig. D1.40).

A significant percentage of *anaplastic astrocytomas* (33.1%) have the same CT appearance as fibrillary and protoplasmic astrocytomas on unenhanced scans. Even postcontrast scans fail to differentiate these tumors in 17% of cases due to absence of enhancement.

Differential diagnosis can be especially difficult in patients with *basal and high parietal tumors.* CT scans of high parietal tumors may demonstrate only the *accompanying edema* while failing to disclose the tumor itself. The hypodense edema, in turn, may be mistaken for an astrocytoma. Misinterpretations of this kind can be avoided by continuing the scans to the level of the vertex or by taking coronal projections.

Misinterpretation can also occur with *small basal meningiomas,* which may incite extensive perifocal edema. The identity of the lesion can usually be established by scanning in another projection and by administering contrast medium (see Fig. D2.17).

Phlegmonous encephalitis can resemble astrocytoma on noncontrast scans, and consideration must be given to the history and clinical findings in order to make a diagnosis. Meningoencephalitis is occasionally encountered, and late cases may demonstrate contrast enhancement in the cortical band (see Fig. F12). Abscesses developing from encephalitis produce extensive glial scars that appear as hypodensities (status spongiosus).

Recent as well as older lesions of *multiple sclerosis* may appear as hypodense areas that can be mistaken for astrocytoma in MS patients who do not present with a typical history.

MR is only sometimes helpful in solving *problems of differential diagnosis.* Intracerebral hematomas in the resorption phase can be distinguished by their demonstrability even on T1-weighted images and by the typical signal pattern of older hemorrhages. Phlegmonous encephalitis and multiple sclerosis generally produce multifocal abnormalities on MR images.

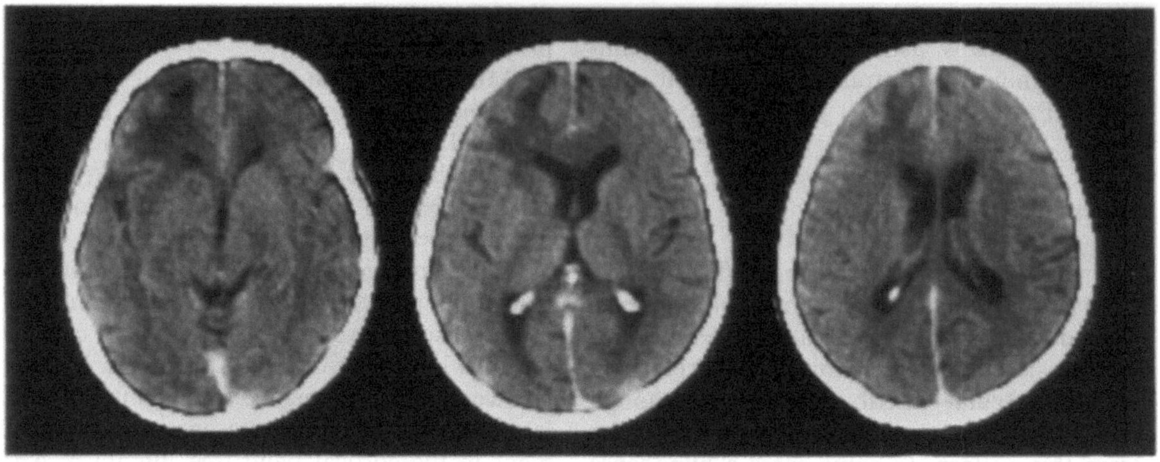

Fig. D 1.1. Astrocytoma of the left frontal lobe extending through the anterior corpus callosum to the right side in a 65-year-old man. The diffuse growth pattern mimics the appearance of perifocal edema. The tumor shows no enhancement on these postcontrast CT scans

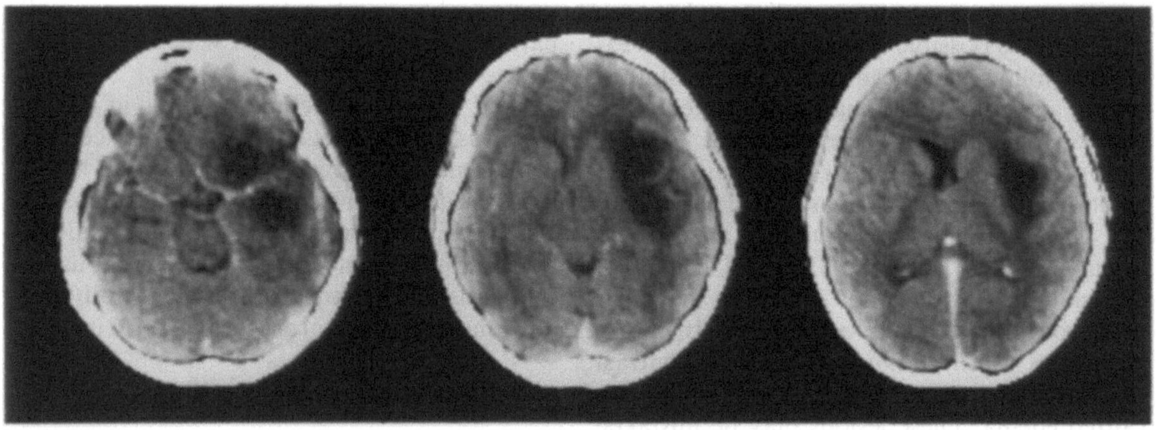

Fig. D 1.2. Diffusely growing astrocytoma of the right frontotemporal region in a 34-year-old woman with seizures. The right middle cerebral artery, encased by tumor, is clearly visible in the left CT scan. There is incipient uncal herniation with mild compression of the brainstem. No enhancement, moderate mass effect

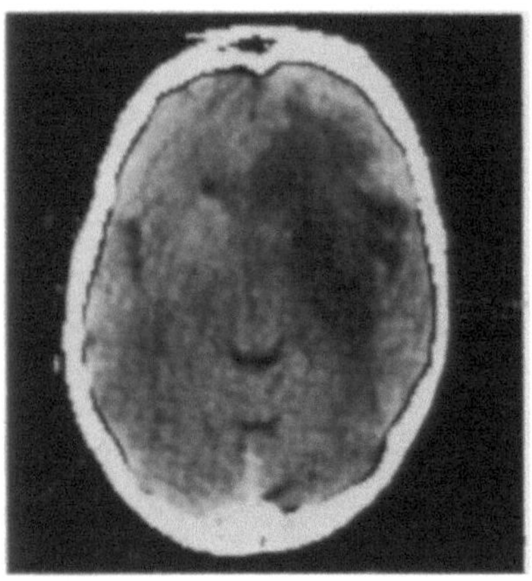

◀ **Fig. D 1.3.** Extensive astrocytoma diffusely involving the white matter of the right hemisphere in a 40-year-old woman with a 10-year history of cerebral seizures. The tumor does not show significant contrast enhancement

Fig. D 1.5. Large astrocytoma in the white matter of the right hemisphere with extension along the lateral ventricle. As the patient is only 5 years old, the tumor has caused marked bulging of the calvarium. Perifocal edema is evident around the hypodense tumor, unusual since the edema associated with low-grade astrocytomas is usually indistinguishable from the tumor itself. There is evidence of possible tumor growth around the left frontal horn

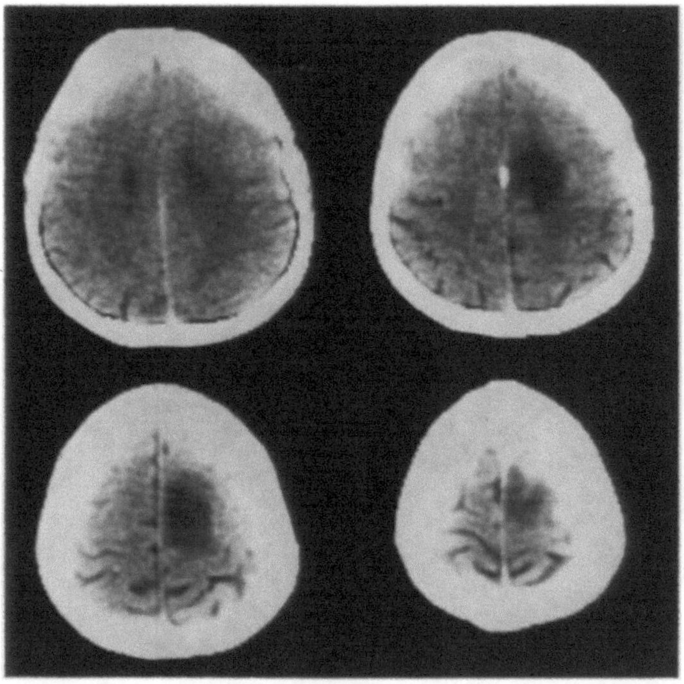

Fig. D 1.4. Astrocytoma of the right central region bordering on the interhemispheric fissure in a 36-year-old man. The clear delineation of the adjacent sulci shows that the mass effect is minimal. The tumor does not enhance. The small hyperdensity at the medial border of the tumor represents a calcification of the falx

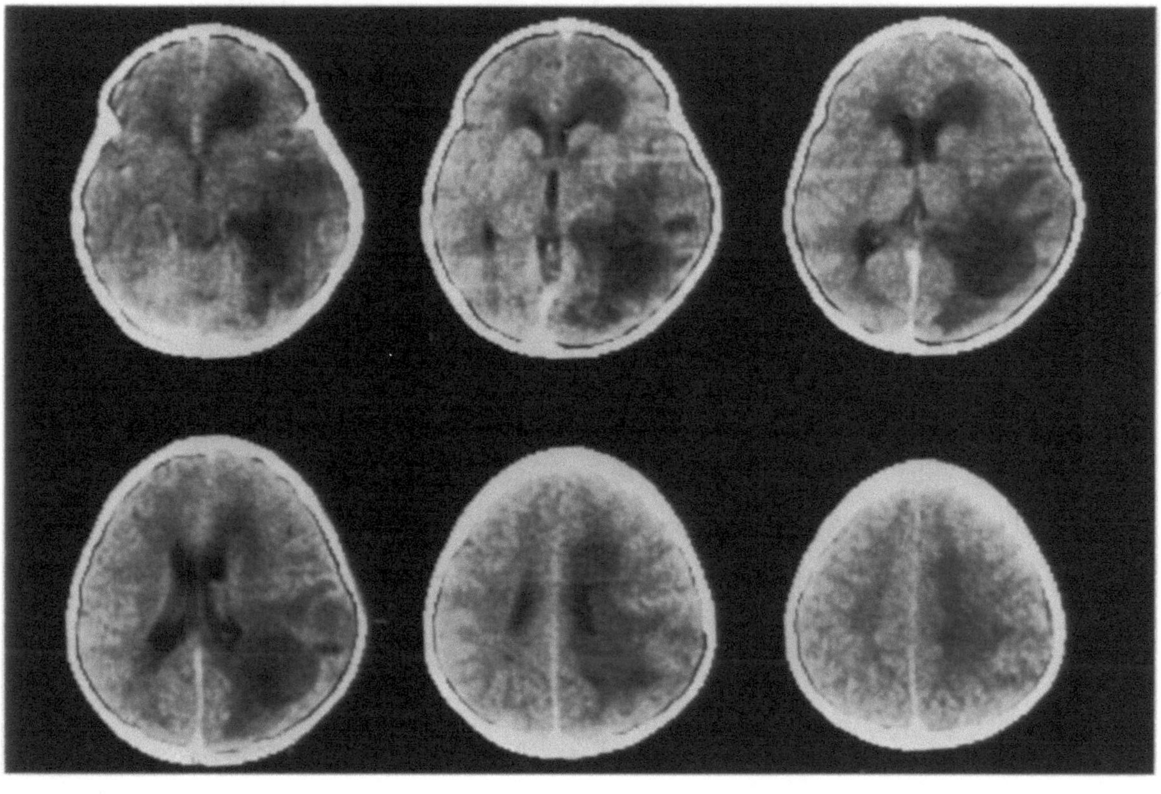

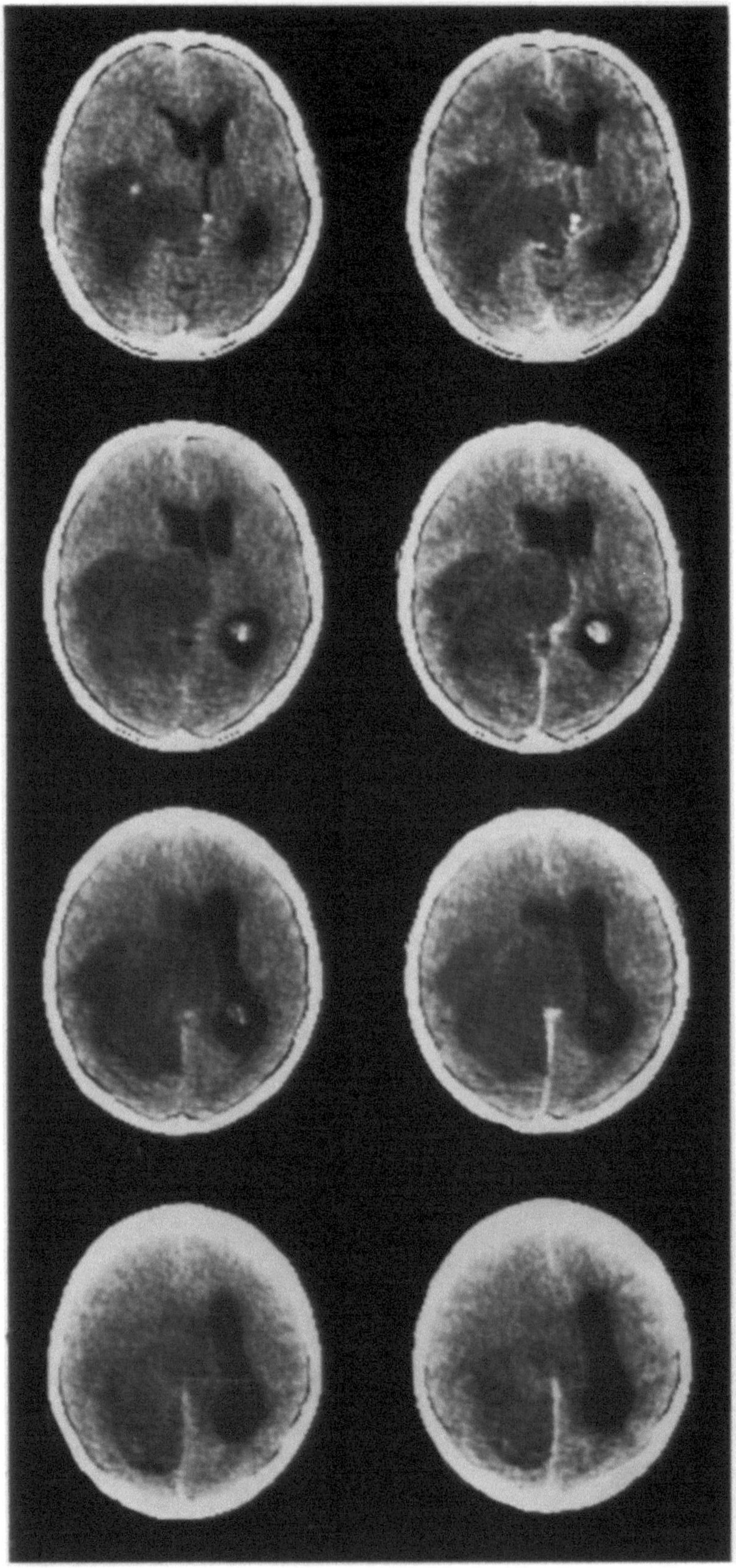

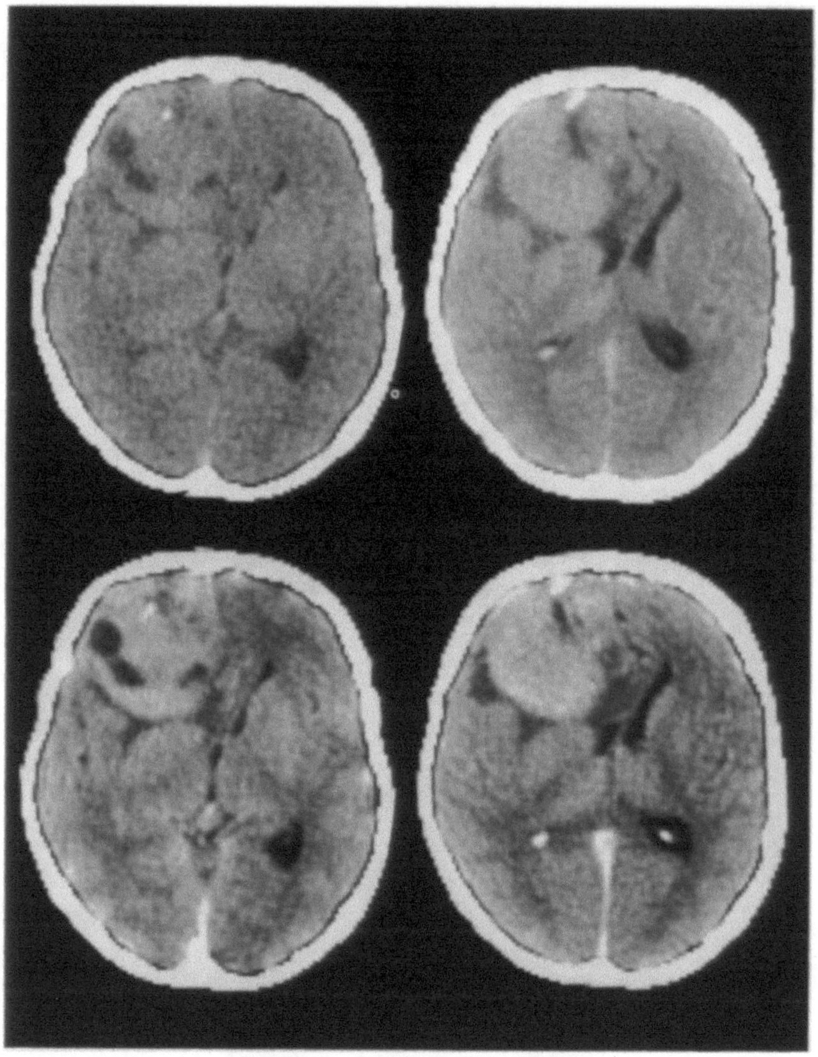

Fig. D 1.7. Gemistocytic astrocytoma in the left frontal lobe of a 35-year-old man. On plain scans the tumor is predominantly isodense with small cystic voids and small foci of calcification. Slight perifocal edema is present (*top*). Postcontrast scans demonstrate the tumor to greater advantage (*bottom*). Its appearance differs markedly from the CT features of the other, nonmalignant astrocytomas. Gemistocytic astrocytomas are prone to malignant transformation

Fig. D 1.6. Very large astrocytoma of the left cerebral hemisphere extending into the basal ganglia in a 37-year-old man with headache and papilledema. Ventricular distention on the right side is caused by CSF obstruction. CT shows no visible change in the hypodense tumor after the injection of contrast medium (postcontrast scans on the *right*), although digital analysis reveals an increase of 2–3 HU

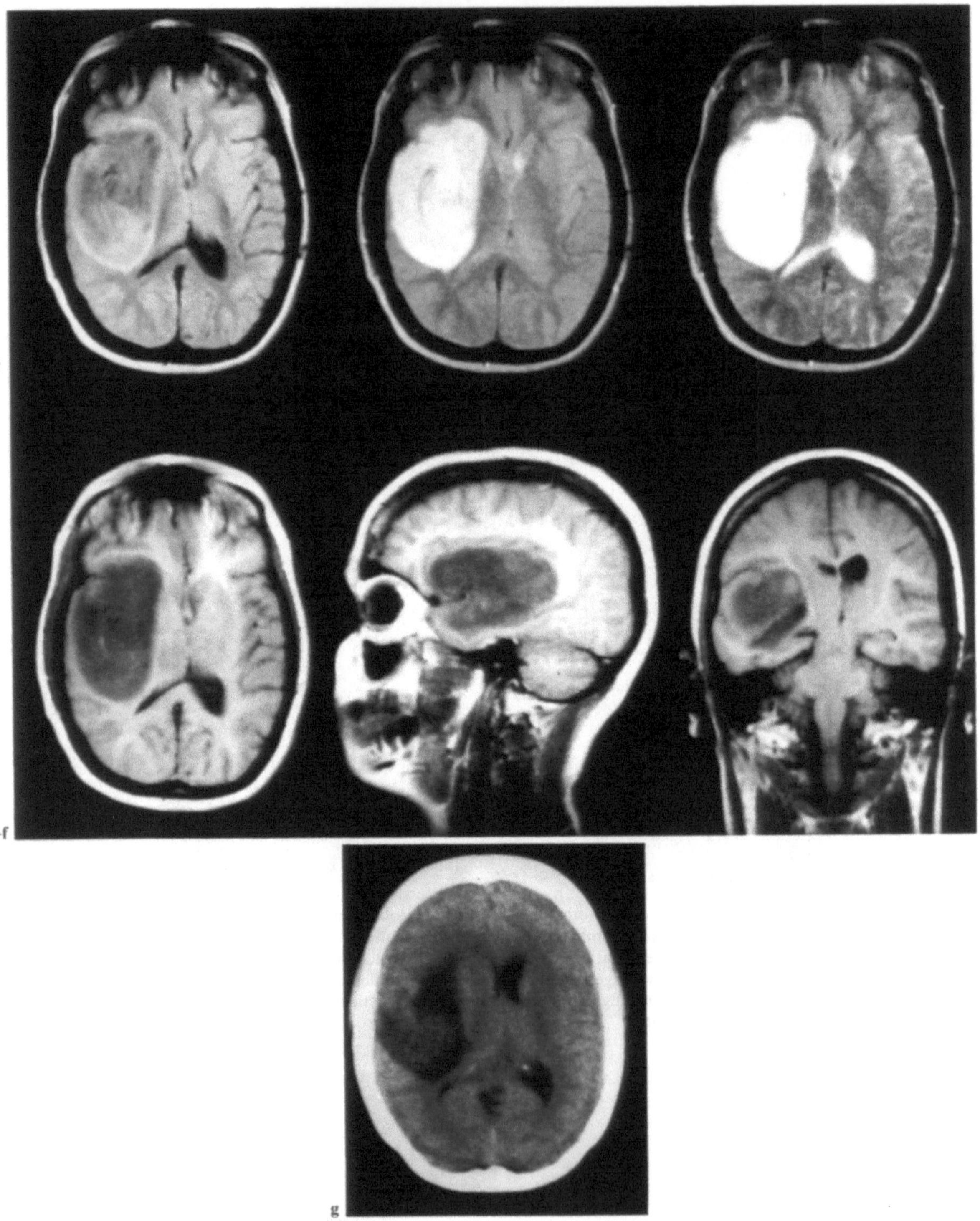

a–c

d–f

g

Fig. D 1.8 a–g. Grade II astrocytoma of the left temporal region. The 36-year-old woman presented with a 4-month history of psychomotor seizures and a 3-month history of headaches. Neurologic exam was negative. MR: **a** SE 1600/30, **b** SE 1600/90, **c** SE 1600/150, **d–f** SE 400/30 axial, sagittal, coronal. CT: **g** noncontrast scan. The T1-weighted images (**d–f**) demonstrate a tumor of low signal intensity causing marked ventricular compression and displacement. On the proton-density image (**a**), the tumor margins appear brighter than surrounding brain. As T2 weighting is increased, the entire lesion becomes very bright and sharply delineated (**b, c**). CT demonstrates a hypodense mass of equal size

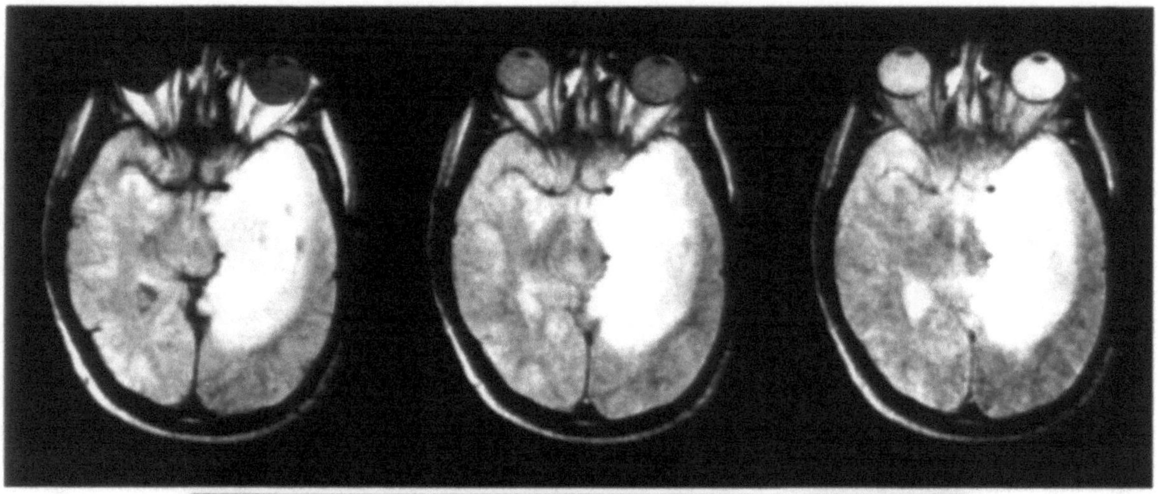

a–c

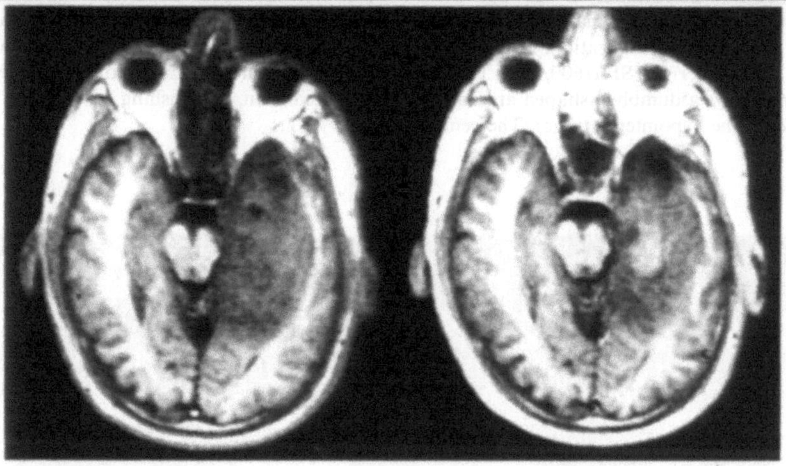

d, e

Fig. D 1.9 a–e. Suspected grade II–III astrocytoma in the right temporo-occipital region, no operation. The 42-year-old man presented with a 20-year history of headaches. Neurologic exam was negative. MR: **a** SE 1600/35, **b** SE 1600/70, **c** SE 1600/105, **d** IR 1500/400/35 noncontrast, **e** post-Gd-DTPA IR sequence. The proton-density and T2-weighted images show a hyperintense, well-defined tumor compressing and displacing the brainstem. The tumor is also well defined on the T1-weighted IR scan, appearing hypointense (**d**). There is moderate central enhancement with Gd-DTPA (**e**)

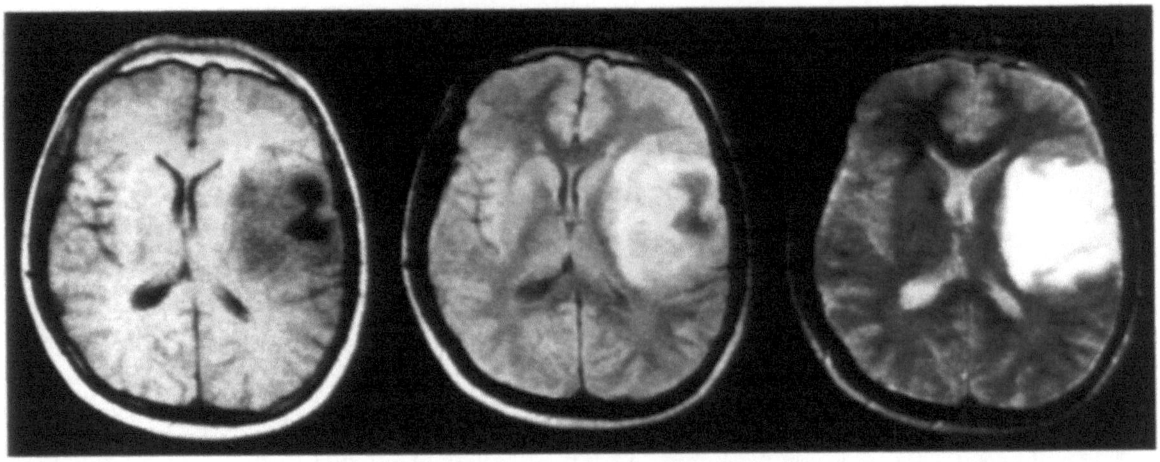

Fig. D 1.10. Grade II–III astrocytoma in the right temporoparietal region. The 30-year-old man presented with focal seizures and secondary generalization. MR: *left* SE 400/35, *center* SE 1600/35, *right* SE 1600/120. The T1-weighted image (*left*) shows a dumbbell-shaped area of signal void at the center of the hypointense tumor. The ventricular system is compressed from the right side. T2 weighting (*center* and *right*) clearly delineates the tumor, which gives a more intense signal as the echo time is increased (*right*). The central hypointensity is no longer visible on the heavily T2-weighted scan, establishing its identity as an intratumoral cyst

a–c

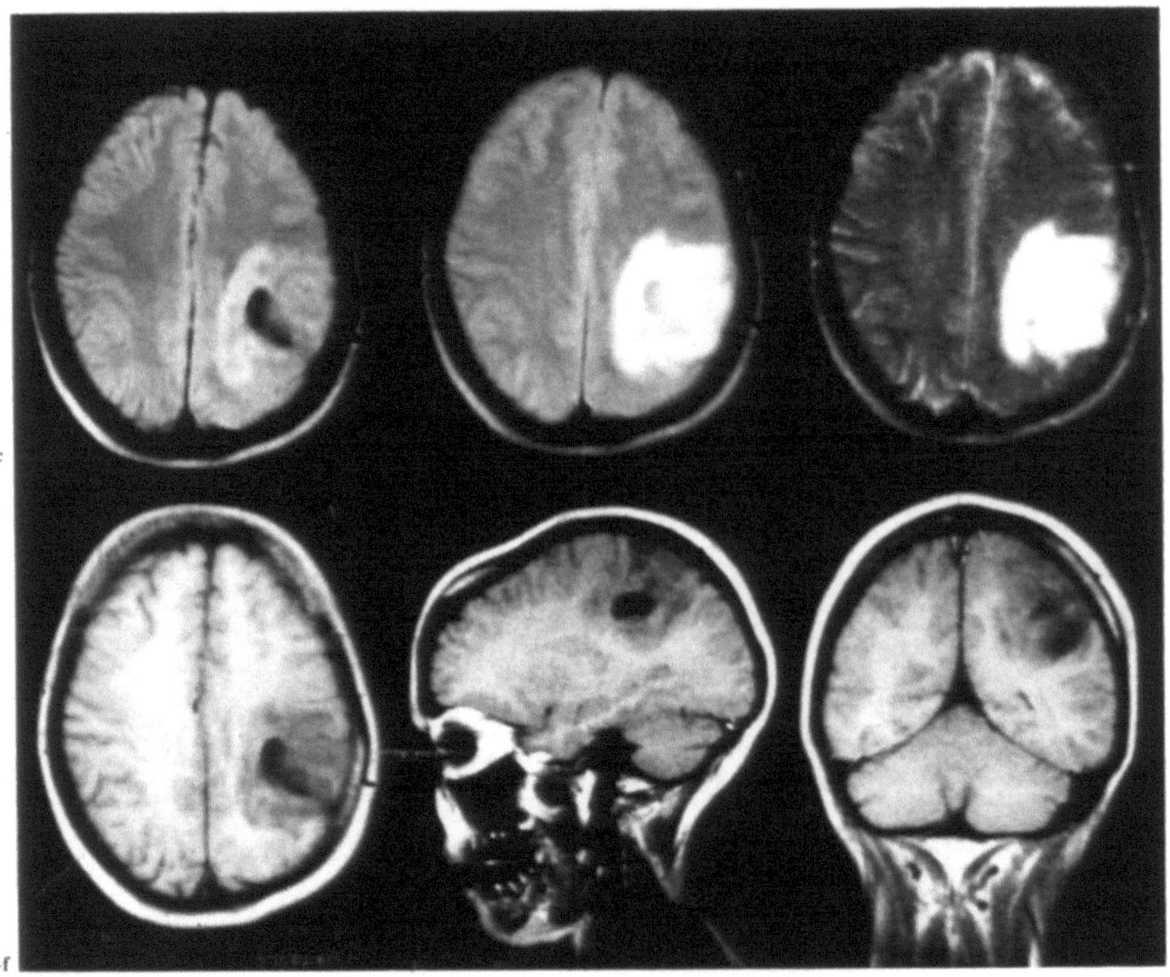

d–f

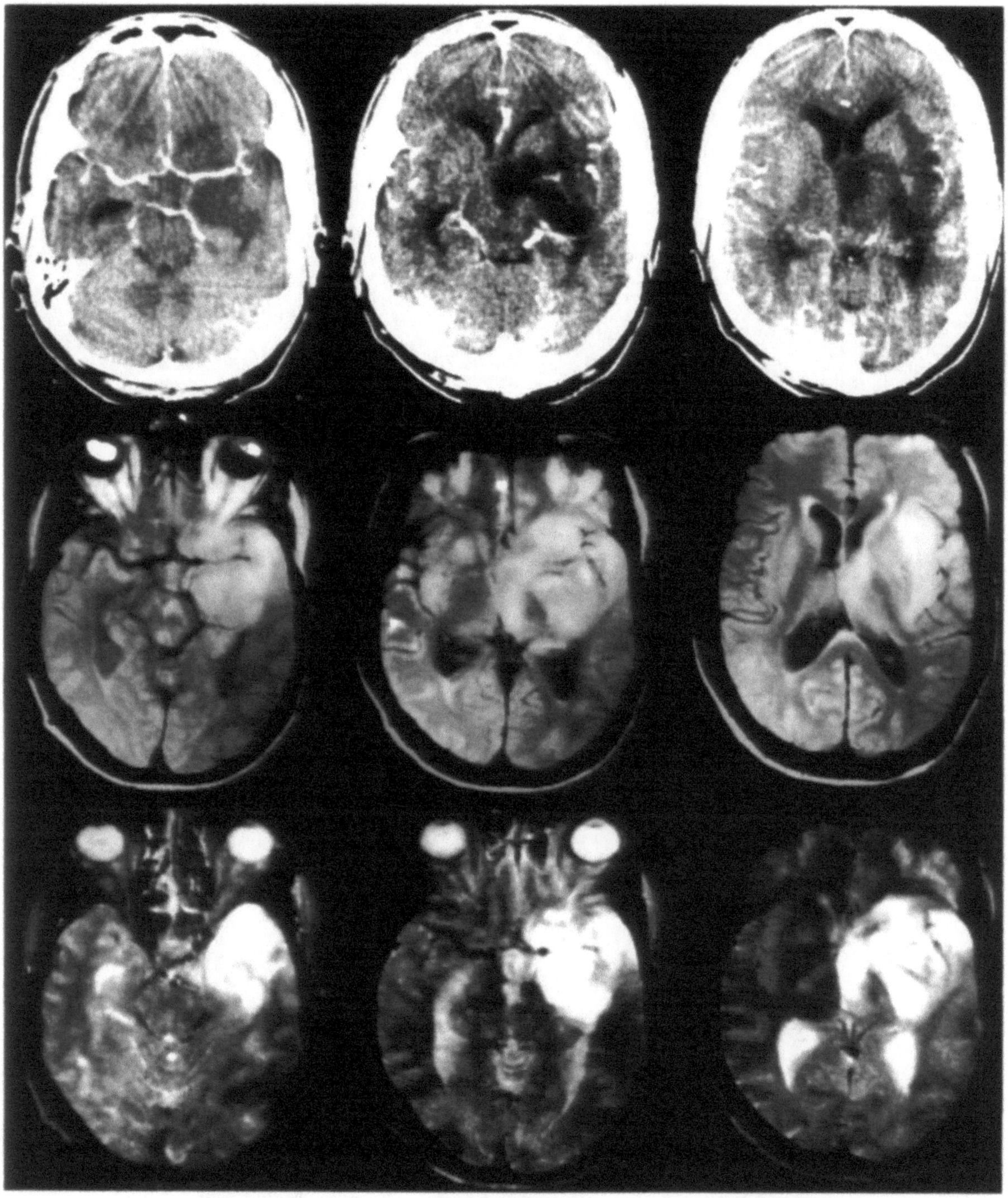

a–c

d–f

g–i

◀ **Fig. D 1.11 a–f.** Suspected grade II–III astrocytoma in the right parietal region, no operation. The 37-year-old woman presented with a 7-year history of focal seizures. Neurologic exam was negative. MR: **a** SE 1600/30, **b** SE 1600/90, **c** SE 1600/180, **d** SE 400/30, **e** SE 400/30 sagittal, **f** SE 400/30 coronal. The proton-density (**a**) and T1-weighted (**d–f**) images show a central, well-defined area of low signal intensity. As T2 weighting is increased (**b, c**) the entire hyperintense lesion is delineated with great clarity. The central hypointensity, presumably a cyst, is not depicted on the T2-weighted images

▲

Fig. D 1.12 a–i. Grade II astrocytoma in the right temporal region of a 44-year-old man with seizure disorder. CT: **a–c** postcontrast scans. MR: **d–f** SE 2500/30, **g–i** SE 2500/120. The CT scans show only minimal lateral enhancement. On the T1-weighted MR scans (**d–f**) the tumor gives a slightly higher signal than the brain parenchyma in its basal portions and is markedly hyperintense on the scan at the highest level (**f**). The T2-weighted images demonstrate a very bright tumor involving the brainstem and corpus callosum (**g–i**)

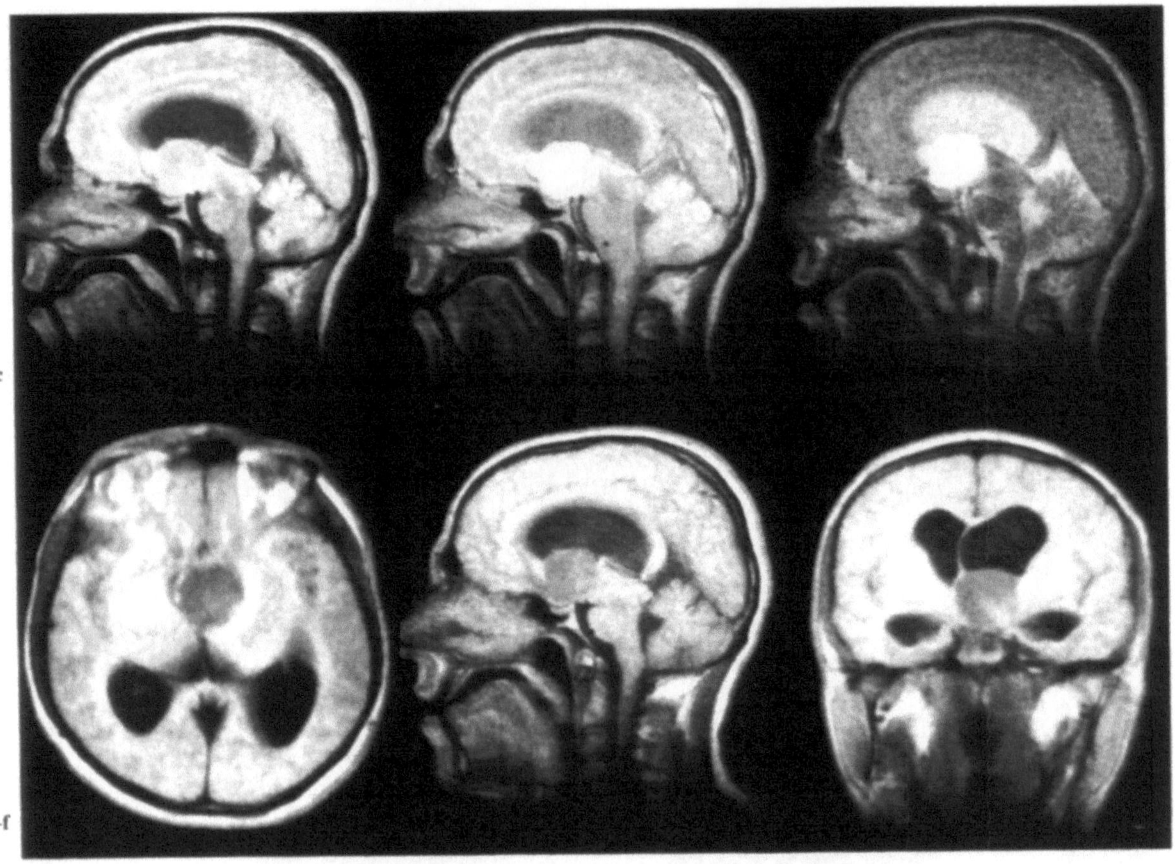

a–c

d–f

D1.13

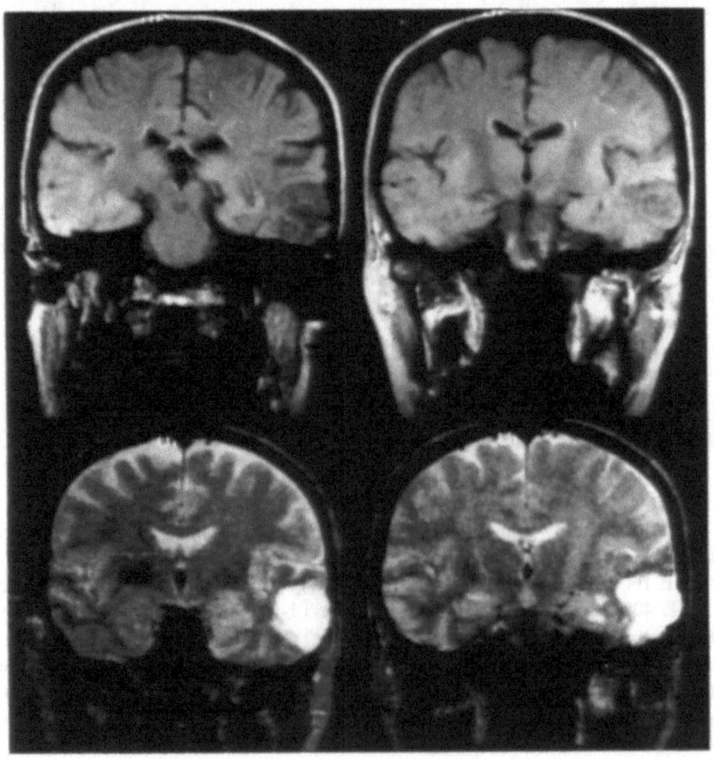

D1.14

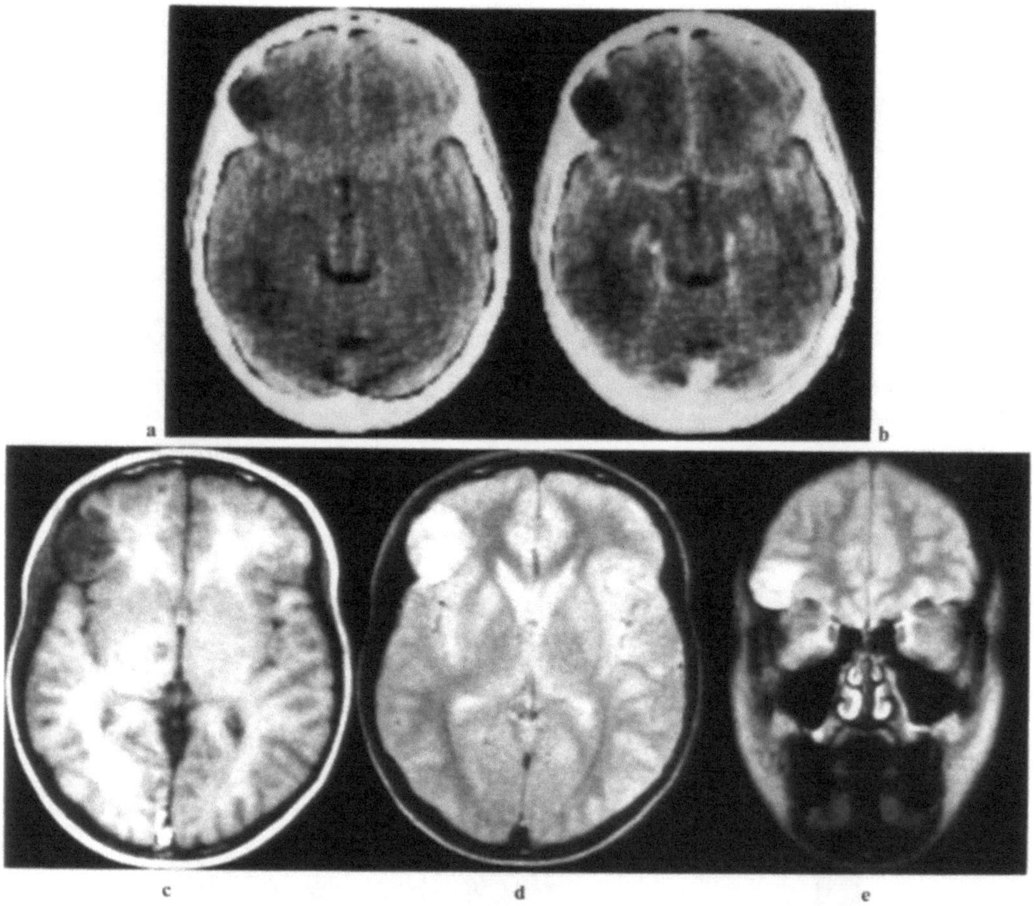

Fig. D 1.15 a–e. Grade II astrocytoma in the left frontolateral region of a 22-year-old man with late epilepsy. CT: **a** precontrast, **b** postcontrast. MR: **c** SE 400/35, **d, e** SE 1600/70 axial, coronal. The hypodense tumor does not enhance on the CT scan. The tumor appears hypointense on the T1-weighted image (**c**), while both the T2-weighted images show a hyperintense tumor equal in size to the mass depicted by CT

Fig. D 1.13 a–f. Grade II astrocytoma in the suprasellar region of a 22-year-old man with a 3-week history of increased intracranial pressure. MR: **a** SE 1600/30, **b** SE 1600/60, **c** SE 1600/150, **d–f** SE 400/35 axial, sagittal, coronal. The tumor gives an increasingly intense signal from the proton-density image (**a**) to the T2-weighted sequence (**b, c**). Marked obstructive hydrocephalus is present. The tumor appears hypointense on the T1-weighted scans, and edema is not visualized in either of the sequences (**d–f**)

Fig. D 1.14. Grade II astrocytoma of the right temporal region in a 44-year-old woman with a history of epileptic seizures for several years. MR: *top* SE 2000/30 coronal, *bottom* SE 2000/120 coronal. The hypointense tumor is almost indistinguishable from brain tissue on the T1-weighted scans. T2-weighted scans at the same levels provide very sharp contrast between the hyperintense tumor and brain tissue

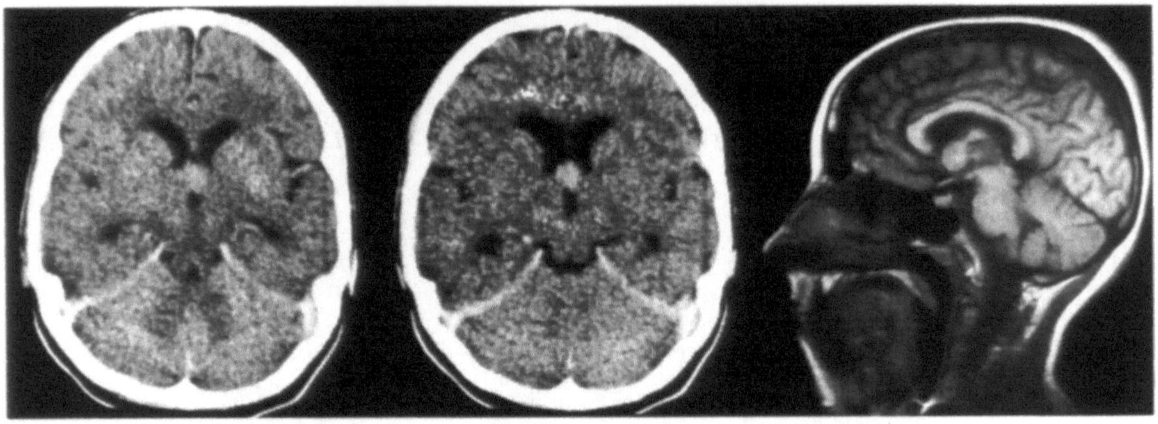

Fig. D 1.16. Fibrillary astrocytoma of the anterior third ventricle, confirmed at operation, in a 15-year-old girl with transitory diabetes insipidus. CT: *left* and *center*, postcontrast. MR: *right* SE 500/30 sagittal. There is no enhancement of the mass on CT. The T1-weighted MR image (*right*) shows a well-defined lesion that is slightly hyperintense to surrounding tissues. A small finger of tumor projects upward and backward

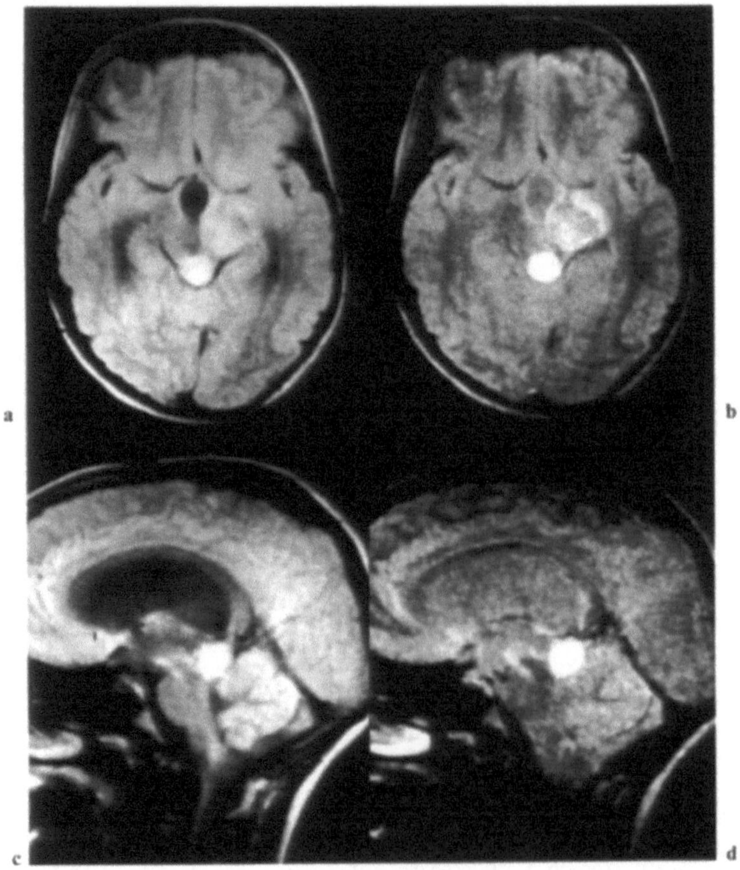

Fig. D 1.17 a–d. Fibrillary astrocytoma with pilocytic components in the region of the pineal body and right basal ganglia. The 15-year-old boy presented with a 5-year history of progressive fine motor deficit in the left hand and dysdiadochokinesia on the left side. MR: **a** SE 1600/35, **b** SE 1600/70, **c** SE 1600/35 sagittal, **d** SE 1600/70 sagittal. On the proton-density images (**a, c**) the tumor appears hyperintense with relatively sharp demarcation. T2 weighting reveals involvement of the basal ganglia and a high-intensity area representing perifocal edema (**b, d**)

b) Anaplastic Astrocytomas

Incidence	Approximately 4% of all brain tumors
Age predilection	35–55 years
Sex predilection	Slight preponderance in males
Typical sites	Frontal, frontoparietal, temporal, temporoparietal
Main clinical features	Seizures, neurologic deficits varying with tumor site, headache
Angiography	Evidence of mass effect; capillary blush is uncommon
CT	
Noncontrast scan	Very heterogeneous; hypodense or isodense areas usually seen, often together in same lesion
Contrast enhancement	Positive in great majority of cases
Postcontrast appearance	Variable: ringlike or solid masses, some with large cysts; may resemble grade II astrocytoma; slight to moderate perifocal edema is common
MR	
Noncontrast scan	Highly variable: low signal on T1-weighted images; high signal on T2-weighted images, often appears larger than on CT scan; signal intensity altered by presence of cysts
Gadolinium enhancement	Generally positive
Post Gd-DTPA appearance	Gd-DTPA often demonstrates solid tumor elements or ring enhancement on T1-weighted image

Differential diagnosis

Glioblastoma
Anaplastic oligodendroglioma without calcifications
Solitary metastasis
Ependymoma
Malignant lymphoma
Pilocytic astrocytoma
Astrocytoma (if tumor does not enhance)

More rarely: brain abscess, acute disseminated encephalomyelitis, leukemic deposits, older intracerebral hematoma

Anaplastic astrocytoma comprised 4.0% of the intracranial tumors in our population. It can occur at any age but is most prevalent between the ages of 35 and 45 years, showing a slight predilection for males. Prognostically the tumor is classified as grade III.

Typical Sites

The most common sites of occurrence are the frontal, frontoparietal, temporal, and temporoparietal regions. The lesions may also affect the parietal lobe, thalamus, and pons. Cerebellar involvement is rare (see Figs. D 1.18–32, 148).

Main Clinical Features

The predominant clinical features are seizures, localized neurologic deficits, and headache.

Additional Diagnostic Procedures

The main finding on cerebral angiography is a mass effect. Tumor vessels are rarely discerned except in more malignant growths, where they can be seen in the center of the tumor. A capillary blush may also be observed. Large cysts appear as avascular spaces.

Computed Tomography

(Figs. D 1.18–23, 25, 26, 30, 31, 148)

Noncontrast Scan

Since the group of anaplastic astrocytomas is considered to include all astrocytomas that contain highly malignant elements, even if the bulk of the tumor is slow-growing, the findings in this group are *exceedingly variable.*

Solid tumor tissue may appear hypodense, isodense, or hyperdense, or any combination of these patterns may coexist in the same lesion (see Figs. D 1.24, 25). Plain scans may demonstrate smooth-bordered cysts (see Fig. D 1.20) with densities of 15–22 HU depending on the protein content of the cystic fluid.

A few *primarily isodense anaplastic astrocytomas may produce minimal indirect tumor signs on the unenhanced CT scan and are easily overlooked* (see Fig. D 1.21 and Table 2, p. 22–23).

Slight to moderate *perifocal brain edema* was present in 67.5% of the anaplastic astrocytomas in our series. In some cases the tumor and accompanying edema caused significant displacement of midline structures. Grade III edema is rare with these tumors (5.1%). The tumor itself usually appears as an isodense area surrounded by low-density edema (Fig. D 1.25). In other cases the tumor and edema are both hypodense and cannot be distinguished on noncontrast scans.

Postcontrast Scan

Contrast enhancement was observed in 83% of the 157 patients in our series; 17% of the anaplastic astrocytomas did not enhance. The latter were primarily hypodense tumors that showed evidence of anaplasia on histologic examination. These varying enhancement patterns suggest that the nonenhancing hypodense tumors may represent a transitional stage between astrocytoma and anaplastic astrocytoma (see above).

The *appearance of anaplastic astrocytomas after contrast injection is highly variable*, but our experience indicates that the following *typical patterns* are encountered:

a) A narrow ring, sometimes discontinuous, enclosing a well-defined hypodensity, usually a cyst. A solid, enhancing tumor nodule may appear at the periphery of the cyst (see Fig. D.120)
b) A hypodense, well-defined area with a subtle, nonhomogeneous, often streaklike pattern of enhancement (see Fig. D 1.19).

In larger, solid, isodense tumor nodules with a density of 32–40 HU on the plain scan, quantitative analysis of the postcontrast scan indicates an average density increase of 11 HU (range 8–16 HU) following a standard dose of contrast medium.

Magnetic Resonance Imaging

(Figs. D 1.24, 27–29, 32)

Noncontrast Scan

As in CT, anaplastic astrocytomas do not present typical or characteristic features on MR images. The T1-weighted image shows a hypo- to isointense mass that may contain a large cyst, which will appear brighter than the tumor itself on the T2-weighted scan. Anaplastic astrocytoma invariably appears larger on T2-weighted images than on CT scans. It is hyperintense and generally has ill-defined borders. Perifocal edema is clearly demonstrated but cannot always be separated from tumor.

Post-Gadolinium Scan

Contrast enhancement may reveal solid, nodular, cystic, or ringlike tumor structures, much as in postcontrast CT. If enhancement does not occur, the appearance is comparable to that of a grade II astrocytoma. Perifocal edema may be visualized and involves a somewhat larger area than on CT scans. It gives a slightly higher signal than the tumor itself.

MR is more sensitive than CT in its ability to detect the tumor and demonstrate its extent. T2-weighted sequences are more valuable in the rare instances of multifocal growth.

Differential Diagnosis

Various differential diagnoses will have to be considered depending on the CT appearance of the anaplastic astrocytoma.

A **hypodense tumor** should mainly arouse suspicion of a low-grade *astrocytoma* or an oligodendroglioma without calcifications. We noted in our series that the hypodense area in anaplastic tumors was generally larger than that seen in other astrocytomas (see also Fig. D1.19).

When **ringlike structures** are observed in the tumor, consideration should be given to *glioblastoma, brain abscess,* and *metastasis. Pilocytic astrocytomas* can produce similar findings (see also p. 130ff.).

A **solid, homogeneously enhancing mass** that does not contain a large hypodensity is consistent with *malignant lymphoma, solitary brain metastasis, ependymoma, leukemic infiltrate,* or *acute disseminated encephalomyelitis.*

MR imaging has not contributed greatly to solving problems of differential diagnosis, although it is more sensitive than CT in the detection of multifocal disease. Differentiation of anaplastic astrocytoma from glioblastoma is especially problematic.

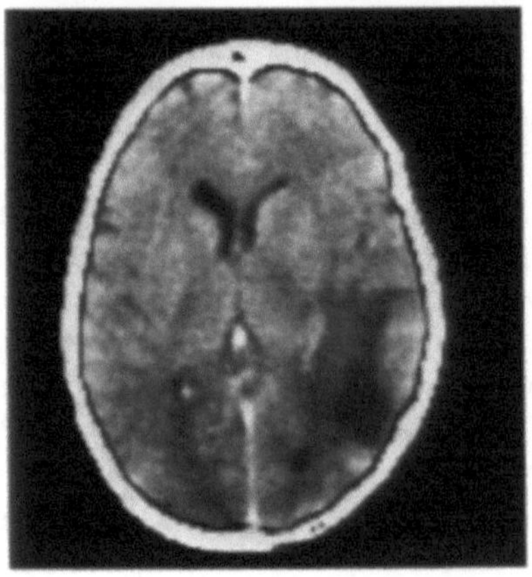

Fig. D 1.18. Anaplastic astrocytoma in the right posterior temporal region of a 51-year-old woman. The lesion contains elements of varying density and shows nonhomogeneous enhancement

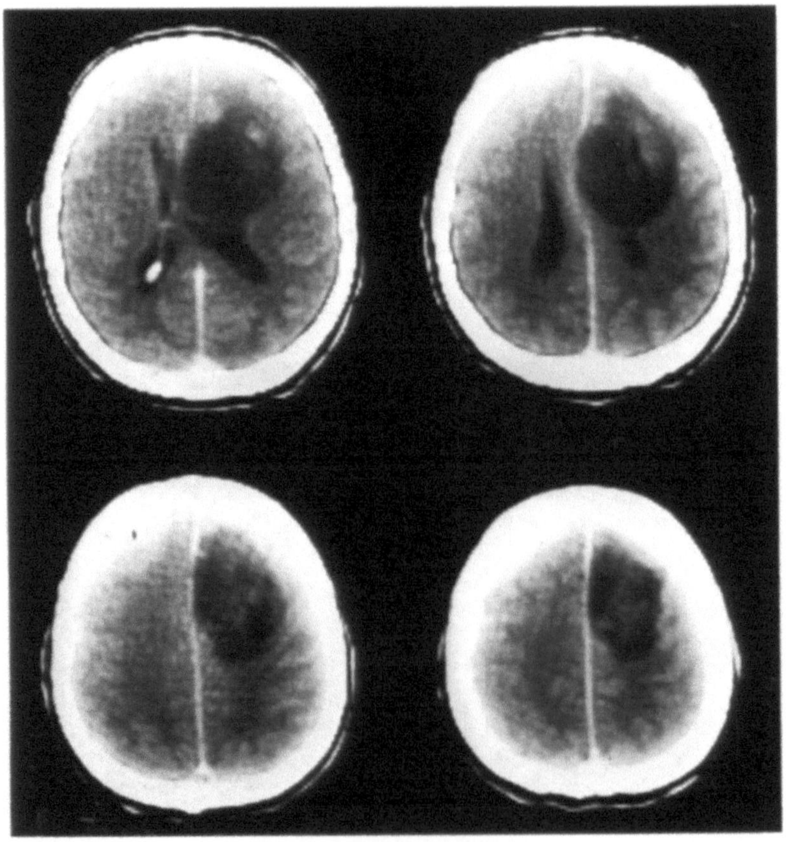

Fig. D 1.19. Large anaplastic astrocytoma in the right frontoprecentral region with extension into the right lateral ventricle in a 40-year-old man with a history of seizures and progressive left-sided hemiparesis in previous years. The hypodense, well-defined tumor shows a faint, patchy enhancement pattern consistent with anaplasia

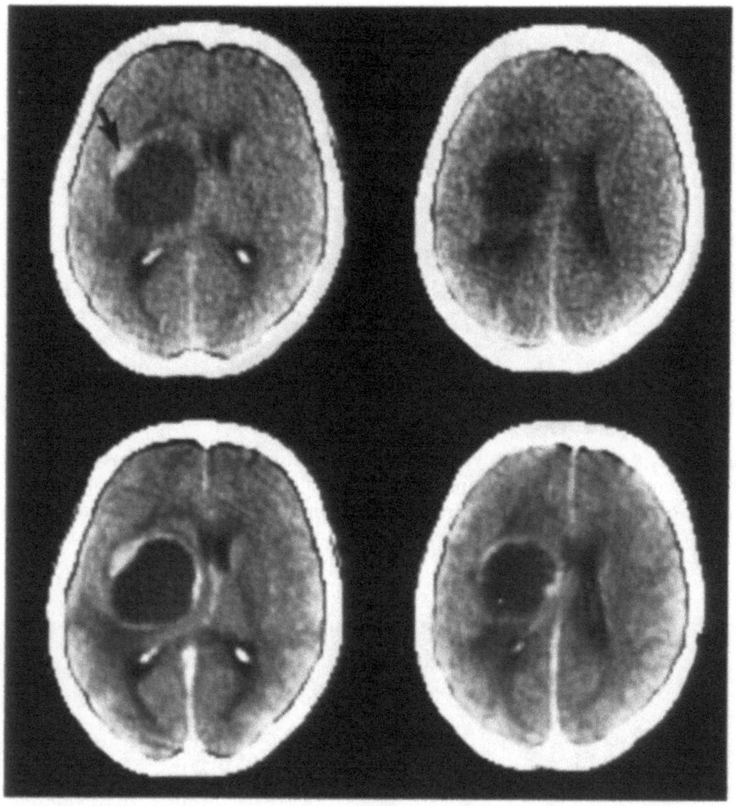

Fig. D 1.20. Anaplastic astrocytoma in the region of the left basal ganglia in a 58-year-old woman. Large tumor cyst, faint peripheral rim enhancement in the solid tumor components. A small hematoma is visible in the anterior wall of the cyst (*arrow*). This tumor could be mistaken for a pilocytic astrocytoma. *Upper* CT scans are precontrast, *lower* are postcontrast

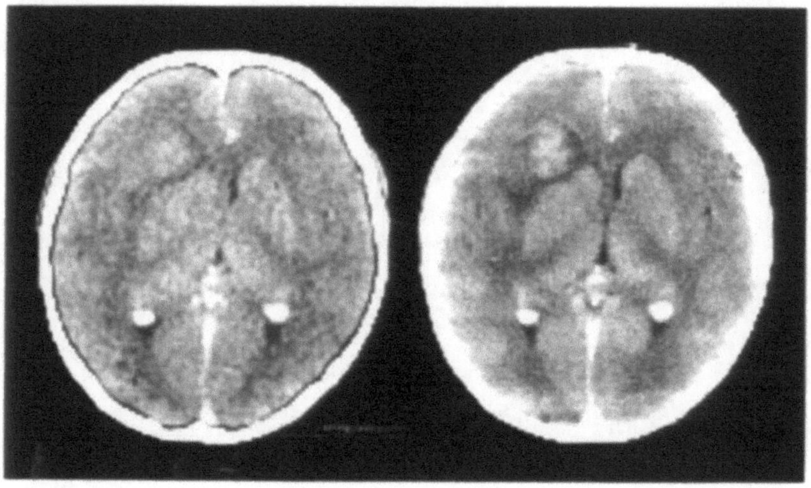

Fig. D 1.21. Anaplastic astrocytoma deep in the frontal white matter of a 36-year-old man with psychomotor seizures. Plain CT scan (*left*) shows a small, semicircular hypodensity at the medial border of the isodense neoplasm. Postcontrast scan (*right*) shows slight, nonhomogeneous enhancement within the tumor

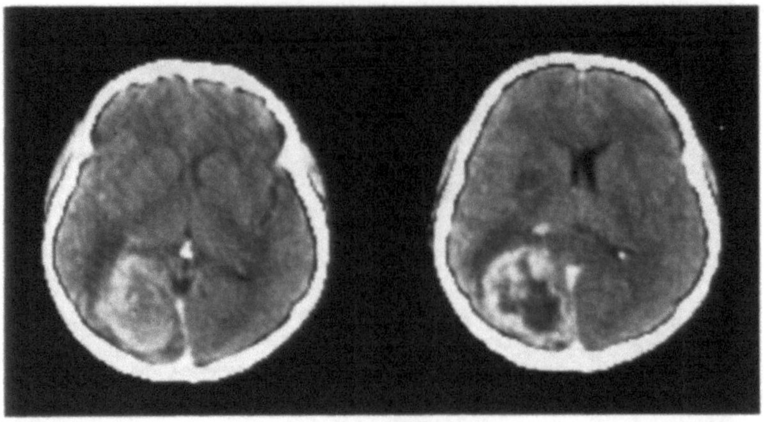

Fig. D 1.22. Anaplastic astrocytoma in the left occipital lobe of a 50-year-old man. The postcontrast CT findings are consistent with glioblastoma. Anaplastic astrocytoma is often indistinguishable from glioblastoma even by histologic examination

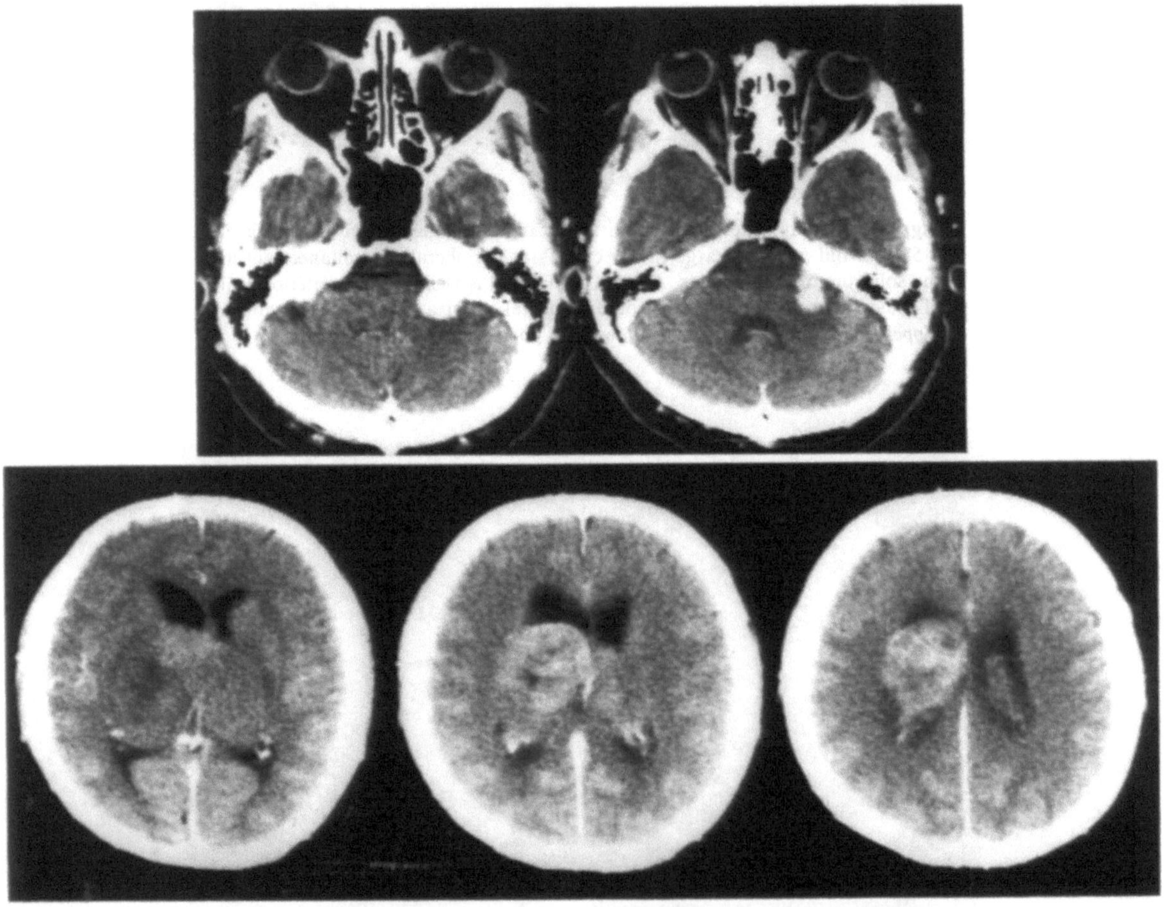

Fig. D 1.23. Anaplastic astrocytoma of the left basal ganglia (confirmed by biopsy). The 40-year-old man presented with a history of mental changes and loss of drive. Besides the basal ganglion pathology, postcontrast CT shows evidence of a meningioma. Differentiation from a neurinoma of the right pyramidal apex is required

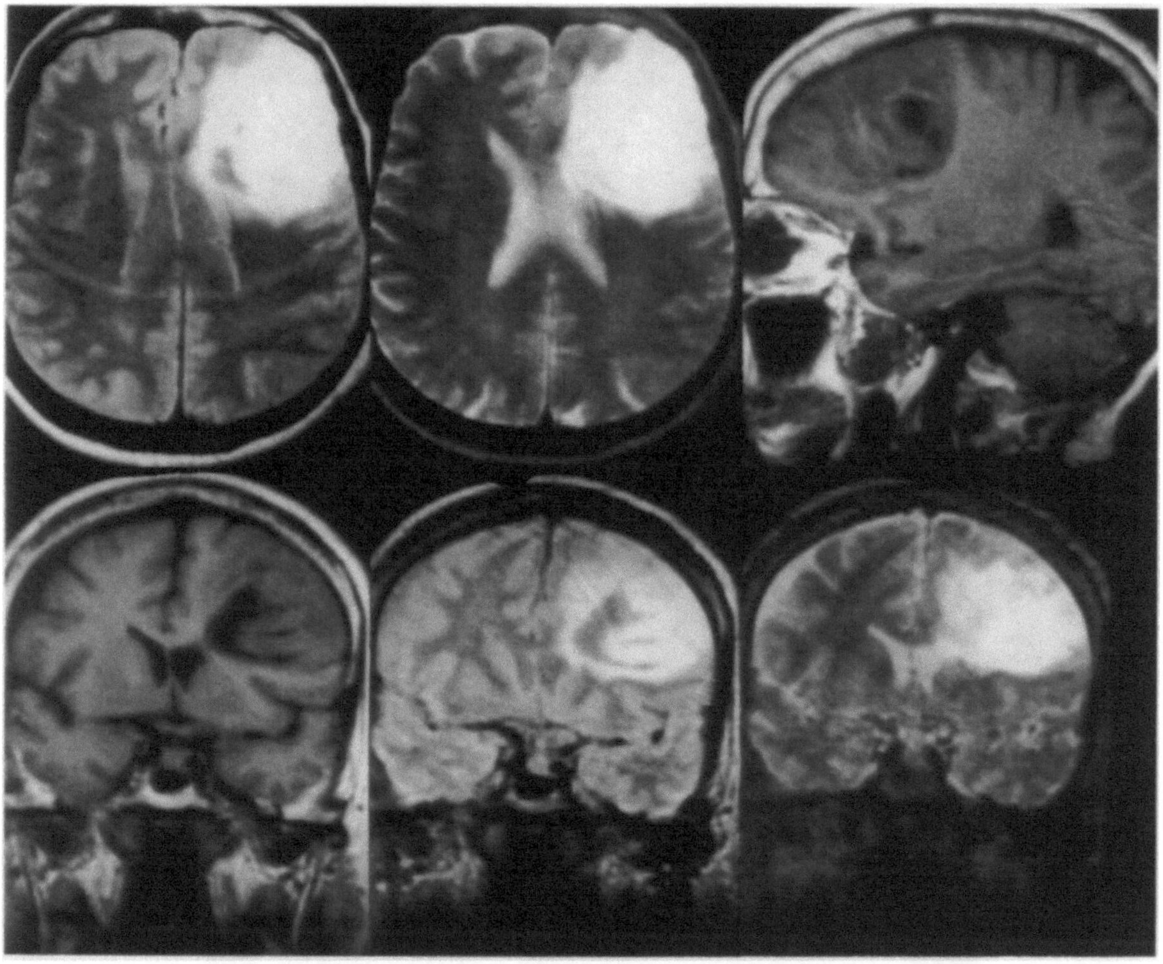

a–c

d–f

Fig. D 1.24 a–f. Anaplastic astrocytoma of the right frontal region in a 69-year-old woman with epileptic seizures and altered mental status. MR: **a** SE 3000/30, **b** SE 3000/90, **c** SE 500/30 sagittal, **d** 500/30 coronal, **e** SE 3000/30 coronal, **f** SE 3000/90 coronal. The tumor appears minimally hypointense on the T1-weighted images (**c, d**) and contains a medial, comma-shaped area of signal void. The tumor is clearly delineated on the T2-weighted images

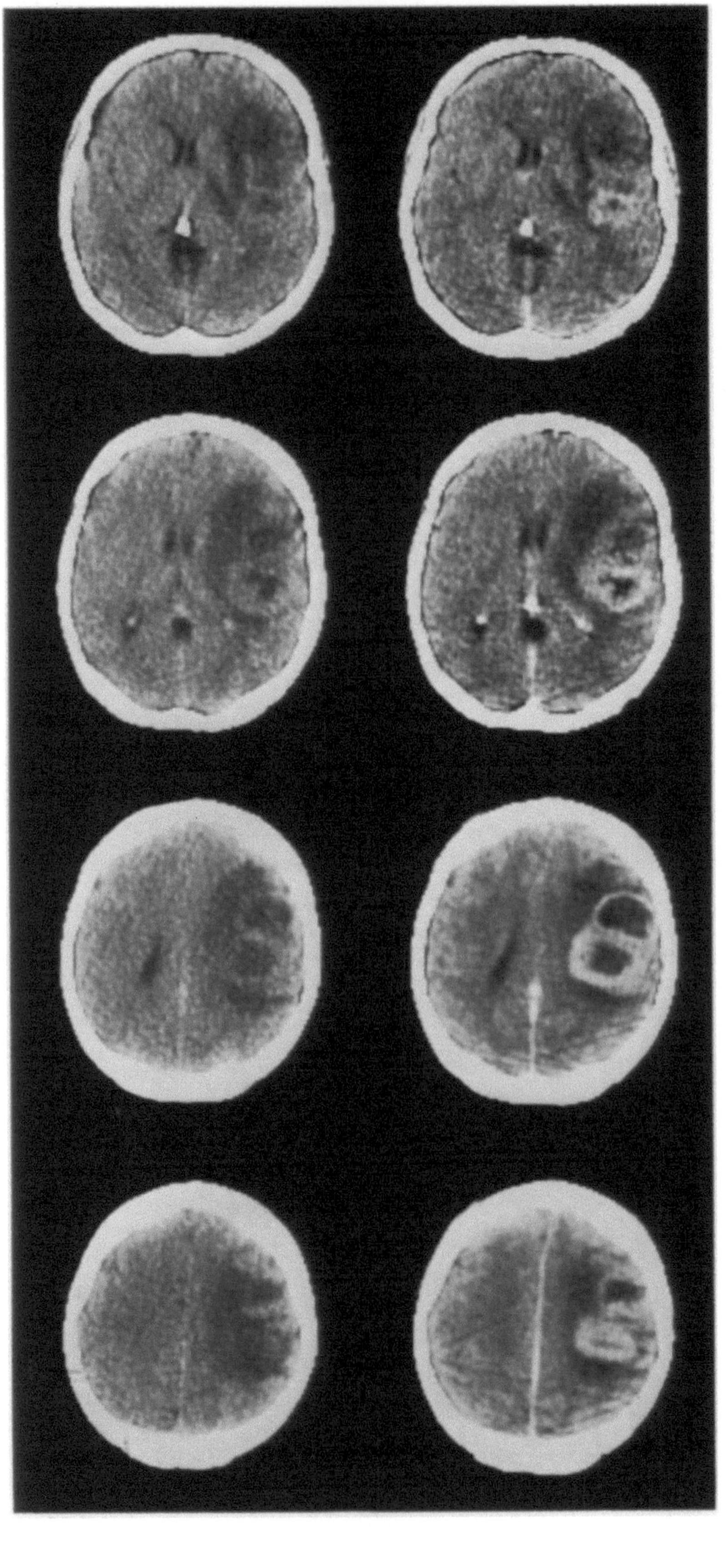

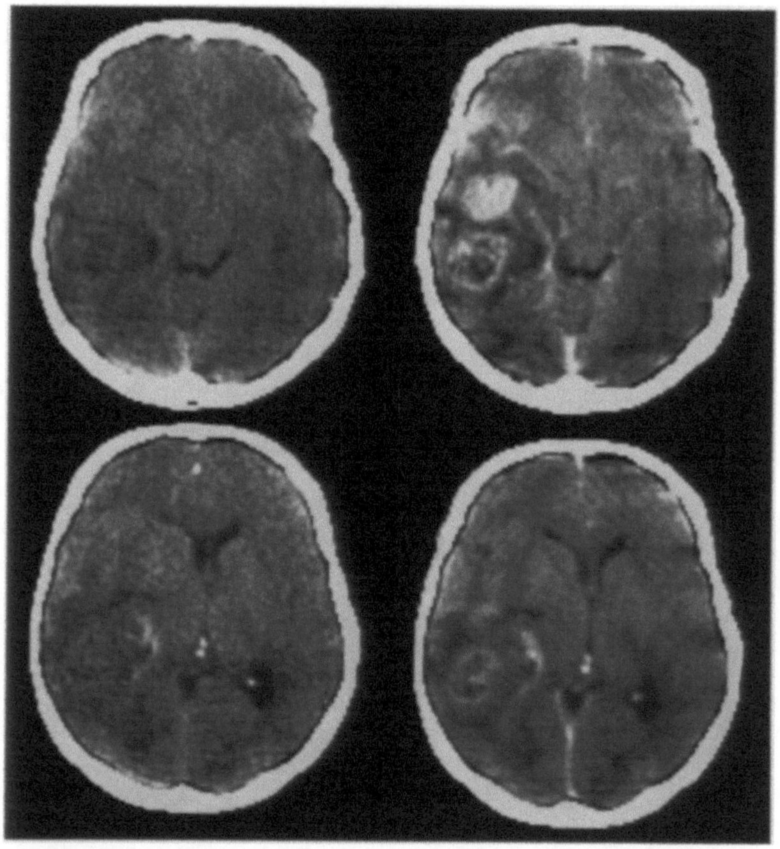

Fig. D 1.26. Anaplastic astrocytoma in the left central and posterior temporal region consisting of two separate tumor nodules with different CT features. There is minimal perifocal edema (36-year-old male). *Left* precontrast scans, *right* postcontrast scans

Fig. D 1.25. Anaplastic astrocytoma with transition to glioblastoma in a 60-year-old man. The plain CT scans (*left*) demonstrate a mass composed of several rings in the right temporoparietal region. The lesion shows dense enhancement on the postcontrast scans (*right*) with improved resolution of tumor from perifocal edema

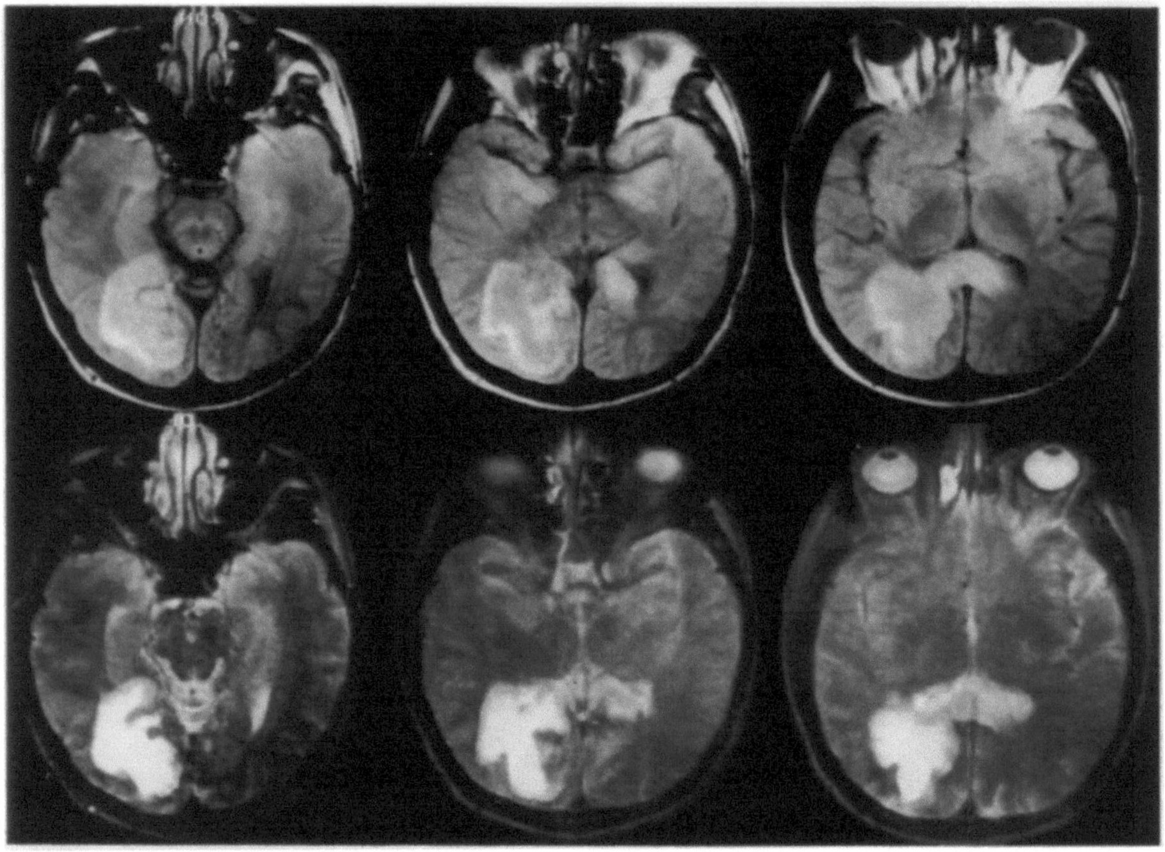

Fig. D 1.27. Anaplastic astrocytoma of the left occipitobasal region in a 44-year-old man with a 6-week history of headaches and seizures; right homonymous hemianopia. MR: *top* SE 2500/30, *bottom* SE 2500/120. The proton-density images (*top*) show the slightly hyperintense tumor extending through the posterior corpus callosum to the right side. This is even more conspicuous on the T2-weighted sequences

Fig. D 1.28 a–d. Giant grade III astrocytoma of the left frontotemporoparietal region in a 60-year-old woman with a 3-week history of right hemiparesis, aphasia, and altered mental status. MR: **a** SE 3000/30, **b** SE 3000/90, **c** SE 700/30 coronal, **d** SE 3000/90 coronal. The T1-weighted image (**c**) shows an area of mixed signal intensity in the basolateral portion of the mass. Above this is a smooth-bordered area of signal void. Separation of tumor from edema is easily accomplished on the T2-weighted scans (**b, d**). Comparing **c** and **d**, we note a signal reversal with the former signal void appearing bright; this establishes the lesion as a cyst

Fig. D 1.29 a–d. Anaplastic astrocytoma in the high right frontal region of a 52-year-old man with a 1-year history of generalized seizures. Neurologic exam was negative. MR: **a** IR 1500/400/35, **b** SE 400/35, **c** SE 1600/35, **d** SE 1600/70. The tumor is hypointense on the T1-weighted image (**a**) and gives a brighter signal with increased T2 weighting

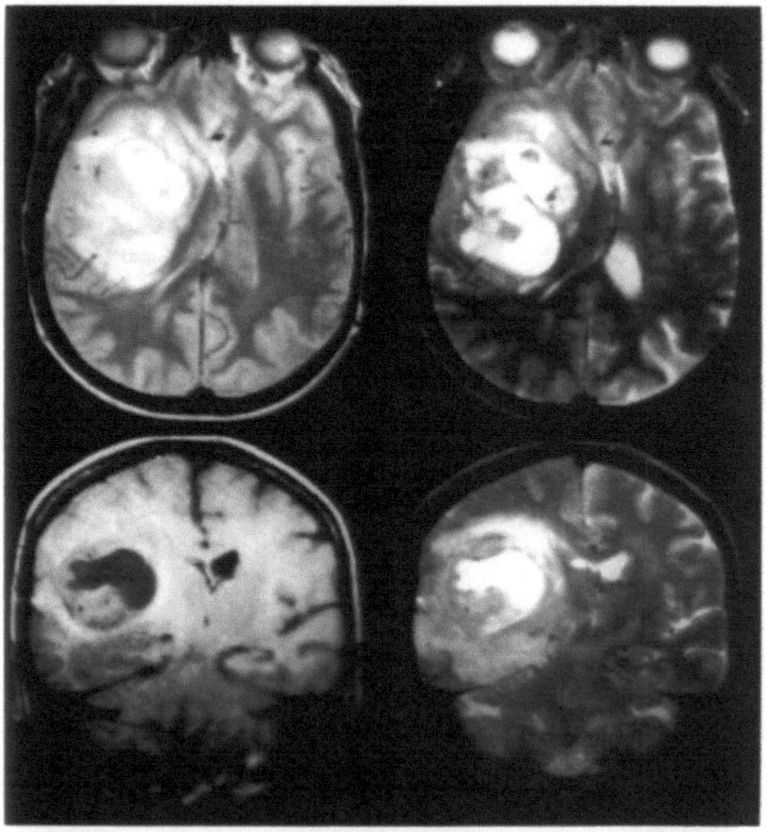

a b c d D 1.28

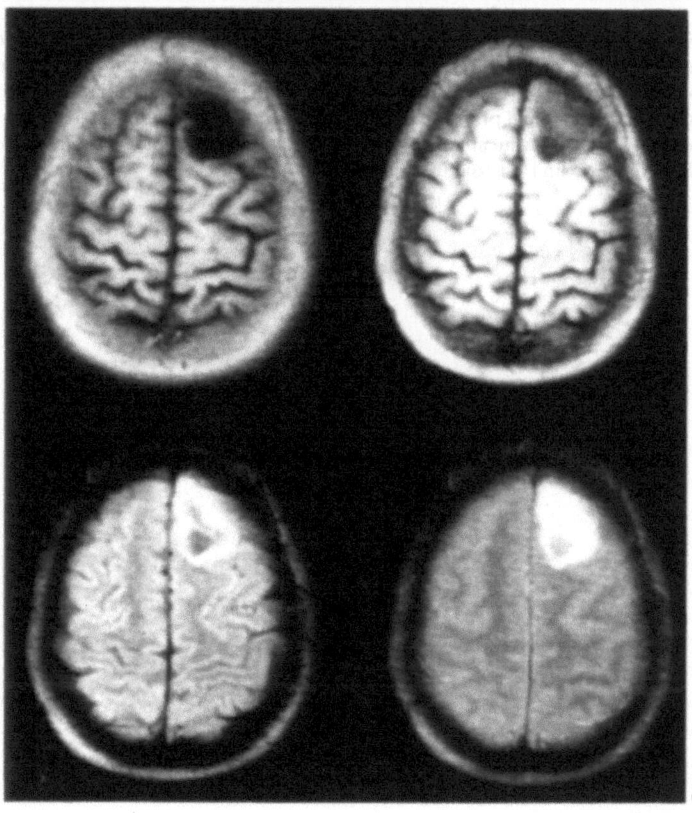

a b c d D 1.29

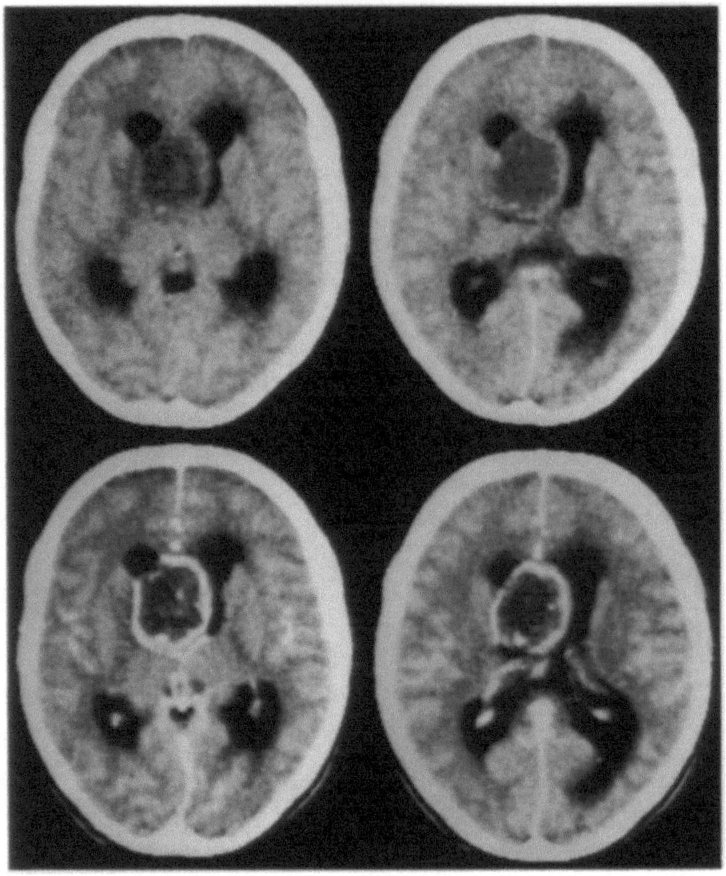

Fig. D 1.30. Anaplastic astrocytoma of the third ventricle with obstructive hydrocephalus, arising from the corpus callosum. The 24-year-old woman presented with a 1-year history of mental changes, emotional lability, and increased intracranial pressure. CT: *top* precontrast scans, *bottom* postcontrast scans. Ring enhancement is seen around the hypodense tumor located in the third ventricle and obstructing the foramen of Monro

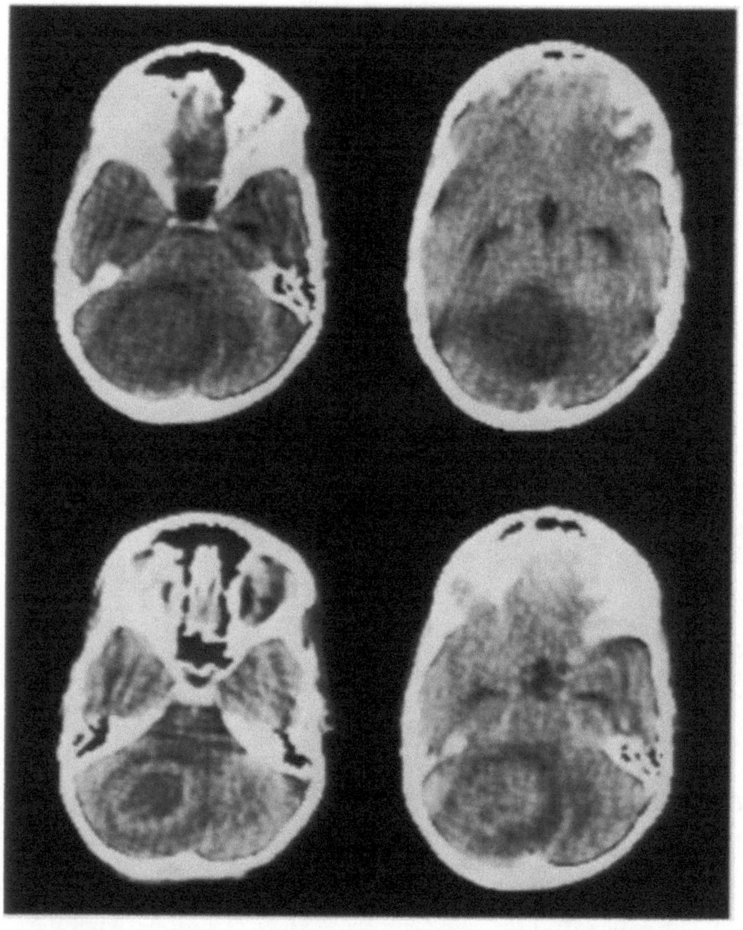

Fig. D 1.31. Cerebral-type anaplastic astrocytoma occurring in the left hemisphere of the cerebellum. The tumor appears iso- to hypodense on the plain CT scans (*top*) and shows ring enhancement on the postcontrast scans (*bottom*) (11-year-old boy with cerebellar symptoms). This lesion may be confused with pilocytic astrocytoma, which has an identical CT appearance

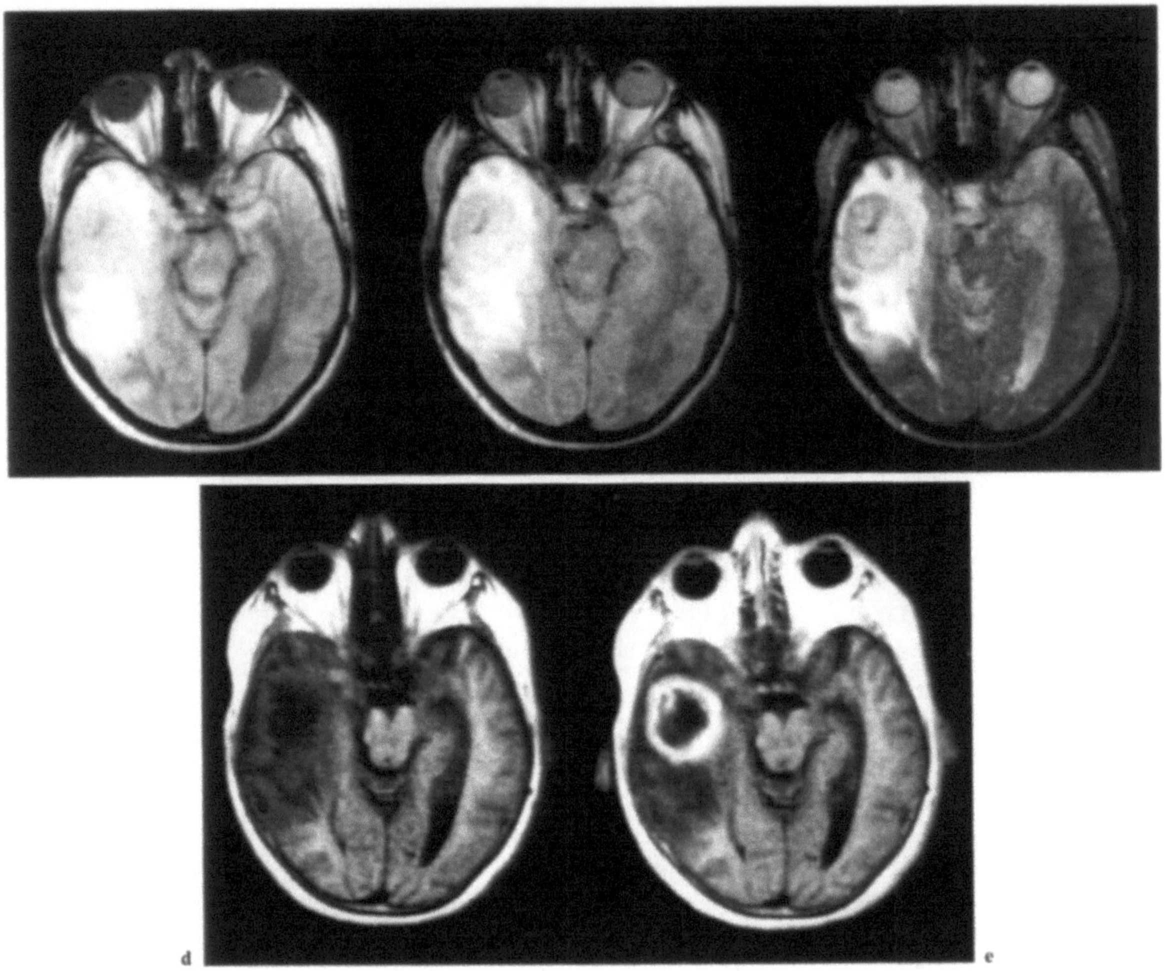

a–c

d

e

Fig. D 1.32 a–e. Astroblastoma of the left temporal region in a 54-year-old woman with a 9-year history of headaches and latent right-sided hemiparesis. MR: **a** SE 1600/35, **b** SE 1600/60, **c** SE 1600/120, **d** IR 1500/400/35, **e** IR 1500/400/35 post Gd-DTPA. Separation of the high-signal tumor from edema is not possible in the proton-density image (**a**), but heavier T2 weighting demonstrates the central, rounded tumor as an area of decreased signal (**b, c**). The post Gd-DTPA IR image shows ring enhancement with central necrosis

c) Oligodendrogliomas

Incidence	2%–10% of all brain tumors
Age predilection	30–55 years
Sex predilection	Slight preponderance in males
Typical sites	Frontal, frontoparietal, frontotemporal, temporal
Main clinical features	Seizures, often existing for some years
Skull X-ray	Faint intracranial calcifications in many cases
Angiography	Evidence of mass effect with all larger tumors, which usually appear hypovascular; higher-grade malignancies show diffuse staining in capillary phase
CT	
Noncontrast scan	Most tumors show irregular areas of extremely high density (calcification); otherwise findings similar to astrocytoma and anaplastic astrocytoma
Contrast enhancement	Only in anaplastic oligodendrogliomas (grade III)
Postcontrast appearance	Mixed-density pattern corresponding to heterogeneous structure of lesion; perifocal edema usually minimal
MR	
Noncontrast scan	Calcifications appear as signal voids if sufficiently large. Lesions bright and well defined on T2-weighted images, appearing larger than with CT. Separation of tumor from edema difficult
Gadolinium enhancement	Only in anaplastic oligodendrogliomas (grade III)
Post Gd-DTPA appearance	Further differentiation not possible with low-grade oligodendrogliomas

Differential diagnosis

If uncalcified, astrocytoma (and its differential diagnoses)
Pilocytic astrocytoma of cerebrum
Gangliocytoma
Calcified meningioma
Ependymoma
Calcified angioma
Sturge-Weber syndrome
Tuberculoma
Cysticercosis
Mixed glioma

Reports on the incidence of oligodendrogliomas in the literature vary greatly [Cushing (1932) 1.3%, Kernohan and Sayre (1952) 5%, Zülch (1986) 9.6%, our series 4.6%]. Most cases occur between the ages of 30 and 55 years, with males affected somewhat more frequently than females. Lesions range from well-circumscribed, calcified grade I tumors to grade III anaplastic growths.

Typical Sites

Oligodendrogliomas affect the cerebrum almost exclusively, occurring typically in the frontal, frontoparietal, frontotemporal, temporal, temporoparietal, and temporo-occipital regions, the thalamus, and the corpus callosum. Involvement of the optic chiasm is uncommon.

Main Clinical Features

The great majority of patients with oligodendroglioma have focal or generalized seizures as their only symptom. Paralytic signs appear only in later stages.

Additional Diagnostic Procedures

Plain skull radiographs in some patients show faint intracranial calcifications that present either a stippled or a garland-like pattern resembling cerebral gyri. Other adjunctive studies are not helpful in establishing a pathologic diagnosis.

Computed Tomography
(Figs. D 1.33–44, 47, D 6.5)

Noncontrast Scan
Calcification is a major feature of oligodendrogliomas and is demonstrable in some 70% of cases (Figs. D 1.33–39, 42, 47). The calcifications may be limited to a few small flecks but more commonly appear as larger, irregular areas of very high density which occasionally follow the course of a gyrus (see Fig. D 1.34). Not infrequently, these calcific foci are surrounded by hypodense tumor. However, surrounding tissue may also appear isodense so that the true extent of the tumor cannot be appreciated (see Fig. D 1.34). In several cases we found a much larger tumor at operation than had been suggested by the extent of visible calcifications on the CT scan.

A few oligodendrogliomas are homogeneously isodense on plain scans and consequently escape detection. Oligodendrogliomas seldom contain cysts that are demonstrable with CT (see Fig. D 1.42).

About one-fourth of the oligodendrogliomas in our series have the hypodense appearance of a fibrillary or protoplasmic astrocytoma on unenhanced CT scans (see Fig. D 1.40).

Calcifications are far less common in anaplastic oligodendrogliomas, which usually contain a mixture of iso- and hypodense areas on CT scans (see Fig. D 1.41). Entirely isodense and slightly hyperdense anaplastic oligodendrogliomas may also be seen (Fig. D 1.43). The edema associated with anaplastic oligodendrogliomas is discussed below.

Intratumoral hemorrhage is a very rare occurrence in anaplastic oligodendrogliomas (see Fig. D 1.44).

Postcontrast Scan
Low-grade oligodendrogliomas do not enhance, whereas anaplastic and pleomorphic oligodendrogliomas (grade III) show marked enhancement in their solid, uncalcified portions (see Figs. D 1.37, 41–43). The enhancement is usually homogeneous, although ring patterns may be seen, and the enhanced area may be surrounded by a perifocal edema that occasionally involves the entire hemisphere. Perifocal edema is observed in 70%–80% of anaplastic oligodendrogliomas. With low-grade oligodendrogliomas, CT usually fails to resolve the margin between the perifocal edema and the hypodense tumor.

Magnetic Resonance Imaging
(Figs. D 1.38, 39, 45, 46, 48)

Noncontrast Scan
The tumors appear hypointense or possibly isointense on T1-weighted images. Calcifications, when large, appear as areas of very low signal intensity. Oligodendrogliomas give a high signal on T2-weighted images, with larger calcifications appearing as hypointense areas within the tumor. Perifocal edema is rarely visualized.

Post-Gadolinium Scan

Grade II neoplasms do not show significant enhancement. Only the malignant forms enhance, giving a pattern similar to that produced by anaplastic astrocytomas on CT and MR.

MR is far more sensitive than CT in the detection of oligodendrogliomas, but CT is more specific owing to its ability to demonstrate even very small foci of calcification. Multifocal growths are better appreciated with MR. CT and MR provide complementary information in the diagnosis of oligodendroglioma.

Differential Diagnosis

When a *pathologic supratentorial calcification* is noted on the CT scan, the following lesions should be considered in addition to oligodendroglioma:

1. Pilocytic Astrocytoma of the Cerebrum. This tumor usually occurs in the temporal region and is often associated with cyst formation. It may also occur in the parietal and occipital regions and may show homogeneous calcification (see Figs. D1.119, 120).

2. Gangliocytoma. This is a very rare tumor usually affecting the temporobasal region, although frontal and parietal sites are known. Calcification and cyst formation are common.

3. Meningioma. Occasionally these tumors develop calcifications resembling those of oligodendroglioma. Differentiation can usually be accomplished with contrast enhancement.

4. Ependymoma. These tumors typically occur at the junction of the parietal, temporal, and occipital lobes. Calcifications and large cysts are usually present. Ependymomas are predominantly tumors of childhood and adolescence.

5. Arteriovenous angioma. Angiomas may resemble oligodendrogliomas on the plain CT scan, but larger angiomas can almost always be identified after contrast enhancement. MR demonstrates the angiomatous vessels as areas of signal void. Final proof of diagnosis is established by cerebral angiography.

6. Sturge-Weber Syndrome (*angioma capillare et venosum calcificans*). Generally this diagnosis is suggested by a facial naevus in the distribution of the second and third trigeminal nerve divisions and by the very extensive garland-like calcifications seen in the temporo-parieto-occipital region on CT scans. Diagnosis may be difficult if the facial naevus is absent or if intracranial calcifications are limited in their extent (see Fig. F93).

7. Tuberculoma. Circumscribed, solitary calcifications may be seen in tuberculoma. Today these lesions are very rare in Central Europe.

8. Cysticercosis. The multifocal calcifications of this parasitism are easily recognized. Again, this disease is very rare at our latitudes.

9. Other Calcifications. Old intracerebral hematomas may calcify in rare cases. Conservatively treated brain abscesses also may undergo calcification. MR generally contributes little to the differential diagnosis of calcifying intracranial lesions.

The differential diagnosis of hypodense oligodendrogliomas is discussed in the section on grade II astrocytomas (see p. 51).

d) Mixed Gliomas

In addition to astrocytomas and oligodendrogliomas, there are mixed tumors that contain elements of both tumor types and are referred to as "mixed gliomas" or "oligoastrocytomas."

Iglesias (1987), in a retrospective study of 447 astrocytomas and oligodendrogliomas, was able to show that 22% of the tumors classified as astrocytomas were in fact mixed gliomas. This figure approaches 55% in the case of oligodendrogliomas. Rubinstein suggested in 1972 that approximately half of tumors diagnosed as oligodendrogliomas were actually oligoastrocytomas.

A tumor may be classified as a mixed glioma only if it consists of equal parts of astrocytic and oligodendroglial elements. Based on the results of recent studies, it is reasonable to conclude that approximately one-third of all astrocytomas and oligodendrogliomas are in reality mixed gliomas.

The mixed gliomas in our population showed a peak incidence between the ages of 30 and 50 years and predominated in males by a 2:1 ratio. The major clinical manifestation was cerebral seizures, which occurred in 80% of cases. Half the patients displayed mental changes or headache, and one-third suffered neurologic deficits which varied with the location of the tumor. On average the diagnosis was made 3 years after onset of the initial symptoms. Fifty percent of patients with mixed glioma died within 8 years.

Computed Tomography

In Table 2 the mixed gliomas are grouped with the oligodendrogliomas because they have a variable CT presentation (solid isodense or hypodense areas, calcifications, occasional cysts) much like that of oligodendroglioma. Illustrative CT scans are shown in Figs. D 1.49–52.

Occasional mixed gliomas are anaplastic and therefore enhance on administration of contrast (Figs. C 5, D 1.49, 51, 52).

Magnetic Resonance Imaging

As in CT, the MR features of mixed gliomas are largely identical to those of oligodendrogliomas. Calcifications must be fairly large to produce a signal void on MR, so CT scans should always be obtained. MR is superior to CT, however, in its ability to detect these tumors and define their true extent. Illustrative MR scans are shown in Figs. D 1.49, 52, and 53.

e) Diffuse Gliomatosis

Diffuse gliomatosis of the brain is a very rare condition marked by the unbounded growth of astrocytic or oligodendrocytic tumor cells in one or both cerebral hemispheres. Brainstem involvement is also possible. The condition may be described as "cerebral astrocytomatosis" or "cerebral oligodendrogliomatosis" depending on the predominant cell type. Foci of anaplasia resembling glioblastoma may occur.

Artigas et al. (1985) reviewed 10 of their own cases and 48 cases from the literature in a comprehensive clinical neuropathologic study. They found that cerebral gliomatosis develops chiefly in middle age. The history of cerebral seizures, altered mentation, and diffuse headaches closely resembles the presentation of low-grade gliomas. Clinical diagnosis is extremely difficult.

When diffuse gliomatosis is unilateral, **CT** shows a general expansion of the affected cerebral hemisphere. In two such cases we observed no density alteration in the brain tissue, and contrast enhancement was negative (see Figs. D 1.54, 55). The CT findings most closely resemble an isodense chronic subdural hematoma, although the latter can usually be identified with CT after the administration of a high contrast dose. Another patient had gliomatosis involving both cerebral hemispheres. There were calcifications within the diseased area and foci of anaplasia that enhanced with contrast medium (see Fig. D 1.54).

It appears that **MR** can greatly facilitate the clinical diagnosis of diffuse gliomatosis. The lesions are visualized in high contrast on T2-weighted images and are more easily detected than the possible hypodensity on CT.

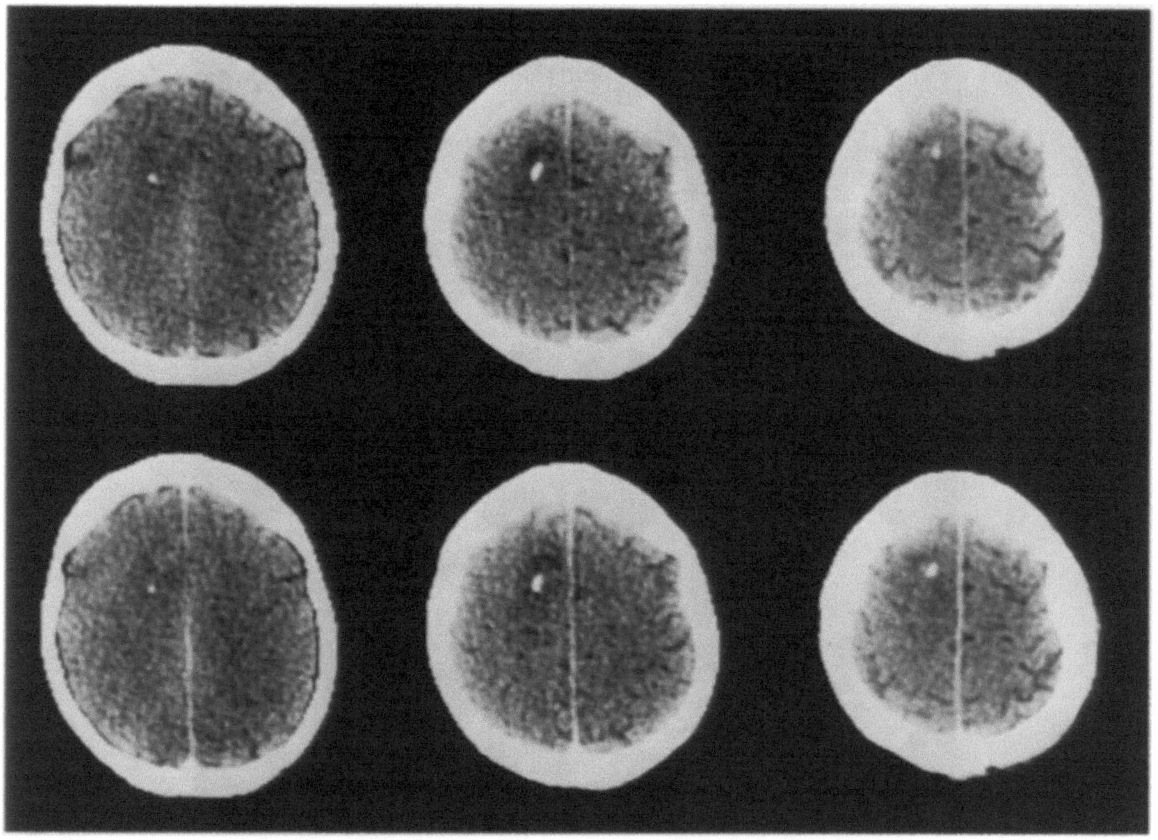

Fig. D 1.33. Oligodendroglioma situated near the left cortical margin in a 30-year-old man with cerebral seizures. The tumor is mildly hypodense and is not clearly demarcated from surrounding brain. Stippled calcifications are seen at the center of the tumor, which does not enhance on the postcontrast scans (*bottom*)

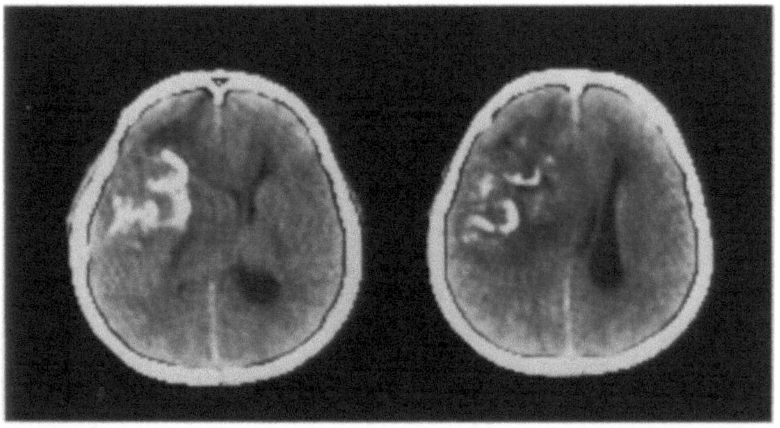

Fig. D 1.34. Oligodendroglioma in the left frontotemporal region of a 51-year-old woman. Garland-like calcifications are seen within an area of iso- and hypodense attenuation values. Mass effect is significant. The tumor does not enhance. These features are typical for oligodendroglioma

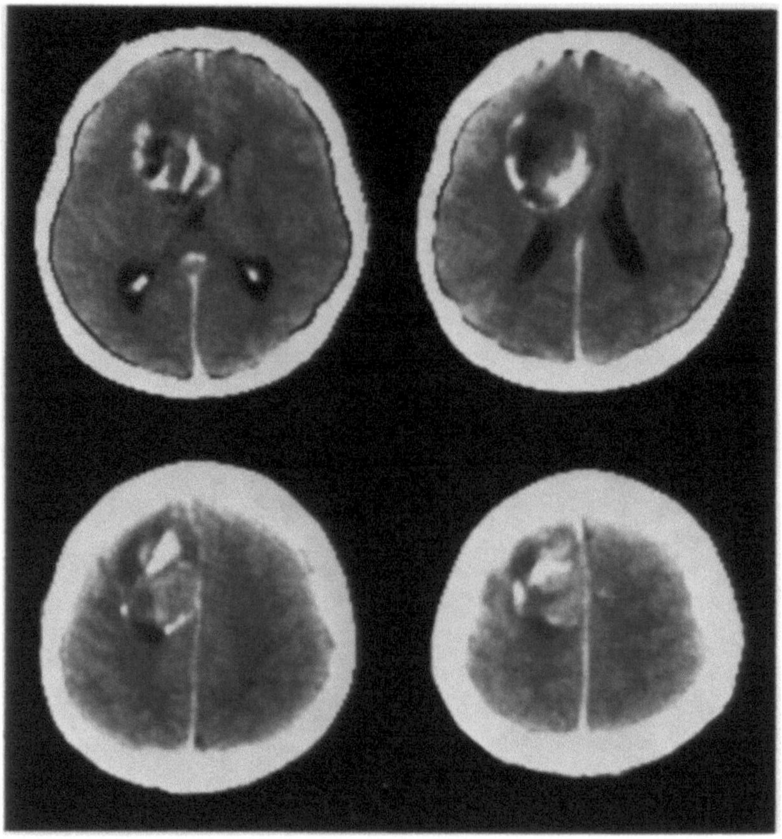

Fig. D 1.35. Oligodendroglioma with anaplastic components in the left fronto-precentral region of a 25-year-old woman. We see a typical CT pattern with shell-like calcifications and areas of iso- and hypodensity. The tumor has reached the corpus callosum in the area of the septum pellucidum. There is no significant contrast enhancement (all scans are postcontrast)

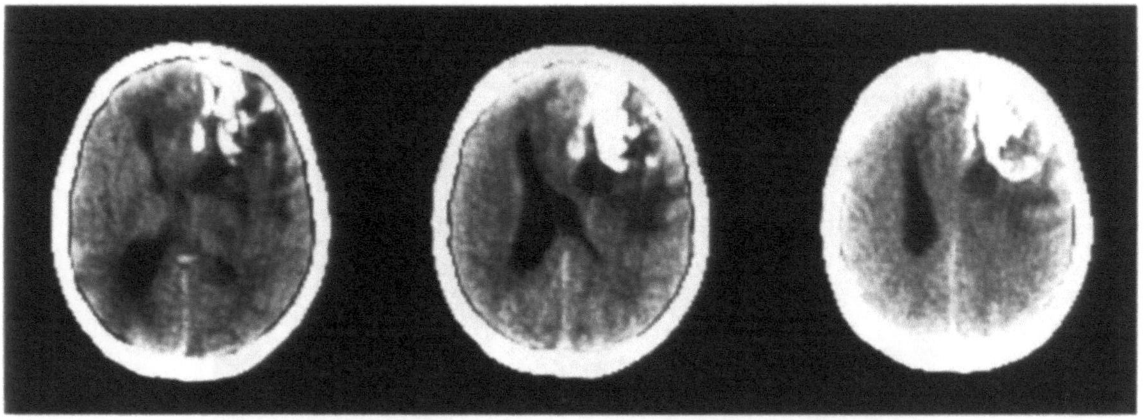

Fig. D 1.36. Large anaplastic oligodendroglioma in the right frontoprecentral region. The mass is markedly heterogeneous with garland-like and shell-like calcifications, cysts, and isodense components. It has reached the anterior part of the corpus callosum and the septum pellucidum. Perifocal edema is marked. The frontomedial portions of the tumor show mild contrast enhancement (*center* scan)

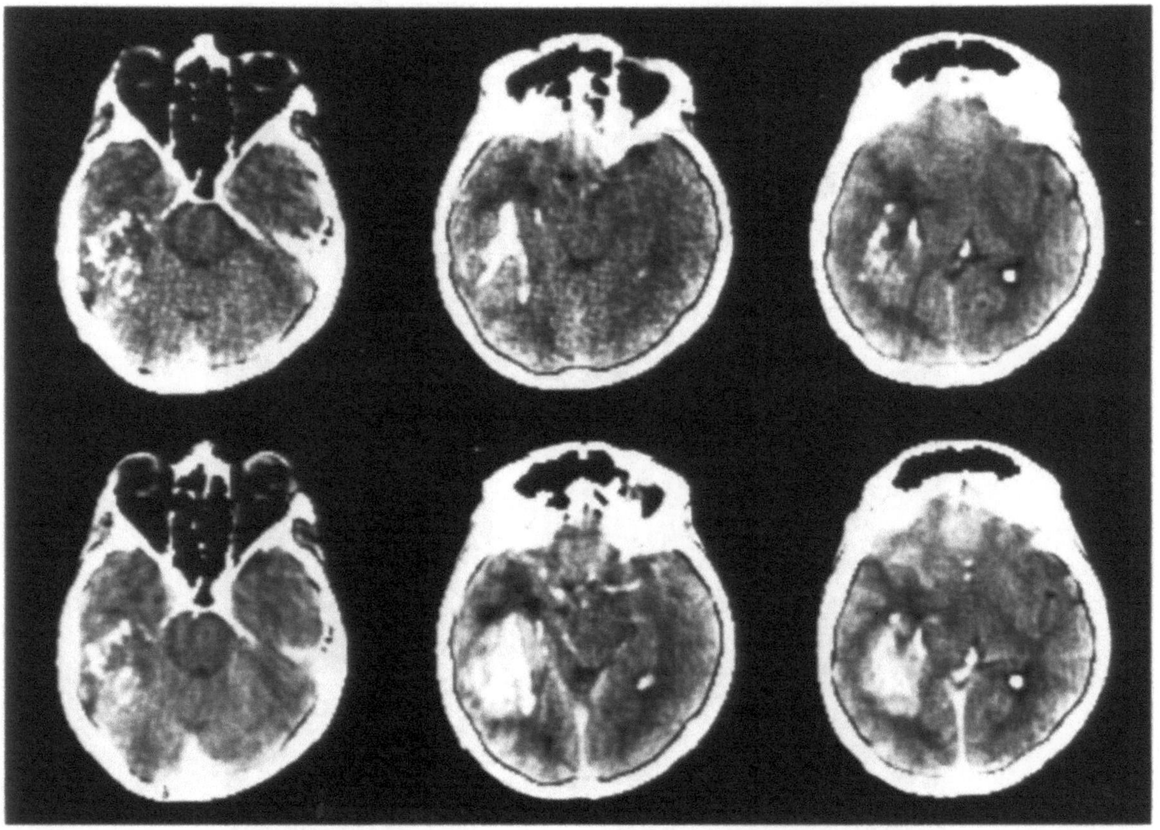

Fig. D 1.37. Anaplastic oligodendroglioma at the junction of the parietal, temporal, and occipital lobes. CT shows typical garland-like and streak-like calcifications within an iso- to hypodense area on noncontrast scans (*top* row). The postcontrast scans (*bottom* row) show marked enhancement of the solid, uncalcified tumor components, and the true extent of the neoplasm is appreciated. There is improved delineation of perifocal edema

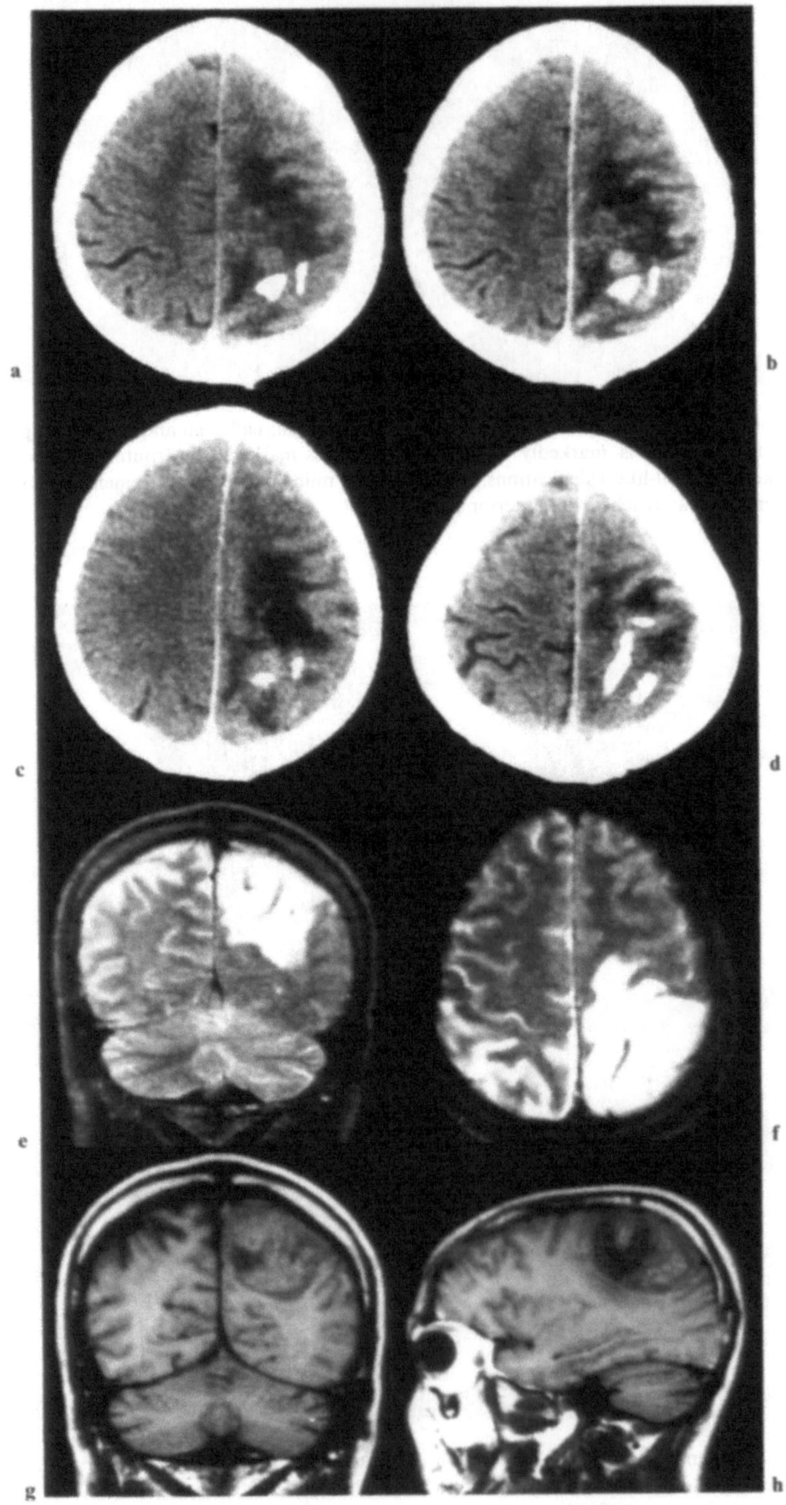

Fig. D 1.38 a–h. Grade III oligodendroglioma of the right parietal area in a 38-year-old man with jacksonian seizures. CT: **a–d** postcontrast. MR: **e** SE 2500/120 coronal, **f** SE 2500/120 axial, **g** SE 500/30 coronal, **h** SE 500/30 parasagittal. CT scans show typical, conspicuous calcifications with no definite enhancement. The tumor is well delineated on the T1-weighted images (**g, h**) but cannot be differentiated on the T2-weighted images, which show the tumor edema as a hyperintense area (**e, f**). Calcium deposits are faintly visible as signal voids

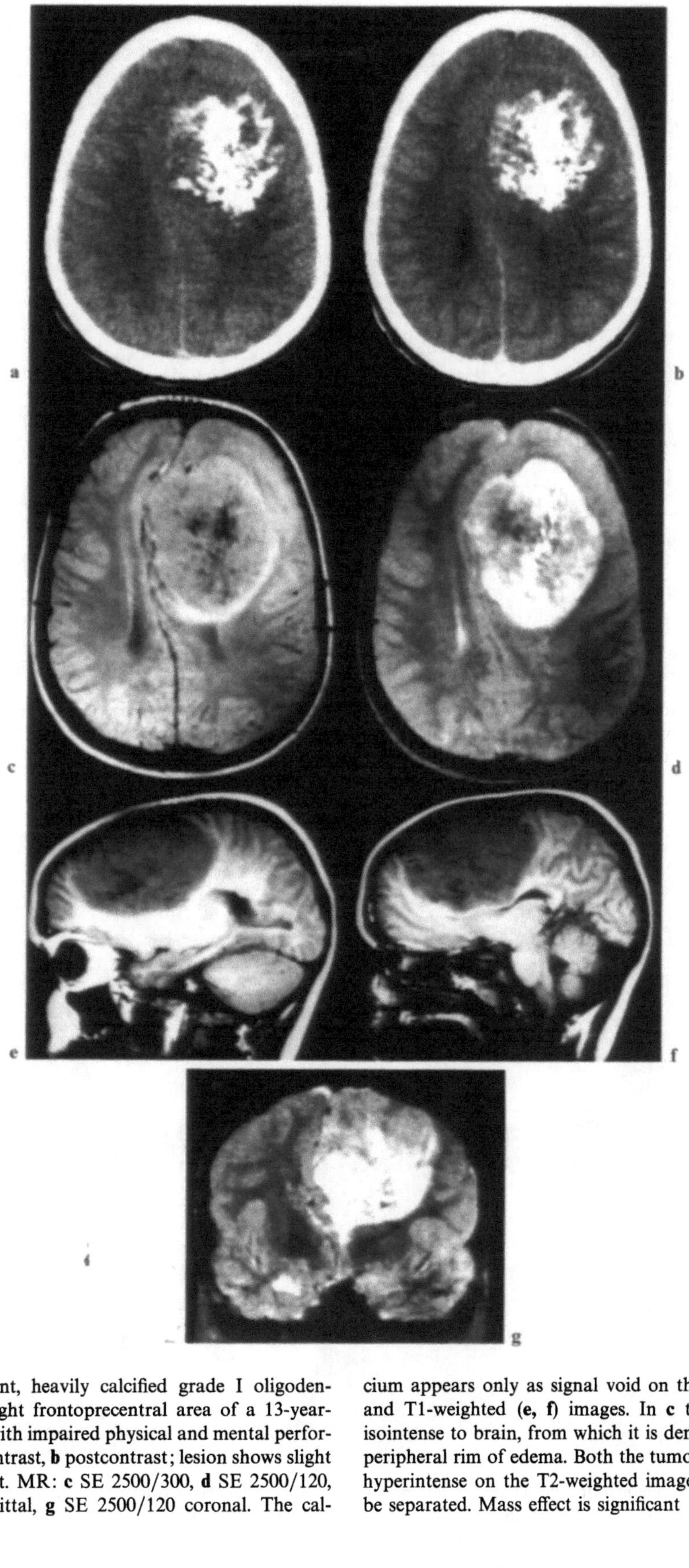

Fig. D 1.39 a–g. Giant, heavily calcified grade I oligodendroglioma in the right frontoprecentral area of a 13-year-old girl presenting with impaired physical and mental performance. CT: **a** precontrast, **b** postcontrast; lesion shows slight medial enhancement. MR: **c** SE 2500/300, **d** SE 2500/120, **e, f** SE 500/30 sagittal, **g** SE 2500/120 coronal. The calcium appears only as signal void on the proton-density (**c**) and T1-weighted (**e, f**) images. In **c** the tumor is almost isointense to brain, from which it is demarcated by a bright peripheral rim of edema. Both the tumor and edema appear hyperintense on the T2-weighted images (**d, g**) and cannot be separated. Mass effect is significant

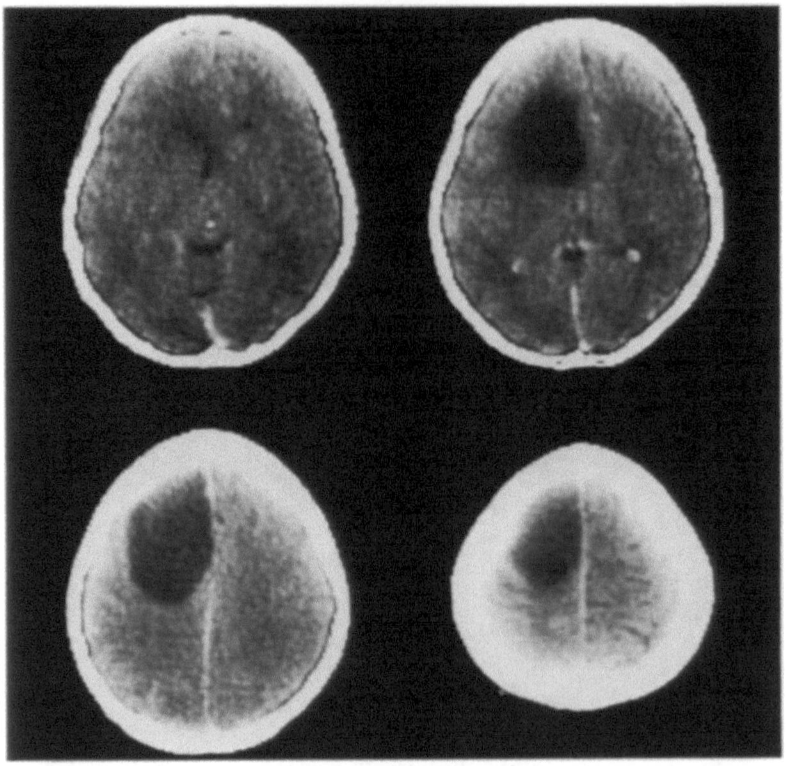

Fig. D 1.40. Oligodendroglioma of the left frontoprecentral region in a 31-year-old woman. The absence of calcifications and the homogeneous tumor density do not permit differentiation from astrocytoma. The tumor shows no significant enhancement on these postcontrast CT scans

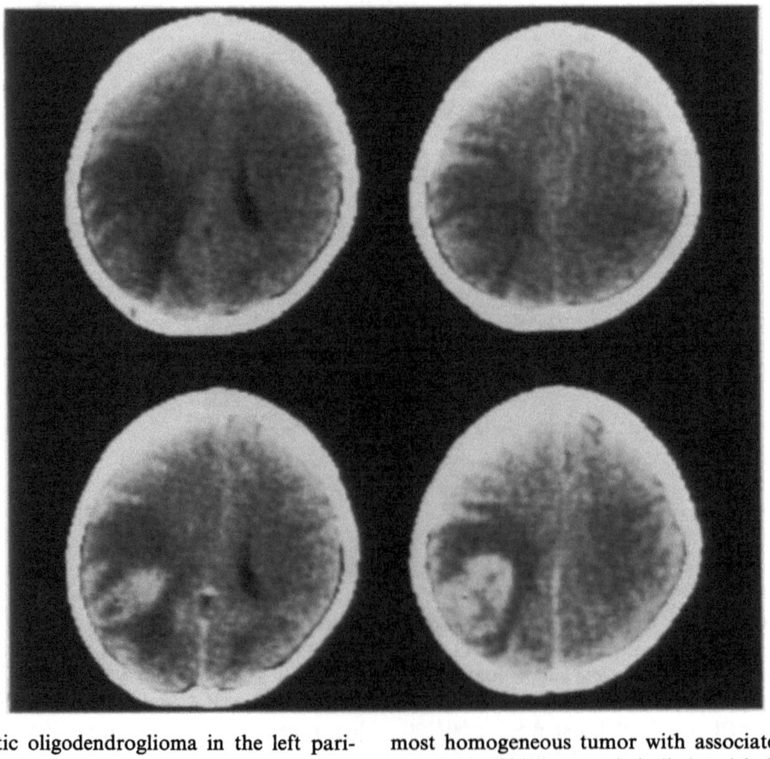

Fig. D 1.41. Anaplastic oligodendroglioma in the left parietal region of a 42-year-old man. The plain scans (*top* row) show a large hypodense area with isodense inclusions. The postcontrast scans (*bottom* row) demonstrate a large, almost homogeneous tumor with associated grade II perifocal edema. This pattern is indistinguishable from anaplastic astrocytoma, glioblastoma, or metastasis

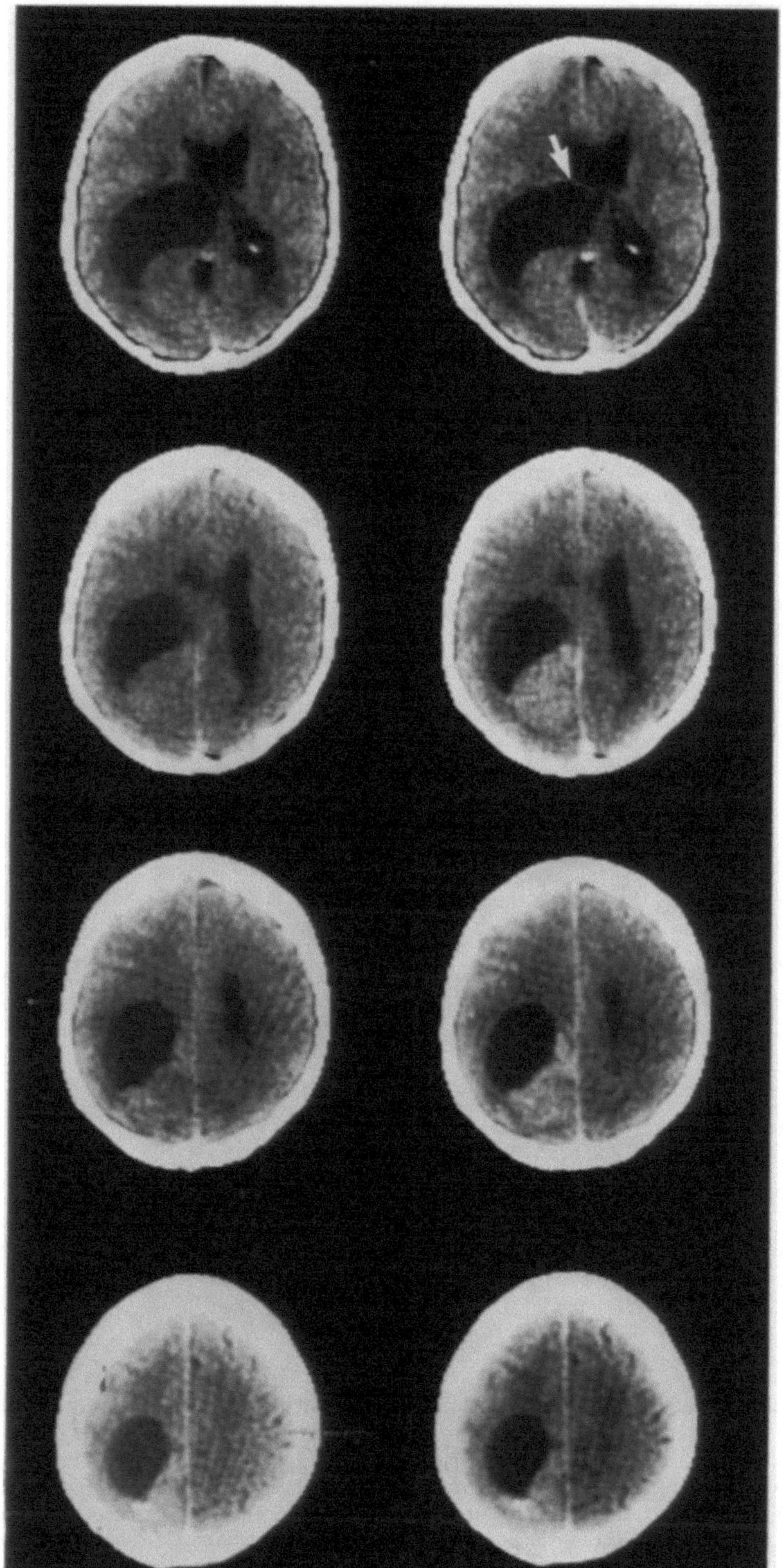

Fig. D 1.42. Very large anaplastic oligodendroglioma in the central and posterior portions of the left cerebral hemisphere in a 36-year-old man. Isodense, hypodense, and hyperdense components (representing solid tumor, cyst, and calcification respectively). The solid tumor components enhance strongly, and the slight enhancement at the rim of the cyst clearly demarcates it from the left lateral ventricle (*arrow*). Plain scans are on the *left*, postcontrast scans on the *right*

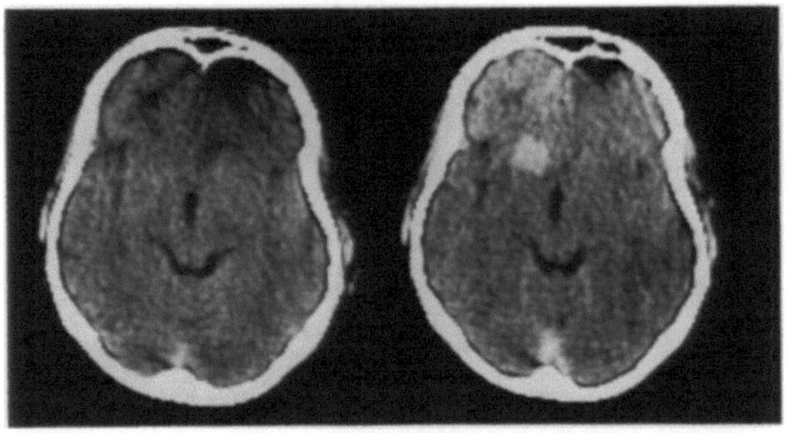

Fig. D 1.43. Primarily isodense, anaplastic oligodendroglioma in the region of the left basal ganglia in a 32-year-old man. The plain CT scan (*left*) shows no direct evidence of tumor mass effect or perifocal edema. The postcontrast scan shows a homogeneously enhancing tumor lying below the head of the caudate nucleus

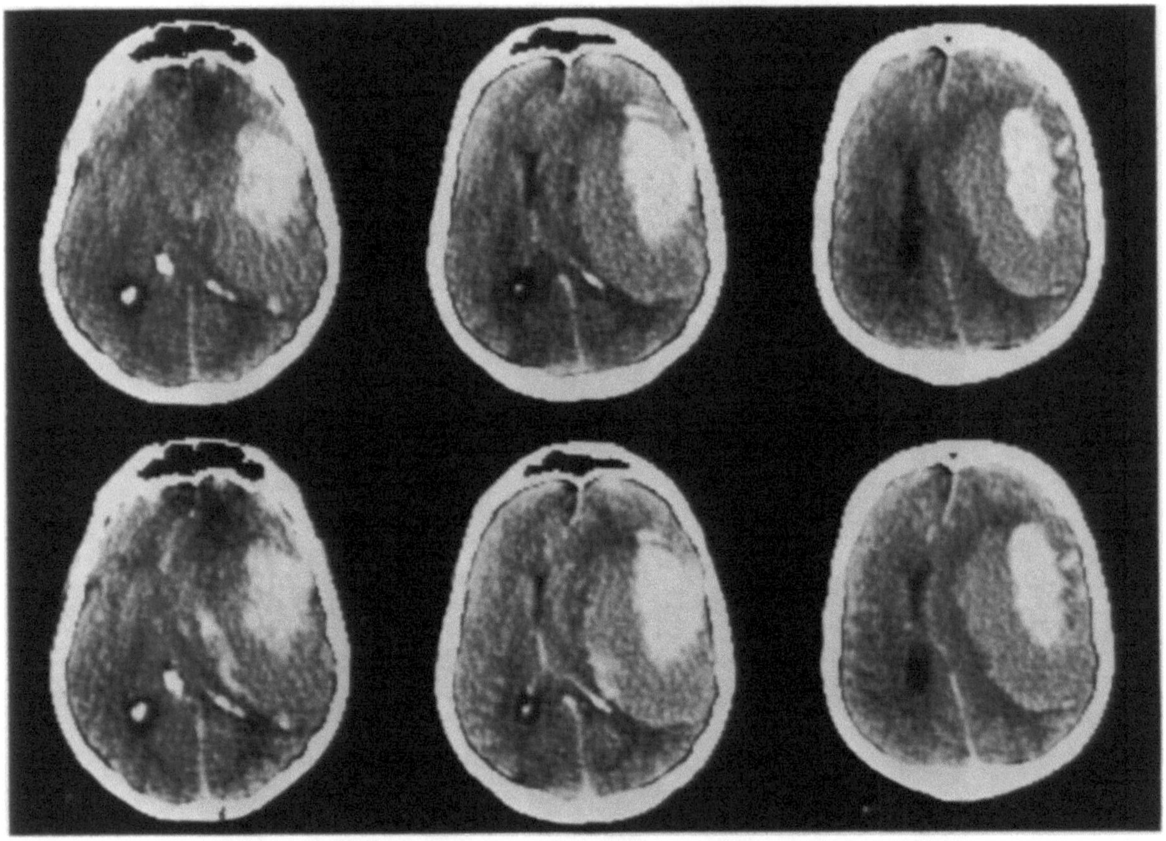

Fig. D 1.44. Large anaplastic oligodendroglioma in the midportion of the right cerebral hemisphere with extensive fresh hemorrhage in a 60-year-old man with disease of abrupt onset. On the plain scans (*top* row) the hemorrhagic component is clearly outlined within the hyperdense portion of the tumor. Postcontrast scans (*bottom* row) show peripheral enhancement in the medial parts of the tumor near the wall of the lateral ventricle, consistent with the diagnosis of tumoral hemorrhage. There is mass effect with marked displacement of midline structures. CT diagnosis of fresh hemorrhage is based on the very high density values (+80 to +84 HU)

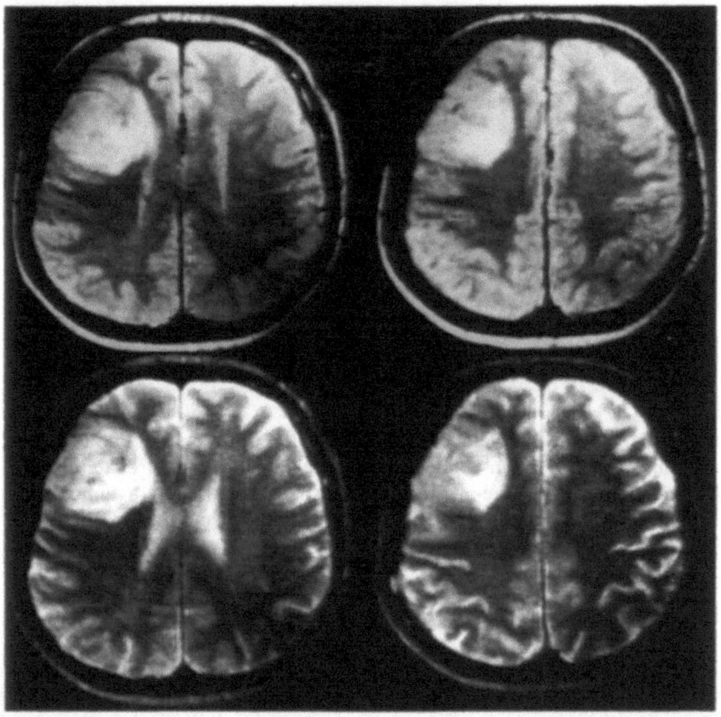

Fig. D 1.45. Grade II/III oligodendroglioma involving the left frontoprecentral region and basal ganglia. The 56-year-old man presented with a 4-month history of right-sided hemiparesis and seizures. MR: *top* SE 3000/30, *bottom* 3000/90. As T2 weighting is increased, the tumor gives a more intense signal and is clearly delineated

a b

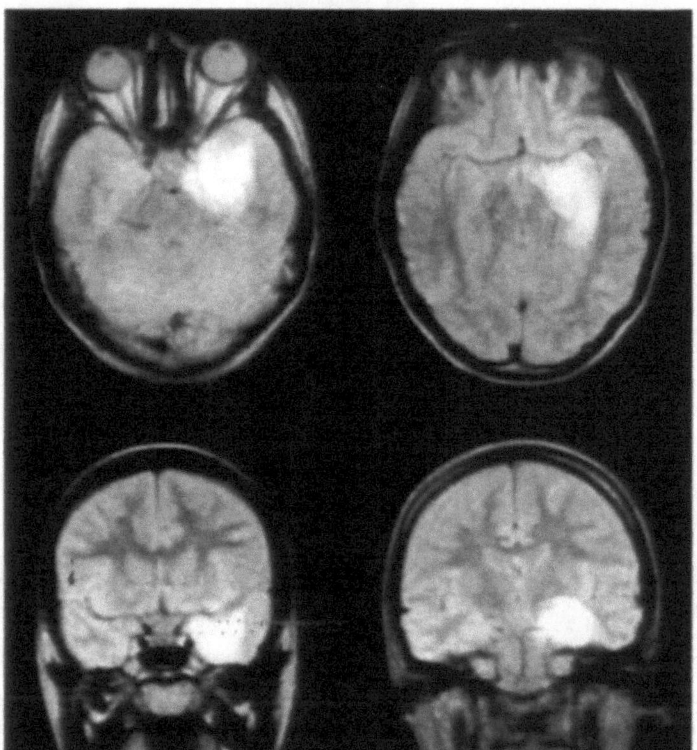

c d

Fig. D 1.46 a–d. Oligodendroglioma of the right medial temporobasal region in a 19-year-old female with temporal lobe seizures of increasing frequency and intensity. MR: **a, b** SE 1600/70, **c, d** SE 1600/70 coronal. Scans demonstrate a uniformly hyperintense mass

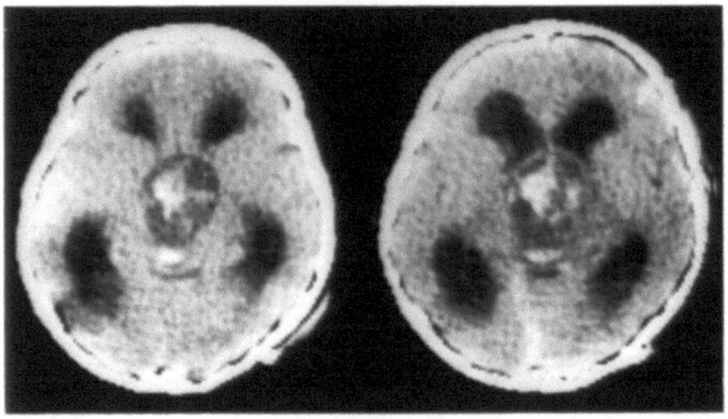

Fig. D 1.47. Grade III oligodendroglioma of the third ventricle in a 5-year-old child with symptoms of increased intracranial pressure, bilateral papilledema, and ataxia. Pre- and postcontrast CT scans show a tumor with irregular calcium deposits and faint peripheral rim enhancement. Obstructive hydrocephalus is present

a b c d

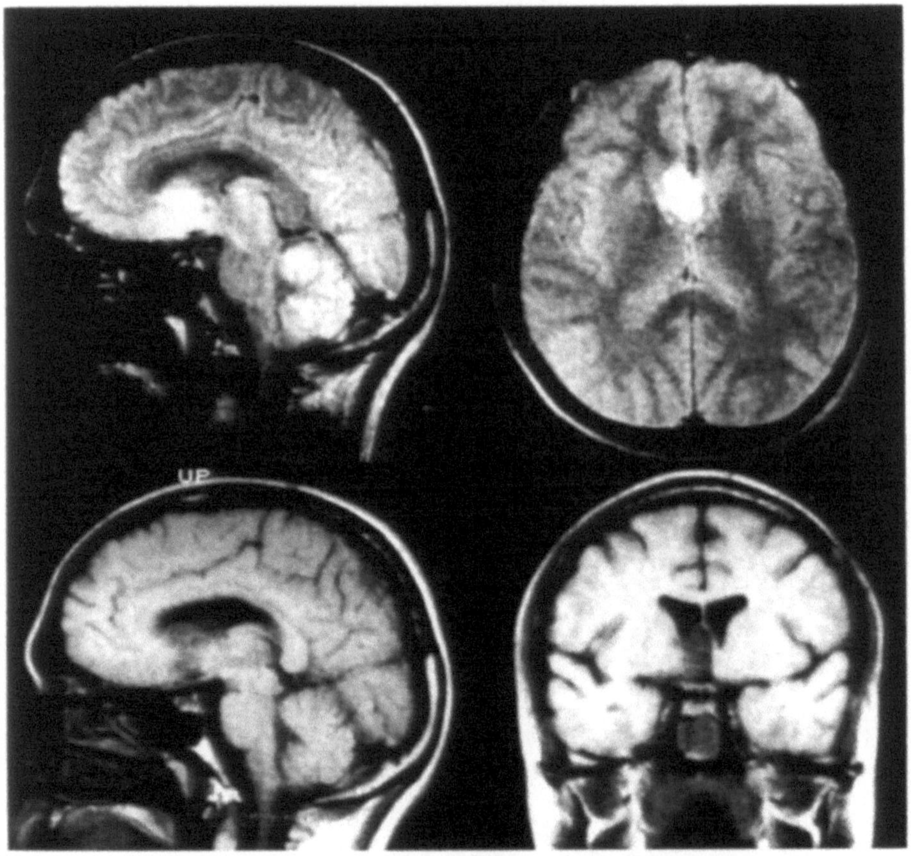

Fig. D 1.48 a–d. Oligodendroglioma in the area of the septum pellucidum and hypothalamus in a 38-year-old man with a 1-year history of generalized seizures and subjective diplopia. Neurologic exam was negative. MR: **a** SE 1600/35, **b** SE 1600/70, **c, d** SE 400/35 sagittal, coronal. The proton-density (**a**) and T2-weighted (**b**) images show a well-defined mass lesion that is hyperintense to brain parenchyma. The T1-weighted images (**c, d**) show a hypointense lesion extending from the septum pellucidum to the hypothalamus

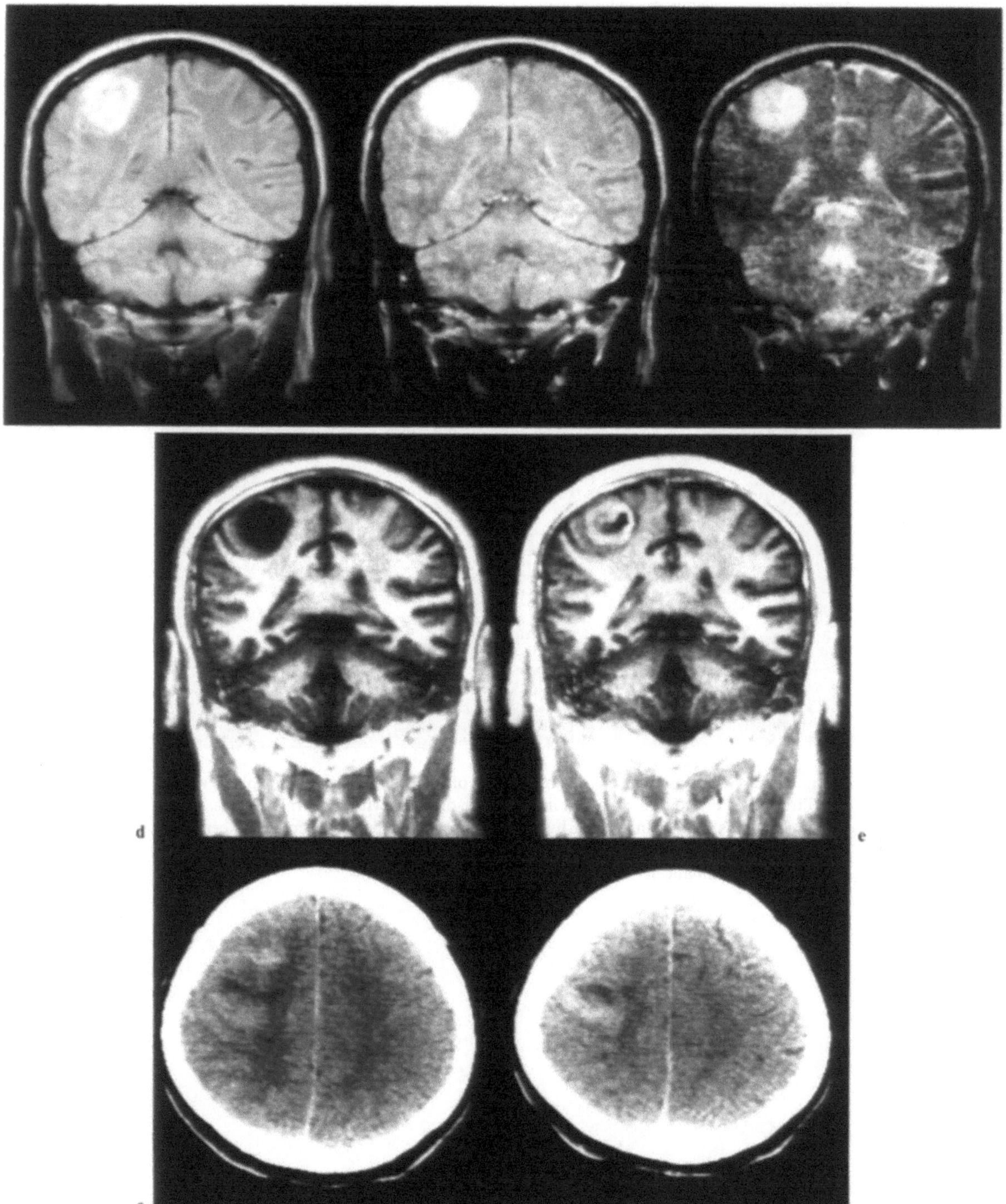

a–c

d

e

f

g

Fig. D 1.49 a–g. Malignant grade III–IV oligoastrocytoma of the left precentral region in a 64-year-old man with a 3-month history of right-sided hemiparesis especially affecting the brachiofacial and distal portions of the body. MR: **a** SE 1600/30, **b** SE 1600/90, **c** SE 1600/180, all coronal; **d, e** IR 1500/400/35 before and after Gd-DTPA enhancement. CT: **f, g** pre- and postcontrast scans. The rounded tumor is displayed to increasing advantage from the proton-density to the T2-weighted sequence **(a–c)**. It appears as a signal void on the noncontrast IR image and shows ring enhancement with Gd-DTPA. The CT scans **(f, g)** demonstrate an ill-defined mass with peripheral enhancement

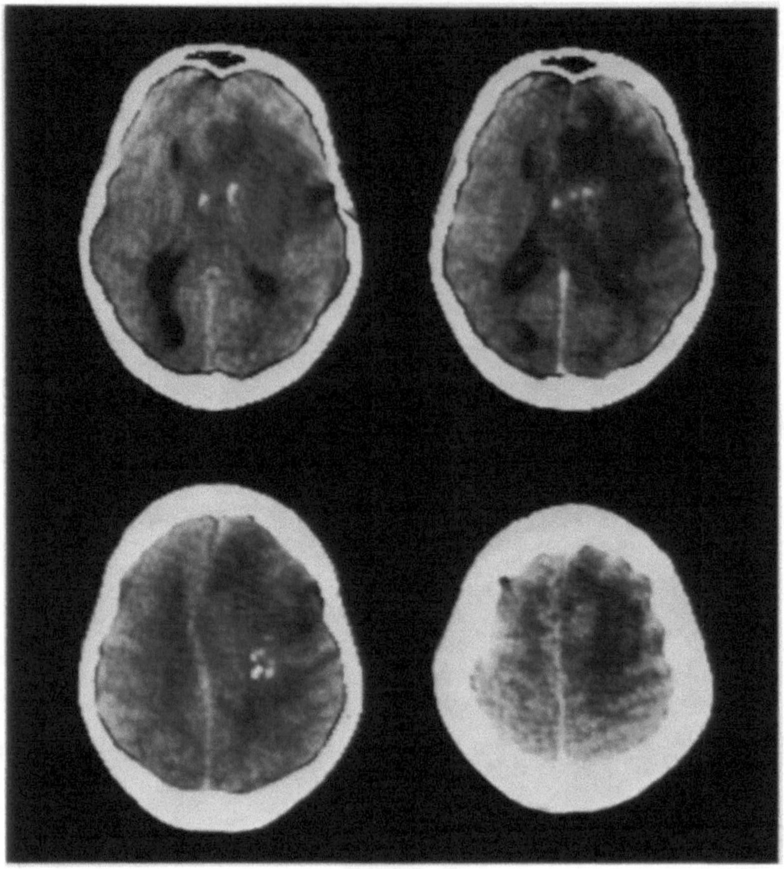

Fig. D 1.50. Mixed glioma (oligoastrocytoma) of the right cerebral hemisphere with infiltration of the corpus callosum in a 30-year-old man with cerebral seizures. The tumor consists predominantly of hypodense areas. Calcific foci increase its central density. The CT findings are the same as in oligodendroglioma. The tumor shows no significant enhancement. Postcontrast scans

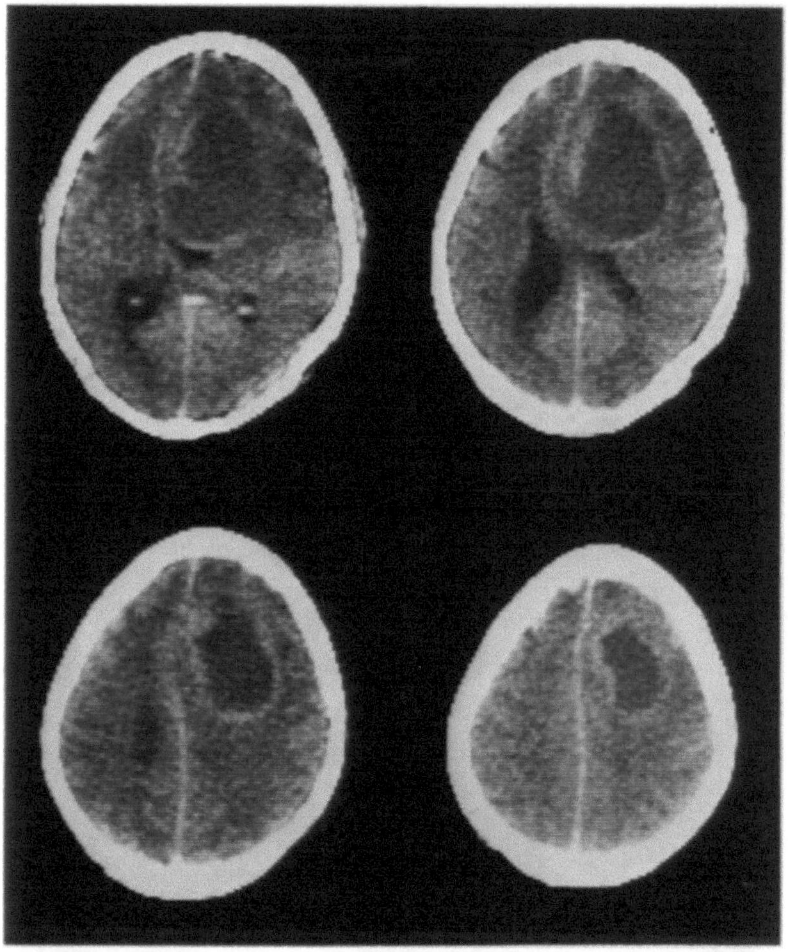

Fig. D 1.51. Mixed glioma of the right frontoprecentral region with involvement of the corpus callosum in a 23-year-old man with altered mental status and cerebral seizures. The CT pattern is consistent with a large cystic tumor. The peripheral enhancement is like that seen in glioblastoma. The tumor was classified histologically as anaplastic oligoastrocytoma. Postcontrast scans

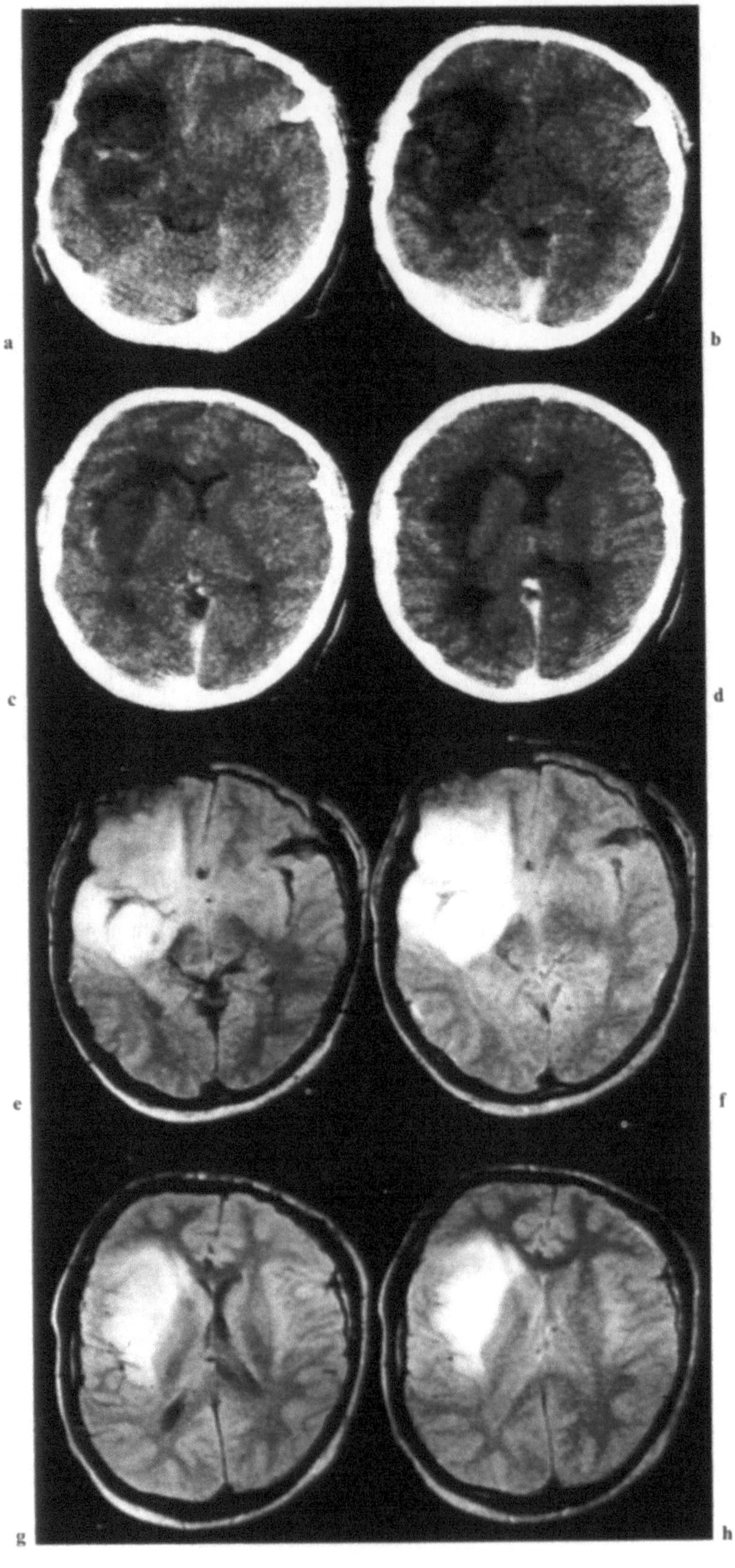
a
b
c
d
e
f
g
h

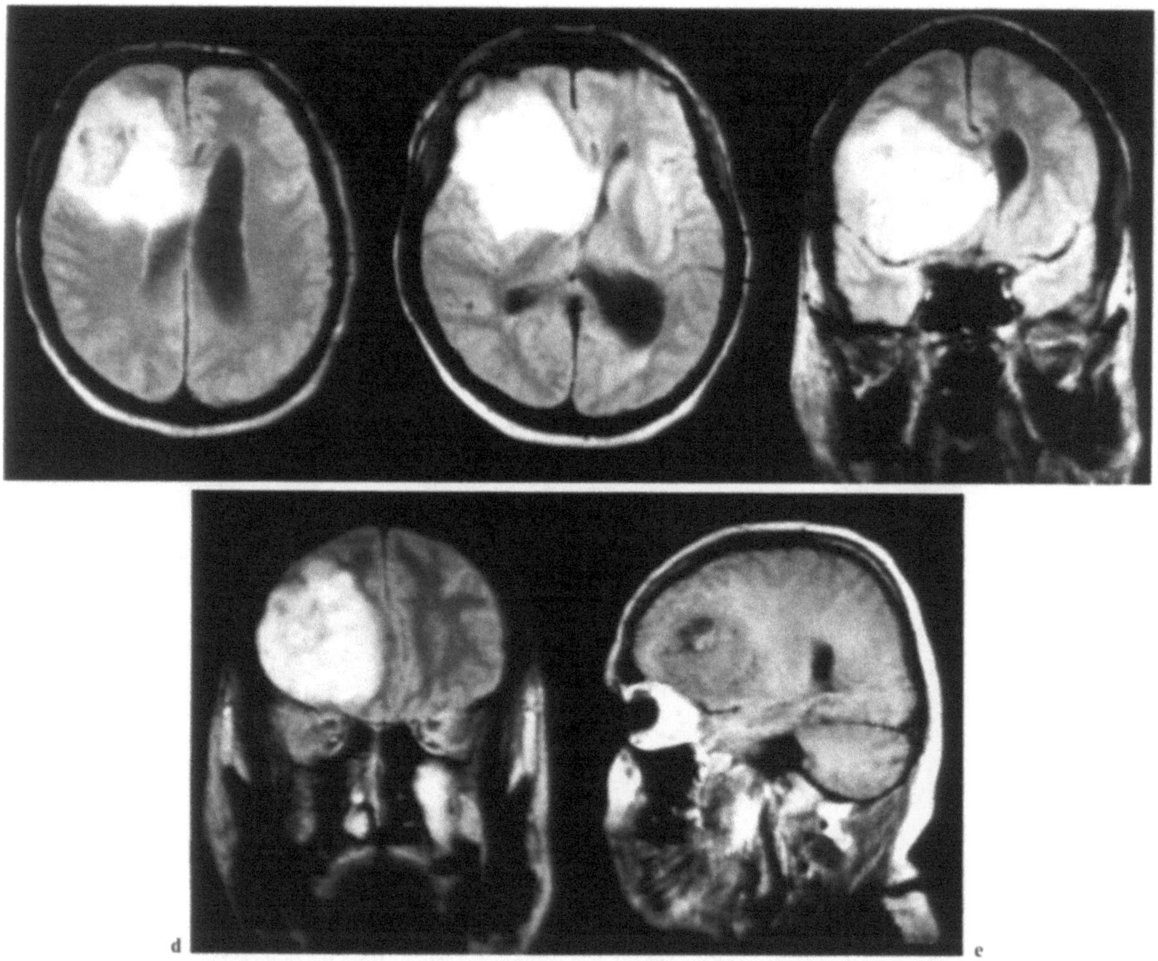

Fig. D 1.53 a–e. Giant grade III mixed glioma of the left frontotemporal region in a 39-year-old man with a 1-year history of headaches; patient presented with mild right-sided hemihypesthesia. MR: **a, b** SE 1600/35, **c** SE 1600/35, **d** SE 1600/70 coronal, **e** SE 400/35 parasagittal. The tumor contrasts poorly with brain parenchyma on the T1-weighted image (**e**), while the proton-density and T2-weighted images show a hyperintense tumor with significant mass effect (**c!**) obstructing the foramen of Monro

Fig. D 1.52 a–h. Oligoastrocytic mixed glioma of the left frontotemporal region. The 29-year-old man with congenital cranial asymmetry presented with a brief history of two generalized seizures. Neurologic and psychologic exam were negative. CT: **a–d** Postcontrast scans. MR: **e** SE 1600/35, **f** SE 1600/70, **g** SE 1600/35, **h** SE 1600/70. CT shows an ill-defined hypodensity with peripheral flecks of calcification. The proton-density images (**e, g**) show homogeneous hyperintense areas. The tumor extent on the T2-weighted image is the same as on the CT scans but is defined more clearly as an area of high signal intensity

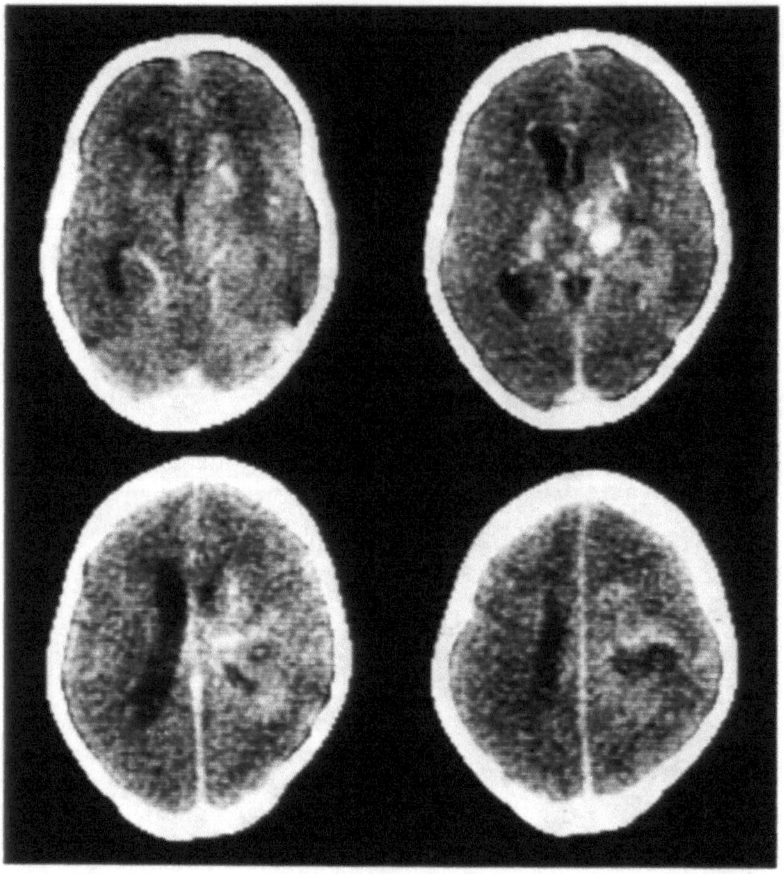

a

Fig. D 1.54. a Diffuse gliomatosis of both cerebral hemispheres with multifocal anaplasia and calcifications in a 12-year-old girl with cerebral seizures. The tumor shows marked contrast enhancement. **b–d** Pathologic sections from the same patient show the diffuse tumor growth in both hemispheres

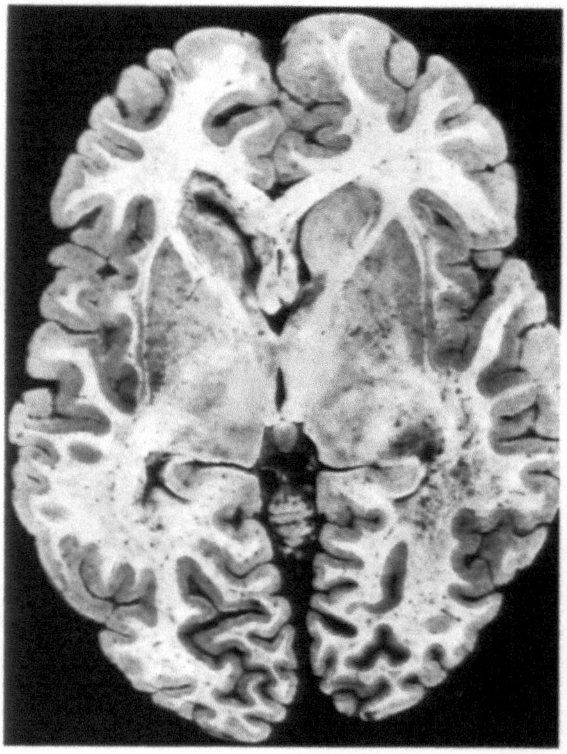
b

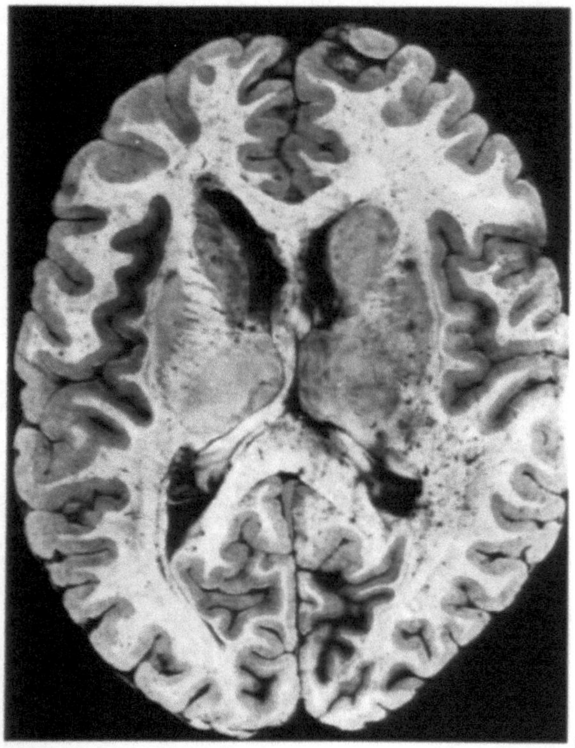
c

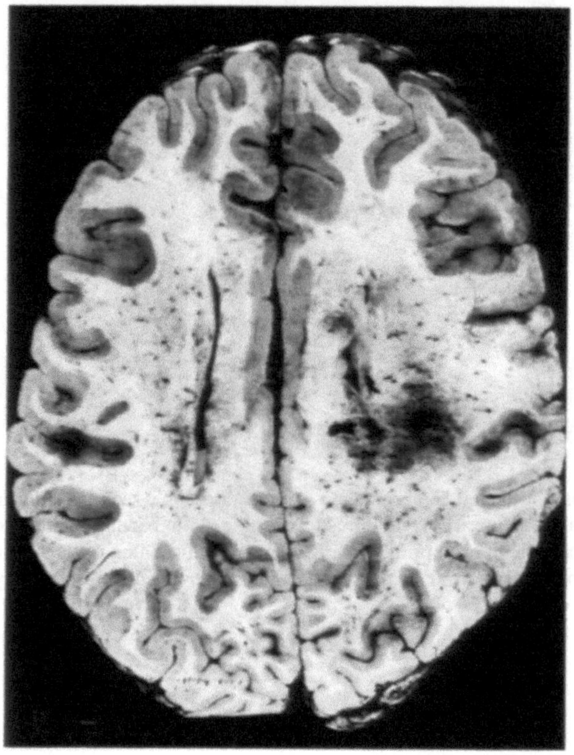
d

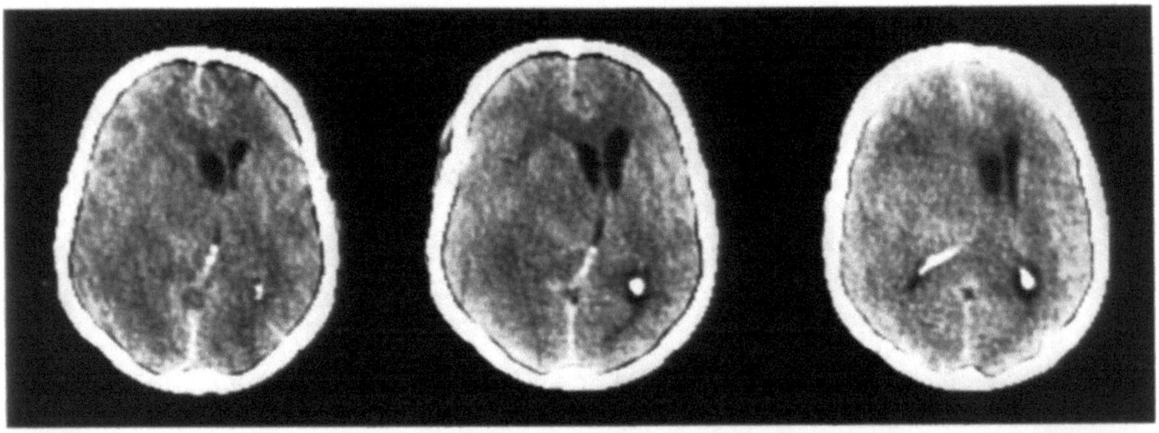

a

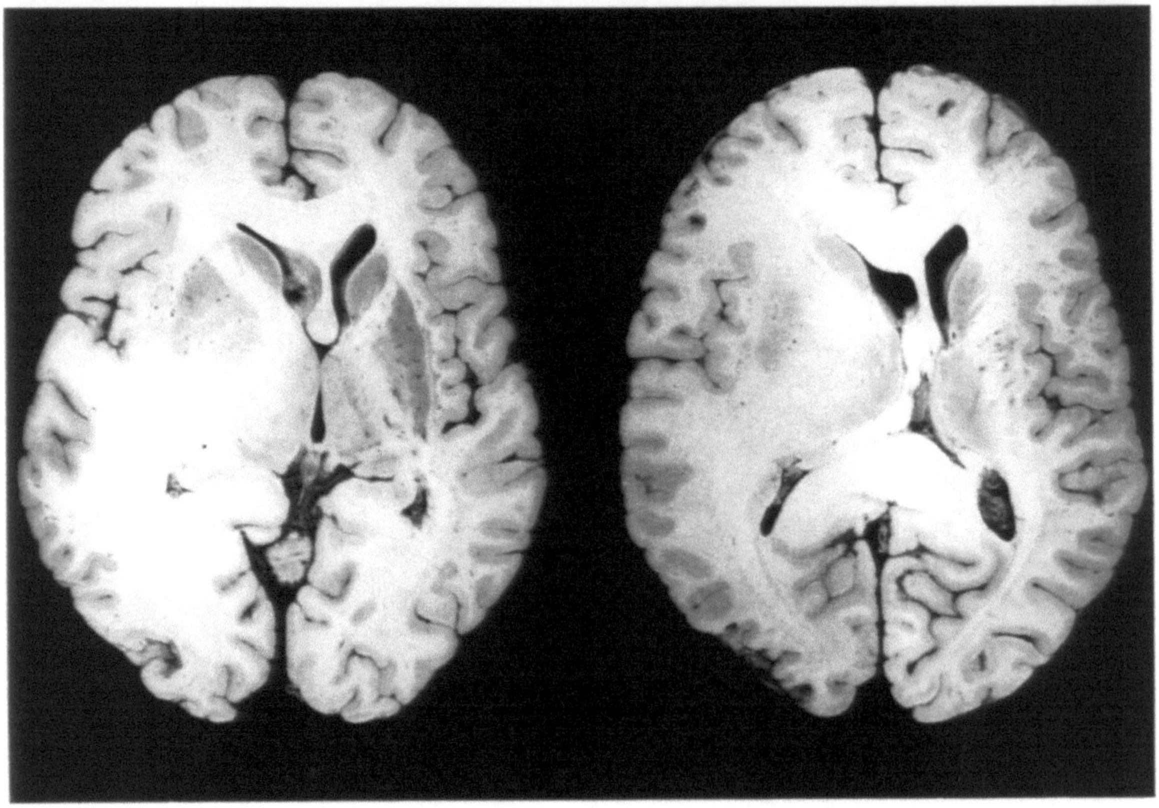

b

Fig. D 1.55 a, b. Diffuse gliomatosis of the left cerebral hemisphere in a 72-year-old man. **a** CT shows only a diffuse enlargement of the entire left hemisphere, prompting an initial misdiagnosis of isodense chronic subdural hematoma. **b** Macroscopic sections show a distended left cerebral hemisphere with partial obliteration of the basal ganglia and marked thickening of the corpus callosum. Histologic examination revealed diffuse astrocytic gliomatosis

f) Glioblastomas

Incidence	12%–20% of all brain tumors
Age predilection	40–65 years
Sex predilection	Almost a 2:1 male preponderance
Typical sites	Frontal, frontomedial, frontolateral, frontodorsal, temporal, temporomedial including the basal ganglia, temporo-parieto-occipital, corpus callosum (butterfly glioma), occipital
Main clinical features	Short history, signs of increased intracranial pressure, marked neurologic deficits, altered mentation
Angiography	Evidence of mass effect with visualization of typical tumor vessels, arteriovenous shunts, sinusoid vessels; 10% of tumors appear avascular due to necrotic changes
CT	
Noncontrast scan	Combination of iso- and hypodense areas, pronounced mass effect, occasional hemorrhagic components
Contrast enhancement	Nearly always positive
Postcontrast appearance	Ring or garland enhancement pattern is frequent; central hypodensities (necrosis, cysts); perifocal edema, usually very conspicuous
MR	
Noncontrast scan	Tumors slightly hypointense, central necrosis often more so, on T1-weighted images. T2-weighted images show a mixed hyperintensity, which with heavier T2 weighting displays a tripartite division into a bright necrotic core, a mildly hyperintense tumor zone with a hypointense ring, and bright peripheral edema
Gadolinium enhancement	Positive
Post Gd-DTPA appearance	T1-weighted images show hyperintense solid or garland-like tumor elements; CT and MR features very similar

Differential diagnosis

Anaplastic astrocytoma
Oligodendroglioma and ependymoma
Brain abscess
Intracranial metastasis
Gliosarcoma
Pilocytic astrocytoma of the cerebrum
Atypical meningioma
Brain infarct in stage of disruption of blood-brain barrier
Older intracerebral hematoma with ring enhancement

Glioblastomas are the most common autochthonous neoplasm of the brain, accounting for 10.3% of the tumors in Cushing's series, 12.2% of the 9000 brain tumors in Zülch's series, and 15% of the 8516 tumors in our population. Glioblastoma is most common in middle-aged and elderly individuals with a peak incidence between 40 and 65 years. It is very rare in children. Males predominate by almost 2:1.

Glioblastomas grow by infiltration and destroy the brain substance. Typically there are extensive areas of necrosis and hemorrhage at varying stages of organization, creating an extremely diverse macroscopic appearance. Pronounced perifocal edema is very common. The tumors are classified as grade IV lesions.

Typical Sites

Glioblastomas occur at all sites in the cerebrum, basal ganglia, and brainstem. Zülch (1986) states that the following sites are typical: frontolateral, frontodorsal, frontobasal, parietolateral, parietodorsal, temporolateral, temporomedial (including the basal ganglia), occipitolateral, and occipitobasal. The tumor may also involve the corpus callosum, creating a "butterfly" pattern, the thalamus, the quadrigeminal area, and the pons. Cerebellar involvement is rare. Multifocal occurrence is possible and has an incidence ranging from 1% to 10% in the literature; Russell and Rubinstein (1977) report 4.5%.

Main Clinical Features

The length of clinical history with glioblastoma is usually very short, with a maximum of 3–4 months. Signs of raised intracranial pressure develop very rapidly, and severe neurologic deficits appear according to the location of the tumor. Altered mentation is a common finding. A cerebral seizure is the initial presenting symptom in many patients.

Additional Diagnostic Procedures

Angiography demonstrates a conspicuous tumor blood supply. Arteriovenous fistulae and typical tumor vessels comprise the angiographic picture of glioblastoma and may be considered pathognomonic for that lesion. In our series over 70% of histologically confirmed glioblastomas were correctly identified from angiographic findings. Similar figures are reported by Krayenbühl and Yasargil (1965).

Computed Tomography

(Figs. D 1.56–68, 70–73, 75, 77, 79–83, 85, 86, 88–94)

Noncontrast Scan

Glioblastoma presents a *very nonhomogeneous density pattern* on CT scans, consistent with its varied macroscopic appearance. Iso- and hypodense areas predominate and are produced by a combination of viable tumor tissue, necrosis, and perifocal edema. Seventy-one percent of the glioblastoma patients in our series displayed mixed absorption on plain CT scans. The remaining 29% were distributed fairly evenly among the remaining absorption patterns.

The slight hypo- or hyperdensity of solid, non-necrotic tumor tissue relative to brain results from the varied histology of the neoplasm and especially from its pathologic blood supply. Our analysis indicates that the solid tumor elements have average density values of 33–34 HU, with individual tumors displaying values up to 4 HU more or less.

Glioblastomas very often contain *necrotic areas*, and *cysts* are commonly found. The density values of cystic and necrotic areas range from 16 to 23 HU, with lower values being more characteristic of cysts. Cysts generally are more clearly defined than necrotic areas. Mean density values range from 16 to 20 HU for cysts and from 19 to 23 HU for necrosis, resulting in an overlap. Calcifications are extremely rare in glioblastomas (oligodendrocytic glioblastoma).

Noncontrast CT scans failed to detect the presence of a tumor in only 2.3% of our material. In some of these cases the glioblastoma became visible with contrast medium, and some tumors were detected only in repeat scans (see Table 2).

Markedly hyperdense areas in glioblastomas should arouse suspicion of a fresh or older intratumoral hemorrhage (glioma apoplecticum, see Figs. D 1.62–65). However, the tumor is not always evident when hemorrhage is detected in the initial CT scan (see Fig. D 1.65). Absorption values in a hyperdense hemorrhage will depend on the age of the hemorrhage. They may range from 70 to 90 HU in a fresh tumoral hemorrhage and are considerably lower in older hemorrhages.

Postcontrast Scan

The great majority of glioblastomas (96.5%) enhance. Absence of enhancement is seen only in necrotic tumors or in intratumoral hemorrhage. The average density increase with our standard intravenous contrast dose was 12.6 ± 5.8 HU. Tumor enhancement is rapid, becomes very marked within a few minutes, and increases with further passage of time. Enhancement is most intense 10–20 min after contrast injection. This prolonged enhancement is due to the breakdown of the blood-brain barrier in the tumor area. Enhancement remains at a high level for about 1 h and then gradually declines.

Contrast medium improves the visualization of glioblastoma and often is necessary to differentiate tumor from surrounding edema, which can be very pronounced (see Fig. D 1.56). Contrast enhancement also makes it easier to distinguish solid tumor tissue from cystic or necrotic elements. About 1 h after contrast injection, marked enhancement is observed in the necrotic area and occasionally even in tumor cysts (see below).

Ring or garland patterns of contrast enhancement are very often seen in CT projections of glioblastomas (Figs. D 1.56, 58, 67, 70–72, 80, 81, 83, 85). Enhancing ring patterns, including complex forms, were seen in 83.9% of our patients with glioblastoma. Some glioblastomas also contain larger solid structures that appear as nodules on CT. We have *rarely seen an exclusively nodular pattern of tumor enhancement* since the introduction of thinner slices and higher density resolution (see Fig. D 1.57).

Approximately 5% of glioblastomas contain *large cysts* with a relatively thin, enhancing peripheral ring or mural nodule (see Fig. D 1.68). Occasionally *contrast medium may enter the cyst and form a visible fluid level* (Fig. D 1.77). This phenomenon serves to distinguish a cyst from a central necrotic core (cf. Afra et al. 1980).

Glioblastoma in statu nascendi appears simply as a hypodense zone: enhancement is not clearly appreciable. Repeat examinations are essential in these cases and, in a period of days or weeks, will disclose a circumscribed mass showing definite contrast enhancement.

Brain edema is a very common finding associated with glioblastoma, occurring in 91.7% of the cases in our series. The extent of the edema was as follows: grade I 24.5%, grade II 57.7%, grade III 17.8%.

The size of the glioblastoma does not influence the extent of edema. Thus, a relatively small tumor may incite edema involving the entire hemisphere, whereas a large tumor may be surrounded by a very thin edematous rim.

The combination of clinical and CT findings enabled us to diagnose glioblastoma correctly in 70% of cases, and glioblastoma was included among the probable differential diagnoses in an additional 12% (Steinhoff et al. 1977). With the availability of improved density resolution, we have increased our diagnostic accuracy rate to better than 80% in the last 100 glioblastoma patients evaluated by CT.

The following features have proved to be highly characteristic of glioblastoma:

1. An irregular ring or garland pattern. The density of the ring tends to diminish over the course of prolonged corticoid therapy.
2. Single or multiple, irregular, central areas of low density, representing necrosis.
3. Typical sites of occurrence (e.g., corpus callosum, basal ganglia, frontal region, temporal region).

Magnetic Resonance Imaging
(Figs. D 1.60, 61, 69, 74–76, 78, 84, 87)

Noncontrast Scan
The tumor tissue gives a low signal on T1-weighted MR images and often cannot be separated from surrounding brain parenchyma. Perifocal edema is poorly visualized. Large cysts or sites of necrotic liquefaction appear hypointense, and hemorrhage appears hyperintense. T2-weighted images are far superior and demonstrate a heterogeneous mass composed of hypo-, iso-, and hyperintense areas. Frequently the tumor contains or adjoins structures which represent pathologic vessels. Heavy T2 weighting often resolves a bright, central

core of necrosis surrounded by slightly hyperintense tumor tissue with a low-intensity rim, surrounded in turn by a peripheral area of hyperintense edema. Large cysts and necrotic areas give a high signal on T2-weighted sequences.

Today MR can detect incipient glioblastomas at an earlier stage than CT, although very early-stage glioblastomas are indistinguishable from astrocytomas. Multiple foci are detected with increasing frequency owing to the high sensitivity of MR. We have found that a second focus is still missed in some cases with CT. MR is equally sensitive in detecting infiltration of the corpus callosum.

Post-Gadolinium Scan

Solid and garland-like tumor components are displayed with high intensity on the post Gd-DTPA image. Tumor and edema can be differentiated. The appearance of glioblastoma is very similar on contrast-enhanced CT and MR images.

Differential Diagnosis

The differential diagnosis of glioblastoma should include all lesions that show a ring pattern of contrast enhancement (except in the posterior fossa, where glioblastomas are extremely rare; there was only one case in our series). Table 7 shows the percentage incidence of ring enhancement observed on CT scans for the most common intracranial tumors and for brain abscess (Kazner et al. 1978).

Table 7. Frequency of ring enhancement in CT studies of intracranial tumors and brain abscesses. (After Kazner et al. 1978)

Diagnosis	Number of patients examined	Ring enhancement (not including complex patterns)	
		n	%
Pilocytic astrocytoma	76	25	33
Anaplastic astrocytoma	109	25	22.9
Oligodendroglioma	117	12	10.3
Glioblastoma	523	282	53.9
Ependymoma	37	5	14
Meningioma	410	8	2.0
Neurinoma	138	13	9.4
Pituitary adenoma	243	12	4.9
Hemangioblastoma	30	4	13
Craniopharyngioma	67	4	6
Other brain tumors	468	24	5.1
Metastases	363	102	28.1
Total	2581	516	20.0
Brain abscess	44	38	86

1. Brain Abscess. The history and clinical findings are of decisive importance in establishing a diagnosis of brain abscess. A brain abscess is difficult or impossible to identify on CT scans if the history is not characteristic. The ring of the abscess, representing the richly vascularized capsule, almost always presents a smooth, rounded, or oval shape of uniform thickness. This pattern is rarely seen with glioblastoma. Garland-like patterns and "nubbins" projecting inward from the peripheral ring are typical of glioblastoma but not of brain abscess. It should be noted that with a multilocular abscess, a slice through the capsule can simulate the appearance of a nodular tumor and steer the overall diagnosis in the wrong direction. Very thin rings favor a diagnosis of tumor rather than brain abscess.

MR does not aid in the differentiation of glioblastoma from abscess. Cerebral angiography is helpful in this regard only if typical glioblastomatous vessels are visualized or there is characteristic staining of the abscess capsule. *Doubtful cases should be resolved by needle biopsy.*

2. Intracranial Metastases. Here differential diagnosis is a simple matter if the primary tumor is known, although it has been our experience that the possibility of a primary brain tumor should be considered even when there is a known primary in a different organ. Multiplicity of lesions should arouse suspicion of metastases even if there is no evidence of a primary neoplasm. *Multifocal glioblastomas* are known to occur but are uncommon (see Figs. D 1.88–91), accounting for only about 1% of the glioblastomas in our series. An irregular ring or garland pattern is an extremely rare CT finding with metastases. Hence two intracranial tumors that show a garland pattern of enhancement should primarily arouse suspicion of multifocal glioblastoma.

MR is of greatest help in differentiating multiple metastases from multicentric glioblastoma when it is able to detect three or more lesions not yet visible on the CT scan.

3. Anaplastic Astrocytoma. Ring patterns appearing on the CT scan of anaplastic astrocytoma are frequently narrow and enclose a cyst (see Fig. D 1.20). This is very unusual with glioblastoma. A homogeneous nodular mass containing no hypodense necrotic components is characteristic of anaplastic astrocytoma but is rare in glioblastoma. However, some anaplastic astrocytomas have a CT appearance identical to that of glioblastoma (Figs. D 1.22, 23, 25, 30).

MR does not contribute further to the histopathologic diagnosis of this tumor.

4. Brain Infarction. This lesion may closely resemble glioblastoma on the contrast-enhanced CT scan at the stage where there is marked disruption of the blood-brain barrier (2nd and 3rd weeks after infarction) (see Fig. F 105). The history, clinical findings, and absence of significant mass effect at 3 weeks post infarction should direct suspicion toward a vascular lesion. Doubts are resolved by repeat CT scans and clinical follow-up.

MR does not aid diagnosis in the luxuriant perfusion stage of a cerebral infarction.

5. Other Space-Occupying Lesions. *Meningioma with an atypical CT presentation – usually a malignant form showing ring enhancement – cannot be confidently distinguished from glioblastoma on the basis of clinical or CT findings.* Plain skull radiographs, serial radionuclide scans, and angiography are valuable diagnostic adjuncts in these cases. Glioblastomas located near the interhemispheric fissure may be mistaken for an atypical falx meningioma, and vice versa. Zimmerman et al. (1977) observed ring enhancement in *intracerebral hematomas in the course of resorption*, and Weisberg (1980) states that this pattern is consistently seen. *Gliosarcomas* cannot be differentiated from glioblastomas by angiography or CT (see Fig. D 1.94). Cerebral pilocytic astrocytoma can occasionally mimic the CT appearance of a typical glioblastoma. The same is true of highly malignant ependymomas.

The MR features closely resemble those on CT, so the same problems of differential diagnosis are encountered.

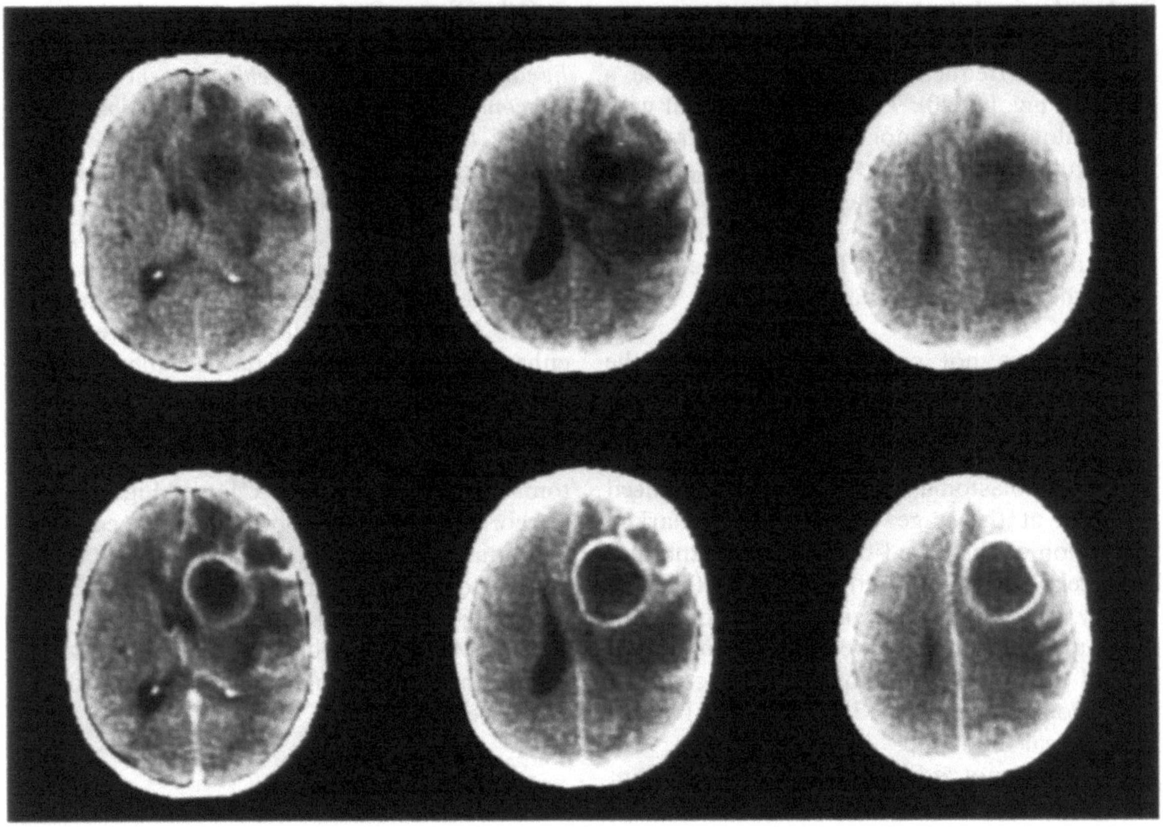

Fig. D 1.56. Glioblastoma of the right frontal-precental region with extension to the basal ganglia in a 65-year-old woman. Plain CT scans (*top*) show a heterogeneous density pattern with no definite tumor outline. Postcontrast scans (*bottom*) show two well-defined, contiguous rings. CT findings are consistent with a multilocular brain abscess or glioblastoma. The central hypodensity is caused by intratumoral necrosis. The density at the core of the lesion is approximately 20 HU

Fig. D 1.57. Glioblastoma deep in the frontal white matter bordering on the basal ganglia in a 42-year-old man with symptoms of increased intracranial pressure. The plain CT scans (*top*) demonstrate the tumor as an iso- to slightly hyperdense, almost circular area (mean density 44 HU) surrounded by edema. Homogeneous, "nodular" enhancement is seen on the postcontrast scans (*bottom*). The density increase is 18 HU with a standard contrast dose

Fig. D 1.58. Glioblastoma in the left temporal region of a 72-year-old woman. The tumor is mostly solid and appears hyperdense even on the plain CT scan (*upper left*). Intense enhancement is seen with contrast medium. A meningioma with regressive changes cannot be excluded on the basis of these findings. Grade III perifocal edema

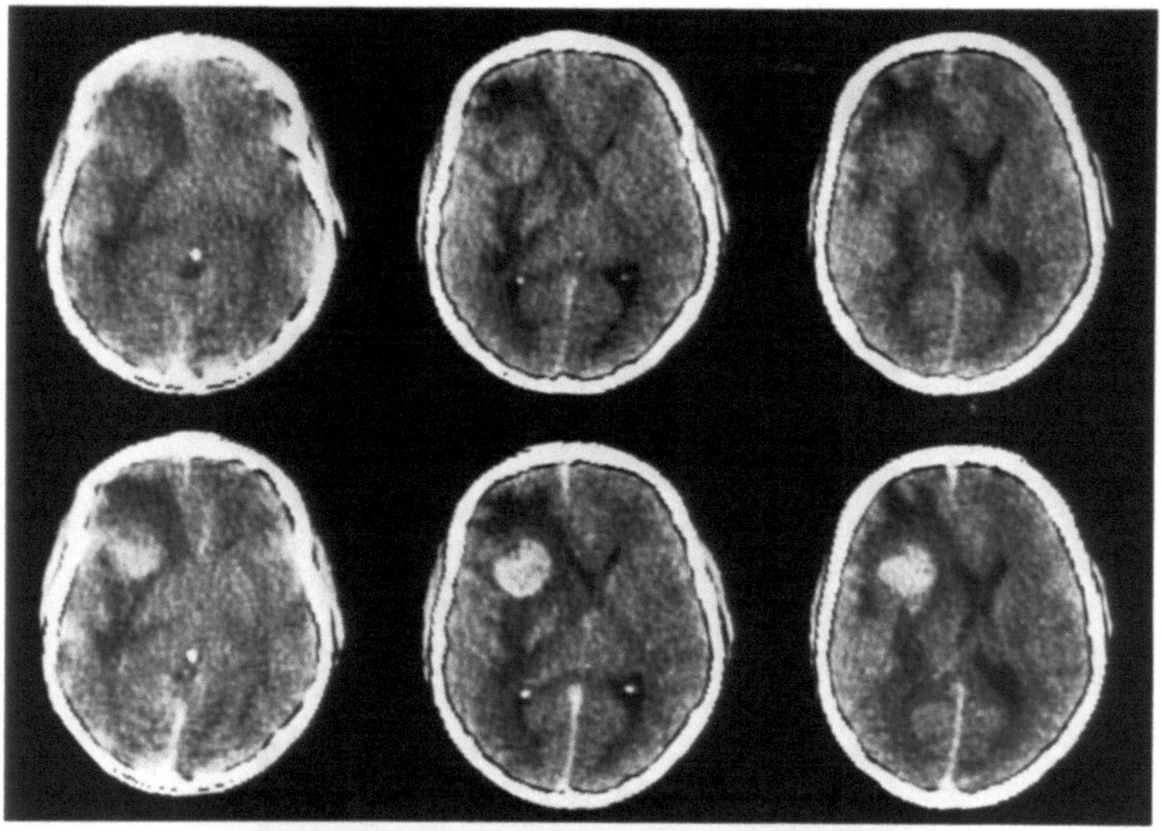

D 1.57

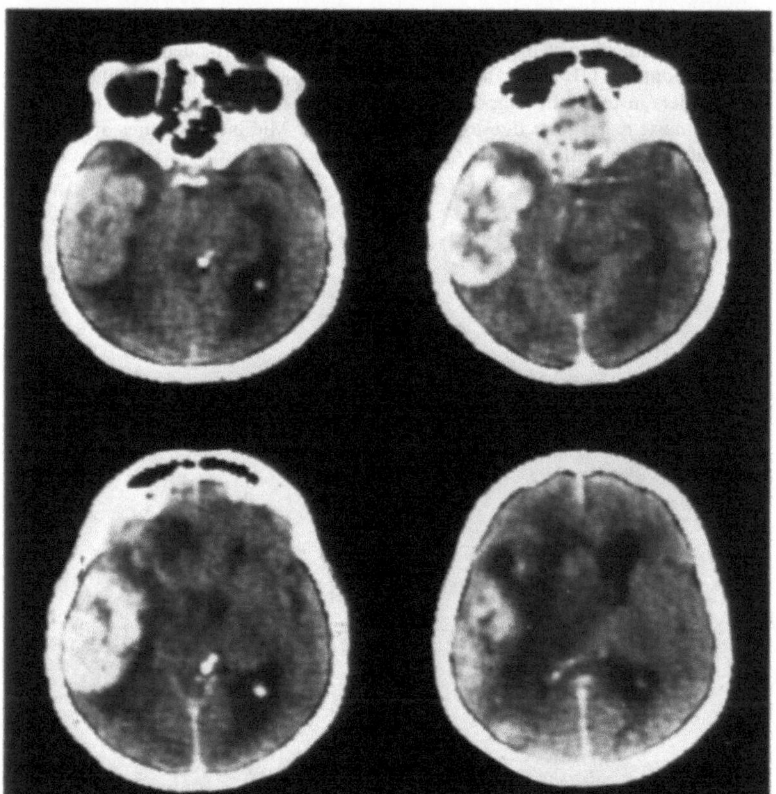

D 1.58

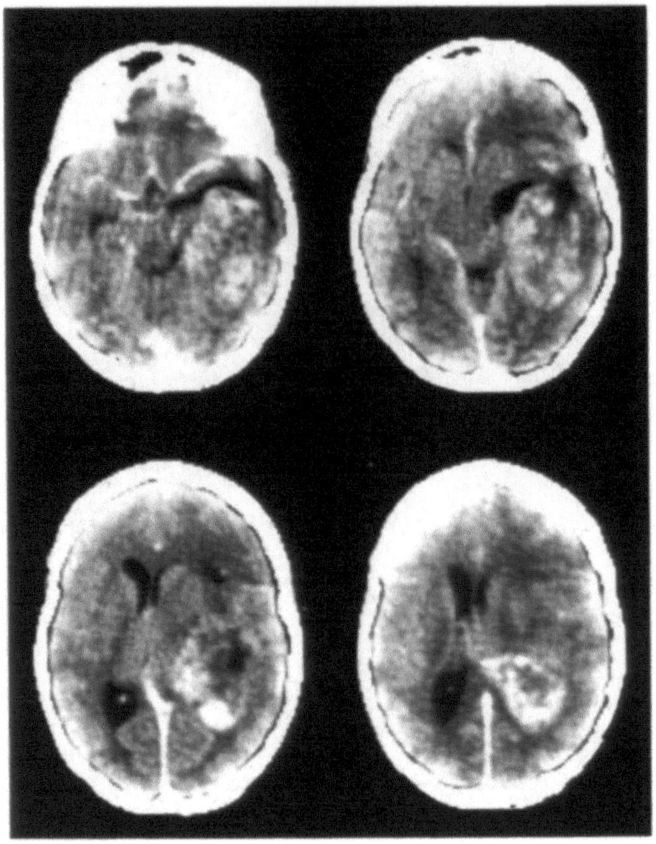

Fig. D 1.59. Glioblastoma multiforme in a 37-year-old woman with a 2-month history of headaches and progressive left-sided paresis. Postcontrast CT shows a strongly enhancing tumor with irregular borders in the right temporo-parieto-occipital region. The density of the mass is irregular due to necrotic changes. Midline structures are shifted to the left

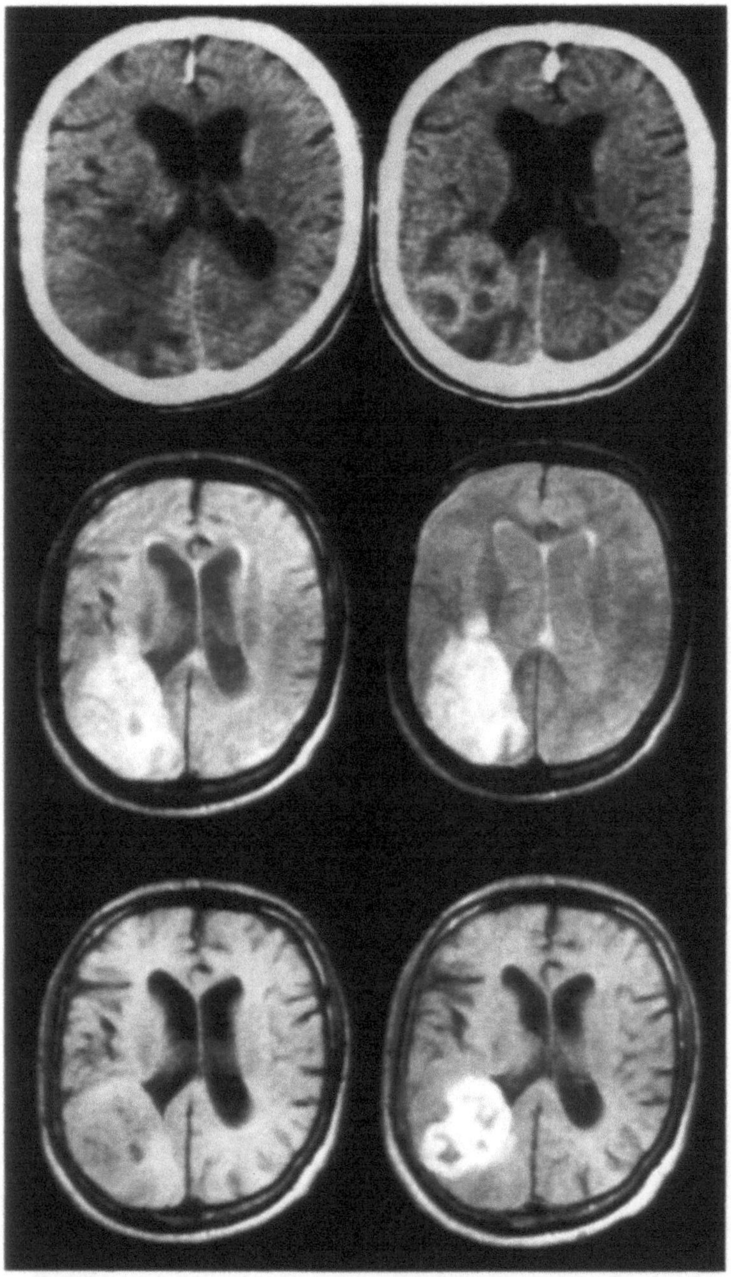

Fig. D 1.60 a–f. Glioblastoma of the left parieto-occipital region in a 71-year-old man with amnestic aphasia and right homonymous hemianopia. CT: **a** precontrast, **b** postcontrast. MR: **c** SE 1600/35, **d** SE 1600/70, **e** SE 800/35, **f** SE 800/35 post Gd-DTPA. A bunch-of-grapes pattern of tumor enhancement is seen on the postcontrast CT scan, with compression and amputation of the left occipital horn. The proton-density and T2-weighted images show a hyperintense mass having the same extent as on the CT scan (**c, d**). The pattern on the gadolinium-enhanced scan (**f**) is identical to the postcontrast CT pattern

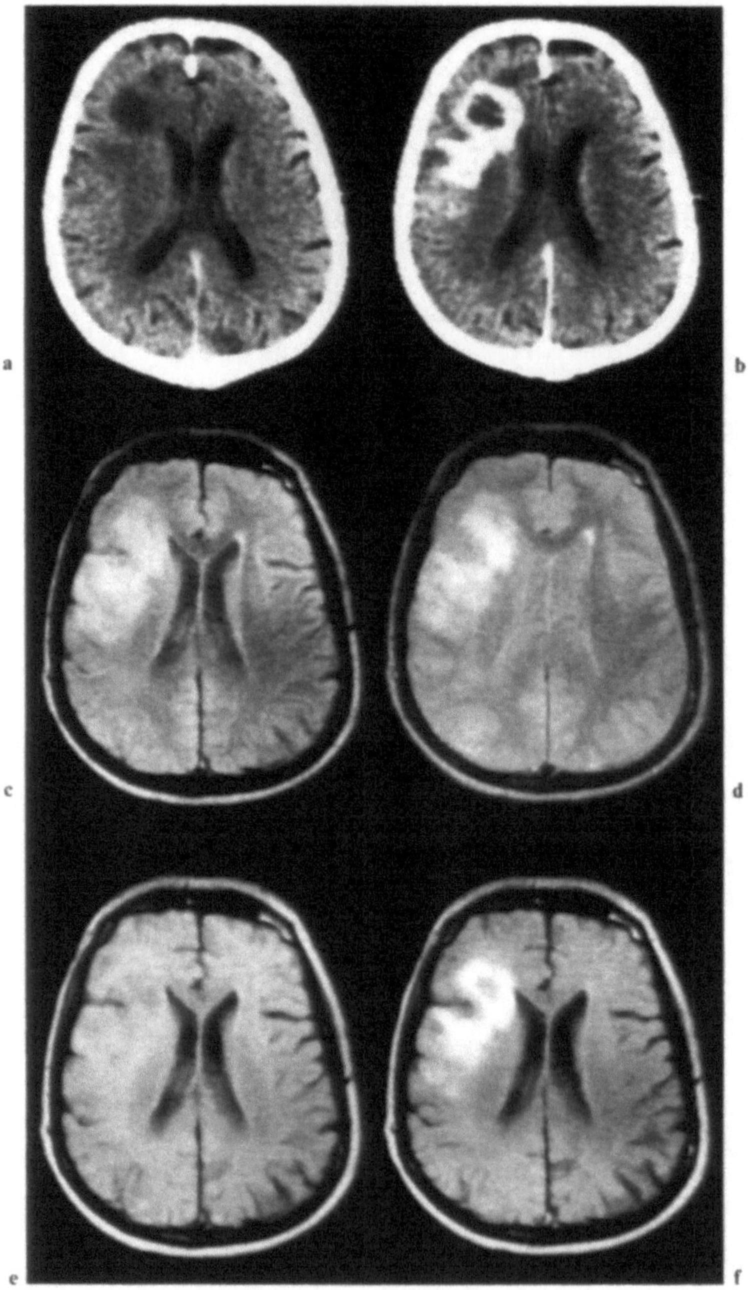

Fig. D 1.61 a–f. Paraventricular glioblastoma of the left frontal region in a 65-year-old man with a 1-year history of increasing loss of drive and fatigability. Patient suffered one grand mal seizure and presented with latent right-sided hemiparesis. CT: **a** precontrast, **b** postcontrast. MR: **c** SE 1600/35, **d** SE 1600/70, **e** SE 800/35, **f** SE 800/35 post Gd-DTPA. Postcontrast CT shows a strongly enhancing lesion with irregular borders and central necrosis (**b**). The tumor is slightly to moderately hyperintense to brain on the proton-density and T2-weighted images (**c, d**) and is not well defined. Only the gadolinium-enhanced scan provides tumor visualization comparable to the CT scan

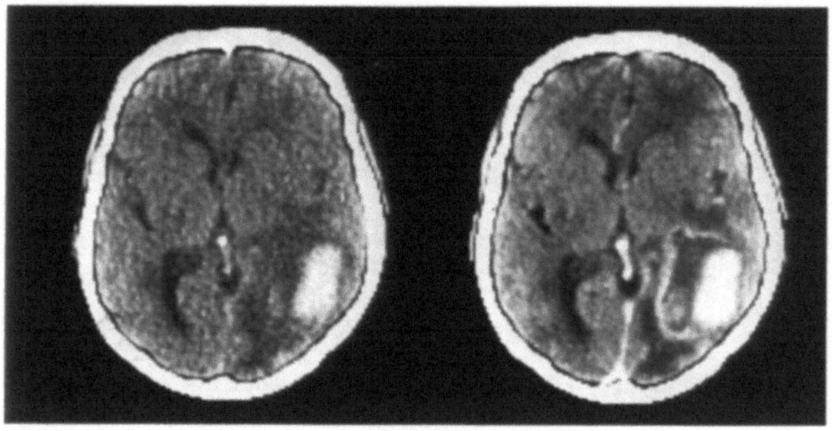

Fig. D 1.62. Hemorrhage within a glioblastoma (glioma apoplecticum) in a 65-year-old man with disease of abrupt onset. Plain CT shows a hyperdense area with density values around 80 HU consistent with freshly clotted blood. There is an extensive hypodense area adjacent to the hemorrhage (*left*). These findings are not typical for recent spontaneous intracerebral hematoma. Postcontrast CT (*right*) reveals the cause of the bleeding: a ring to garland pattern of enhancement surrounding the hemorrhage. This confirms the diagnosis of intratumoral hemorrhage

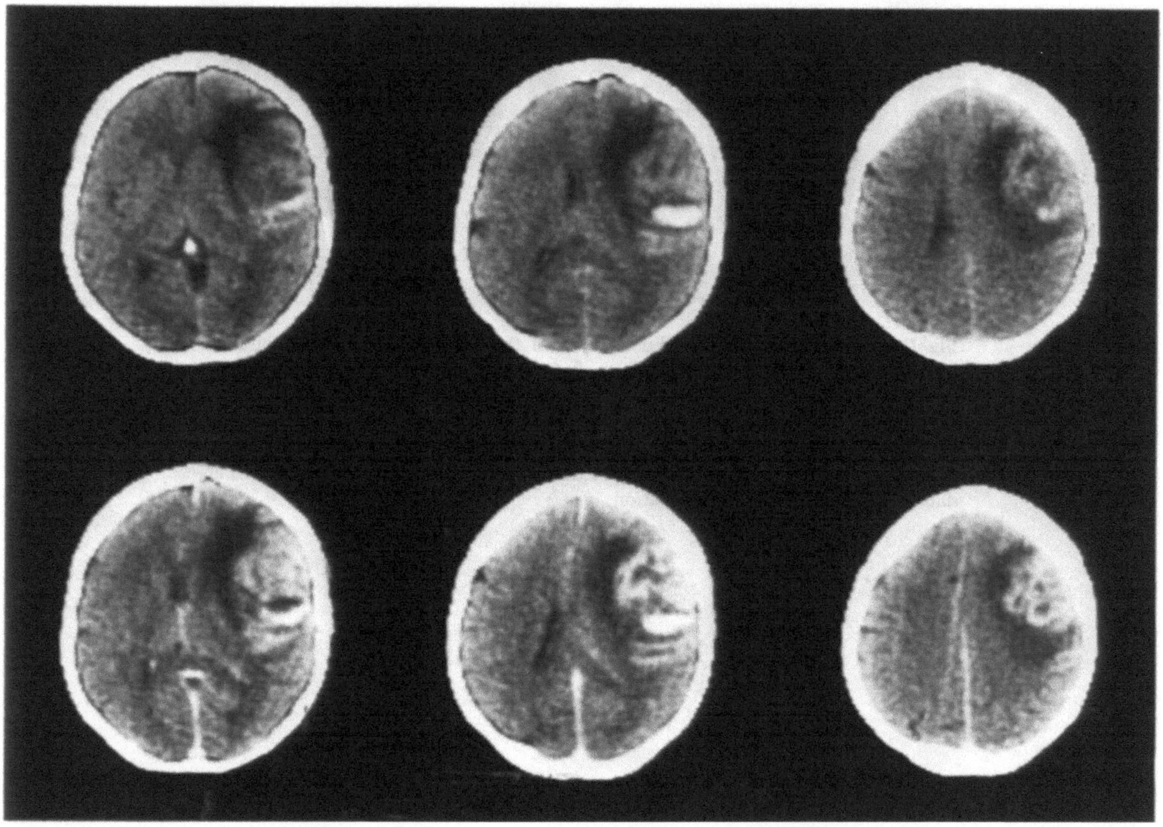

Fig. D 1.63. CT findings several days after hemorrhage within a glioblastoma of the right fronto-precentral region in a 69-year-old woman. Plain scans (*top*) demonstrate a hyperdense area with a fluid level. Postcontrast scans (*bottom*) show intense enhancement of viable tumor tissue with scattered, hypodense foci of necrosis. Grade II perifocal edema

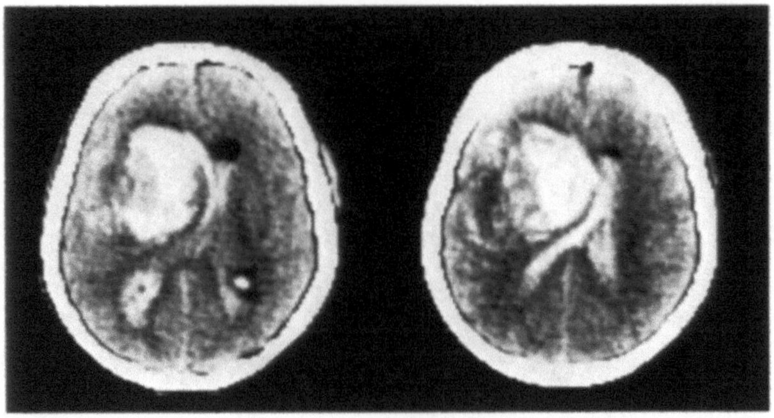

Fig. D 1.64. Massive hemorrhage from a glioblastoma has penetrated the ventricular system in this 62-year-old man. A glioblastoma deep in the left temporal lobe had been diagnosed a short time previously by angiography

13.7.1978

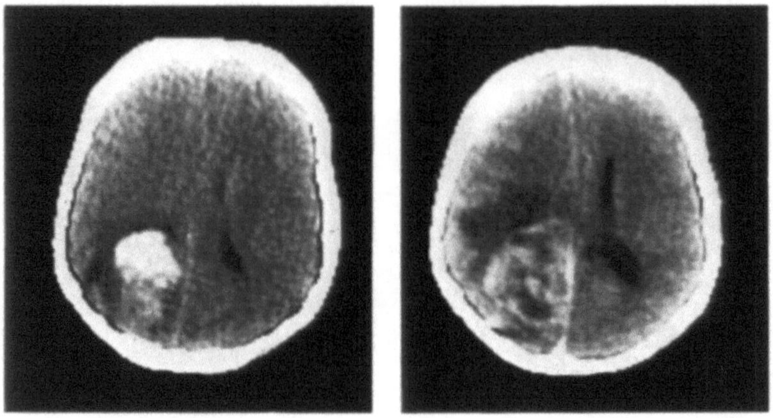

10.10.1979

Fig. D 1.65. Hemorrhage in a glioblastoma of the left parieto-occipital region in a 54-year-old man. The initial CT scan (*left*) shows a massive hemorrhage in the left parieto-occipital area. The hemorrhage was surgically evacuated and examined histologically, with no evidence of tumor. Fifteen months later the patient presented with gradually progressive right-sided hemiparesis and dysphasia. The follow-up scan (*right*) shows a heterogeneous mass that was interpreted as glioblastoma. This diagnosis was confirmed at operation

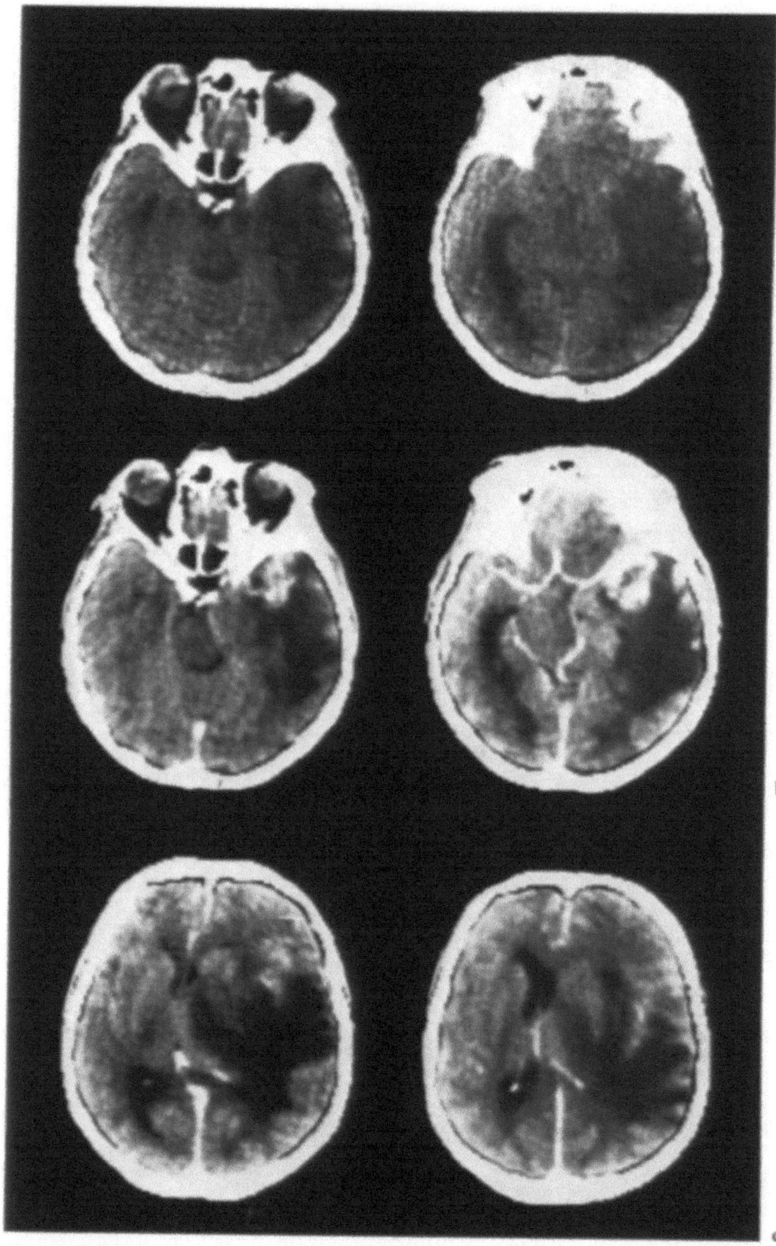

a

b

c

Fig. D 1.66 a–c. Glioblastoma in the right temporal lobe of a 44-year-old man. **a** Plain CT scans show a large hypodense area in the right temporal lobe, but the actual tumor nodule is not defined. **b** These contrast-enhanced scans show a relatively small, centrally necrotic tumor at the right temporal pole causing marked displacement of midline structures with transtentorial herniation of the medial portions of the right temporal lobe and its vessels. **c** Contrast scans show grade III perifocal edema extending throughout the right cerebral hemisphere

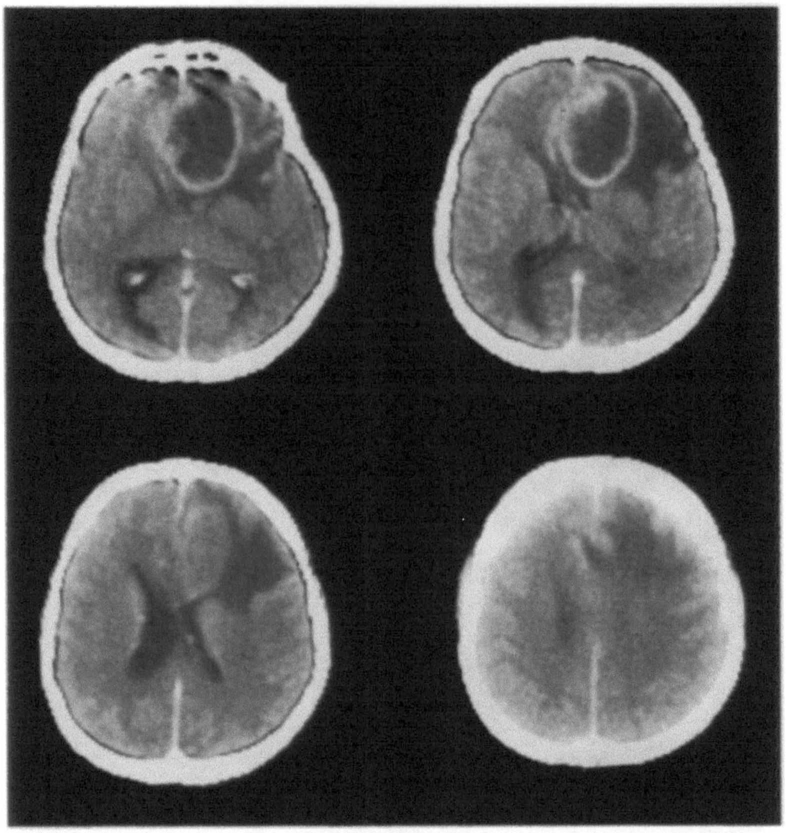

Fig. D 1.67. Large right frontal glioblastoma with ring enhancement and typical frontal edema with a tail-like termination in the area of the basal ganglia. The well-defined hypodensity at the center of the tumor was identified at operation as necrotic tissue. The CT pattern is consistent with glioblastoma or abscess. Postcontrast scans

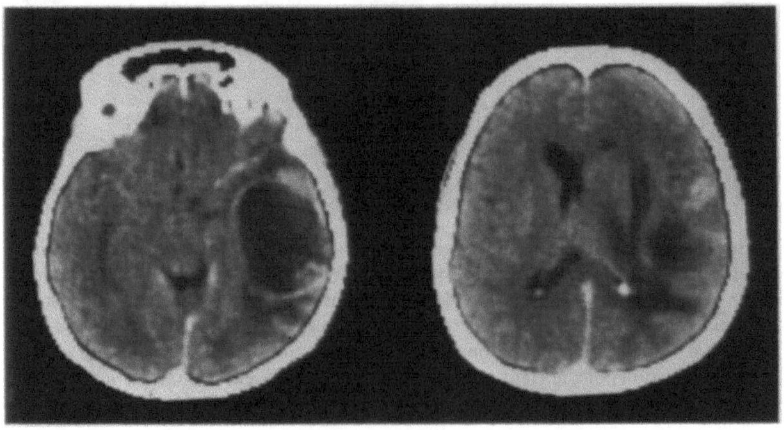

Fig. D 1.68. Large cystic glioblastoma in the right temporal lobe of a 67-year-old woman. The postcontrast CT scan on the *left* shows thin peripheral enhancement with multiple intramural tumor nodules. There is marked displacement of the midbrain with compression of the right ambient cistern. The enhanced scan on the *right* shows a typical "finger" of edema on the midventricular plane, which traverses a small portion of the neoplasm

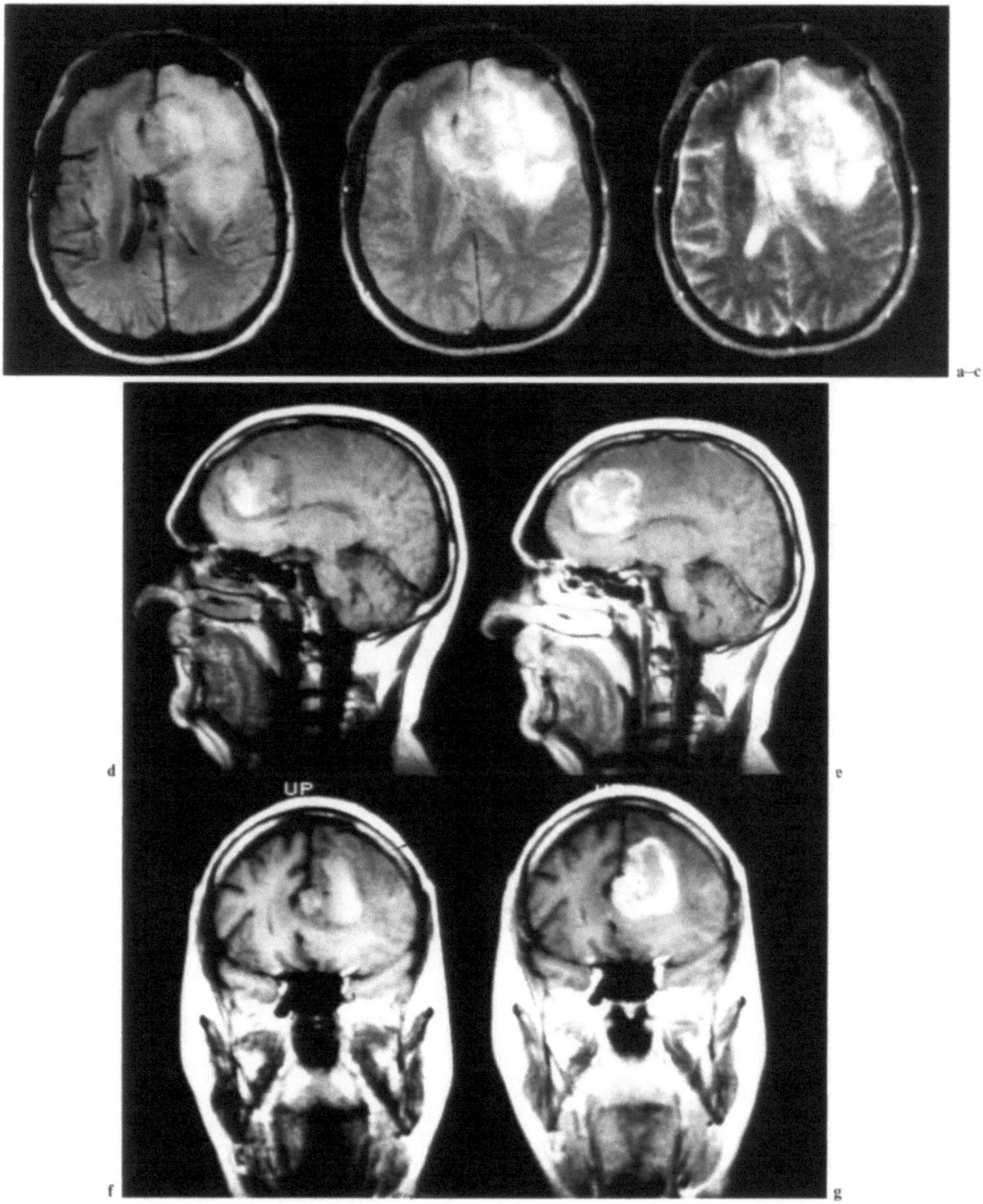

Fig. D1.69a–g. Isomorphous glioblastoma of the right frontal region in a 59-year-old man with headache, concentration difficulties, and altered mental status. MR: **a** SE 1600/30, **b** SE 1600/90, **c** SE 1600/180, **d** SE 400/30 sagittal, **e** SE 400/30 sagittal post Gd-DTPA, **f** SE 400/30 coronal, **g** SE 400/30 coronal post Gd-DTPA. The tumor gives an increasingly bright signal from the proton-density image to the T2-weighted image (**a–c**) but cannot be differentiated further. A garland pattern of enhancement is seen on the postcontrast scans (**e, g**)

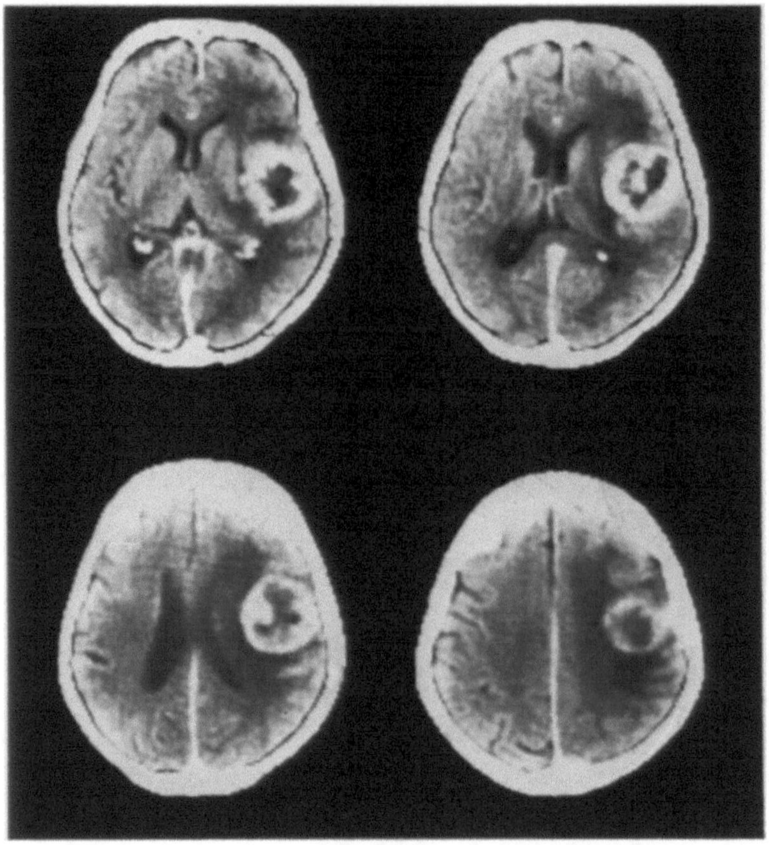

Fig. D 1.70. Typical glioblastoma of the right temporo-parietal region with extensive perifocal edema in a 63-year-old man. Mass effect is relatively slight. The very intense enhancement of solid tumor results from an increased contrast dose

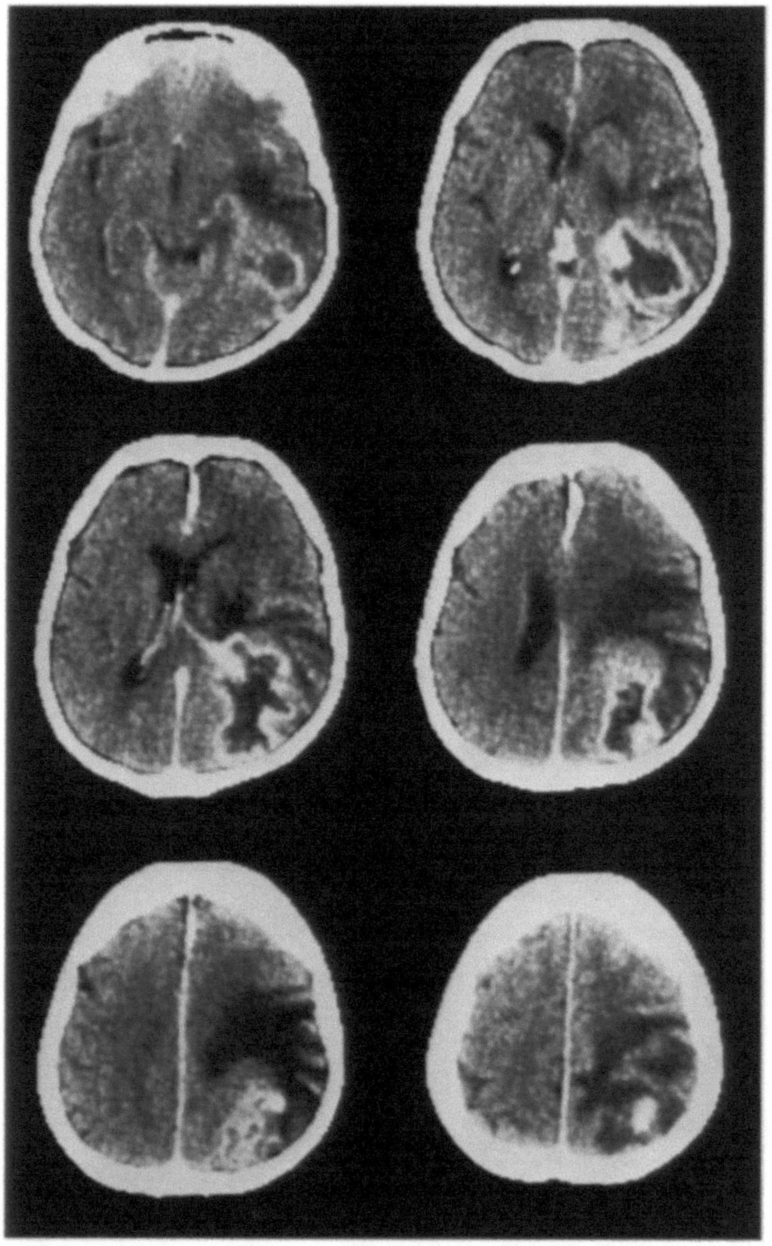

Fig. D 1.71. Typical CT appearance of a glioblastoma at the junction of the right temporal, parietal, and occipital lobes in a 56-year-old man. The tumor extends to the right lateral ventricle and choroid plexus in the region of the trigone. Grade II perifocal edema

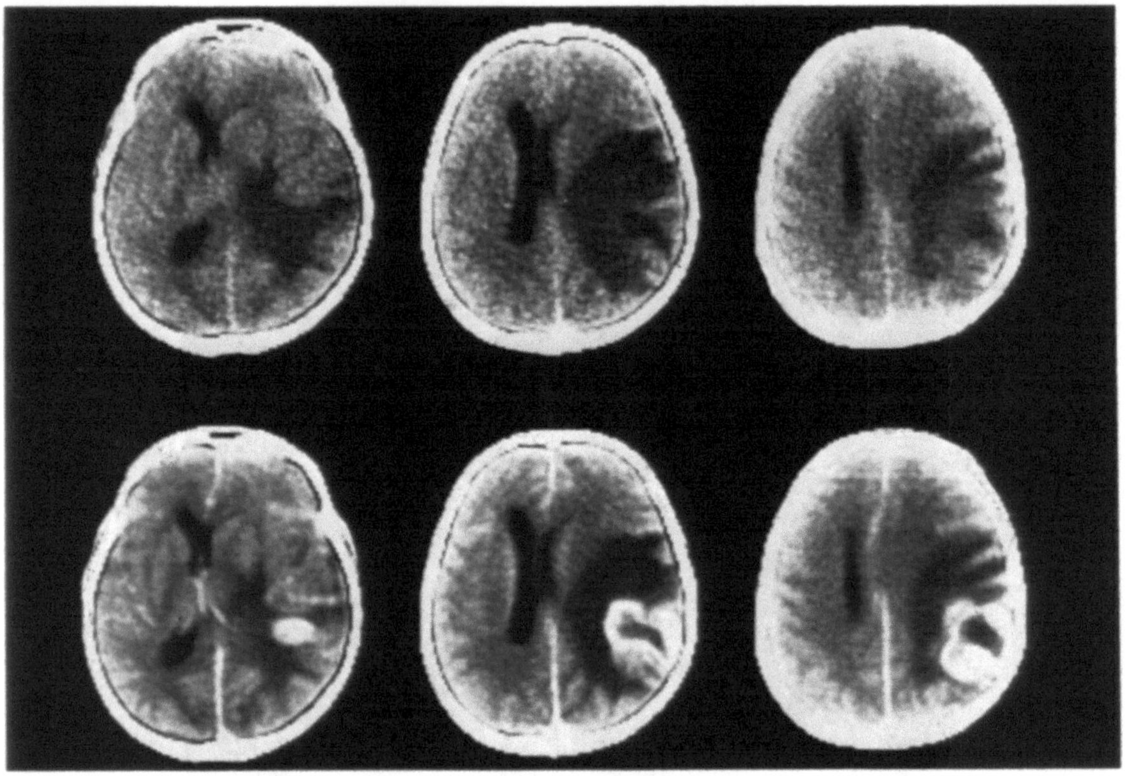

Fig. D 1.72. Glioblastoma near the cortex in the right temporo-parieto-occipital region of a 47-year-old man. The tumor is difficult to separate from the hypodense peritumoral edema on the unenhanced scans (*top*). The post-contrast scans (*bottom*) disclose a large mass composed of ringlike and nodular segments. A similar pattern may be seen with metastases and rarely with a meningioma of the convexity

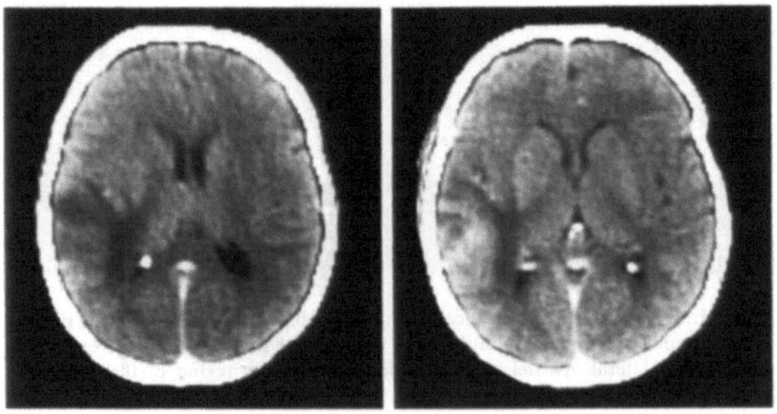

Fig. D 1.73. Glioblastoma in the left posterior temporal region of a 56-year-old woman. The initial CT scan taken on 1/26/79 (*left*) shows an isodense area bounded medially by a faint finger of edema. Midline structures do not appear shifted, although the left choroid plexus is displaced medially. Right-sided hemiparesis of acute onset led to the diagnosis of a previous hemorrhage. A follow-up scan performed on 6/16/79 (*right*) following dexamethasone therapy showed regression of the perifocal edema and choroid plexus displacement. The scan demonstrates a lightly enhancing area near the cortex in the left posterior temporal region. A tumor was diagnosed and identified at operation as a glioblastoma

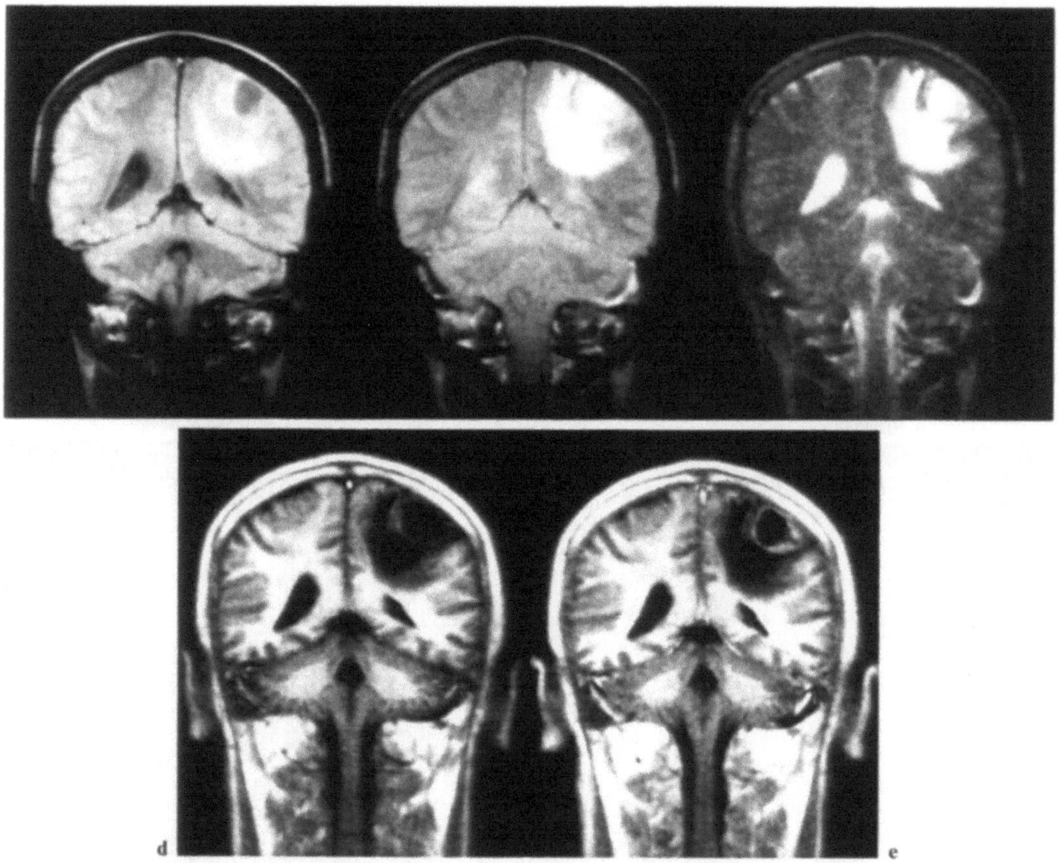

Fig. D 1.74 a–e. Glioblastoma of the right parietal area in a 50-year-old man with progressive memory loss, right-left confusion, and left-sided hemiparesis. MR: **a** SE 1600/30, **b** SE 1600/90, **c** SE 1600/210, all coronal; **d** IR 1500/400/35, **e** IR 1500/400/35 post Gd-DTPA. The initially low-signal core (**a**) becomes more intense (**c**) as T2 weighting is increased. The finger-shaped area of edema (**c**) is distinguishable from tumor. Ring enhancement is apparent on the post-gadolinium IR image (**e**)

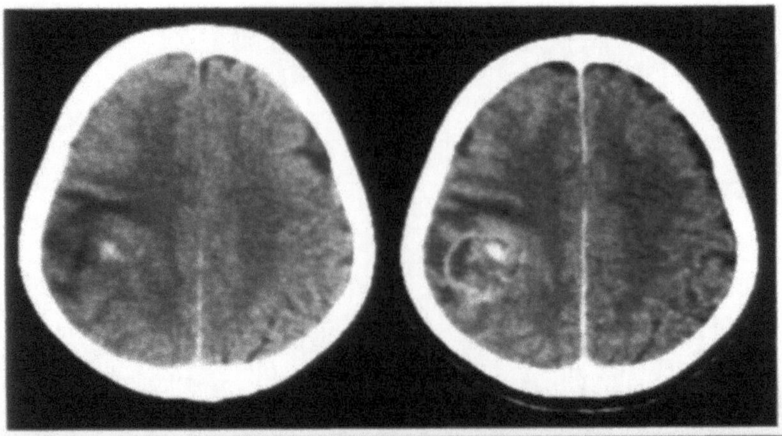

a b

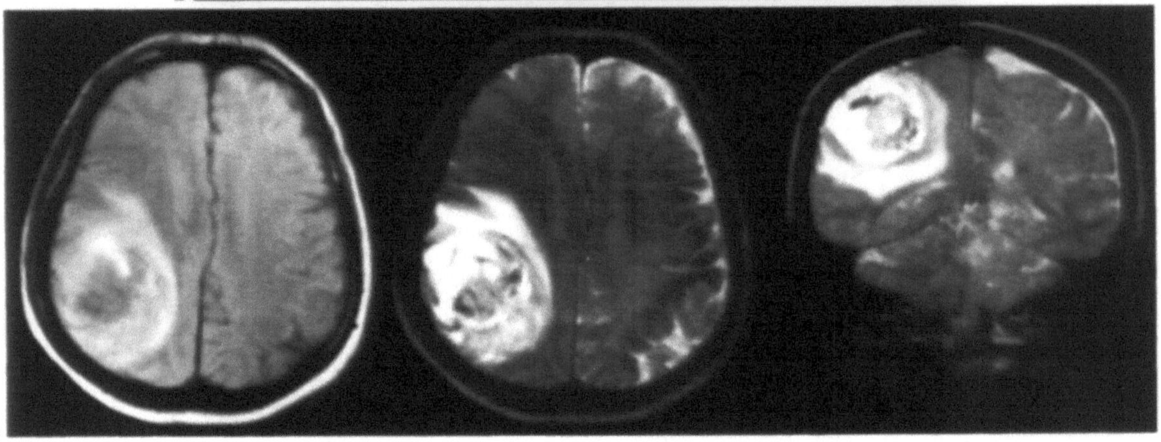

c–e

Fig. D 1.75 a–e. Glioblastoma of the left parietal area in a 62-year-old woman with altered mental status and right-sided hemiparesis. CT: **a** precontrast, **b** postcontrast. MR: **c** SE 2500/30; **d, e** SE 2500/120 axial, coronal. CT shows thin peripheral ring enhancement (**b**). The proton-density MR image shows a ring-shaped hyperintense tumor with a central hypointense area (**c**). T2 weighting shows a complex, partly shell-like structure with a heterogeneous density pattern. The border between tumor and edema can be resolved. The tumor contains structures that appear to be pathologic vessels

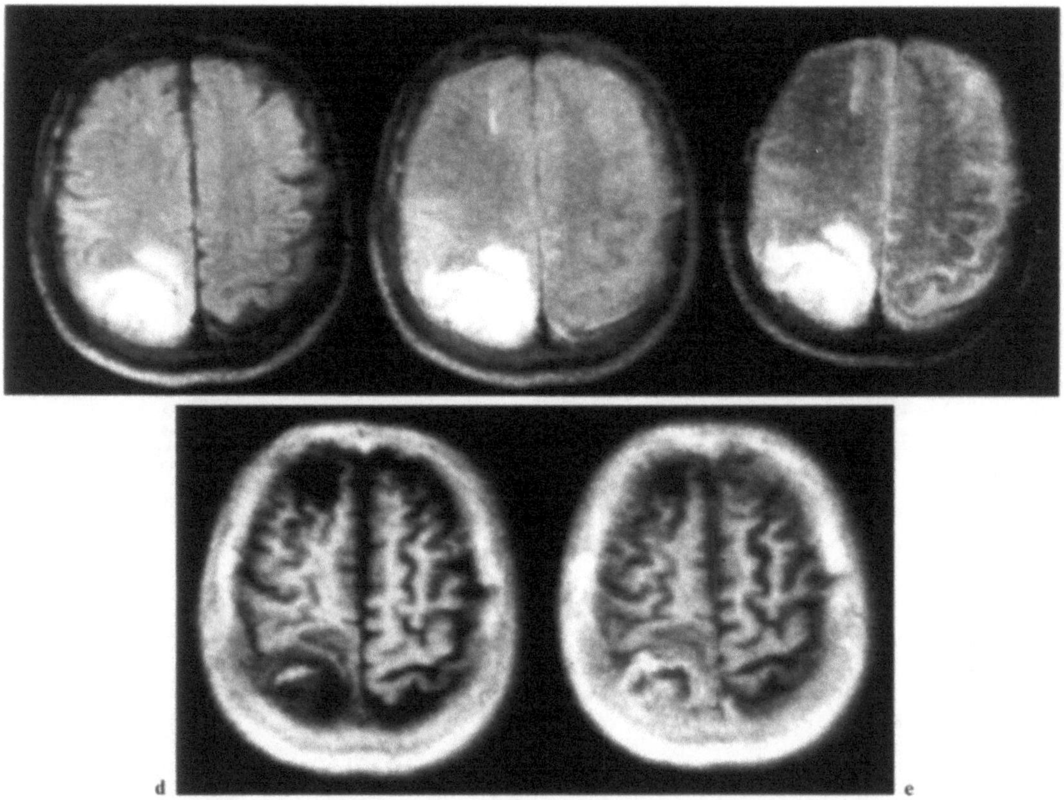

Fig. D 1.76 a–e. Glioblastoma of the left parieto-occipital region in a 70-year-old man with a 4-month history of grand mal seizures and concentration difficulties. Latent right-sided hemiparesis, right-sided hemihypesthesia. MR: **a** SE 1600/35, **b** SE 1600/70, **c** SE 1600/105, **d** IR 1500/400/35, **e** IR 1500/400/35 post Gd-DTPA. The plain IR scan shows a predominantly low-signal area which displays ring enhancement with Gd-DTPA. Findings are consistent with a left frontal arachnoidal cyst

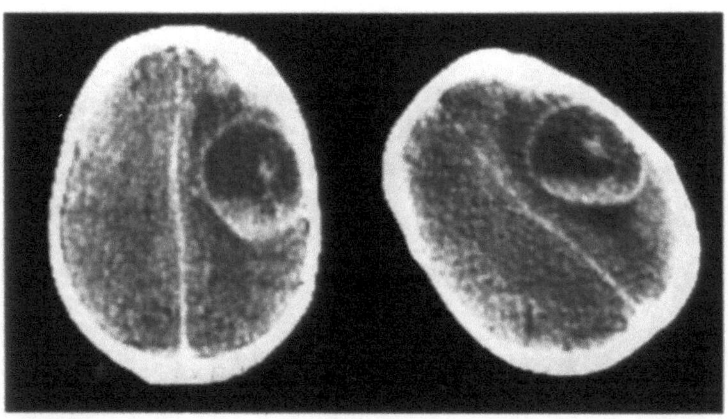

Fig. D 1.77. Glioblastoma in the right precentral region with a large cyst. Postcontrast CT shows ring enhancement of the peripheral, solid tumor components and reveals a small tumor nodule within the cyst, which contains contrast medium. A repeat scan in the oblique position demonstrates gravity-dependent sedimentation of contrast material within the cyst fluid

a–c

d–f

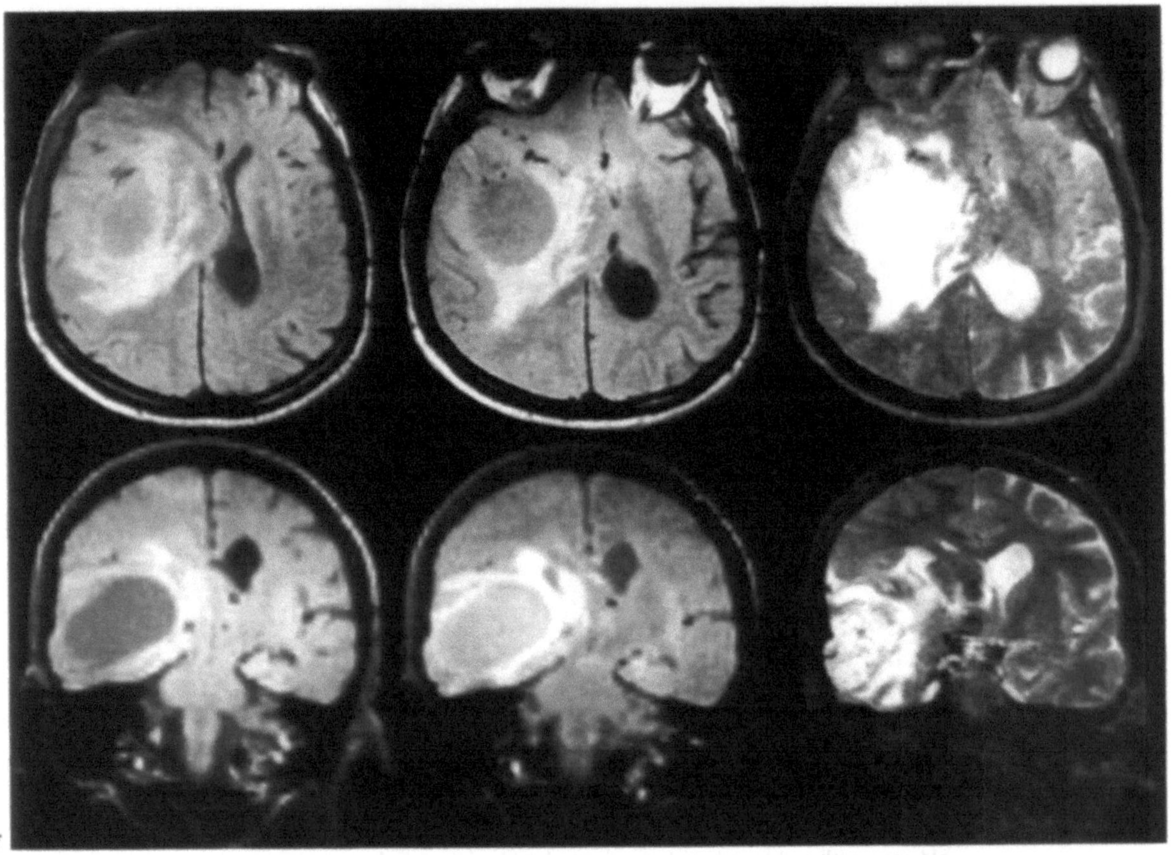

Fig. D 1.78 a–f. Large cystic glioblastoma of the left temporal region in a 56-year-old man with altered mental status and a 3-week history of headaches. MR: **a, b** SE 2500/30, **c** SE 2500/120, **d** SE 2500/30 coronal, **e** SE 1500/60 coronal, **f** SE 1500/120 coronal. The proton-density image shows a large basal lesion of mixed signal intensity, which at a lower level (**b, d**) is seen to contain a round, cystic area of relatively low signal intensity. The T2-weighted image (**c**) shows a marked homogeneous signal increase. The cyst is no longer distinguishable from its surroundings (**c**). In **f** the tumor is well delineated by a relatively hypointense zone. It is surrounded by a high-signal area representing edema

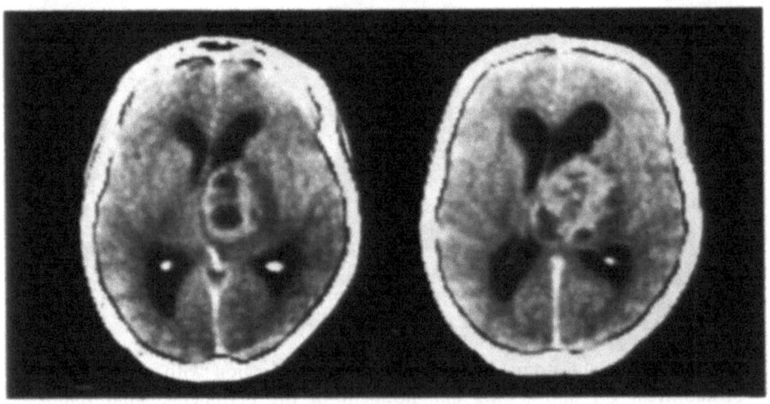

Fig. D 1.79. Large glioblastoma of the right basal ganglion region with obstruction of CSF flow in a 56-year-old male. There is minimal development of perifocal edema due to lack of contact with the cerebral white matter. Postcontrast CT

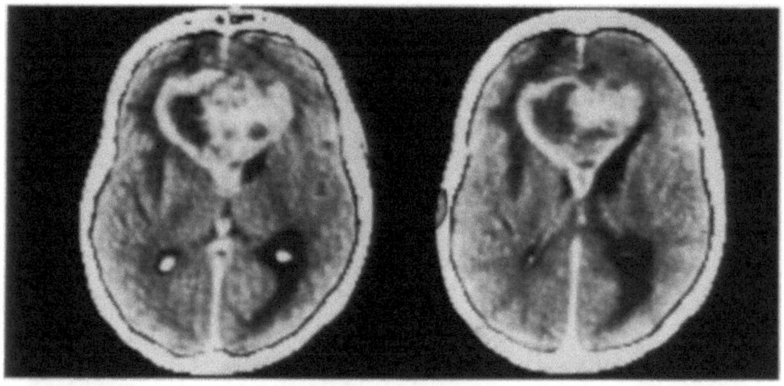

Fig. D 1.80. Butterfly glioblastoma in the area of the anterior corpus callosum with involvement of the septum pellucidum. The tumor displays a mixed density pattern on the unenhanced CT scan with slight evidence of peripheral calcification. The postcontrast scan demonstrates the entire extent of the neoplasm, which contains numerous foci of necrosis

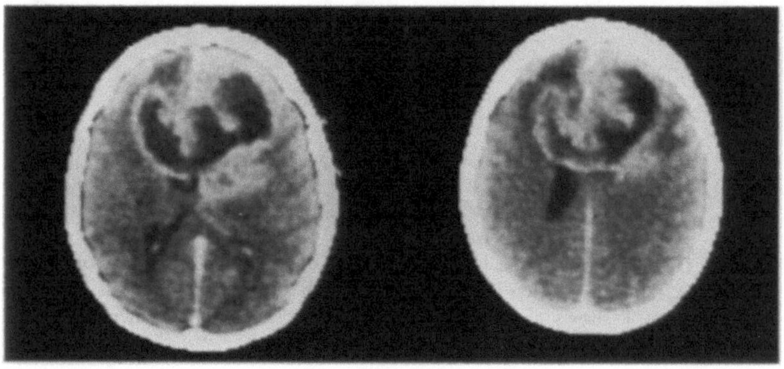

Fig. D 1.81. Butterfly glioblastoma in the anterior portions of the corpus callosum in a 64-year-old woman with altered mental status (postcontrast scans). The solid parts of the tumor show intense contrast enhancement, while central necrotic areas do not enhance

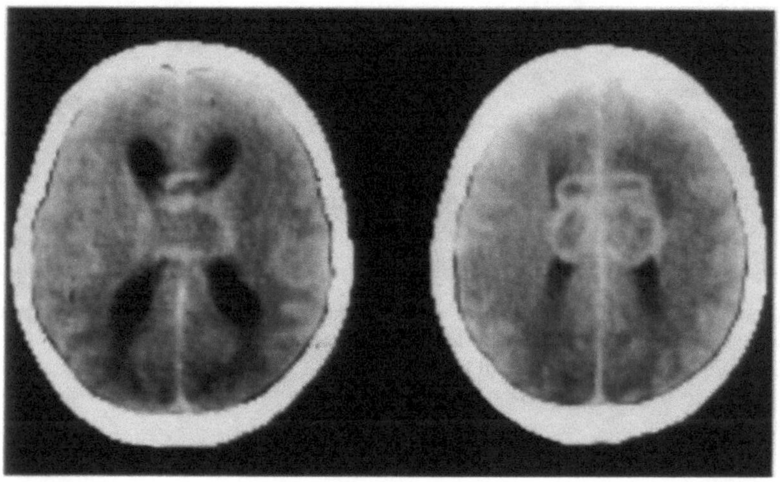

Fig. D 1.82. Glioblastoma in the central portions of the corpus callosum showing a typical garland pattern of contrast enhancement

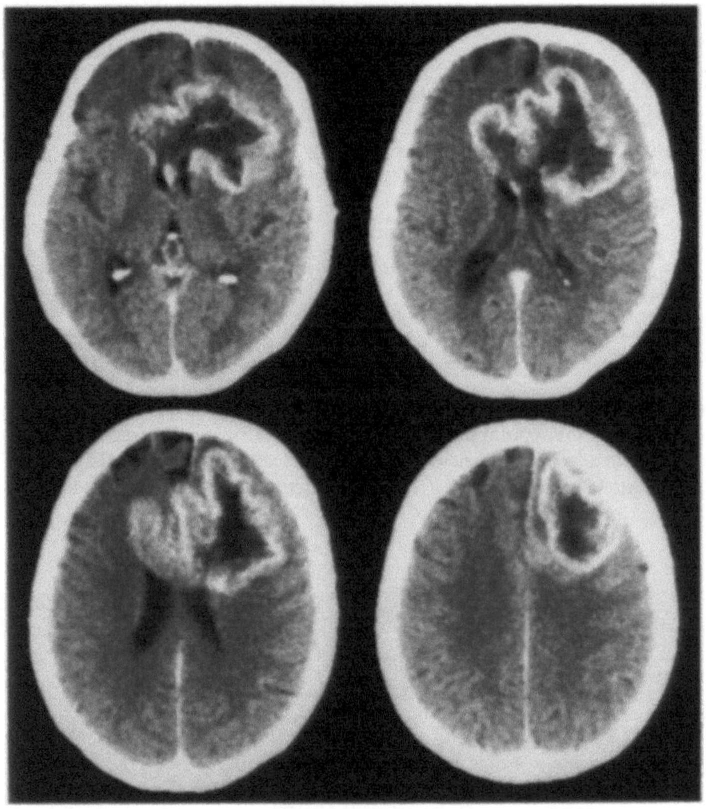

Fig. D 1.83. Glioblastoma involving mainly the right anterior part of the corpus callosum in a 66-year-old woman with altered mental status. Postcontrast CT shows a peripheral, garland pattern of enhancement at all levels; central necrosis

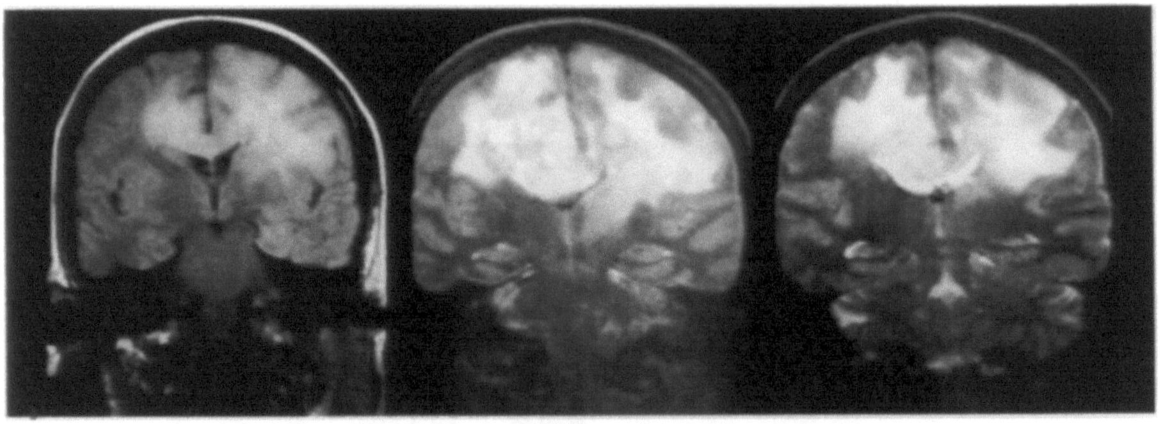

Fig. D 1.84. Glioblastoma of the corpus callosum in a 50-year-old woman with altered mental status. MR: *left* SE 2500/30, *center* SE 2000/90, *right* SE 1500/120, all coronal. The tumor gives a very intense signal as T2 weighting is increased

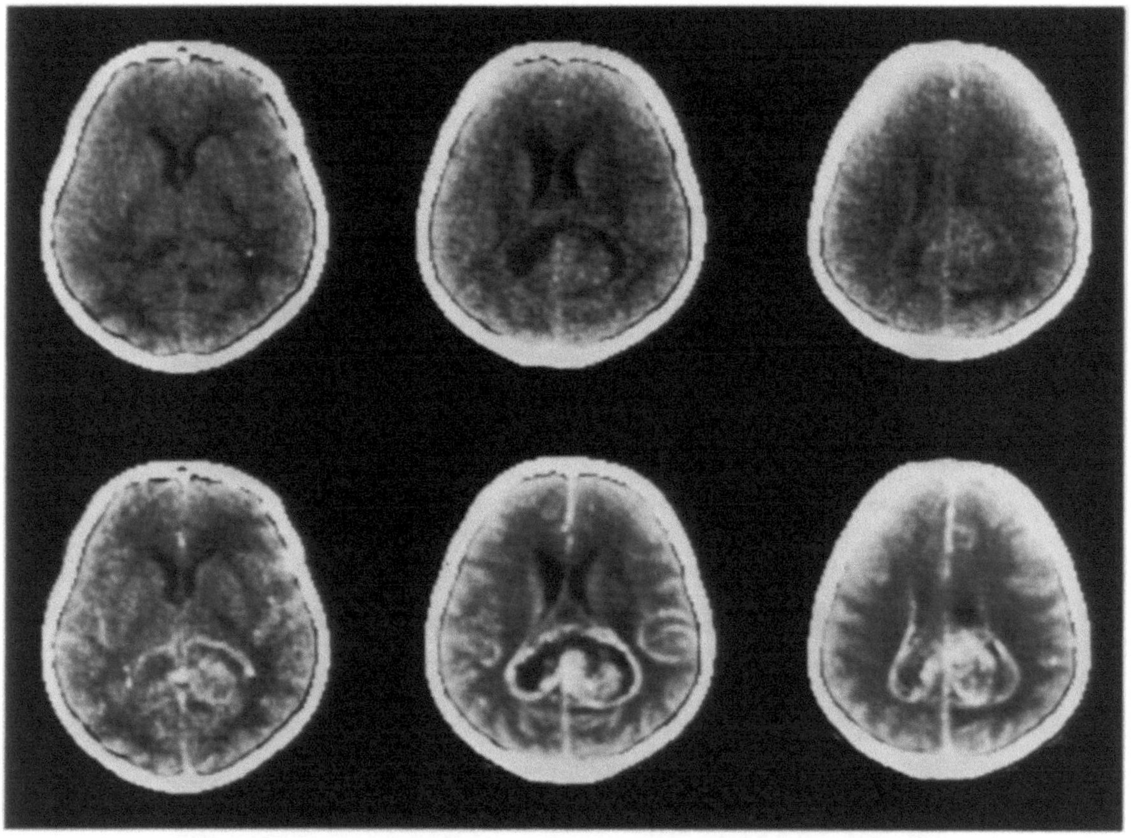

Fig. D 1.85. Glioblastoma of the posterior corpus callosum and quadrigeminal region in a 58-year-old man. The enhancement pattern on the postcontrast scans (*bottom* row) is typical of glioblastoma

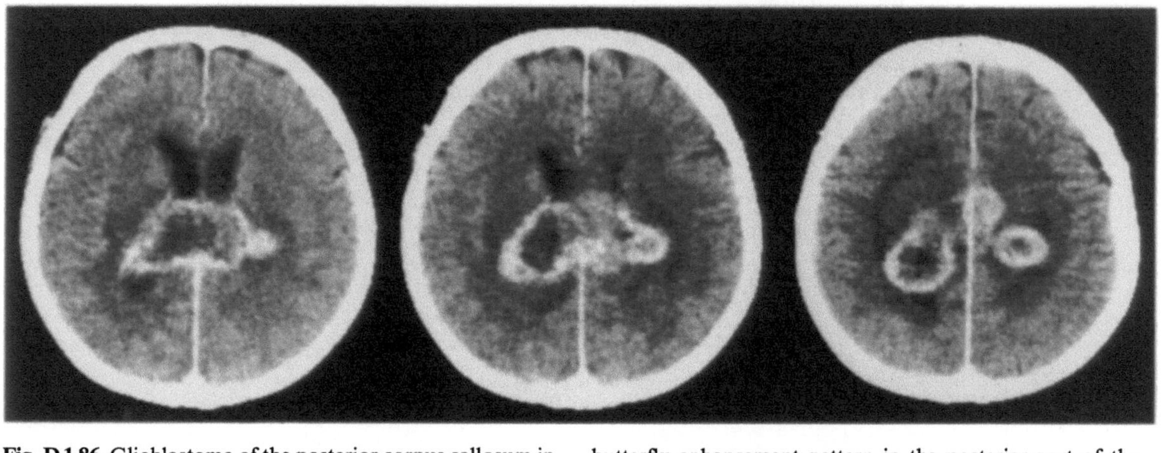

Fig. D 1.86. Glioblastoma of the posterior corpus callosum in a 40-year-old woman with progressive altered mental status. Neurologic exam was negative. Postcontrast CT shows a butterfly enhancement pattern in the posterior part of the corpus callosum. The hypodense areas represent necrotic tumor components

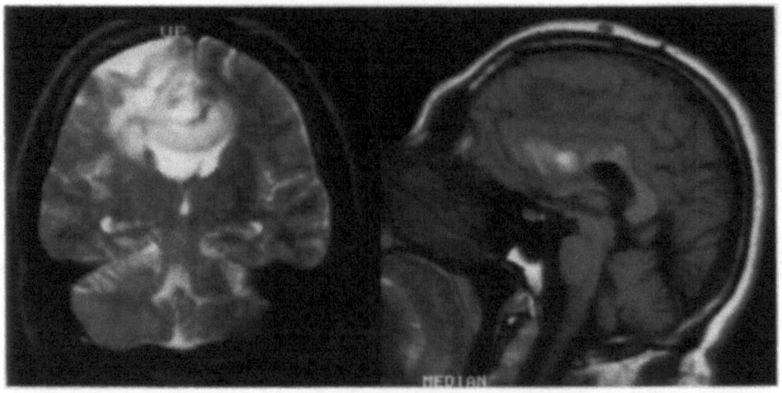

Fig. D1.87. Glioblastoma of the anterior corpus callosum in a 46-year-old man with headaches and altered mental status. MR: *left* SE 2500/100 coronal, *right* SE 500/17 midsagittal. The anterior part of the corpus callosum, infiltrated and expanded by tumor, is clearly appreciated on the T2-weighted scan (*left*). Intratumoral hemorrhage is apparent (*right*)

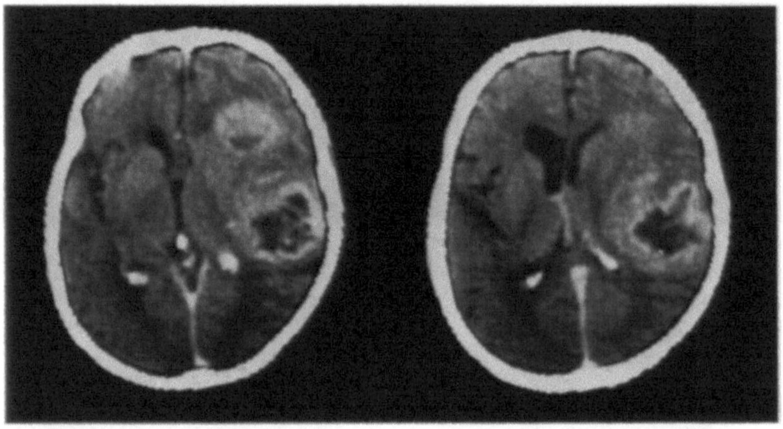

Fig. D1.88. Multifocal glioblastoma. The discrete tumor nodules are clearly delineated in the right frontal white matter and right temporal lobe. Diagnosis was confirmed histologically. Postcontrast CT

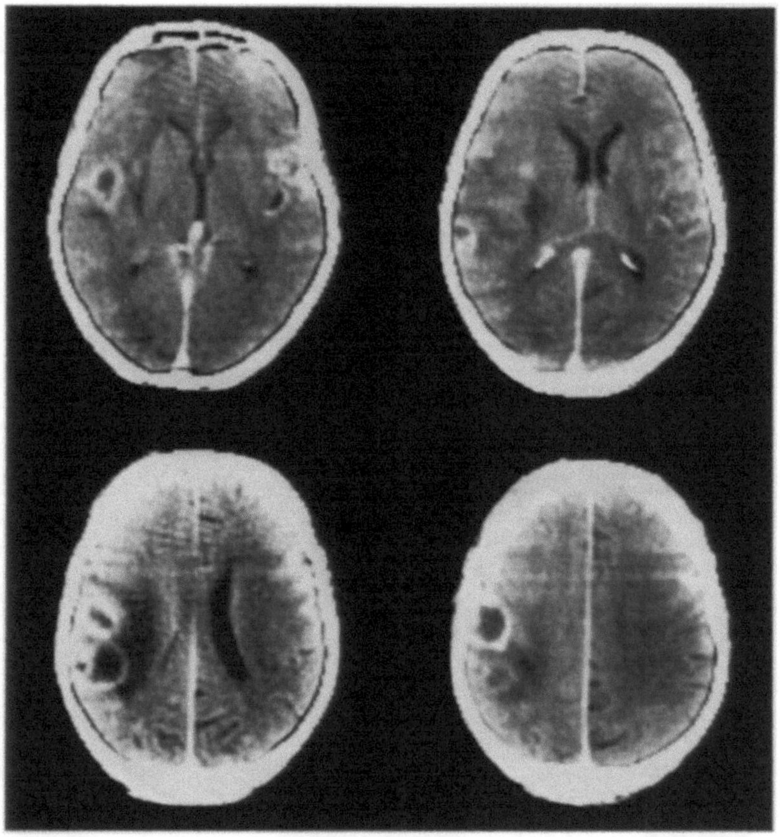

Fig. D 1.89. Multifocal glioblastoma of the left temporoparietal region and right temporal lobe in a 60-year-old woman. CT findings are consistent with multiple metastases. Diagnosis was confirmed by histologic examination. Postcontrast study

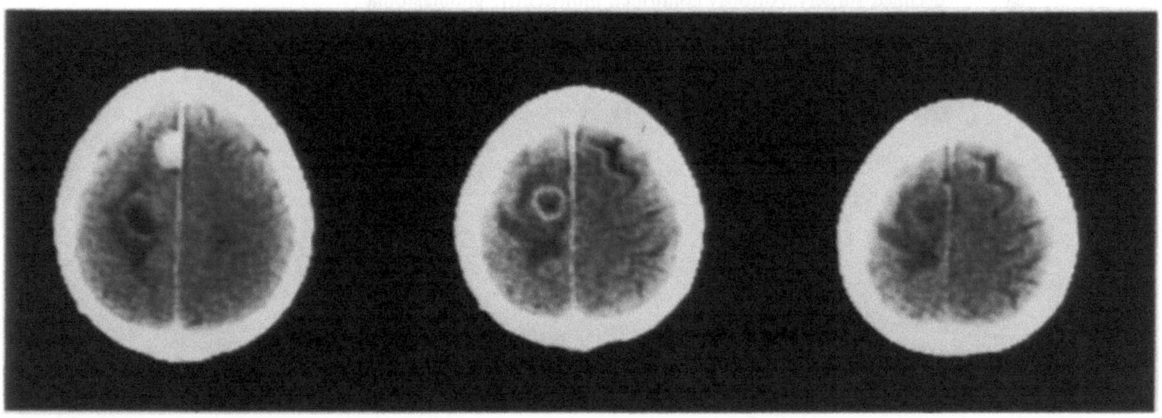

Fig. D 1.90. Multiple tumors of the left hemisphere adjacent to the interhemispheric fissure in an 85-year-old woman with slowly progressive right-sided hemiparesis. Postcontrast CT shows a small glioblastoma in the left central region with ring enhancement and associated grade I–II perifocal edema. Anterior to it is a small, homogeneously enhancing falx meningioma producing no symptoms. Both diagnoses were confirmed histologically

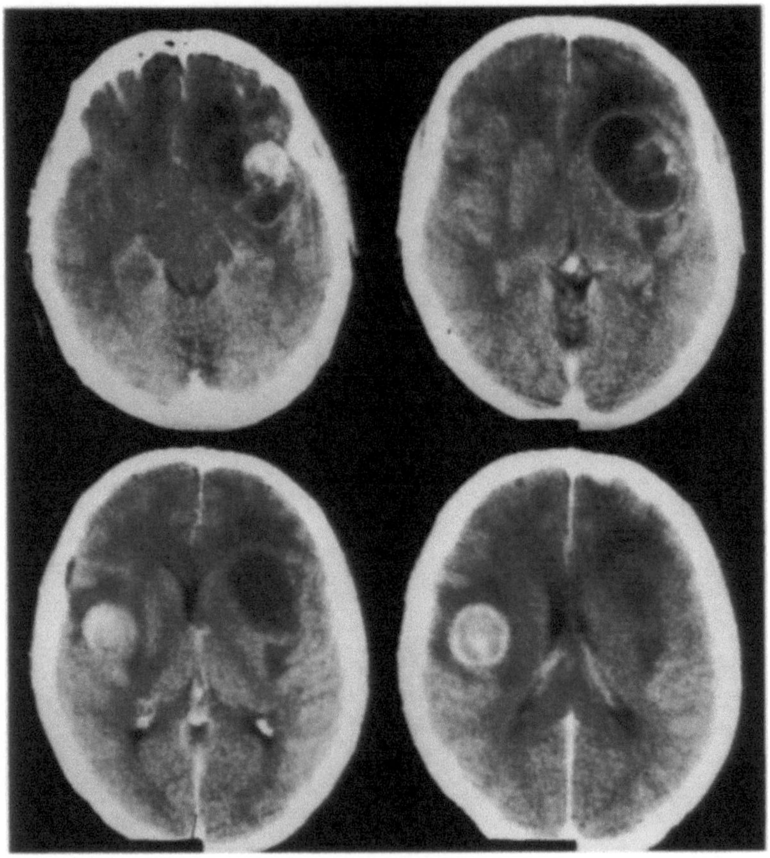

Fig. D1.91. Multicentric glioblastoma multiforme in a 69-year-old man with facial paresis, dysphagia, and dysarthria. Postcontrast CT demonstrates partly hypodense and partly hyperdense, circumscribed lesions in the right fronto-central and left parietal regions with marked perifocal edema. The patient declined surgery. Autopsy confirmed multicentric glioblastoma

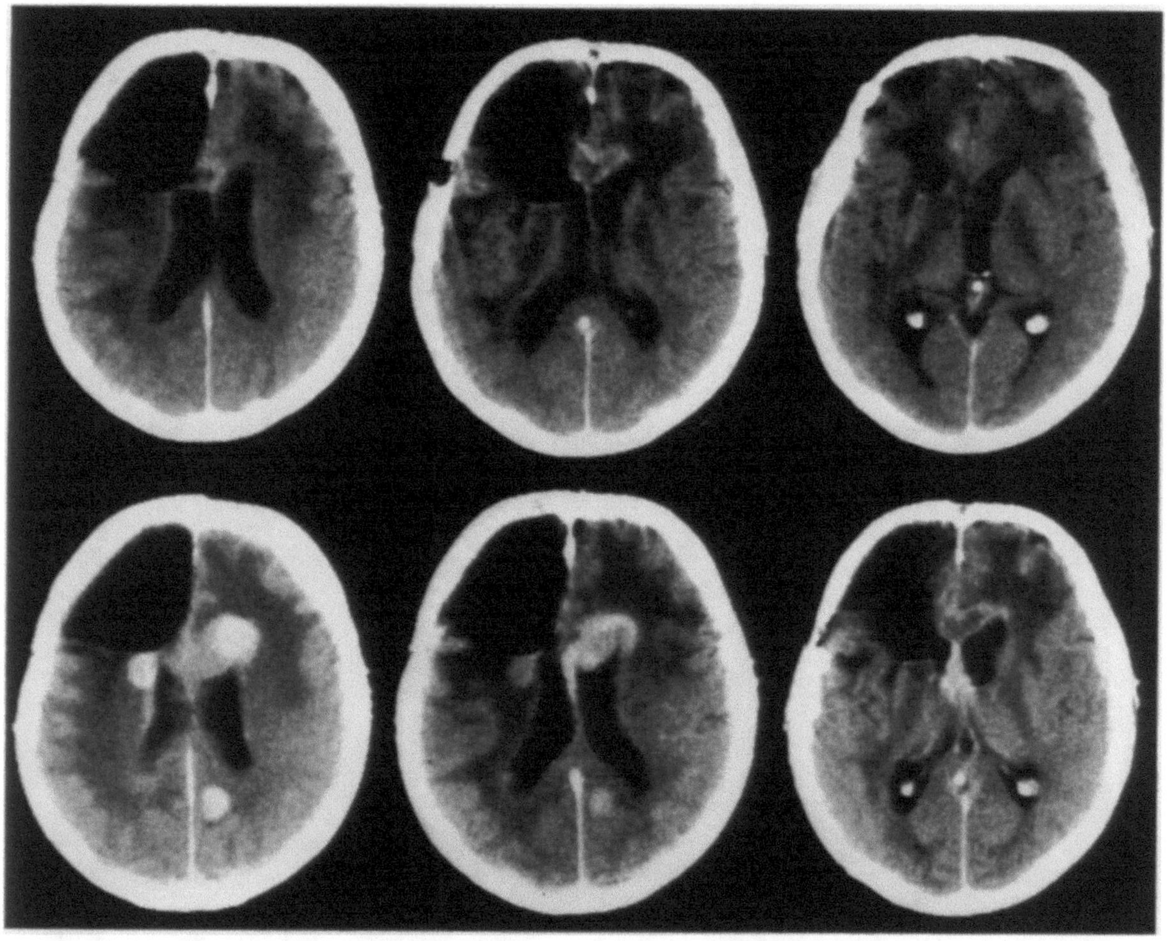

Fig. D 1.92. Recurrence of glioblastoma in the left frontal region of a 49-year-old man with right-sided hemiparesis. CT: *top row* postcontrast, *bottom row* postcontrast 2 months later. Adjacent to the large extirpation defect we observe continued tumor growth through the anterior corpus callosum toward the right side. Follow-up scans reveal further expansion along the ventricle wall and septum pellucidum with increased contrast enhancement. The scan at *lower left* demonstrates an additional tumor in the right parasagittal area

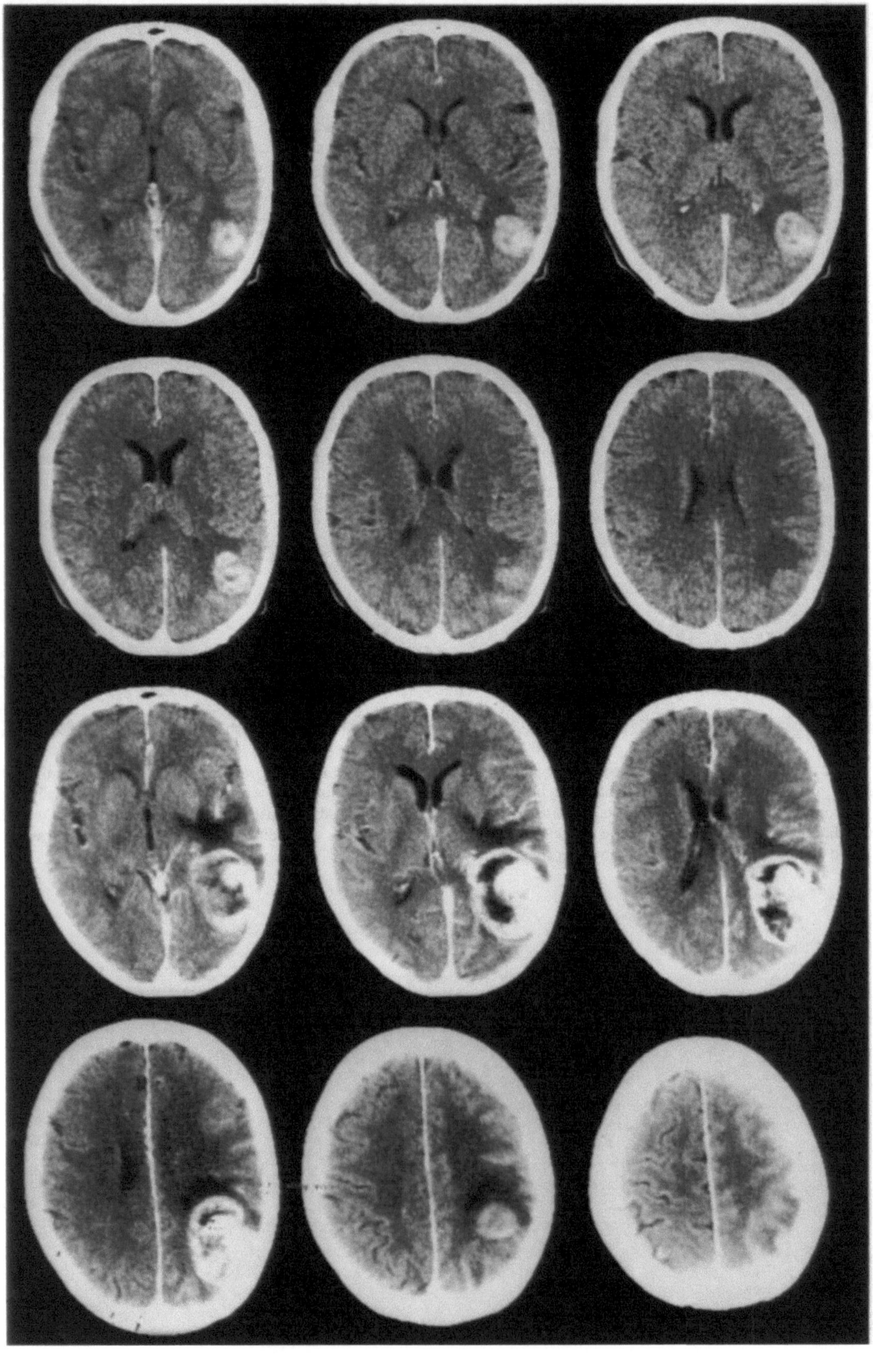

a–c

d–f

g–i

j–l

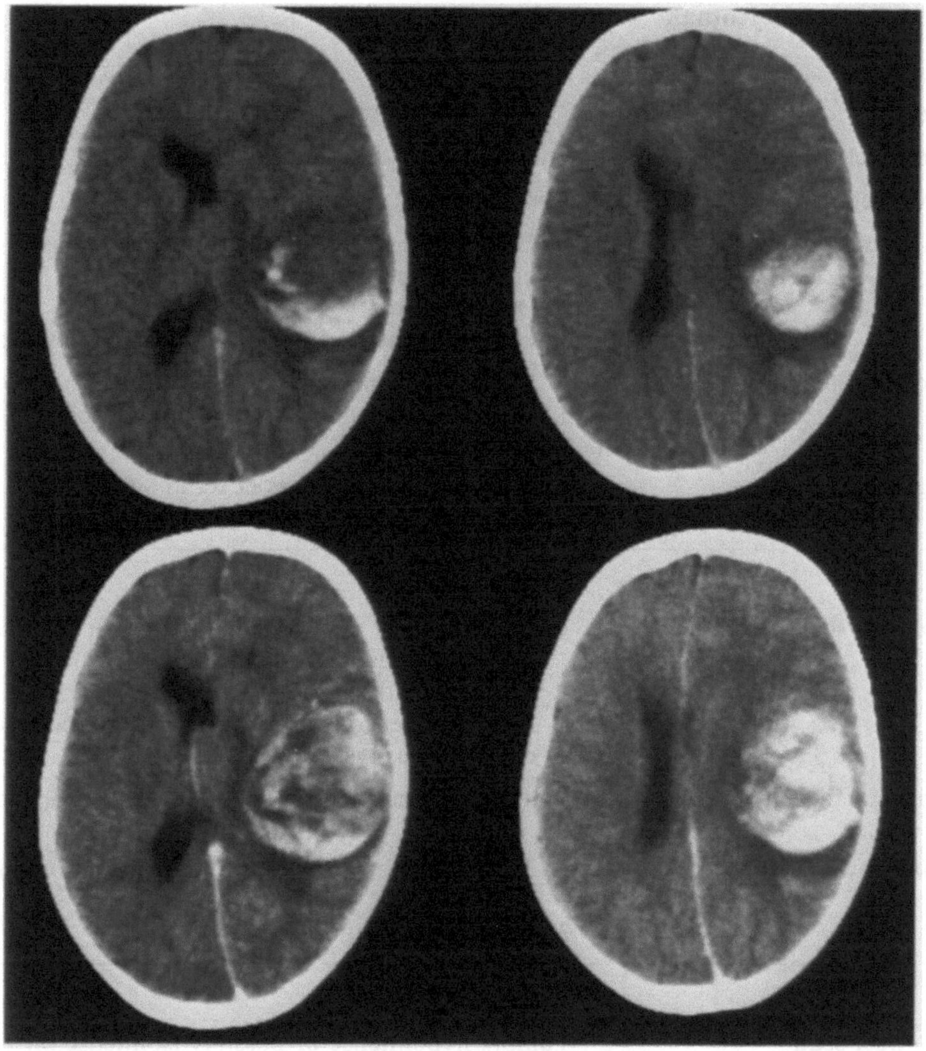

Fig. D 1.94. Gliosarcoma in a 7-year-old boy whose leukemia had responded well to therapy for 3 years. Patient was admitted with left-sided hemiparesis and somnolence of sudden onset. Plain CT scans (*top*) demonstrate a large mass lesion in the right temporal region. Hemorrhage is apparent within the mass. Postcontrast CT (*bottom*) shows marked enhancement of the tumor with mild perifocal edema

◄

Fig. D 1.93 a–l. Glioblastoma multiforme in a 57-year-old woman with left-sided paresis and altered mental status. The initial postcontrast CT examination in October of 1986 (**a–f**) shows an enhancing, circumscribed mass in the right parietal area with moderate associated edema in the right hemisphere. The patient declined surgical treatment. She was readmitted in February of 1987 with marked clinical deterioration and increased paresis. Postcontrast scans at that time (**g–l**) showed significant enlargement of the mass, which enhanced more intensely. A hypodense necrotic area is visible within the tumor. Edematous changes in the right hemisphere are more pronounced, and there is obvious mass effect

g) Pilocytic Astrocytomas

Incidence	3%–6% of all brain tumors
Age predilection	First and second decades of life
Sex predilection	Approximately equal distribution
Typical sites	1. Cerebellum, vermis, fourth ventricle, pons, quadrigeminal region 2. Optic chiasm 3. Less frequently, cerebrum (especially temporal lobe)
Main clinical features	Site 1. Headache, vomiting, ataxia Site 2. Visual impairment, hypothalamic deficits Site 3. Seizures
Angiography	Nonspecific signs of mass effect at sites 1 and 3; tumors at site 2 visualized only if large
CT	
Noncontrast scan	1. Hypodense or rarely isodense area, or combination of both; occasional calcification 2. Predominantly iso- or hyperdense 3. Nonhomogeneous absorption pattern, occasional calcification, cysts
Contrast enhancement	Marked enhancement in solid, uncalcified portions of the tumor
Postcontrast appearance	1., 3. Solid tumor nodules, some with cyst or ring formation 2. Usually solid tumor pattern
MR	
Noncontrast scan	Tumors hypointense or possibly isointense on T1-weighted images. T2-weighted images show increasing signal intensity, with cysts appearing uniformly bright; calcifications appear as signal void
Gadolinium enhancement	Moderate to good
Post Gd-DTPA appearance	Homogeneous enhancement of solid tumor components

Differential diagnosis

Site 1. Atypical medulloblastoma, ependymoma
Angioblastoma
Cerebellar abscess

Site 2. Craniopharyngioma
Pituitary adenoma

Site 3. Anaplastic astrocytoma
Glioblastoma
Oligodendroglioma
Gangliocytoma
Metastasis

Tumors previously described under the following headings are now grouped together as pilocytic astrocytoma because of their common histologic features: *cystic and solid cerebellar astrocytoma, cerebellar spongioblastoma, polar spongioblastoma, optic nerve glioma, hypothalamic glioma, juvenile-type astrocytoma, and infundibuloma.*

Total removal of pilocytic astrocytoma from the cerebral hemispheres or cerebellum is curative, hence the tumor is classified as grade I.

An incidence of 6%–7% is reported for pilocytic astrocytoma in the literature (Zülch 1975; Cushing 1932). The incidence in our series was only 2.7%. Pilocytic astrocytomas occur at all ages but show a predilection for children and adolescents. Males and females are affected with about equal frequency.

Typical Sites

Pilocytic astrocytomas occur most commonly in the *cerebellar region* (vermis, cerebellar hemispheres, fourth ventricle, caudal brainstem). They are the third most common neoplasm of the *chiasmal* region. Less common sites are the *cerebral hemispheres*, especially the medial portions of the temporal lobes, the *basal ganglia*, and the *quadrigeminal region.*

Main Clinical Features

Various symptoms may predominate depending on the location of the tumor: headache, vomiting, and ataxia are characteristic of cerebellar lesions. Visual disturbances indicate involvement of the optic nerve or optic chiasm, while spread to the hypothalamus produces diencephalic disturbances with cachexia, especially in early childhood. Seizures are characteristic of cerebral tumors.

Additional Diagnostic Procedures

Plain skull radiographs show general signs of intracranial hypertension only when the tumor is located in the posterior fossa. Tumor calcifications are occasionally seen.

Angiograms can demonstrate vascular displacement caused by pilocytic astrocytoma but cannot contribute to the pathologic diagnosis.

Computed Tomography

(Figs. D 1.95–101, 103–107, 113–116, 118–121, 124–126, D 6.8)

Noncontrast Scan

The density pattern of pilocytic astrocytomas varies greatly as a result of frequent cyst formation and calcification.

1. Posterior Fossa, Pons and Quadrigeminal Region (Figs. D 1.95–101, 103–107, 125, 126). Scans typically show a large, smooth-bordered hypodensity in which solid tumor components are identifiable even without contrast enhancement. These solid areas are usually hypodense and occasionally isodense to surrounding cerebellar tissue.

The more hypodense areas usually represent cysts (18–20 HU) or perifocal edema (18–26 HU). Areas of very high density signify intratumoral hemorrhage or calcification (Figs. D 1.103, 107).

The fourth ventricle is usually compressed and is often displaced laterally by the neoplasm. With low-sited tumors the ventricle may appear enlarged or deformed on the upper cerebellar scans. When the tumor extends quite high, the fourth ventricle may not be visible on the CT scan. Tumors occasionally appear within the fourth ventricle, completely surrounded by CSF (see Fig. D 1.104). In these cases the origin of the tumor is not appreciated. Usually the ventricular system is greatly expanded, and it is common to see periventricular lucency, especially around the frontal horns.

2. Chiasmal Region (Figs. D 1.116, G 16). In most isodense pilocytic astrocytomas of this region, the suspicion of tumor rests mainly on the absence or partial visualization of the opticochiasmatic cistern or third ventricle on the plain CT scan. Calcifications may be present, and small cysts are occasionally observed. If the tumor extends far upward, unilateral or bilateral ventricular expansion will be seen due to obstruction of the foramen of Monro. Perifocal edema is absent. A tumor that spreads from the chiasm to the optic nerve, or vice versa, will produce corresponding optic nerve changes that are clearly displayed on the CT scan (see Figs. G 14–16).

3. Cerebral Hemispheres and Basal Ganglia (Figs. D 1.113–115, 118–121, 124). The density pattern is extremely diverse and ranges from hypodense in cystic tumors to isodense in solid tumors and hyperdense in calcified lesions. Solid, isodense tumors are visible on plain scans only if they coexist with perifocal edema or calcifications or if a tumor of the quadrigeminal region has produced hydrocephalus. However, *perifocal brain edema is seen in only 25% of pilocytic astrocytomas, less frequently than in any other tumors of the cerebral hemispheres.*

Postcontrast Scan

With few exceptions, pilocytic astrocytomas show marked contrast enhancement in their solid, uncalcified portions. The density increase after a standard contrast dose ranges from 12 to 14 HU. The enhancement persists for some time.

Enhancement of the solid, uncalcified tumor components makes it easier to recognize cystic elements and perifocal edema. Ring patterns may be observed (see Fig. D 1.118).

It is our experience that *pilocytic astrocytomas of the cerebellum may present any of the following three patterns*:

1. Large cyst with a peripheral tumor nodule
2. Large solid tumor with a cyst and a peripheral ring of variable thickness
3. Solid, relatively small tumor without a cyst

Magnetic Resonance Imaging

(Figs. D 1.101, 102, 108–112, 117, 122, 123)

Noncontrast Scan

Variations in the histologic structure of pilocytic astrocytoma lead to the appearance of hypo-, iso-, and hyperintense areas on T1- and T2-weighted images which represent cystic and solid tumor components. Large calcifications appear as signal voids.

1. Posterior Fossa, Pons, Quadrigeminal Region (Figs. D 1.101, 102, 108–112, 117). Cystic components appear as well-defined hypointensities on T1-weighted images and as very hyperintense areas on T2-weighted sequences. An advantage of MR over CT is its ability to demonstrate the exact spatial relationship of the tumor to neighboring structures, especially the pons, fourth ventricle, and quadrigeminal plate. CSF spaces give a bright signal on heavily T2-weighted sequences.

2. Chiasmal Region. The tumor usually gives a low signal and causes amputation or obstruction of the opticochiasmatic cistern or third ventricle. Sagittal and paramedian scans greatly facilitate diagnosis compared with CT.

3. Cerebral Hemispheres and Basal Ganglia (Figs. D 1.122, 123). The patterns are the same as in CT, although additional information can be gained by scanning in projections not available with CT.

Postcontrast Appearance

The patterns on post Gd-DTPA scans are the same as on enhanced CT scans but are improved by the spatial information yielded by MR. Contrast enhancement is moderate to good.

Differential Diagnosis

It should be stated at the outset that MR contributes little, compared with CT, to solving the problems of differential diagnosis.

1. Posterior Fossa. The main lesion to be differentiated in this region is atypical *medulloblastoma* with primarily isodense or even hypodense absorption values. These tumors are very rare, however. Medulloblastomas and pilocytic astrocytomas show about equal degrees of contrast enhancement, but their washout kinetics differ markedly (see p. 189).

Pilocytic astrocytomas of the fourth ventricle can be difficult to distinguish from *ependymoma* when the latter is uncalcified. We found no case in our series where a calcified pilocytic astrocytoma was located in the fourth ventricle.

Angioblastomas can present identical CT features, but these tumors mainly affect middle-aged individuals and are decidedly rare in the pediatric age group (only 2 of 41 angioblastomas in our population). Angioblastomas enhance much more densely than pilocytic astrocytomas owing to their rich vascularity.

Cerebellar abscesses can simulate the CT appearance of a pilocytic astrocytoma with ring enhancement (see Fig. F 4). Differentiation relies on the history and clinical findings.

2. Chiasmal Region. CT is of little help in differentiating *craniopharyngiomas* of this region from pilocytic astrocytomas when calcification exists. This is true even when clinical parameters (roentgenograms, endocrinology) are taken into account.

Suprasellar *pituitary adenomas* are readily distinguishable from a pilocytic astrocytoma of the optic chiasm or hypothalamus by means of endocrinologic and radiographic studies.

3. Cerebral Hemispheres. Pilocytic astrocytomas of the cerebral hemispheres have such a variety of CT presentations that we can point to no features distinguishing them from other tumors. If the tumor is confined to the medial temporal lobe, differential diagnosis is limited to *gangliocytoma* and *meningioma.*

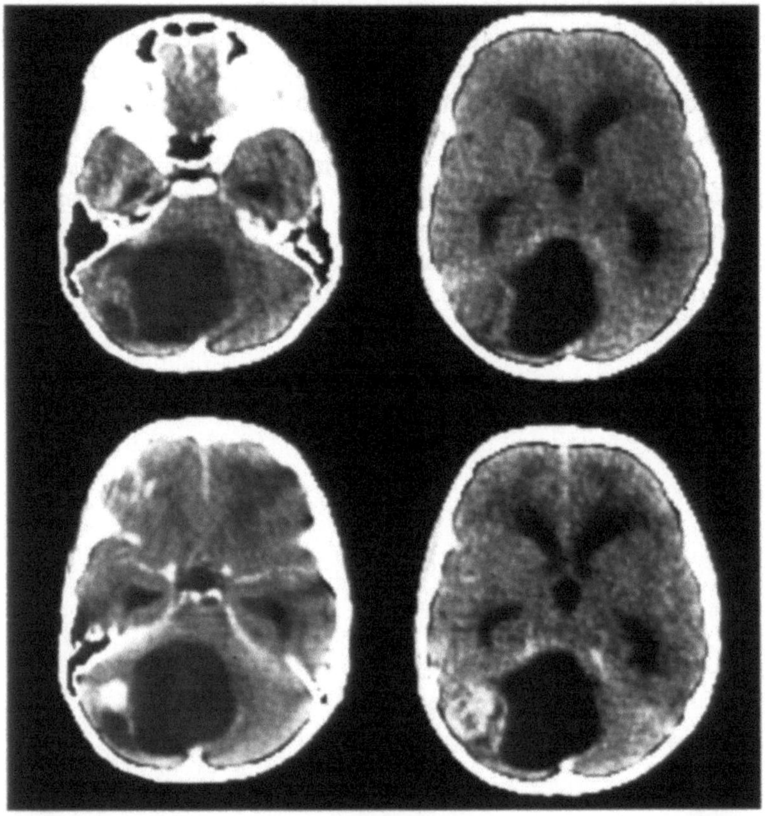

D1.95

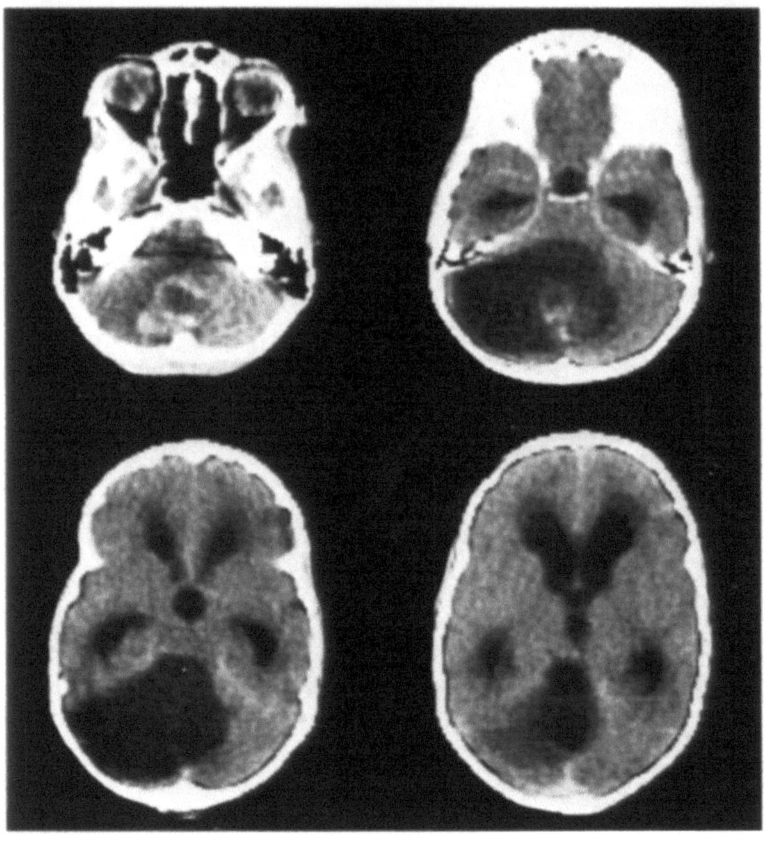

D1.96

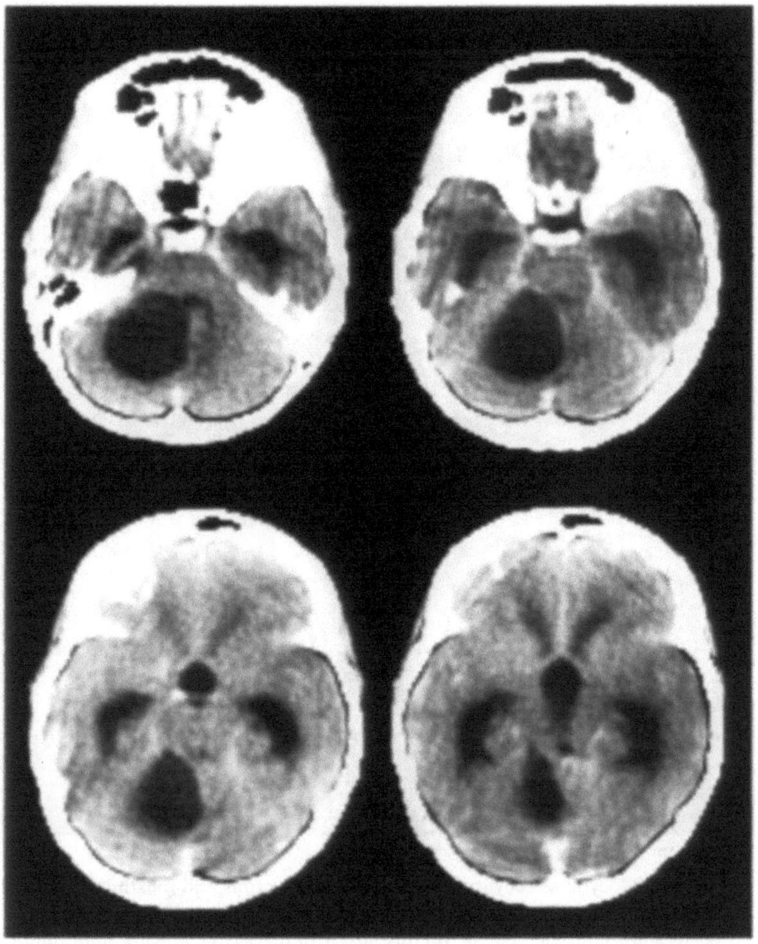

Fig. D 1.97. Pilocytic astrocytoma involving the left cerebellar hemisphere and caudal brainstem in a 30-year-old woman. CT shows a clearly delineated hypodense area representing a cyst but does not reveal the solid tumor nodule that has invaded the caudal brainstem. The most likely misdiagnosis would be angioblastoma. Postcontrast scans

Fig. D 1.95. Pilocytic astrocytoma in a 10-year-old boy with left-sided cerebellar symptoms. Plain CT scans (*top*) show a large cystic lesion in the posterior cranial fossa, mainly involving the left side. Postcontrast scans (*bottom*) show an enhancing solid tumor at the left lateral border of the cyst. The actual tumor tissue exhibits slightly hypodense values on densitometry. There is expansion of the ventricular system and slight periventricular lucency

Fig. D 1.96. Pilocytic astrocytoma of the cerebellum in a 12-year-old girl with cerebellar symptoms. The large cystic mass almost completely fills the left side of the posterior cranial fossa and projects across the midline. Scans at lower levels of the cerebellum demonstrate a nodular mass at the border of the cyst with central hypodensity. The tumor appeared slightly hypodense on the plain CT scans. These postcontrast scans reveal pronounced hydrocephalus with slight periventricular lucency

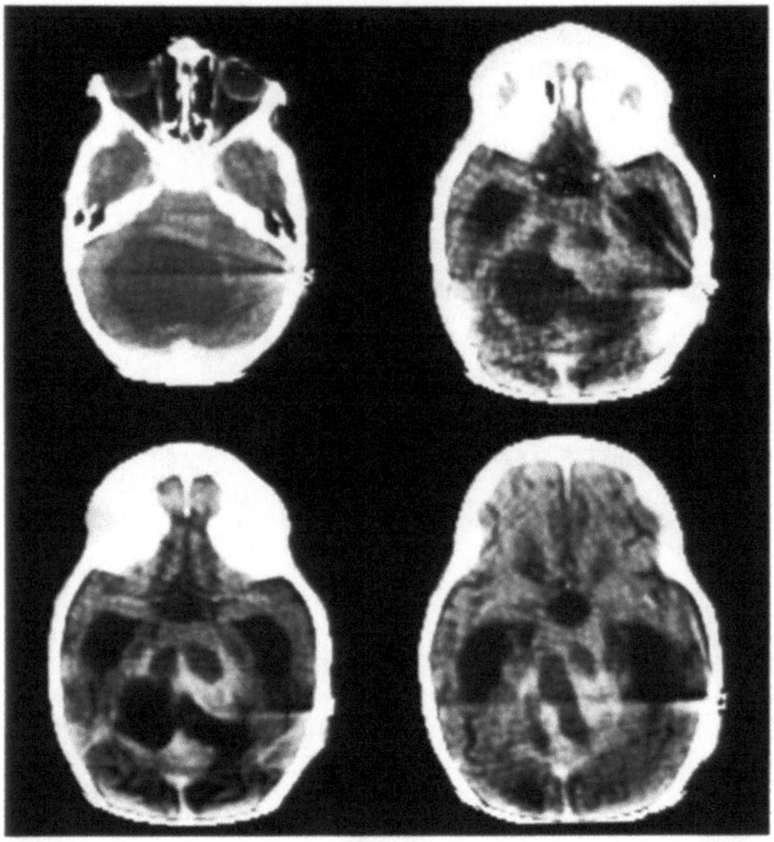

Fig. D 1.98. Pilocytic astrocytoma of the cerebellar vermis and fourth ventricle in an infant 6 months after insertion of a CSF shunt (artifacts). These postcontrast CT scans show multiple cysts of varying size with densely enhancing solid tumor intervening. Differentiation of tumor from brainstem is not possible. The tumor, which originated from the roof of the fourth ventricle, was completely removed at operation. It had greatly expanded and distorted the fourth ventricle but had not infiltrated its floor. Precontrast scans showed only a large hypodensity in the posterior cranial fossa

Fig. D 1.99. Pilocytic astrocytoma of the left cerebellar hemisphere in a 15-year-old boy presenting with headache, nausea, vomiting, angled head carriage, and papilledema. Postcontrast CT scans show a hypodensity extending from the upper spinal canal into the left cerebellar hemisphere as far as the fourth ventricle, left cerebellopontine angle, and prepontine area. The tumor does not enhance but shows massive peripheral calcification

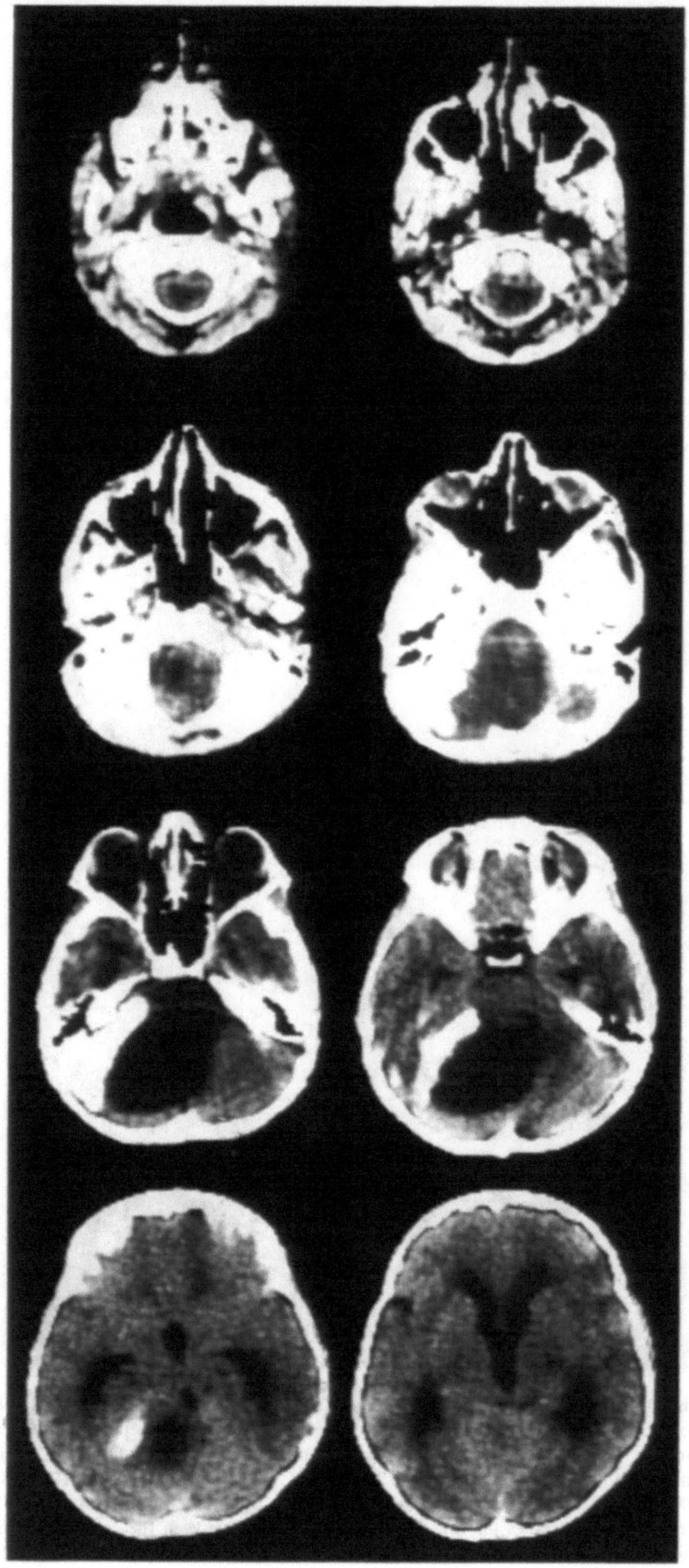

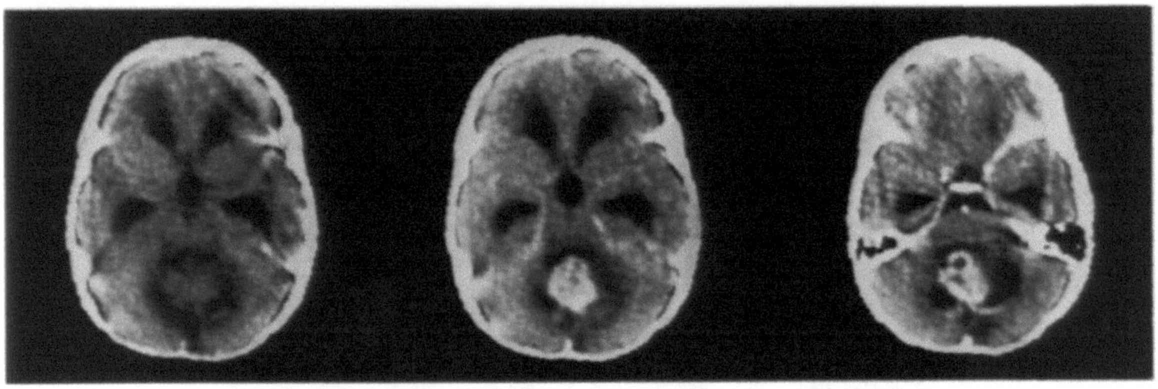

Fig. D 1.100. Pilocytic astrocytoma in the roof of the fourth ventricle and cerebellar vermis in a 9-year-old girl. The plain CT scan (*left*) shows a slightly hypodense mass with perifocal edema. The postcontrast scans (*center* and *right*) show marked enhancement with visualization of adjacent cystic components. There is moderate hydrocephalus with slight periventricular lucency. The plain scan provides the key to histologic diagnosis!

a b

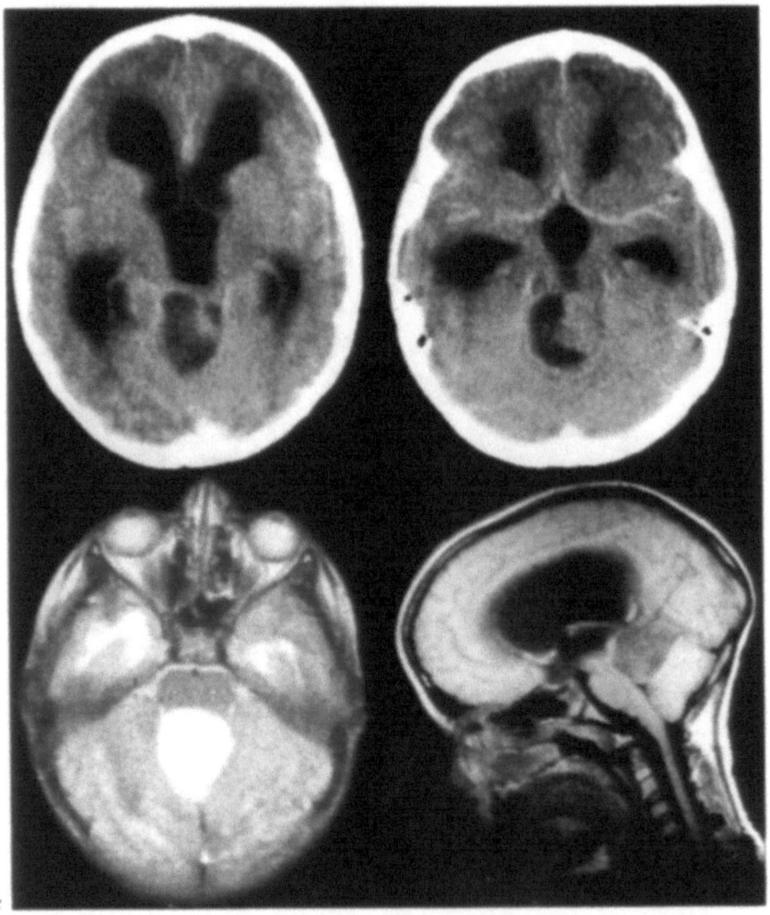

c d

Fig. D 1.101 a–d. Pilocytic astrocytoma of the fourth ventricle in a 14-year-old boy with a history of headaches, vertigo, and tinnitus in the previous several months. Patient presented with bilateral papilledema, right-sided facial paresis, and a tendency to fall toward the left side. CT: **a, b** postcontrast. MR: **c** SE 2000/34, **d** SE 500/34. Extreme hydrocephalus is apparent on all scans. The T1-weighted image shows the low-signal tumor situated between the cerebellum and third ventricle and constricting the aqueduct. Image **c** demonstrates the cystic component with high intensity. CT shows a partly solid and partly cystic mass

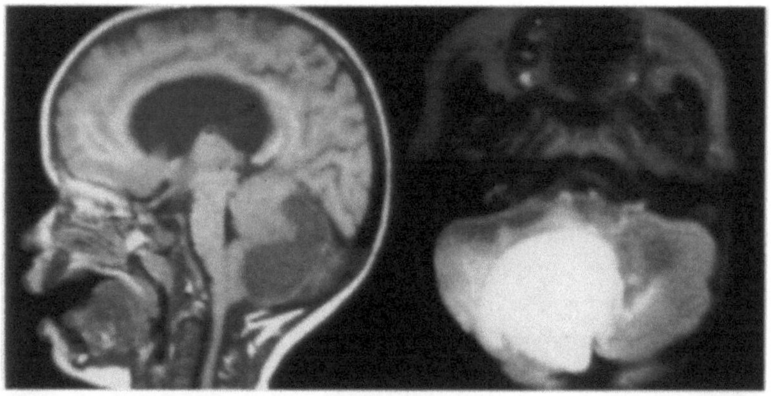

Fig. D 1.102. Grade I (!) astrocytoma of the cerebellum with a large cyst, left cerebellar hemisphere. The 6-month-old child was admitted with progressive ataxia and signs of increased intracranial pressure. MR: *left* SE 500/30, *right* SE 3000/90. The T1-weighted sagittal image (*left*) shows a clearly delineated, hypointense tumor which appears uniformly hyperintense on the T2-weighted sequence (*right*)

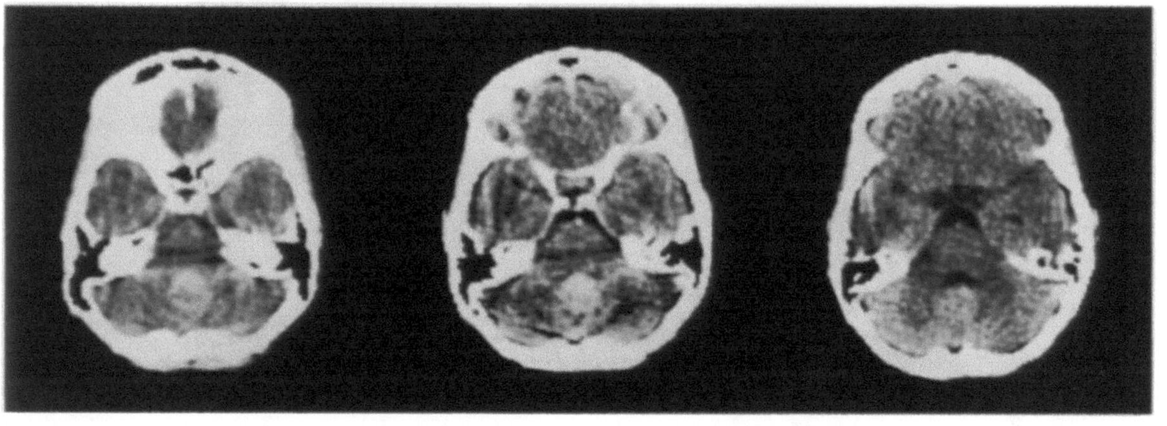

Fig. D 1.103. Pilocytic astrocytoma with hemorrhage in a 15-year-old girl presenting with symptoms of an acute subarachnoid hemorrhage. Scans demonstrate a round, cherry-size hyperdensity at the outlet of the fourth ventricle that shows no significant contrast enhancement. At operation, solid tumor was found only at the periphery of the lesion; the rest consisted of old blood

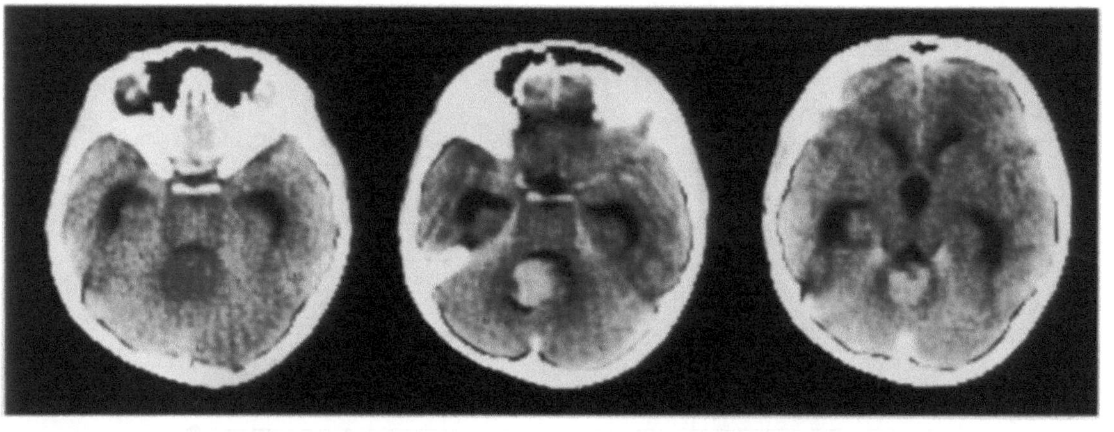

Fig. D 1.104. Pilocytic astrocytoma in an 8-year-old boy. The primarily hypodense tumor (*left*) enhances homogeneously with contrast medium. It appears to be surrounded by CSF (*center*), and its site of origin cannot be determined from CT findings. The density pattern is sufficient to suggest a histologic diagnosis. At operation the tumor was found to arise directly from the brainstem in the lower portion of the rhomboid fossa

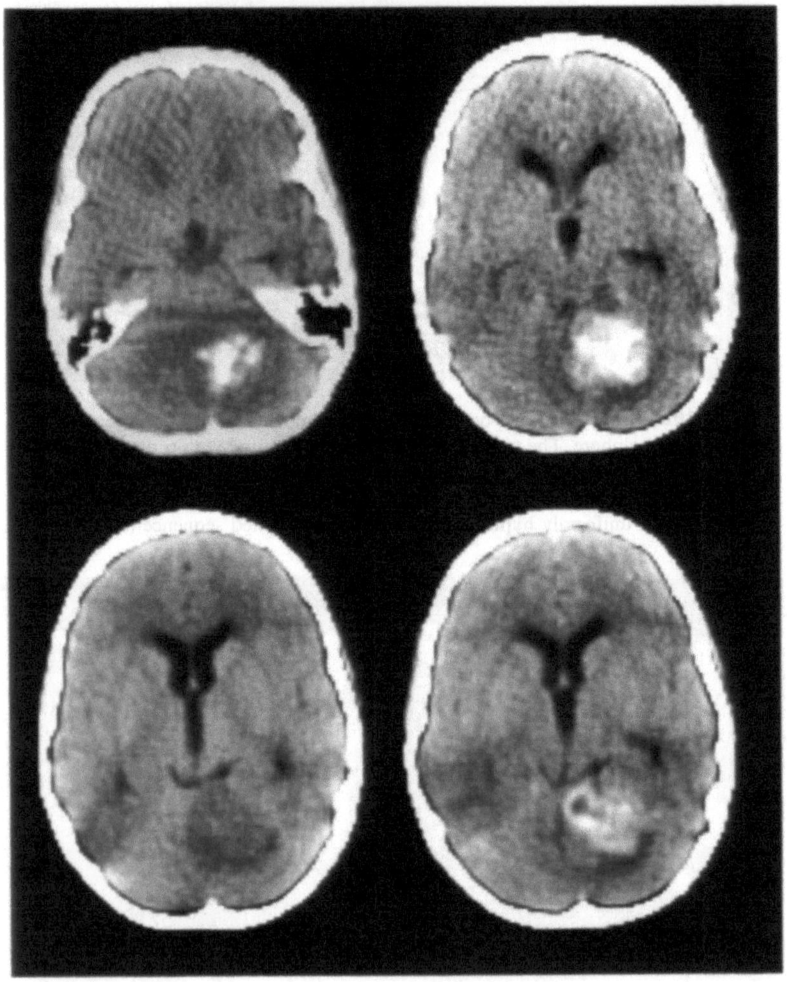

Fig. D 1.105. Pilocytic astrocytoma in the right cerebellar hemisphere of a 13-year-old girl with cerebellar symptoms. The tumor appears partly hypodense and partly calcified on the plain CT scans (*left*). The solid, uncalcified tumor components enhance very strongly with contrast medium (*right*)

Fig. D 1.107. Pilocytic astrocytoma. The 11-year-old boy presented with about a 4-week history of progressive ataxia, vomiting, and headaches. Noncontrast CT scans show an irregularly shaped mass of calcific density with a central lucency in the region of the fourth ventricle, which cannot be discerned

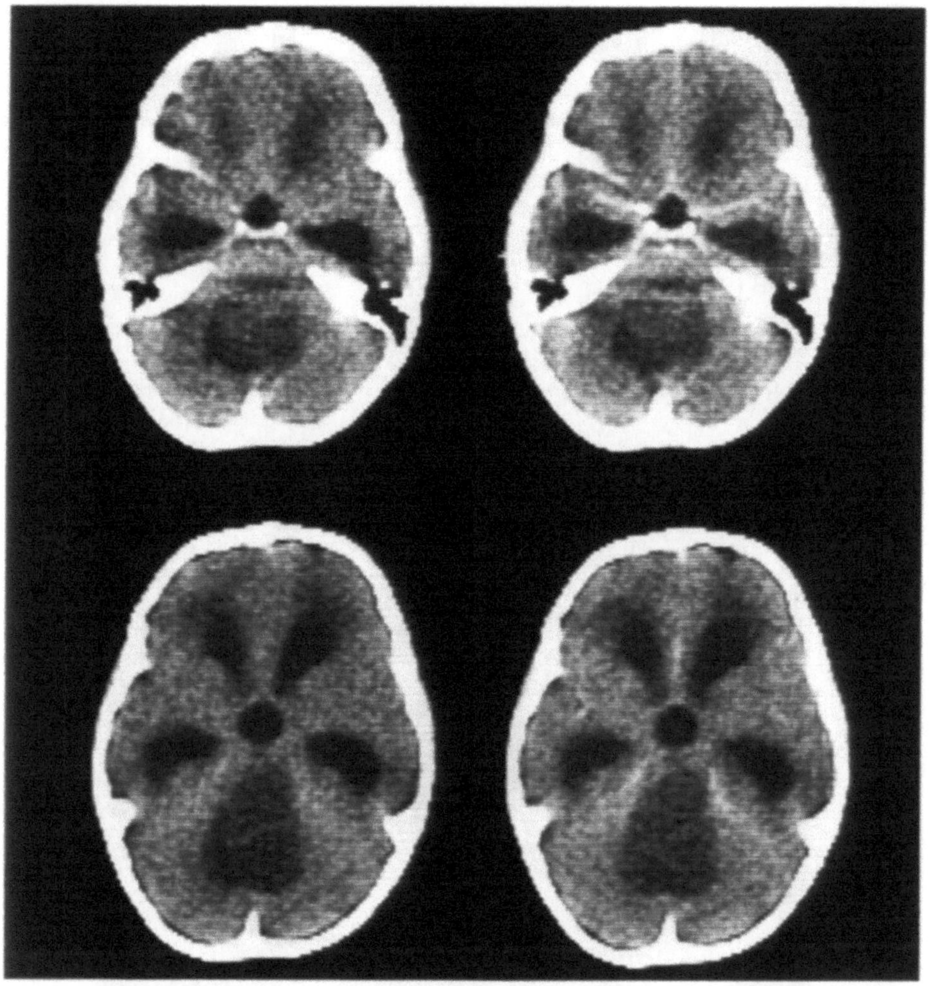

Fig. D 1.106. Variant of pilocytic astrocytoma in a 7-year-old boy. The tumor is located in the vermis and extends to the midbrain. It appears consistently hypodense on the pre- and postcontrast CT scans. A solid, glassy tumor was removed at operation and identified histologically as a variant of pilocytic astrocytoma

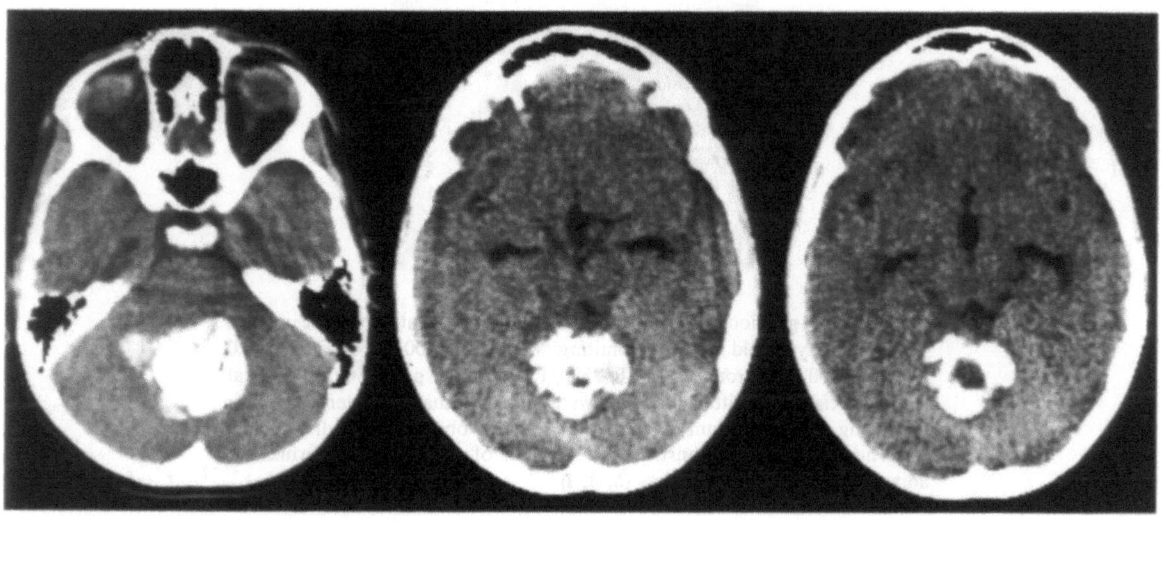

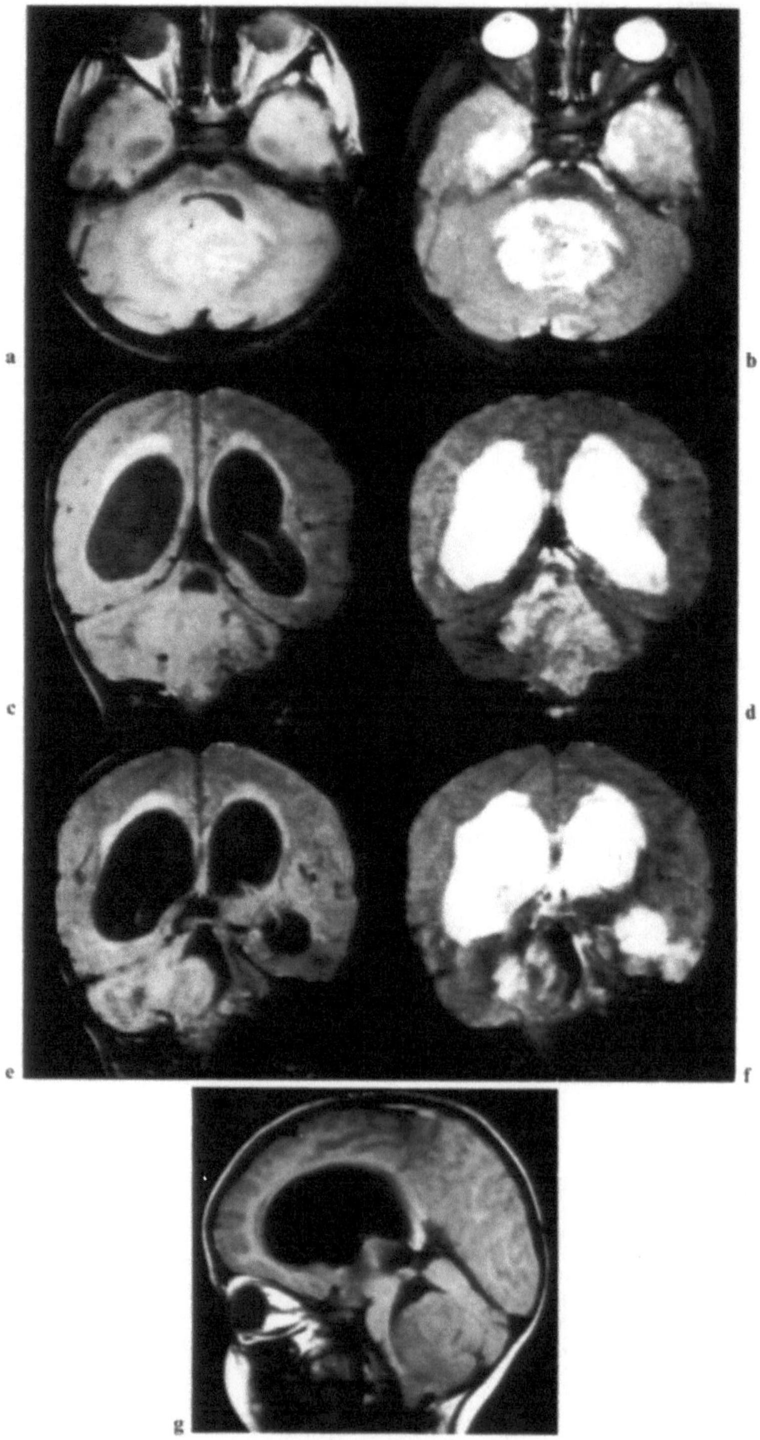

Fig. D 1.108 a–g. Pilocytic astrocytoma of the fourth ventricle and cerebellar vermis in a 2-year-old boy with vomiting. MR: **a** SE 2500/30, **b** SE 2500/120, **c, e** SE 2500/30 coronal, **d, f** SE 2500/120 coronal, **g** SE 800/30 sagittal. The T1-weighted sagittal image shows a spherical mass isointense to brain displacing the cerebellum upward and causing obstructive hydrocephalus (**g**). The T2 images demonstrate involvement of the cerebellar vermis and adjacent cerebellar hemispheres (**b, d, f**)

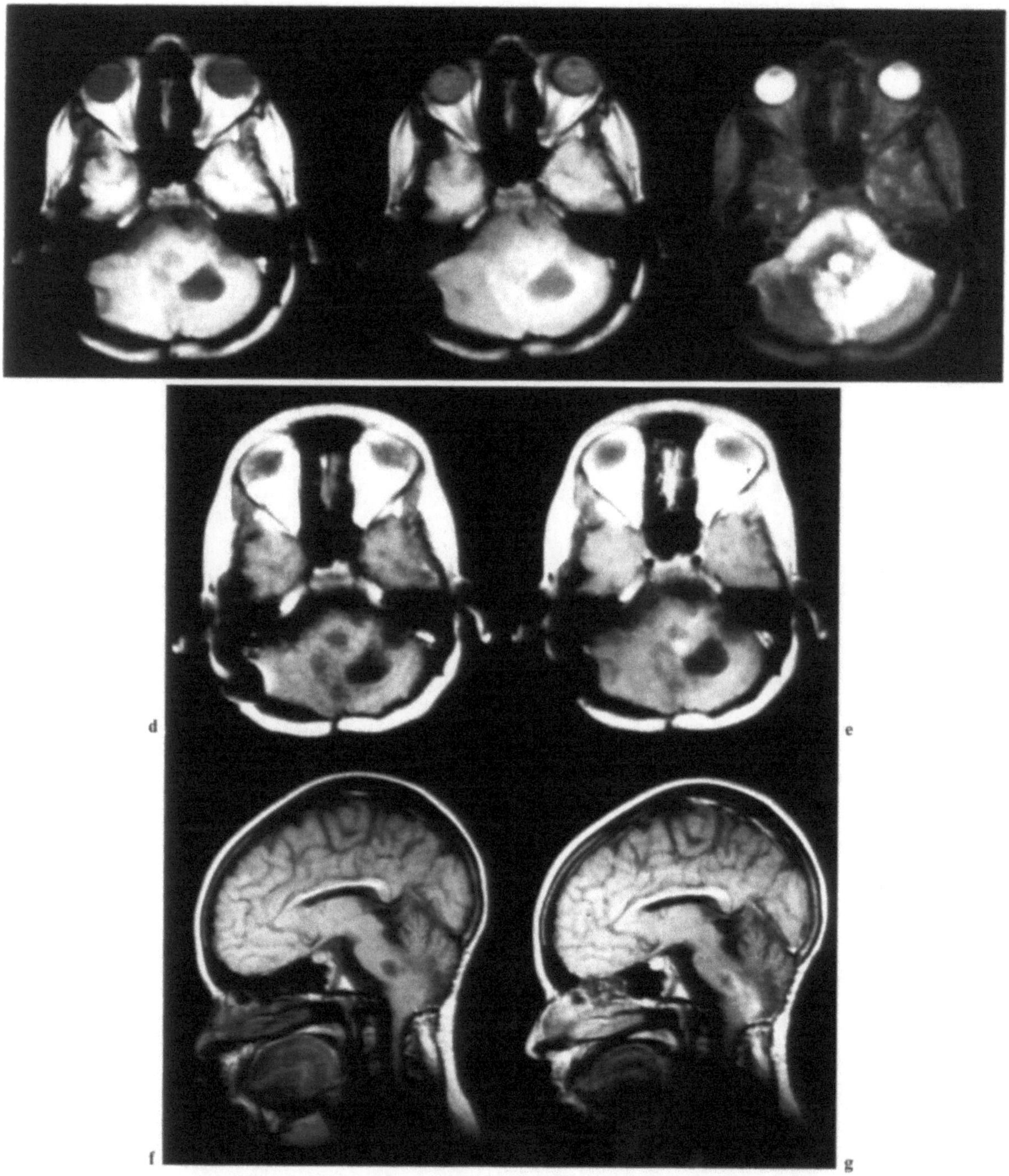

Fig. D 1.109 a–g. Recurrence of a pilocytic astrocytoma of the right cerebellar hemisphere in a 15-year-old girl initially operated at 7 years of age. The patient presented with recurring symptoms of increased intracranial pressure, complete horizontal gaze paresis, vertical nystagmus, right-sided facial paresis, and predominantly left-sided cerebellar ataxia. MR: **a** SE 1600/30, **b** SE 1600/60, **c** SE 1600/240, **d** SE 400/30, **e** SE 400/30 post Gd-DTPA, **f** SE 400/30 sagittal, **g** SE 400/30 post Gd-DTPA sagittal. The proton-density image (**a**) demonstrates even the low-signal portion of the tumor in the left cerebellar hemisphere. Increased T2 weighting brings out areas of high signal involving the right cerebellar hemisphere (**b, c**). A cystic component is discriminated from surrounding tissue on the T2-weighted image (**c**). Mild, diffuse enhancement is seen on the post-gadolinium scans

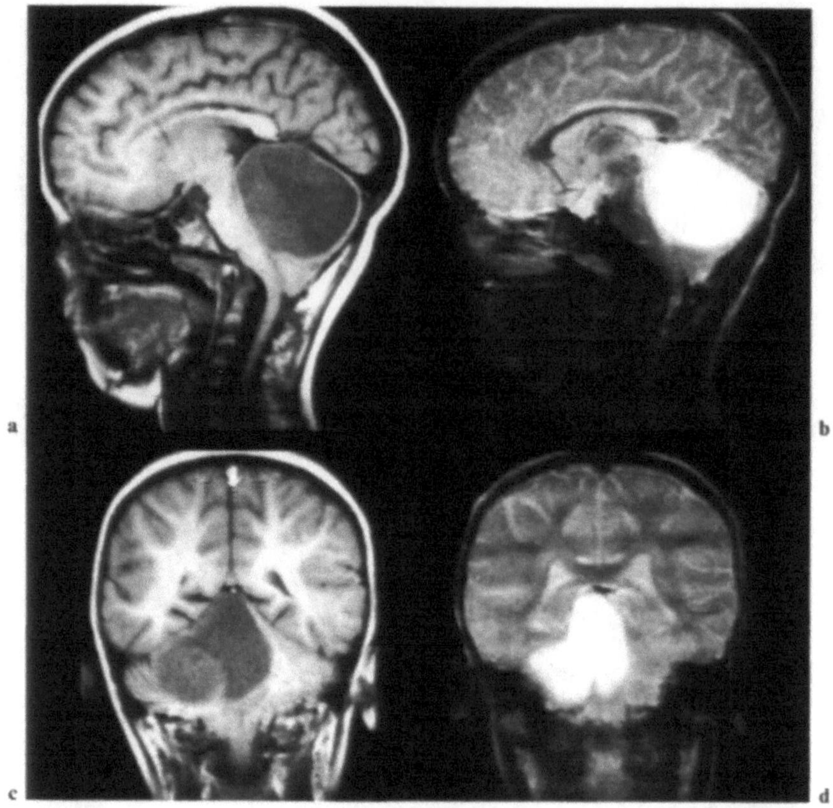

Fig. D1.110a–d. Pilocytic astrocytoma of the cerebellum in a 7-year-old girl with headache, vomiting, and ataxia. MR: **a, c** SE 400/30, **b, d** SE 2000/120; **a, b** sagittal, **c, d** coronal. The T1-weighted images (**a, c**) show a septate, cystic, hypointense tumor. The cyst becomes hyperintense with T2 weighting (**b, d**)

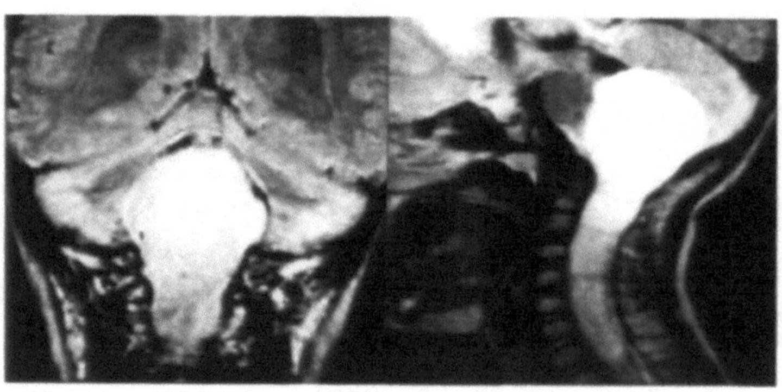

Fig. D1.111. Pilocytic astrocytoma in a 6-year-old boy with a history of encephalitis with right-sided hemiparesis (at age 2) and internal hydrocephalus with a progressive tendency. Now he presented with headaches, vomiting, and incipient papilledema. CT showed pronounced internal hydrocephalus and a 2.5-cm hypodensity in the posterior cranial fossa that enhanced slightly and presented irregular margins on the postcontrast scan (not shown). MR: SE 1600/30. The coronal (*left*) and sagittal (*right*) projections show distention of the brainstem and medulla. The tumor extends to the first thoracic vertebra and gives a bright signal. Anterior to the tumor in the pons area is a low-signal region representing a cystic component

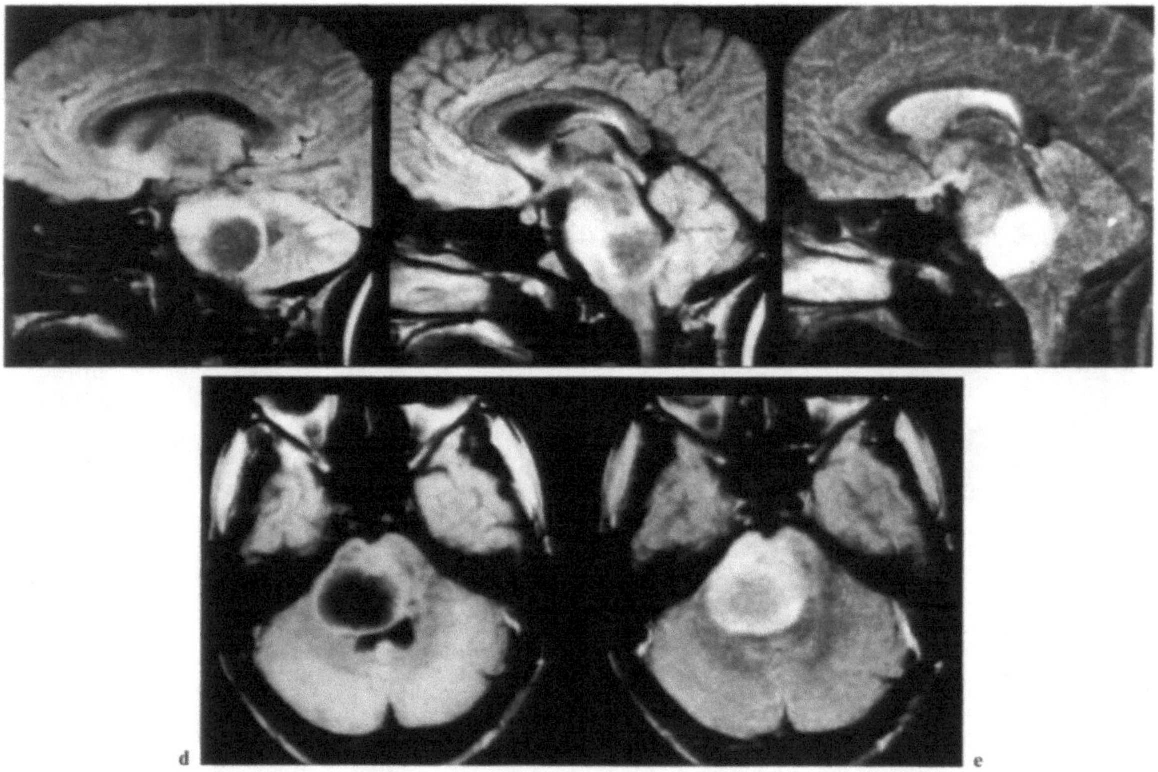

a–c

d e

Fig. D 1.112 a–e. Pilocytic astrocytoma of the pons in a 12-year-old boy with headaches, increasing symptoms of raised intracranial pressure, somnolence, and dysfunction of the lower cranial nerves. MR: **a** SE 1800/30, **b** SE 1800/35, **c** SE 1800/120, **d** SE 1800/30, **e** SE 1800/90. The proton-density image (**a**) demonstrates a hypointense area within a hyperintense ring. The compressed, obstructed fourth ventricle is appreciated on the axial scans. The central cyst is difficult to distinguish from tumor and surrounding edema on the T2-weighted sequences

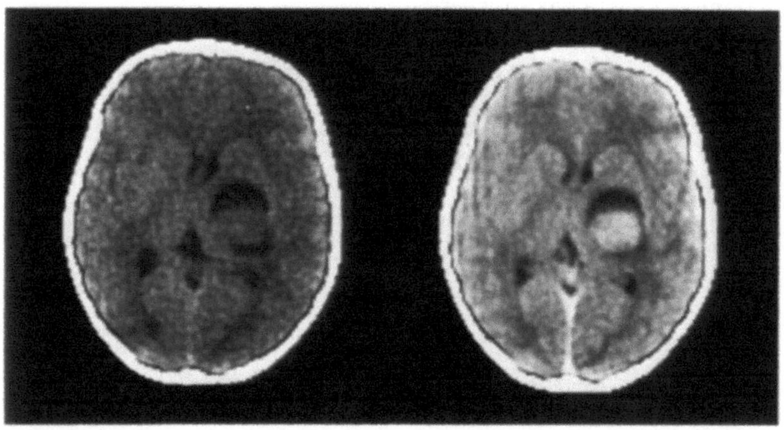

Fig. D 1.113. Pilocytic astrocytoma deep in the right temporal lobe with involvement of the basal ganglia in a 7-year-old boy with progressive left-sided hemiparesis. A solid tumor nodule is demonstrated inside a cyst. The tumor tissue appears slightly hypodense on the plain CT scan (*left*) and enhances strongly with contrast medium (*right*)

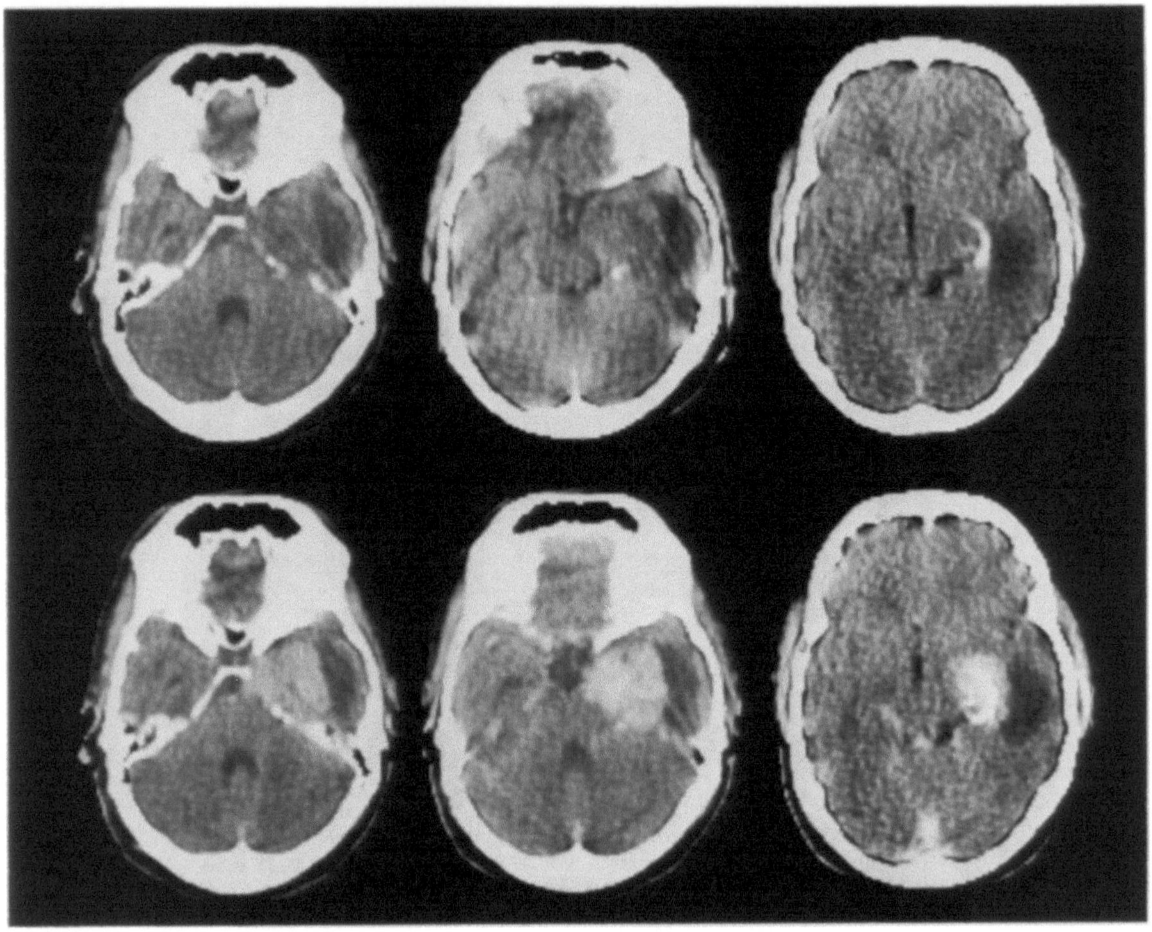

Fig. D 1.114. Pilocytic astrocytoma in the right temporal lobe of a 17-year-old boy with cerebral seizures. The tumor density is very heterogeneous on the plain CT scans (*top*). Solid, slightly hypodense areas of tumor coexist with calcifications and a crescent-shaped area of very low density representing a cyst. The solid tumor components enhance strongly on the postcontrast scans (*bottom*)

Fig. D 1.115. Large tumor of the left basal ganglion region with extension into the left cerebral peduncle and hypothalamus in a 17-month-old child. The lesion appears hypodense and somewhat heterogeneous on the plain scans (*left*), meeting the CT criteria for pilocytic astrocytoma. There is marked ventricular dilatation with periventricular lucency (postcontrast scans on the *right*)

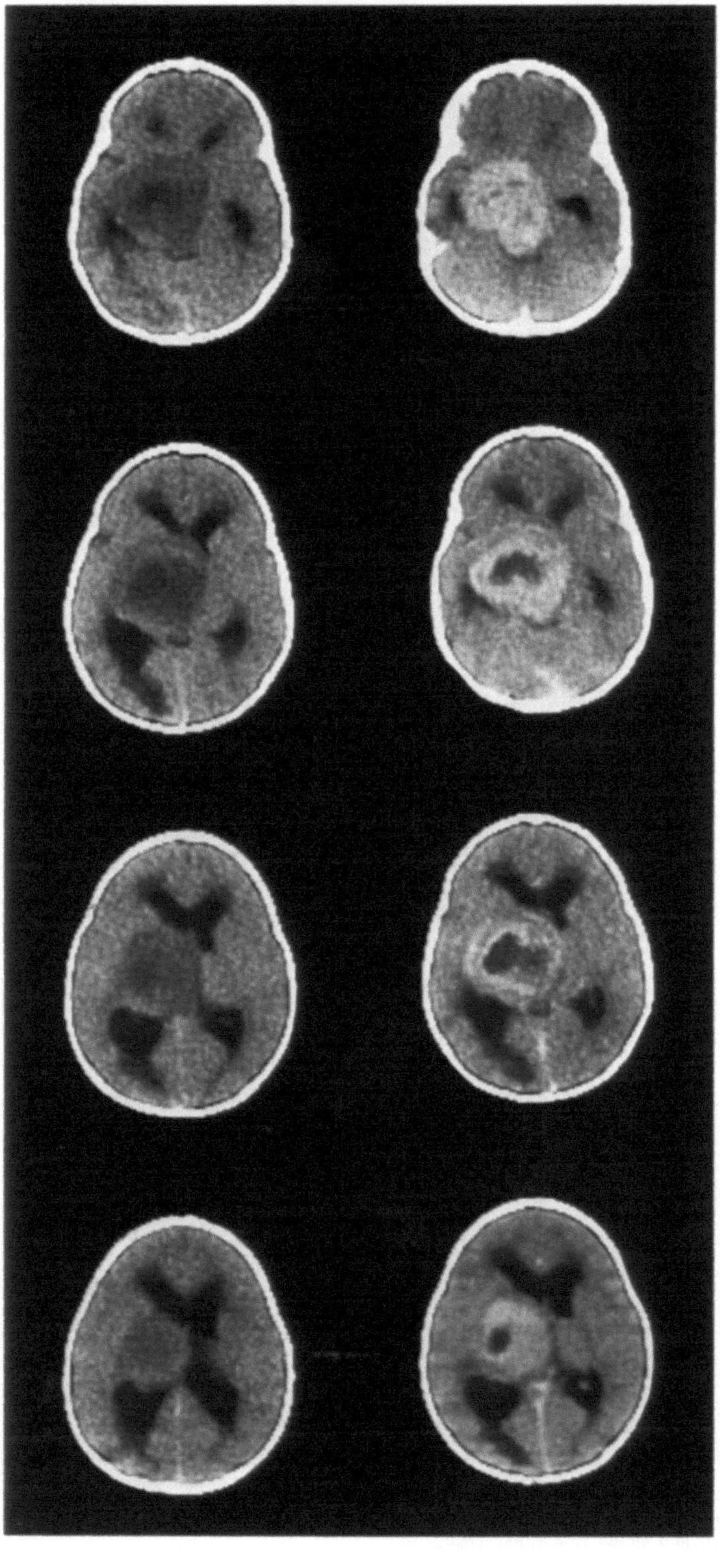

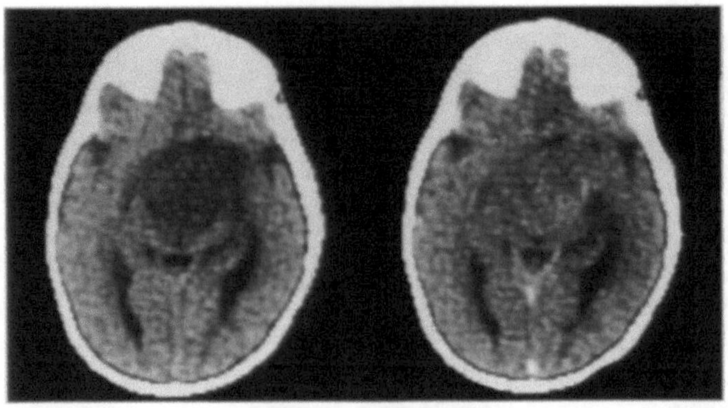

Fig. D 1.116. Grade I pilocytic astrocytoma, juvenile type, in a 4-year-old boy. CT scans before (*left*) and after (*right*) contrast infusion display a large suprasellar mass in the region of the third ventricle obstructing the foramen of Monro. The hypodense tumor extends into the mesencephalon and cisterna venae magnae and laterally to the basal ganglia and insular region

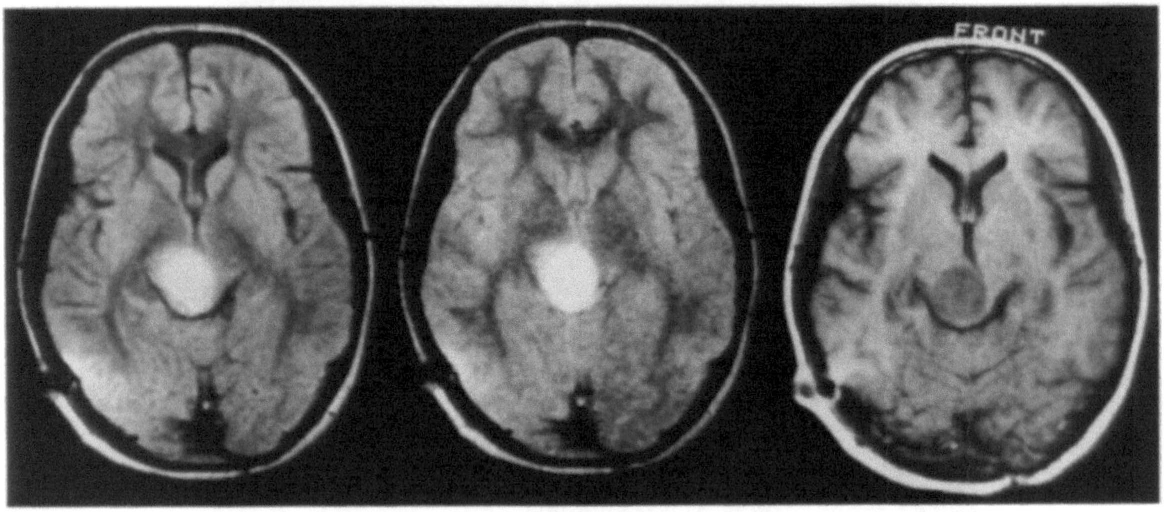

a b c

Fig. D 1.117 a–c. Pilocytic astrocytoma of the brainstem in a 15-year-old boy with symptoms of increased intracranial pressure, photosensitivity, and impaired ocular motility. MR: **a** SE 1600/35, **b** SE 1600/70, **c** SE 400/35. The proton-density and T2-weighted images show a rounded tumor of high signal intensity (**a, b**). The tumor appears hypointense with T1 weighting (**c**)

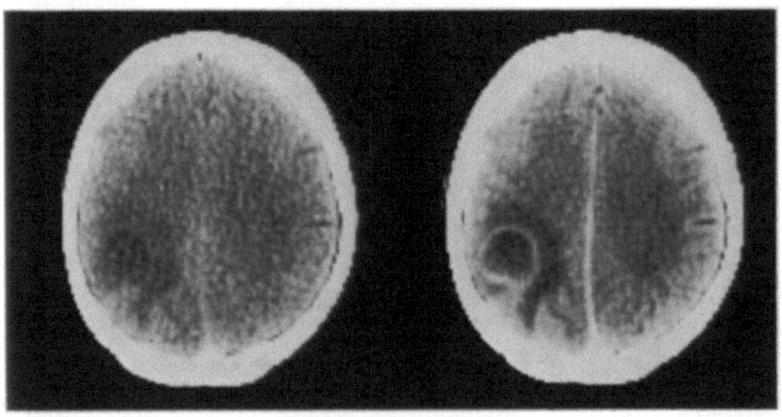

Fig. D 1.118. Pilocytic astrocytoma of the left parietal region in a 38-year-old woman. The lesion appears hypodense on the plain CT scan (*left*) and shows ring enhancement on the postcontrast scan (*right*). Grade I perifocal edema. CT findings are consistent with anaplastic astrocytoma

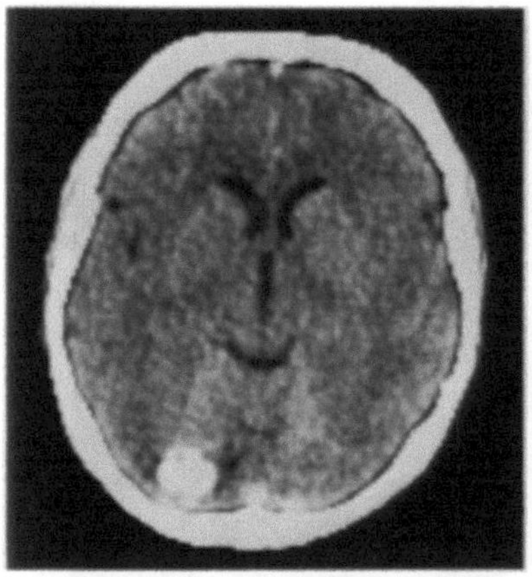

Fig. D 1.119. Pilocytic astrocytoma of the left occipital pole in a 31-year-old man. CT shows a rounded, calcified focus in the left occipital lobe. A thin layer of cortex separates the tumor from the skull. Intracerebral tumors are unlikely to produce such findings. A calcified meningioma arising from the tentorium can give a similar appearance on horizontal projections

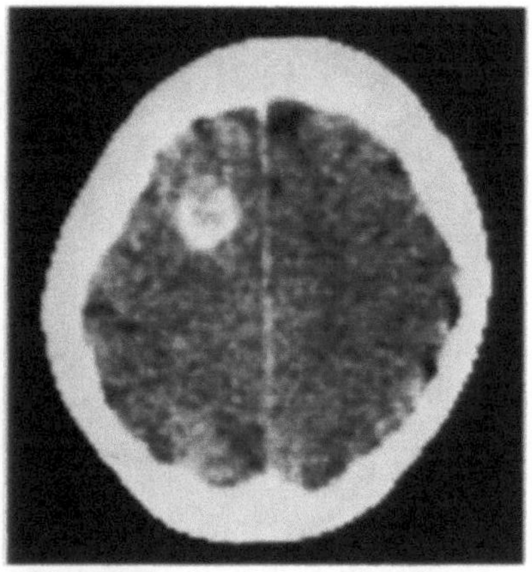

Fig. D 1.120. Pilocytic astrocytoma in the left precentral region of a 66-year-old woman. The tumor is almost entirely calcified. Oligodendroglioma need not be considered in the differential diagnosis

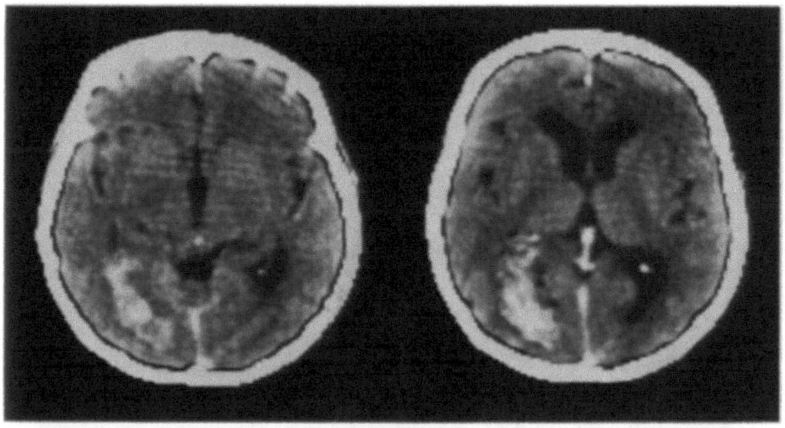

Fig. D 1.121. Pilocytic astrocytoma of the left occipital lobe in a 55-year-old female with intermittent right homonymous hemianopia. The tumor, which is partly intraventricular, presents irregular margins and shows marked contrast enhancement; it was initially diagnosed as an angioma. There is no mass effect or perifocal edema. Postcontrast CT scans

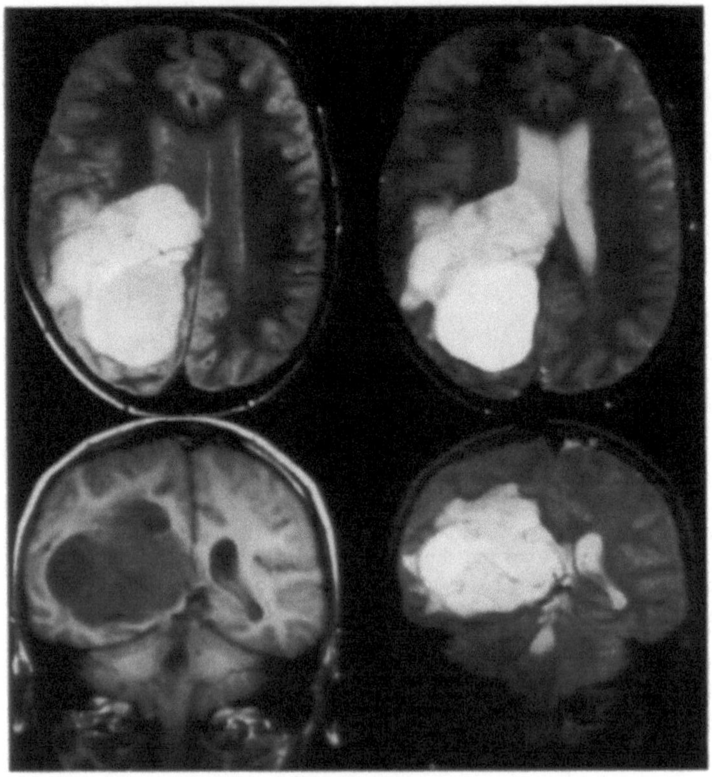

D 1.122

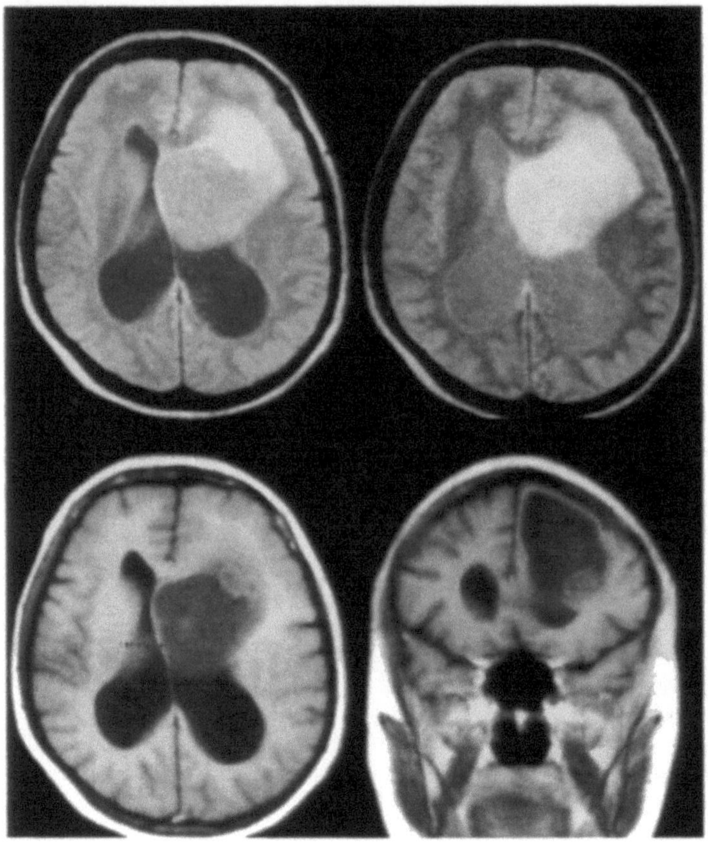

D 1.123

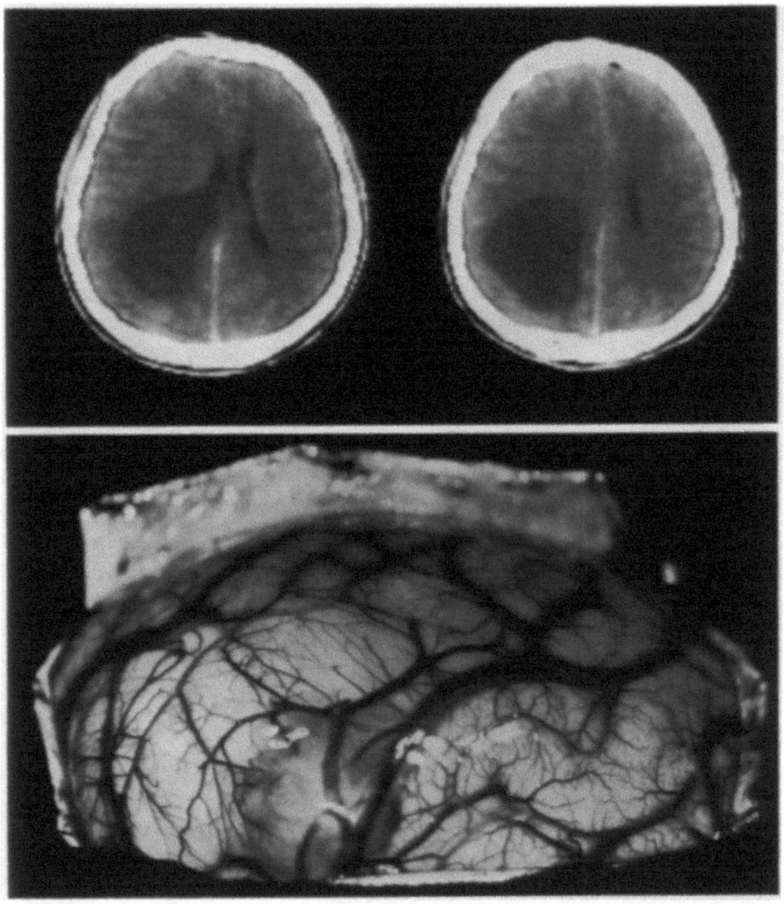

a

b

Fig. D 1.124. a Pilocytic astrocytoma with a large cyst in a 19-year-old male with progressive right-sided paresis. The solid tumor nodule high in the parietal area was not visualized by CT. The cyst fluid was strongly xanthochromic, so its density values are much higher than those of CSF (24–26 HU). **b** Intraoperative photo of the same patient showing a cortical mass 15 mm in diameter located near the interhemispheric fissure

◄

Fig. 1.122a–d. Pilocytic astrocytoma of the left occipital region in a 14-year-old boy with headaches and one generalized seizure. MR: **a** SE 3000/30, **b** SE 3000/90, **c** SE 500/30 coronal, **d** SE 3000/90 coronal. The tumor gives a very high signal on the proton-density image (**a**), and heavier T2 weighting (**b**) further delineates the greatly expanded occipital horn. T1 weighting (**c**) demonstrates a lateral tumor-associated cyst, recognized by its hypointensity

Fig. D 1.123a–d. Pilocytic astrocytoma of the right frontal region in a 45-year-old woman with Recklinghausen's disease. Patient had a history of severe intermittent headaches and subtle alteration in mental status. MR: **a** SE 1600/35, **b** SE 1600/70, **c** SE 400/30, **d** SE 400/30 coronal. Solid tumor gives a bright signal on the proton-density image; the cyst appears only slightly hyperintense to brain. There is compression of the right frontal horn and obstruction of the foramen of Monro with hydrocephalus. The axial and coronal T1-weighted scans (**c, d**) show the tumor, which appeared reddish at operation ("angioglioma"), projecting into the cyst. Tumor and cyst are not differentiated on the T2-weighted image (**b**)

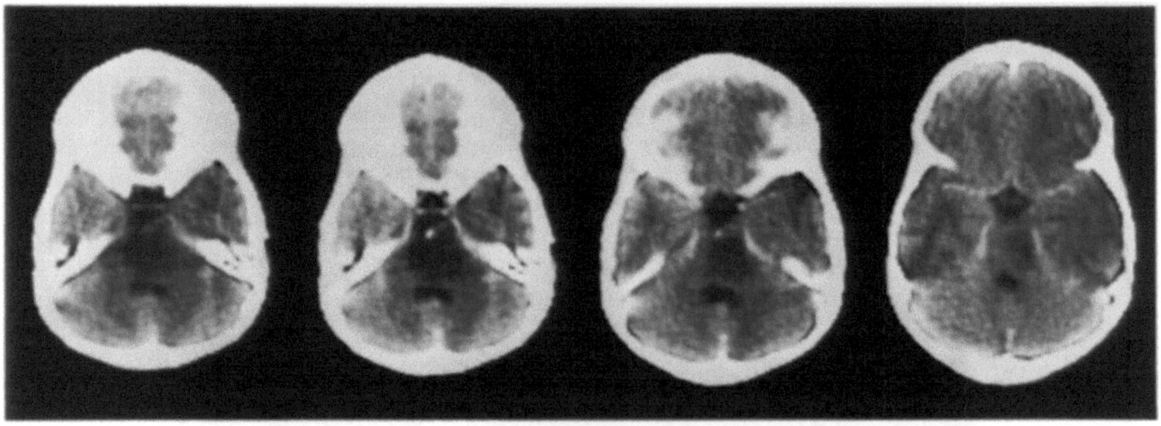

Fig. D 1.125. Bulbopontine astrocytoma in a $4^1/_2$-year-old girl with cranial nerve deficits and involvement of the long tracts. The tumor shows a very low density on the plain CT scan (18 HU, *far left*) and does not enhance significantly (19.5 HU) with contrast medium. The pontine part of the tumor chiefly involves the right side (image at *far right*)

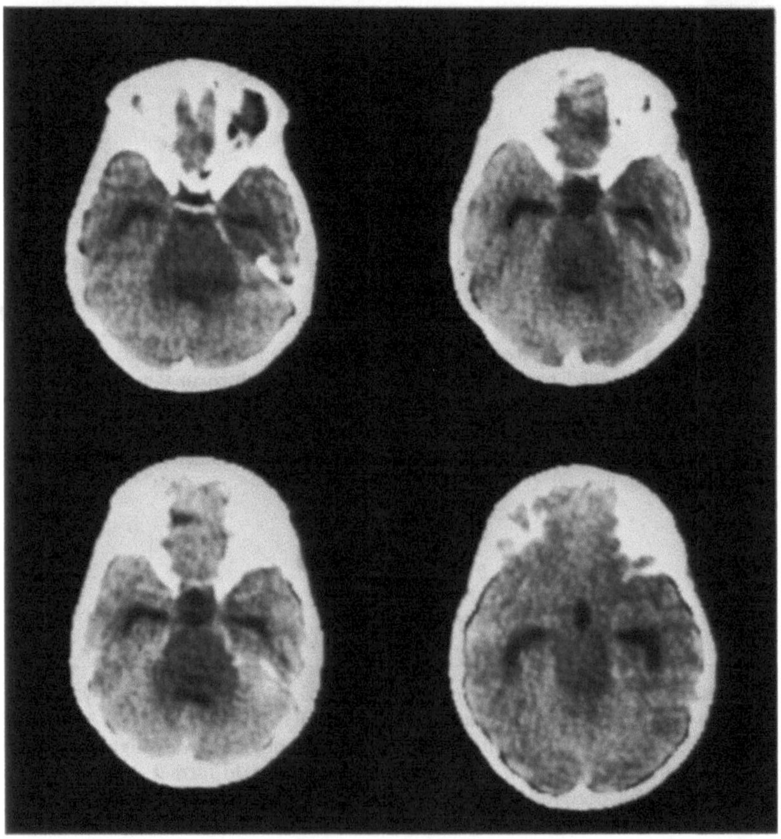

Fig. D 1.126. Astrocytoma of the pons in a 9-year-old girl with cranial nerve deficits, ataxia, and long tract involvement. The pons appears generally expanded and is markedly hypodense. The fourth ventricle is displaced posteriorly. The inferior horns are dilated as an expression of moderate hydrocephalus. Postcontrast CT (*lower left*) shows no appreciable tumor enhancement relative to the plain scans. Diagnosis was confirmed histologically

h) Pontine Gliomas

Most bulbopontine tumors are slow-growing fibrillary or pilocytic astrocytomas. Anaplastic astrocytomas and glioblastomas are less common. Medulloblastomas develop infrequently in the pontine region. These tumors mainly affect children under 10 years of age. Most pontine neoplasms in adults are metastases, a few are primary glioblastomas. Pontine tumors are rare, constituting only about 1% of all intracranial neoplasms.

Pontine tumors frequently cause cranial nerve deficits and disturbances of the motor and sensory pathways. The slow-growing gliomas increase the intracranial pressure only in later stages when hydrocephalus has developed. CSF circulation may be preserved for a very long time. Fast-growing tumors, on the other hand, cause obstructive hydrocephalus at a relatively early stage with associated symptoms of intracranial hypertension.

Before the advent of CT, the primary modality for diagnosing pontine neoplasms was pneumoencephalography, which revealed bowing or more circumscribed dorsal displacement of the aqueduct and fourth ventricle signifying tumor-related distention of the pons.

With larger pontine tumors, angiography can demonstrate the stretching of the posterior cerebral arteries and venous displacement caused by pathologic expansion of the pons. Other adjunctive studies do not disclose signs specific for pontine tumors.

Computed Tomography (Figs. D 1.125–128)

Noncontrast Scan

The plain CT scan is diagnostic for the majority of pontine tumors. Distention of the pons causes some degree of dorsal displacement of the fourth ventricle, which appears on the unenhanced scan as a narrow, well-defined hypodensity with an irregular shape bordering on the posterior aspect of the tumor. Some pontine tumors also cause narrowing of the interpeduncular cistern and indent the pentagon from behind.

Most pontine gliomas appear hypodense on the unenhanced scan (19–26 HU). In our experience this applies to slightly more than half of all pontine neoplasms. The rest present an isodense, slightly hyperdense, or mixed-density pattern. Cysts appear as well-defined voids within the pons.

Pontine tumors are often associated with mild to moderate ventricular expansion, but occasionally the ventricles appear normal in size. Larger pontine gliomas that have obstructed CSF flow by displacement of the aqueduct and fourth ventricle may incite a severe hydrocephalus.

Postcontrast Scan

It is our experience that approximately 60% of pontine gliomas show contrast enhancement in their solid portions. This is especially helpful in delineating primarily isodense lesions from normal brain parenchyma. Approximately half of primarily hypodense pontine gliomas demonstrate ring or nodular enhancement or a combination of both patterns. The enhanced scan is also helpful in determining whether a tumor has spread to involve one of the cerebral peduncles or the thalamus.

Pontine tumors are occasionally missed on initial CT examination, as was the case in 3 of our 44 patients. The best view of these tumors is obtained by using the standard projection for posterior fossa examinations. We have also had good results with the projection used for orbital scanning, in which case the brainstem is perpendicular to the scan plane and troublesome artifacts emanating from the petrous bones are reduced (see Fig. D 1.127).

The majority of hypodense, nonenhancing pontine tumors are *fibrillary astrocytomas*. In tumors showing a ring or nodular pattern of enhancement, it is not possible to distinguish between a *pilocytic astrocytoma* and *anaplastic astrocytoma* on the basis of CT findings.

Medulloblastoma of the pons is characterized by a largely homogeneous, intense enhancement of the pons as a whole.

Metastases in the pons may present a variety of patterns corresponding to their presentation in other brain regions.

Magnetic Resonance Imaging
(Figs. D 1.129, 130)

MR has contributed greatly to the diagnosis of pontine neoplasms. A major advantage over CT is the absence of bony artifact, making it possible to acquire vertical and midline projections that demonstrate the true extent of brainstem tumors. It has been found that the tumors almost always display a greater extent on MR images than on CT scans. It is not unusual to detect tumor extension into the spinal canal or upward extension into the thalamus.

Noncontrast Scan
T1-weighted images furnish little useful information. The tumors appear slightly hypo- to isointense and are recognized by the expanded condition of the pons. T2-weighted images are a rich source of information, and pontine gliomas give an intense signal on these sequences. MR is almost invariably positive in cases where CT findings are equivocal.

Post-Gadolinium Scan
Gd-DTPA is unnecessary in the majority of cases, although moderate to intense enhancement is observed depending on the tumor histology.

MR has a leading role in the diagnostic evaluation of suspected pontine glioma, taking precedence over CT. However, it is unable to differentiate among the various histologic forms of astrocytoma or distinguish them from other tumors such as medulloblastoma or metastases.

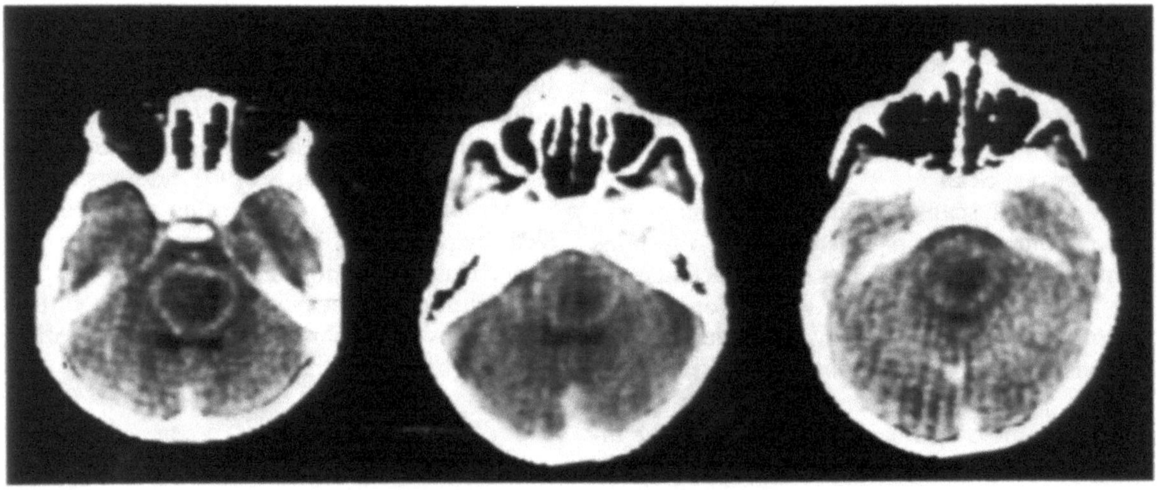

Fig. D 1.127. Pontine glioma with ring enhancement in a 2-year-old child. Anaplastic or pilocytic astrocytoma. The standard CT projection (*left*) is compared with scans taken with the head extended (*center* and *right*)

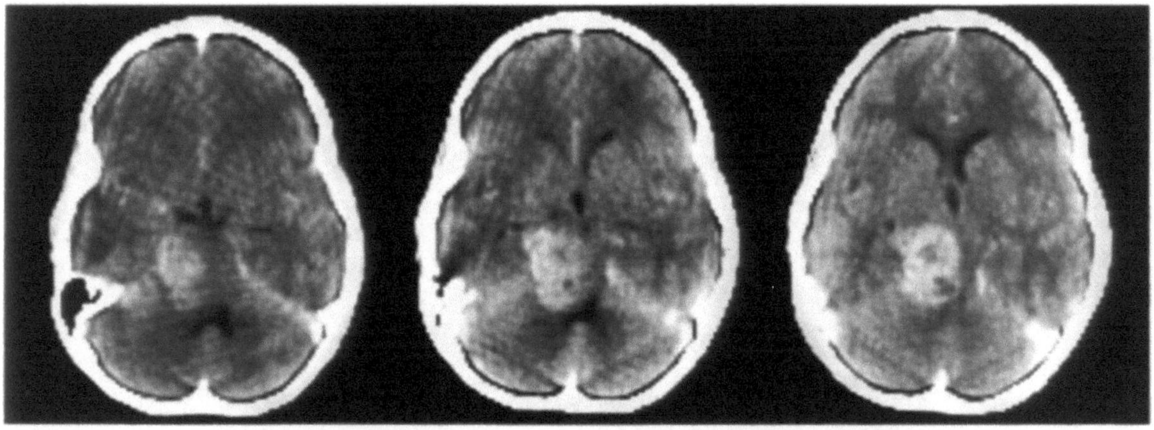

Fig. D 1.128. High pontine tumor extending into the left cerebral peduncle and thalamus of a 7-year-old girl with rapidly progressive hemiparesis and cranial nerve dysfunction. The primarily isodense tumor shows marked contrast enhancement with two small nonenhancing areas that may represent necrosis. Postcontrast scans. The rapid clinical course with left-sided cranial nerve dysfunction and right-sided hemiparesis suggested a diagnosis of anaplastic astrocytoma or glioblastoma

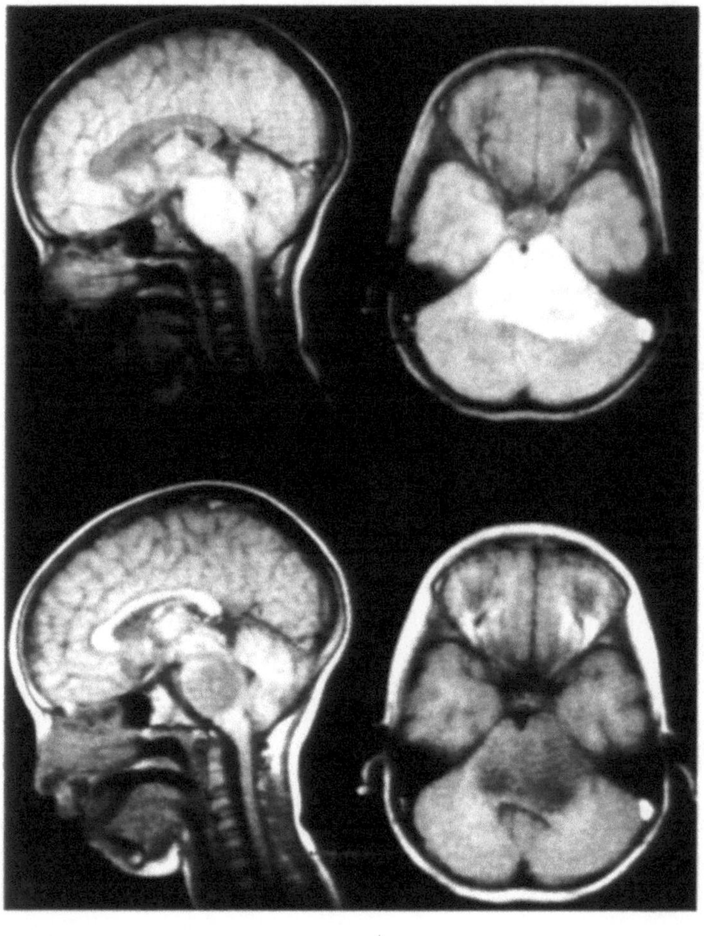

a b c d

Fig. D 1.129 a–d. Pontine glioma in a 7-year-old girl with a 6-month history of headaches. She presented with diplopia and ocular torticollis, a coarse gaze nystagmus with a rotatory component, facial paresis, and gait ataxia. MR: **a** SE 1600/35 sagittal, **b** SE 1600/60, **c** SE 400/35 sagittal, **d** SE 400/35. Distention of the brainstem is evident on the sagittal and axial views and gives a high signal on the T2-weighted sequence (**b**). The T1-weighted images demonstrate the rounded, hypointense tumor (**c, d**)

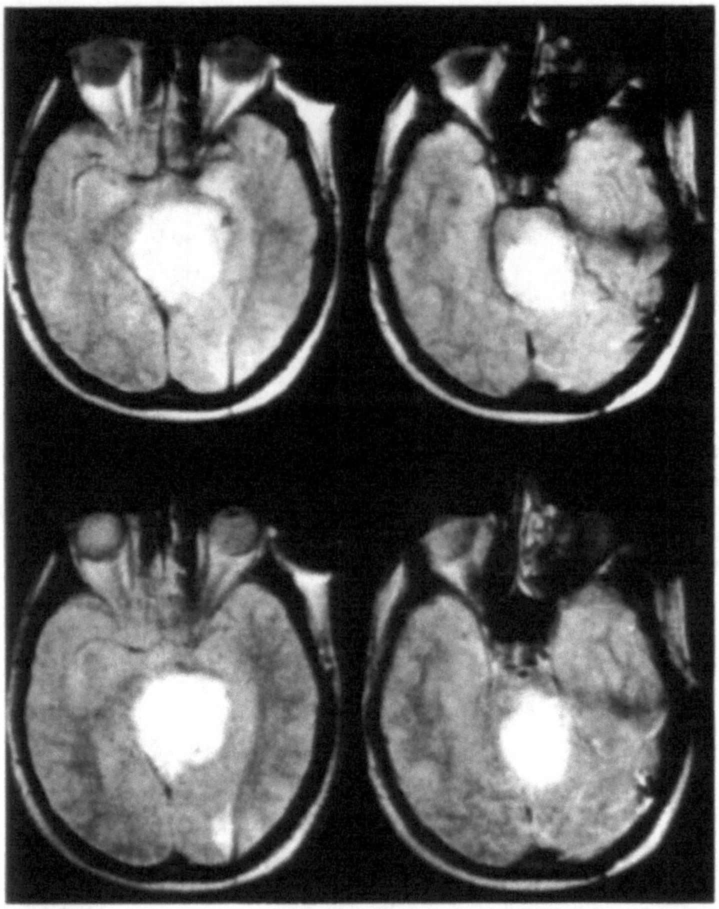

Fig. D 1.130. Pontine glioma in a 32-year-old man with altered mental status and left-sided hemiparesis mainly affecting the lower extremity. MR: *top* SE 1600/35, *bottom* SE 1600/70. The tumor appears equally hyperintense on the proton-density images (*top*) and T2-weighted images (*bottom*)

i) Ependymomas

Incidence	1%–4% of all brain tumors
Age predilection	First and second decades of life
Sex predilection	Male preponderance
Typical sites	Fourth ventricle, lateral ventricle, third ventricle; cerebral hemispheres in children; temporo-parieto-occipital and frontal regions
Main clinical features	Fourth ventricle tumors usually cause only vomiting; all may produce various symptoms of increased intracranial pressure
Angiography	Usually negative for tumors in fourth ventricle; often shows extreme vascular displacement in cerebrum; may show increased vascularization with irregular vessels
CT	
Noncontrast scan	Often shows area of slightly increased density, possibly with calcific features. Large hypodensities may be seen in cerebral tumors (cysts)
Contrast enhancement	Moderate enhancement of solid tumor components
Postcontrast appearance	Tumor with flecks of calcification, often contrasting poorly with caudal brainstem; cerebral ependymomas in small children may contain large cysts and occasional calcifications. Moderate perifocal edema around cerebral tumors
MR	
Noncontrast scan	Tumors hypointense on T1-weighted images, most conspicuous on proton-density and slightly T2-weighted images owing to their slight hyperintensity, indistinguishable from CSF on heavily T2-weighted sequences
Gadolinium enhancement	Positive
Post Gd-DTPA appearance	T1-weighted images show hyperintense mass with irregular Gd-DTPA enhancement

Differential diagnosis

Fourth ventricle tumors: medulloblastoma, choroid plexus papilloma

Lateral ventricle tumors: choroid plexus papilloma, subependymal giant cell astrocytoma

Third ventricle tumors: pineal tumors, pilocytic astrocytoma, choroid plexus papilloma, colloid cyst

Cerebral tumors: pilocytic astrocytoma, anaplastic astrocytoma, glioblastoma, monstrocellular sarcoma, gangliocytoma

An incidence of 1%–4% is reported for ependymomas in the literature, and we encountered 163 ependymomas in the 8516 tumors in our series (1.9%). They are predominantly tumors of childhood and adolescence but also occur in adults. Males are predominantly affected, the ratio being 3:2 according to Zülch (1986).

Extraventricular cerebral ependymomas in children, like anaplastic ependymomas in adults, are highly malignant tumors (grade III–IV). Ependymomas of the fourth ventricle also may be malignant, especially in children ("ependymal medulloblastoma"). All other ependymomas are classified as grade I or II.

A subgroup is the grade I subependymoma, which develops within the ventricles. According to our analysis these tumors comprise approximately 15% of all ependymomas.

Typical Sites

Typical sites are the lateral ventricle with predilection for the area of the foramen of Monro, the floor of the fourth ventricle, and the third ventricle, with most tumors growing within the ventricular cavity. In some cases, and especially with recurrent growths, tumor deposits may seed to multiple intracranial sites via the CSF.

Cerebral ependymoma is the most common cerebral tumor of children and adolescents. It develops in the paraventricular white matter and extends to the surface of the cerebrum. The junction of the parietal, temporal, and occipital lobes is a common site of occurrence, and we have found a number of these lesions in the frontal lobes. The tumors occur in very close relation to the lateral ventricles. Most contain large cysts, and a few show calcification. Fine calcifications may also be found in intraventricular ependymomas.

Main Clinical Features

The major symptom in children with a fourth ventricle tumor is vomiting, caused by encroachment of the lesion on the area postrema. Other intraventricular ependymomas obstruct the flow of CSF and produce obstructive hydrocephalus with its associated symptoms (headache, vomiting).

Cerebral ependymomas may precipitate seizures in young patients, but signs of increased intracranial pressure often predominate due to the potentially great size of these tumors. By contrast, pronounced neurologic deficits are uncommon.

Additional Diagnostic Procedures

Plain skull films reveal secondary signs of increased intracranial pressure such as separation of the sutures in small children or accentuation of the gyric impressions. Calcification is occasionally seen in cerebral ependymomas.

Angiograms can demonstrate intraventricular tumors large enough to cause vascular displacement. Cerebral ependymomas also cause significant vascular displacement. Neovascularization is rarely observed, although some tumors may resemble glioblastomas and show a faint blush in the capillary phase. Large cysts appear as avascular spaces.

Computed Tomography
(Figs. D 1.131–139, 142, 147)

Noncontrast Scan

Ependymomas often appear slightly hyperdense on the unenhanced scan, regardless of their location. Calcific densities scattered throughout the tumor are especially common in tumors of the fourth ventricle and of the caudal brainstem. Cerebral ependymomas frequently demonstrate large, low-density areas representing cysts (see Fig. D 1.134). Calcifications are not an unusual finding even in cerebral ependymomas (see Fig. D 1.138). These tumors present a mixed-density pattern on noncontrast scans.

Contrast Enhancement

Ependymomas usually enhance following contrast injection (see Figs. D 1.135, 136). This was observed in 41 of the 49 patients examined (83.7%). Tumors of the fourth ventricle appear to enhance less than cerebral ependymomas, which show an average density increase of 14 HU with a standard dose of contrast medium.

Postcontrast Appearance

Ependymomas of the fourth ventricle show a characteristic pattern on enhanced scans (Fig. D 1.131). Their size is variable. *A residual pocket of CSF is frequently seen behind the tumor within the ventricle.*

CT scans may occasionally show the characteristic cauliflower-like structure of ependymomas that is familiar to neuropathologists. The site of tumor origin on the floor of the fourth ventricle often cannot be discerned. However, this origin may be inferred if the tumor is not clearly demarcated from the pons and medulla oblongata, and CSF is visible behind the neoplasm. A scan performed through a very low site of tumor attachment can give the impression that the lesion is surrounded by CSF on all sides. This is only a projection effect, however.

Ependymomas of the third ventricle most often occur in its posterior portion. They compress and displace the quadrigeminal plate and often cannot be distinguished from thalamus on the lateral side (see Fig. D 1.133).

Ependymomas of the lateral ventricle tend to occur in the area of the foramen of Monro and generally cause unilateral obstruction to the flow of CSF. We have encountered a few of these tumors in the region of the trigone and occipital horn (see Figs. D 1.134, 135).

The CT presentation of *anaplastic ependymomas of the cerebrum* varies with the age of the patient. In *children* the tumors most commonly occur at the junction of the parietal, temporal, and occipital lobes and frequently contain very large cysts or calcifications in addition to their solid components (Figs. D 1.136–138). Intratumoral hemorrhage is occasionally present. Cysts and calcifications are less common in *adults*, but the trilobar junction still forms an area of predilection.

Perifocal edema is not demonstrated around ependymomas occurring in the CSF pathways. Cerebral ependymomas, by contrast, are frequently surrounded by edema, usually grade I (61%).

Magnetic Resonance Imaging

(Figs. D 1.139–147, 221)

Noncontrast Scan

Ependymomas appear hypo- to isointense on the T1-weighted image. T2 weighting increases the signal intensity of the tumor, which is readily distinguishable from brain and CSF. Lightly T2-weighted and proton-density images show the tumor to best advantage, since heavier T2 weighting causes the tumor to become isointense to CSF and edema. When very long echo times are used, the tumor can again be differentiated from the very high-intensity CSF.

Small calcifications are not detected by MR. Large calcifications appear as areas of low signal intensity.

Post-Gadolinium Scan

Solid tumor components show moderate, heterogeneous enhancement with Gd-DTPA, analogous to the pattern on postcontrast CT scans.

MR is superior to CT in its ability to delineate a tumor with respect to its surroundings, especially when the tumor is located in the area of the lateral ventricle, foramen of Monro, pineal body, or fourth ventricle. MR is also superior to CT in demonstrating infratentorial lesions owing to the absence of artifact emanating from bone. It can differentiate tumor from brainstem tissue in the rhomboid fossa with far greater accuracy than CT.

Differential Diagnosis

Medulloblastoma and *choroid plexus papilloma* are the primary alternative diagnoses to be considered for a fourth ventricle neoplasm. Medulloblastomas generally are outlined more clearly relative to the brainstem than ependymomas on the postcontrast CT scan, and calcifications are very rare. Medulloblastomas usually enhance more strongly than ependymomas, and they present smoother borders.

Choroid plexus papilloma of the fourth ventricle is rounded, well-defined, and presents numerous surface tuberosities which distinguish it from ependymoma. It enhances very intensely on postcontrast scans. Calcifications may be observed. Angioblastomas develop very rarely in the fourth ventricle, and pilocytic astrocytomas are also unusual (see Figs. D 1.100, 101, 107, 108). In two patients we observed ectopic pinealomas occurring inside the fourth ventricle (Fig. D 1.220).

An *ependymoma of the lateral ventricle* may be simulated by a *subependymal giant cell astrocytoma*, which has the same site of attachment near the foramen of Monro at the head of the caudate nucleus (Figs. D 1.150, 151). Calcifications in the ventricle wall favor a diagnosis of subependymal giant cell astrocytoma. *Subependymomas* of the lateral ventricle are usually hypodense on plain CT scans and show little contrast enhancement.

Central and posterior lateral ventricle neoplasms may represent choroid plexus papilloma, subependymoma (most common in children), or an intraventricular meningioma (most common in middle-aged and elderly patients). Differentiation between choroid plexus papilloma and subependymoma can be extremely difficult (see Figs. D 1.143, 217).

The differential diagnosis of *anterior third ventricle neoplasms* should include colloid cysts in the area of the foramina of Monro (see Figs. D 6.25–27). *Posterior third ventricle neoplasms* include tumors of the quadrigeminal region such as pinealomas, germinomas, teratomas, and pilocytic astrocytomas.

Pinealoma and *germinoma* are indistinguishable from ependymoma on CT scans. They are isodense or slightly hyperdense and show intense contrast enhancement. These tumors are readily distinguishable from *pineal teratoma*, which has a very heterogeneous structure and includes components of extremely low density. *Pilocytic astrocytomas* (spongioblastomas) of the quadrigeminal plate are difficult to distinguish from a posterior third ventricle ependymoma on CT scans, although the presence of a cystic component should direct suspicion toward astrocytoma.

The differential diagnosis of *cerebral ependymomas in children and adolescents* should include the following:

1. Pilocytic astrocytoma with a large cyst
2. Monstrocellular sarcoma
3. Gangliocytoma

All the foregoing tumors may contain cysts and calcifications, and their similarities may preclude a reliable CT differentiation in any given case. Nevertheless, we found that the ependymomas in our series tended to be quite large compared with pilocytic astrocytomas and gangliocytomas.

Cerebral ependymomas in adults may present the same CT features as anaplastic astrocytomas and glioblastomas. It is noteworthy, however, that the solid components of ependymomas were markedly larger than those of the other tumor groups in our patients. Age at diagnosis is another factor to be considered, since most of the cerebral ependymomas in our series were diagnosed at about 20 years of age.

MR does not contribute any additional information that would be helpful in establishing a pathologic diagnosis.

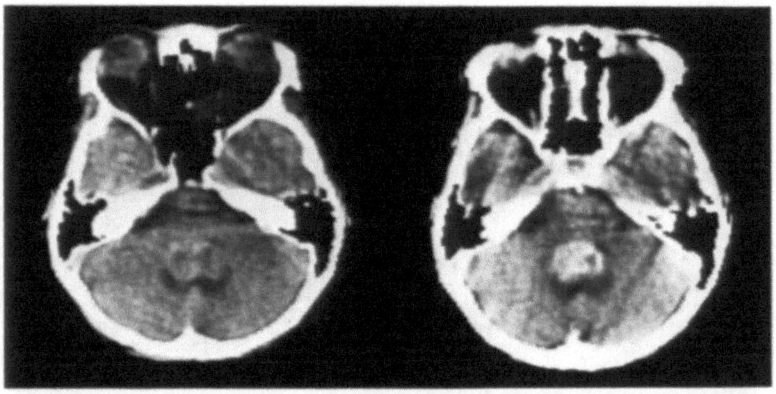

Fig. D 1.131. Ependymoma of the fourth ventricle in a 46-year-old man. Plain CT shows a mixed-density lesion causing marked posterior displacement of the fourth ventricle. Dense enhancement is seen on the postcontrast scan (*right*). Note the small CSF pocket on the right anterior aspect of the tumor

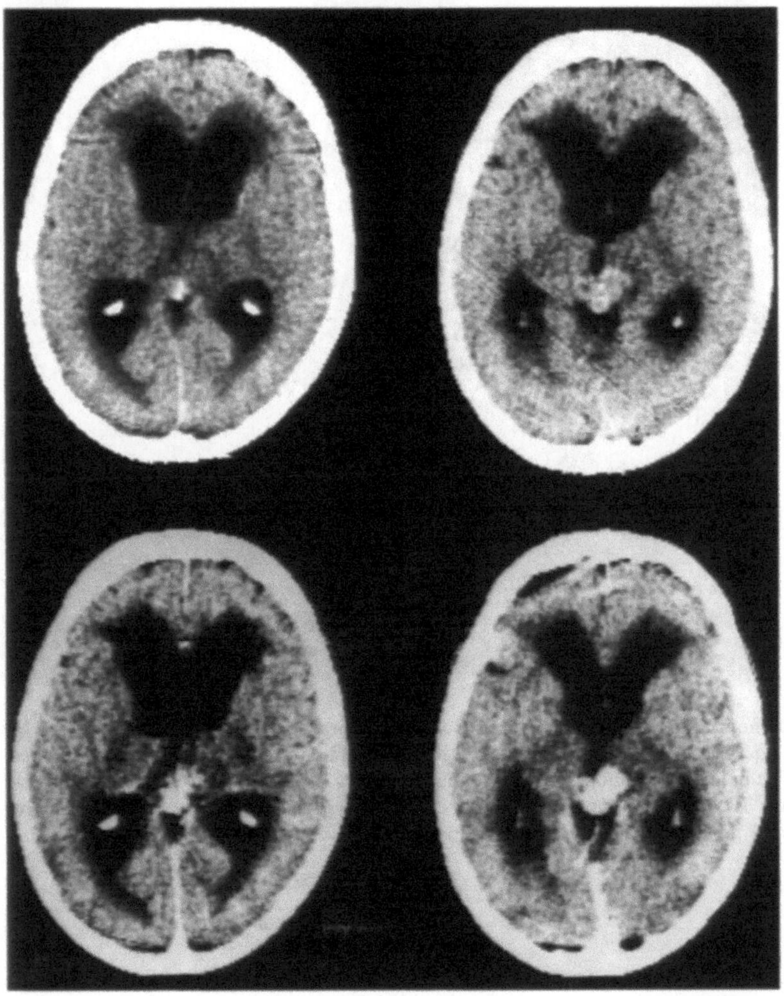

Fig. D 1.132. Primarily hyperdense ependymoma of the pineal region and posterior third ventricle with extension into the right thalamus in a 44-year-old woman with paresis of upward gaze and symptoms of increased intracranial pressure. Postcontrast scans (*bottom*) show a densely enhancing tumor with severe associated hydrocephalus and periventricular lucency

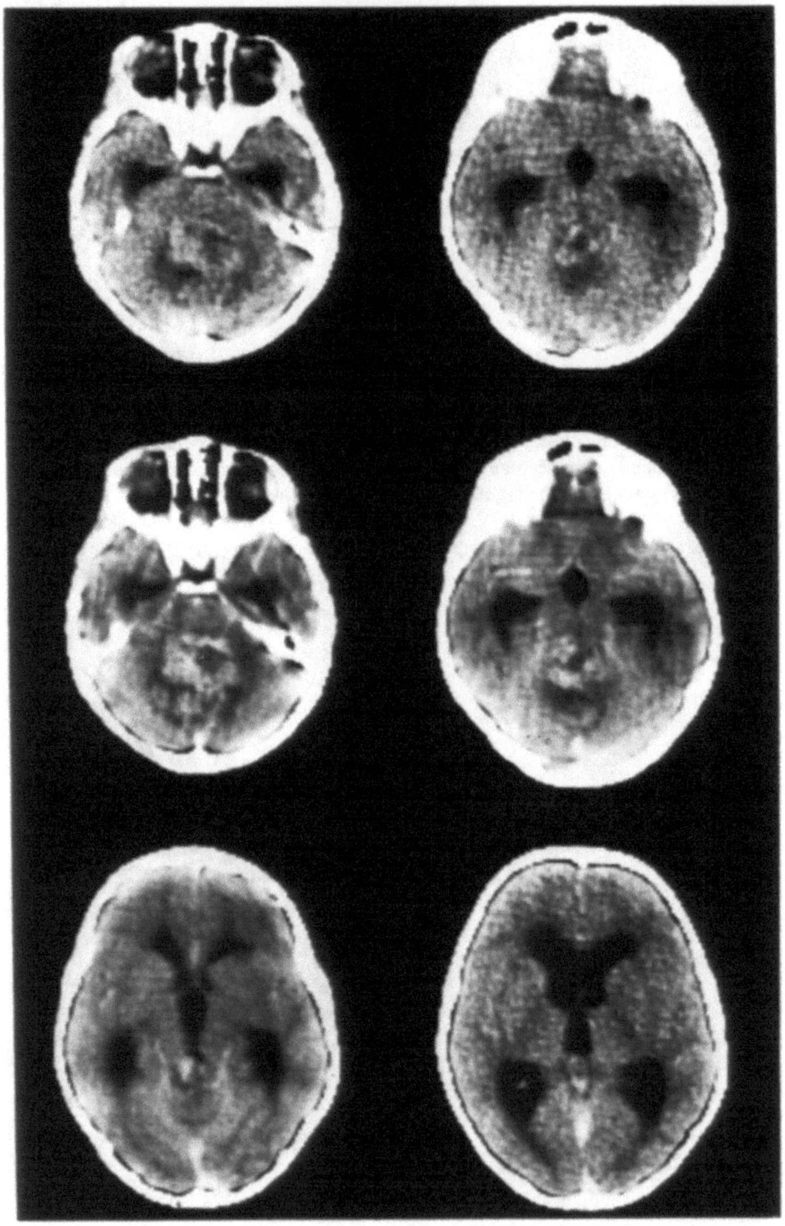

Fig. D 1.133. Ependymoma extending from the fourth ventricle through the aqueduct into the third ventricle in a 10-year-old child. The bulk of the tumor is inside the fourth ventricle. The tumor is very nonhomogeneous with central necrosis and mild perifocal edema. Solid tumor tissue appears slightly hyperdense on the plain CT scans (*top*). Mild contrast enhancement is observed. The part of the tumor protruding into the third ventricle is clearly displayed (*lower right*). There is severe obstructive hydrocephalus with periventricular lucency

Fig. D 1.134. Subependymoma of the left trigone and occipital horn in a $6^1/_2$-year-old girl. Postcontrast scans (*right*) show a narrow, mildly enhancing solid tumor component in the wall of the cyst

Fig. D 1.135. Papillary ependymoma of the right lateral ventricle in an 11-month-old infant. The tumor tissue is hyperdense on the plain CT scans (*top*) and shows a further density increase with contrast medium (*bottom*). The CT pattern is indistinguishable from choroid plexus papilloma (cf. Figs. D 1.207–210)

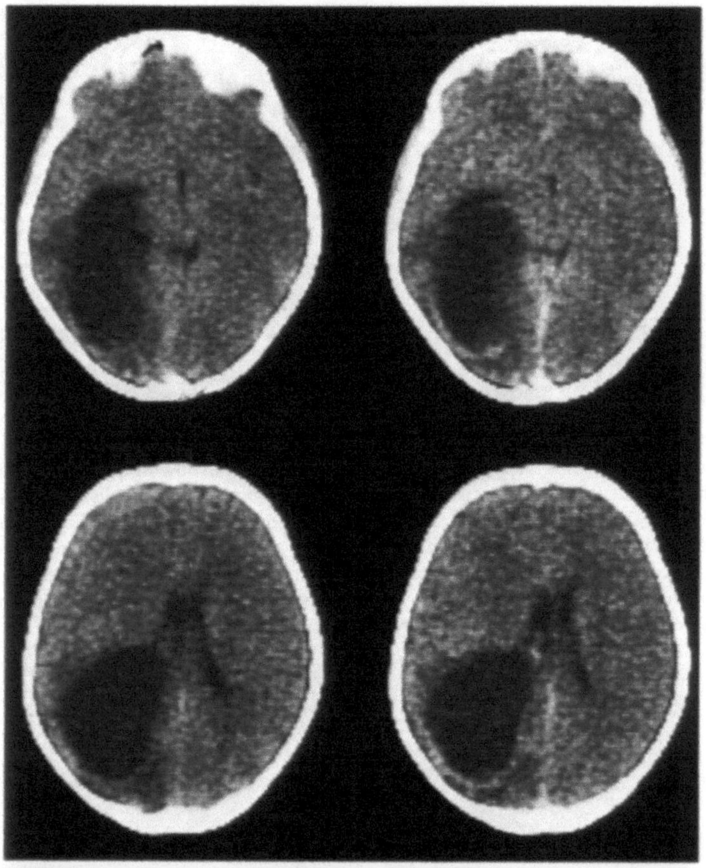

D 1.134

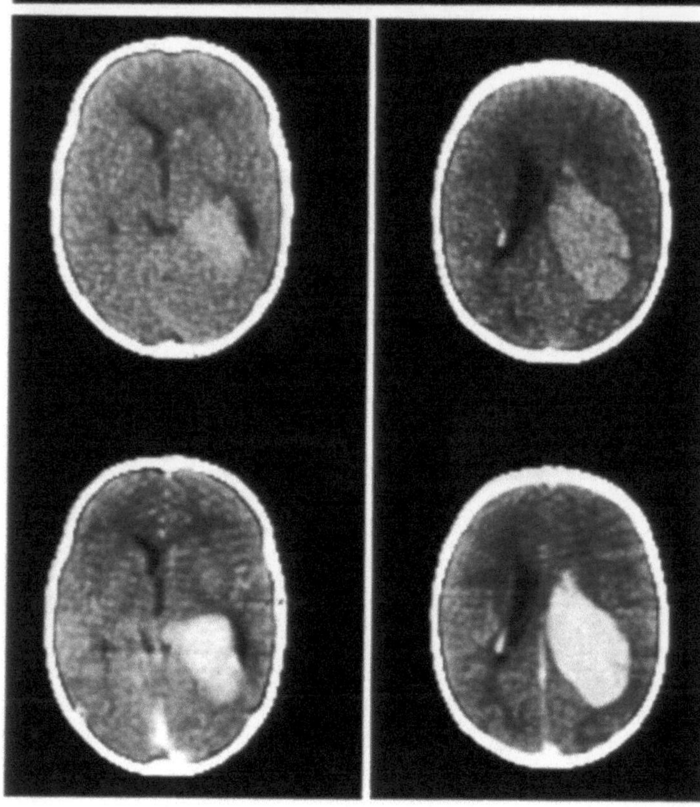

D 1.135

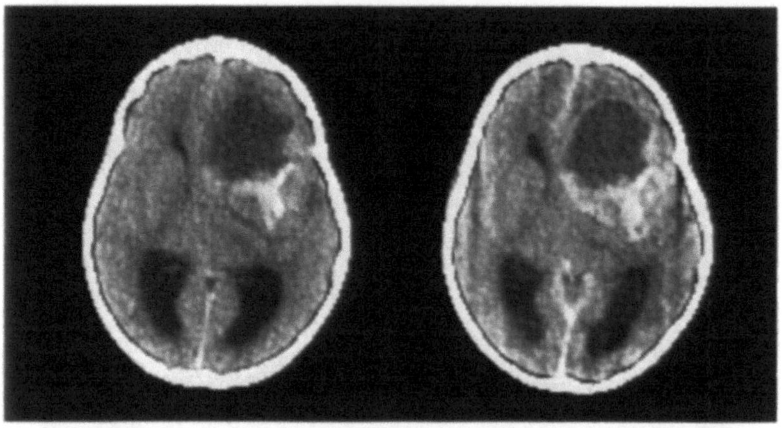

a

Fig. D1.136a, b. Cerebral ependymoma in a 7-year-old girl. **a** Initial CT examination demonstrates a partly cystic, partly calcified mass showing marked contrast enhancement (*right*) in the right frontotemporal region. The tumor is compressing the right frontal horn and obstructing the foramen of Monro with consequent dilatation of both occipital horns. CT findings are consistent with ependymoma. **b** CT scans 3 months later after subtotal tumor removal disclose a large recurrent growth that is slightly hyperdense on the plain scans (*upper* panel) and enhances markedly with contrast medium (*lower* panel)

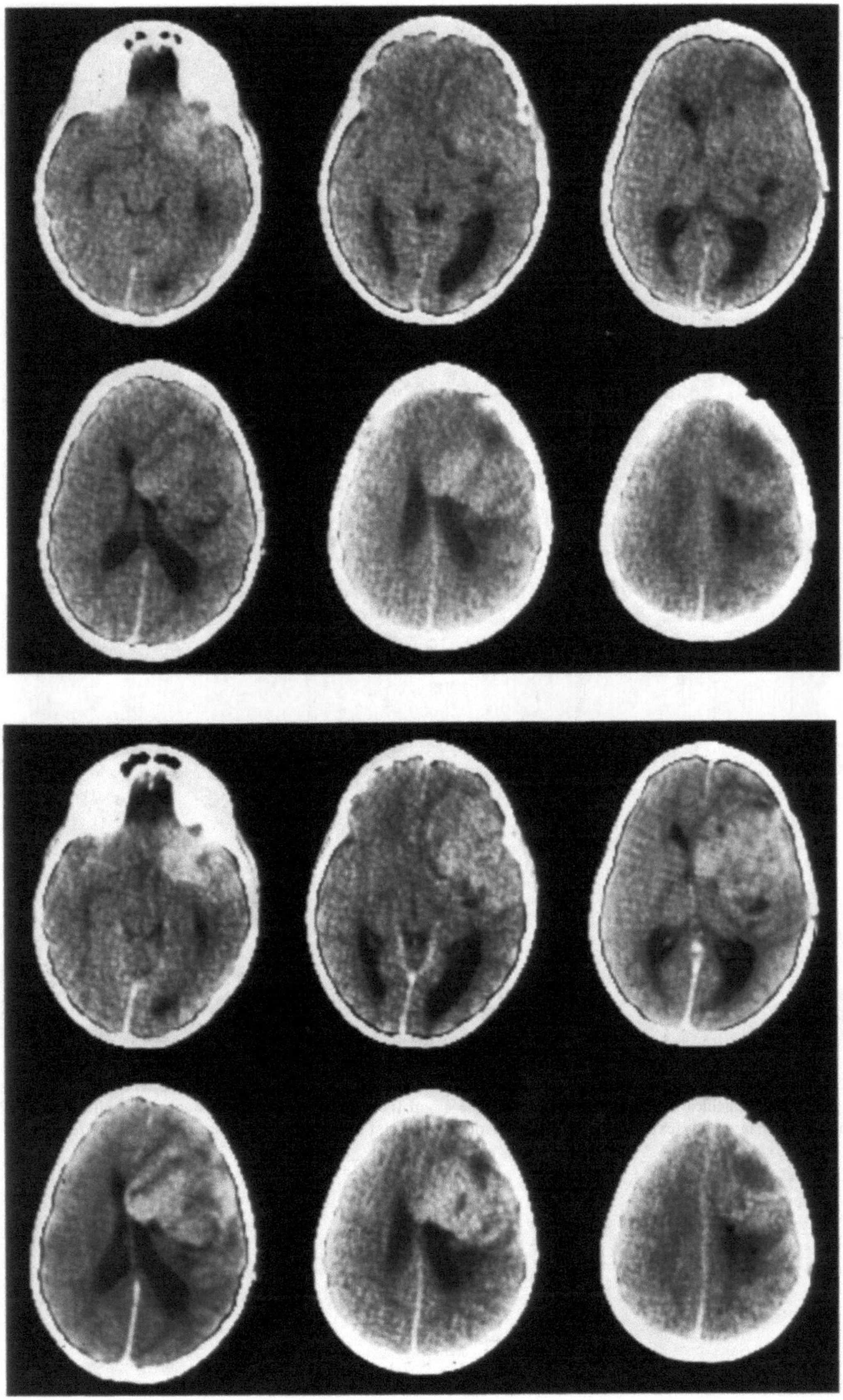

D1.136b

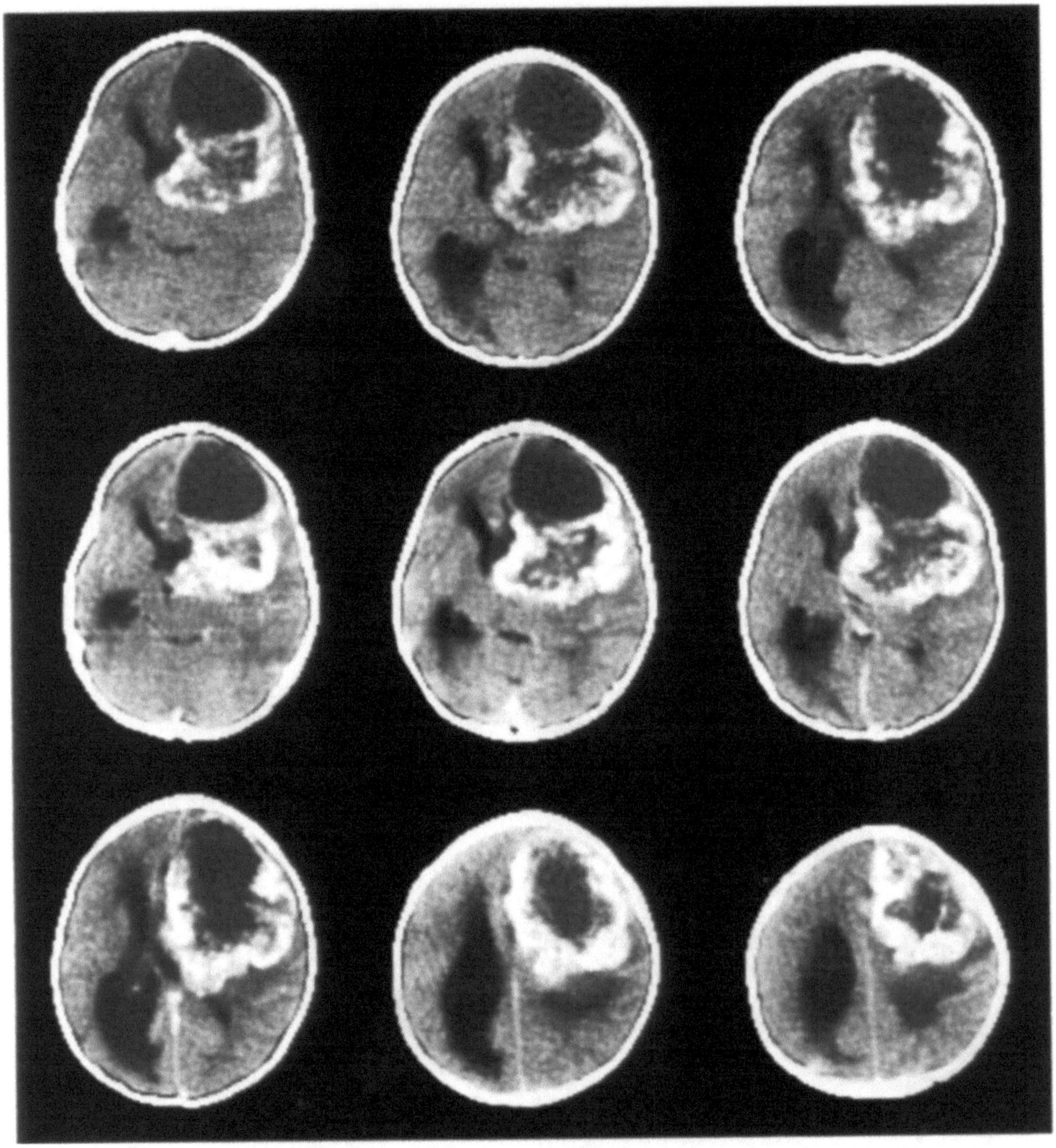

Fig. D 1.137. Cerebral ependymoma with a large cyst and extensive garland-like calcifications in a 2-year-old boy. The left lateral ventricle is greatly expanded secondary to obstruction of the foramen of Monro. Perifocal edema is seen on the higher-level scans through the white matter. (Plain scans at *top*, contrast scans at *center* and *bottom*)

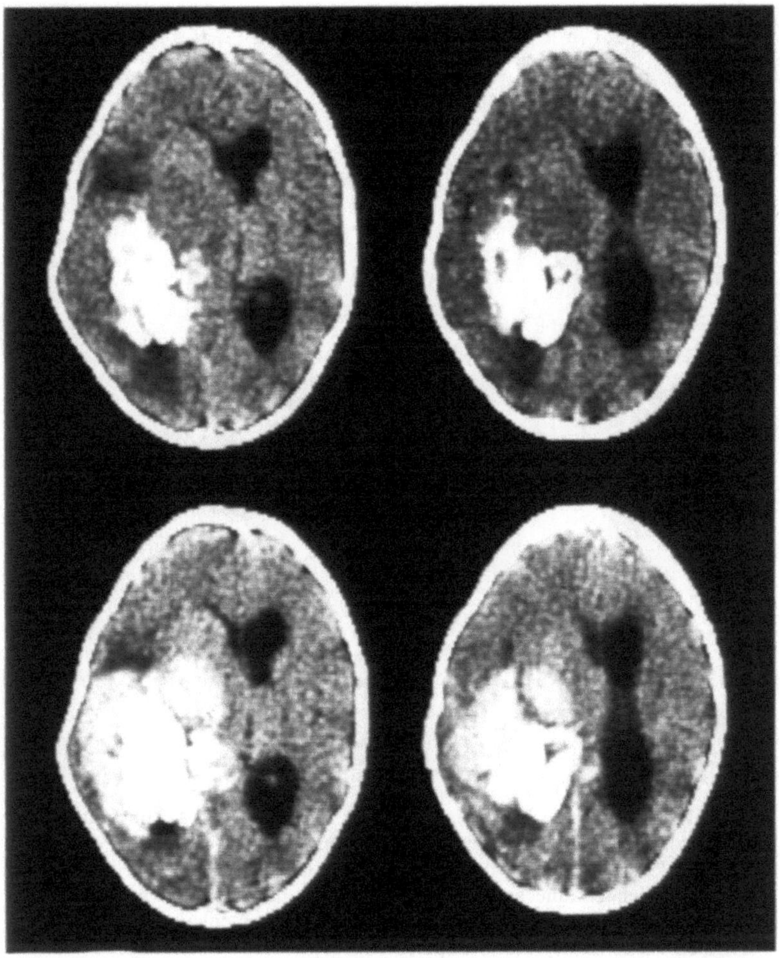

Fig. D1.138. Giant tumor with extensive calcifications in the left cerebral hemisphere of a 14-year-old girl. The minimally hypodense tumor areas around the calcifications on the plain scans (*top*) show very intense enhancement with contrast medium (*bottom*). The calvarium bulges outward over the neoplasm as an expression of the slow tumor growth. The tumor could not be definitively classified on histologic examination; some parts were characteristic of ependymoma and others of pilocytic astrocytoma

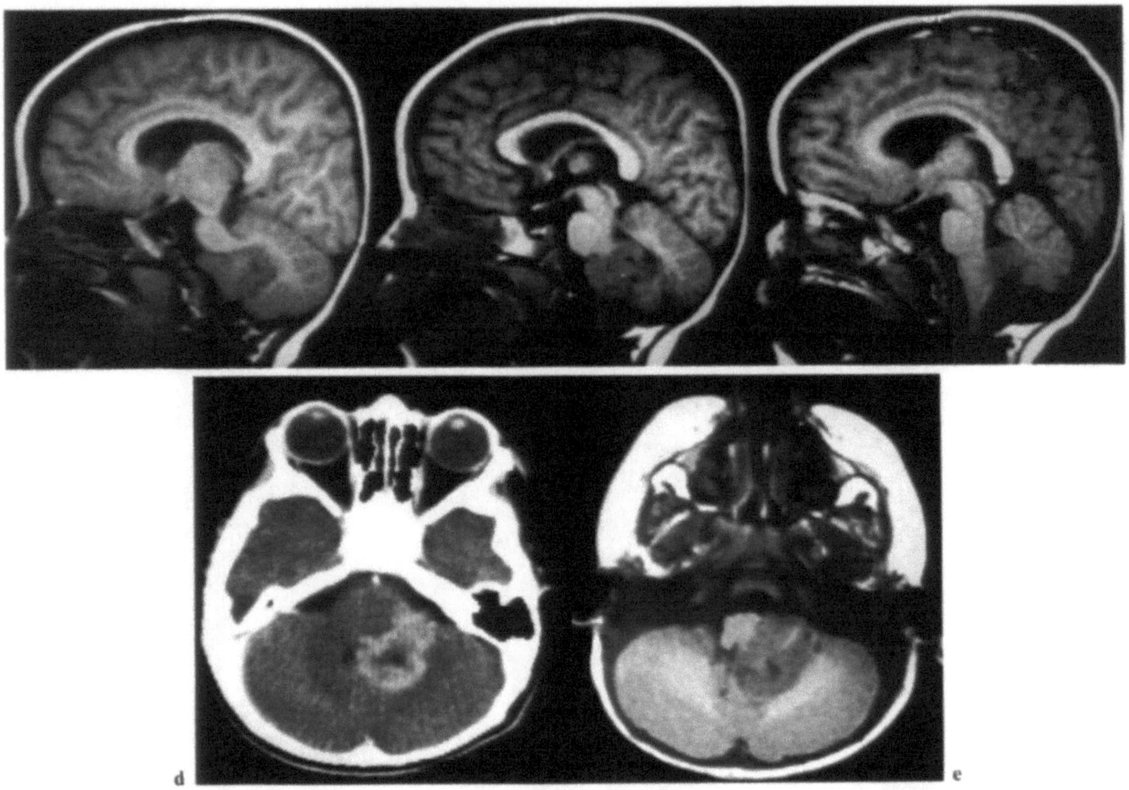

a–c d e

Fig. D 1.139 a–e. Grade III–IV ependymoma in a 16-month-old boy with a 14-day history of progressive ataxia and vomiting. MR: **a–c** SE 500/30 sagittal, **e** SE 700/30. CT: **d** contrast-enhanced. Scans show a mass lesion in the area of the cerebellopontine angle compressing and displacing the brainstem. CT demonstrates a peripheral, garland pattern of tumor enhancement. The T1-weighted image clearly shows displacement of the medulla and right cerebellar peduncle by the tumor, which is hypointense to surrounding brain

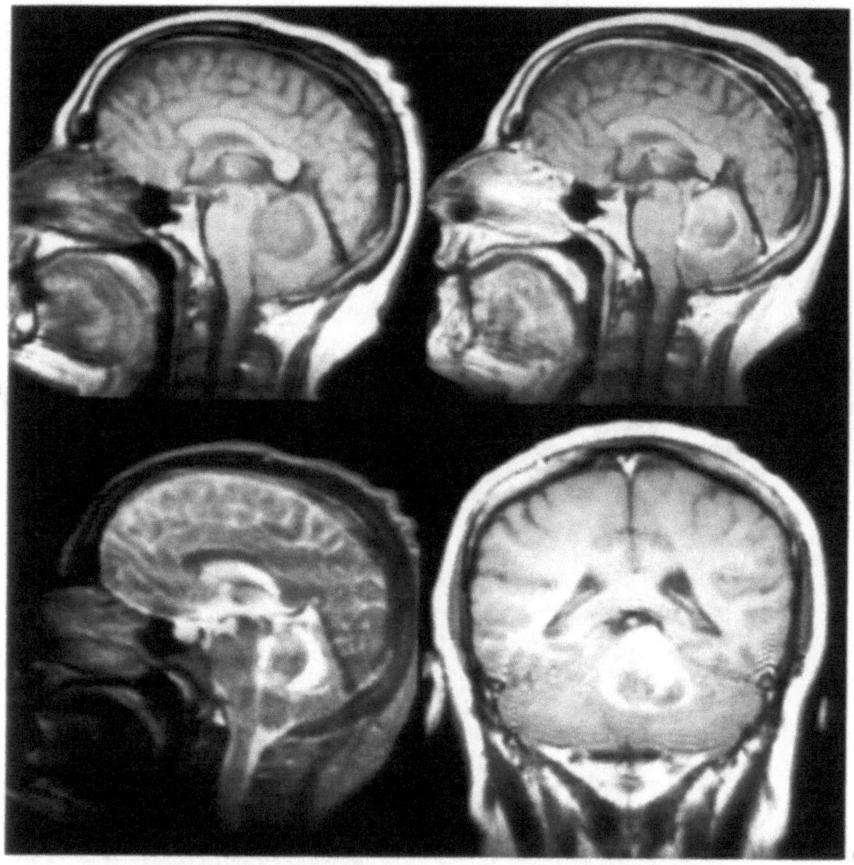

a b c d

Fig. D 1.140 a–d. Ependymoma of the right cerebellar region, originating from the fourth ventricle. The 30-year-old woman presented with progressive ataxia. MR: **a** SE 400/30, **b** SE 400/30 post Gd-DTPA, both parasagittal; **c** SE 2000/120 sagittal; **d** SE 400/30 post Gd-DTPA. The tumor is predominantly hypointense on the T1-weighted image (**a**) and shows a combination of ring and homogeneous enhancement with Gd-DTPA (**b, d**). The T2-weighted image (**c**) shows marked perifocal edema of high intensity

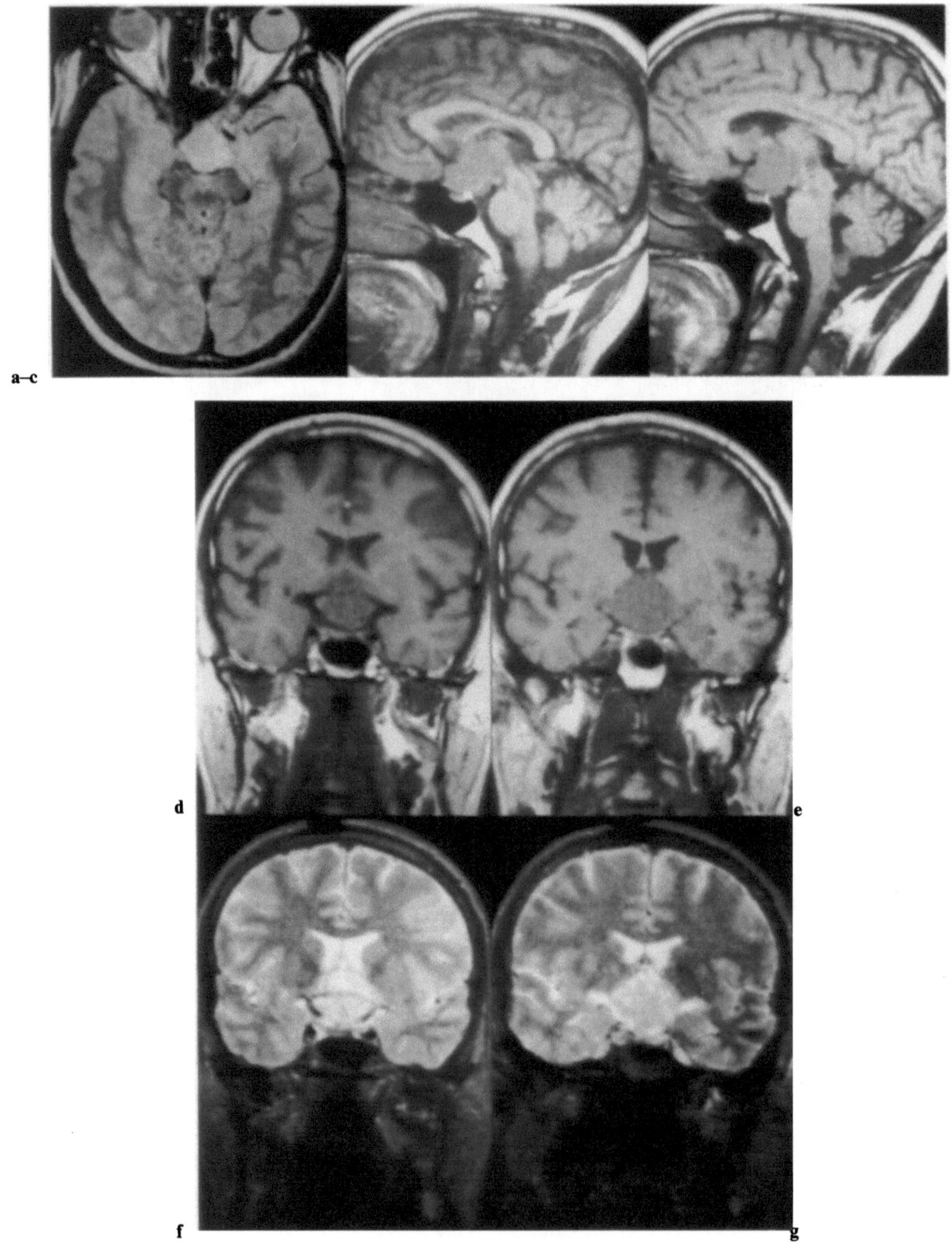

Fig. D 1.141 a–g. Recurrence of suprasellar ependymoma in the right lateral ventricle and fourth ventricle. The 30-year-old man had been operated 3 years previously for an ependymoma of the cauda equina. He presented with a 6-month history of visual acuity loss and 4-week history of altered mental status and paraparesis of the lower limbs. MR: **a** SE 3000/30 axial, **b, c** SE 500/30 sagittal, **d, e** SE 500/30 coronal, **f, g** SE 3000/90 coronal. The axial proton-density image shows a hyperintense mass in the sellar region (**a**). The sagittal views show the isodense, heterogeneous tumor projecting from the sella into the lateral ventricle and a coexisting tumor in the fourth ventricle (**b–d**)

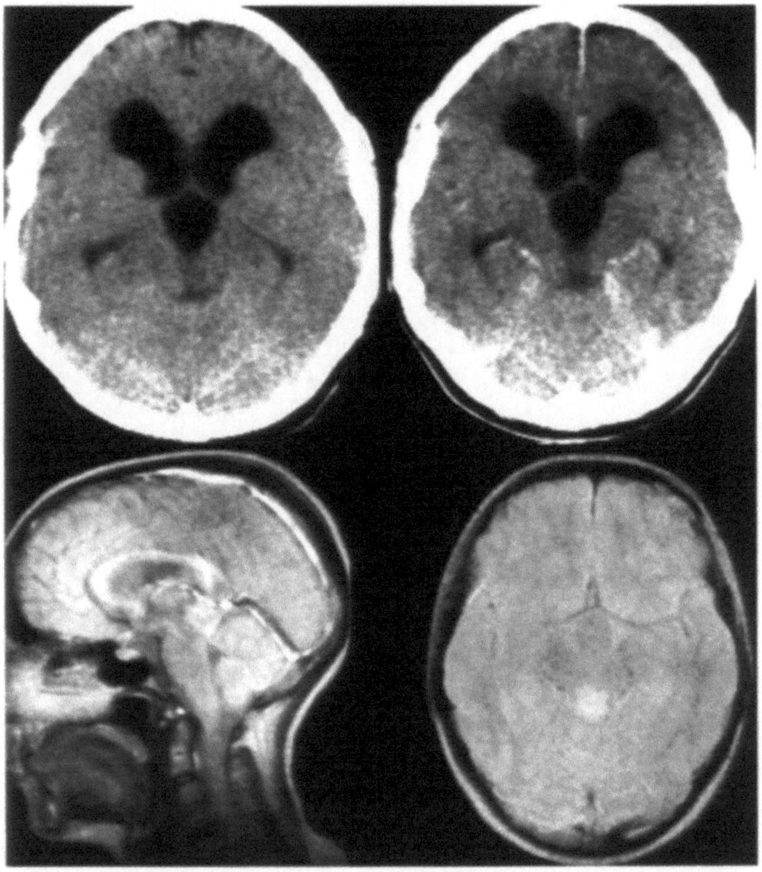

Fig. D 1.142 a–d. Subependymoma of the pineal region in a 30-year-old woman with a 1-year history of headaches. CT: **a** precontrast, **b** postcontrast. MR: **c, d** SE 1600/70. CT shows obstructive hydrocephalus with evidence of a slightly hypodense lesion that does not enhance. The T2-weighted image clearly demonstrates the juxtapineal tumor as an area of increased signal intensity

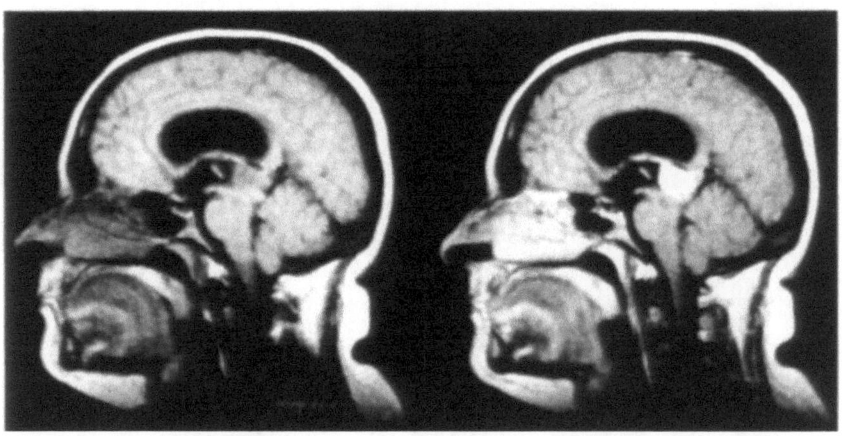

Fig. D 1.143. Subependymoma of the pineal region in a 49-year-old woman with a 4-year history of occipital headaches and increasing fatigue. She presented with ataxia and spastic left-sided hemiparesis mainly affecting the lower limb. MR: *left* SE 400/35 sagittal, *right* SE 400/35 post Gd-DTPA. The T1-weighted image shows the isodense tumor with associated obstructive hydrocephalus. The post Gd-DTPA image (*right*) shows marked tumor enhancement

D1.144

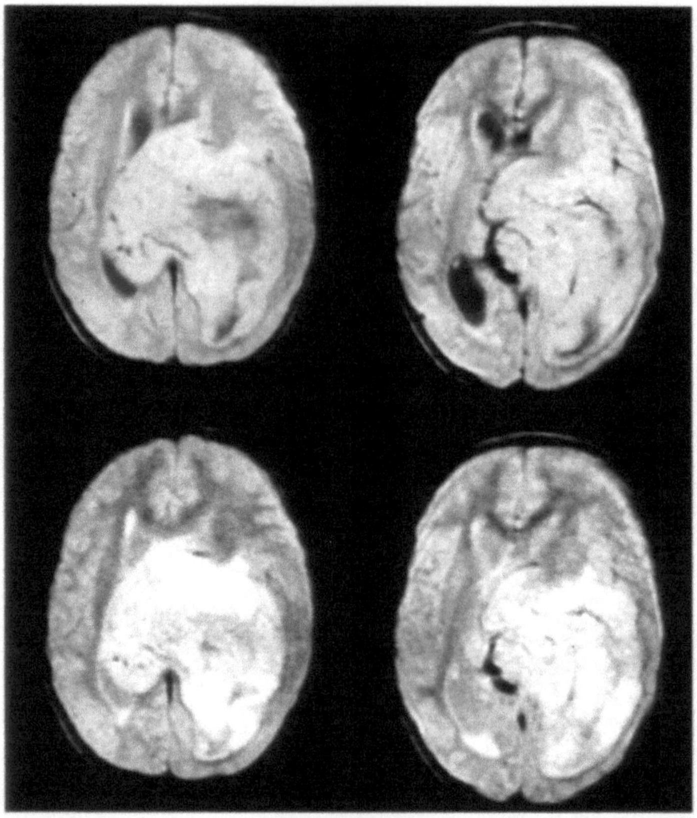

a b c d

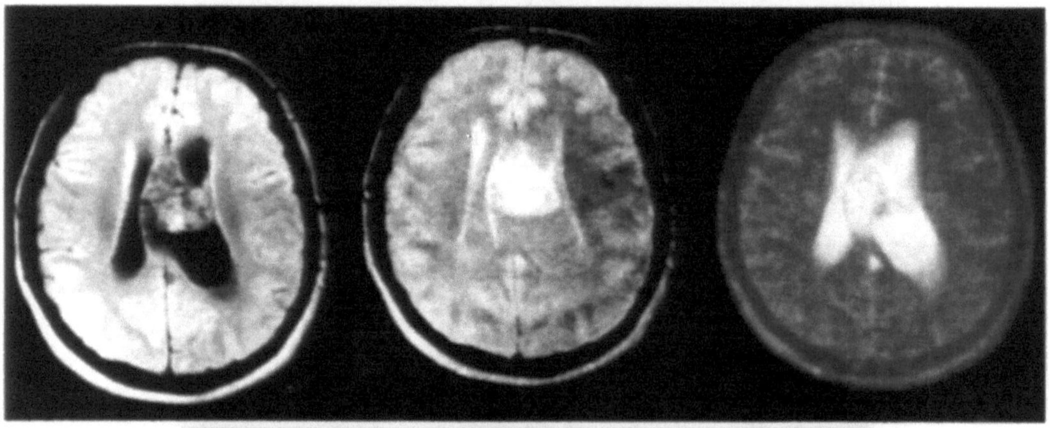

a–c

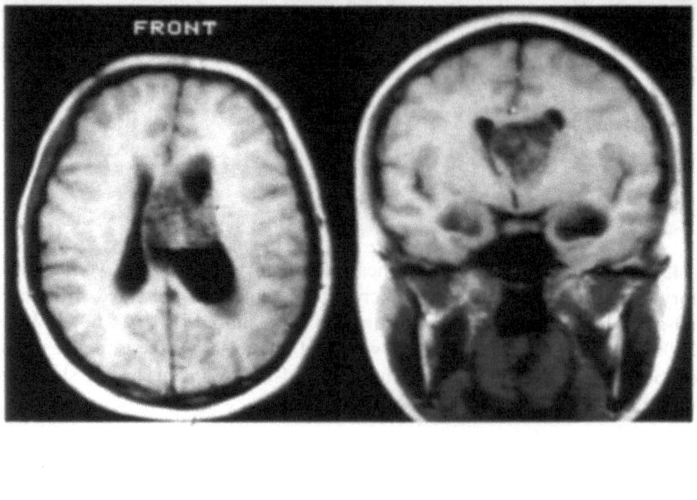

D1.145 d e

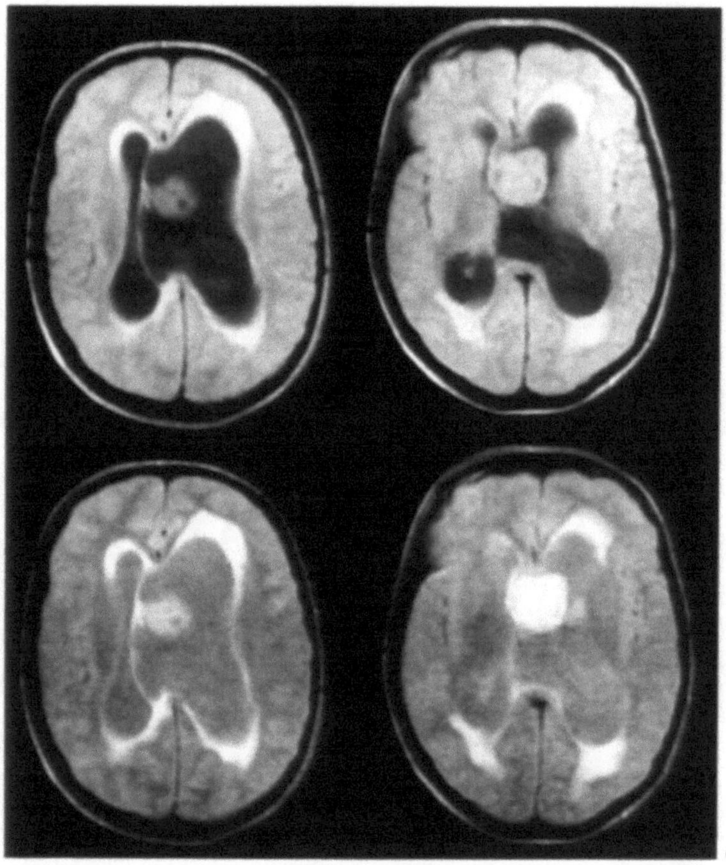

a b c d

Fig. D 1.146 a–d. Ependymoblastoma of the right lateral ventricle in a 23-year-old woman with a 1-year history of parietal headaches and concentration difficulties. MR: **a, b** SE 1600/35, **c, d** SE 1600/70. The tumor appears hyperintense on the proton-density images (**b**). The T2-weighted images show the hydrocephalus-associated periventricular edema as bandlike areas of high intensity

Fig. D 1.144 a–d. Giant ependymoblastoma of the right occipital horn with extension toward the left side. The 5-year-old patient was admitted with intermittent symptoms of increased intracranial pressure and mild left-sided hemiparesis. MR: **a, b** SE 1600/35, **c, d** SE 1600/70. The heavily T2-weighted images (**c, d**) show the hyperintense tumor filling and expanding the right lateral ventricle and protruding into the left lateral ventricle

Fig. D 1.145 a–e. Subependymoma of the right lateral ventricle in a 19-year-old girl with progressive headaches, right abducent paresis, and papilledema on the left side. MR: **a** SE 1600/30, **b** SE 1600/90, **c** SE 1600/240, **d** SE 400/35, **e** SE 400/35 coronal. The structural details of the tumor are appreciated on the proton-density image (**a**). The lesion becomes isointense to CSF, and thus less conspicuous, as T2 weighting is increased (**b, c**). Marked obstructive hydrocephalus is present

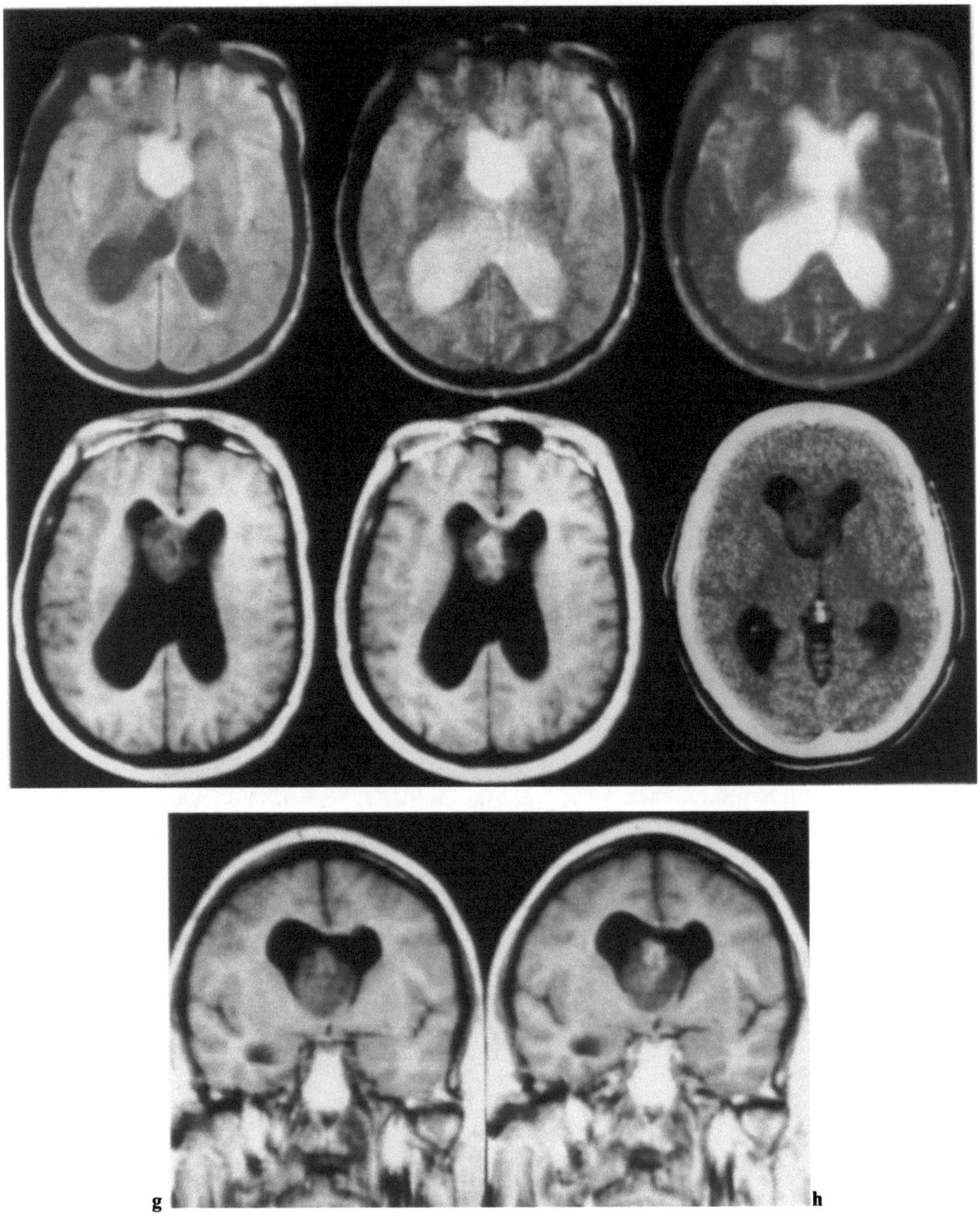

a–c

d–f

g h

Fig. D 1.147 a–h. Myxoid ependymoma in the left frontal horn of a 53-year-old man with a 3-month history of motor dysphasia, concentration difficulties, and loss of balance; latent right-sided hemiparesis. MR: **a** SE 1600/60, **b** SE 1600/120, **c** SE 1600/240, **d** SE 400/30, **e** SE 400/30 post Gd-DTPA, **g** SE 400/30 coronal, **h** SE 400/30 coronal post Gd-DTPA. Noncontrast CT (**f**) demonstrates a rounded mass of slightly lower density than brain. The tumor is slightly hypointense on the T1-weighted images (**d, g**) and shows central, nonhomogeneous enhancement with Gd-DTPA (**e, h**). Only the slightly T2-weighted sequence (**a**) clearly delineates the tumor with respect to brain parenchyma and CSF. The tumor is isointense to CSF on the heavily T2-weighted sequence (**c**)

j) Subependymal Giant Cell Astrocytomas

The very rare subependymal giant cell astrocytoma (0.32% in our series) is most commonly encountered in the setting of tuberous sclerosis. Symptoms of the tumor almost always appear in childhood or adolescence, and our observations indicate that males and females are affected with about equal frequency.

Typical Sites

The tumor most commonly occurs in the lateral ventricle. When situated between the foramen of Monro, the septum pellucidum, and the head of the caudate nucleus, subependymal giant cell astrocytoma can obstruct one or both foramina of Monro and produce severe hydrocephalus with symptoms of increased intracranial pressure. This may occur with very sudden onset and create a life-threatening situation. Many affected children experience cerebral seizures and display characteristic facial skin changes (sebaceous adenoma).

Subependymal giant cell astrocytoma is a grade I tumor and is not known to recur after complete removal.

Additional Diagnostic Procedures

Procedures other than CT and MR usually disclose only nonspecific abnormalities. Diagnosis is currently based almost entirely on CT findings.

Computed Tomography
(Figs. D1.148–153)

Noncontrast Scan
Even on the unenhanced CT scan, subependymal giant cell astrocytoma has a very characteristic appearance. The tumor is usually found in the frontal horn (see Figs. D1.148–151) and appears isodense or slightly hyperdense with respect to surrounding brain. Calcifications are occasionally seen within the tumor itself (Fig. D1.151a), and it is common to find ventricular wall calcifications entirely separate from the tumor (see Figs. D1.149–151b).

Hydrocephalus is almost always present with subependymal giant cell astrocytoma and helps to delineate the tumor from the surrounding CSF, even when the lesion has the same density as brain tissue. The tumors are walnut-size on average but may attain a huge size, especially in children with CSF shunts.

Contrast Enhancement
Even a standard contrast dose will produce 20–30 HU of tumor enhancement. Peak enhancement is recorded shortly after injection of the medium, and washout is prolonged. Most of these tumors enhance homogeneously.

Postcontrast Appearance
The intense contrast enhancement increases the conspicuousness of the lesion and helps delineate it from the head of the caudate nucleus.

Magnetic Resonance Imaging (Fig. D1.151 b)

Noncontrast Scan
The tumors appear hypo- to isointense on T1-weighted sequences. Their intraventricular location makes it easy to define the tumor boundaries. T2-weighted images demonstrate a highly intense mass whose extent corresponds to that on the CT scan. The tumor origin is demonstrated better with MR owing to its greater flexibility in the selection of image planes. CT offers about the same or perhaps better overall quality of diagnostic information than MR, as it is able to demonstrate even very small subependymal calcifications with exceptional clarity.

Post-Gadolinium Scan
Contrast enhancement is homogeneous, as on the CT scan.

Differential Diagnosis

Intraventricular *ependymomas* and *subependymomas* occur very rarely in the same region. One *astroblastoma* in our series occurred at a site typical for subependymal giant cell astrocytomas (see Fig. D1.148). We have found that *choroid plexus papillomas* tend to occur closer to the central part of the lateral ventricle. *Colloid cysts* of the foramen of Monro never transgress the boundary of the third ventricle. Most of these lesions appear hyperdense on plain CT scans and do not enhance. Moreover, they affect adults almost exclusively.

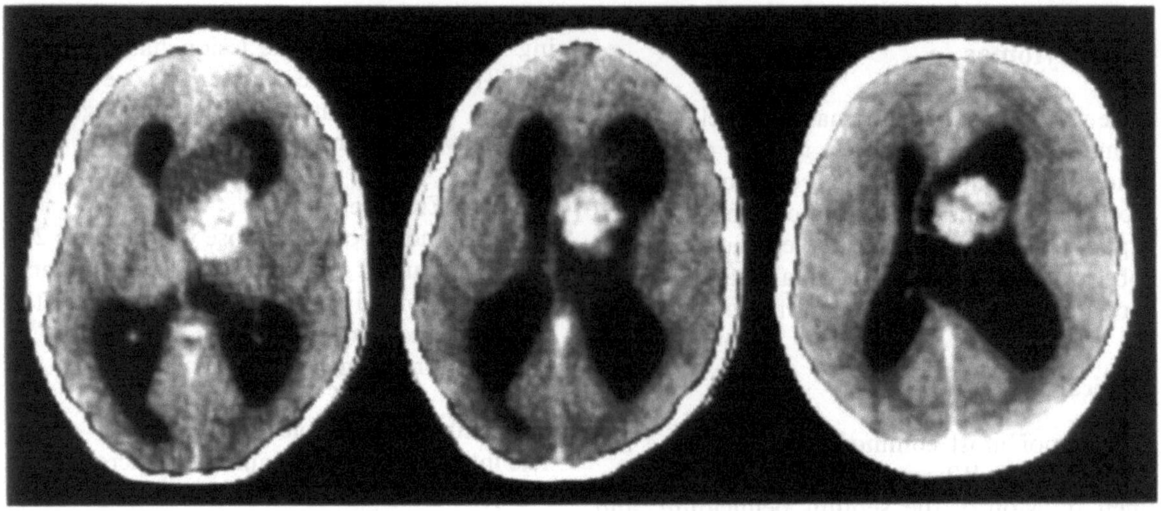

Fig. D 1.148. Astroblastoma with calcifications and a cyst occurring in the right frontal horn between the foramen of Monro, the septum pellucidum, and the head of the caudate nucleus. Obstructive hydrocephalus is more pronounced on the right side. The septum pellucidum is bowed to the left (*right* scan). The most likely diagnosis was thought to be subependymal giant cell astrocytoma. This tumor cannot be differentiated from astroblastoma with confidence on the basis of CT findings, even though the large tumor cyst and absence of ventricular wall calcifications are not characteristic of giant cell astrocytoma. All scans are contrast-enhanced

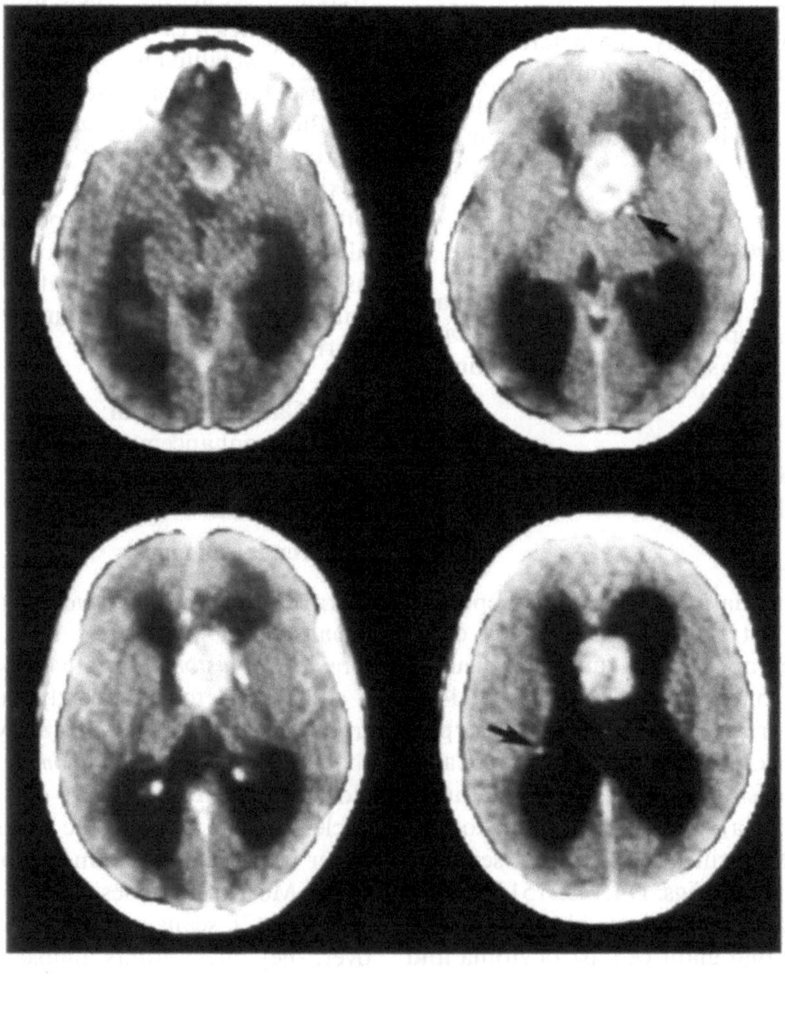

D 1.149

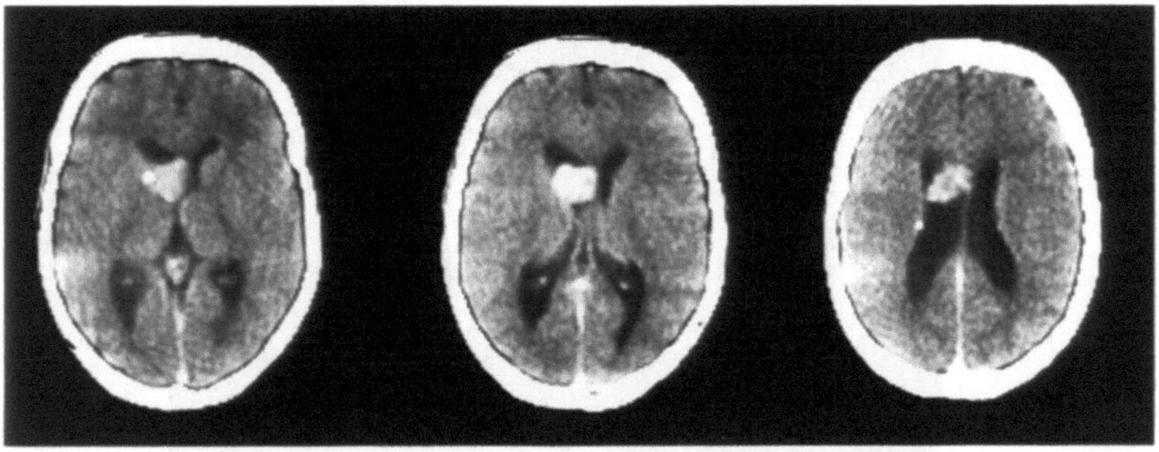

Fig. D 1.150. Subependymal giant cell astrocytoma at its typical site in the left frontal horn of a 17-year-old girl with the complete picture of tuberous sclerosis (cerebral seizures, sebaceous adenoma, ventricular wall tumors). Again a small calcification is seen on the central wall of the left lateral ventricle (all scans postcontrast)

Fig. D 1.149. Subependymal giant cell astrocytoma at its typical site in the right frontal horn of a 17-year-old girl with tuberous sclerosis. There is severe associated hydrocephalus. In addition to the tumor we observe two small calcifications on the ventricular wall (*arrows*) consistent with tuberous sclerosis, which frequently coexists with subependymal giant cell astrocytoma

Fig. D 1.151 a (see p. 178). Serial CT scans from a $5^1/_2$-year-old girl with a subependymal giant cell astrocytoma in the setting of tuberous sclerosis. Examination on December 19, 1977 shows a large tumor at a typical site in the left lateral ventricle between the foramen of Monro, septum pellucidum, and basal ganglia. The tumor presents isodense and slightly hyperdense absorption values (calcifications) on the precontrast scans. Note the many calcified tubers on the ventricular walls as an expression of the underlying disease. Follow-up examination on November 28, 1978 demonstrates considerable tumor enlargement in an 11-month period. Surgery was withheld because of oligophrenia. Plain scans are on the *left*, contrast scans on the *right*

Fig. D 1.151 b (see p. 179). Subependymal giant cell astrocytoma in a 13-year-old boy with debility, sebaceous adenoma, headache, and incipient right-sided hemiparesis. Postcontrast CT. MR: SE 3000/90 axial, SE 700/30 coronal and parasagittal. CT demonstrates right and left frontal intraventricular masses with involvement of the third ventricle and left trigone region. There is a coexisting cyst with mass effect. Hydrocephalus has developed from obstruction of the foramen of Monro. Subependymal calcifications are apparent. The tumors appear isointense on the T1-weighted MR images and hyperintense on the T2-weighted images, with CSF and cyst contents appearing bright

19.12.1977

28.11.1978

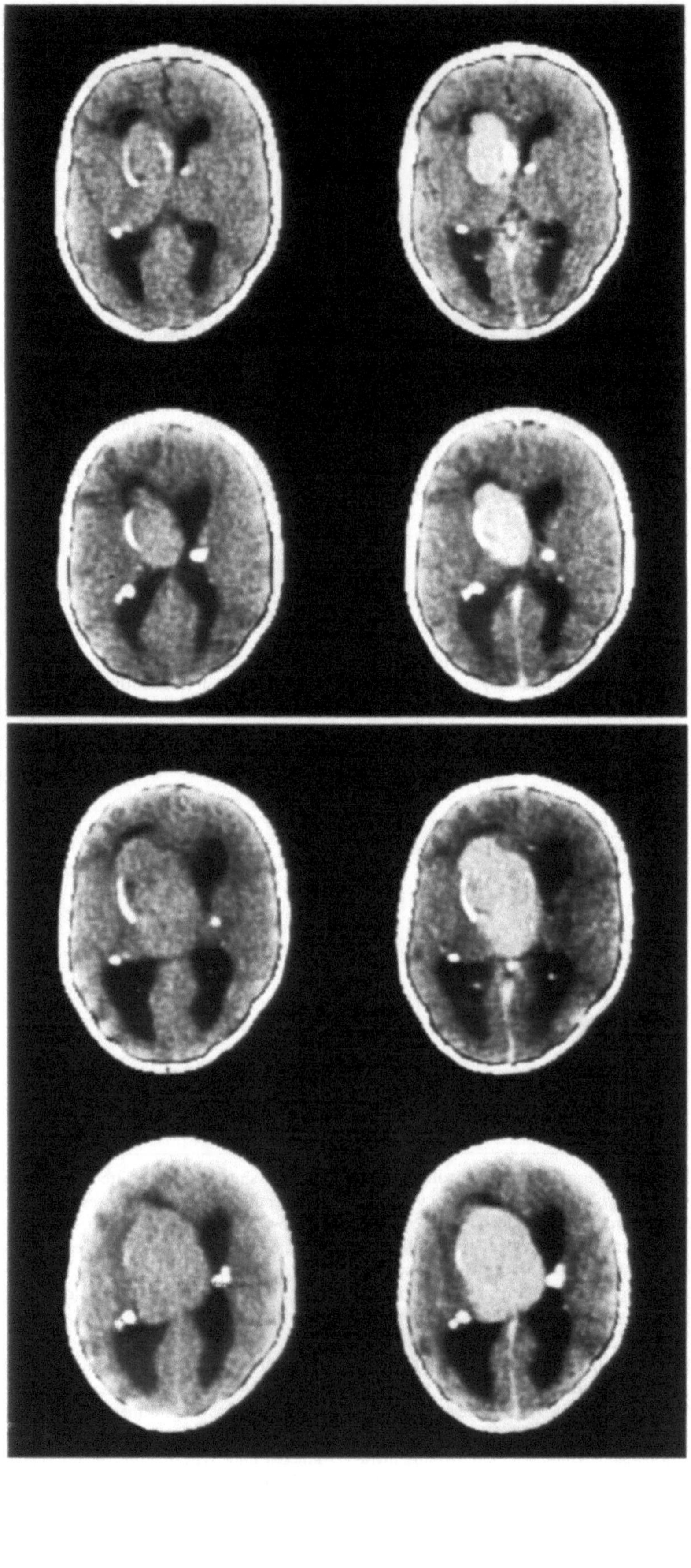

D1.151a
(Legend see p. 177)

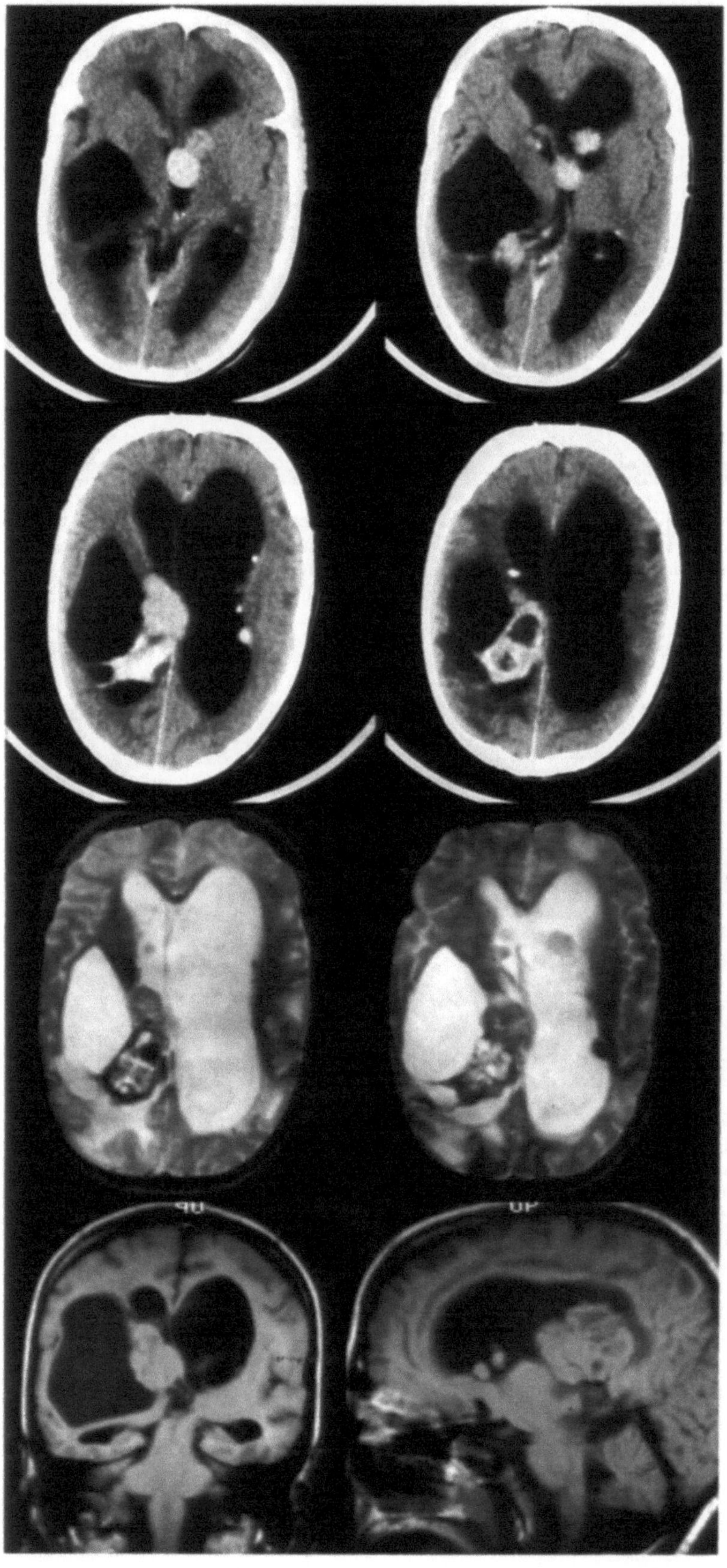

D1.151b
(Legend see p. 177)

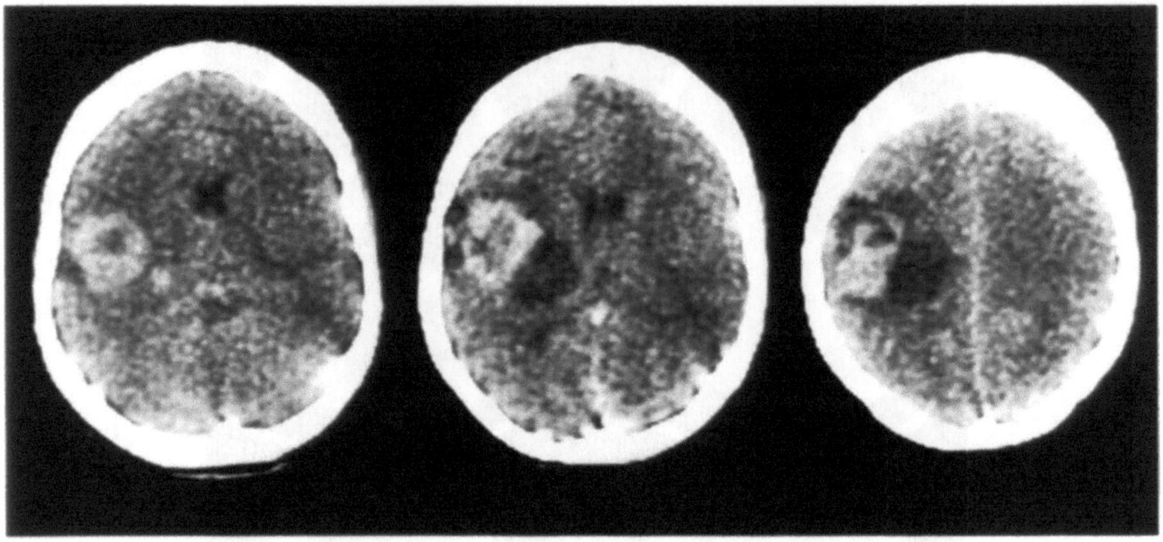

Fig. D 1.152. Subependymal giant cell astrocytoma in the left temporal lobe of a 24-year-old woman. Noncontrast CT shows a mixed-density lesion, while enhanced scans show a heterogeneous tumor with an adjacent cyst. The tumor itself contains lucent areas that were found to be cysts at operation. A specific diagnosis could not be made from CT findings. Because of its unusual CT appearance, the lesion was thought to be a rare brain tumor

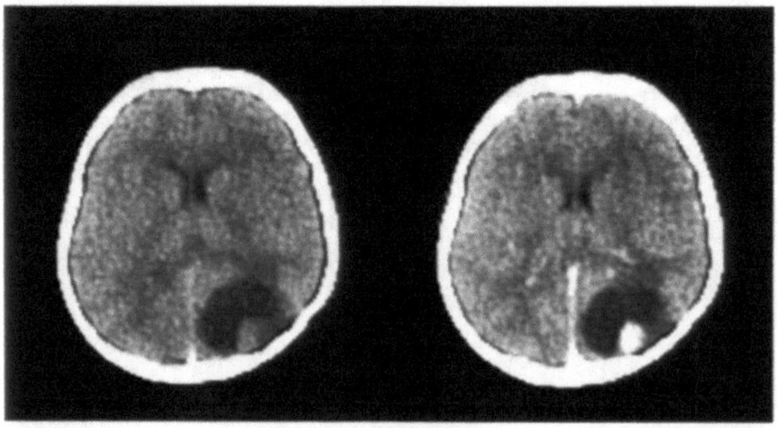

Fig. D 1.153. Subependymal giant cell astrocytoma in the right occipital lobe of a 13-year-old girl with infrequent cerebral seizures. Noncontrast CT (*left*) demonstrates a large, hypodense, smooth-bordered lesion with a peripheral isodense area. This area enhances intensely with contrast medium (*right*). Operative exposure disclosed a large cyst with a cherry-size tumor nodule on its wall, later identified as a subependymal giant cell astrocytoma. The CT appearance is atypical, and the lesion was originally thought to be a pilocytic astrocytoma

k) Nerve Cell Tumors

Nerve cell tumors are very rare, making up only 0.5% of all intracranial neoplasms. The following tumor types derived from ganglion cells and other nerve cells are recognized:

1. Dysplastic gangliocytoma (grade I)
2. Ganglioglioma (gangliocytoma) (grade II)
3. Anaplastic ganglioglioma (ganglioneuroblastoma) (grade III)
4. Neuroblastoma (grade IV)

The grade II and grade III tumors occur predominantly in the first three decades of life and appear to affect males with greater frequency. Neuroblastomas grow very rapidly in the brain tissue and do not present well-defined boundaries. Children and adolescents are most commonly affected. In the literature the tumors are grouped with medulloblastomas and medulloepitheliomas under the heading of "primitive neuroectodermal tumors" (PNET).

Sites of Predilection

Dysplastic gangliocytomas occur in the cerebellum, where they produce a circumscribed "blastomatous" area marked by hyperplastic-appearing cerebellar gyri (Lhermitte and Duclos 1920; Zülch 1956, 1980). Most ganglion cell tumors occur in the cerebrum, displaying a preference for the medial temporal lobe, the tuber cinereum region, the thalamus, and the mesencephalon (Zülch 1956). We have also found these tumors close to the midline in the frontal and parietal lobes (Figs. D 1.154–159). Cysts and calcifications are common.

Main Clinical Features

The main symptom of cerebral ganglion cell tumors is seizures, which may be present for some years. Neurologic deficits are rare and are seen only with larger neoplasms.

Gangliocytomas in the posterior fossa produce signs referrable to cerebellar dysfunction. Dysfunctions of the cranial nerves may also be present.

Computed Tomography
(Figs. D 1.154–160, 162)

Noncontrast Scan
Most gangliocytomas are easily recognized as mass lesions on the plain CT scan owing to the presence of calcifications and/or cysts. The same applies to gangliogliomas. We have found that the combination of a large cyst and intratumoral calcifications is highly characteristic of a gangliocytoma or related tumor on the unenhanced CT scan (Figs. D 1.157, 158).

Most of the neuroblastomas in our population were isodense to normal brain tissue or only slightly different in density.

Postcontrast Scan
Solid, uncalcified tumor components may enhance with contrast medium, though this is not always the case. Usually very little difference is noted between the pre- and postcontrast CT scans.

Magnetic Resonance Imaging
(Figs. D 1.161, 163, 164)

Noncontrast Scan
The tumors are hypointense on the T1-weighted image and hyperintense on T2-weighted sequences.

Post-Gadolinium Scan
Some of these tumors enhance with Gd-DTPA.

Differential Diagnosis

The tumors most closely resembling gangliocytomas on CT scans are *oligodendrogliomas*. However, the latter are unlikely to contain large cysts. The differential diagnosis should also include *pilocytic astrocytomas* as well as *hamartomas* of the temporal lobe. Cerebellar tumors with calcifications in adults should always arouse suspicion of a gangliocytoma. Unless the foregoing typical patterns are recognized, there is little likelihood of diagnosing a ganglion cell tumor on the basis of CT findings, especially if calcifications are absent.

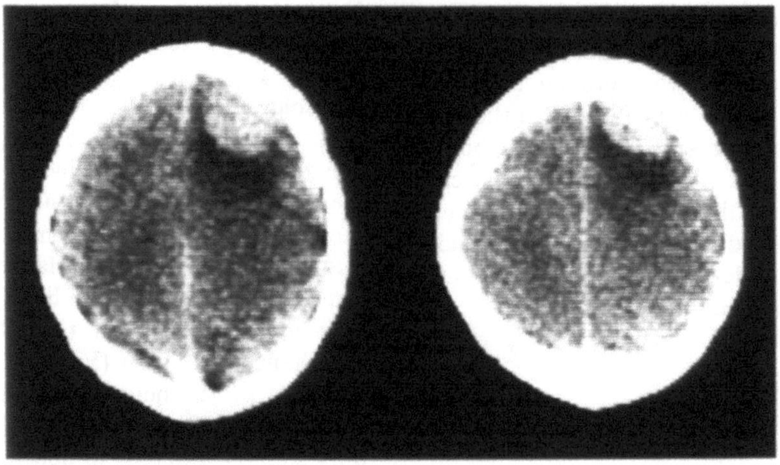

Fig. D 1.154. Gangliocytoma of the right fronto-precentral region in a 37-year-old man. Postcontrast CT shows a solid, enhancing nodular tumor within a clearly delineated hypodensity (cyst). The initial suspicion was of meningioma

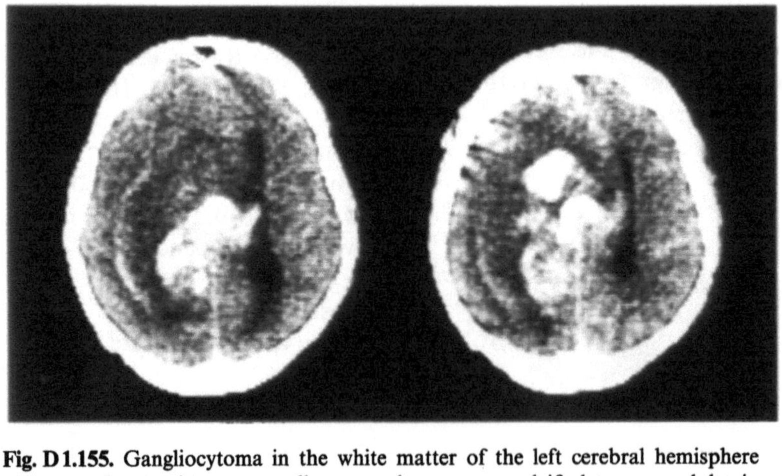

Fig. D 1.155. Gangliocytoma in the white matter of the left cerebral hemisphere with extension to the corpus callosum and numerous calcified tumor nodules in a 32-year-old man with cerebral seizures and dysphasic disturbances. Postcontrast CT

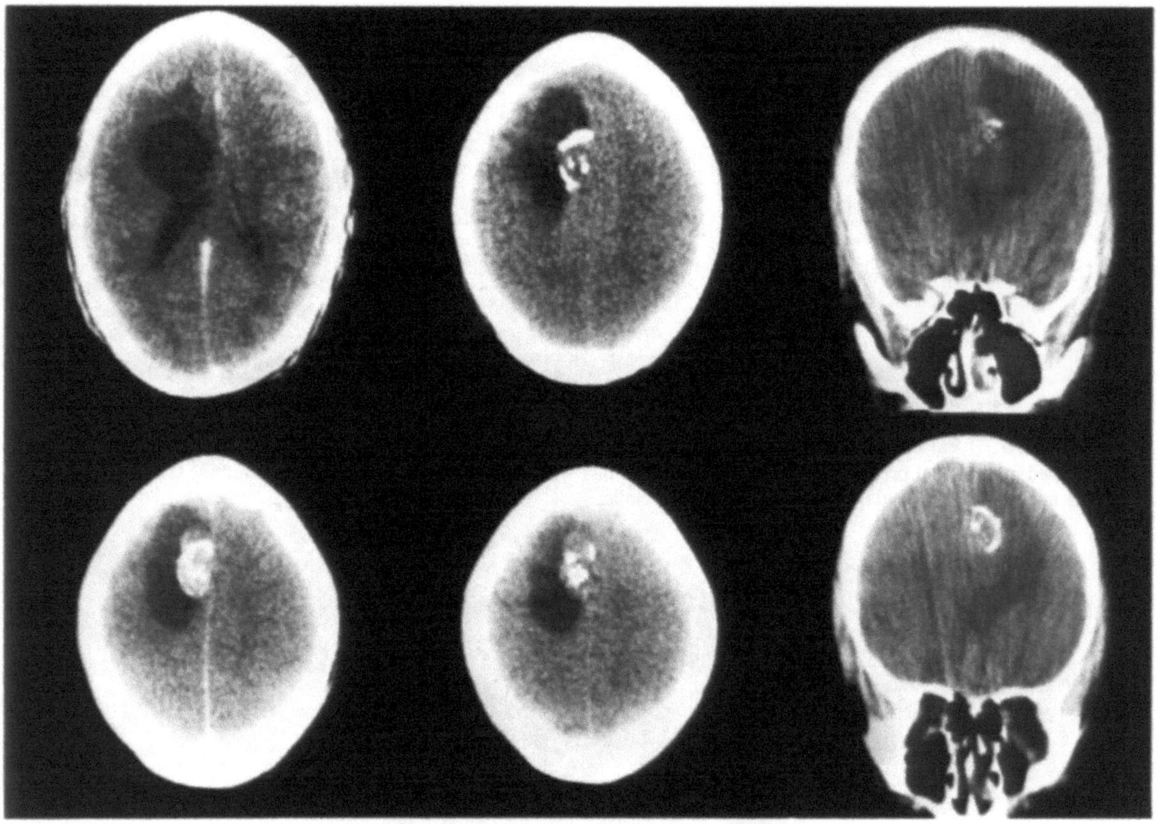

Fig. D 1.156. Ganglioglioma of the left precentral region, bordering on the interhemispheric fissure, in an 18-year-old male. On postcontrast CT the tumor consists of faintly enhancing solid tissue and of calcified components on the wall of a large cyst. The coronal scans show extension of the cyst into portions of the left cerebral cortex

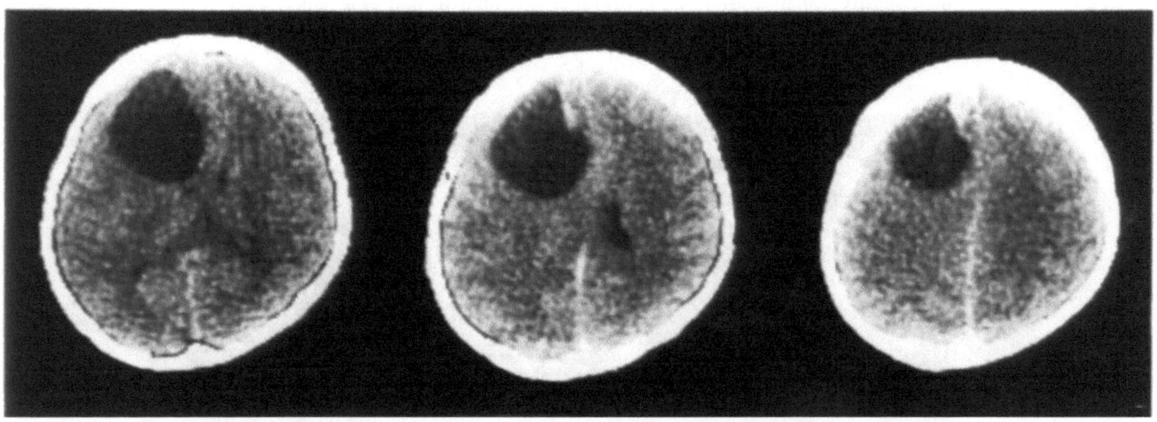

Fig. D 1.157. Ganglioneuroblastoma in a 27-year-old man with seizures. Scans show a large cystic mass with solid, markedly enhancing tumor components on the medial cyst wall (postcontrast scans at *center* and *right*). The density of the cystic component is 19.5 HU

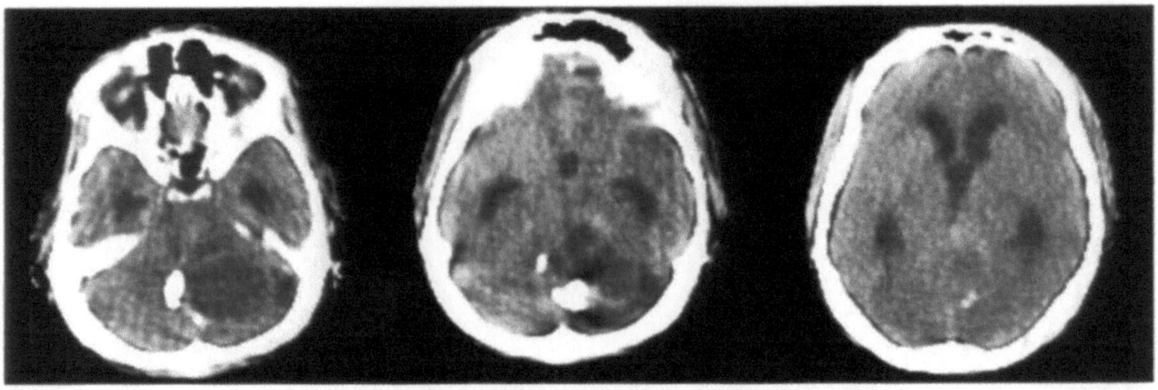

Fig. D 1.158. Ganglioneuroblastoma of the right cerebellar hemisphere in a 37-year-old man with ataxia and symptoms of incereased intracranial pressure. The nerve cell tumor appears as a ring-shaped, partially calcified mass. The solid, uncalcified tumor components show little contrast enhancement. There is displacement of the fourth ventricle and obstructive hydrocephalus. Postcontrast CT

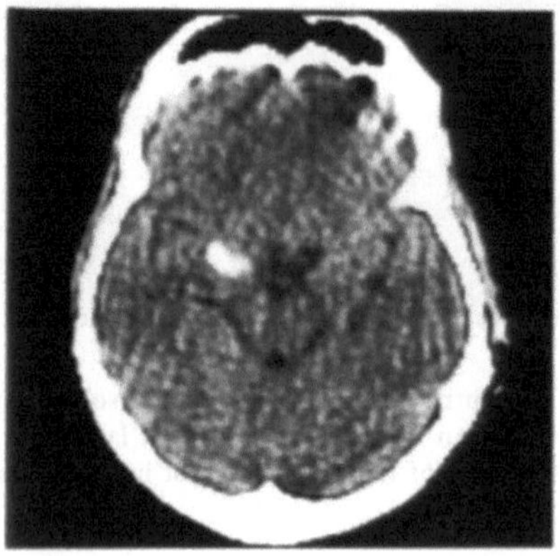

Fig. D 1.159. Gangliocytoma in the uncus of the left temporal lobe in a 25-year-old man with temporal lobe seizures. CT shows only a comma-shaped area of very high density (calcification). The appearance is similar to that of a hamartoma

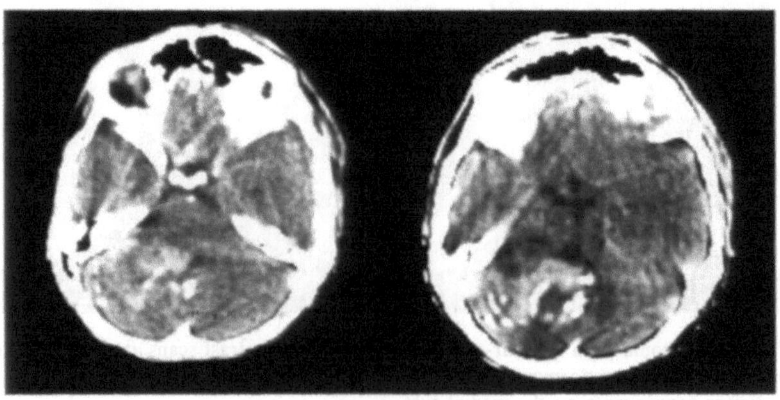

Fig. D 1.160. Large gangliocytoma of the left cerebellar hemisphere in a 32-year-old man with loss of dexterity in the left hand and visual disturbances. Scans show numerous calcium flecks in the mass with mildly enhancing solid components and slight perifocal edema

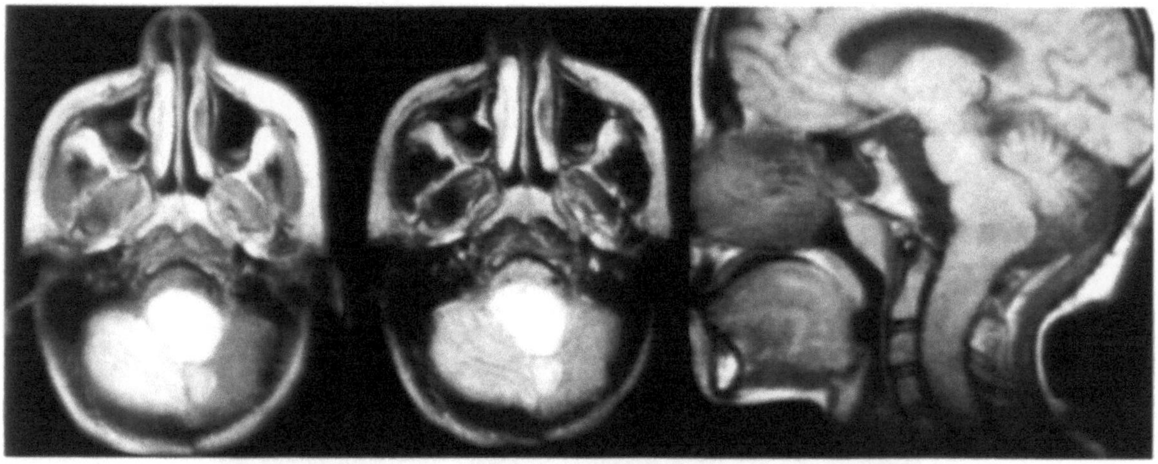

Fig. D 1.161. Gangliocytoma of both cerebellar hemispheres, with greater involvement of the left side. The 13-year-old girl presented with ataxia, spastic right-sided hemiparesis, and dysfunction of the lower cranial nerves. She underwent an initial subtotal tumor resection at 7 years of age, at which time the tumor had infiltrated the cerebellum, pons, and medulla oblongata. MR: *left* SE 1600/35, *center* SE 1600/70, *right* SE 400/35 sagittal. The proton-density and T2-weighted images show hyperintense tumor components in the left cerebellar hemisphere with smaller components in the right hemisphere and medulla oblongata. Expansion of the pons and medulla is evident on the sagittal image (*right*)

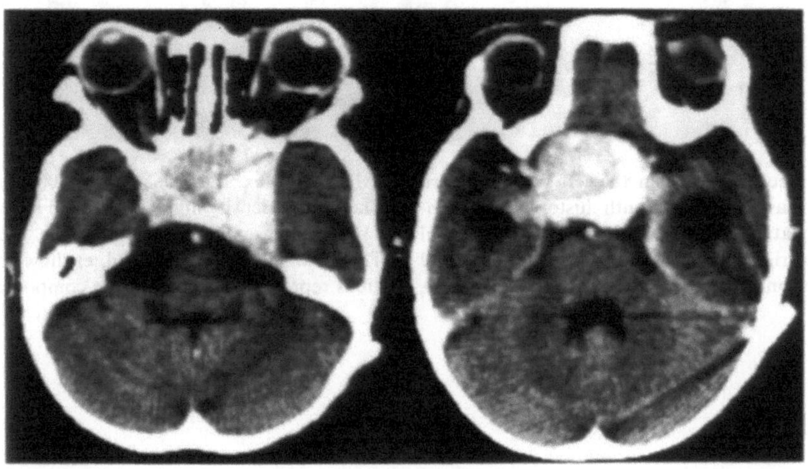

Fig. D 1.162. Intra- and parasellar neuroblastoma in a 2-year-old boy with severe, progressive loss of vision. Postcontrast CT shows marked tumor enhancement in the sellar and parasellar areas with calcium inclusions

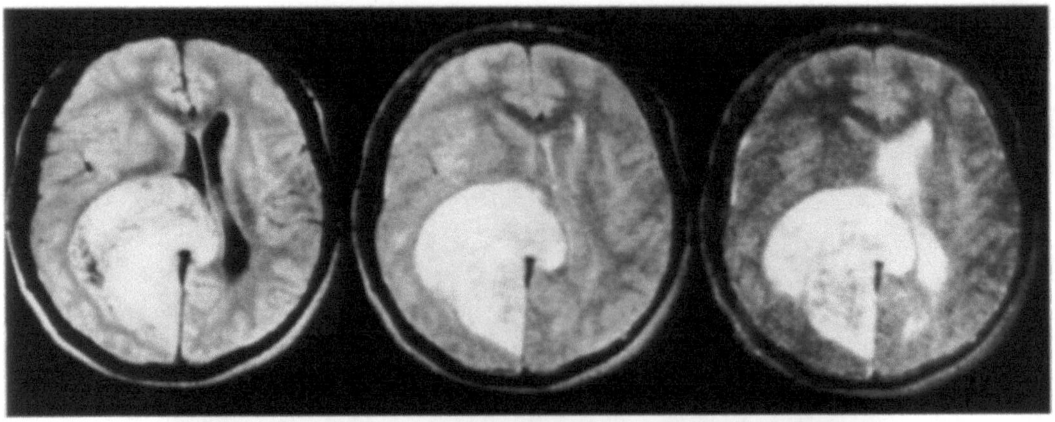

a–c

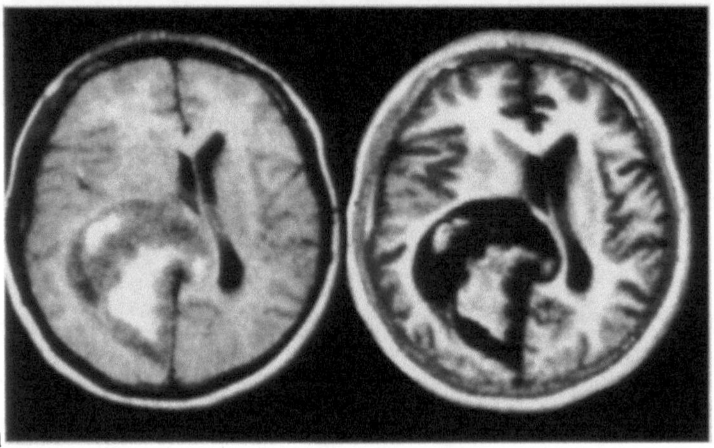

d e

Fig. D 1.163 a–e. Neuroblastoma in the left occipital horn of a 19-year-old man with a 3-month history of personality change and fatigue. Patient presented with bilateral papilledema, lower right quadrant anopsia, anisocoria, and latent hemiparesis on the right side. MR: **a** SE 1600/30, **b** SE 1600 /90, **c** SE 1600/150, **d** SE 400/35, **e** IR 1500/400/35. The proton-density and T2-weighted sequences demonstrate a hyperintense mass expanding the occipital horn (**a–c**). The T1-weighted sequences (**d, e**) show central hyperintense areas representing hemorrhagic components

a b c d e f
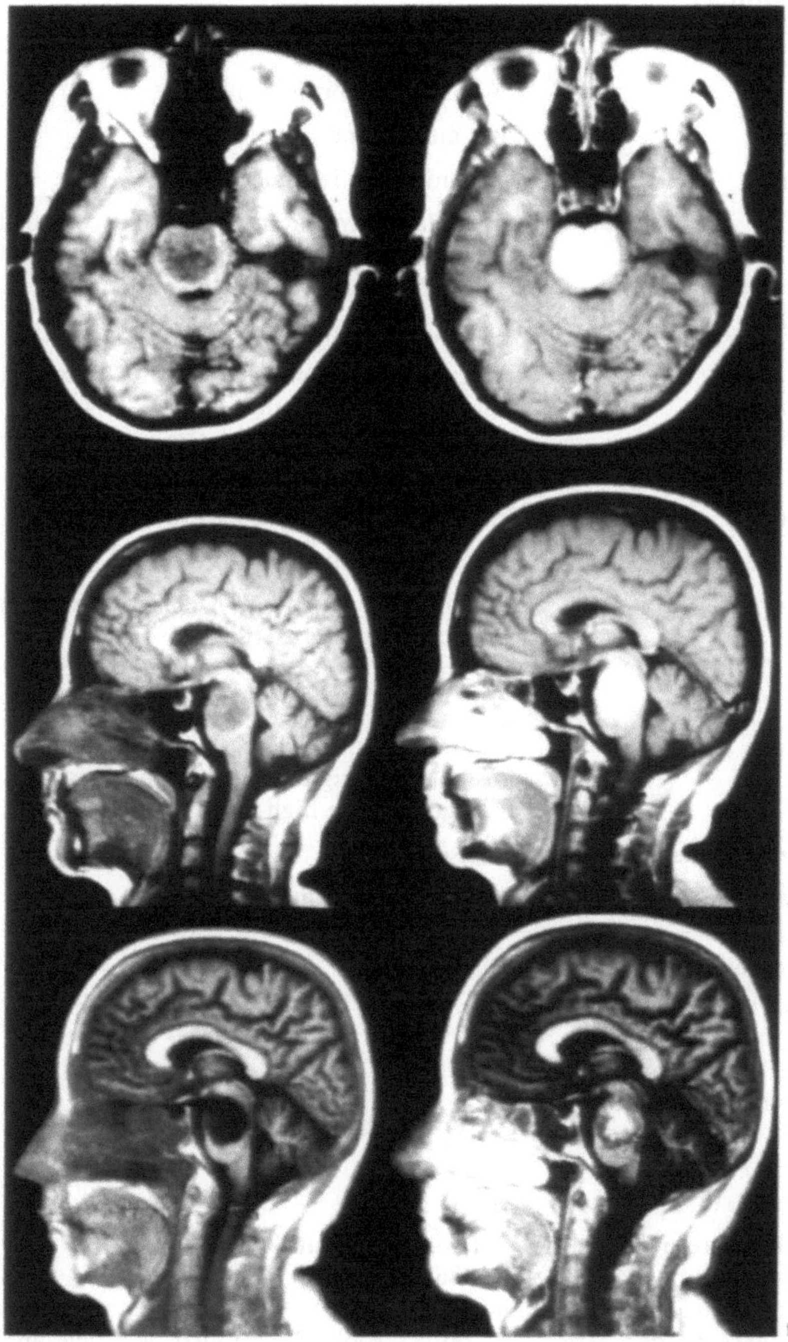

Fig. D 1.164 a–f. Neuroblastoma of the pons in a 47-year-old woman with intermittent headaches and diplopia. MR: **a** SE 400/30, **b** SE 400/30 post Gd-DTPA, **c** SE 400/30, **d** SE 400/30 post Gd-DTPA sagittal, **e** IR 1500/400/35, **f** IR 1500/400/35 post Gd-DTPA. The tumor, hypointense without contrast medium, enhances markedly with Gd-DTPA on the axial and sagittal T1-weighted images (**b, d**). The tumor appears hypointense with clear borders on the T1-weighted IR sequence (**e**) and again shows bright central enhancement with Gd-DTPA (**f**)

l) Medulloblastomas

Incidence	2%–6% of all brain tumors
Age predilection	First and second decades of life
Sex predilection	Preponderance in males
Typical sites	Cerebellar vermis, fourth ventricle, cerebellar hemispheres, caudal brainstem; can metastasize to all sites in CSF pathways
Main clinical features	Headache, vomiting, ataxia
Angiography	Evidence of mass effect; may show fine pathologic vessels and tumor staining
CT	
Noncontrast scan	Tumor appears hyperdense or occasionally isodense
Contrast enhancement	Generally positive
Postcontrast appearance	Solid homogeneous tumor in majority of cases; slight perifocal edema not unusual
MR	
Noncontrast scan	Tumors hypointense on T1-weighted images, hyperintense on T2-weighted images and may be difficult to distinguish from high-signal edema
Gadolinium enhancement	Intense
Post Gd-DTPA appearance	Homogeneous enhancement
Differential diagnosis	
Pilocytic astrocytoma	
Ependymoma	
"Pseudotumor vermis" (only on CT scan)	
Cerebellar angioma (on MR scan)	

Varying incidences are reported for medulloblastoma in the literature: 4.2% (Zülch 1986), 4.5% (Cushing 1932), 6.5% (Ringertz and Tola 1950). The incidence in our series was only 1.5% overall and showed a tendency to decline in recent years.

Medulloblastoma is the most common brain tumor of childhood, with a peak incidence between 5 and 15 years of age. A small percentage occur in adults. Males are affected more than twice as often as females. The tumor is classified as grade IV.

Typical Sites

The most common sites of occurrence are the roof of the fourth ventricle and the cerebellar vermis, from which the tumor may spread in all directions. A medulloblastoma filling the cavity of the fourth ventricle may extend through the foramen of Magendie into the cisterna magna and spinal canal, through the foramina of Luschka into the cerebellopontine angle, or upward through the aqueduct into the third ventricle. Confinement of tumor to one cerebellar hemisphere is unusual. Medulloblastomas occasionally arise from the caudal brainstem.

The tumor is highly malignant and can metastasize throughout the ventricles and subarachnoid space. Fortunately it is highly radiosensitive, and 5-year survival rates of 60%–70% are reported.

A variant of medulloblastoma described by Foerster and Gagel is *cerebellar arachnoidal sarcoma*, which typically occurs in the cerebellar hemispheres. Russell and Rubinstein call this tumor *desmoplastic medulloblastoma*. The patients' average age is slightly higher than with medulloblastoma, and the prognosis is somewhat more favorable (grade III–IV).

Main Clinical Features

In addition to local symptoms such as ataxia and dysdiadochokinesia, almost all patients experience headaches and vomiting secondary to the increase in intracranial pressure caused by obstruction to CSF flow. Not infrequently the head is carried at an angle due to irritation of the uppermost cervical nerve roots.

Additional Diagnostic Procedures

Angiography shows nonspecific evidence of a mass lesion in the posterior cranial fossa and occasionally demonstrates pathologic vessels and tumor staining.

Computed Tomography
(Figs. D 1.165–176, 178–180)

Noncontrast Scan
Medulloblastoma presents in about two-thirds of cases as a hyperdense, smooth-bordered mass in the region of the vermis or fourth ventricle. Mixed density is observed in about one-fifth of cases due to the presence of necrotic or hemorrhagic components (Fig. D 1.167 a). Solid isodense medulloblastomas are less common and comprise only about 10% of the cases in our series (Fig. D 1.174). In two of our cases the tumor was almost completely necrotic. Intratumoral hemorrhage appears as an area of exceptionally high density (Fig. D 1.170).

The hypodense areas surrounding medulloblastoma represent perifocal edema, present in 46% of our cases. Cysts are extremely rare in these tumors (Fig. D 1.171).

Contrast Enhancement
Viable tumor components always show marked enhancement, averaging 11–12 HU with a standard contrast dose. Enhancement is maximal a short time after contrast injection and fades rapidly.

Postcontrast Appearance
The total extent of the tumor is usually defined more clearly on the postcontrast scan. Very often the tumor enhances homogeneously (Fig. D 1.165). Less frequently, necrotic components will be present that appear as nonenhancing voids (see Figs. D 1.166, 167). Perifocal edema appears more vivid on the postcontrast scan.

With meningeal seeding, enhancement is observed in the CSF spaces that are involved by tumor (Figs. D 1.178–180). Retrograde metastasis may result in the appearance of giant supratentorial masses, which tend to be located within the ventricles.

Magnetic Resonance Imaging
(Figs. D 1.176, 177)

Noncontrast Scan
The lesion appears hypointense on T1-weighted images, hyperintense on T2-weighted images, and usually presents smooth borders. The tumor is not clearly delineated, however, in the region of the rhomboid fossa. The margin between tumor and edema can be resolved on the unenhanced MR scan. The advantage of MR over CT is its ability to demonstrate the relationship of the tumor to surrounding structures without artifact (fourth ventricle, cerebellar vermis, pons, medulla oblongata).

Post-Gadolinium Scan
As a rule, medulloblastomas enhance intensely with Gd-DTPA. Findings on the T1-weighted image correspond to those on the postcontrast CT scan. Again, MR is superior in its ability to demonstrate the topography of the lesion.

Differential Diagnosis

The main entity requiring differentiation from medulloblastoma is *pilocytic astrocytoma* (spongioblastoma). In our experience, pilocytic astrocytoma of the cerebellum appears hyperdense on plain CT scans only in the presence of intratumoral hemorrhage. Otherwise the lesion is almost always hypodense, and this serves to distinguish it from medulloblastoma. The tumors are indistinguishable from each other on contrast-enhanced scans. A cystic component in children almost invariably signifies pilocytic astrocytoma. Perifocal edema is far less common with pilocytic astrocytoma, but this in itself is not a useful criterion for differentiation. Unlike classic medulloblastomas, pilocytic astrocytomas tend to be lateralized and in that sense resemble desmoplastic medulloblastoma.

MR can contribute little to the differential diagnosis of pilocytic astrocytoma versus ependymoma.

Studies on enhancement kinetics indicate that pilocytic astrocytomas retain their contrast enhancement considerably longer than medulloblastomas (Kazner et al. 1977). An *ependymoma* of the fourth ventricle is not always distinguishable from medulloblastoma. Calcifications favor a diagnosis of ependymoma but are occasionally seen in medulloblastomas as well (see Fig. D1.168). The intensity of contrast enhancement is similar. Posterior displacement of the fourth ventricle by extension from the rhomboid fossa would favor a diagnosis of ependymoma.

Another condition requiring differentiation from medulloblastoma is *pseudotumor vermis.* The cerebellar vermis is composed chiefly of gray matter and is enclosed by the cerebellar white matter, which has a slightly lower radiographic density on CT scans. The vermis enhances slightly (by about 4 HU) with contrast medium and can simulate a cerebellar tumor. At the same time, an early-stage medulloblastoma not yet causing CSF obstruction may be misinterpreted as pseudotumor vermis.

MR can solve the problem of pseudotumor vermis owing to its superior sensitivity. The suspicious area can be identified as physiologic or pathologic by appropriate selection of the MR image plane.

Special diagnostic problems can arise when aqueductal stenosis is combined with pseudotumor vermis, as this may create the erroneous impression that the pseudotumor is the cause of the hydrocephalus. Doubts can be resolved by the judicious use of MR.

A homogeneously enhancing *cerebellar angioma* can be mistaken for a medulloblastoma or other cerebellar tumor, as two of our own observations have shown. However, the typical angiomatous pattern with vascular signal voids is easily appreciated on MR images.

In infants and small children whose hydrocephalus is managed with an implanted shunt, portions of the cerebellum may herniate into the tentorial incisure and simulate a high-sited cerebellar tumor. The cerebellar tissue within the tentorial incisure consists mostly of gray matter, which appears significantly more dense than its surroundings. MR can solve this problem by identifying the tissue as non-neoplastic.

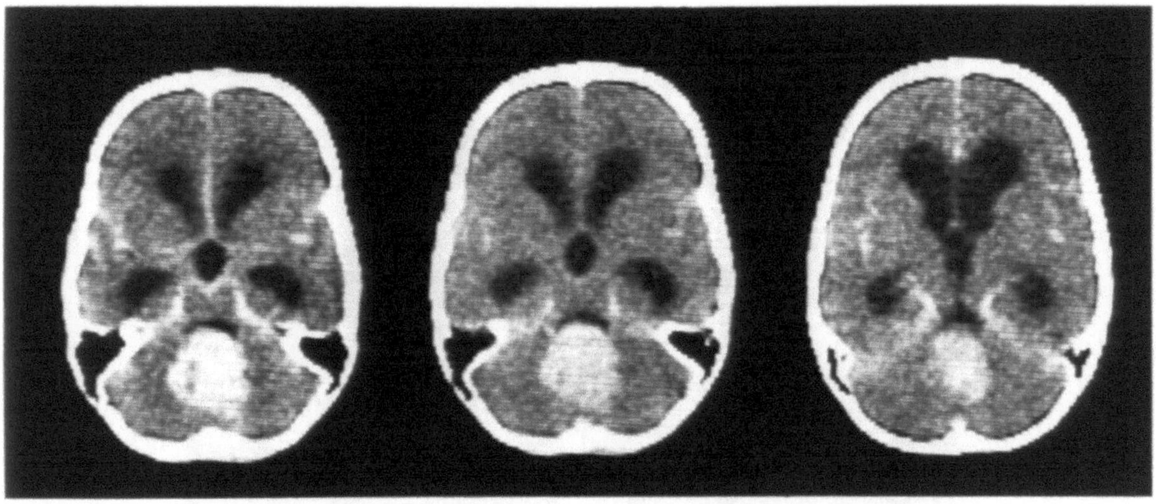

Fig. D 1.165. Large medulloblastoma in the cerebellar vermis of a 6-year-old boy. The tumor, which appeared slightly hyperdense on the plain scan (not shown), enhances almost homogeneously and is surrounded by slight edema. A CSF pocket at the roof of the fourth ventricle demarcates the tumor from the brainstem. Hydrocephalus is pronounced. Postcontrast CT

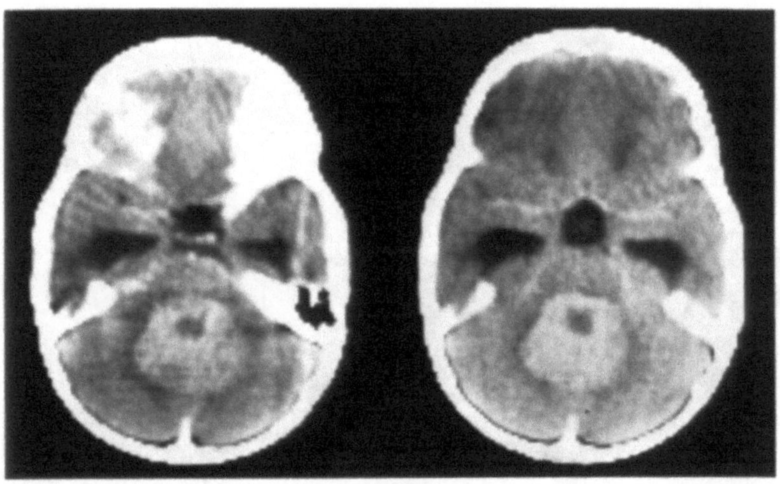

Fig. D 1.166. Symmetric medulloblastoma of the cerebellar vermis in a 3-year-old boy with cerebellar symptoms. The primarily hyperdense tumor shows marked contrast enhancement. A small necrotic focus does not enhance. The tumor has caused significant compression and thinning of the brainstem. Peritumoral edema is minimal, and obstructive hydrocephalus is present. Postcontrast CT

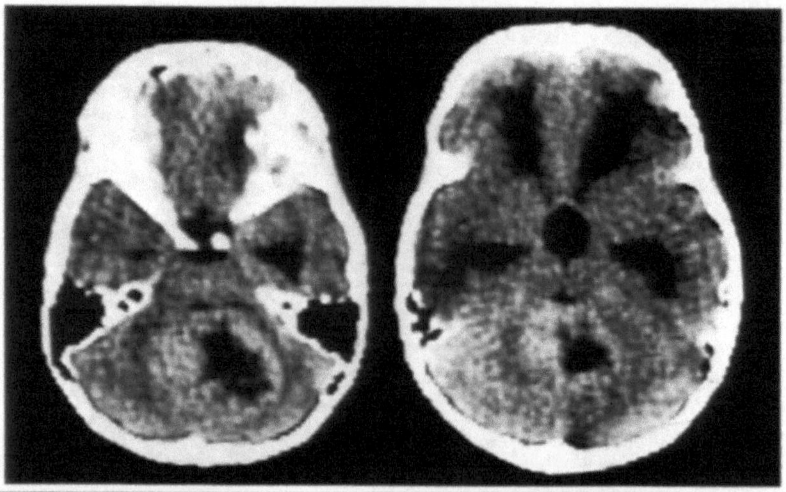
a

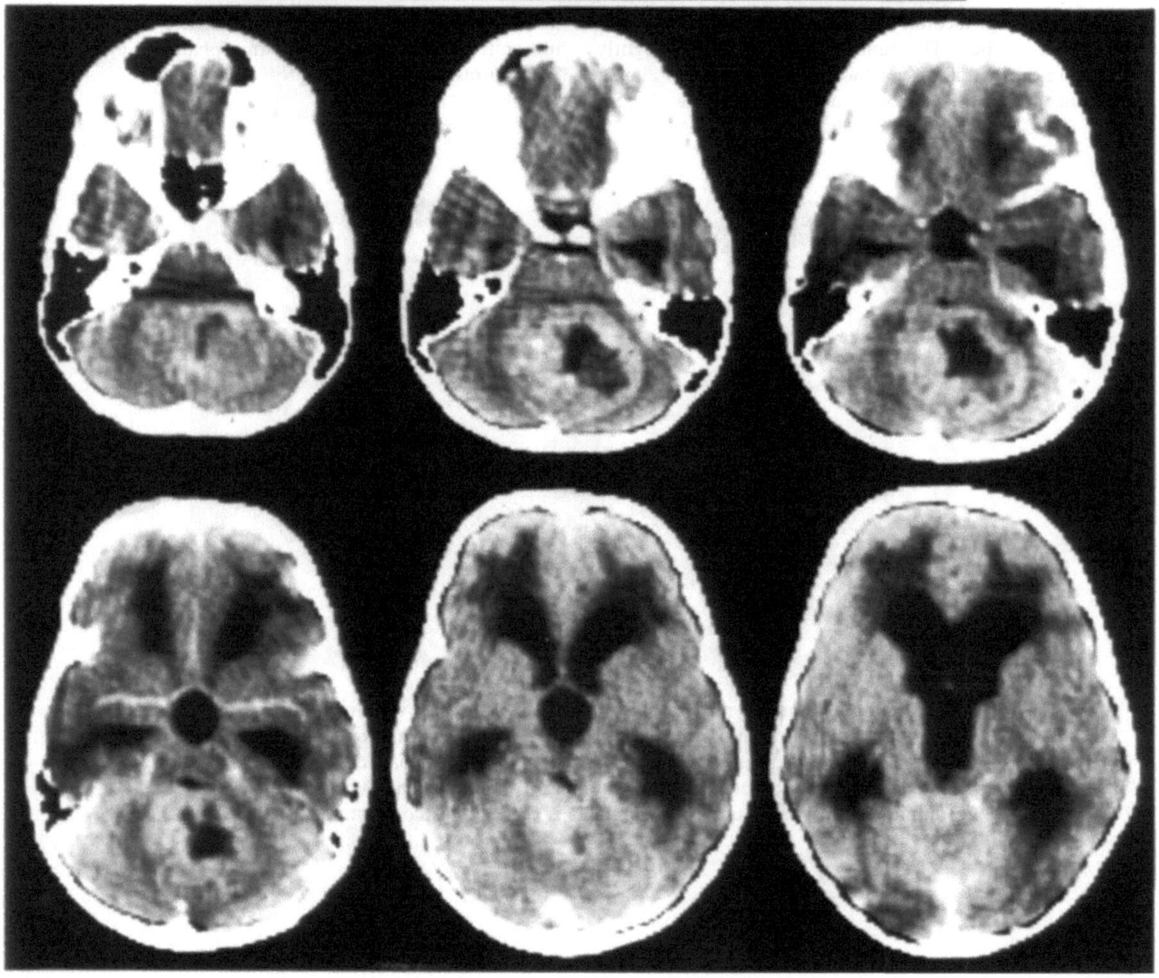
b

Fig. D 1.167 a, b. Very large medulloblastoma in a 7-year-old girl. The tumor arises from the roof of the fourth ventricle and extends far into both cerebellar hemispheres. **a** The solid tumor tissue appears markedly hyperdense on the plain CT scans and contains a large hypodense area of necrosis. A small CSF pocket demarcates the tumor from the brainstem. **b** Postcontrast views of the same tumor demonstrate its extent from the foramen magnum to the supracerebellar cistern. There is marked periventricular lucency as a result of hydrocephalus. [Scans were taken with a large window width (200 HU) for better visualization of transependymal passage of CSF; hence tumor enhancement is less pronounced than it otherwise would be]

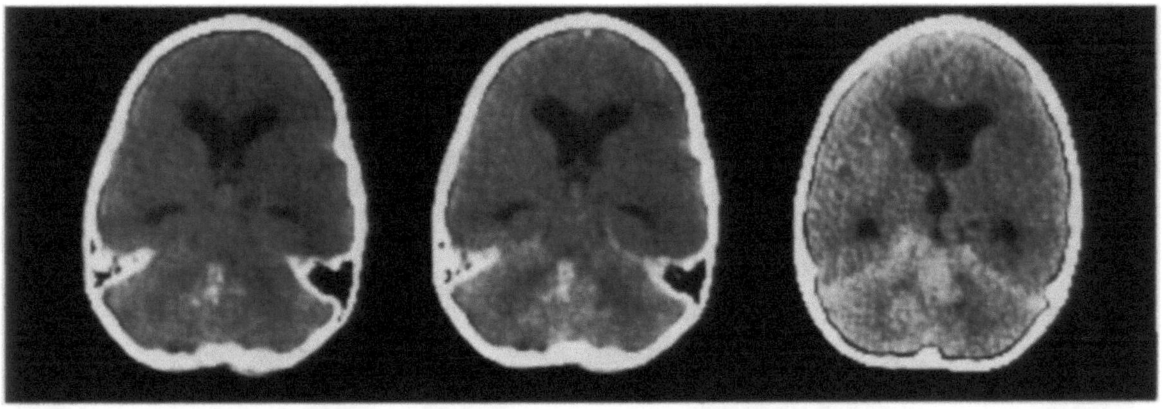

Fig. D 1.168. Medulloblastoma of the cerebellar vermis with numerous small calcifications, meningeal seeding, and a metastasis in the third ventricle. *Left* precontrast CT, *center* and *right* postcontrast scans. The *right* scan shows tumor tissue filling the supracerebellar and ambient cisterns. Differential diagnosis would include ependymoma

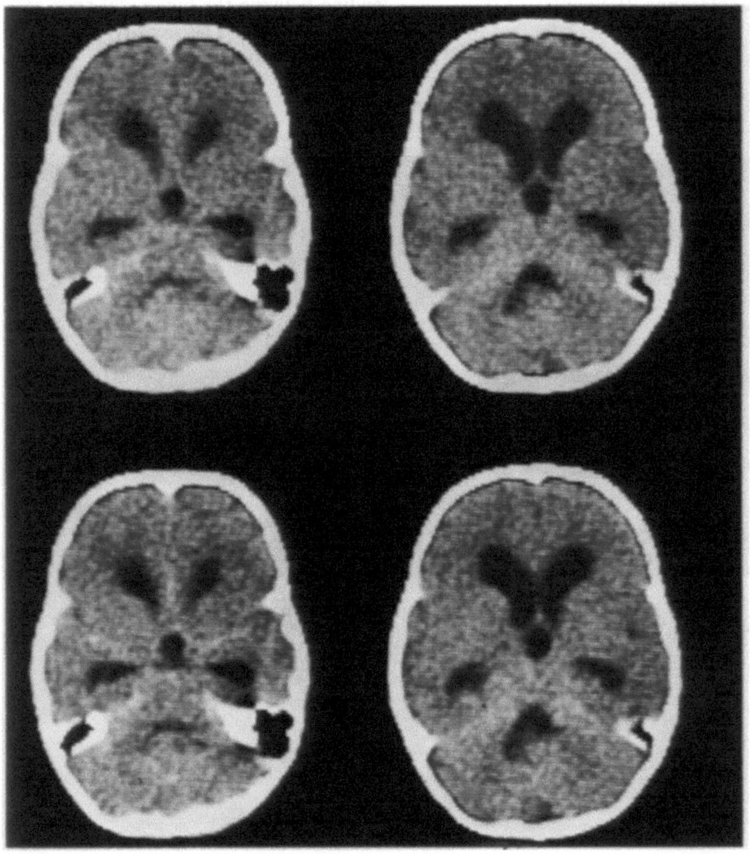

Fig. D 1.169. Isodense medulloblastoma of the cerebellar vermis in a 7-year-old boy with cerebellar symptoms. The tumor tissue does not enhance due to recent, total necrosis (confirmed at operation). The tumor was detected by its indentation of the fourth ventricle from the right side. Moderate hydrocephalus is present. CT scans before (*top*) and after (*bottom*) contrast medium

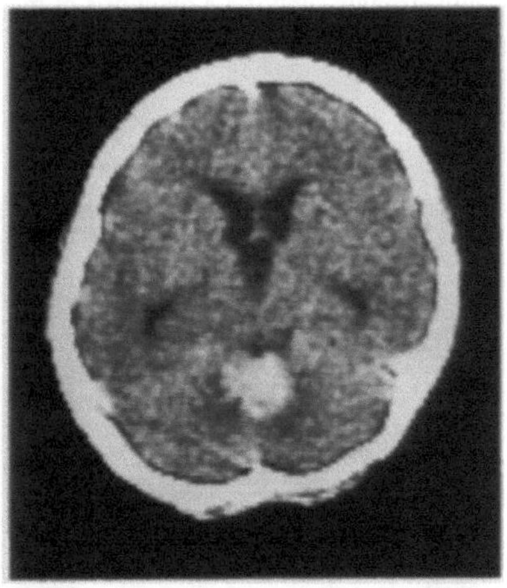

Fig. D 1.170. Medulloblastoma in the superior vermis of a 14-year-old boy with cerebellar symptoms of apoplectiform onset. Noncontrast CT shows a hyperdense area in the superior vermis with density values like those of a fresh hemorrhage. Operation disclosed a walnut-size medulloblastoma with a hemorrhagic component. Similar hemorrhages occur in pilocytic astrocytomas and angiomas

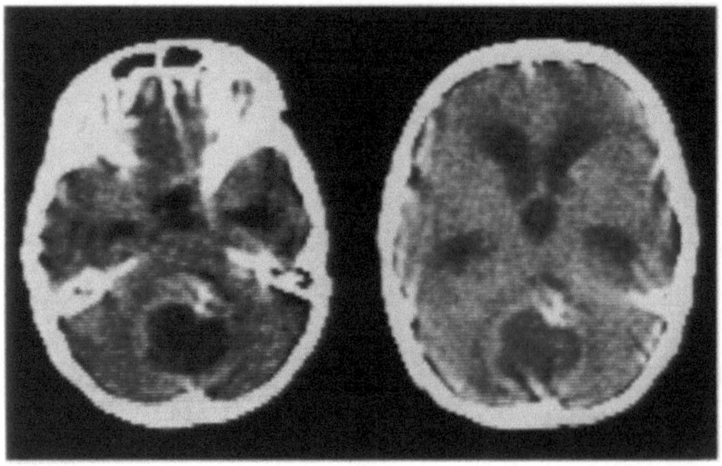

Fig. D 1.171. Atypical medulloblastoma of the cerebellar vermis in a 9-year-old boy with cerebellar symptoms. This is a very unusual CT pattern with a large central cyst and peripheral calcification, consistent with pilocytic astrocytoma. However, the slight hyperdensity of the solid tumor tissue on the unenhanced scan (not shown) is not characteristic of pilocytic astrocytoma and strongly supports a diagnosis of medulloblastoma. Postcontrast CT

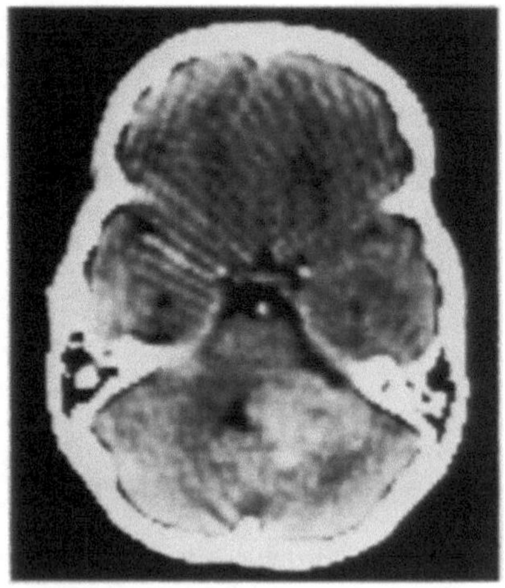

Fig. D 1.172. Desmoplastic medulloblastoma (cerebellar sarcoma) in a 5-year-old girl with facial paralysis and right-sided cerebellar symptoms. Postcontrast CT demonstrates a lateralized mass extending between the pyramidal apex and fourth ventricle. The density pattern is typical for medulloblastoma

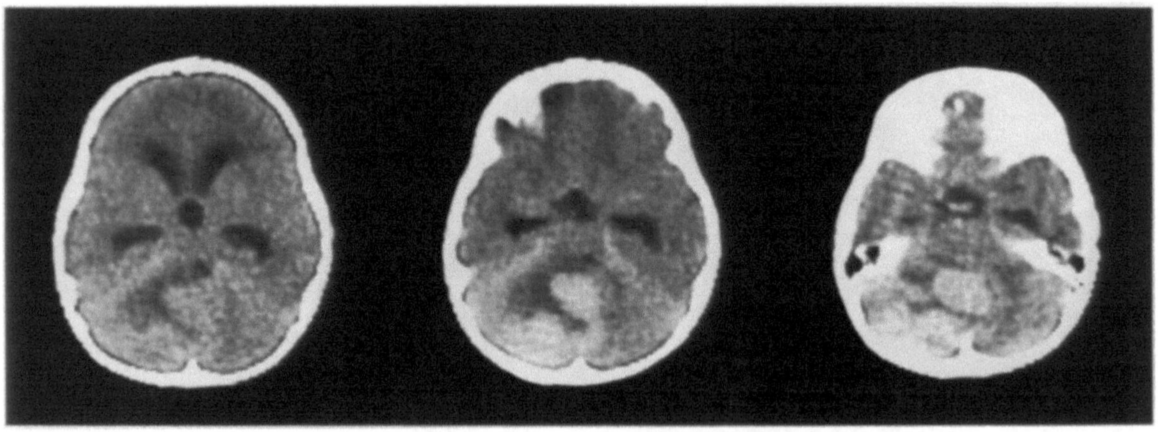

Fig. D 1.173. Large desmoplastic medulloblastoma in a 3-year-old boy with cerebellar symptoms. The predominant unilateral involvement of the cerebellum is unusual for medulloblastoma. There is marked perifocal edema. The tumor is slightly hyperdense on the plain CT scan (*left*) and shows intense contrast enhancement (*center, right*)

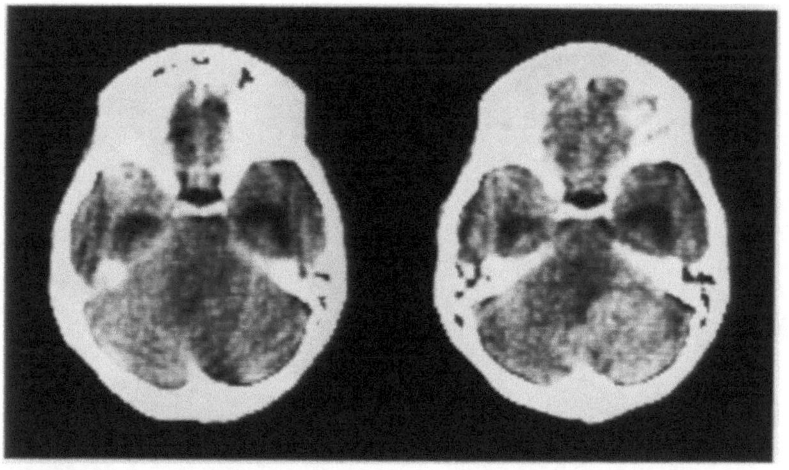

Fig. D 1.174. Desmoplastic medulloblastoma (cerebellar sarcoma) of the right cerebellar hemisphere in a 29-year-old woman with right-sided cerebellar symptoms. The tumor is isodense on the plain CT scan (*left*) and shows marked enhancement with contrast medium (*right*). There is severe hydrocephalus with expansion of the temporal horns

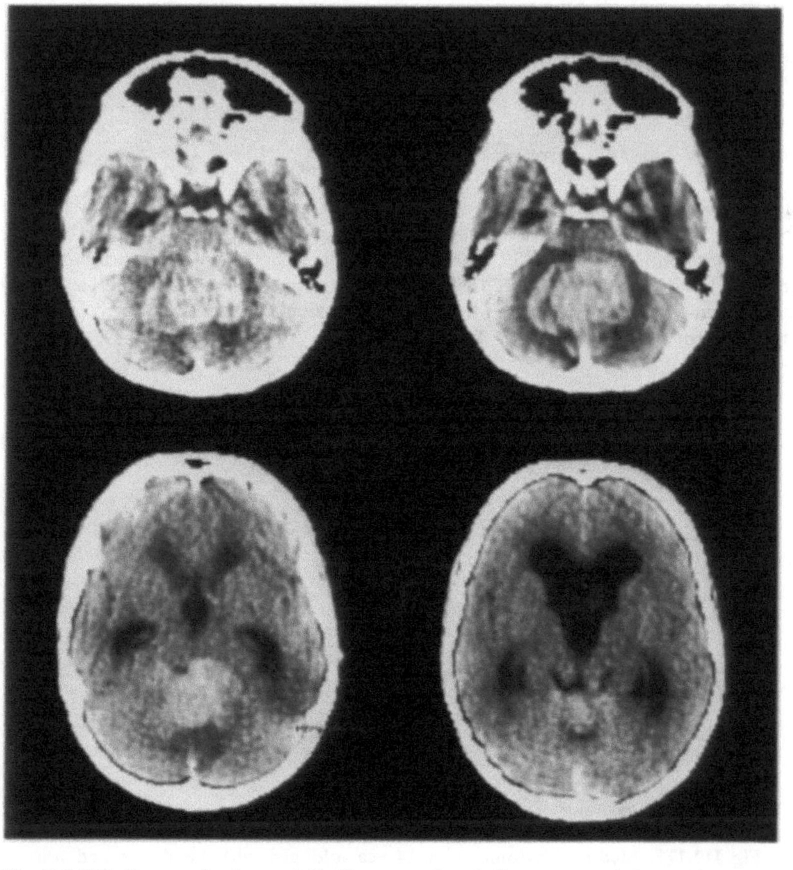

Fig. D 1.175. Desmoplastic medulloblastoma (cerebellar sarcoma) in a 28-year-old woman with truncal ataxia. Postcontrast CT demonstrates a large (primarily hyperdense) tumor filling the vermis region and showing intense enhancement

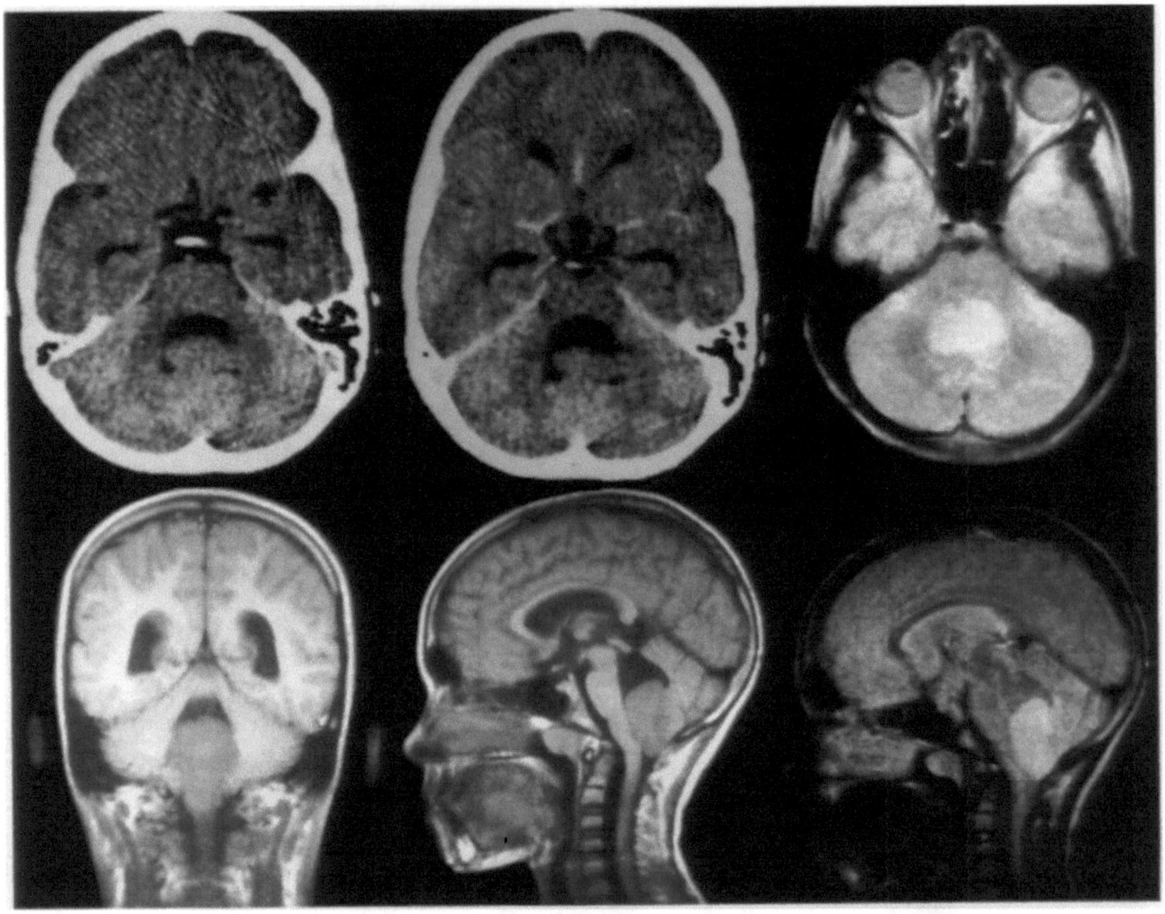

a–c

d–f

Fig. D 1.176 a–f. Medulloblastoma of the cerebellar vermis in an 11-year-old boy with symptoms of increased intracranial pressure. CT: **a, b** postcontrast. MR: **c** SE 1600/90, **d** SE 400/30 coronal, **e** SE 400/30 sagittal, **f** SE 1600/70. CT shows an isodense lesion with slightly hyperdense components and evidence of ventricular expansion. The T1-weighted images (**d, e**) show a hypointense lesion causing massive compression of the cerebellar hemispheres and ventricular expansion. The fourth ventricle is compressed from the occipital side. The tumor appears hyperintense on the T2-weighted sequences (**c, f**)

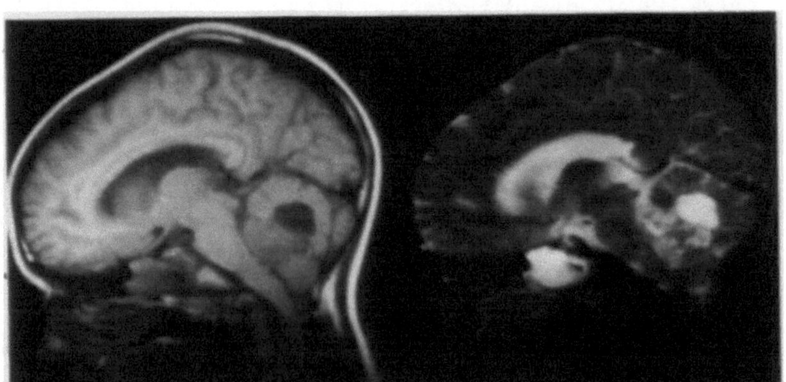

Fig. D 1.177. Medulloblastoma in a 14-year-old girl with headache and ataxia. MR: *left* SE 400/30 sagittal, *right* SE 2000/210 sagittal. Solid tumor is isointense to brain on the T1-weighted image, and the cyst is markedly hypointense (*left*). The cyst gives a very bright signal on the T2-weighted image (*right*)

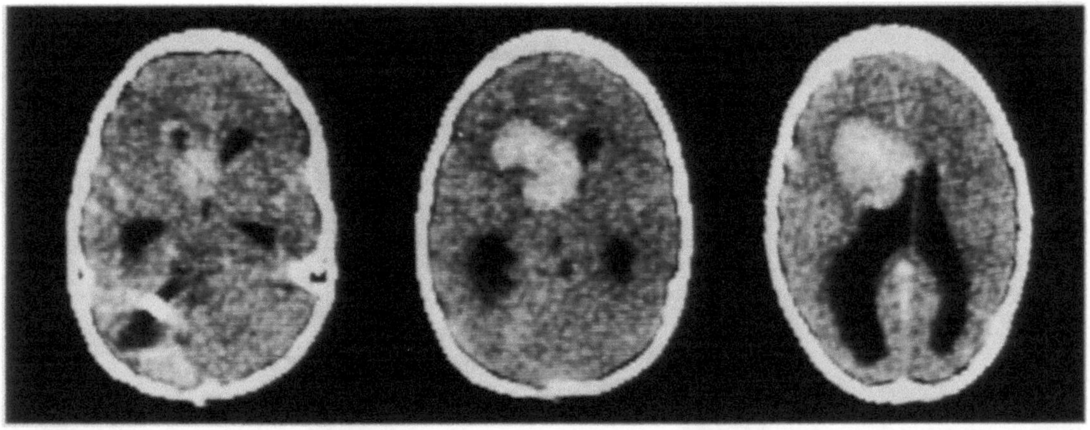

Fig. D 1.178. Intraventricular metastasis from a medulloblastoma previously resected in a 7-year-old girl. The tumor has almost completely obliterated the frontal horn and has occluded the foramen of Monro, causing hydrocephalus. There is equivocal evidence of a recurrence in the posterior fossa next to an artifact emanating from a metallic clip. Postcontrast CT

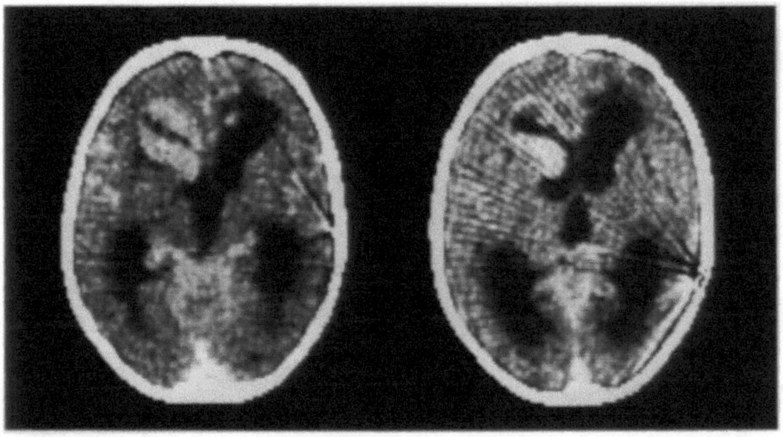

Fig. D 1.179. Meningeal and intraventricular tumor seeding in a 10-year-old boy with previous resection of medulloblastoma. Intense contrast enhancement is seen in the supracerebellar and ambient cisterns and on the wall of the left frontal horn, which is heavily lined with tumor. There is equivocal meningeal infiltration in the area of the left sylvian fissure. Postcontrast CT

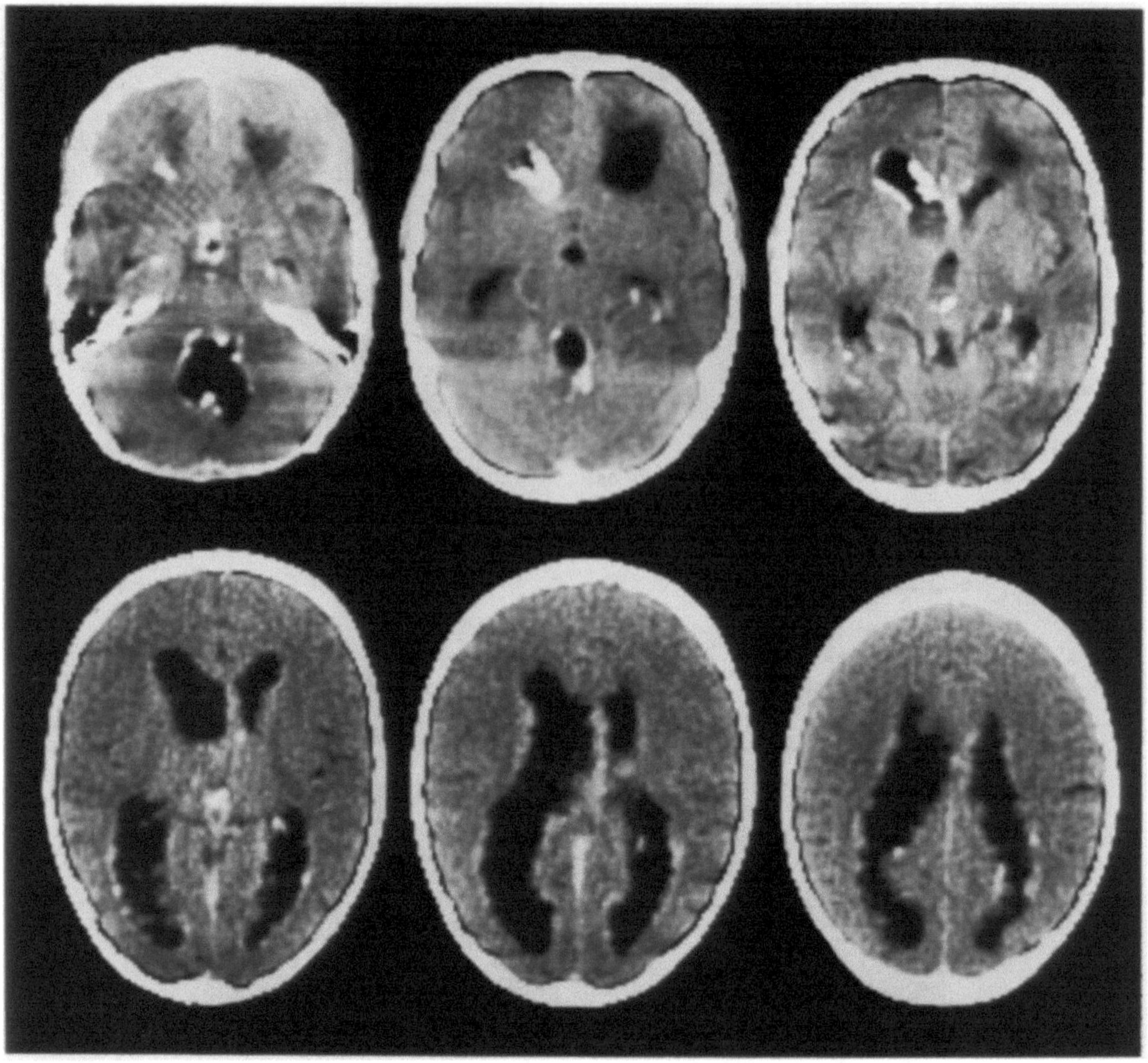

Fig. D 1.180. Status following removal of a medulloblastoma of the cerebellar vermis with subsequent X-irradiation and cytostatic therapy (methotrexate) in a 15-year-old boy. Scans show numerous calcifications and nubbin-like deposits on the ependyma of the lateral ventricles. Findings were interpreted as liquefied and calcified CSF metastases but were not confirmed histologically

m) Malignant Lymphomas

Incidence	0.8%–1.5% of all brain tumors
Age predilection	45–65 years
Sex predilection	Males and females affected about equally
Typical sites	Cerebral hemispheres, basal ganglia
Main clinical features	Depend on tumor location
Angiography	Vascular displacement, tumor staining in some cases
CT	
Noncontrast scan	Lesions often slightly hyperdense, occasionally isodense, usually homogeneous
Contrast enhancement	Generally intense
Postcontrast appearance	Tumors well defined, often indistinguishable from meningioma when located near cortex; perifocal edema common
MR	
Noncontrast scan	Lesions hypointense on T1-weighted images, sharply defined and hyperintense on T2-weighted images
Gadolinium enhancement	Positive
Post Gd-DTPA appearance	Brightly enhancing tumor easily distinguished from edema on T1-weighted sequences
Differential diagnosis	
Meningioma Anaplastic astrocytoma Metastases Disseminated encephalomyelitis Leukemic infiltrates	

"Malignant lymphoma" is a relatively new term applied to a class of primarily intracerebral tumors. This condition was previously described or subsumed under a large variety of headings: lymphosarcoma, reticulosarcoma, leptomeningeal sarcoma, perivascular sarcoma, perithelial sarcoma, periadventitial sarcoma, diffuse sarcoma, round cell sarcoma, reticulum cell sarcoma, microglioma, plasmocytic myeloma, microgliomatosis, diffuse sarcomatosis of the vessels, and "reticulohistiocytic granulomatous encephalitis." Malignant lymphoma is classified as a grade III to grade IV tumor.

Jellinger et al. (1975) report a frequency of 0.8%, and Zimmerman (1975) 1.5%. The incidence in our series was 1.7% and shows a rising trend. The two sexes are affected about equally. The disease is most common between 40 and 70 years of age, with a peak incidence in the sixth decade.

Some cases represent the secondary organic manifestation of a systemic illness. Malignant lymphomas are being detected in AIDS patients with increasing frequency (see pp. 516, 517).

Typical Sites

Malignant lymphomas most commonly occur in the cerebrum and basal ganglia and occasionally involve the brainstem and cerebellum. Multiple tumors are not unusual (see Figs. D1.185, 192). Growth may be circumscribed or diffuse.

Main Clinical Features and Additional Diagnostic Procedures

The clinical manifestations depend on the site of involvement. The prior history is usually short, ranging from a few weeks to several months. Adjunctive studies other than cerebral angiography are not rewarding. Angiograms show varying degrees of vascular displacement, depending on the tumor size. Small, irregular tumor-feeding vessels may be visualized in some cases.

Computed Tomography
(Figs. D181–192, 194–196; E18, 31; F29; G33)

Noncontrast Scan
Solid, nodular growths appear slightly hyperdense on the plain CT scan (38 HU on average, see Fig. D1.183). With diffuse tumor growth, scans show only an area of decreased density resembling astrocytoma or brain edema (see Fig. D1.187).

Contrast Enhancement
Solid tumor nodules show marked, homogeneous enhancement averaging 18.6 HU. Circumscribed enhancement is not seen in diffuse growths. Maximal enhancement is attained rapidly after contrast injection, the level of enhancement being slightly less than that in meningiomas. The enhancement fades slowly over a period of 25 min after the medium is injected (Kazner et al. 1978).

Postcontrast Appearance
Solid tumor nodules of malignant lymphoma appear more conspicuous on postcontrast scans and are easier to distinguish from surrounding structures, although the tumor-brain and tumor-edema boundary is not defined as sharply as with meningioma. Perifocal edema is a very common finding (see Figs. D1.181, 182, 185, 188–192, 194, 195).

Magnetic Resonance Imaging
(Figs. C17, D1.190–193, F29)

Noncontrast Scan
The lesions of malignant lymphoma appear on T1-weighted images as ill-defined areas of low signal intensity. T2-weighted sequences show hyperintense, relatively well-defined tumors with impressive clarity. Multifocal tumors are displayed more clearly than with postcontrast CT.

Post-Gadolinium Scan
Lymphomas enhance with Gd-DTPA and have much the same appearance as on postcontrast CT.

Differential Diagnosis

Malignant lymphoma may be mistaken for meningioma when located near the cortex (see Fig. D1.181). However, angiography does not demonstrate the vascular pattern typical of meningioma. The relatively poor demarcation of many malignant lymphomas was noted previously.

Lymphomas occurring in the brain parenchyma are difficult to distinguish from *anaplastic astrocytoma*. Multifocal lesions are indistinguishable from *metastases* based on CT findings alone. Similarly, *acute disseminated encephalitis* and *leukemic infiltrates* can be differentiated from lymphoma only by referral to the history and other clinical findings.

Leukemic infiltrates may occasionally appear as primarily hyperdense foci that enhance homogeneously and mimic the appearance of malignant lymphoma (see Fig. D1.194). In other cases the edema incited by leukemic infiltration is the predominant feature.

MR offers no advantages over CT in terms of differential diagnosis.

n) Monstrocellular Sarcomas

These are very rare, grade IV malignancies of undetermined origin (gigantocellular or xanthomatous glioblastomas? malignant pleomorphic fibrous histiocytomas?). They affect all age groups and are usually associated with cyst formation.

The tumor usually appears on the **CT scan** as a hypodense area with a peripheral ring of contrast enhancement (Figs. D1.197, 198). The CT findings most closely resemble a cystic anaplastic or pilocytic astrocytoma, and glioblastoma-like or abscess-like patterns may also be seen. Generally a diagnosis of monstrocellular sarcoma cannot be made from CT findings, although cyst formation appears to be a characteristic feature.

o) Fibrous Histiocytomas

These are very rare intracranial tumors that occur in both benign and malignant forms. The few observations that we have to date suggest that fibrous histiocytomas lack a characteristic **CT appearance** (see Figs. D1.199, 200). Our most striking case involved a 48-year-old woman with seizures whose plain CT scan demonstrated a large hypodense mass in the region of the corpus callosum. The mass enhanced intensely with contrast medium and looked very much like a falx meningioma (see Fig. D1.199). The density characteristics of the lesion before and after contrast enhancement did not fit any previously known pattern. At operation a soft, yellowish, well-vascularized tumor about the size of an apple was found in the cistern of the corpus callosum and was identified histologically as a benign fibrous histiocytoma.

The CT features of the *malignant histiocytomas* in our series most closely resembled those of intracranial metastases (Fig. D1.200). One case simulated meningioma. It is our experience that the histologic diagnosis cannot be correctly predicted from the CT scan.

p) Histiocytosis X

Histiocytosis X (formerly called Hand-Schüller-Christian disease, eosinophilic granuloma, and Abt-Letterer-Siwe disease) very rarely involves intracranial structures. The region of the hypothalamus and optic chiasm is a site of predilection. Endocrine disorders and visual disturbances are the most prominent clinical findings, and some patients experience attacks of narcolepsy.

Plain CT scans usually demonstrate a slightly hyperdense lesion partially or completely filling the opticochiasmatic cistern (Figs. D1.201–203). The affected area enhances intensely and homogeneously with contrast medium and presents somewhat ill-defined borders, as in malignant lymphoma. These features preclude pituitary adenoma and suprasellar meningioma but are consistent with pilocytic astrocytoma or ectopic pinealoma (germinoma). Malignant lymphomas at this location are very rare.

T1-weighted **MR images** usually demonstrate the lesion as an area of isointensity or mild hyperintensity. A very strong signal is returned on T2-weighted sequences. MR is more sensitive than CT in the detection of histiocytosis X and makes it easier to evaluate the topography of the lesion owing to the capacity for arbitrary plane selection. However, neither MR nor CT can provide a specific diagnosis.

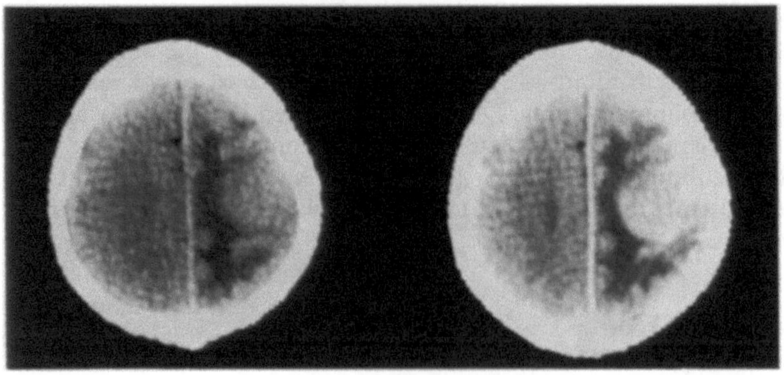

Fig. D 1.181. Malignant lymphoma of the right parietal region in a 79-year-old woman. The density pattern resembles meningioma. Differential diagnosis cannot be accomplished without angiography. *Left* precontrast, *right* postcontrast CT

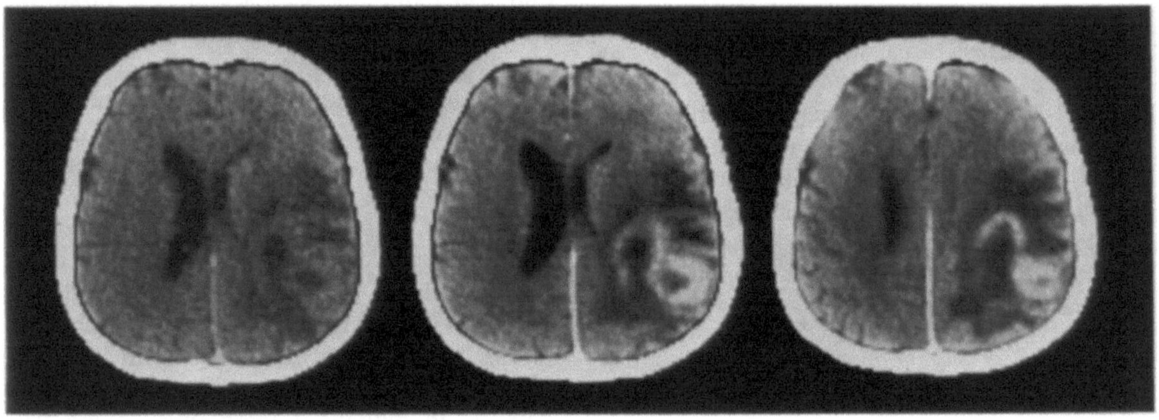

Fig. D 1.182. Malignant lymphoma of the right parietal region in a 65-year-old man. The "open ring" pattern of contrast enhancement is unusual. *Left* precontrast, *center* and *right* postcontrast CT

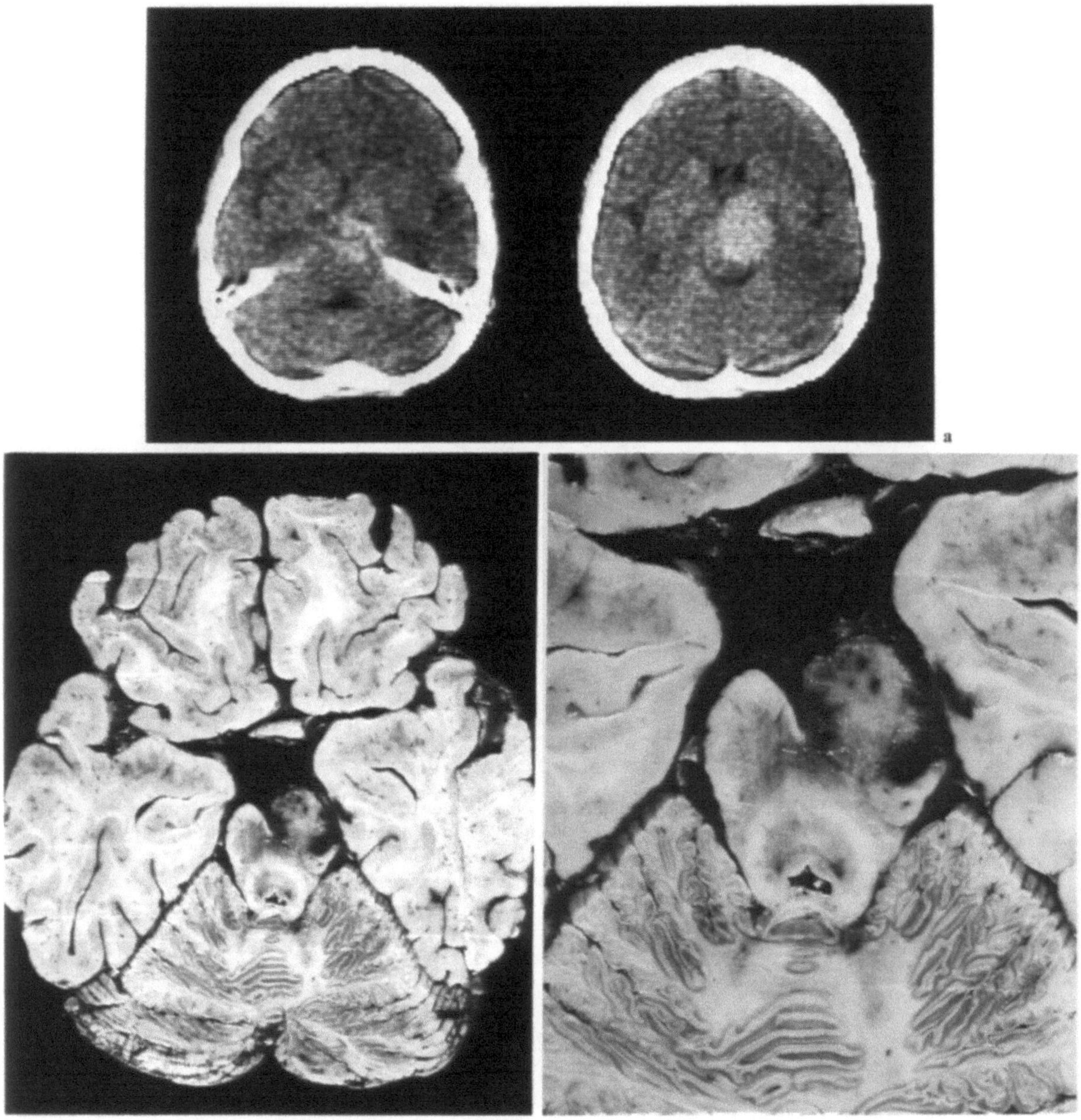

Fig. D1.183 a, b. Malignant lymphoma of the right cerebral peduncle and thalamic region in a 41-year-old woman with vertigo, diplopia, and oculomotor paresis. **a** CT demonstrates a markedly enhancing mass lesion on the floor of the middle fossa with extension into the right thalamus and midbrain. CT findings are consistent with basal meningioma or malignant lymphoma. The latter diagnosis was confirmed by open biopsy. The patient died 4 weeks later. **b** Autopsy disclosed expansion of the right cerebral peduncle and bilateral involvement of the basal ganglia, especially on the right side. Tumor growth was entirely diffuse

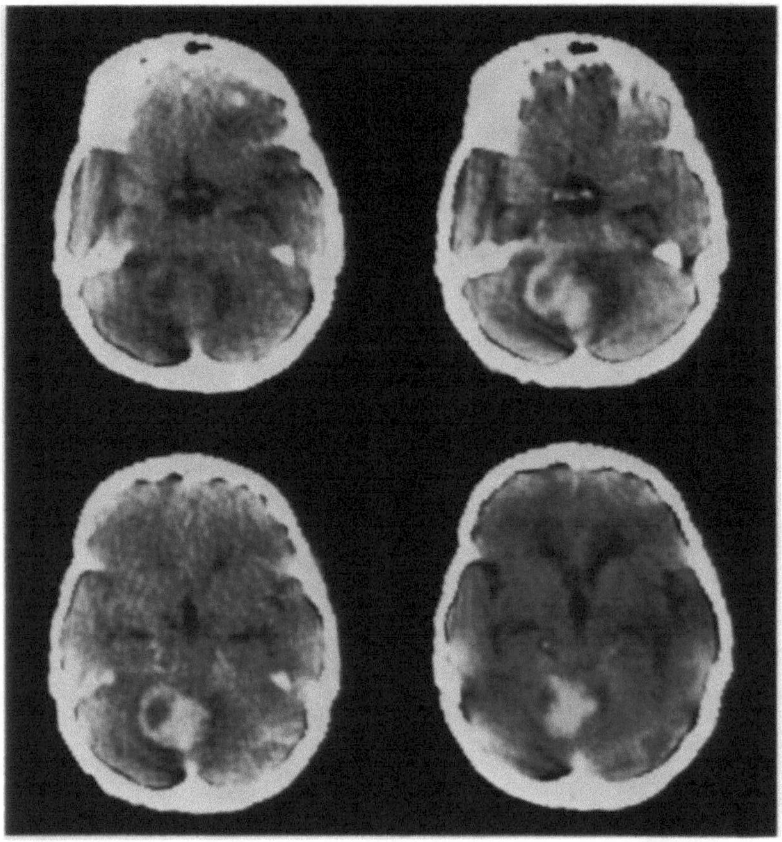

Fig. D1.184. Malignant lymphoma (centroblastic-centrocytic lymphoma) of the cerebellar vermis and left cerebellar hemisphere in a 51-year-old woman with cerebellar symptoms. Plain CT shows an isodense tumor with an eccentric hypodensity. Postcontrast scans show intense enhancement of viable tumor tissue with a discontinuous ring pattern

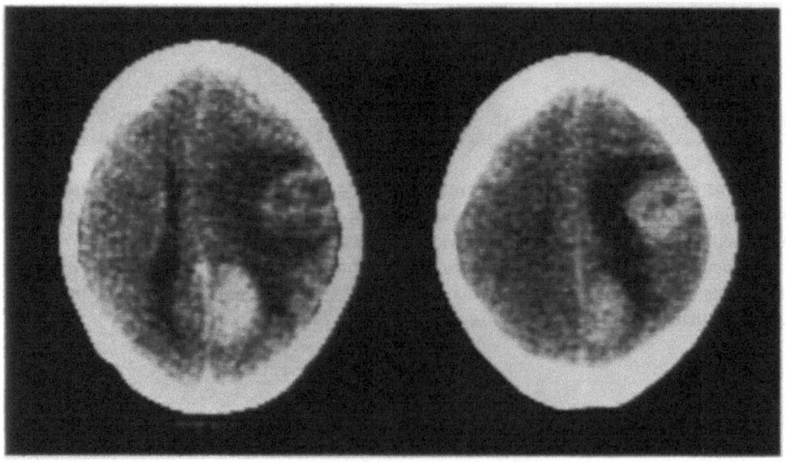

Fig. D1.185. Multifocal malignant lymphoma (lymphoblastic type) in a 39-year-old woman with a 3-month history of progressive weakness in the left hand. CT demonstrates two nodular masses with different features, both of which show marked contrast enhancement and appeared only slightly hyperdense on the plain scan. Findings are consistent with multifocal glioblastoma or multiple intracranial metastases. Postcontrast CT

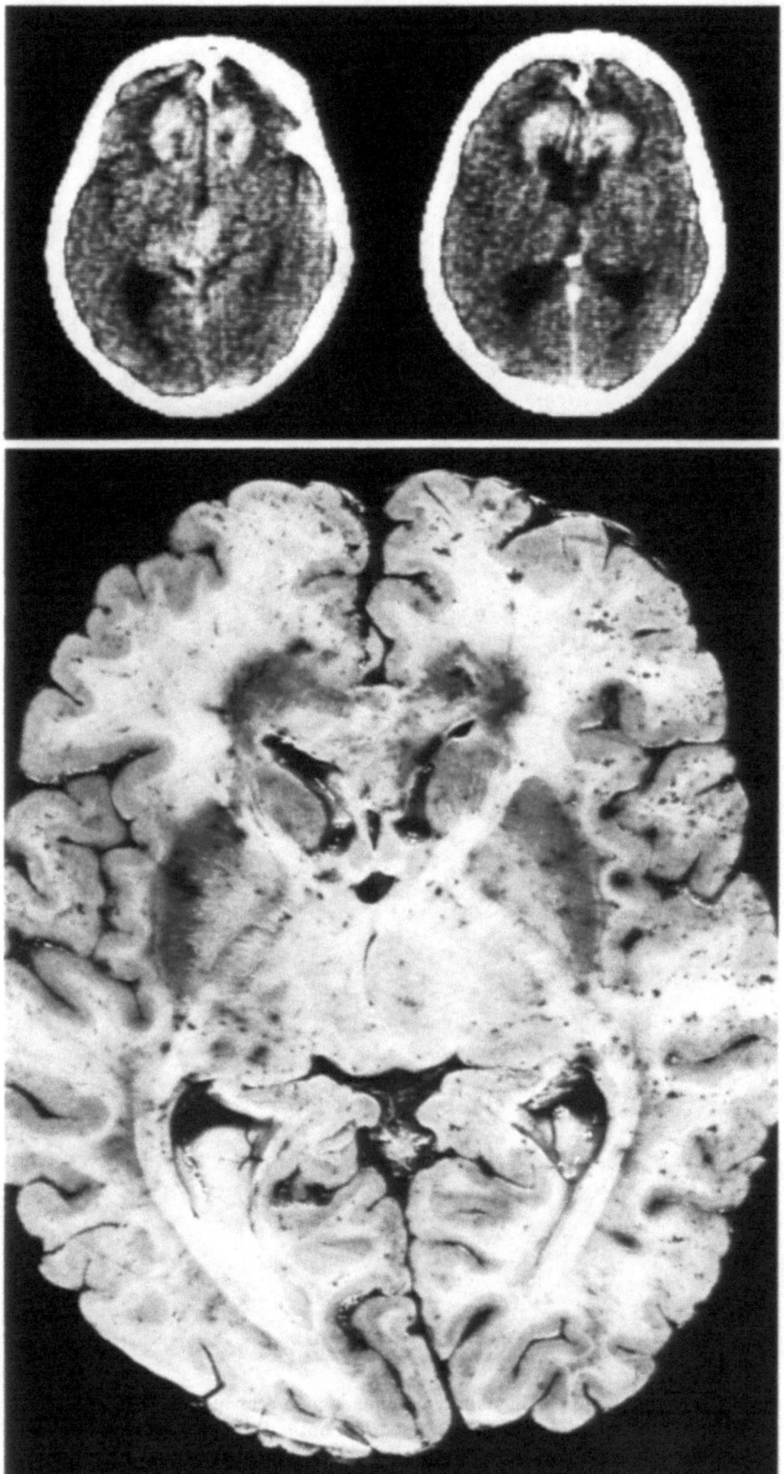

a

b

Fig. D 1.186 a, b. Malignant lymphoma in a 59-year-old woman with headache, vertigo, increasing left-sided hemiparesis, and altered mental status. **a** CT demonstrates multiple tumors bilaterally involving the basal ganglia and quadrigeminal region with an associated periventricular butterfly pattern of tumor spread. Findings are consistent with a butterfly glioma or malignant lymphoma. The patient died 4 weeks after the CT examination. **b** Autopsy disclosed a pattern of tumor growth and spread corresponding to that seen on the CT scans. The lesion was identified as lymphoplasmocytoid lymphoma

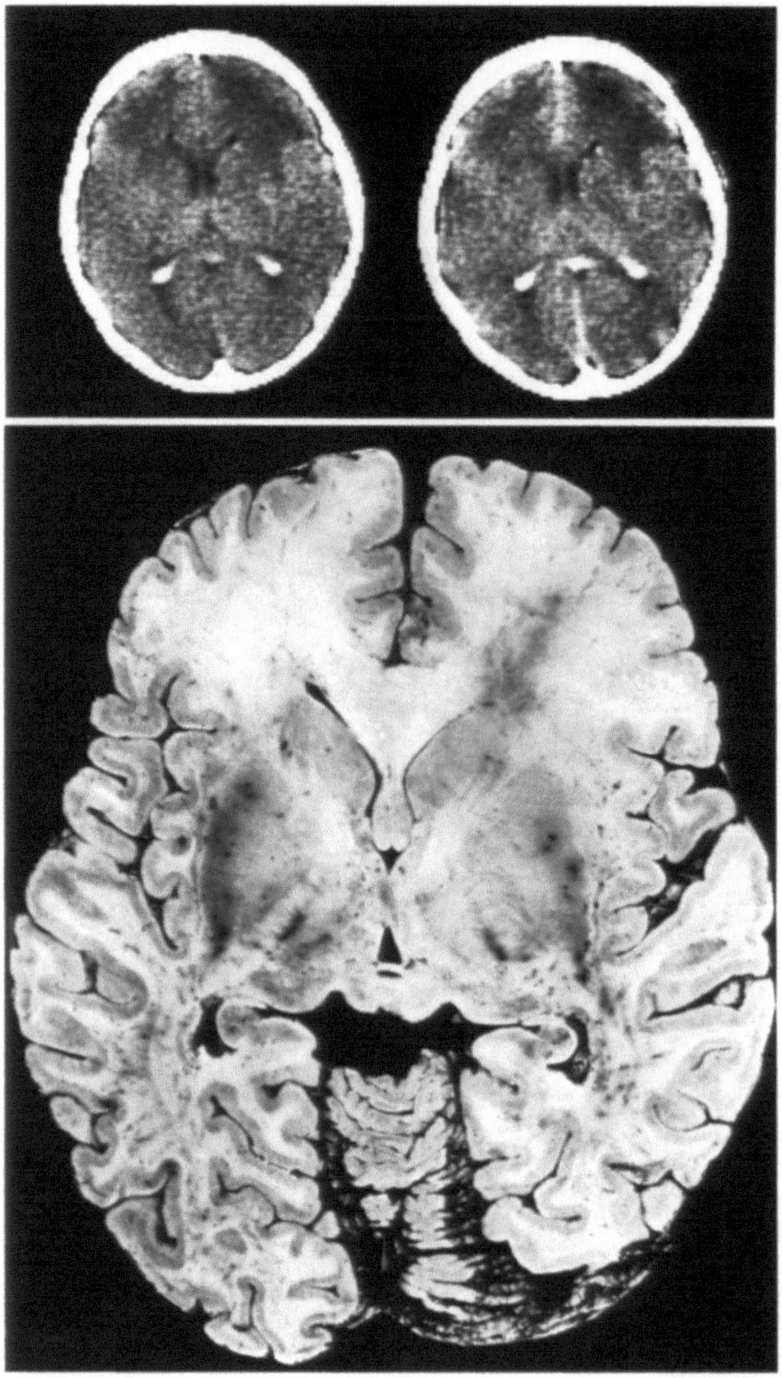

a

b

Fig. D1.187 a, b. Diffuse malignant lymphoma in a 55-year-old man with impaired consciousness of sudden onset that persisted until death. **a** CT demonstrates hypodense, nonenhancing areas in both frontal lobes. **b** Autopsy revealed diffuse tumor growth distending the anterior corpus callosum and diffusely expanding both frontal lobes

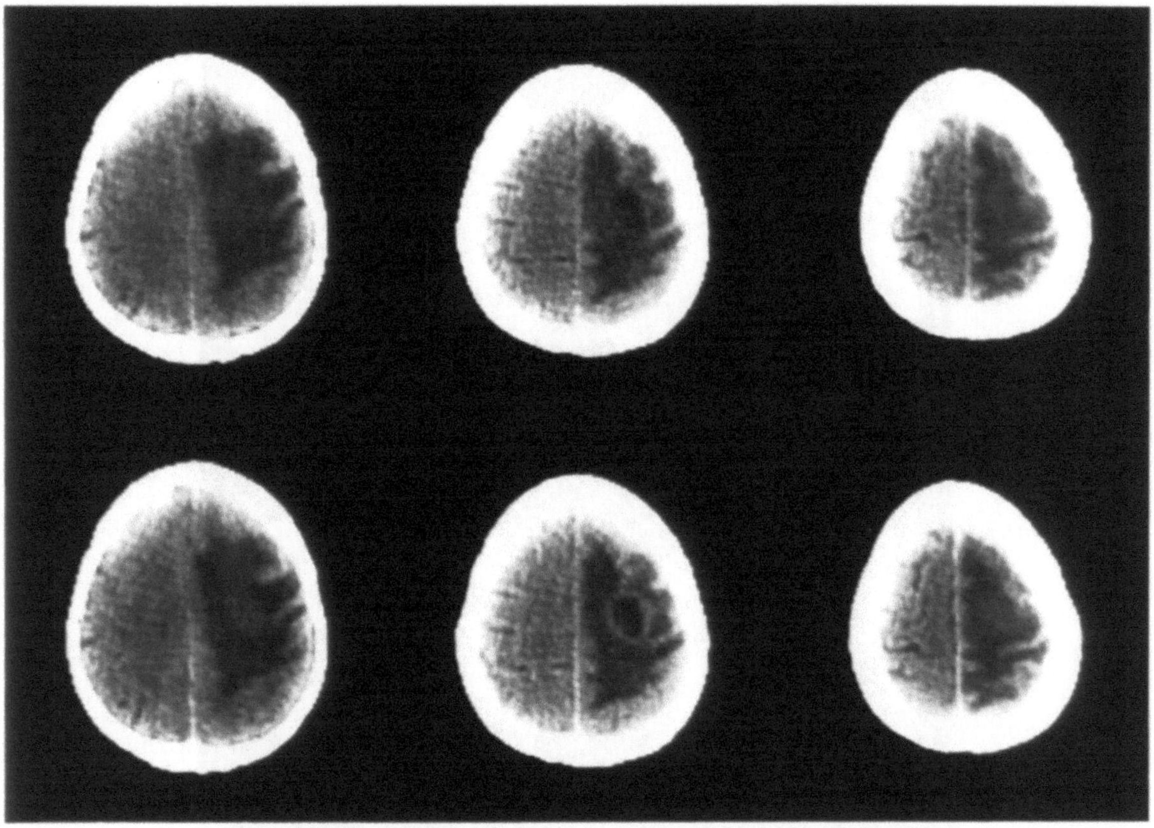

Fig. D 1.188. Metastatic malignant lymphoma of the right central region in a 51-year-old woman who underwent resection of a malignant inguinal lymphoma 9 years earlier. Large hypodense areas are seen on the plain CT scans (*top*). Postcontrast scans (*bottom*) demonstrate a faint ring pattern initially interpreted as malignant glioma. Histologic examination identified the excised tumor as malignant lymphoma

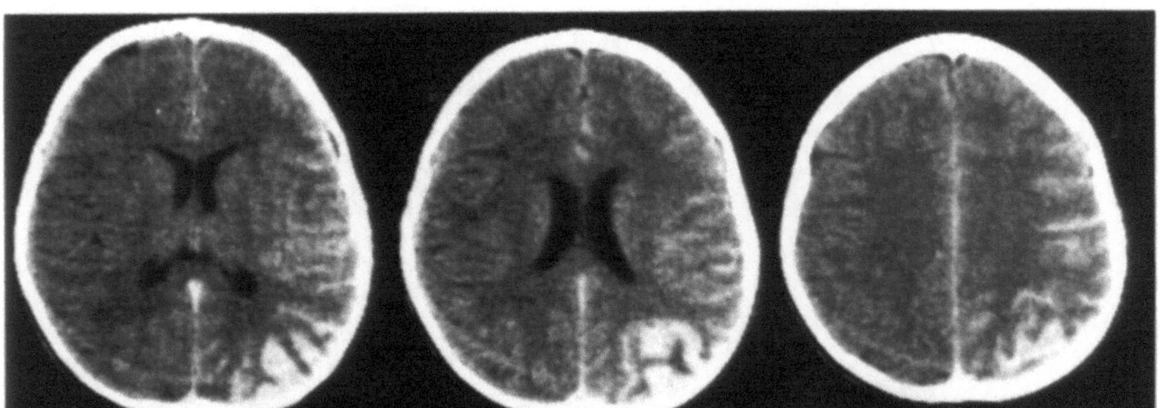

Fig. D 1.189. Burkitt's lymphoma of the right parieto-occipital region with seeding in the subarachnoid space. The 5-year-old patient, with leukemia in remission for 2 years, was admitted with acute impairment of consciousness and left-sided hemiparesis. Postcontrast CT demonstrates the solid tumor component in addition to pronounced gyral infiltration on the right side

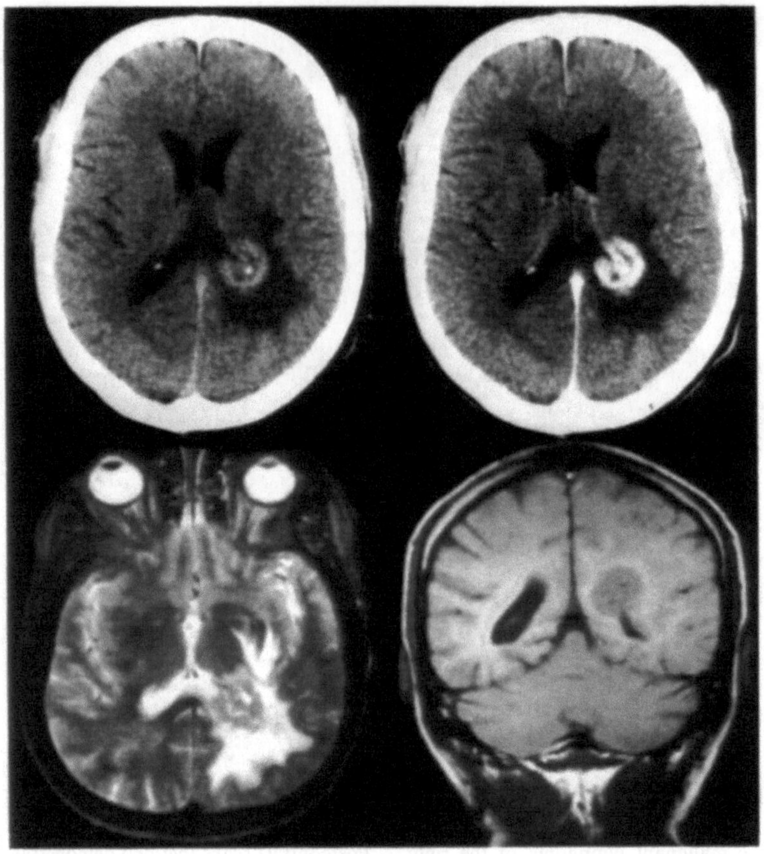

a b c d

D 1.190

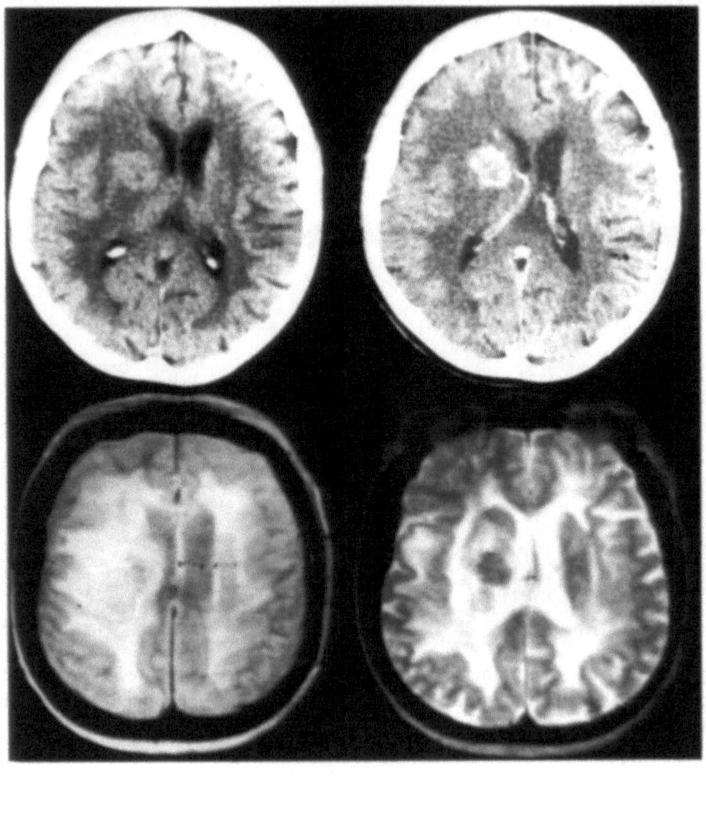

a b c d

D 1.191

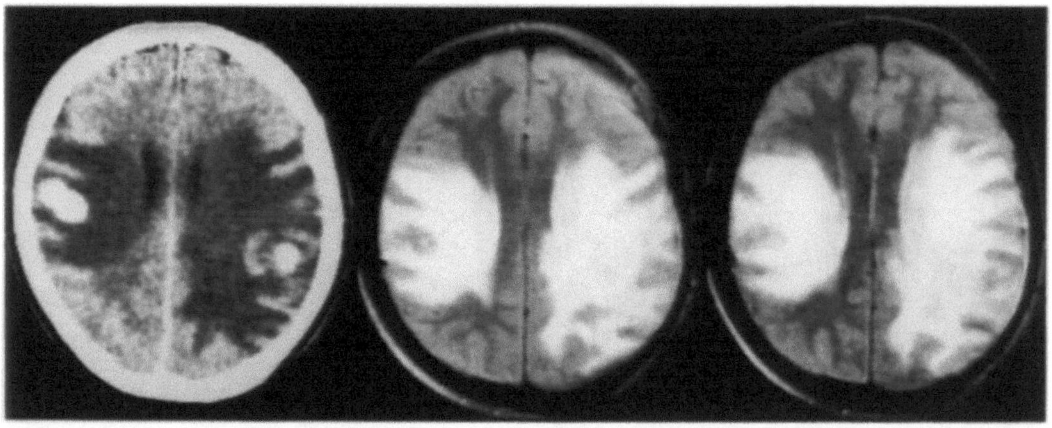

Fig. D 1.192. Malignant lymphoma of the left frontoprecentral and right parietal regions in a 15-year-old boy with personality change, apathy, and right-sided hemiparesis. *Left:* postcontrast CT. *Center* and *right*: SE 1600/60 MR. The tumor in the left frontoprecentral region gives a low signal on the T2-weighted image, while the extensive bilateral edema gives a very intense signal

Fig. D 1.190 a–d. Highly malignant non-Hodgkin's lymphoma of the right occipital horn in a 61-year-old woman with left-sided hemiparesis and left homonymous hemianopia. CT: **a** precontrast, **b** postcontrast. MR: **c** SE 3000/90, **d** SE 700/30. Postcontrast CT shows a brightly enhancing tumor that contrasts well with perifocal edema. The tumor and surrounding hyperintense edema also are conspicuous on the T2-weighted MR sequence (**c**)

Fig. D 1.191 a–d. Malignant lymphoma of the left basal ganglia in a 53-year-old woman with right-sided hemiparesis and altered mental status; lymphoma of the left frontal region had been diagnosed 2 years earlier. CT: **a** precontrast, **b** postcontrast. MR: **c** SE 3000/30, **d** SE 3000/90. The tumor enhances well on the postcontrast CT scan. It is hypointense on the T2-weighted image (**d**) and contrasts well with the hyperintense edema

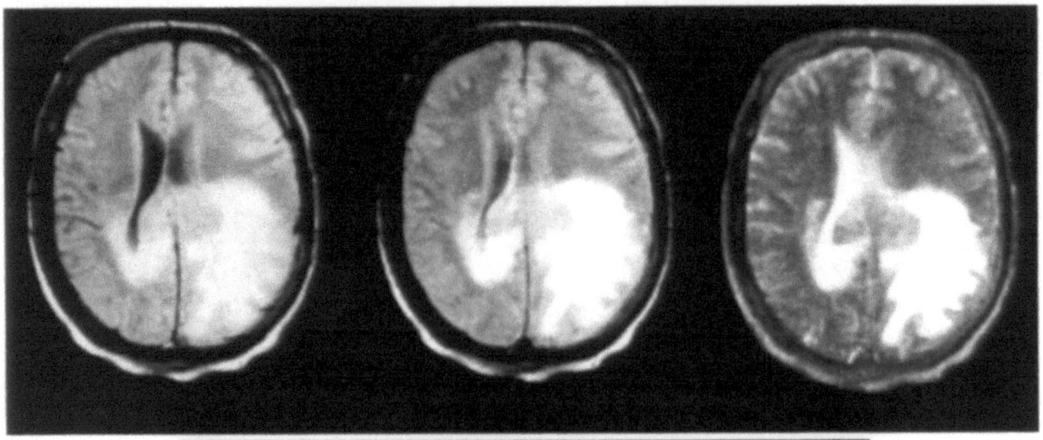

a–c

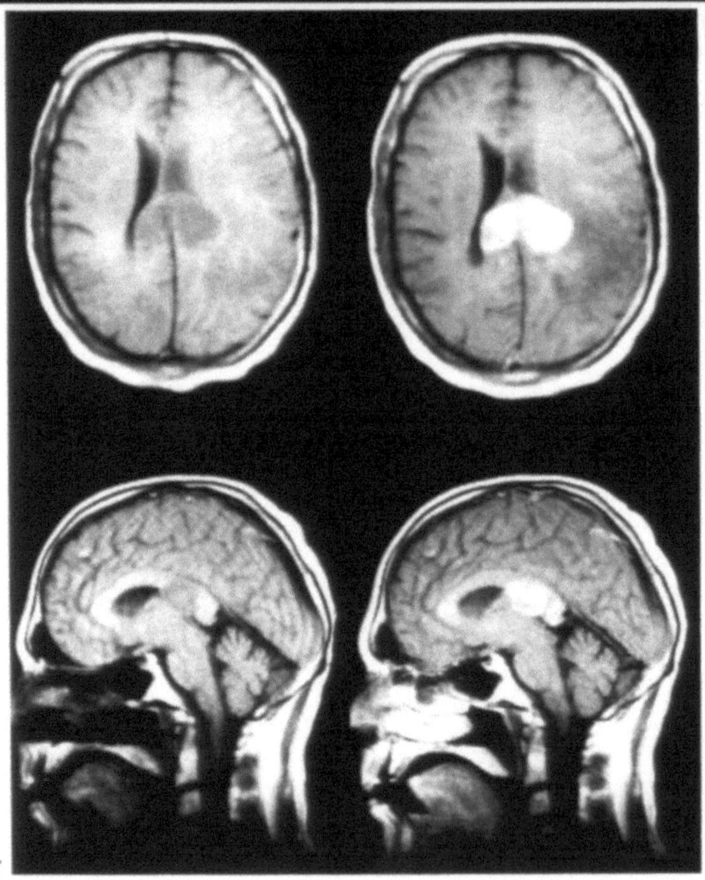

d e f g

Fig. D 1.193 a–g. Malignant lymphoma of the posterior corpus callosum, chiefly involving the right side. The 45-year-old man had a 2-month history of headaches, somnolence, and loss of orientation; he presented with latent left-sided hemiparesis. MR: **a** SE 1600/30, **b** SE 1600/60, **c** SE 1600/180, **d** SE 400/30, **e** SE 400/30 post Gd-DTPA, **f** SE 400/30 sagittal, **g** SE 400/30 sagittal post Gd-DTPA. The boundary between tumor and edema is poorly resolved on the proton-density image (**a**). The heavily T2-weighted image demonstrates the hypointense tumor in higher contrast (**c**). The lesion enhances well with Gd-DTPA

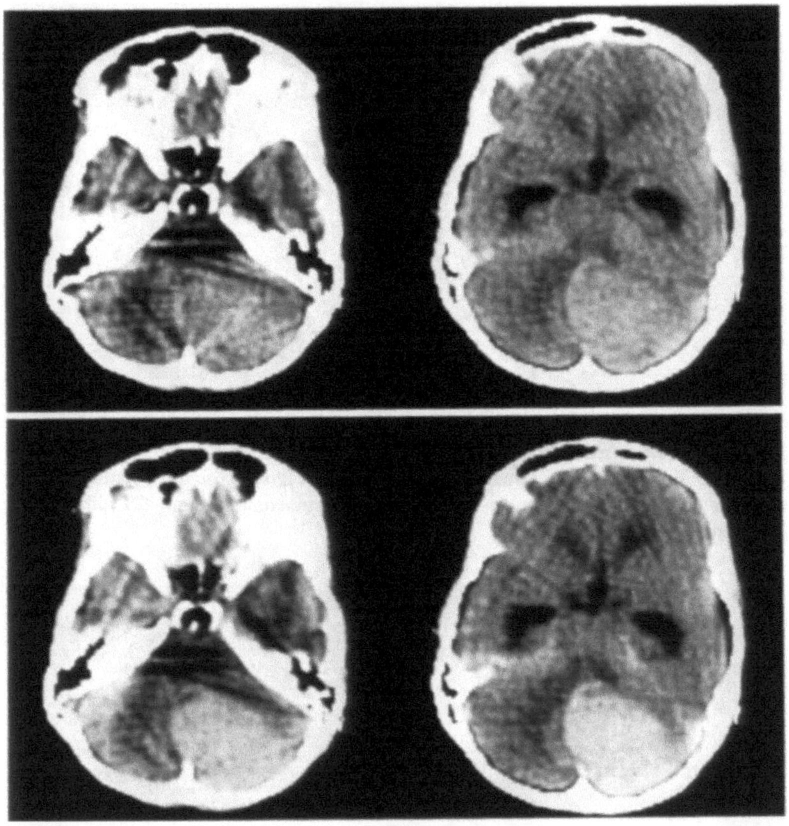

Fig. D 1.194. Leukemic infiltrate in the right cerebellar hemisphere with erosive bone change in a 15-year-old girl undergoing chemotherapy for acute lymphoblastic leukemia. The tumor appears hyperdense on the plain CT scans (*top*) and has incited perifocal edema in the cerebellum in addition to obstructive hydrocephalus. Enhancement is noted on the postcontrast scans (*bottom*)

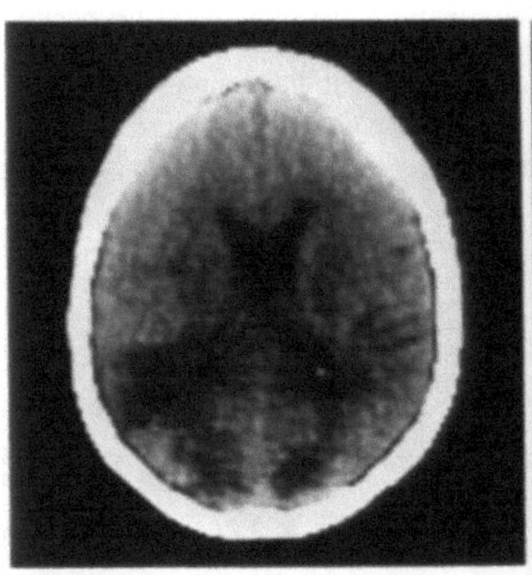

D 1.195

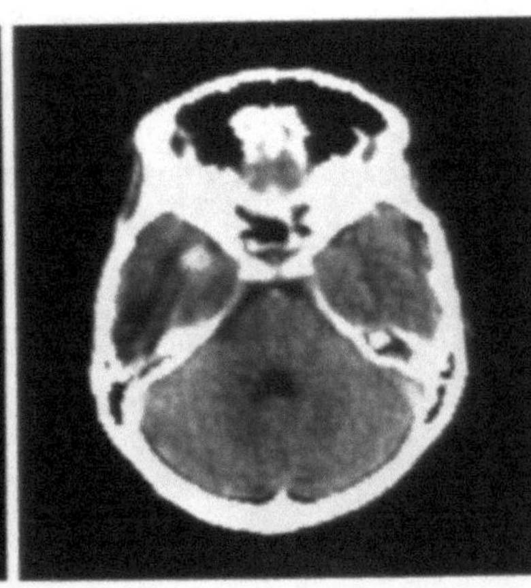

D 1.196

Fig. D 1.195. Hodgkin's lymphoma of the left occipital region in a 53-year-old woman with generalized lymphogranulomatosis. The lesion itself is slightly hyperdense and is surrounded by edema. There is possible involvement of the right occipital lobe, where increased white-matter density is apparent. Noncontrast CT

Fig. D 1.196. Cerebral involvement in a 45-year-old woman with multiple myeloma: a lesion in the mediobasal portion of the left temporal lobe. Postcontrast CT. The tumor appeared slightly hyperdense even on the unenhanced scan.

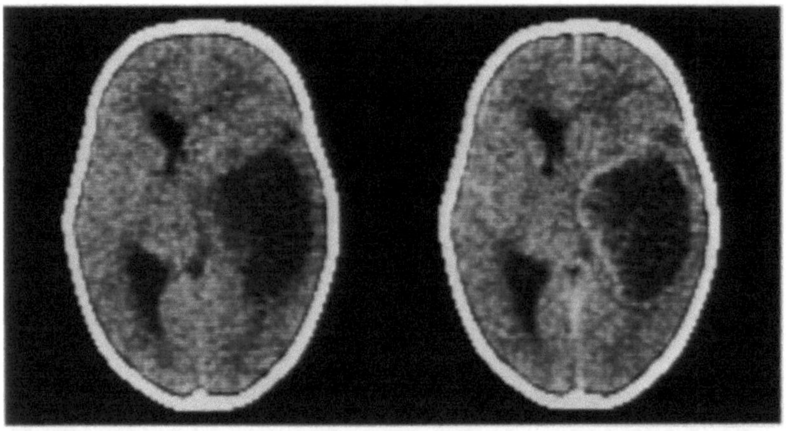

Fig. D 1.197. Huge monstrocellular sarcoma of the right temporal region in a $2^1/_2$-year-old child. The plain CT scan (*left*) shows a large hypodense area. After contrast medium (*right*) the area shows thin peripheral rim enhancement. CT differential diagnosis: ependymoma

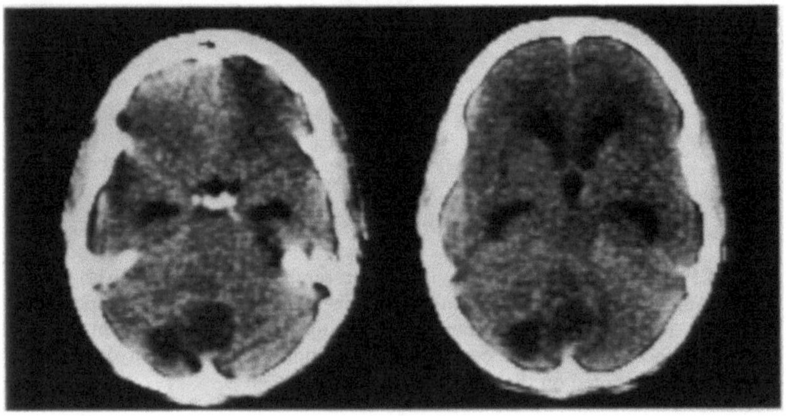

Fig. D 1.198. Monstrocellular sarcoma involving the superior vermis and left cerebellar hemisphere in a 28-year-old man. Solid tumor tissue shows faint peripheral contrast enhancement. The densities within the cystic component of the tumor are much higher than in CSF, signifying a high protein content. Postcontrast CT

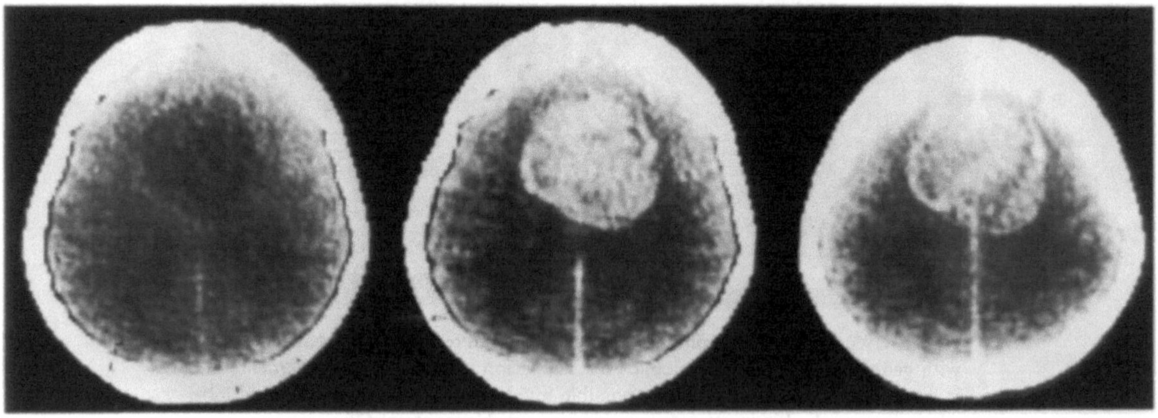

Fig. D 1.199. Histiocytoma in a 48-year-old woman with a brief history of seizures. The tumor appears markedly hypodense on the plain CT scan (*left*) and enhances intensely and nonhomogeneously on the postcontrast scans (*center* and *right*). The primary CT diagnosis was thus falx meningioma. At operation tumor was found on both sides of the falx in the interhemispheric fissure and callosal cistern. The tumor was predominantly well demarcated, yellow in color, and had a neurinoma-like consistency

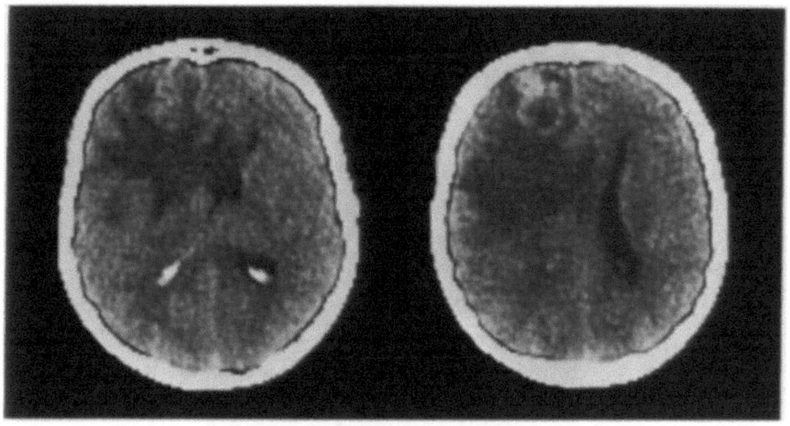

Fig. D 1.200. Malignant histiocytoma of the left frontal lobe with extensive perifocal edema in a 46-year-old man. The tumor presents a combined ring and nodular pattern on CT, indistinguishable from a metastasis. *Left* precontrast, *right* postcontrast

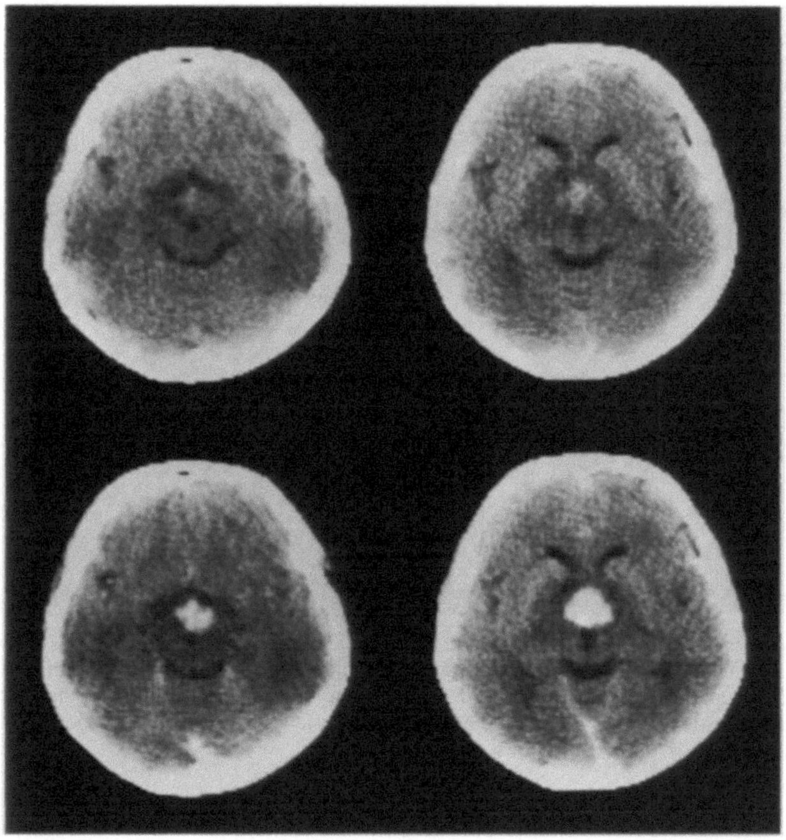

Fig. D 1.201. Histiocytosis X of the optic chiasm and hypothalamus in a 33-year-old woman with narcoleptic attacks. The lesion appears slightly hyperdense on plain CT scans (*top*) and enhances intensely with contrast medium (*bottom*). The tumor is projected onto the chiasmal-hypothalamic region. Massive expansion of the optic chiasm was found at operation. Excisional biopsy identified the lesion as histiocytosis X

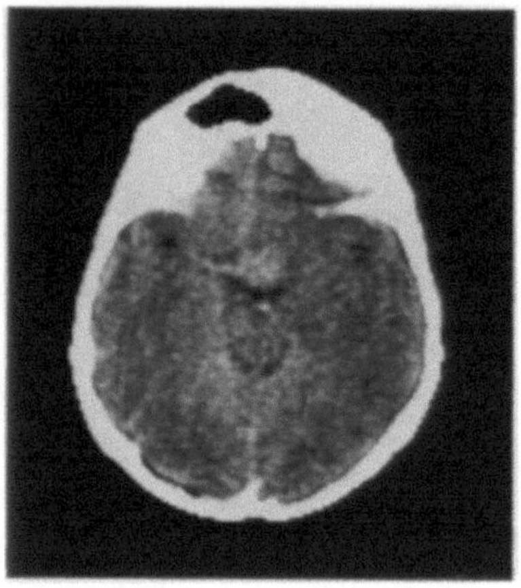

Fig. D 1.202. Histiocytosis X of the optic chiasm-hypothalamic region in a 52-year-old man with visual and endocrine abnormalities. The minimally enhancing tumor completely fills the chiasmatic cistern and shows suprasellar extension. It is indistinguishable from a pilocytic astrocytoma at the same location, although the age of the patient would not support that diagnosis

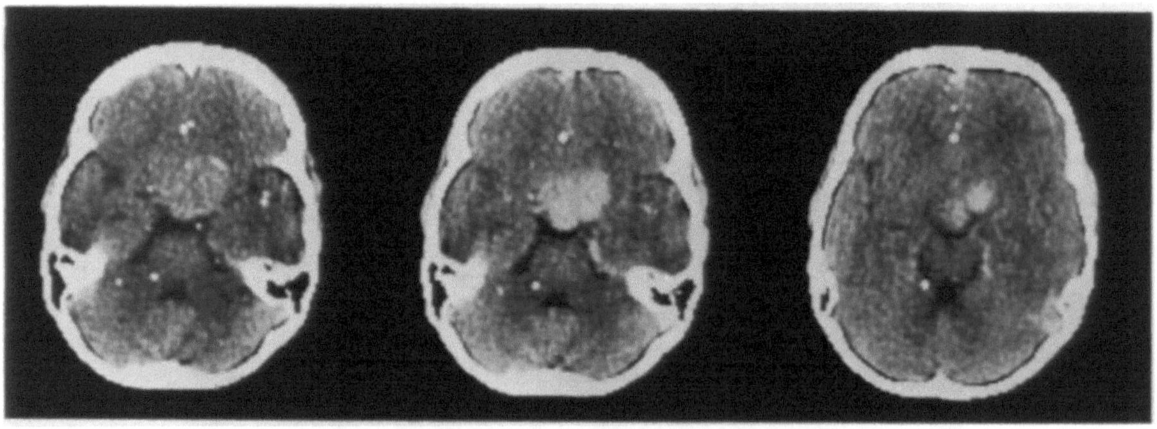

Fig. D 1.203. Histiocytosis X of the optic chiasm-hypothalamic region in a 14-year-old girl. Noncontrast CT (*left*) demonstrates a lesion of markedly increased density filling the chiasmatic cistern and extending far into the suprasellar region. Postcontrast CT (*center* and *right*) shows marked enhancement with discrimination of two separate tumor nodules. CT findings prompted an initial diagnosis of pituitary adenoma. The multiple small, white spots represent dye residues from previous myelography

q) Choroid Plexus Papillomas

Incidence	0.3%–0.6% of all brain tumors
Age predilection	Childhood, adolescence, middle age
Sex predilection	Roughly equal distribution
Typical sites	Fourth ventricle, lateral ventricle (trigone), third ventricle
Skull X-ray	Occasional tumor calcifications
Angiography	Diffuse, homogeneous tumor staining
CT	
Noncontrast scan	Tumor usually slightly hypodense; partially calcified intraventricular mass not uncommon
Contrast enhancement	Intense
Postcontrast appearance	Solid, intraventricular, nodular tumor with knobbly surface
MR	
Noncontrast scan	Tumors hypointense and poorly defined on T1-weighted images, more intense and more clearly defined on T2-weighted sequences
Gadolinium enhancement	Intense
Post Gd-DTPA appearance	Well-defined, homogeneously enhancing mass on T1-weighted sequences
Differential diagnosis	
Ventricular meningioma	
Subependymal giant cell astrocytoma	
Ependymoma	
In fourth ventricle: pilocytic astrocytoma or, very rarely, solid angioblastoma	

This tumor arises from the choroid plexus and is usually benign (grade I). Malignant forms are rare (grade III, choroid plexus carcinoma).

Reports on incidence range from 0.6% (Zülch 1986; Cushing 1932) to 0.3% (Olivecrona 1967). The incidence in our series was 0.38%. Males and females are affected with about equal frequency. We have noted peak incidences of choroid plexus papilloma in early childhood and also in the middle decades.

Typical Sites

The fourth ventricle, the lateral ventricle (especially the trigone), the third ventricle, and the cerebellopontine angle are affected in that order of frequency.

Main Clinical Features

Most patients present with general signs of intracranial hypertension caused partly by the obstruction to CSF flow and partly by the overproduction of CSF. Hydrocephalus with associated cranial deformity is seen in affected infants.

Additional Diagnostic Procedures

Adjunctive studies provide only nonspecific findings. Angiograms often demonstrate a diffuse, homogeneous tumor staining.

Computed Tomography
(Figs. D 1.204–212)

Noncontrast Scan
Choroid plexus papilloma appears as an isodense or slightly hyperdense lesion, which is surrounded by CSF when intraventricular (see Figs. D 1.205–210). Calcifications of varying size may be present (Figs. D 1.206, 211). Cyst formation is very unusual (Fig. D 1.209). We have found that choroid plexus papillomas of the trigone region may be associated with a marked decrease of density in adjacent brain caused by edema and the penetration of CSF into brain tissue (Fig. D 1.208).

Contrast Enhancement
The richly vascularized tumor enhances intensely with contrast medium, similar to meningioma. The enhancement tends to be uniformly distributed throughout the mass (see Figs. D 1.204–209, 212).

Postcontrast Appearance
The intense contrast enhancement aids in delineating the tumor from surrounding CSF and brain. Many tumors present a rough or spiculated surface (Fig. D 1.205).

Magnetic Resonance Imaging
(Fig. D 1.212)

The hypointense tumor is virtually indistinguishable from CSF on the T1-weighted image. T2 weighting increases the relative signal intensity of the tumor, which is more easily recognized and differentiated from CSF. The lesion enhances with Gd-DTPA.

Differential Diagnosis

Lateral ventricular meningiomas present a smoother surface contour than papillomas. All patients with lateral ventricular meningiomas in our series were over 25 years of age.

The proximity of *subependymal giant cell astrocytoma* to the foramen of Monro at the head of the caudate nucleus serves to distinguish that tumor from choroid plexus papilloma, which is not known to occur at that site. Similar considerations apply to *lateral ventricular ependymoma*, which tends to arise near the foramen of Monro.

With a *fourth ventricular tumor* that is surrounded by CSF, *pilocytic astrocytoma* (Fig. D 1.104) and *ependymoma* (Fig. D 1.131) should be considered in differential diagnosis. Usually these tumors present smoother margins than choroid plexus papilloma. The location and morphology of choroid plexus papilloma in the cerebellopontine angle are so characteristic that they are virtually pathognomonic for that entity (Fig. D 1.211).

Intraventricular *angioblastoma* occurs very rarely. This richly vascularized tumor can present CT features closely resembling choroid plexus papilloma.

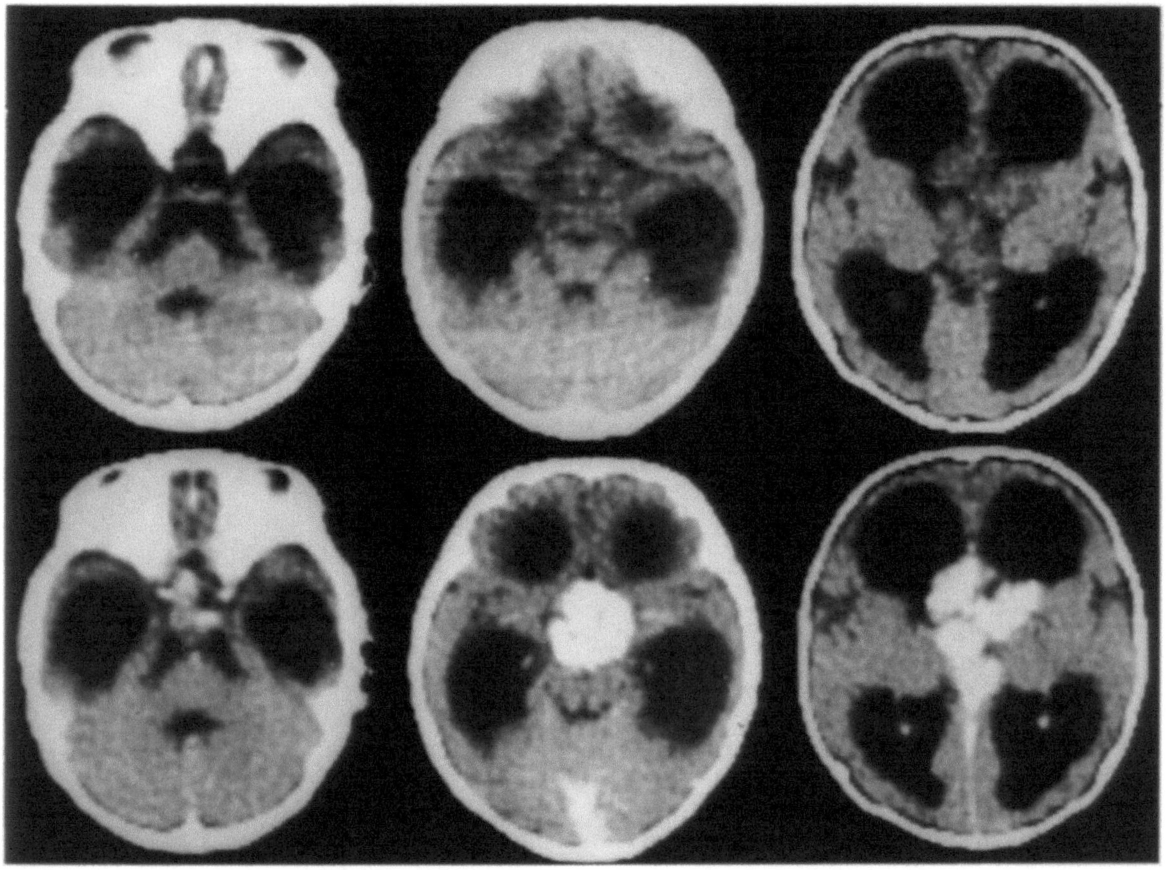

Fig. D 1.204. Choroid plexus papilloma of the third ventricle in a 4-month-old boy. Routine examination disclosed macrocephalus with tense fontanelles and sunset phenomenon. CT: *top* precontrast, *bottom* postcontrast. Scans reveal marked dilatation of both lateral ventricles. On the plain scan the enlarged third ventricle is completely filled with tumor. The tumor enhances markedly with contrast medium and is seen to extend through the foramen of Monro into the lateral ventricles

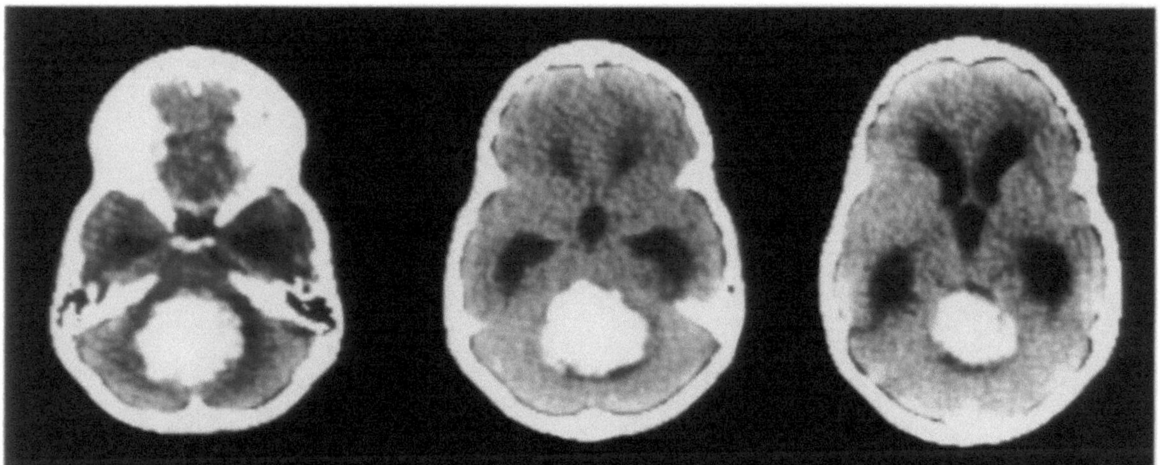

Fig. D 1.205. Choroid plexus papilloma of the fourth ventricle in a 9-year-old boy with ataxia, papilledema, and vomiting. Postcontrast CT shows an intensely enhancing lesion with rough, irregular borders in the region of the fourth ventricle. There is obstructive hydrocephalus with dilatation of the third ventricle and both lateral ventricles

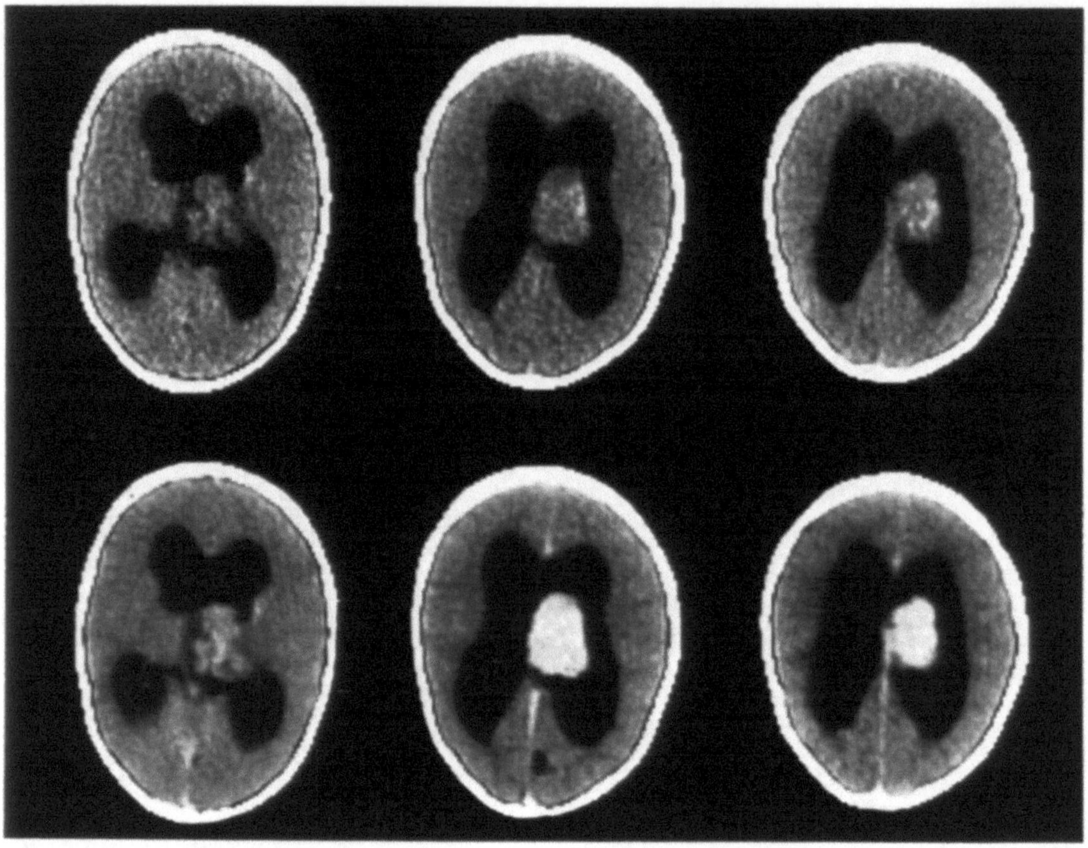

Fig. D 1.206. Choroid plexus papilloma in the central portion of the right lateral ventricle in a 2-year-old child with hydrocephalus. The plain scans (*top*) show a predominantly isodense tumor with interspersed flecks of calcification. The postcontrast scans (*bottom*) show very intense enhancement of the intraventricular tumor. The irregular tumor surface is appreciated most clearly in the *lower left* scan

Fig. D 1.208. Choroid plexus papilloma in the region of the trigone and occipital horn in a 4-month-old infant with rapid cranial enlargement on the left side. The CT scans on the *left* demonstrate the relationship of the partially cystic tumor to the choroid plexus (*arrows*). CSF has infiltrated the brain tissue, simulating peritumoral edema

a, b

c, d

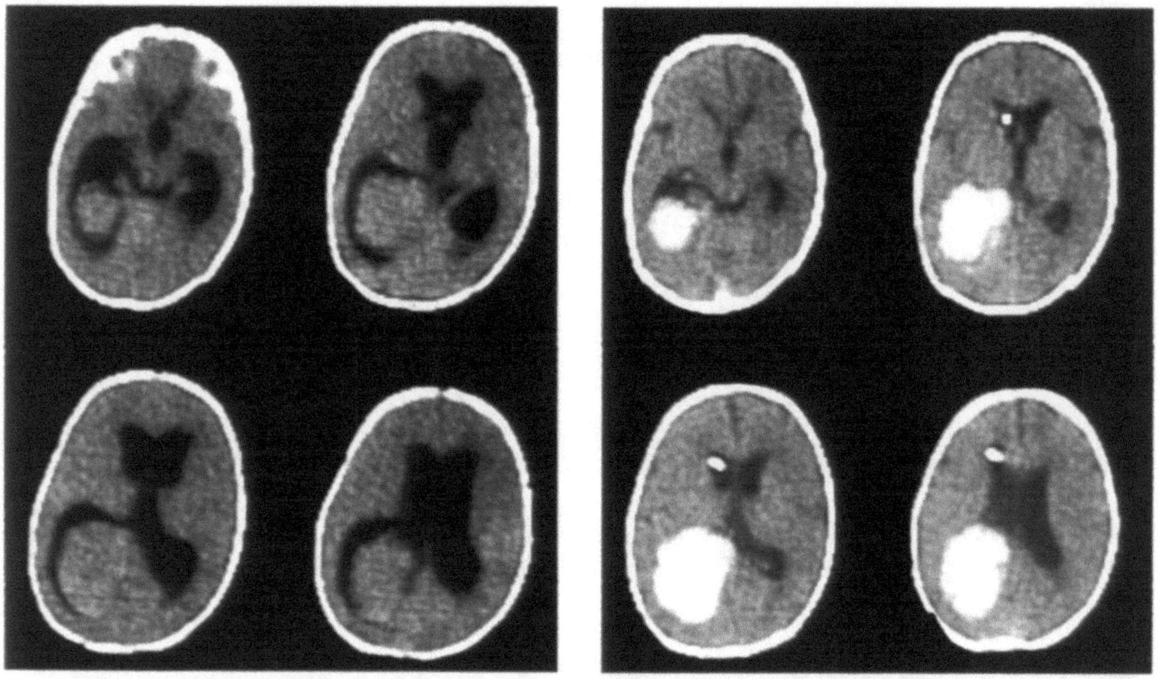

e, f

g, h

Fig. D1.207 a–h. Choroid plexus papilloma of the left occipital horn in a 2-month-old child. A shunt was implanted in the interval between the noncontrast CT examination (**a–d**) and the contrast examination performed several days later (**e–h**). The tip of the shunt is visible in the left frontal horn. The plain scans reveal pronounced internal hydrocephalus. The left frontal horn is displaced laterally and appears indented from the medial side. The contrast scans confirm a large, intensely enhancing tumor almost completely filling the left occipital horn. The tumor is indistinguishable from normal brain tissue on the unenhanced scans

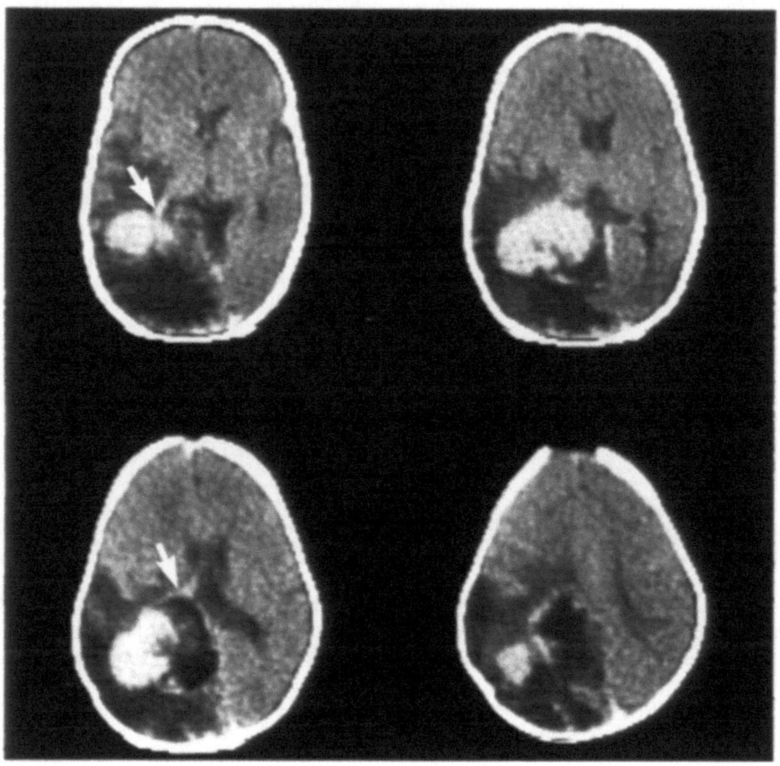

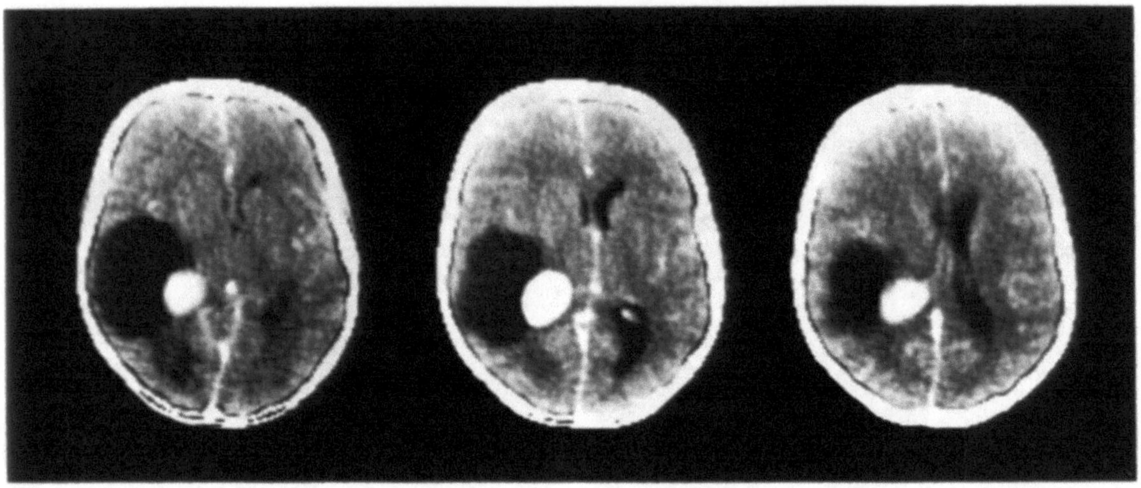

Fig. D 1.209. Walnut-size choroid plexus papilloma in the left trigone of a 25-year-old woman. The tumor is obstructing the left lateral ventricle, causing extreme dilatation of the temporal horn and mimicking a cyst. The tumor was hyperdense on plain scans (not shown) and enhanced with contrast medium

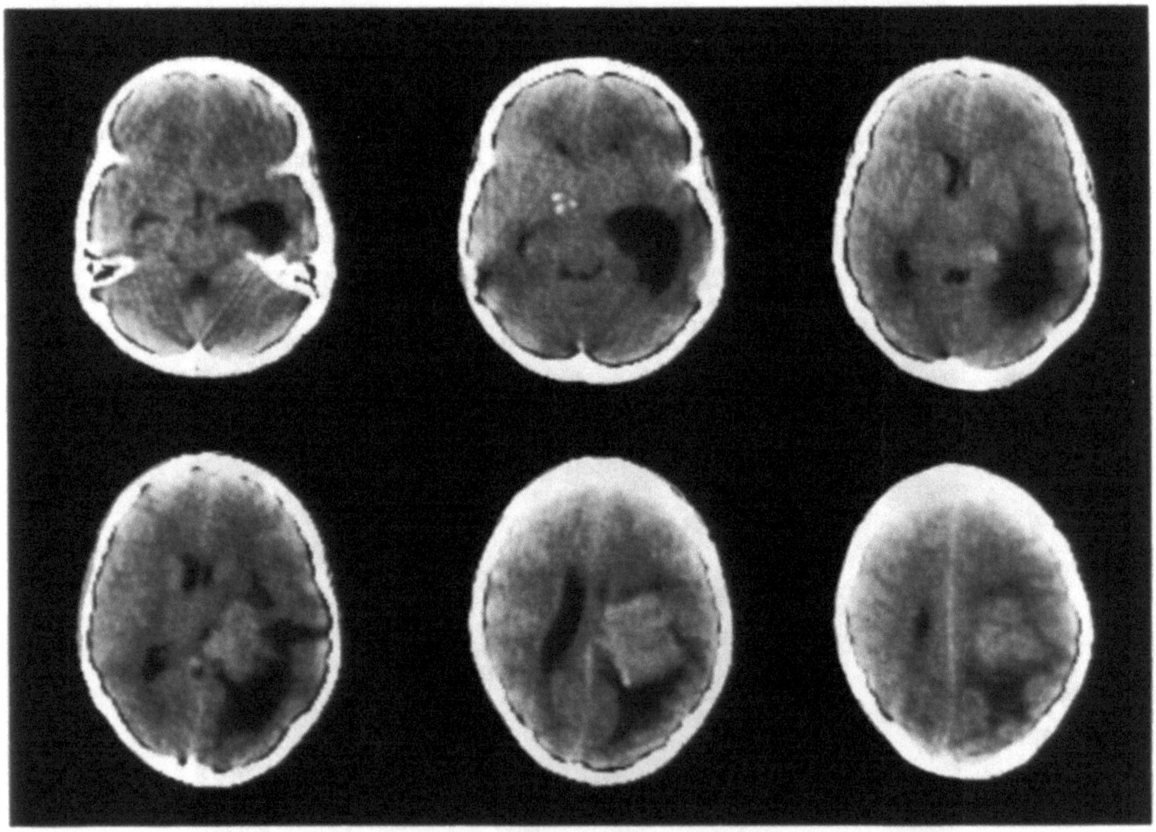

Fig. D 1.210. Choroid plexus carcinoma in the right trigone with expansion of the right temporal horn and penetration of CSF into surrounding brain (*bottom*). The tumor appears hyperdense and lobulated on the plain CT scans. Contrast medium was withheld due to iodine allergy. The flecks of calcification in the left basal ganglia are an incidental finding

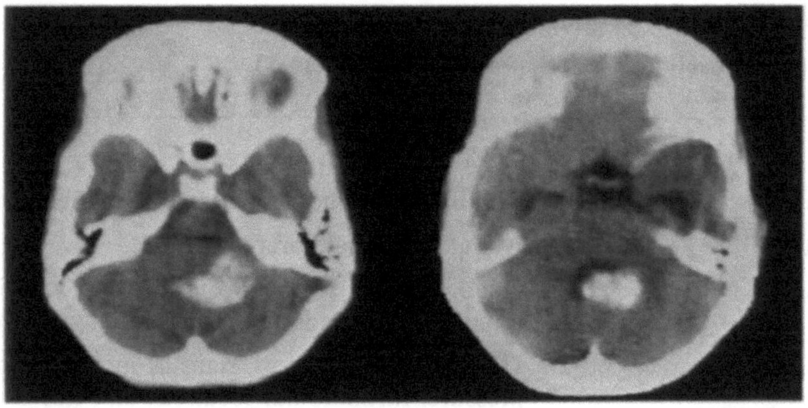

Fig. D 1.211. Calcified choroid plexus papilloma extending from the right cerebellopontine angle through the foramen of Luschka into the fourth ventricle in a 34-year-old woman with symptoms of a cerebellopontine angle lesion. The tumor originates from the pars aperturae lateralis of the choroid plexus

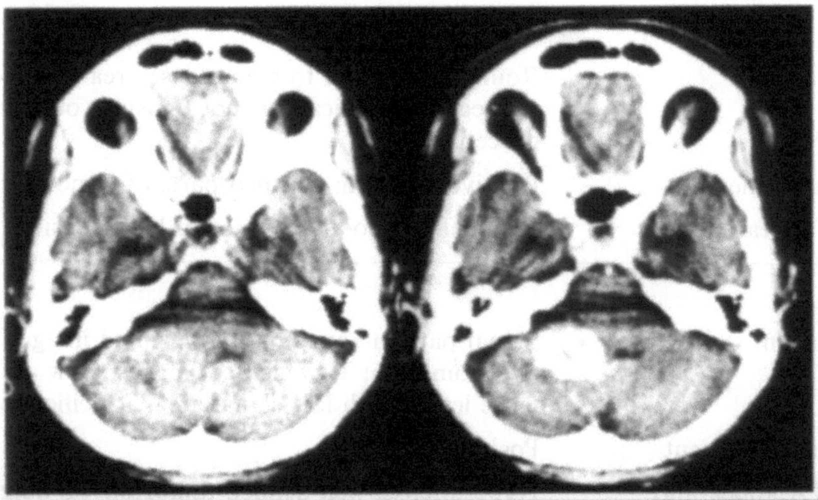

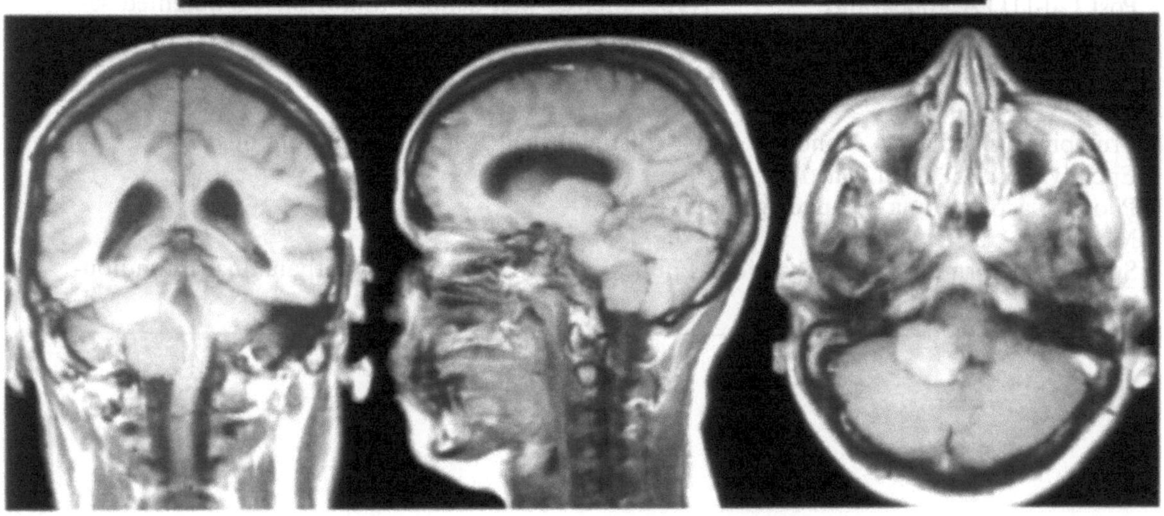

Fig. D 1.212. Choroid plexus papilloma arising from the fourth ventricle and extending into the left cerebellopontine angle in a 35-year-old woman with a 2-month history of diffuse headache, blurred vision, and diplopia. Patient presented with bilateral papilledema, ataxia, and decreased mentation. CT scans at *top*, SE 400/30 MR scans at *bottom*. Plain CT scan shows displacement of the fourth ventricle across the midline toward the right side. Postcontrast scan shows marked circumscribed tumor enhancement. MR shows marked displacement of the pons and medulla by a smoothly delineated mass. The tumor is moderately hyperintense to normal brain

r) Tumors of the Pineal Region

(Including Ectopic Pinealomas and Suprasellar Germinomas)

Incidence	0.5% of all brain tumors
Age predilection	Childhood and adolescence, less frequently in adults
Sex predilection	About a 2:1 male preponderance
Typical sites	Quadrigeminal region, posterior third ventricle. Ectopic form: infundibulum or rarely fourth ventricle
Main clinical features	Upward gaze paralysis, signs of increased intracranial pressure. Infundibular location: diabetes insipidus and visual disturbances
Skull X-ray	Displacement and enlargement of calcified pineal body
Angiography	Tumor vessels rare; signs of hydrocephalus, displacement of internal cerebral veins
CT	
Noncontrast scan	Rounded isodense to hyperdense area in quadrigeminal region; calcifications not unusual; obstructive hydrocephalus
Contrast enhancement	Positive except in calcified parts of tumor
Postcontrast appearance	Well-defined nodular tumor of high density
MR	
Noncontrast scan	Signal pattern varies on T1-weighted images but usually isointense; T2-weighted images show a hyperintense lesion with low-signal areas (calcifications)
Gadolinium enhancement	Positive
Post Gd-DTPA appearance	Hyperintense, well-defined tumor on T1-weighted sequences

Differential diagnosis

True pineal neoplasms cannot be clearly distinguished from other tumors of region:
Ependymoma of third ventricle
Pilocytic astrocytoma of quadrigeminal region
Metastases
Suprasellar form: craniopharyngioma, pilocytic astrocytoma of hypothalamus (infundibuloma)

True pineal tumors consist of **pineoblastoma** (pinealoblastoma), classified as grade IV, and the less malignant **pineocytoma** (pinealocytoma), which ranges from grade I to grade III. Both are very uncommon.

The most common tumor of the pineal region is the **germinoma**, a grade II or grade III germ-cell tumor not derived from the cells of the pineal parenchyma.

Pineal tumors account for 0.5%–0.7% of intracranial neoplasms, with a higher incidence reported in Japan, where Russell and Rubinstein (1977) report a range from 4.5% to 9.3%. The incidence in our series was 0.30% for pineocytomas and pineoblastomas and 0.15% for germinomas. Males are predominantly affected. Most cases occur in childhood and adolescence, although adult cases are not unusual. The typical site of involvement is the region of the pineal gland and quadrigeminal plate. In addition, there are suprasellar *germinomas which tend to occur in the pituitary infundibulum* (Fig. D 1.217) and were formerly identified as ectopic pinealomas. Ectopic pineocytomas occasionally occur in the fourth ventricle (Fig. D 1.220).

Pinealomas can metastasize via CSF pathways (spinal tumors, meningeal seeding, ventricular tumors).

The **pineal region** is the site for a number of other tumors and malformations including *pilocytic astrocytoma of the quadrigeminal plate, posterior third ventricular ependymoma, meningioma of the tentorial incisure, teratoma, epidermoid, dermoid, lipoma of the quadrigeminal plate, arachnoid cyst of the quadrigeminal cistern, aneurysm of the vein of Galen, and metastasis of the quadrigeminal plate.*

Main Clinical Features

The main clinical manifestations of pineal tumors consist of increased intracranial pressure due to CSF obstruction at the outlet of the third ventricle or at the aqueduct and paresis of upward gaze (Parinaud's syndrome).

Additional Diagnostic Procedures

Plain skull X-rays often show secondary signs of increased intracranial pressure with changes in the sella. The pineal gland may be normal or markedly displaced. Importance is attached to enlargement of the calcified pineal body, which signifies involvement by neoplastic disease.

Angiography reveals marked displacement of the posterior choroidal vessels in addition to elevation and flattening of the internal cerebral vein.

Computed Tomography
(Figs. D 1.213–220, 225)

Noncontrast Scan
True pineal tumors are highly cellular and as such appear isodense or slightly hyperdense on plain CT scans. Some show calcification. We have seen instances of cyst formation following radiation therapy (Fig. D 1.213).

Postcontrast Scan
All true pineal tumors enhance intensely unless they are completely calcified. This enhancement demarcates the tumor from surrounding structures and gives an accurate picture of its total extent.

In most cases the enhancement is homogeneous and nodular. Ring patterns are uncommon.

Meningeal seeding may be evidenced by increased density of the cortical band or by enhancement of the cisterns (Figs. D 1.215, 216). Spread to the ventricles may cause the latter to become entirely filled with tumor (Fig. D 1.219). This is most commonly observed in the frontal horns.

Magnetic Resonance Imaging
(Figs. D 1.221–225)

Noncontrast Scan
The tumor usually appears isointense on the T1-weighted image and can be detected on the midsagittal view. The T2-weighted image generally shows a hyperintense mass in which larger calcifications produce areas of low signal. Most of these tumors are well defined.

Post-Gadolinium Scan
Pineal tumors generally show intense enhancement with Gd-DTPA. The postcontrast appearance is the same as on enhanced CT scans.

Differential Diagnosis

The CT and MR features of pinealomas may closely resemble those of pilocytic astrocytoma, ependymoma, meningioma of the tentorial incisure, and intracranial metastasis. It may be impossible to differentiate among these tumors in any given case. Primary cyst formation is most consistent with pilocytic astrocytoma. An *aneurysm of the vein of Galen* projected onto the pineal region can usually be identified by its profound contrast enhancement, its size, and the presence of large draining vessels on the CT scan (see Fig. F 84). MR displays the enlarged vessels as signal voids.

Hypodense tumors and malformations of this region are illustrated on pp. 383–385, 397–398, 406, 530.

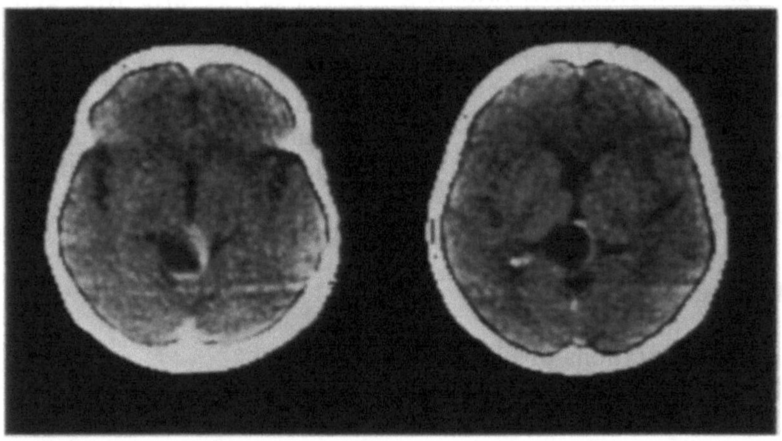

Fig. D 1.213. Pineocytoma of the quadrigeminal region with ring enhancement in a 42-year-old woman with Parinaud's syndrome who had undergone radiotherapy. Prior to radiotherapy the tumor was slightly hyperdense and showed homogeneous enhancement

Fig. D 1.214. Germinoma of the pineal gland in a 22-year-old man. *Right* CT scans are contrast-enhanced. The scans on the *left* are a vertical reconstruction demonstrating the exact relation of the tumor to the tentorium and the cisterns

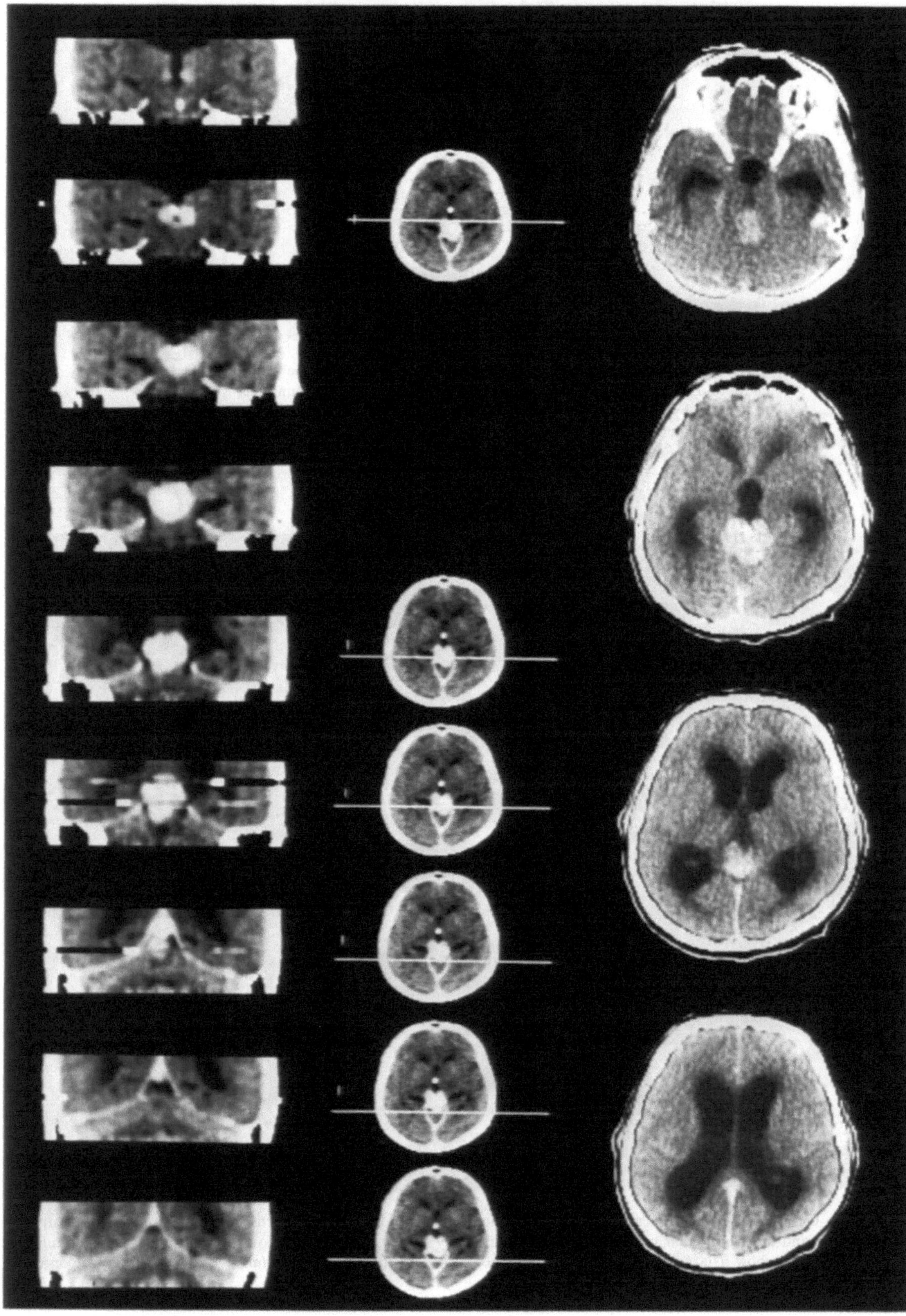

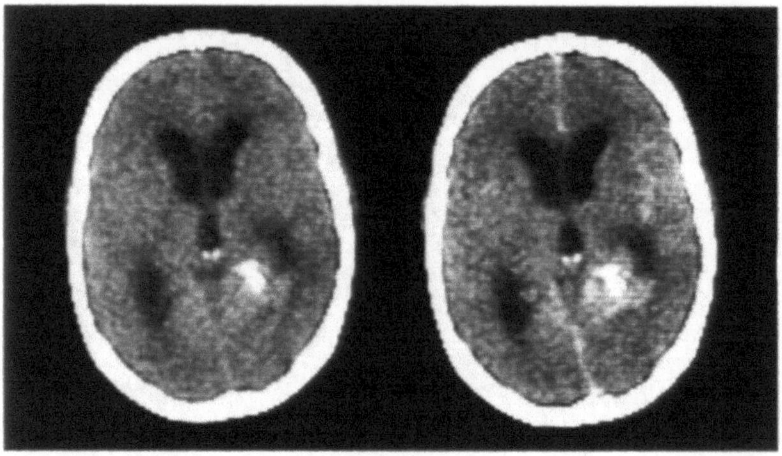

Fig. D 1.215. Pineoblastoma in a 34-year-old man. The tumor arose from the pineal gland and mainly involves the region of the right trigone. The tumor is isodense to slightly hyperdense with calcifications on the plain CT scan (*left*) and shows marked enhancement on the postcontrast scan (*right*). Faint enhancement of the sylvian fissure signifies tumor infiltration of the meninges

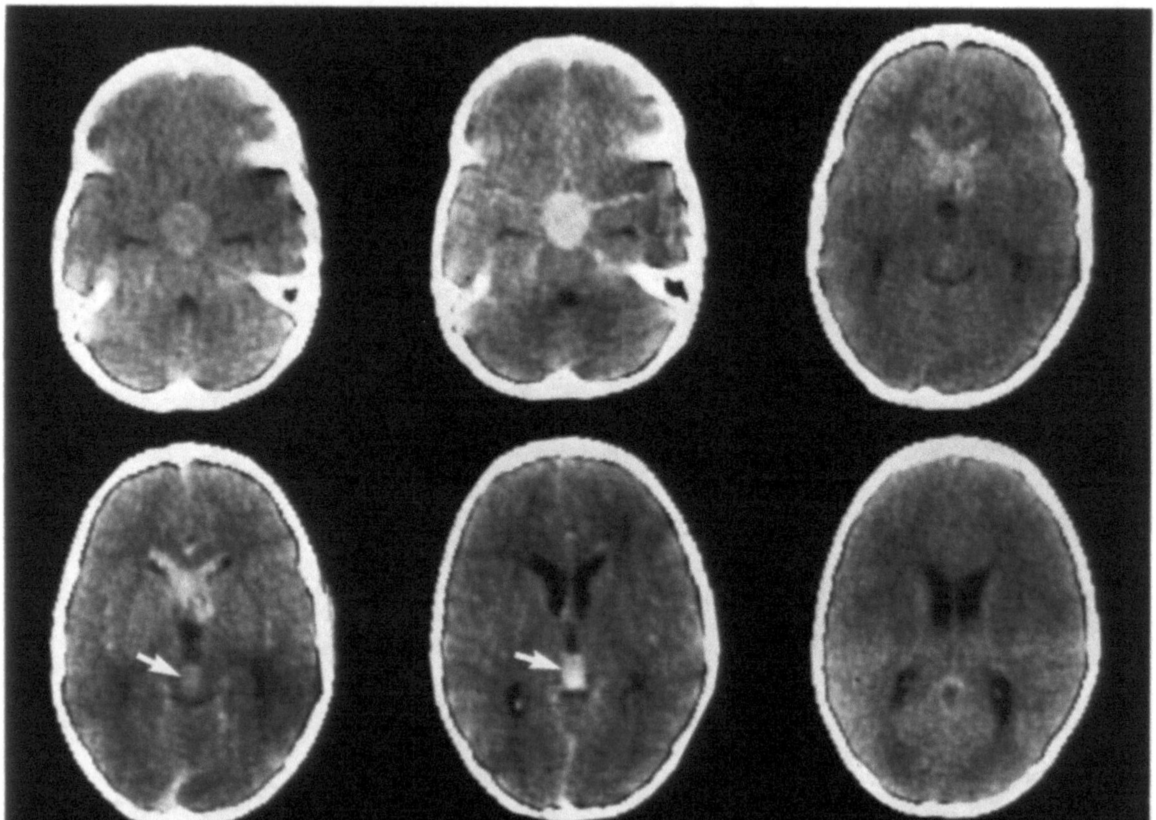

Fig. D 1.216. Germinoma of the pineal gland with ectopic tumor growth and intraventricular metastasis in a 12-year-old boy. CT scans show a large, rounded mass filling the chiasmatic cistern; infiltration of the ventricle wall with tumor in both frontal horns, which are completely occupied by tumor tissue on the lower scans; and a smaller tumor mass in the pineal region (*arrow*). All scans are postcontrast

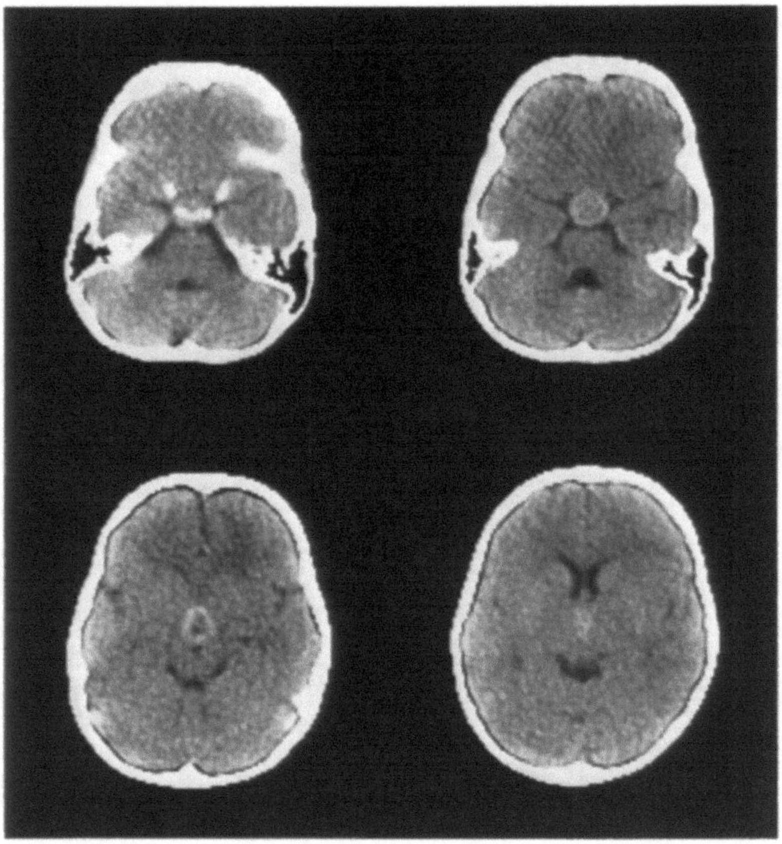

Fig. D 1.217. Ectopic pinealoma (germinoma) of the suprasellar region in a 5-year-old girl. Enhancement is most pronounced in the tumor capsule. Postcontrast CT

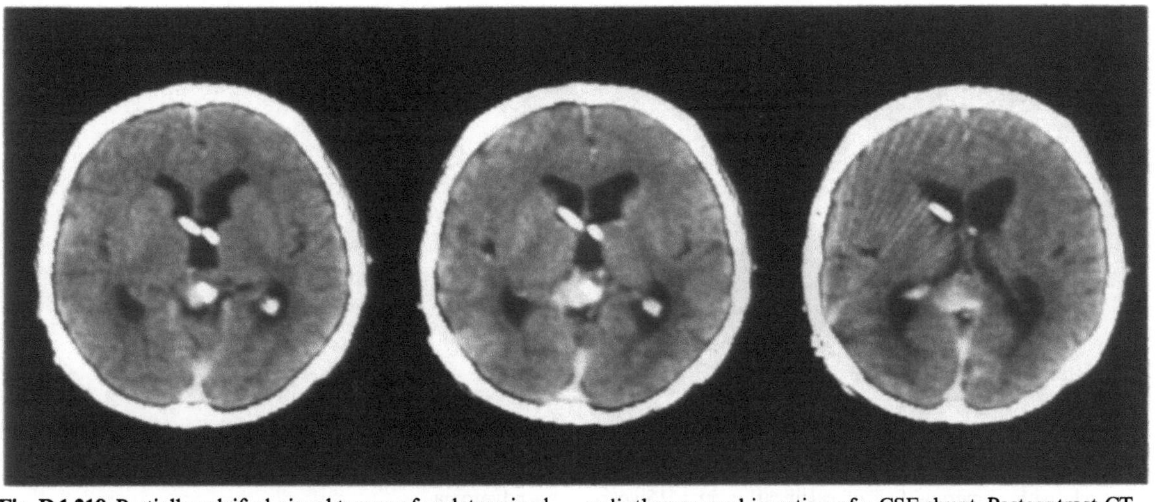

Fig. D 1.218. Partially calcified pineal tumor of undetermined histology (pineocytoma?) in a 54-year-old man 15 years after radiotherapy and insertion of a CSF shunt. Postcontrast CT

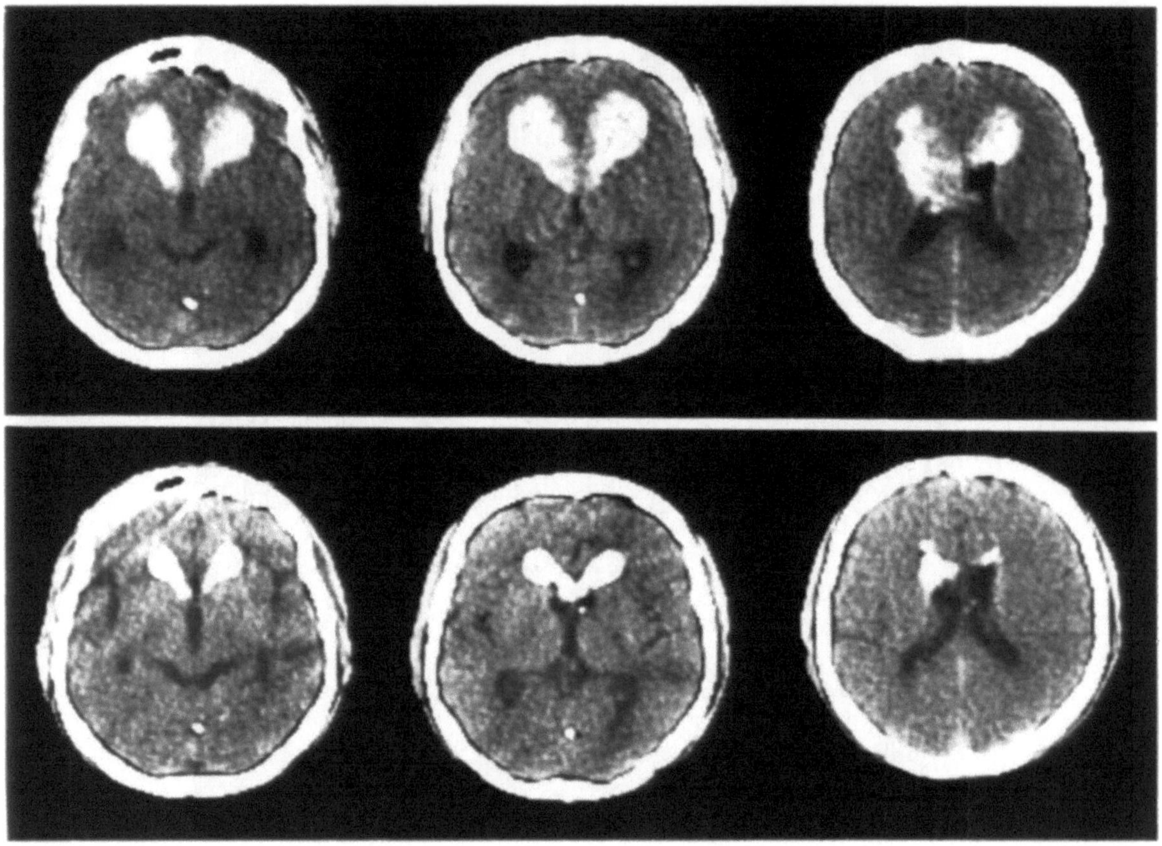

Fig. D 1.219. Serial CT study of a germinoma involving spinal and intraventricular sites in a 19-year-old man initially presenting with symptoms of cord disease. Following resection of a spinal tumor identified as a germinoma, a cranial CT examination was ordered despite the absence of cerebral symptoms. The scans (*top*) demonstrated hyperdense tumor filling both frontal horns. The lesion did not enhance further with contrast medium. Follow-up scans performed 4 months after irradiation with 50 Gy (*bottom*) indicate a marked reduction of tumor size

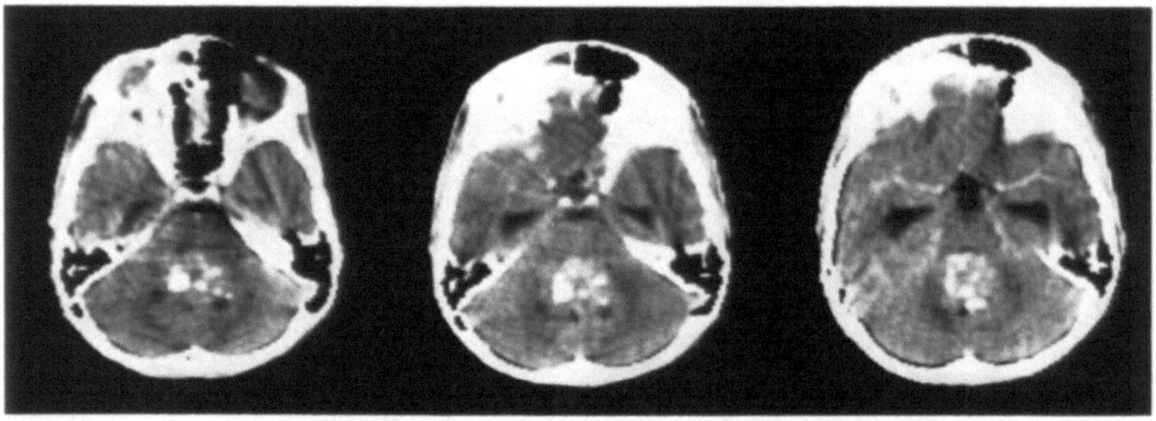

Fig. D 1.220. Anisomorphous pineocytoma of the fourth ventricle with numerous foci of calcification in a 15-year-old boy. CT findings are reminiscent of fourth ventricular ependymoma

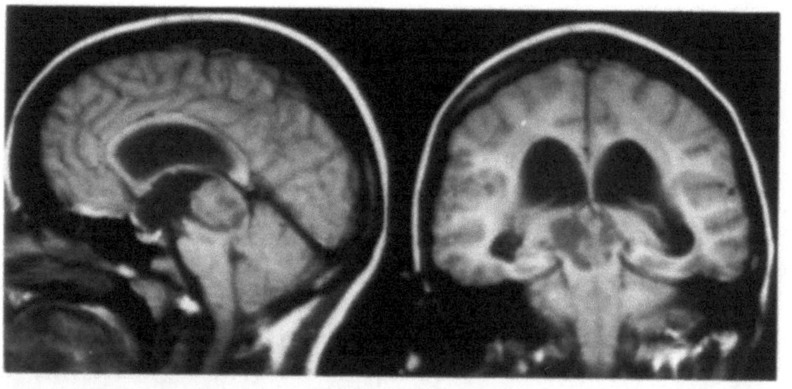

Fig. D 1.221. Ependymoma, presumed to be a pinealoma on the basis of MR findings. The 24-year-old woman presented with headache, lassitude, and Parinaud's syndrome. MR: SE 400/30, *left* sagittal, *right* coronal. The T1-weighted image demonstrates a mixed-intensity lesion

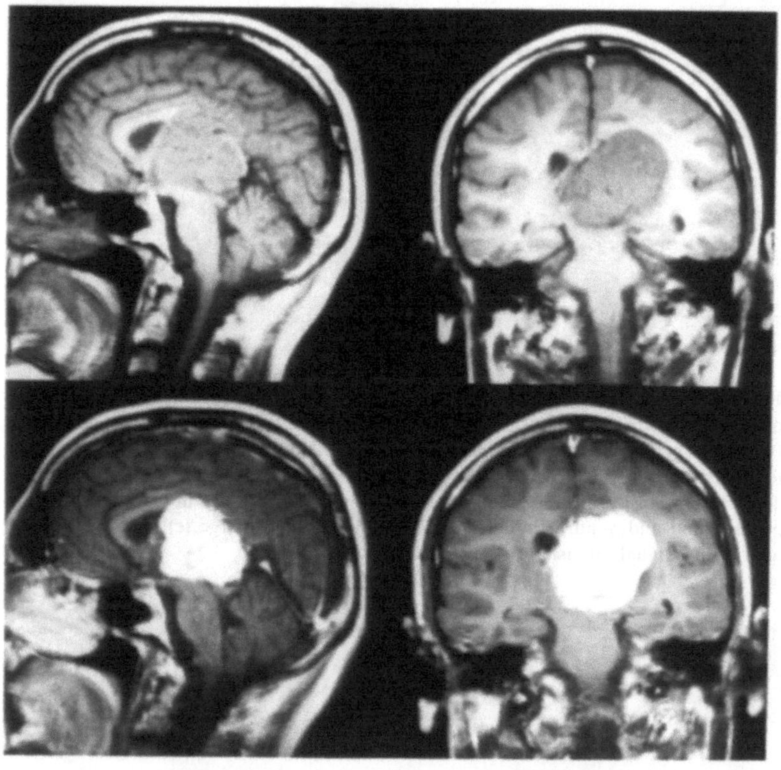

Fig. D 1.222. Giant teratoma, thought to be a pinealoma on the basis of MR findings. The 22-year-old man presented with left-sided hemiparesis and Parinaud's syndrome. MR: *top* SE 400/30 sagittal, coronal; *bottom* SE 400/30 post Gd-DTPA. The tumor is predominantly hypointense on the T1-weighted sequences (*top*). It enhances intensely with Gd-DTPA (*bottom*)

a b c d

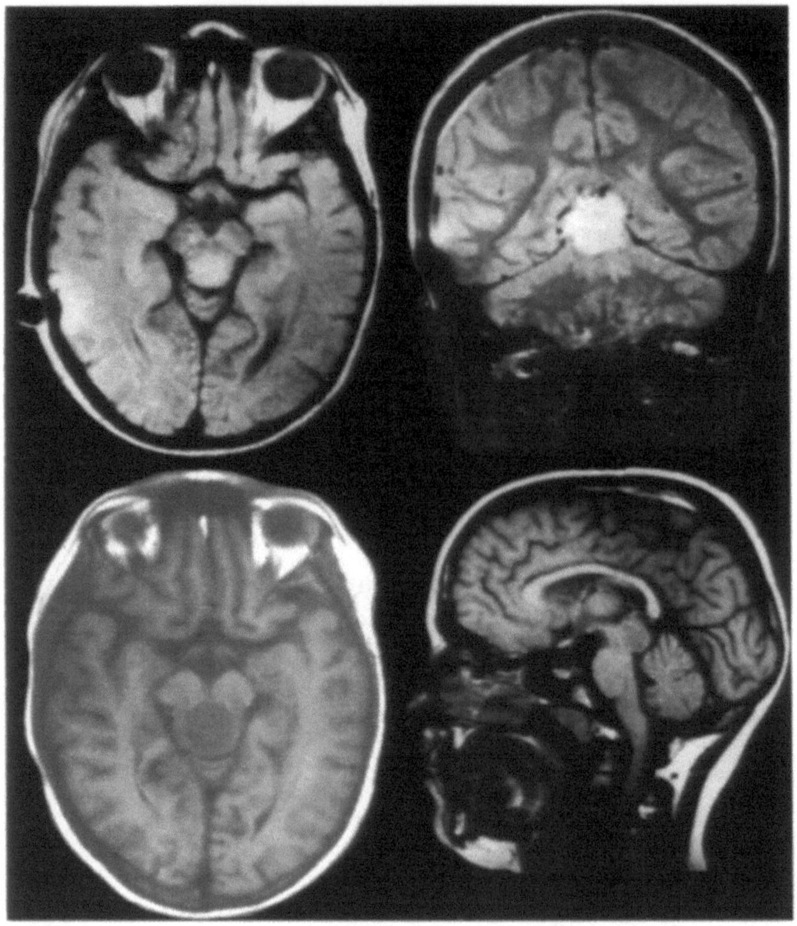

Fig. D 1.223 a–d. Isomorphous pinealoma in a 16-year-old girl with CT-confirmed obstructive hydrocephalus but no evidence of neoplasia. The patient developed Parinaud's syndrome following insertion of a CSF shunt. MR was ordered to screen for tumor: **a** SE 2500/30, **b** SE 3000/30 coronal, **c** SE 500/30, **d** SE 500/30 sagittal. The proton-density images (**a, b**) show a slight hyperintensity in the region of the pineal gland and quadrigeminal plate. The T1-weighted image (**c**) demonstrates an area of low signal intensity at that location

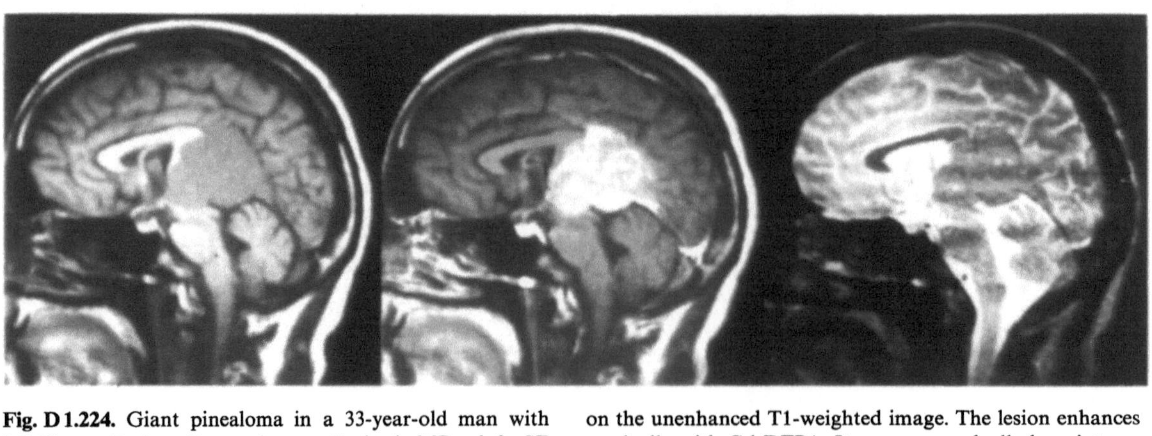

Fig. D 1.224. Giant pinealoma in a 33-year-old man with full-blown Parinaud's syndrome. Sagittal MR: *left* SE 500/30, *center* SE 500/30 post Gd-DTPA, *right* SE 1600/120. The tumor appears homogeneous and isointense to brain on the unenhanced T1-weighted image. The lesion enhances markedly with Gd-DTPA. It appears markedly hypointense on the T2-weighted image (*right*)

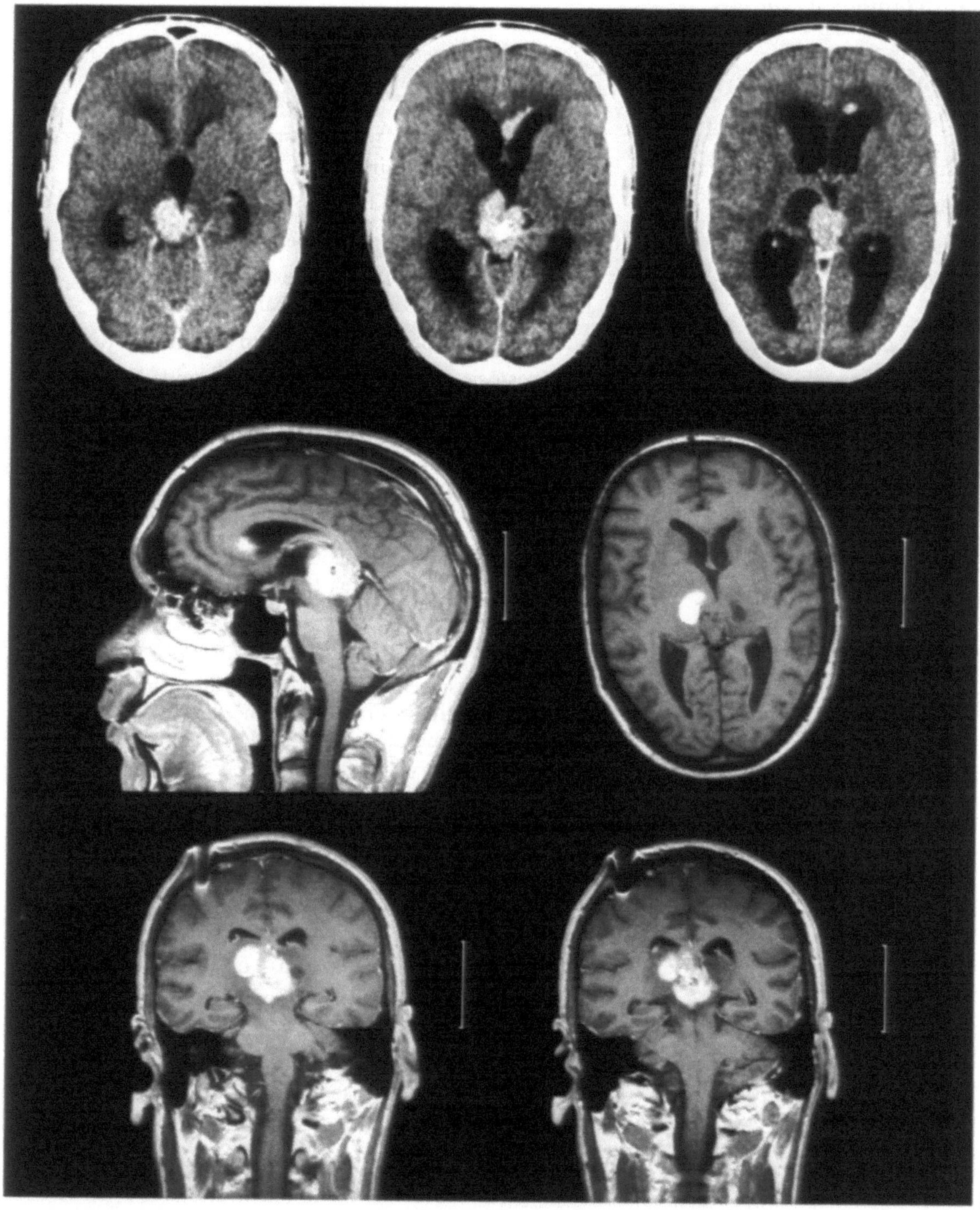

a–c

d, e

f, g

Fig. D 1.225 a–g. Germinoma in a 24-year-old man with a 6-week history of headache and vomiting and a 5-day history of diplopia. Postcontrast CT (**a–c**) shows intense enhancement of solid tumor components and of meningeal metastases in the right frontal horn. A cystic component is visible in the left thalamus. MR **d–g** SE 600/30; **d** sagittal post Gd-DTPA, **e** axial, **f, g** coronal post Gd-DTPA. Blood is visible in the cystic component in the left thalamus following stereotactic biopsy. The borders of the right frontal horn appear irregular due to isointense tumor infiltration of the ependyma (**e**)

2. Meningeal Tumors

a) Meningiomas

Incidence	14%–19% of all brain tumors
Age predilection	35–70 years
Sex predilection	Almost a 2:1 female preponderance
Typical sites	Parasagittal region, falx, convexity, entire skull base, posterior fossa, tentorium, lateral ventricles
Main clinical features	Neurologic symptoms according to location of tumor
Skull X-ray	Hyperostosis, erosive bone change, expanded vascular channels
Angiography	Displacement of intracranial vessels, typical tumor staining
CT	
Noncontrast scan	Predominantly homogeneous, slightly hyperdense or occasionally isodense area that may contain calcifications; frequently, hypodense halo representing edema
Contrast enhancement	Always very intense unless lesion is wholly calcified
Postcontrast appearance	Homogeneous, well-defined tumor, almost invariably related to meninges or cranial bone (cranial vault, skull base); moderate perifocal edema common
MR	
Noncontrast scan	T1-weighted sequences may not distinguish isointense tumor from brain, and detection relies on evidence of mass effect. Both tumor and edema give intense signal on T2-weighted images. T1 and T2 weighting often demonstrate tumor/brain or tumor/edema margin as narrow, hypointense rim. Long echo times aid in resolving tumor from edema, and osteoplastic foci appear hypointense
Gadolinium enhancement	Intense
Post Gd-DTPA appearance	Well-defined hyperintense lesion on T1-weighted sequences

Differential diagnosis

Cerebral convexity and falx	*Floor of middle fossa*
Metastases	Trigeminal neurinoma
Malignant lymphoma	Gangliocytoma
Rarely glioblastoma or	Pilocytic astrocytoma
anaplastic astrocytoma	Carotid aneurysm
	Chondroma
Suprasellar region and floor of anterior fossa	
Pituitary adenoma	Less frequently:
Pilocytic astrocytoma	Chondroma
Carotid aneurysm	Metastatic carcinoma
Chordoma	Malignant lymphoma
Posterior fossa	*Ventricles*
Acoustic neurinoma	Choroid plexus papilloma
Metastasis	Colloid cyst (third ventricle)
Solid angioblastoma	
Malignant lymphoma	
Basilar artery aneurysm	
Glomus tumor	
Clivus chordoma	

Meningiomas are the second most common intracranial tumor after glioblastomas. Cushing (1932) states that meningiomas comprise 13.4% of all brain tumors, while Zülch (1986) reports 16.6% and Olivecrona (1967) 18.2%. Meningiomas accounted for 18.5% of the tumors in our population.

Meningiomas can occur at any age but show a peak incidence between the ages of 35 and 70 years. Females are affected almost twice as frequently as males.

Meningiomas arise from the arachnoid and grow by expansion, displacing the brain tissue from which they are separated by a layer of pia mater. Tumor growth hampers venous drainage and can precipitate ischemic necrosis of the adjacent cerebral cortex, allowing the tumor to come into contact with the white matter. This process is invariably associated with the development of brain edema.

The great majority of meningiomas are slow-growing and benign (grade I). Anaplastic forms with a tendency toward more rapid growth accounted for about 5% of cases in our series. Meningiomas tend to recur if their site of origin cannot be completely extirpated, as may be the case in the region of the skull base.

Typical Sites

Meningiomas characteristically occur in close relation to the meninges or cranial bone. Typical sites are, in order of frequency, the parasagittal region (dura-falx angle) in the middle, anterior, and posterior thirds of the sagittal sinus; the falx; the cerebral convexity; the olfactory groove; the tuberculum sellae; the medial and lateral sphenoid wings; Meckel's cavity; the tentorium; the cerebellopontine angle; the clivus; and the craniospinal junction. The stroma of the choroid plexus is a very rare site of occurrence (lateral ventricular meningioma, third ventricle).

Multifocal occurrence is possible with meningioma and may be associated with diffuse seeding (meningiomatosis), which most often occurs in the "central" form of von Recklinghausen's disease. Besides their typical globular form, meningiomas may exhibit a plaque-like type of growth that is especially common in osteoplastic meningiomas of the sphenoid bone. Meningiomas can invade adjacent cranial bone, causing it to become thickened and producing a visible external bulge. They can also extend into the orbit and occasionally into the paranasal sinuses.

Main Clinical Features

Clinical findings vary greatly with the site of involvement. The patient may present with signs of acute cerebral ischemia or with seizures, which are very common in meningiomas of the convexity. Profound psycho-organic disturbances are most characteristic of olfactory groove meningiomas and lesions involving the frontotemporal region of the dominant hemisphere.

Sphenoid wing meningiomas can produce a bulge in the temporal region and exophthalmos. Basal meningiomas frequently incite cranial nerve deficits. Meningiomas of the posterior fossa often result in signs of chronic intracranial hypertension, possibly combined with cerebellar symptomatology.

Additional Diagnostic Procedures

Skull radiographs demonstrate bone changes in almost half of meningioma patients. Thickening of the cranial vault or skull base at the site of tumor attachment (enostosis) is the most common finding. Osteoplastic sphenoid wing meningiomas can be recognized on plain skull films.

Meningioma may even perforate the skull, giving rise to "spicules," or very fine columns of new bone arranged in a regular pattern, usually oriented at right angles to the surface of the calvarium.

It is common to find marked expansion of the vascular channels in the cranial vault as a result of increased blood flow to the tumor with hypertrophy of the meningeal vessels.

Some intracranial meningiomas are directly visible on plain skull X-rays owing to the presence of calcifications.

Meningiomas derive their blood supply from branches of the internal and external carotid arteries. The parts of the tumor supplied by these vessels can vary in size. Hence it is necessary to opacify each of the vascular trunks separately so that the full extent of the lesion can be appreciated. Angiography reveals a typical pattern with large feeding vessels and almost homogeneous tumor staining that begins in the capillary phase and often persists beyond the venous phase. Meningiomas differ from glioblastomas in that they are very rarely associated with arteriovenous fistulas, so early venous filling generally is not observed.

The smooth or lobulated contours of the tumor, the homogeneous staining persisting to the end of the venous phase, and hypertrophied feeding vessels coursing from the external carotid artery to the tumor are quite characteristic of meningioma and may be considered specific for that lesion.

Computed Tomography
(see also figures in Chap. D1 and D2)

Noncontrast Scan

The great majority of meningiomas appear on plain CT scans as homogeneous, hyperdense lesions (74.7%, see Figs. D2.1, 2). Some contain calcifications (10%–20%, see Figs. D2.4–6), and a few become completely calcified even at infratentorial sites (Figs. D2.67, 72, 73). Osteoplastic sphenoid wing meningioma represents a special form (Fig. D2.49).

Of the meningiomas in our series, 14.4% appeared isodense to brain on the nonenhanced CT scan. Such tumors may be overlooked unless accompanied by evidence of mass effect or perifocal edema. In our experience these associated signs are absent in about 40% of isodense meningiomas. Ten percent of meningiomas are mixed-density lesions (disregarding calcifications within hyperdense tumors). This pattern is usually caused by the development of cysts or other regressive changes (Figs. D2.7, 8, 10, 13). Cysts may occur within the meningioma or adjacent to it (Figs. D2.9, 16, 23). Very few meningiomas appear hypodense on the noncontrast scan (0.9%, see Figs. D2.8, 10, 11, 13).

The diagnosis of meningioma is reinforced by the detection of *enostosis at the site of tumor attachment* (Figs. D2.12, 14). Bony thickening of the adjacent skull vault is sometimes observed (Fig. D2.15).

Perifocal edema is a common finding in meningiomas (61.3%) and can delineate the tumor even on nonenhanced scans. Exceptions are temporobasal and high parietal meningiomas, where plain scans may demonstrate only the edema. Meningiomas of the sylvian fissure can cause *retention of CSF in the insular cistern* (Fig. D2.16).

The dark zone seen at the boundary between the meningioma and surrounding brain is not necessarily perifocal edema and may represent a *fluid film*. Digital analysis of these areas yields Hounsfield values lower than those of brain edema. Operation in these patients discloses a film of CSF-like fluid intervening between the tumor surface and edematous brain. The white matter appears very spongy in these cases, and its water content is greatly increased.

Contrast Enhancement
Unless homogeneously calcified, all meningiomas show visible contrast enhancement. The average degree of enhancement with a standard contrast dose is 18 HU. Only 97% of the meningiomas in our series enhanced. We attribute this to calcification in some cases and in others to the temporobasal or high parietal location of small tumors sometimes obscured by overlying structures or by artifacts.

Peak enhancement of meningioma occurs immediately after contrast injection. The enhancement fades relatively quickly over about a 30-min period.

Postcontrast Appearance
Meningiomas tend to enhance homogeneously with contrast medium. This greatly improves the delineation of the tumor, especially if it was isodense on the plain scan. Meningiomas may be round, oval, or lobulated and usually present smooth, clear borders. Except for intraventricular lesions, meningiomas are always in close relation to the meninges or cranial bone. Malignant meningiomas and en plaque growths may present irregular borders that are less sharply defined.

Visualization of the falx and tentorium can be very helpful in establishing the relation of the tumor to the meninges. Occasionally the topography of the lesion is appreciated better on coronal views, and this projection is essential for demonstrating small en plaque growths at the base of the middle fossa (Fig. D2.17). Contrast medium can improve the delineation of cysts and other regressive changes in meningiomas. Tumors of this kind may show ring enhancement (1.5% of all meningiomas), leading to confusion with other ringlike lesions (see Figs. D2.18, 26).

Vassoulithis and Ambrose (1979) reviewed a series of 102 meningioma patients examined by CT in an effort to correlate CT findings with specific histologic subgroups (transitional, fibroblastic, angioblastic, or syncytial types). While some correlation does exist between CT presentation and meningioma type, it is our experience that CT does not provide reliable criteria for this type of differentiation. A notable exception is malignant meningioma, in which case aggressive growth can often be inferred from the absence of typical CT features of meningioma (see p. 294).

Magnetic Resonance Imaging
(see also figures in Chaps. C, E, and G)

Noncontrast Scan
Meningiomas are poorly demonstrated on T1-weighted images because of their isointensity to adjacent brain. The greatest differences in signal intensity are observed on proton-density images. Perifocal edema is displayed poorly if at all. Generally the tumor presents a homogeneous internal structure, although heterogeneities may result from the presence of psammomatous bodies, cysts, necrosis, or heavy vascularization. However, these changes must attain significant size before they are visualized, and small calcium deposits are not detected with MR. Approximately 30%–40% of meningiomas are surrounded by a thin rim of reduced signal whose intensity is appreciably below that of the meningioma and adjacent brain (with or without brain edema). This feature may represent the tumor capsule with veins and arteries, a thin film of CSF, a gliotic boundary zone, or pressure-atrophied cortex undergoing structural change. The sites of attachment of meningiomas to bone and foci of hyperostosis appear as widened, hypointense areas between the tumor and diploe. Transosseous growth obliterates the low-signal area of the inner table, and the tumor appears to be continuous with the diploe.

If the meningioma attains sufficient size and exerts sufficient mass effect, MR will reveal obvious displacement and distortion of adjacent structures. Plain scans are excellent for demonstrating tumor ingrowth into the venous sinuses and their consequent displacement as well as the encasing of large blood vessels at the skull base.

On T2-weighted images meningiomas appear slightly hyperintense; some are nearly isointense. Adjacent brain edema stands out more clearly than on T1-weighted scans. The tumor is usually homogeneous. T2-weighted images display the heterogeneities of regressive change to better advantage. Cystic and necrotic components of substantial size produce a selective increase of signal, while circumscribed fibrotic areas and calcifications give a very low signal. These features should be of help in determining the histologic type of meningioma, although Spagnoli et al. (1986) were unable to find a correlation between MR findings and tumor pathology.

Post-Gadolinium Scan

Gadolinium-enhanced MR is comparable to postcontrast CT in its depiction of meningiomas. The tumors enhance very brightly on T1-weighted sequences and are readily distinguished from hypointense edema. The enhancement peaks very rapidly and remains at a high level for 30 min to 1 h. Calcified areas do not enhance. Gd-DTPA diffuses slowly into cysts. It should be noted that adjacent dura may enhance brightly with Gd-DTPA, and that this does not necessarily signify involvement by tumor.

Small meningiomas less than 1.5–2 cm in diameter can be detected with MR only when they are enhanced with Gd-DTPA.

When contrast medium is not used, CT is somewhat superior to MR in the detection and evaluation of meningiomas. But when contrast medium is administered, MR is advantageous for the diagnosis of medial sphenoid wing meningiomas, en plaque meningiomas, recurrent tumors, tentorial extension of meningiomas, and meningiomas at the craniospinal junction.

Fig. D 2.1. Large olfactory groove meningioma in a 45-year-old man with frontal headache and olfactory disturbances. The tumor appears markedly hyperdense on the plain CT scans (*left*). It contains small central calcifications and is associated with bifrontal edema that is more pronounced on the left side. The frontal horns are greatly displaced and narrowed by tumor. Enhancement on the postcontrast scans (*right*) is intense

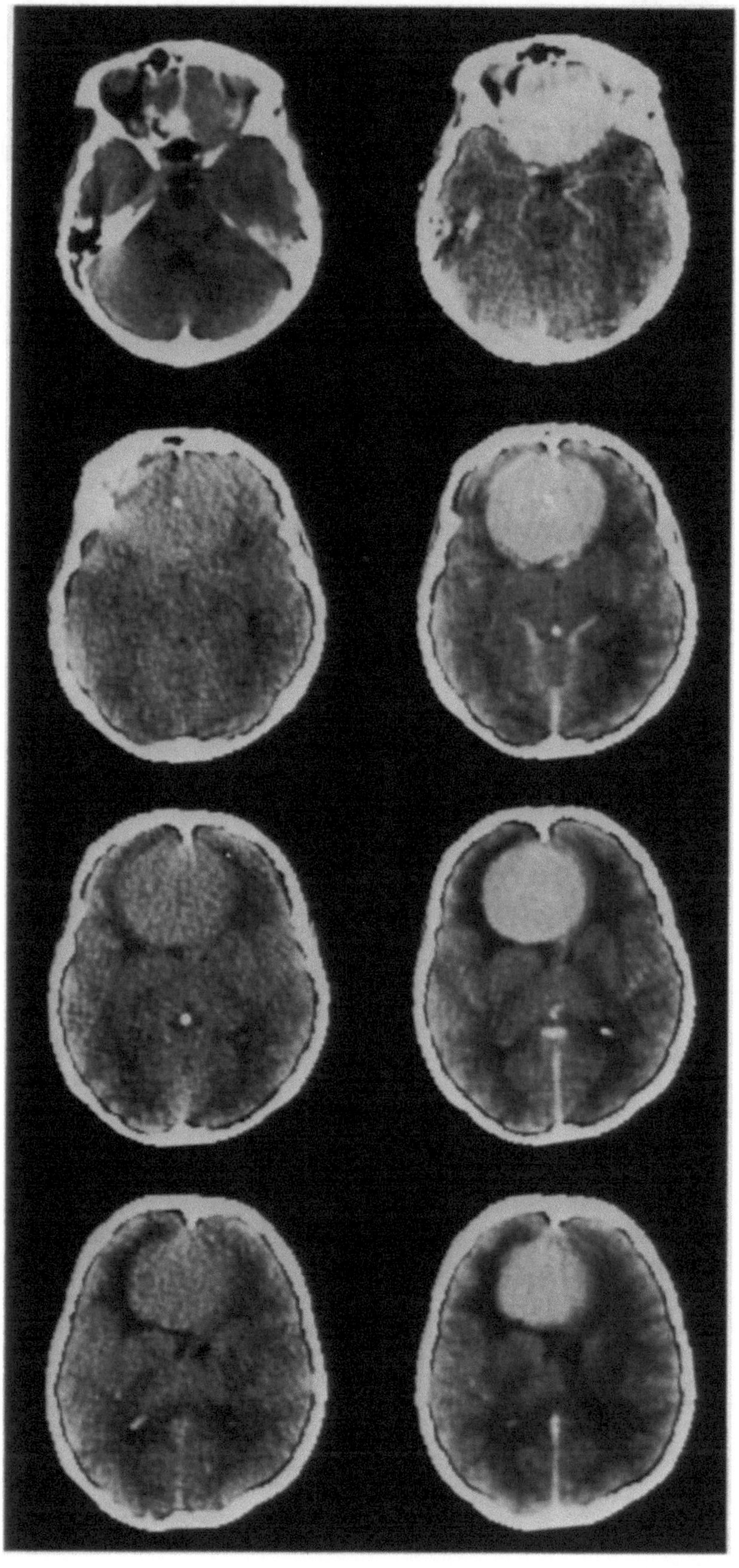

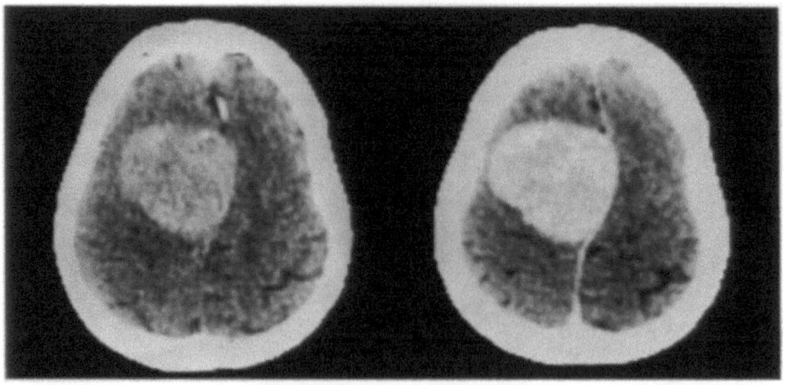

Fig. D 2.2. Middle-third falx meningioma in a 61-year-old woman. The tumor is hyperdense on the plain scan (*left*) and shows bright contrast enhancement (*right*). The central falx is displaced toward the right side

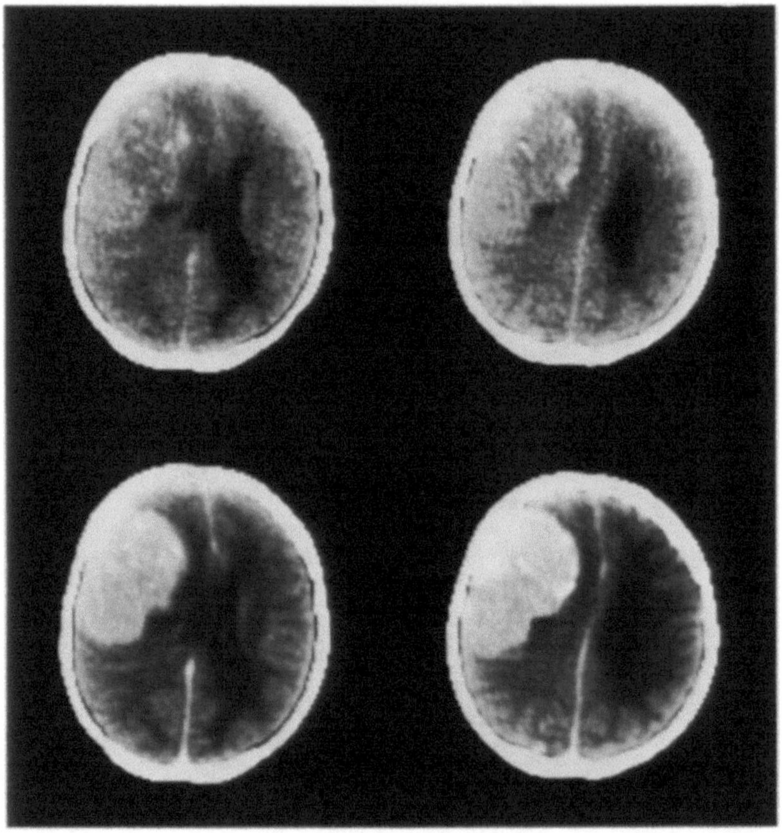

Fig. D 2.3. Large meningioma of the frontoprecentral convexity showing mixed densities on plain CT (*top*) with numerous flecks of calcification. Contrast enhancement is intense, homogeneous, and sharply defined (*bottom*). There are signs of intracranial mass effect with displacement of the ventricular system and falx in their lower, central portions

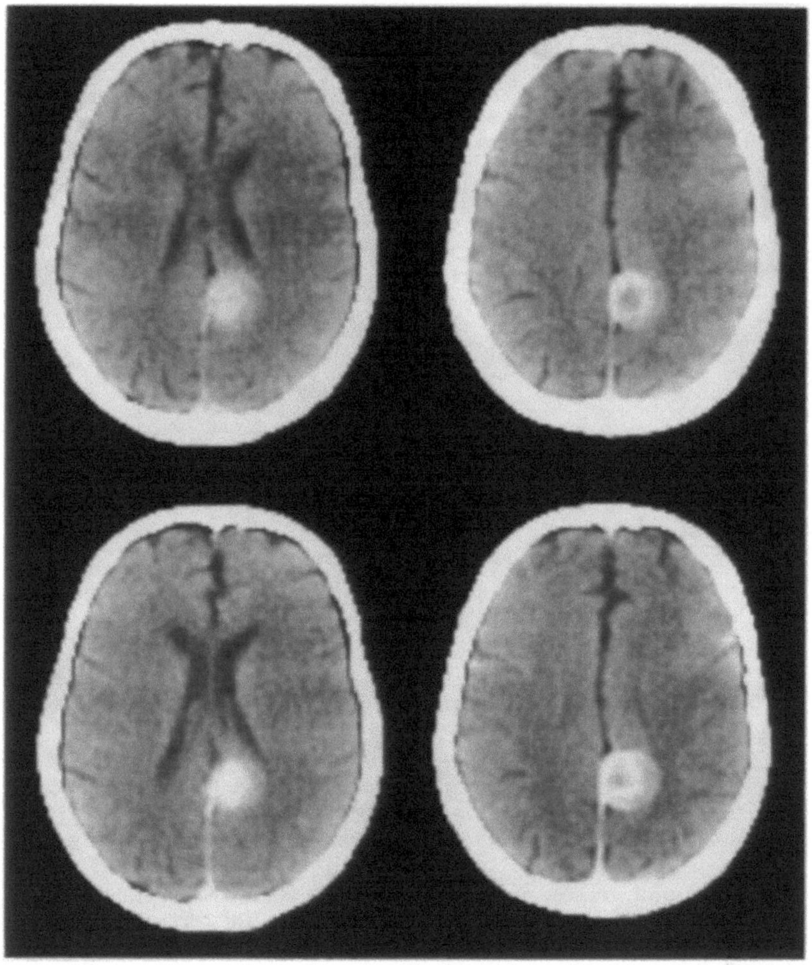

Fig. D 2.4. Small, partially calcified meningioma on the lower border of the falx at the junction of its middle and posterior thirds. The tumor density is very high on the plain CT scans (*top*) and shows minimal enhancement with contrast medium (*bottom*)

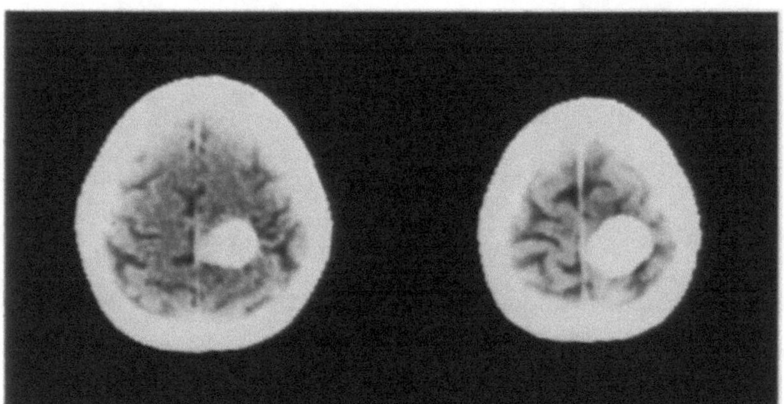

Fig. D 2.5. Totally calcified parasagittal meningioma at the level of the middle third of the sagittal sinus in a 73-year-old woman. The gyral pattern is appropriate for age on these nonenhanced scans and is not obliterated by the tumor. There is no evidence of perifocal edema

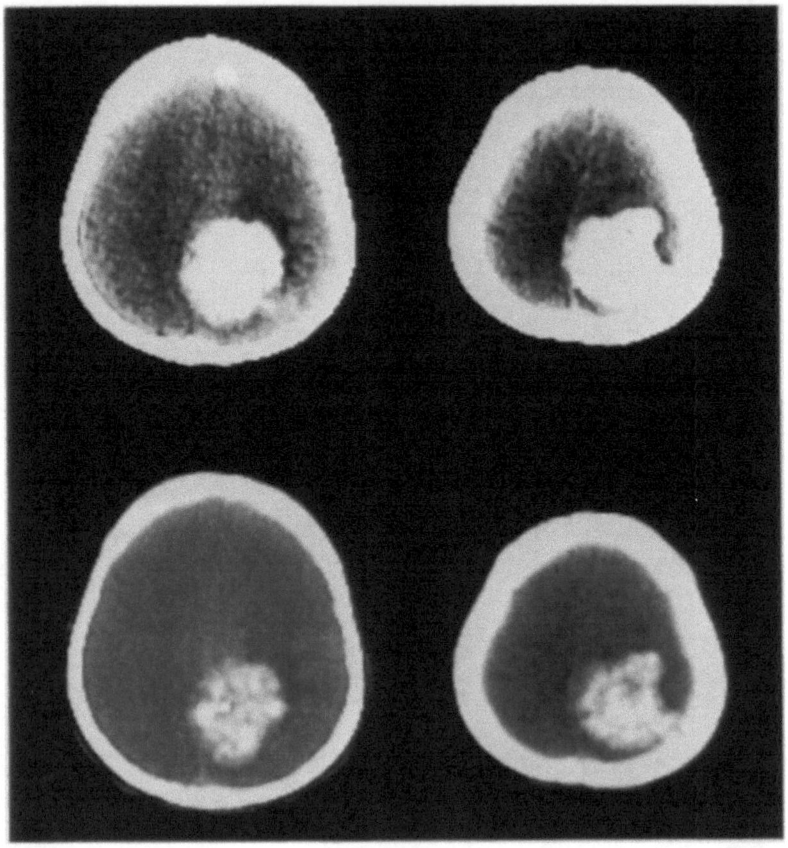

Fig. D 2.6. Heavily calcified parasagittal meningioma at the junction of the middle and posterior thirds of the sinus in a 54-year-old woman. The calcification pattern within the tumor is not defined on the routine scans (*top*) but is brought out by increasing the window width (*bottom*)

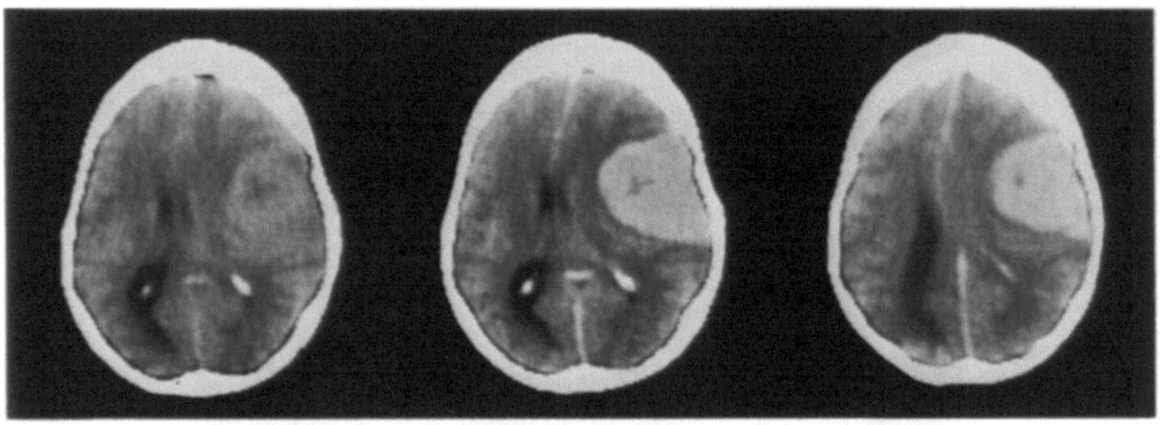

Fig. D 2.7. Large convexity meningioma on the right sphenoid wing in a 26-year-old man. Plain CT demonstrates a mixed-density lesion (*left*) which contains an eccentric nonenhancing area on the postcontrast scans (*center* and *right*), signifying regressive change

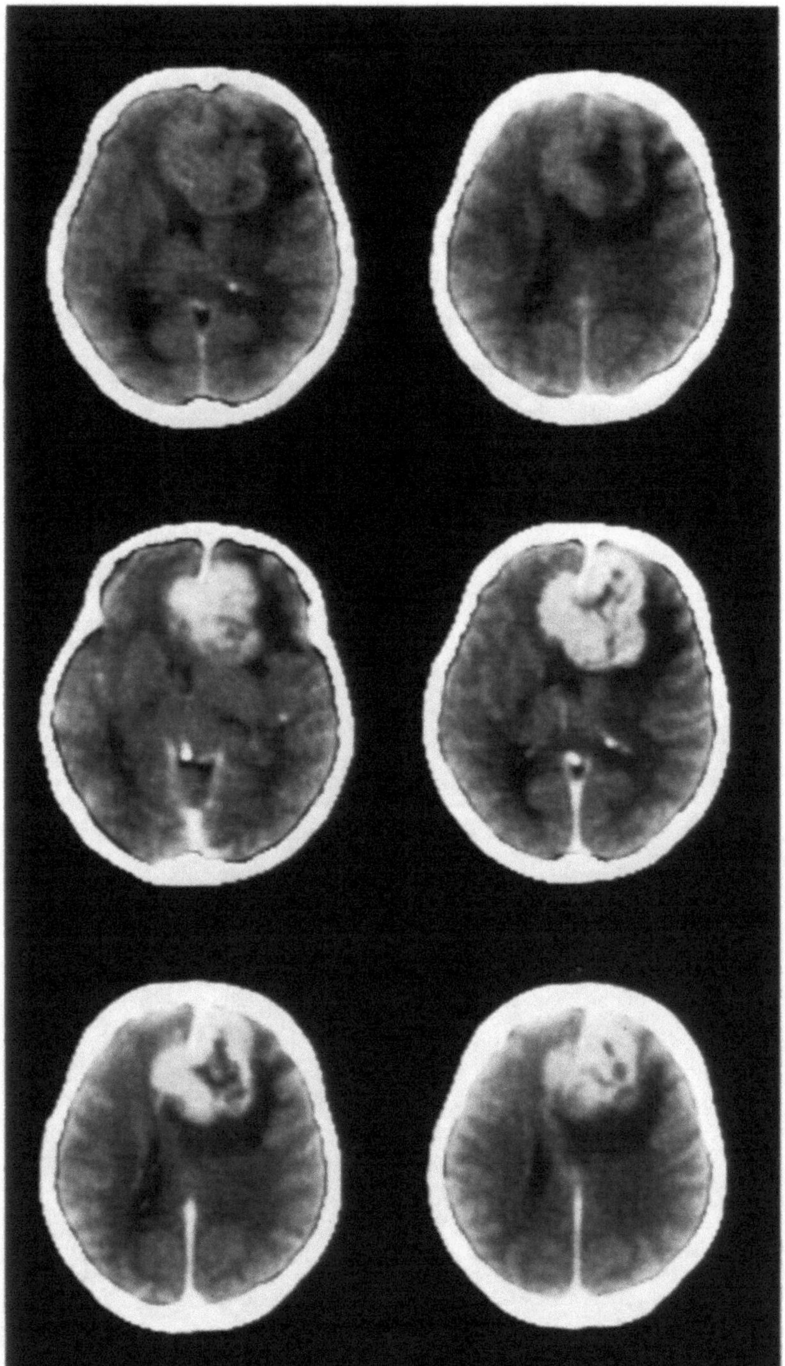

Fig. D 2.8. Anterior-third falx meningioma chiefly involving the right side in a 53-year-old woman. The tumor exhibits isodense and hypodense components on the plain CT scans (*top*). The postcontrast scans (*center* and *bottom*) give a clearer impression of the regressive changes in the lobulated mass. Perifocal edema on the plain scans clearly demarcates the tumor from its surroundings

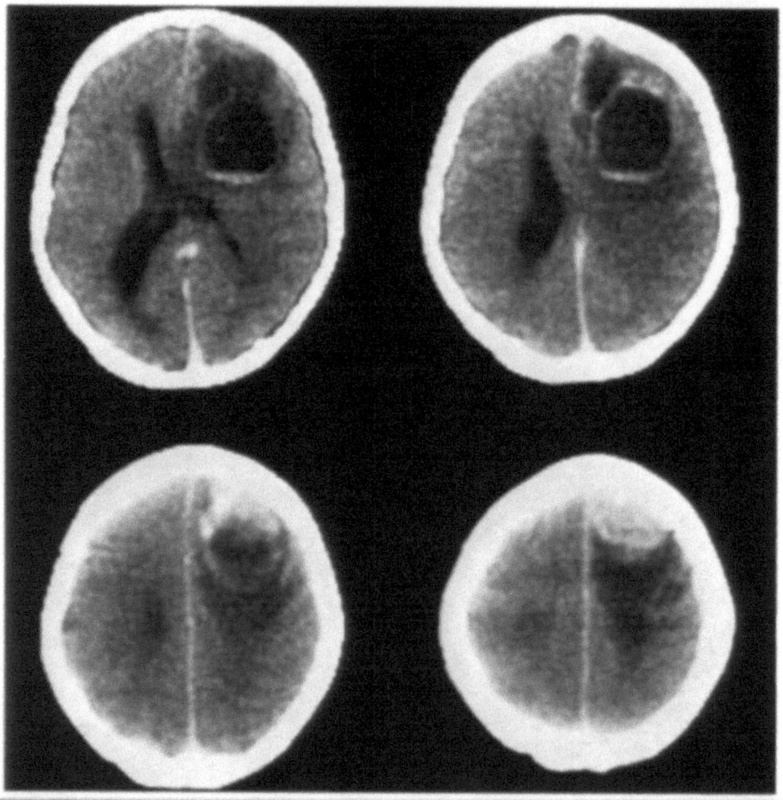

a

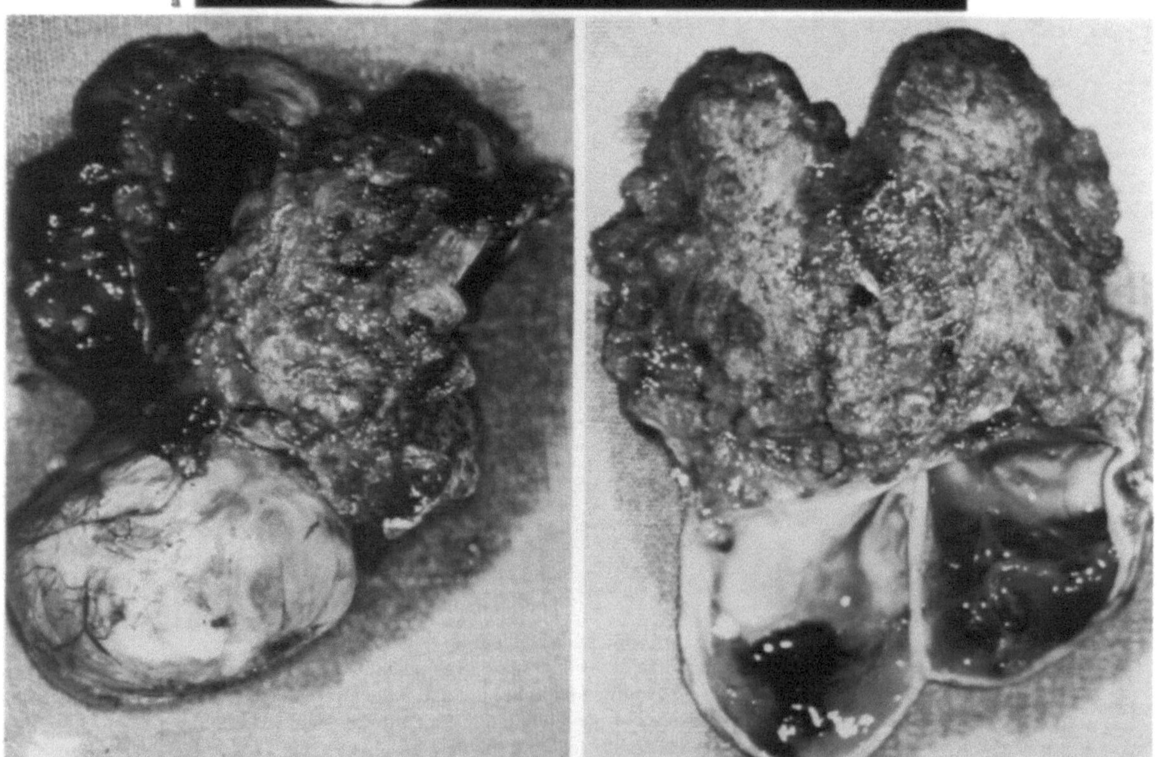

b

Fig. D 2.9 a, b. Atypical meningioma of the right fronto-precentral convexity with a large cyst in a 71-year-old woman. **a** Postcontrast CT (*top*) demonstrates a partly solid, partly cystic mass adjacent to the calvarium showing faint ring enhancement and a sedimentation effect in the posterior part of the cyst. **b** Surgical specimen with a large peripheral cyst

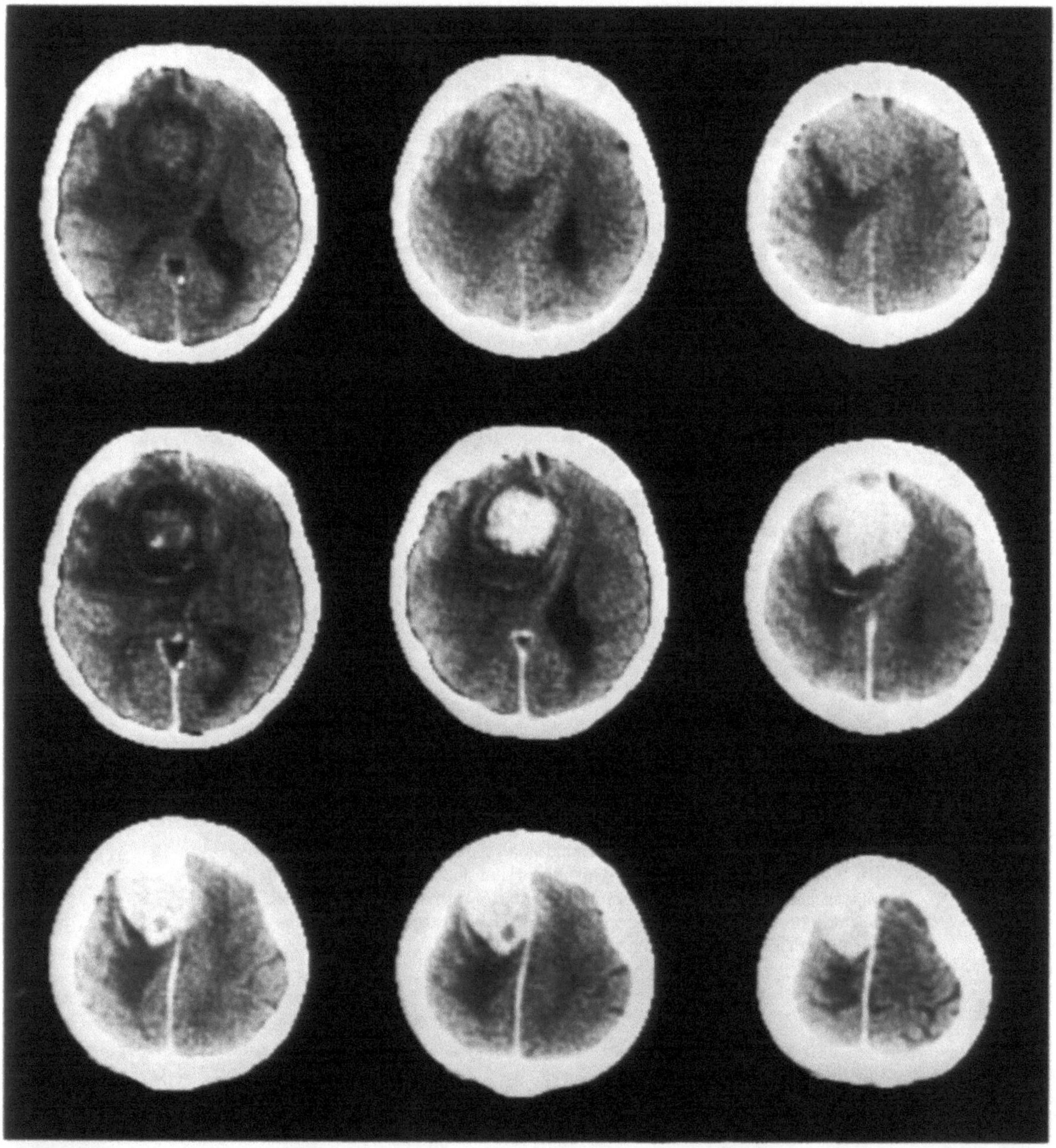

Fig. D 2.10. Atypical anterior-third falx meningioma in a 67-year-old woman. Plain CT scans (*top*) show a mixed-density lesion whose full extent is appreciated only on the postcontrast scans (*center* and *bottom*). Despite its atypical appearance, meningioma was diagnosed by virtue of its location between the cranial vault and falx and the largely homogeneous enhancement of its solid components. The bull's-eye pattern seen in the basal parts of the tumor (*left* and *center* scans, *center* row) is caused by extensive regressive changes. There is significant intracranial mass effect and grade II–III perifocal edema

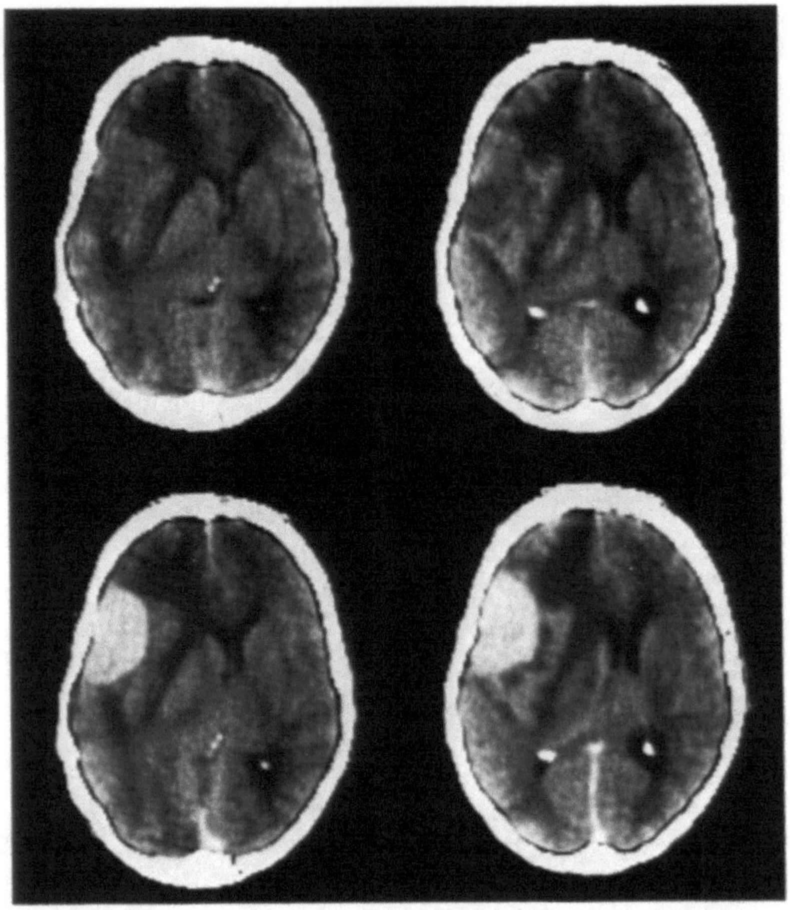

Fig. D 2.11. Primarily hypodense meningioma of the left frontotemporal convexity in a 37-year-old man with a 4-year history of mental changes culminating in dysphasia. The extent of the tumor is poorly appreciated on the plain CT scans (*top*) despite marked peritumoral edema. The contrast-enhanced scans (*bottom*) display the typical meningioma pattern

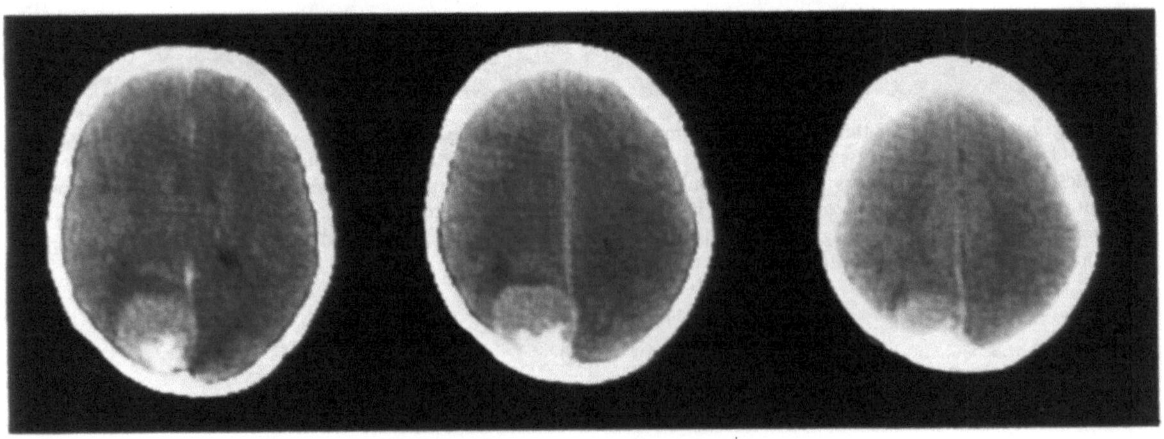

Fig. D 2.12. Posterior-third parasagittal meningioma in a 51-year-old woman. There is marked enostosis of the cranial bone with calcifications in contiguous parts of the tumor. The low contrast of the meningioma results from the large window width

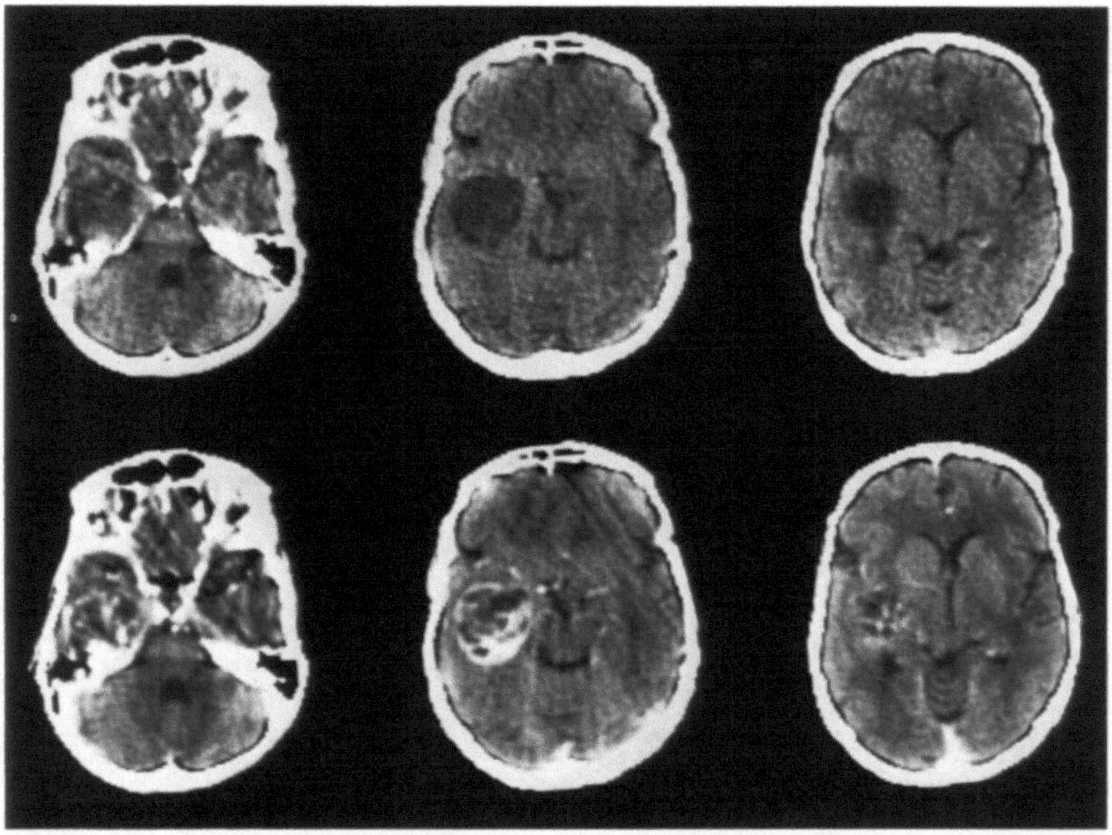

Fig. D2.13. Meningioma at the base of the left middle fossa in a 59-year-old man. The tumor, hypodense on the plain scans (*top*), enhances nonhomogeneously with contrast medium (*bottom*). Nevertheless the smooth borders of the lesion strongly support a diagnosis of meningioma. The central lucencies in the tumor are foci of regressive change

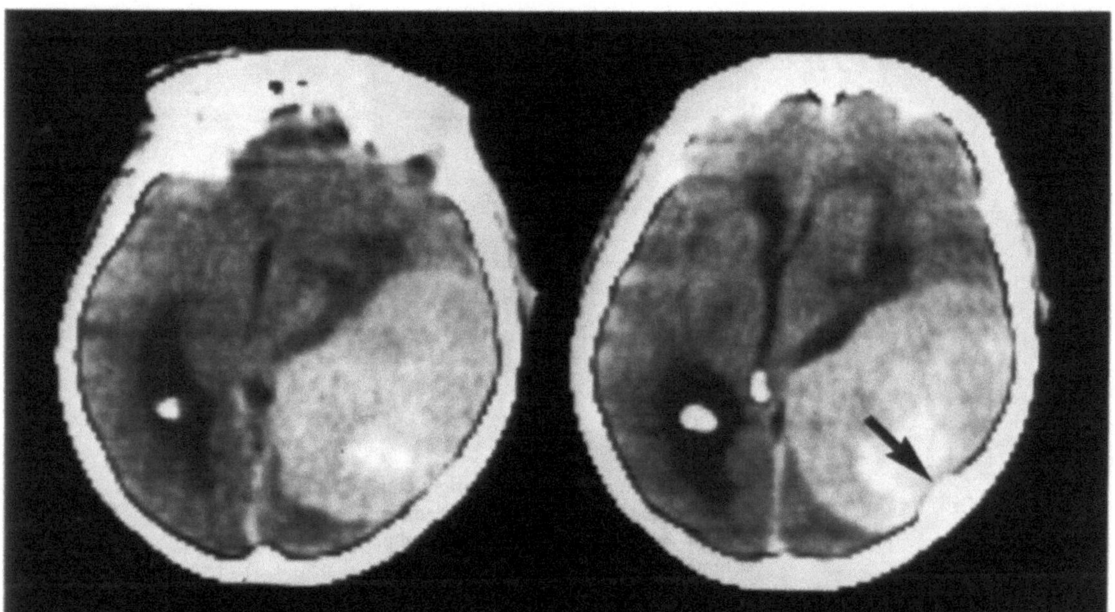

Fig. D2.14. Very large meningioma of the right temporo-parieto-occipital convexity with marked bony enostosis at the site of tumor attachment (*arrow*). The tumor contains large calcifications opposite the enostosis (postcontrast CT)

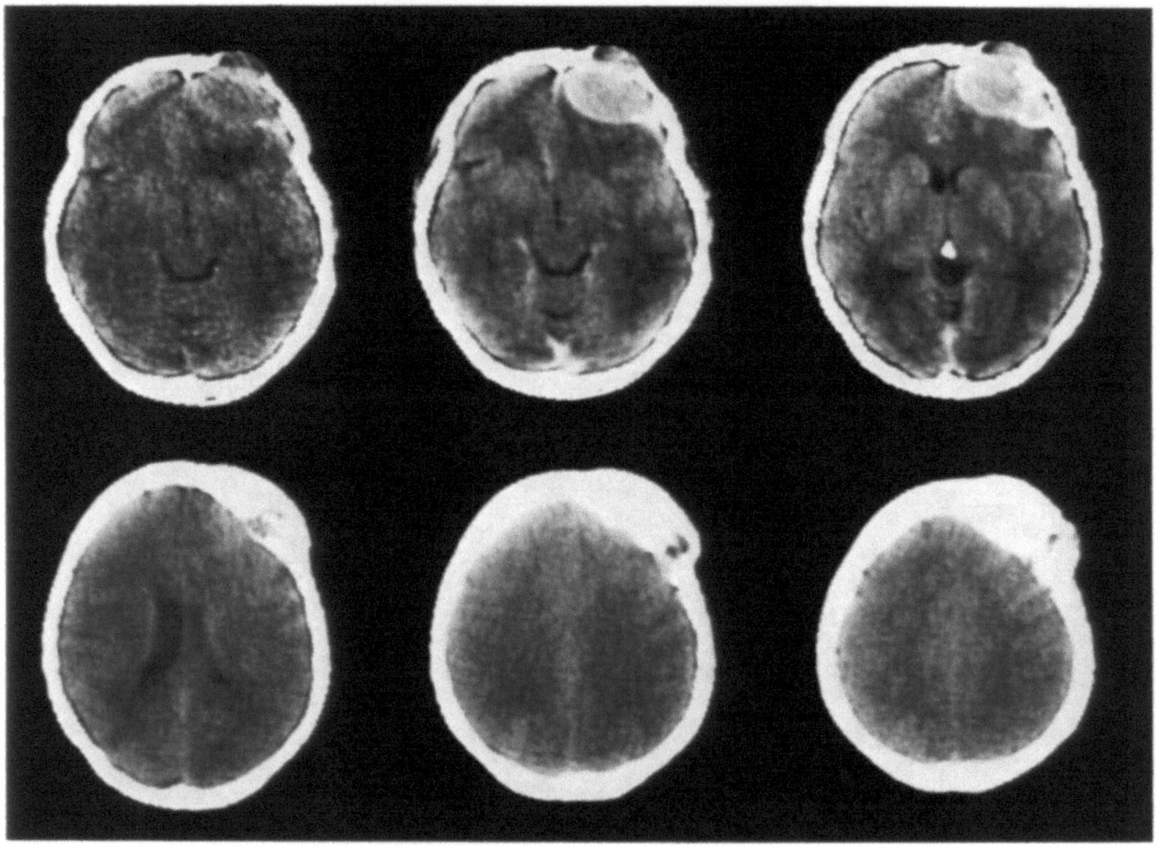

Fig. D 2.15. Right frontal meningioma with expansion of the cranial vault, which is penetrated by soft tumor tissue in the frontal region. Soft portions of the tumor projecting into the cranial cavity are visible only on the contrast-enhanced scans (*center* and *right* scans, *top* row). CT findings are typical for meningioma

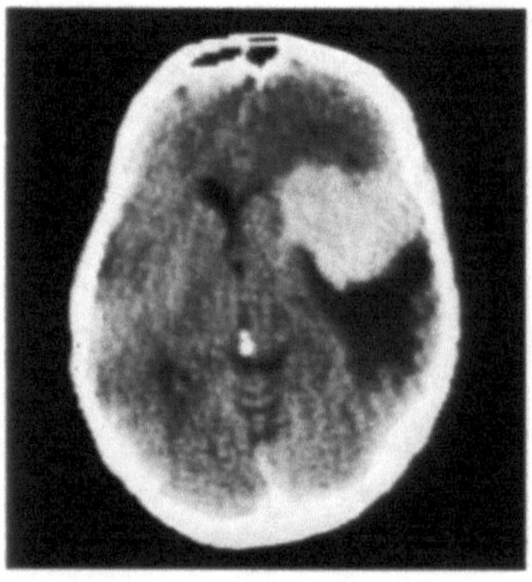

Fig. D 2.16. Meningioma of the right convexity in the region of the sylvian fissure in a 46-year-old man. The tumor is bounded posteriorly by a large hypodensity identified at operation as the obstructed cistern of the sylvian fissure

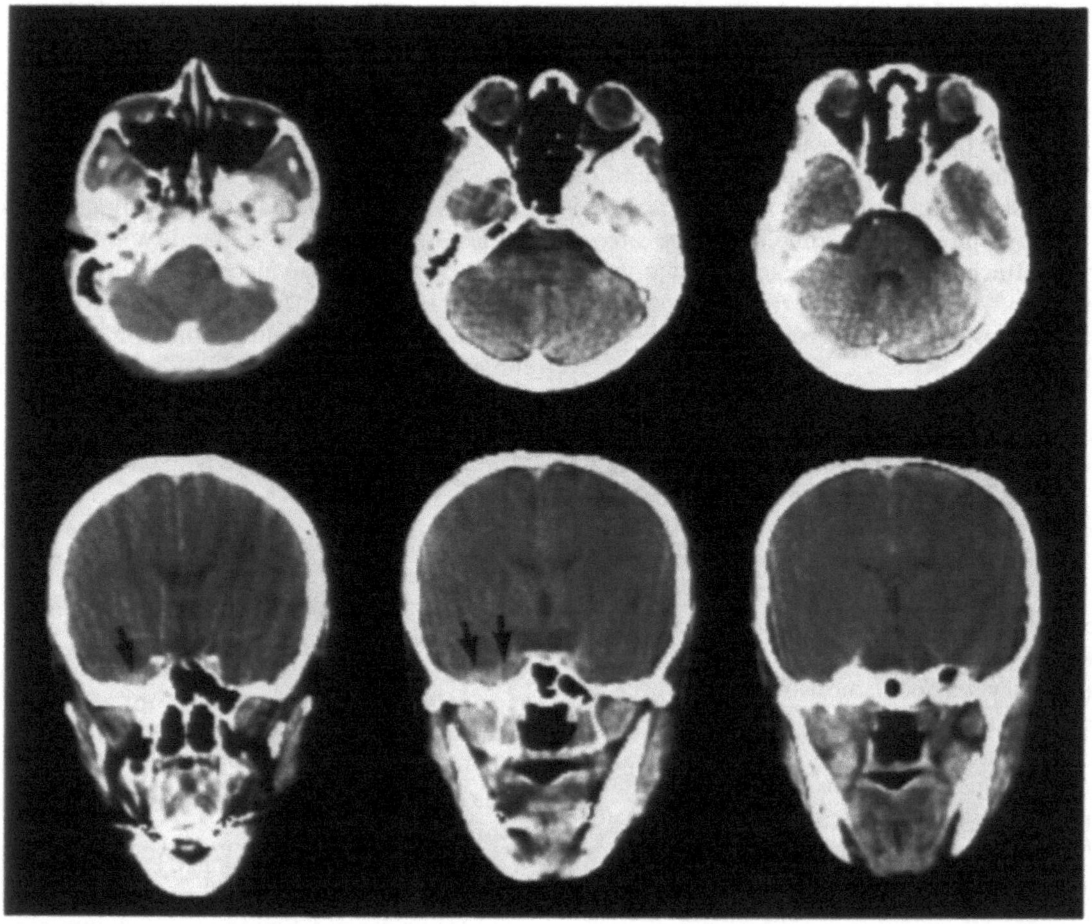

Fig. D 2.17. Plaque-like meningioma at the base of the right middle fossa in a 52-year-old woman. The carpet-like growth is poorly displayed on the transverse scans (*top*) but is well demarcated from the skull base on the coronal scans (*arrows*)

Parasagittal and Falx Meningiomas

CT finding alone are often insufficient for differentiating between parasagittal meningiomas arising from the meninges adjacent to the sagittal sinus and meningiomas attached to the falx itself. Usually this question can be resolved by angiography, but in some cases the site of tumor attachment can be established only at operation. As mentioned earlier, topographic relationships may be appreciated best on coronal scans.

Parasagittal meningiomas are cherry- to apple-size lesions usually adjoining the middle third of the sagittal sinus, less commonly the anterior third, and rarely the posterior third (Figs. D.2.18–26). Small meningiomas located at the junction of the anterior and middle thirds of the sagittal sinus may be missed on CT scans when obscured by the curvature of the cranial vault. They will be demonstrated, however, by coronal scans.

Falx meningiomas can have a variety of CT appearances depending on their location. Involvement may be unilateral or bilateral, and small extensions toward the opposite side are easily detected with CT. The lower the site of tumor attachment to the falx, the greater the likelihood of bilateral, symmetrical tumor growth. Meningiomas arising from the anterior portions of the falx can attain a very large size and cause an extreme mass effect in the region of the septum pellucidum and frontal horns (Fig. D2.22).

Meningiomas arising from the inferior border of the falx near the central portion of the inferior sagittal sinus can obstruct CSF flow and precipitate hydrocephalus when the tumor attains sufficient size (see also Meningiomas of the Tentorial Incisure, p. 277, and Fig. D2.76).

MRI aids in evaluating the topography of the lesion owing to its capability for arbitrary plane selection. It can also establish the patency of the superior sagittal sinus without the need for angiography. Small meningiomas require enhancement with Gd-DTPA before they can be visualized with MR.

Differential Diagnosis

All homogeneously enhancing tumors of this region can simulate meningioma, especially parasagittal metastases, malignant lymphomas, and grade III gliomas. Meningiomas having a mixed-density pattern due to the presence of regressive components are apt to be confused with glioblastoma or a ringlike metastasis. Other less common lesions to be considered are chondroma, tuberculoma, and histiocytoma.

The only contribution of MR to differential diagnosis is its ability to distinguish an extra-axial lesion from a tumor of the glioma series.

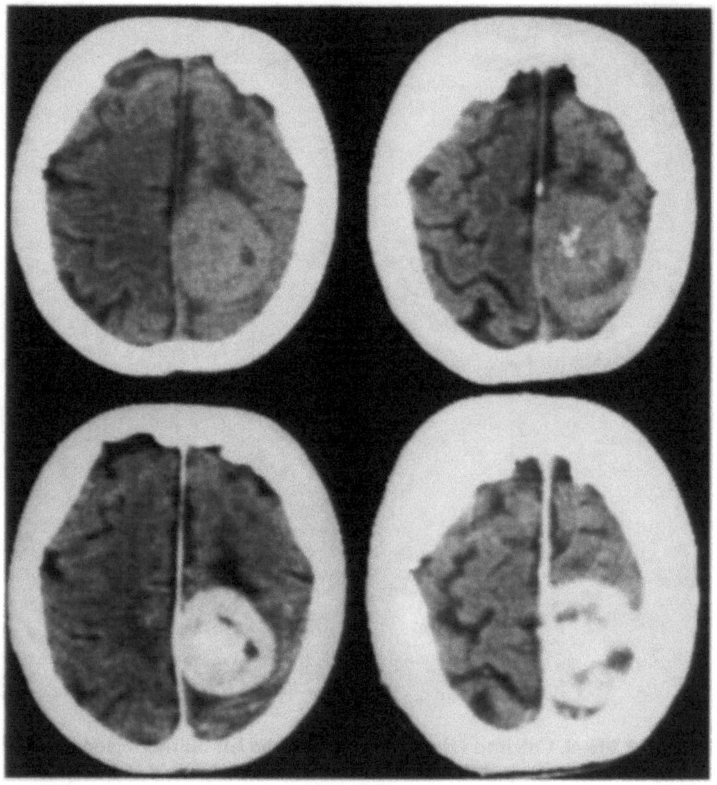

Fig. D 2.18. Right posterior-third falx meningioma in an 83-year-old woman with a 3-year history of intermittent left-sided hemiparesis. CT: *top* noncontrast, *bottom* postcontrast. The plain scans demonstrate flecks of calcification and hypodense areas within the mass. The hypodense areas do not enhance with contrast medium, identifying them as foci of regressive change

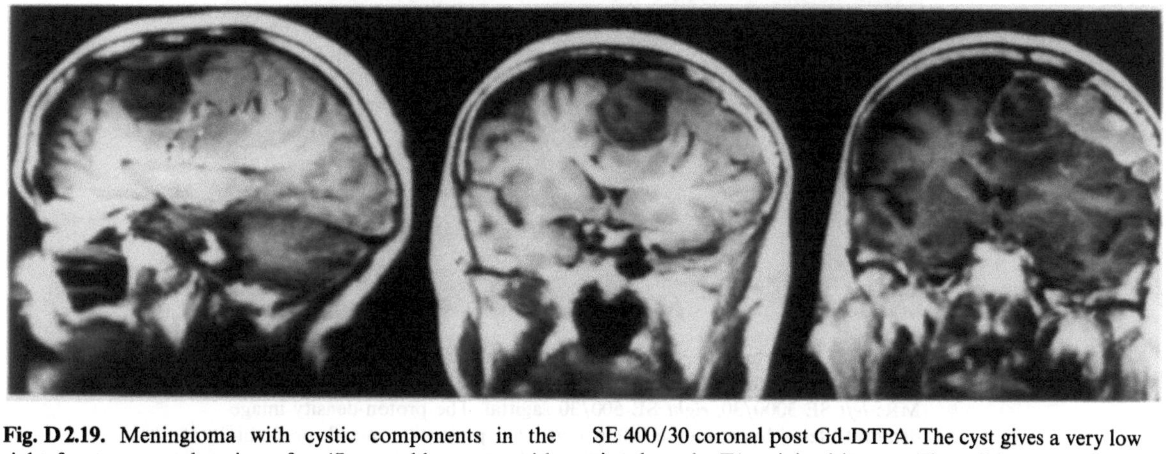

Fig. D 2.19. Meningioma with cystic components in the right frontoprecental region of a 47-year-old woman with headaches, jacksonian seizures, and left-sided hemiparesis. MR: *left* SE 400/30 sagittal, *center* SE 400/30 coronal, *right* SE 400/30 coronal post Gd-DTPA. The cyst gives a very low signal on the T1-weighted images. The solid tumor component enhances brightly on the post-Gd-DTPA coronal image and is well delineated

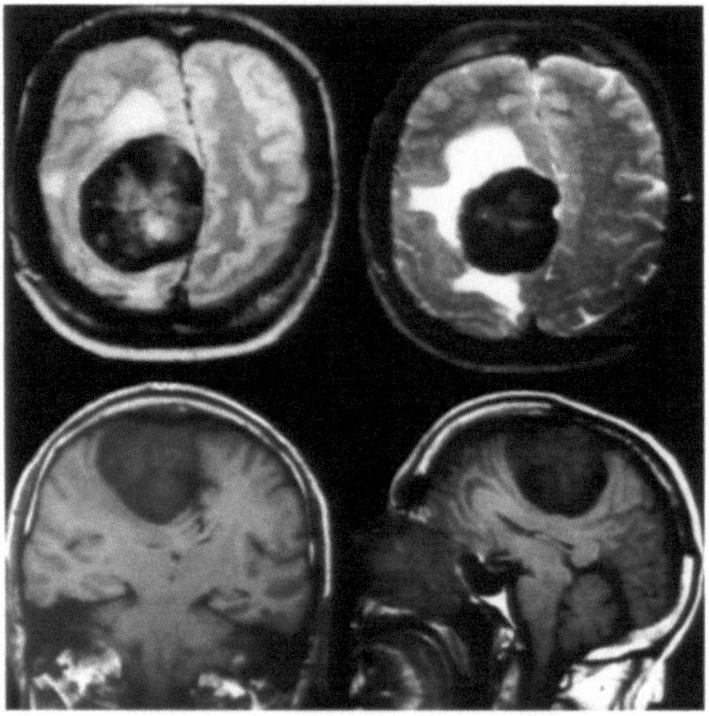

a b c d

Fig. D 2.20 a–d. Calcified falx meningioma of the left central region in a 65-year-old man with jacksonian seizures and latent right-sided hemiparesis. MR: **a** SE 2500/30, **b** SE 2500/120, **c** SE 500/30 coronal, **d** SE 500/30 sagittal. The tumor is hypointense to brain on the T1- and T2-weighted scans and is sharply defined. The hyperintense edema is most conspicuous on the T2-weighted sequence (**b**)

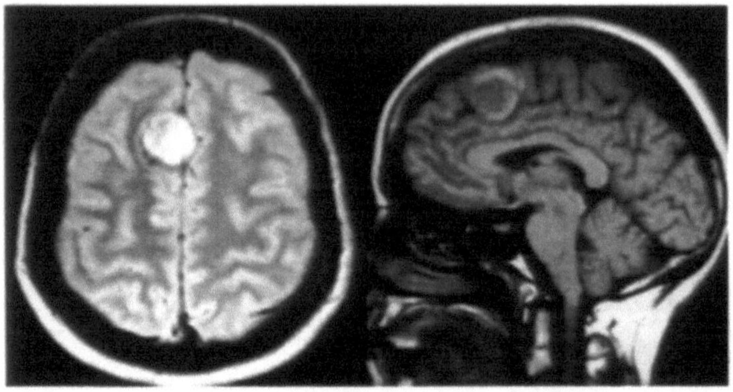

Fig. D 2.21. Left anterior-third falx meningioma in a 54-year-old woman with a 1-year history of altered mental status and right-sided hemiparesis. MR: *left* SE 3000/30, *right* SE 500/30 sagittal. The proton-density image demonstrates a hyperintense lesion (*left*) that presents a mixed, predominantly hypointense pattern on the T1-weighted sequence

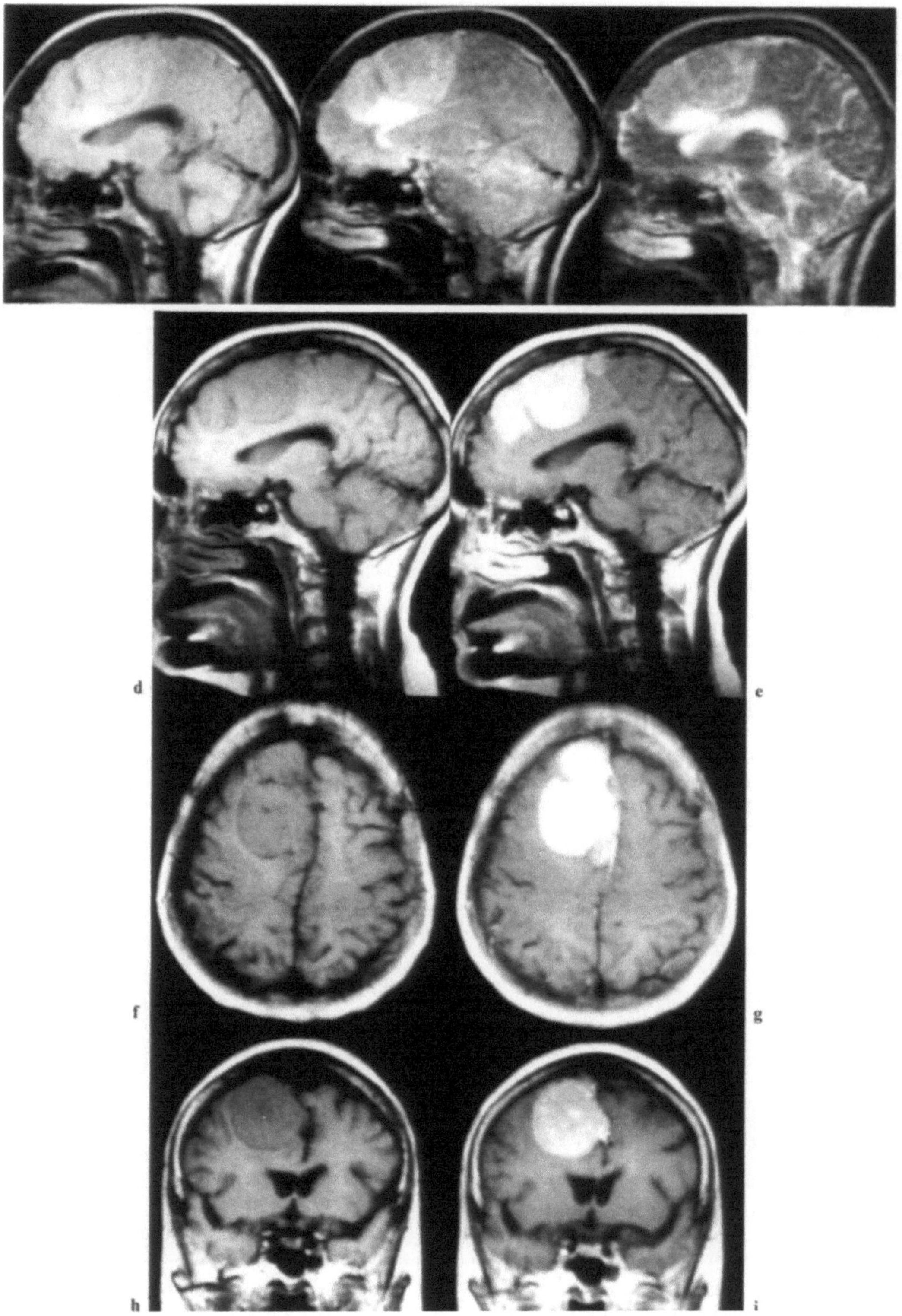

a–c d e f g h i

Fig. D 2.22 a–i. Left anterior-third falx meningioma in a 72-year-old woman with a 2-month history of headaches, attacks of vertigo, and unsteady gait. MR: **a** SE 1600/30, **b** SE 1600/60, **c** SE 1600/150, parasagittal; **d** SE 400/30, **e** SE 400/30 post Gd-DTPA, parasagittal; **f** SE 400/30, **g** SE 400/30 post Gd-DTPA, axial; **h** SE 400/30, **i** SE 400/30 post Gd-DTPA, coronal. The T2-weighted image (**c**) clearly distinguishes the slightly hyperintense tumor from the surrounding hyperintense edema. The enhanced T1-weighted images (**e, g, i**) show a very intense tumor that is displacing the expanded left lateral ventricle downward and is broadly attached to the falx, which is greatly displaced toward the right side

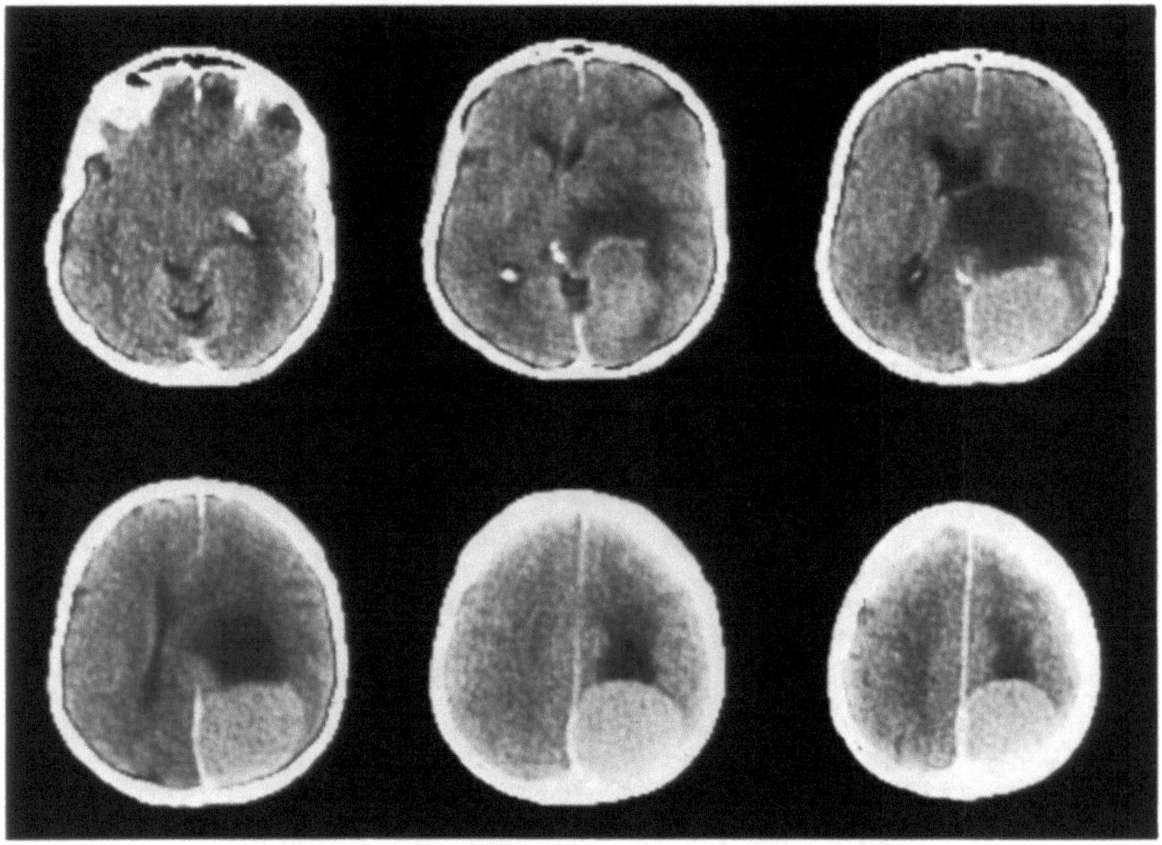

Fig. D 2.23. Right posterior-third parasagittal meningioma in a 67-year-old woman. Postcontrast CT demonstrates a large tumor at the angle between the falx and the dura of the convexity. Contrast enhancement is intense and homogeneous. The tumor is bordered anteriorly by a large cyst appearing as a smooth-bordered hypodensity. Perifocal edema is slight. The choroid plexus of the right lateral ventricle is displaced forward (*upper left* scan)

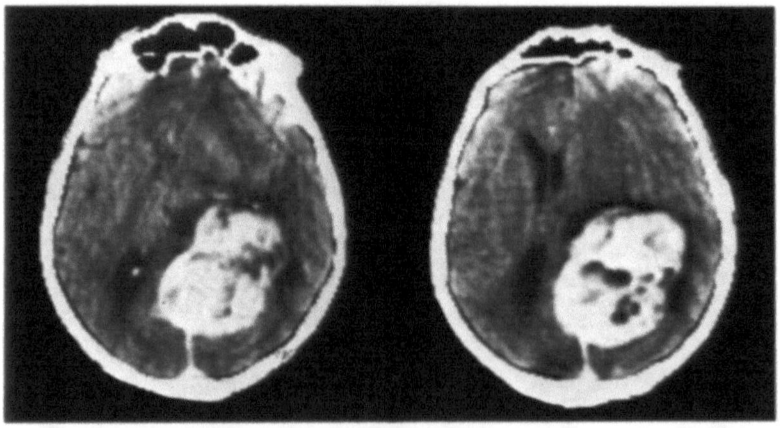

Fig. D 2.24. Huge meningioma arising from the inferior border of the falx and mainly involving the right side. Postcontrast CT scans show a typical pattern with central hypodensities representing regressive changes. The relations of the tumor to the falx are clearly appreciated, confirming the diagnosis of meningioma

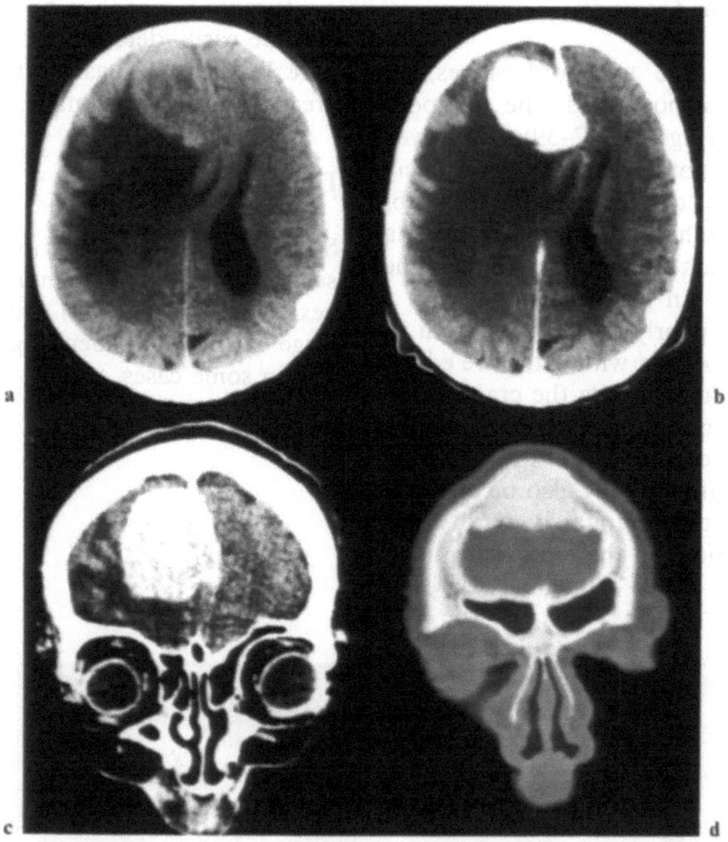

Fig. D 2.25 a–d. Multiple meningiomas of the left frontal and right parietal areas in a 67-year-old woman with increasing concentration difficulties and one generalized seizure. CT: **a** noncontrast; **b** postcontrast, **c** postcontrast coronal; **d** bony window, coronal. The frontal, anterior-third tumor is causing an extreme shift of midline structures toward the right side, and the entire left hemisphere is edematous. The coronal scan (**d**) shows massive tumor infiltration of the cranial vault

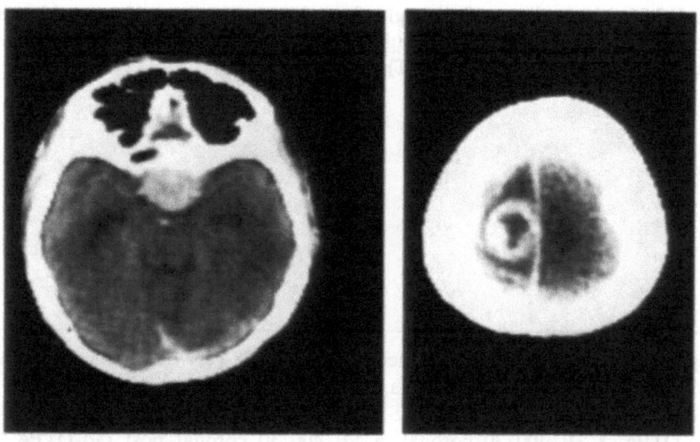

Fig. D 2.26. Multiple meningiomas in a 47-year-old woman. While the tuberculum sellae meningioma enhances homogeneously, a second, left parasagittal meningioma shows a ring pattern of enhancement resembling a glioblastoma or metastasis. Both tumors were identified as meningiomas at operation

Meningiomas of the Convexity

Typical sites are the sphenoid ridges, the frontoprecentral region, and the temporo-occipital region (Figs. D2.27–39). Even very small meningiomas of the convexity can precipitate seizures. Most of these tumors are visible only on contrast-enhanced scans, appearing as a hemispheric mass contiguous to the inner table of the skull. En plaque meningiomas of the convexity are poorly demarcated from the brain and are associated with extensive edema.

Meningiomas that invade the cranial vault can greatly expand the bone and give it a rarefied appearance (see Fig. D2.25). Concurrent intracranial growth may also be observed. Meningiomas of the occipital convexity may demonstrate relations to the tentorium on the coronal scan.

Tumors larger than about 2–3 cm in diameter are easily detected with **CT** and also with **MR**. Diagnosis is easier with MR owing to its greater capacity for image plane selection.

Differential Diagnosis

Superficial malignant lymphomas can have the same CT features as meningiomas of the convexity (see Fig. D1.181). Differentiation from a large calcified oligodendroglioma may be difficult in some cases.

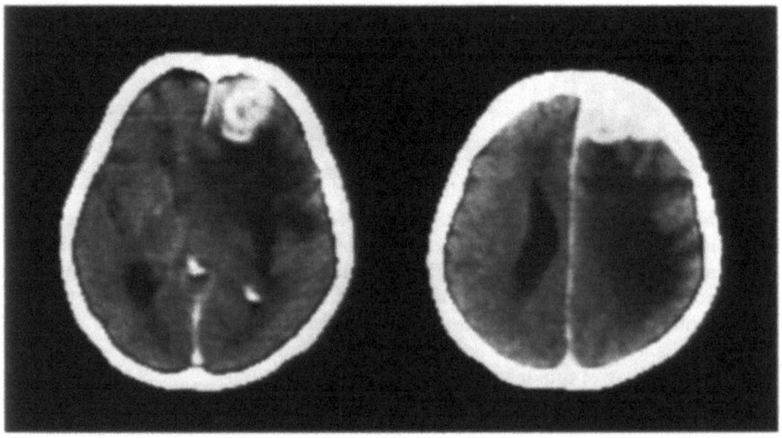

Fig. D2.27. Meningioma of the right frontal convexity in a 63-year-old woman. Brain edema is unusually severe (grade III) and has caused a marked shift of midline structures (postcontrast CT)

Fig. D2.28a–i. Large left frontal meningioma in a 38-year-old man with headaches, two generalized seizures, hyposmia, and subtle alterations in mental status. MR: **a** SE 1600/30, **b** SE 1600/90, **c** SE 1600/150, **d** SE 400/30, **e** SE 400/30 post Gd-DTPA, **f** SE 400/30 coronal, **g** SE 400/30 coronal post Gd-DTPA, **h** SE 400/30 parasagittal, **i** SE 400/30 parasagittal post Gd-DTPA. The demarcation between tumor and edema is poorly resolved on the proton-density and T2-weighted images (**a–c**). Tumor enhancement is very intense on the post-gadolinium T1-weighted images. The frontal location of the mass is shown to good advantage on the parasagittal scans

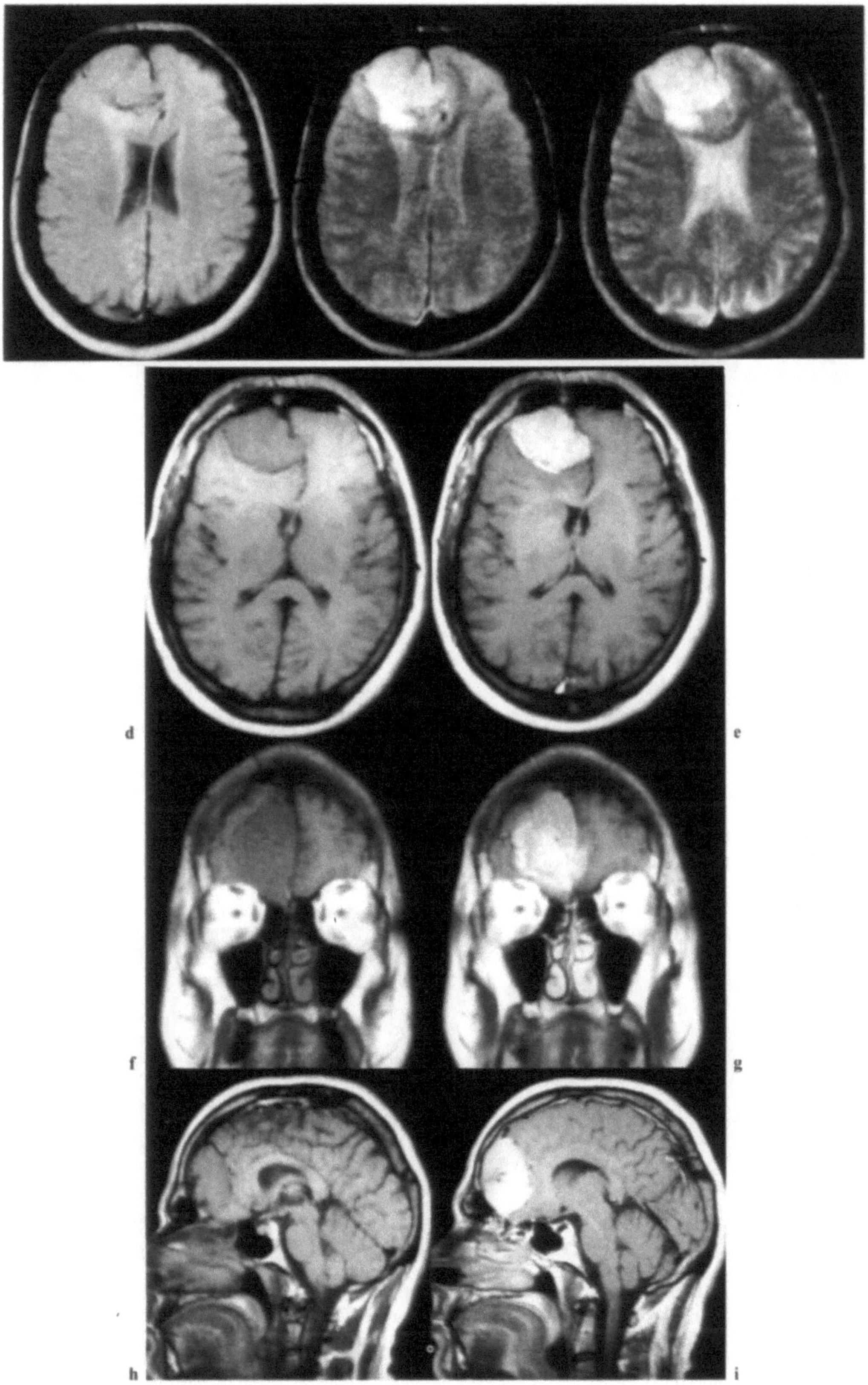

a–c d e f g h i

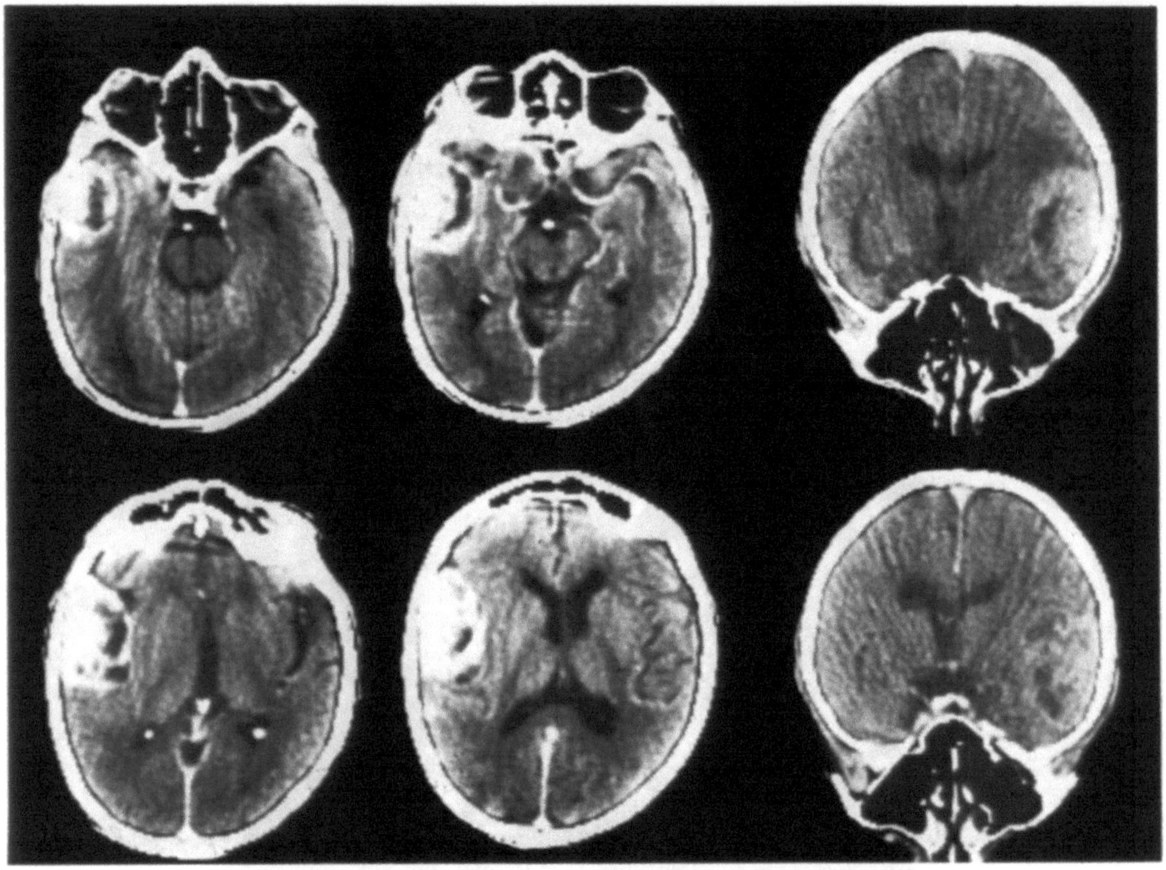

Fig. D 2.29. Meningioma of the left temporal convexity in a 46-year-old man. CT scans show an intensely enhancing, smoothly bordered lesion with peripheral nonenhancing foci of regressive change. Perifocal edema is absent, so there is very little midline displacement. The left ambient cistern is narrowed by incipient uncal herniation. The coronal views demonstrate the entire craniocaudal extent of the tumor and its relation to the convexity. Again, there is minimal evidence of midline displacement. All scans are contrast-enhanced

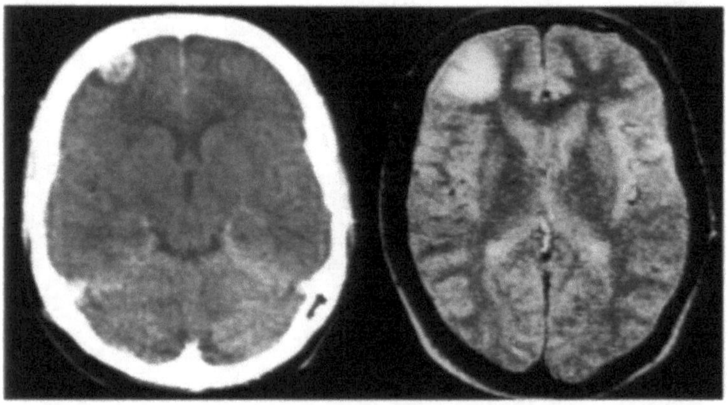

Fig. D 2.30. Fibrous meningioma of the left frontal region in a 42-year-old woman who experienced a generalized seizure. *Left*: postcontrast CT. *Right*: SE 1600/70 MR image. Tumor and edema can be separated on the CT scan, and a pathologic diagnosis can be made. The T2-weighted MR image demonstrates the entire hyperintense lesion but cannot establish its identity

a 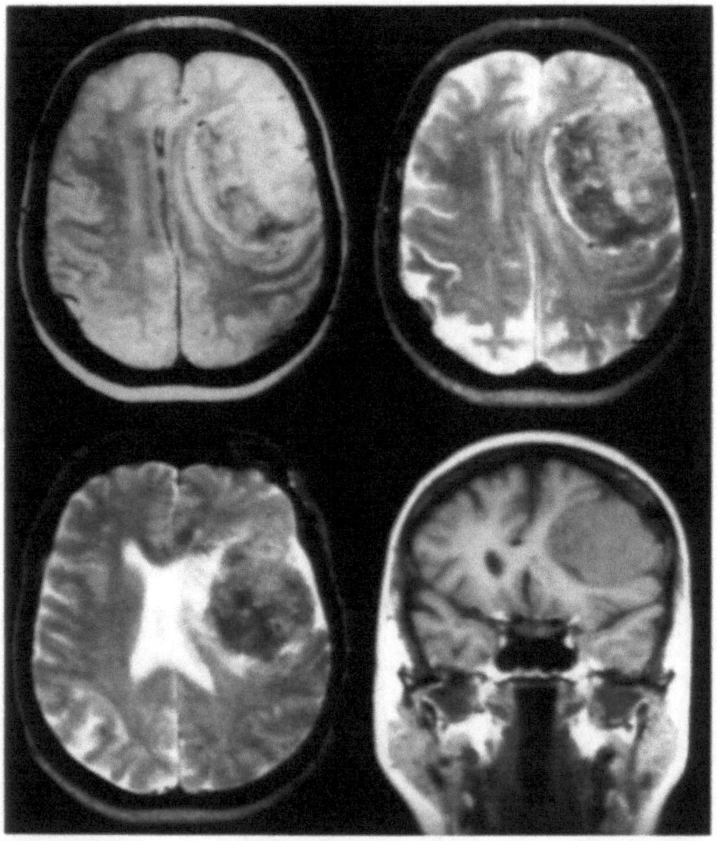 b

c d

Fig. D 2.31 a–d. Right frontoparietal meningioma in a 65-year-old man with altered mental status and increasing left-sided hemiparesis. MR: **a** SE 3000/30, **b** SE 3000/90, **c** SE 3000/90, **d** SE 500/30 coronal. The T1-weighted image (**d**) demonstrates a hypointense tumor causing significant mass effect. The proton-density image (**a**) shows a well-defined lesion with a heterogeneous signal pattern. A small area of hyperintense perifocal edema is evident on the T2-weighted scan (**c**)

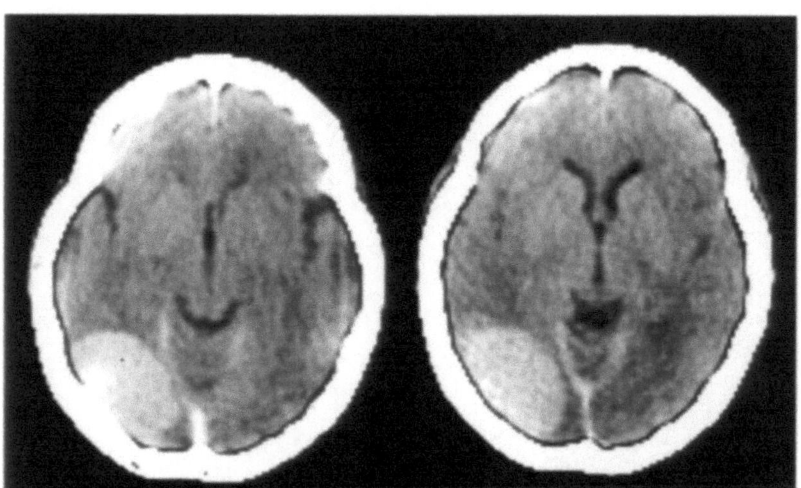

Fig. D 2.32. Meningioma of the left occipital convexity in a 52-year-old woman. The cranium over the tumor is thickened (*left*), a finding which excludes the tentorium as the site of tumor origin. Postcontrast CT

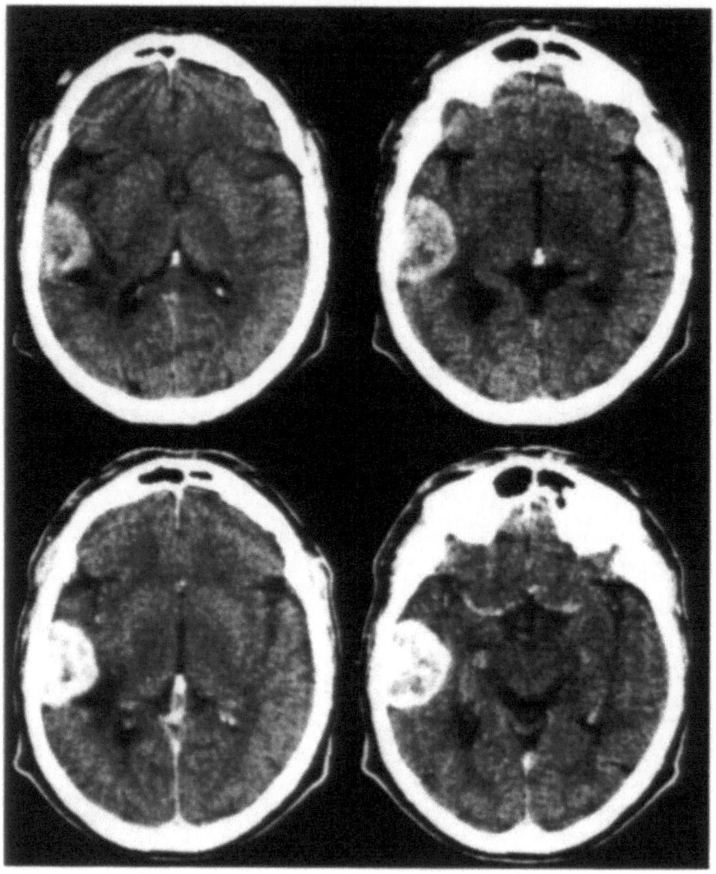

Fig. D 2.33. Meningioma of the left temporal convexity in a 40-year-old man who experienced a generalized seizure. CT *top* precontrast, *bottom* postcontrast. Plain scans show a hyperdense lesion containing hypodense foci of regressive change. These foci remain hypodense on the postcontrast scans while the rest of the tumor enhances brightly

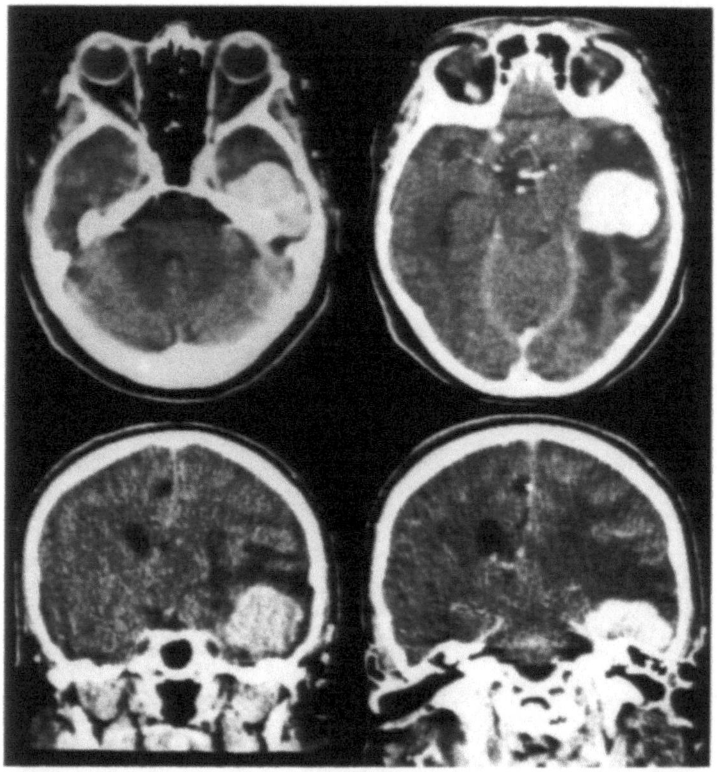

Fig. D 2.34. Large temporobasal meningioma in a 62-year-old woman with a 6-month history of seizures and mildly progressive left-sided hemiparesis. CT *top* postcontrast, *bottom* coronal. There is marked evidence of mass effect with compression and displacement of the ventricular system toward the left side. Edema is pronounced

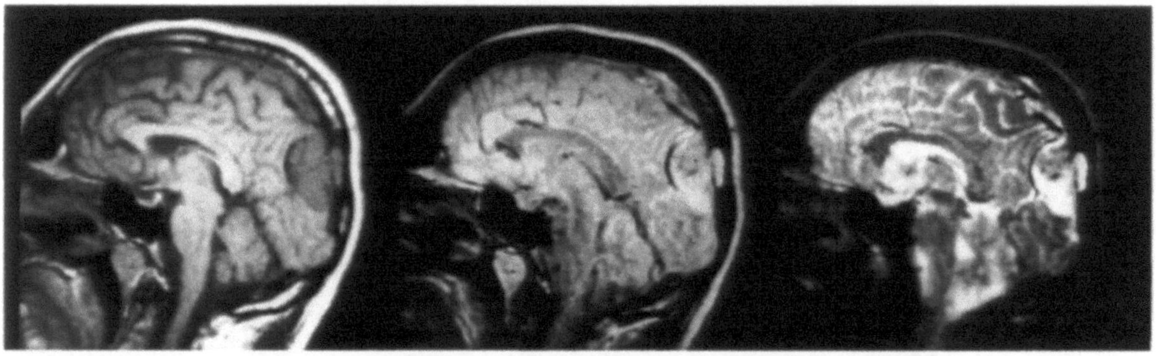

Fig. D 2.35. Left occipital meningioma in a 42-year-old alcoholic male who experienced two generalized seizures. MR: *left* SE 500/30, *center* SE 3000/30, *right* SE 3000/90, all sagittal. The T1-weighted image (*left*) demonstrates a hypointense, clearly delineated tumor displacing the tentorium and cerebellum downward and invading the adjacent skull. Tumor and edema are poorly differentiated on the T2-weighted image

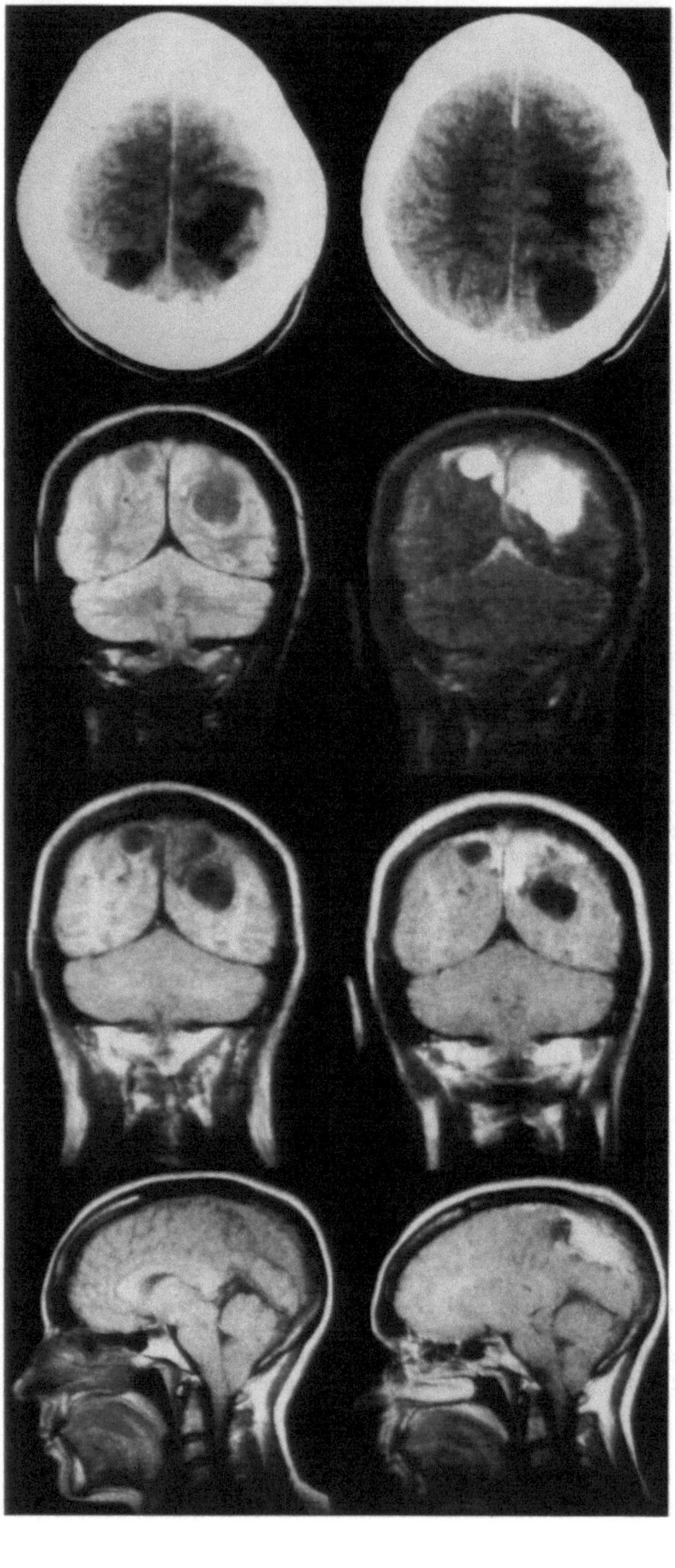

a b c d e f g h

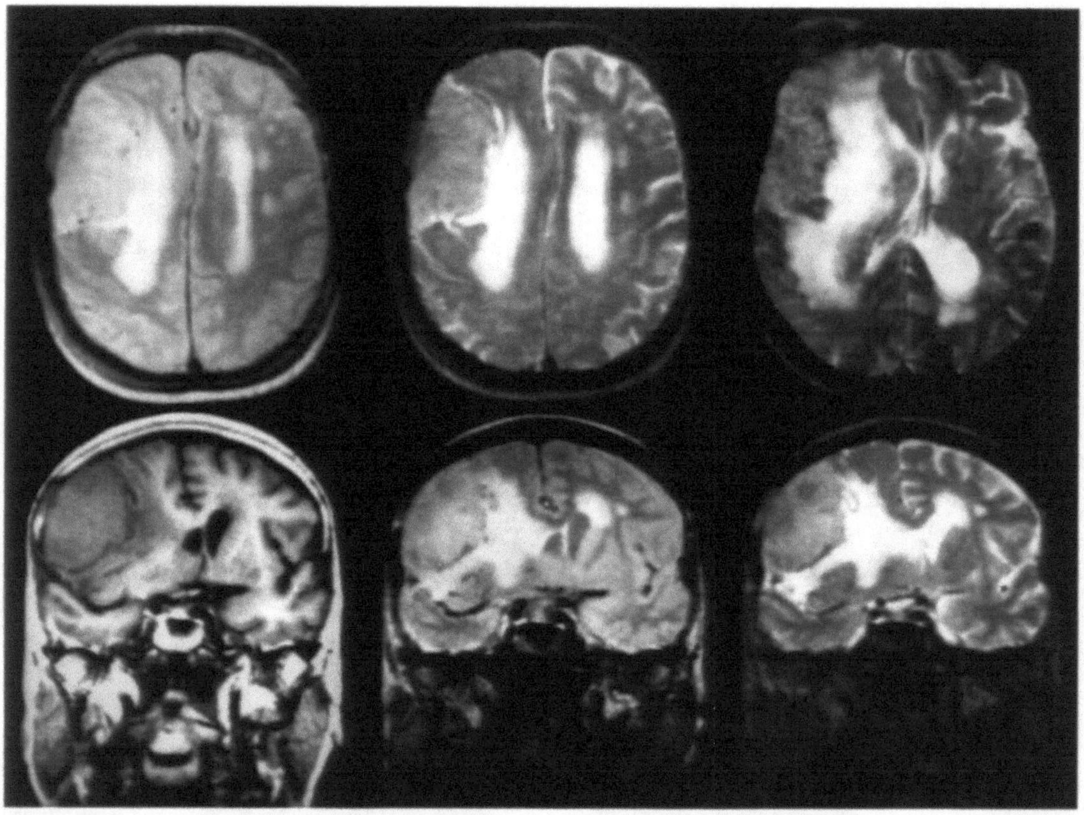

a–c

d–f

Fig. D 2.37 a–f. Meningioma of the left parietal convexity in a 79-year-old woman with changing right-sided hemiparesis and mild dysphasia. MR: **a, b** SE 3000/30, **c** SE 3000/90, **d** SE 500/30, **e** SE 3000/30, **f** SE 3000/90 (**d–f** coronal). The meningioma is shown to best advantage on the T1-weighted sequence (**d**), appearing as a hypointense mass with a peripheral rim of signal void

Fig. D 2.36 a–h. Biparietal-occipital falx meningioma chiefly involving the right side in a 45-year-old woman with a history of frontal headaches for many years. She presented with mild alteration of mental status; neurologic exam was negative. CT: **a, b** postcontrast. MR: **c** SE 1600/30, **d** SE 1600/180, **e** SE 400/35, **f** SE 400/35 post Gd-DTPA, all coronal; **g** SE 400/35, **h** SE 400/35 post Gd-DTPA, both right parasagittal. Postcontrast CT demonstrates only the hypodense, cystic components of the tumor; a specific diagnosis cannot be made. MR demonstrates low-signal cystic areas in addition to solid, intensely enhancing tumor components (**f, h**) at the falx and convexity

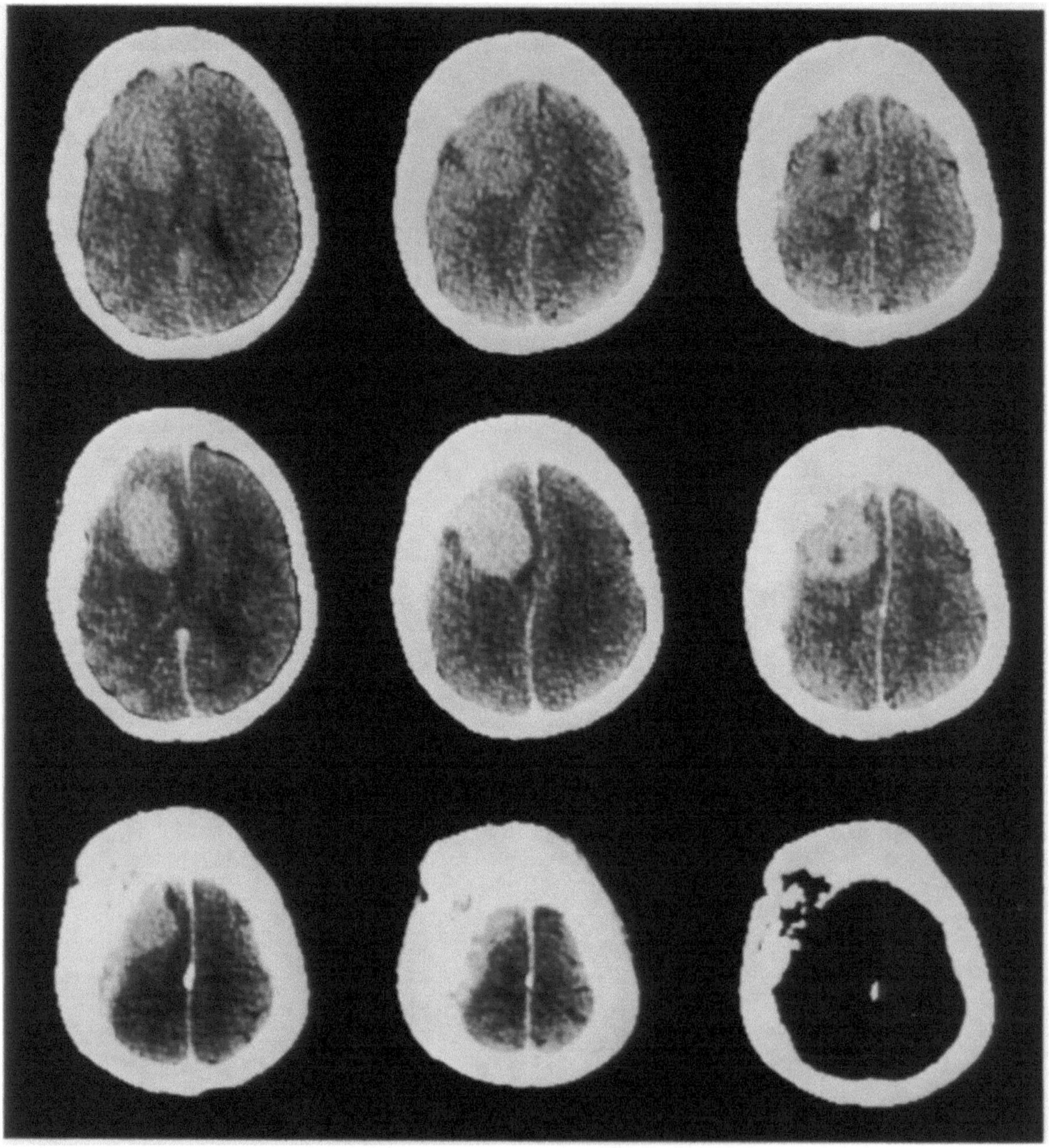

Fig. D 2.38. Meningioma of the left frontoprecentral convexity in a 67-year-old woman. Involvement of the cranium, a large area of which is expanded by the tumor. The intracranial tumor components are isodense to slightly hyperdense on the plain CT scans (*top*) and enhance intensely with contrast medium (*center*). Plaque-like tumor growth is evident in the higher slices (*bottom left*). Osteoplastic tumor growth coexists with bone destruction, which is disclosed by the appropriate window setting (*bottom right*)

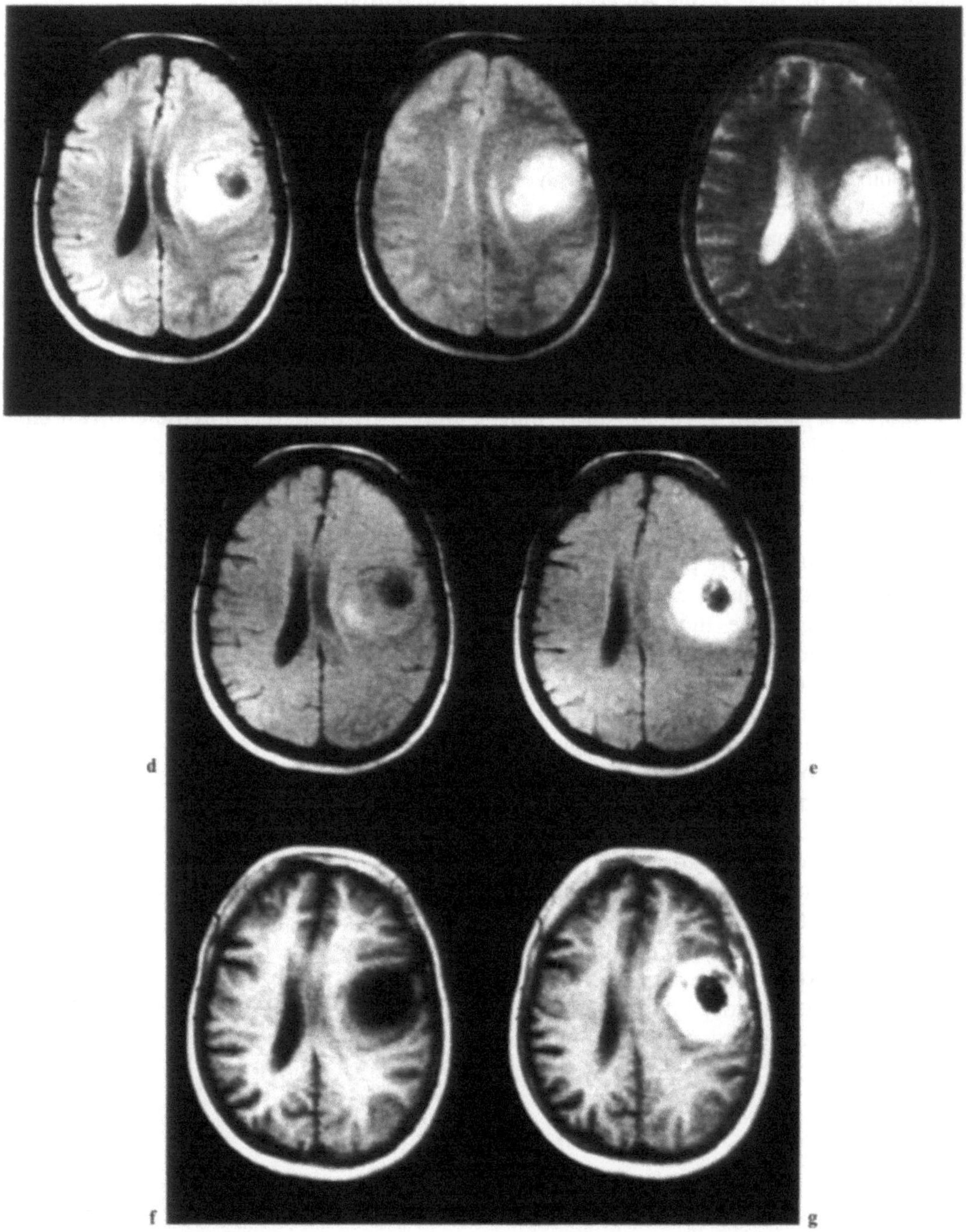

Fig. D 2.39 a–g. Right frontoprecentral meningioma in a 45-year-old woman with a history of concentration difficulties for 1 year and impaired fine motor control in the left hand. MR: **a** SE 1600/30, **b** SE 1600/90, **c** SE 1600/240, **d** SE 800/35, **e** SE 800/35 post Gd-DTPA, **f** IR 1500/400/35, **g** IR 1500/400/35 post Gd-DTPA. The proton-density sequence (**a**) reveals a tumor with a hyperintense periphery and low-signal core compressing the ventricular system on the right side. A thick ring of enhancement appears with Gd-DTPA (**e**), even on the IR sequence (**g**). The central area of regressive change is not appreciated on the heavily T2-weighted image (**c**)

Meningiomas at the Base of the Anterior Cranial Fossa

The CT findings of *frontobasal meningiomas* are quite characteristic: a rounded, central mandarin- to apple-size tumor mass associated with bifrontal white-matter edema. Very large olfactory groove meningiomas may be accompanied by minimal edema due to extreme compression of the white matter by the tumor. Coronal scans can demonstrate the broad area of tumor attachment on the anterior skull base. Extension into the ethmoid cells is occasionally noted. Many of these tumors contain calcifications (Figs. D2.1, 40–43). Predominantly unilateral frontobasal meningiomas arise from the meninges on the skull base adjacent to the olfactory groove or over the orbital roof.

Suprasellar meningiomas are projected over the area of the opticochiasmatic cistern and show anterior extension. Some tumors grow large enough to obstruct the foramen of Monro, and retrosellar extension is occasionally seen. Most suprasellar meningiomas originate from the area of the tuberculum sellae or planum sphenoidale. Tumors arising from the dorsum sellae extend in suprasellar direction and as far as the clivus (Fig. D2.45).

Midsagittal and parasagittal **MR** images provide the operator with extremely helpful localizing information for neoplasms on the midline. Gadolinium enhancement can demonstrate the tumor extent on the skull base, sometimes with far greater clarity than postcontrast CT (see Figs. D2.42–44).

Differential Diagnosis

Olfactory groove meningiomas present no problems of differential diagnosis.

Suprasellar meningiomas are most likely to be mistaken for *pituitary adenomas* on the CT scan. Differentiation is accomplished by obtaining radiographic views of the sella and by evaluating for endocrine abnormalities (see diagrams in Fig. D4.30). Other tumors of this region may occasionally have a CT appearance similar to meningioma. *Large aneurysms* projecting into the suprasellar space are distinguished by their peripheral calcifications and/or by their very intense contrast enhancement (see Figs. F74–79, 81).

The MR signal characteristics of pituitary adenomas do not reliably distinguish them from meningiomas, and differentiation relies mainly on the topography of the lesion. A large suprasellar, nonthrombosed aneurysm is easily recognized on MR images by the complete absence of signal.

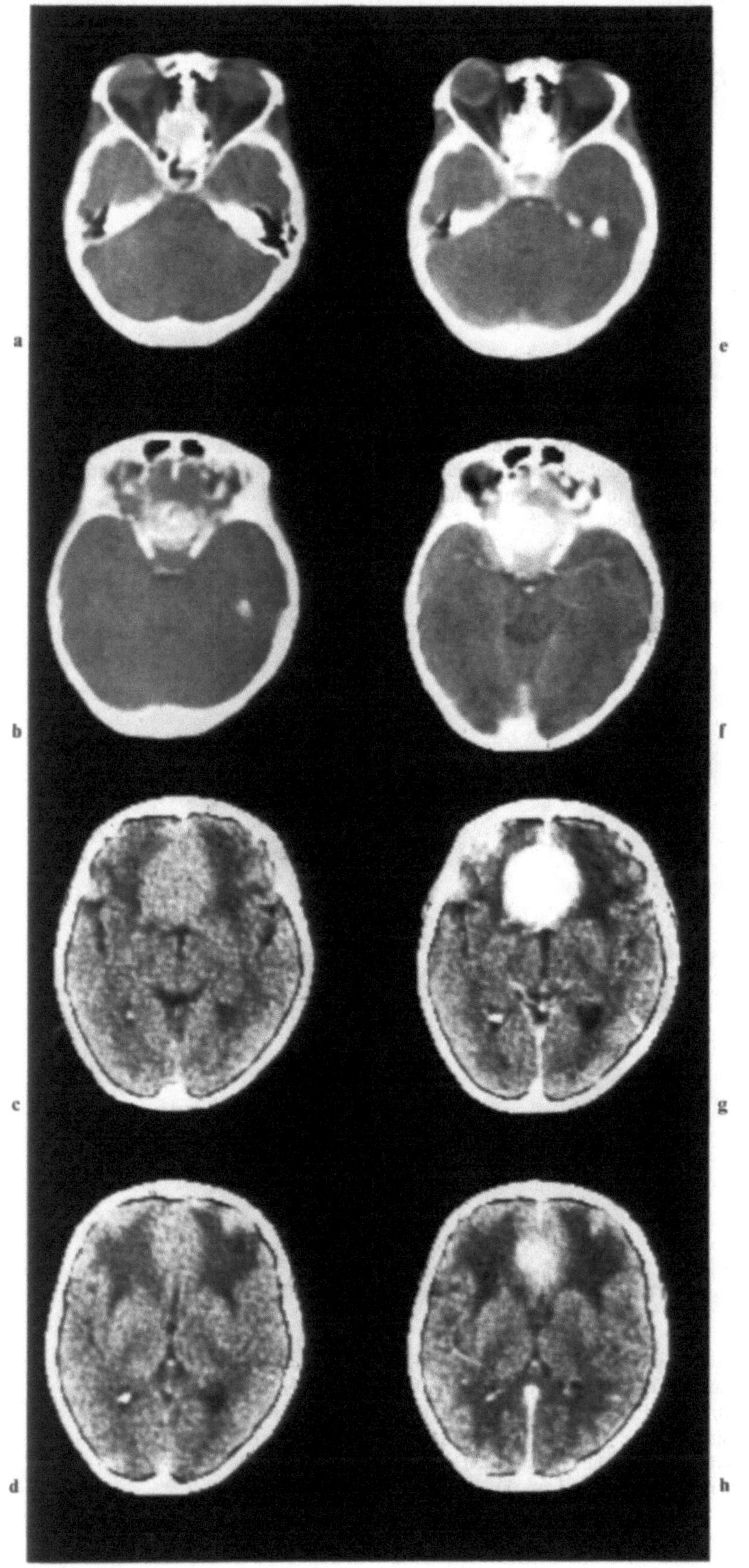

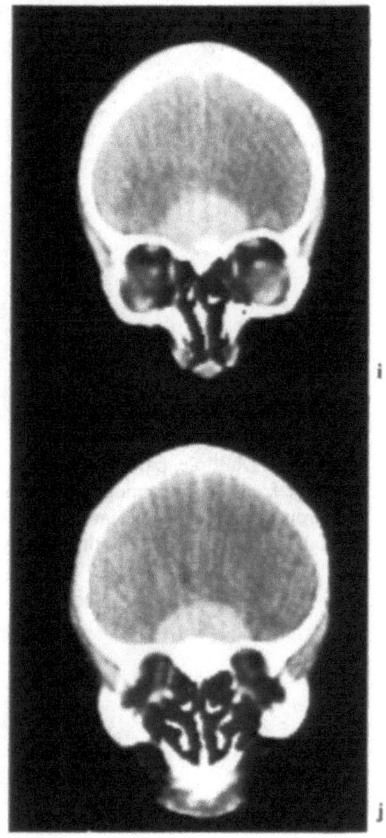

Fig. D 2.40 a–j. Olfactory groove meningioma in a 62-year-old man. Plain CT scans disclose a slightly hyperdense to isodense soft-tissue mass (**c, d**) with basal calcification (**a, b**). The solid tumor component enhances intensely with contrast medium (**e–h**). There is typical bifrontal white-matter edema. The site of tumor origin in the olfactory groove is clearly appreciated on both the axial and coronal views. The planum sphenoidale is greatly thickened (**i, j**)

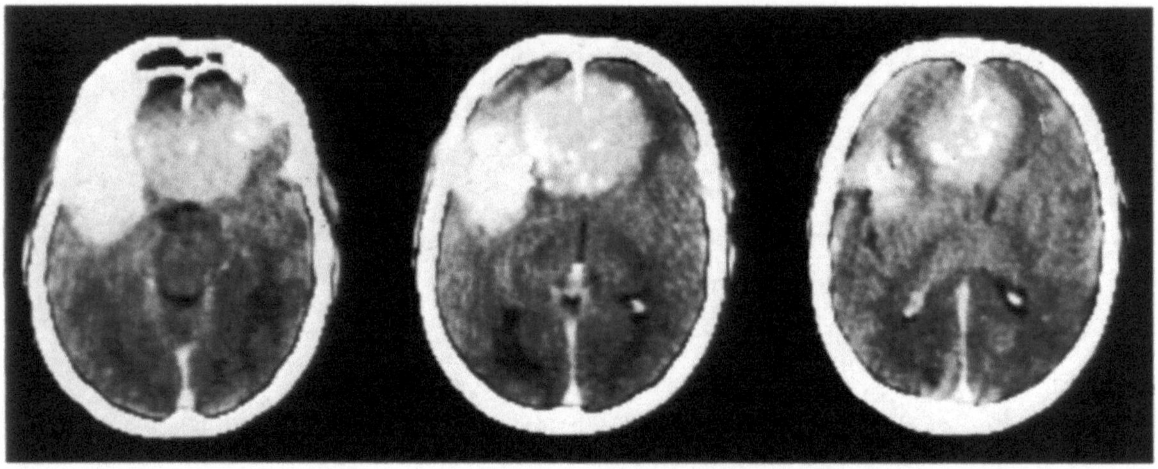

Fig. D 2.41. Multiple, partially calcified meningiomas. There is a large frontobasal meningioma on the midline containing numerous flecks of calcification and showing relation to the falx. It is bordered on the left by a heavily calcified meningioma arising from the sphenoid wing. The frontal horns are compressed and are displaced backward and to the right. Postcontrast CT

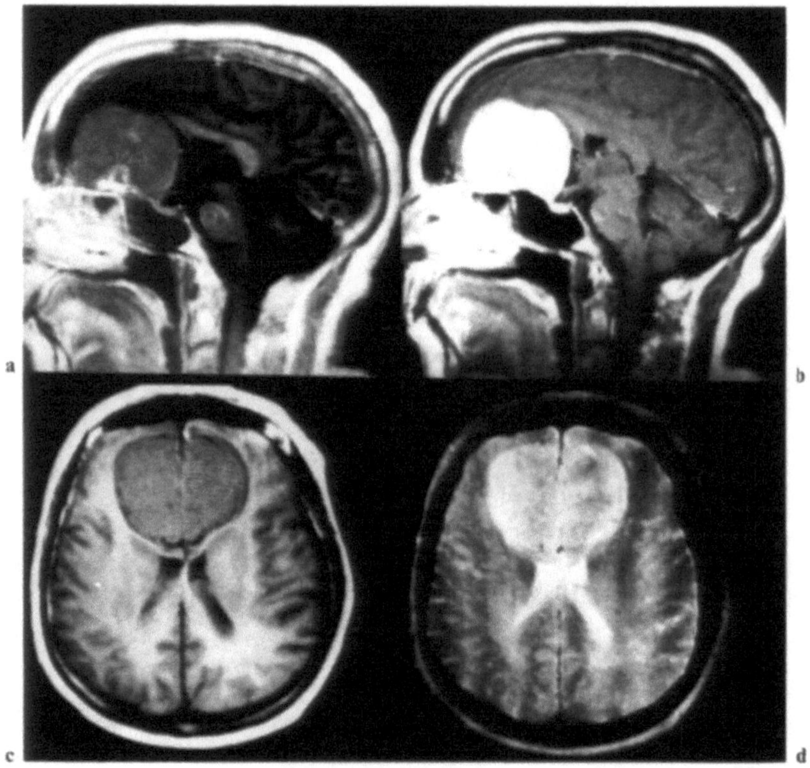

Fig. D 2.42 a–d. Giant olfactory groove meningioma in a 60-year-old woman with altered mental status and anosmia. MR: **a** SE 400/30 sagittal, **b** SE 400/30 sagittal post Gd-DTPA, **c** SE 1600/30, **d** SE 2000/120. The proton-density image (**c**) shows a hypointense tumor causing massive posterior displacement of the frontal horns. The lesion appears hyperintense on the T2-weighted image (**d**). The intensely enhancing neoplasm rides upon the frontal base (**b**)

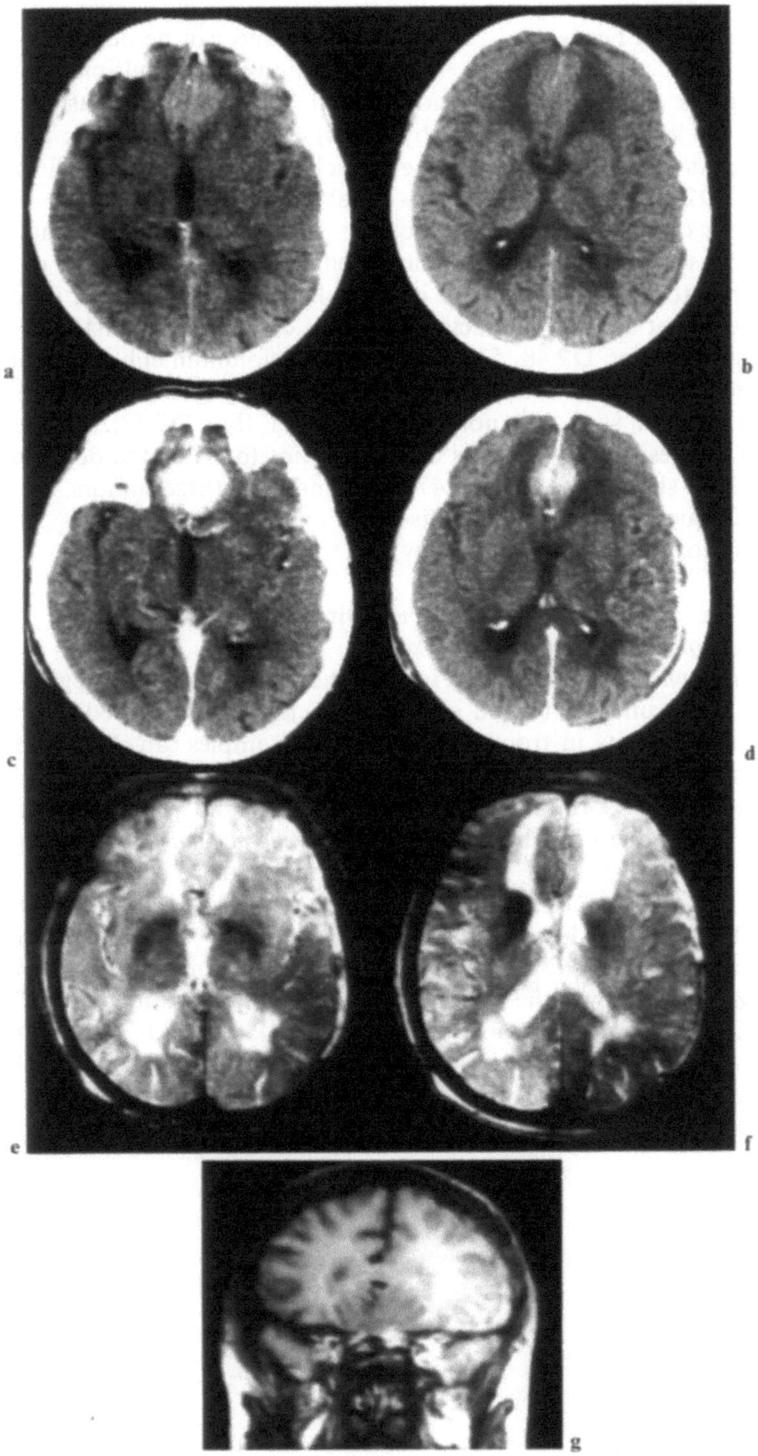

Fig. D 2.43 a–g. Olfactory groove meningioma in a 79-year-old woman with a 2-year history of altered mental status and seizures. CT: **a, b** precontrast, **c, d** postcontrast. MR: **e** SE 2500/120, **f** SE 2500/120, **g** SE 500/30 coronal. The lesion enhances brightly on the postcontrast CT scans (**c, d**). On the T2-weighted MR image, the tumor is demarcated only by the surrounding hyperintense edema. CT is superior to MR in the detection of meningiomas in cases where Gd-DTPA enhancement is not employed

Meningiomas of the Sphenoid Wing and the Base of the Middle Cranial Fossa

The sphenoid ridge is a site of predilection for meningiomas. The lesions are described by their location as *medial or lateral sphenoid wing meningiomas* (Figs. D2.44, 46, 47–57). Extension into the anterior cranial fossa or even the posterior fossa is observed (Fig. D2.48). The relation of the tumor to the skull base and its upward and medial extent are best appreciated on coronal projections (Figs. D2.48, 54). Appearance of the internal carotid artery within the tumor area on the axial scan does not necessarily mean that the vessel is encased, as our own observations have shown (see Fig. D2.47). In many cases this question cannot be satisfactorily resolved prior to operation, even by angiography.

Osteoplastic bone involvement is common with sphenoid meningiomas and can cause marked expansion of the sphenoid wing (see Figs. D2.49, 54, E2). It is not unusual to find additional soft tumor components in front of and below the temporal pole, below the temporal muscle, and on the lateral orbital wall (see Figs. G7 and 10). En plaque growths may escape detection by CT.

Meningiomas confined to the base of the middle fossa are rare (Fig. D2.13). Meningiomas in the Meckel's cave area may spread forward to the sphenoid wing, medially over the tentorial margin to the brainstem, or into the posterior fossa. Contrast injection in these cases produces very dense enhancement of the ipsilateral tentorial margin (Fig. D2.53).

Parasellar meningiomas frequently grow en plaque and can be detected only by very careful scanning on multiple axial planes near the skull base (meningiomas of the cavernous sinus). Orbital projections have proven useful. Such tumors are also well displayed on coronal views (Fig. D2.17).

MR imaging is advantageous in that it demonstrates the relation of the tumor to the skull base, large vessels, cavernous sinus, and optic chiasm better than CT (see Figs. D2.55, 57). Gadolinium enhancement can reveal other tumor components that are difficult to visualize with CT (Fig. D2.52). MR may sometimes be superior to CT in the detection and evaluation of many of these tumors.

Differential Diagnosis

Other tumors of this region include *pilocytic astrocytomas* of the medial temporal lobe; noncystic examples can resemble meningioma. Differentiation is also required from *trigeminal neurinoma* and *gangliocytoma*. A partially calcified *chondroma* likewise can simulate a basal meningioma.

Large carotid aneurysms may resemble meningiomas on CT scans (see Figs. F77 and 79). Partial thrombosis of the aneurysm produces a highly distinctive bull's-eye pattern (see Fig. F81). But if the aneurysm is not thrombosed, MR will demonstrate a signal void that positively distinguishes the lesion from meningioma (see Fig. F80).

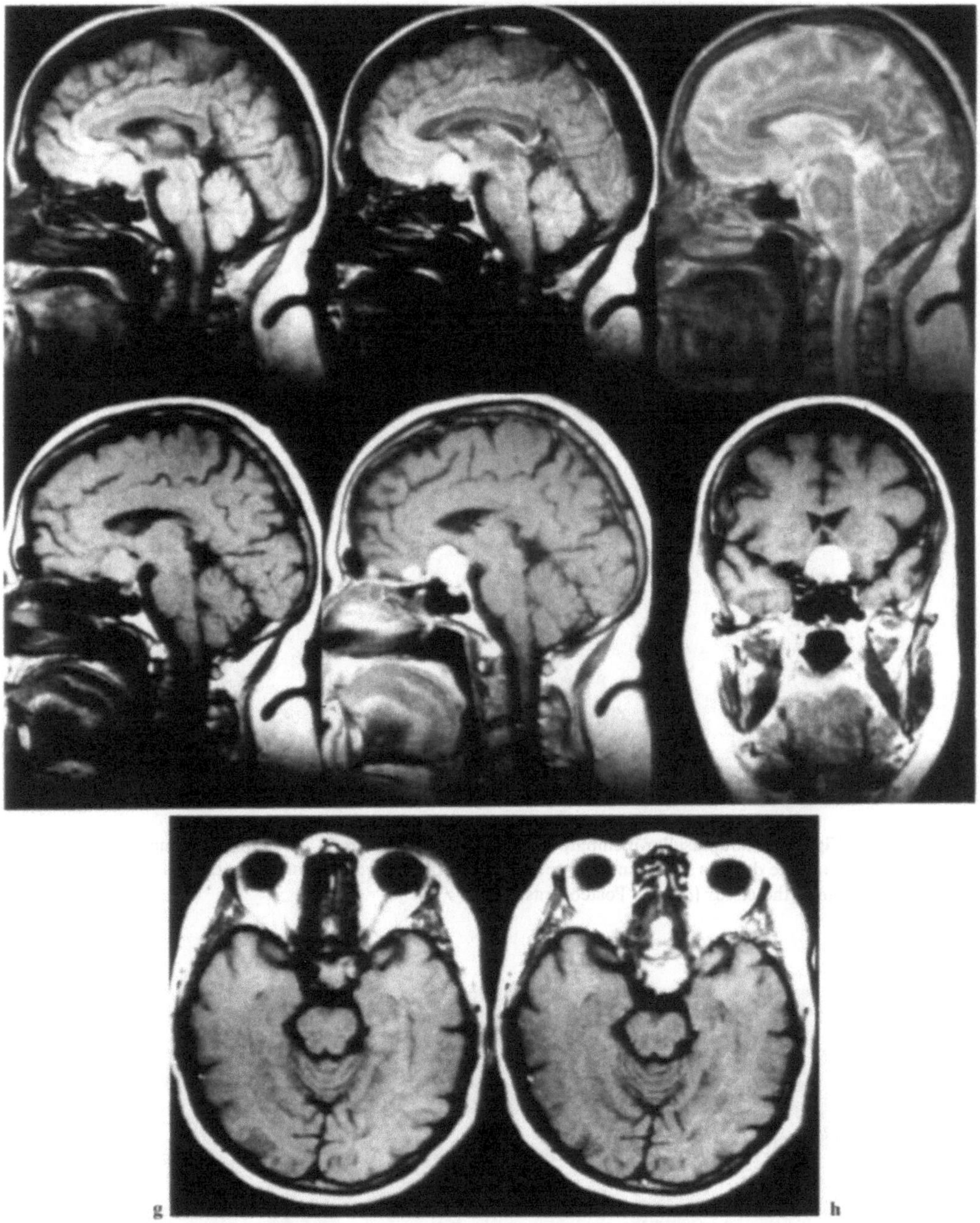

a–c

d–f

g

h

Fig. D 2.44 a–h. Meningioma of the tuberculum sellae and left medial sphenoid wing in a 55-year-old woman with a 3-month history of visual acuity loss and left hemianopia. MR: **a** SE 1600/30, **b** SE 1600/60, **c** SE 1600/150, **d** SE 400/30, **e** SE 400/30 post Gd-DTPA (all sagittal), **f** SE 400/30 post Gd-DTPA coronal, **g** SE 400/30, **h** SE 400/30 post Gd-DTPA. The contrast-enhanced T1-weighted images (**e, f, h**) demonstrate several small frontobasal tumor components arising from the tuberculum sellae

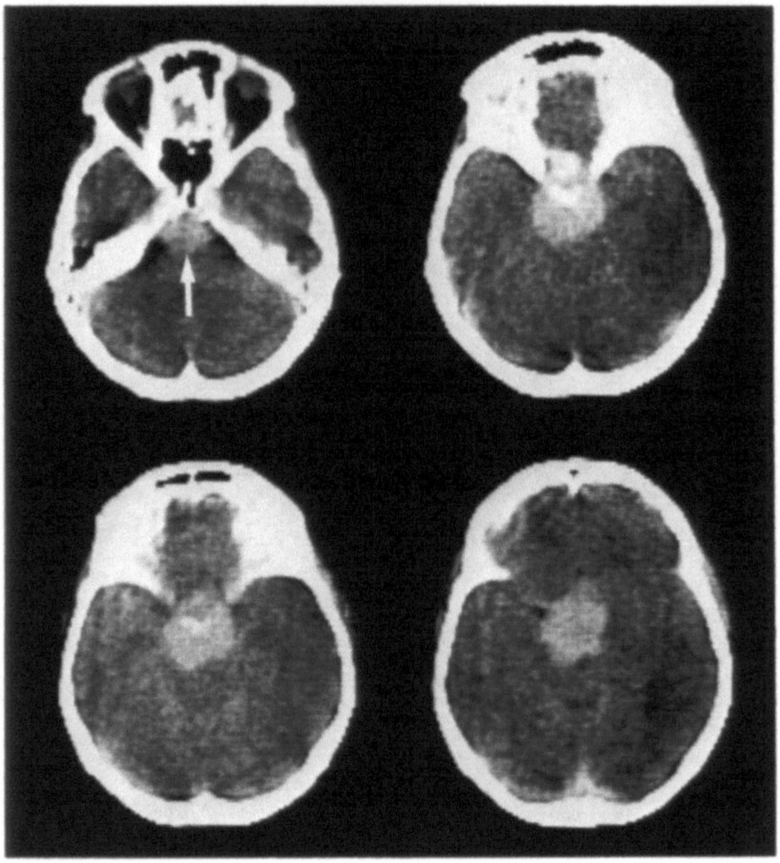

Fig. D 2.45. Suprasellar meningioma in a 55-year-old woman. The tumor originates from the dorsum sellae and has spread above the sella and into the posterior fossa along the clivus (*arrow*). Postcontrast CT

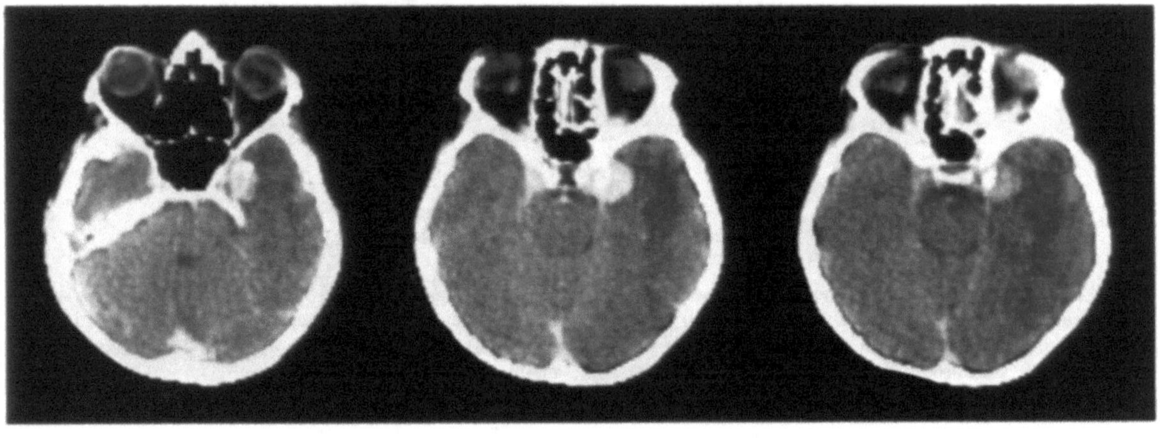

Fig. D 2.46. Small meningioma of the right medial sphenoid wing in a 57-year-old woman. The tumor was slightly hyperdense on plain CT scans (not shown) and enhances intensely with contrast medium. CT does not disclose its relation to the internal carotid artery. There is marked perifocal edema in the right temporal lobe. Postcontrast CT

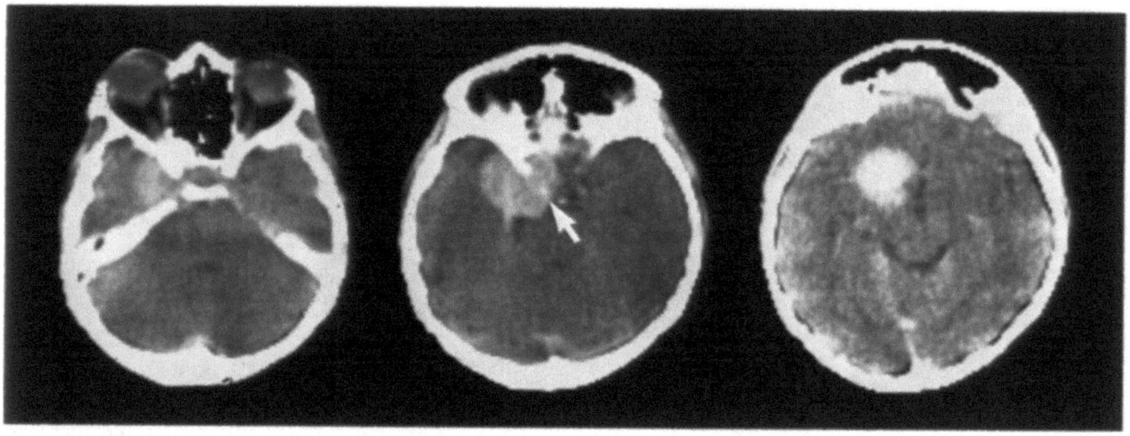

Fig. D 2.47. Medial sphenoid wing meningioma in a 57-year-old woman. Increasing the window width demonstrates the left internal carotid artery in cross-section within the tumor mass (*arrow*). At operation it was found that the tumor lay against the vessel but did not envelop it. Postcontrast CT

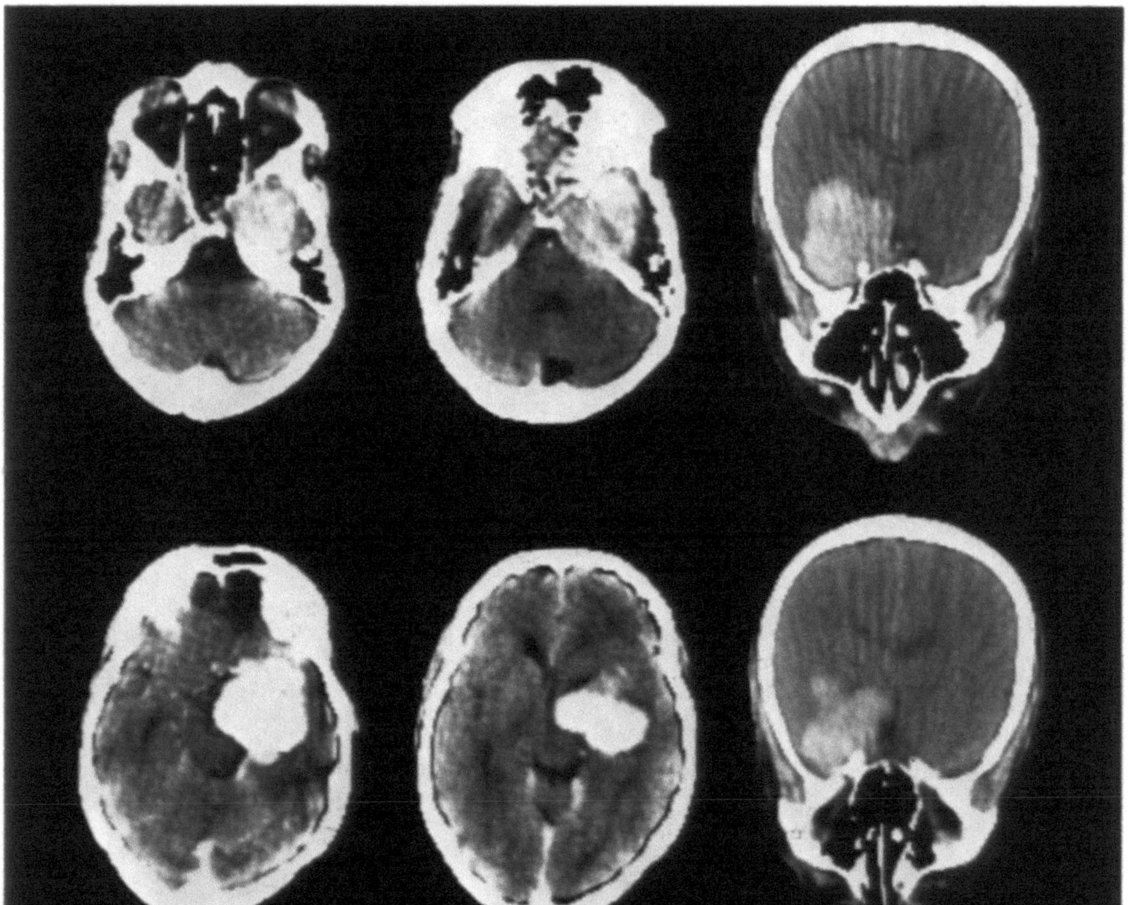

Fig. D 2.48. Very large meningioma at the base of the middle fossa with extention into the chiasmatic cistern, posterior fossa, and basal ganglion region in a 50-year-old man. The postcontrast CT scans show very intense, largely homogeneous enhancement of the tumor. The coronal view clearly demonstrates the craniocaudal extent of disease

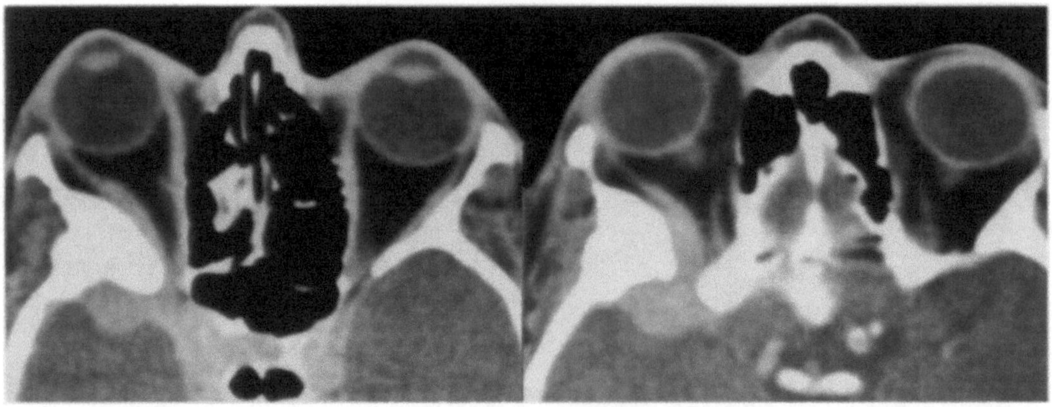

Fig. D 2.49. Osteoplastic left sphenoid meningioma expanding the sphenoid wing and transgressing the optic foramen in a 47-year-old woman with headache and left-sided exophthalmos. The sphenoid expansion was visible externally. Postcontrast CT

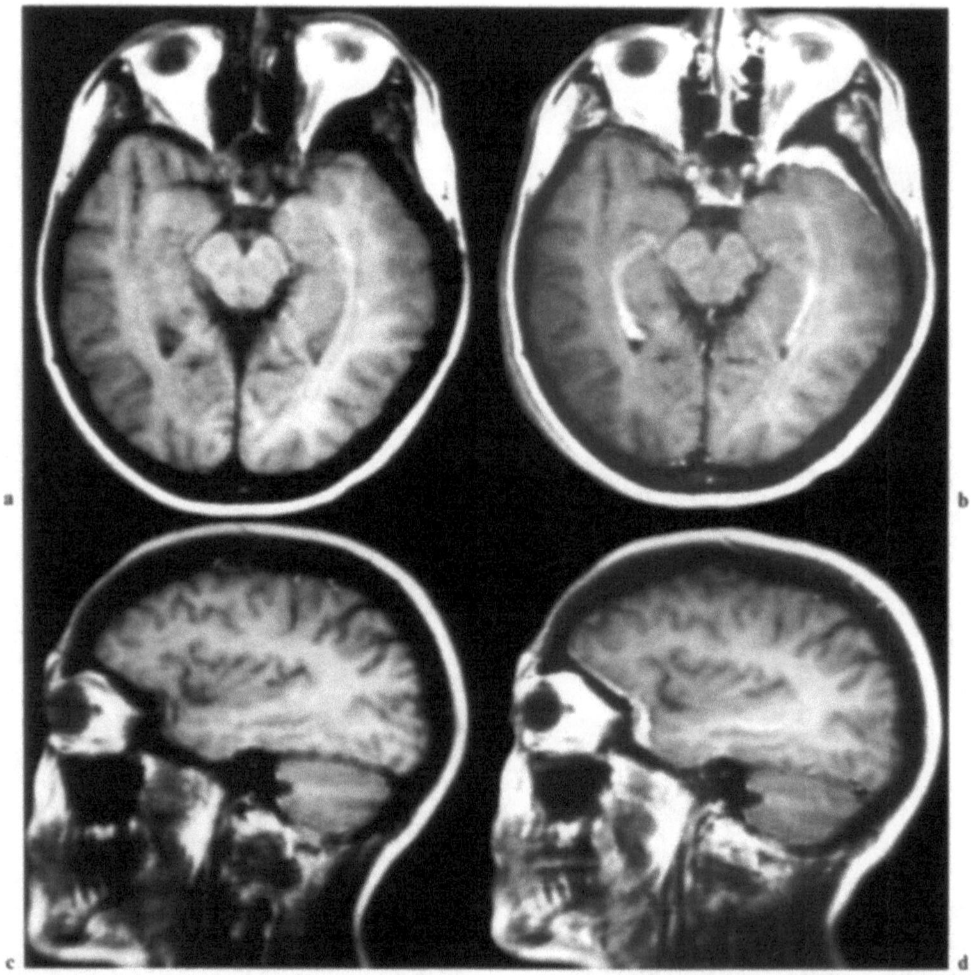

Fig. D 2.50 a–d. Meningioma en plaque involving the temporal calvarium, sphenoid wing, and orbital roof. The 43-year-old woman presented with a 1-year history of slowly progressive exophthalmos on the right side. Postcontrast CT showed only a reactive hyperostosis of the right sphenoid wing but gave no direct evidence of tumor. MR: **a–d** SE 400/30; **a, c** before Gd-DTPA, **b, d** post Gd-DTPA. The post-gadolinium scans demonstrate a plaque-like area of enhancement along the sphenoid wing and orbital roof. The plain scans demonstrate widening of the adjacent bone, which gives no signal. Histologic examination identified the lesion as endotheliomatous meningioma

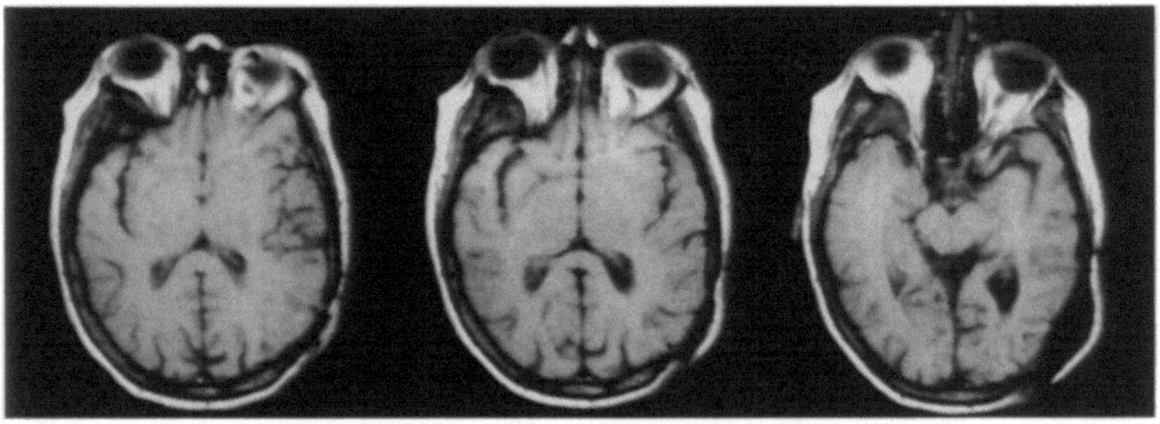

Fig. D 2.51. Osteoplastic meningioma of the left sphenoid wing in a 65-year-old woman with a 1-year history of exophthalmos. She had undergone resection of a parieto-occipital meningioma 20 years previously. MR: SE 400/30. Tumor involving the bone is poorly demonstrated, but the soft tumor tissue, which appears hypointense on the T1-weighted image, is seen compressing the orbit and optic nerve from the lateral side. The signal void between the brain tissue and right parieto-occipital galea is a residuum of the old operation

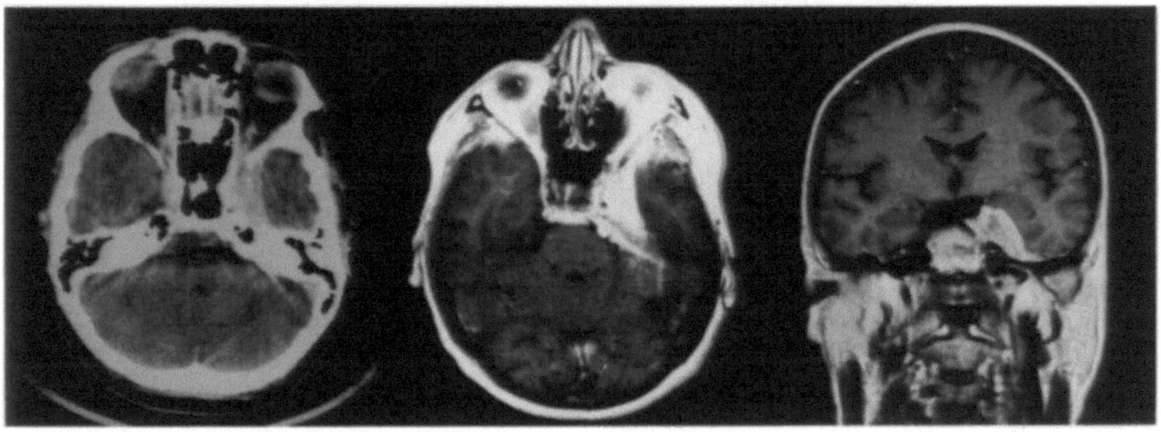

Fig. D 2.52. Meningioma infiltrating the sphenoid sinus from the right medial temporobasal region in a 56-year-old man who experienced a generalized seizure. CT *left* postcontrast. MR: *center* and *right* SE 300/17 post Gd-DTPA, axial and coronal. The post-Gd-DTPA T1-weighted image gives a coronal view of the hyperintense tumor invading the cavity of the sphenoid sinus

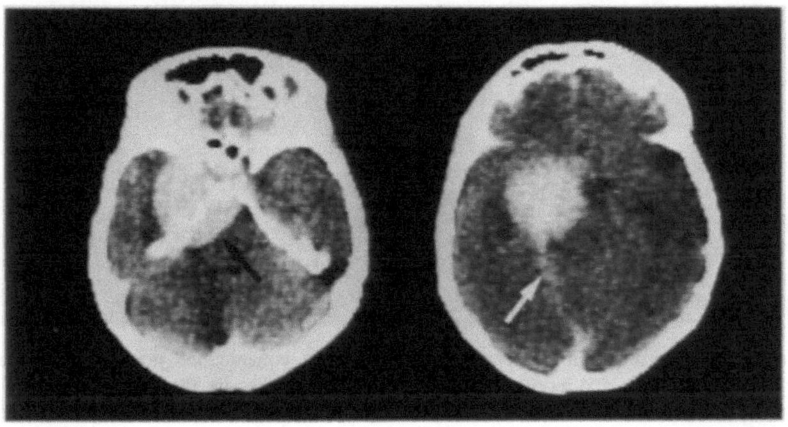

Fig. D 2.53. Meningioma arising from the dura over Meckel's cave and extending past the tentorial margin into the posterior fossa (*black arrow*). The richly vascularized tentorial margin behind the tumor shows marked contrast enhancement (*white arrow*). Postcontrast CT

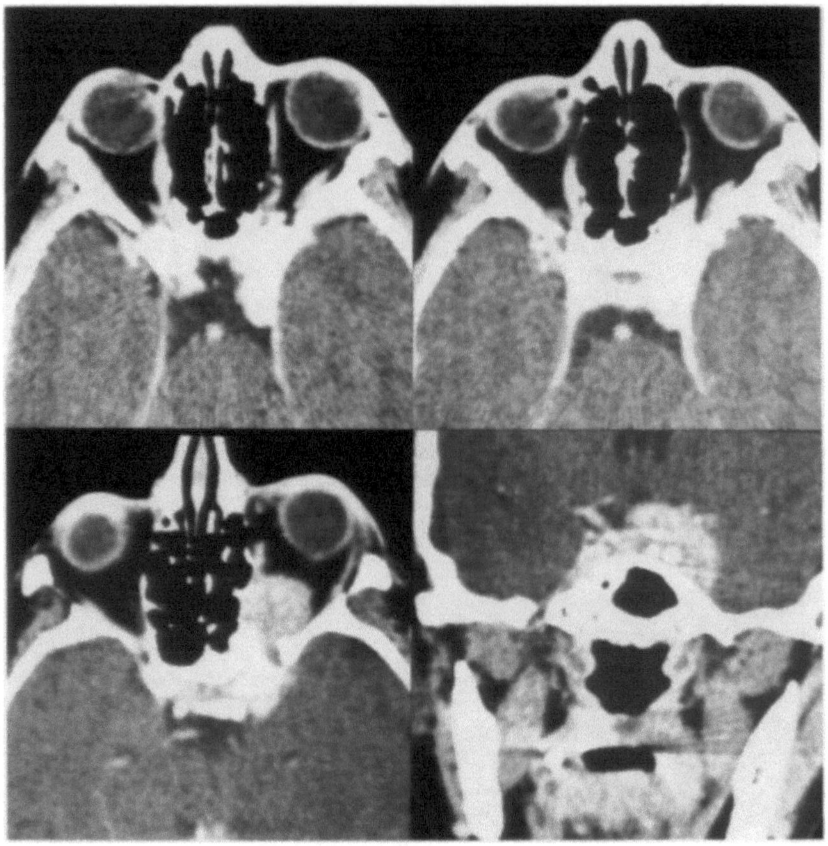

Fig. D 2.54. Right parasellar sphenoid meningiona invading the orbit in a 7-year-old boy (!) with exophthalmos, decreased visual acuity in the right eye, and right-sided oculomotor paresis. Postcontrast CT

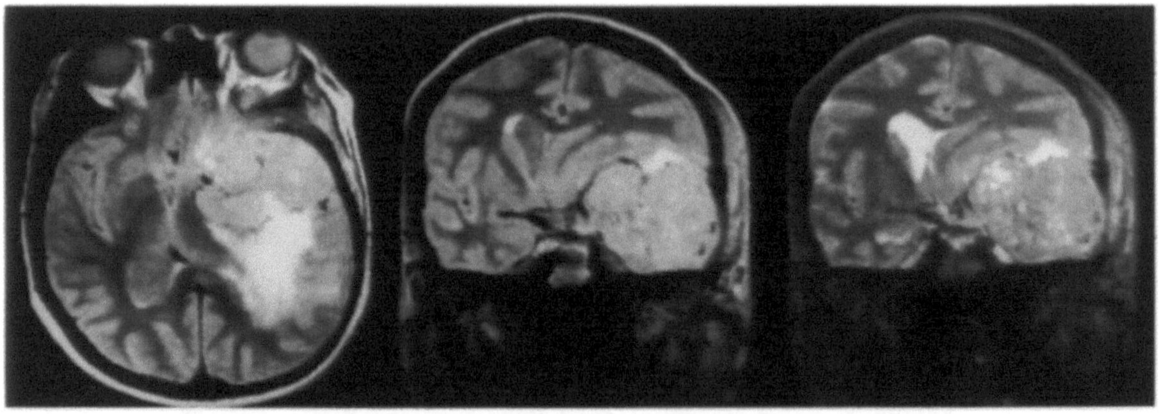

Fig. D 2.55. Large sphenoid wing meningioma invading the orbit in a 61-year-old woman with a 4-month history of marked alteration of mental status. MR: *left* SE 3000/30 axial, *center* SE 3000/30 coronal, *right* SE 3000/90 coronal. The tumor is slightly hyperintense to brain on the proton-density and T2-weighted images. The hyperintense edema is most conspicuous posteriorly and appears as multiple bright patches on the coronal plane of section (*right*). The middle cerebral artery is displaced and appears as signal void. Tumor vessels give the same appearance in the richly vascularized meningioma

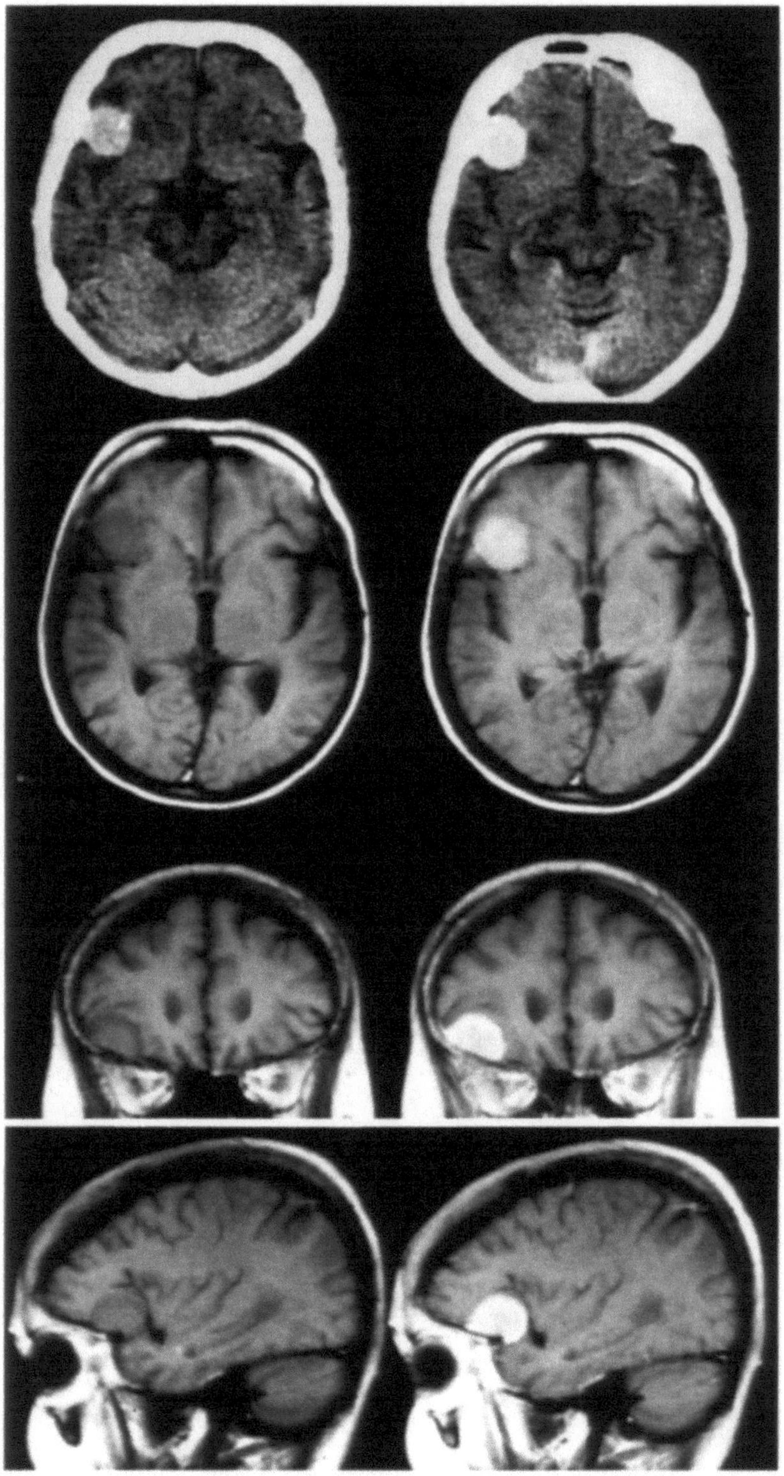

a b c d e f g h

Fig. D 2.56 a–h. Lateral meningioma of the left sphenoid in a 62-year-old woman with frequent migraine-like headaches; neurologic exam was negative. CT: **a** precontrast, **b** postcontrast. MR: **c** SE 400/30, **d** SE 400/30 post Gd-DTPA, **e** SE 400/30 coronal, **f** SE 400/30 coronal post Gd-DTPA, **g** SE 400/30 parasagittal, **h** SE 400/30 parasagittal post Gd-DTPA. The lesion enhances intensely on the postcontrast CT scan. The tumor is nearly isointense to brain on the T1-weighted image and enhances brightly with Gd-DTPA (**d, f, h**)

a–c

d–f

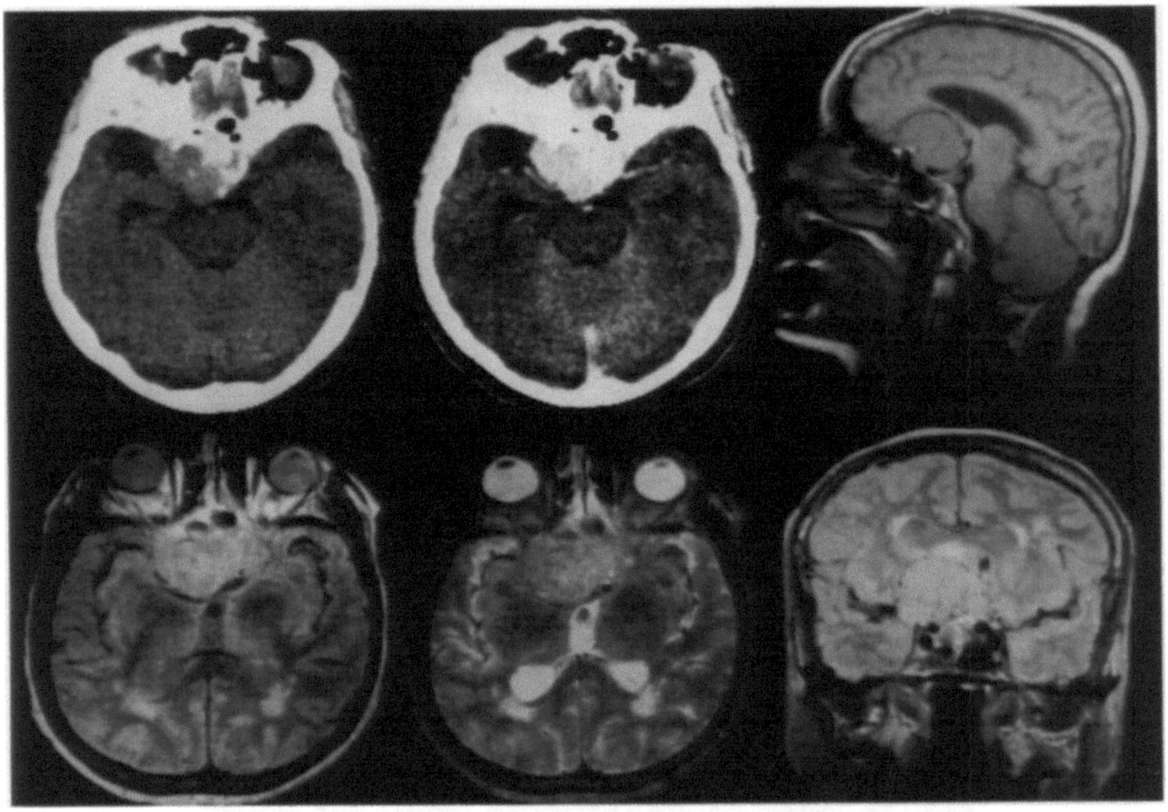

Fig. D 2.57 a–f. Left medial sphenoid meningioma in a 60-year-old woman with a long history of chiasmatic disturbances, chiefly on the left side. CT: **a** precontrast, **b** postcontrast. MR: **c** SE 700/30 sagittal, **d** SE 3000/30, **e** SE 3000/90, **f** SE 3000/30 coronal. CT shows marked contrast enhancement of the medial tumor, which is seen to extend across the midline. T1-weighted MR shows a predominantly isointense but clearly delineated tumor riding on the skull base (**c**). The proton-density image (**d**) displays as signal voids the displaced anterior cerebral artery and middle cerebral artery at the border of the tumor. The coronal image (**f**) shows marked extension of the slightly hyperintense tumor toward the right side. Small, bright areas of edema are visible above the lesion

Tentorial Meningiomas

Meningiomas originating from the tentorium may be *supratentorial or infratentorial* in location (Figs. D2.58–62, 64, 65) or a combination of both (Figs. D2.69, 74). Relations to the tentorium are clearly depicted only on coronal views. Tentorial meningiomas that are projected into the supratentorial space on axial sections may actually be infratentorial lesions causing circumscribed elevation of the tentorium. This can be confirmed on coronal scans.

A meningioma abutting directly on the tentorium can simulate an intracerebral growth (Fig. D2.60). Its infratentorial location is indicated by a straight, diagonal tumor border paralleling the edge of the petrous pyramid (Figs. D2.68, 72).

Growth of a meningioma around the tentorial margin is signified by indentation of the tumor by the free border of the tentorium (Fig. D2.74).

MR can define the topographic relations of the tumor with much greater accuracy than **CT** owing to its capacity for variable plane selection. MR is superior in its ability to define the relation of the meningioma to the tentorium and check for obstruction of the sigmoid and transverse sinuses. Tentorial meningiomas can almost always be distinguished from intracerebral growths.

Meningiomas of the Cerebellopontine Angle

Meningiomas occurring medially near the internal acoustic pore at the border of the petrous pyramid are called cerebellopontine angle meningiomas (Fig. D2.66–71). They are prone to calcification (Fig. D2.67). The acoustic pore is not enlarged.

The early clinical features of these lesions are headache and vertigo, followed later by a slowly progressive hypacusis and cerebellar symptoms. By contrast, hearing loss is a very early feature of acoustic neurinoma.

Meningiomas of the Cerebellar Convexity

The site of tumor origin cannot be identified on CT scans, so these lesions often are indistinguishable from tentorial meningiomas. **MR** is of great help in solving this problem owing to its multiplanar capabilities.

Meningiomas in the Tentorial Incisure

These lesions cause hydrocephalus by exerting pressure on the aqueduct from above and on the posterior part of the third ventricle. Pineal tumors also occur at this site, but dense contrast enhancement of the tentorial margin in contact with the tumor helps to identify the lesion as a meningioma (Fig. D2.76).

MR can establish the site of tumor origin with great accuracy and can delineate the displaced structures within the tentorial incisure (Fig. D2.74).

Meningiomas of the Clivus and Craniospinal Junction

These tumors are difficult to visualize on axial scans. Slices at the level of the craniospinal junction will occasionally demonstrate a nubbin of tumor on the side of the foramen magnum facing the clivus. Involvement of the clivus by mediobasal meningiomas is not uncommon (Figs. D2.43, 77–79).

This is a case where **MR** is decidedly superior to **CT**. A plane can be selected which demonstrates the relationship of the meningioma to surrounding structures with exceptional clarity. Displacement of the pons and medulla is readily appreciated (Figs. D2.75, 77–79).

Differential Diagnosis

It is unlikely that a large infratentorial meningioma will be mistaken for any other tumor. We encountered problems of differentiation only in the case of a large, circumscribed *malignant lymphoma* and a *cerebellar sarcoma* (desmoplastic medulloblastoma), both of which presented the CT features of meningiomas (see Fig. D1.174).

Glomus tumors in the cerebellopontine angle may resemble meningioma, but characteristic bone changes serve to differentiate them (see p. 462).

Certain *acoustic neurinomas* can be very difficult to distinguish from a meningioma of the same region. Differential diagnosis in these cases is based largely on neuro-otologic findings. **MR** is helpful if the tumor has filled and expanded the acoustic pore, but otherwise it is not. Even the hypointense ring that surrounds many meningiomas has been observed around acoustic neurinomas growing in extra-axial locations.

A solid *angioblastoma* may also simulate meningioma, and there are no reliable CT criteria for distinguishing between them. In the case of *metastases*, the history will usually provide sufficient grounds for a presumptive diagnosis. *Large, laterally projecting aneurysms of the basilar artery* are distinguished by their smooth borders, their spherical or oval shape, and their very intense contrast enhancement unless partial thrombosis has occurred. Calcifications are occasionally seen in the vessel wall (see p. 556).

Clivus chordomas and clivus meningiomas often have an identical appearance on CT scans. There is no measurable CT difference between a calcified meningioma and an osteoma in the cerebellopontine angle, since the density values in a calcified meningioma can closely approximate those in an osteoma.

MR cannot distinguish between a calcified meningioma and an osteoma, or between a meningioma and a chordoma, in the region of the clivus or craniospinal junction. Large *basilar artery aneurysms* are readily identified as areas of signal void.

Intraventricular Meningiomas

Meningiomas of the lateral ventricles most commonly occur in the area of the trigone, where they adhere firmly to the choroid plexus from which they arise. They appear on the CT scan as a large, rounded or oval mass with uniformly well-defined borders (Figs. D2.80–82). There may be dilatation of the temporal horn. A focus of calcification adjacent to the medial tumor surface represents the displaced glomus of the choroid plexus.

MR provides better information on the exact location of the intraventricular tumor. We found that the tumors appeared slightly hyperintense on T2-weighted sequences and contrasted extremely well with the surrounding CSF. Paramedian and vertical projections are the best source of information (see Fig. D2.81).

Meningiomas occur very rarely in the third or fourth ventricle, arising from the choroid plexus on the floor of the ventricle affected (Fig. D2.82).

Differential Diagnosis

Choroid plexus papilloma should always be considered in the differential diagnosis of lateral ventricle tumors, but as this lesion occurs predominantly in children and adolescents while lateral ventricle meningiomas affect adults almost exclusively, the age of the patient should serve to differentiate the lesions.

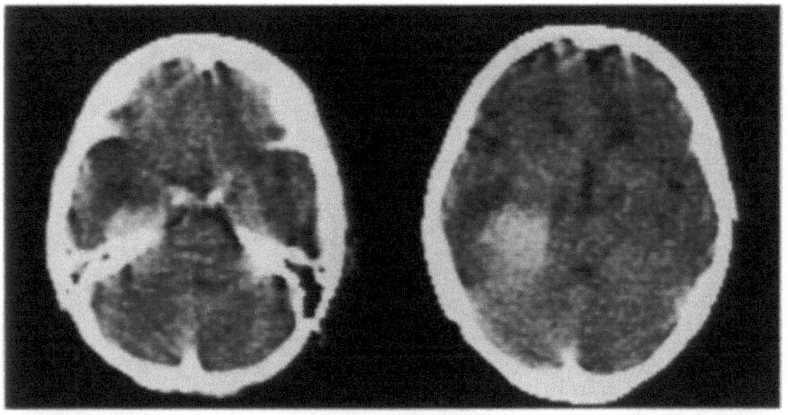

Fig. D 2.58. Supratentorial meningioma arising from the left tentorium in a 60-year-old woman. The straight medial demarcation of the tumor by the tentorial margin (*right*) indicates the site of tumor origin and thus its site of attachment. Postcontrast CT

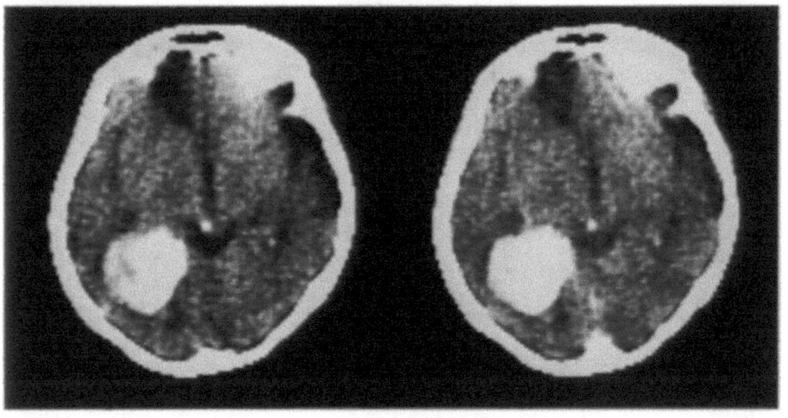

Fig. D 2.59. Supratentorial, densely calcified meningioma of the left tentorium situated below the trigone and occipital lobe in an 80-year-old woman. CT: *left* precontrast, *right* postcontrast. The lesion does not enhance significantly

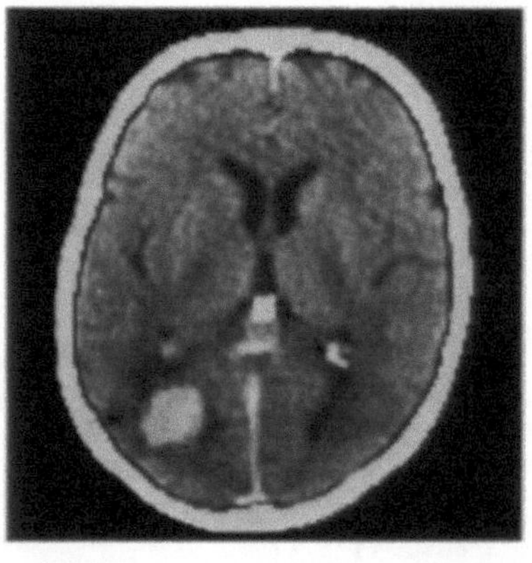

Fig. D 2.60. Small left supratentorial meningioma in a 66-year-old woman. There is slight evidence of an intracranial mass lesion with amputation of the occipital horn. The tumor appears to be intra-axial. Its site of origin cannot be ascertained on the axial scan

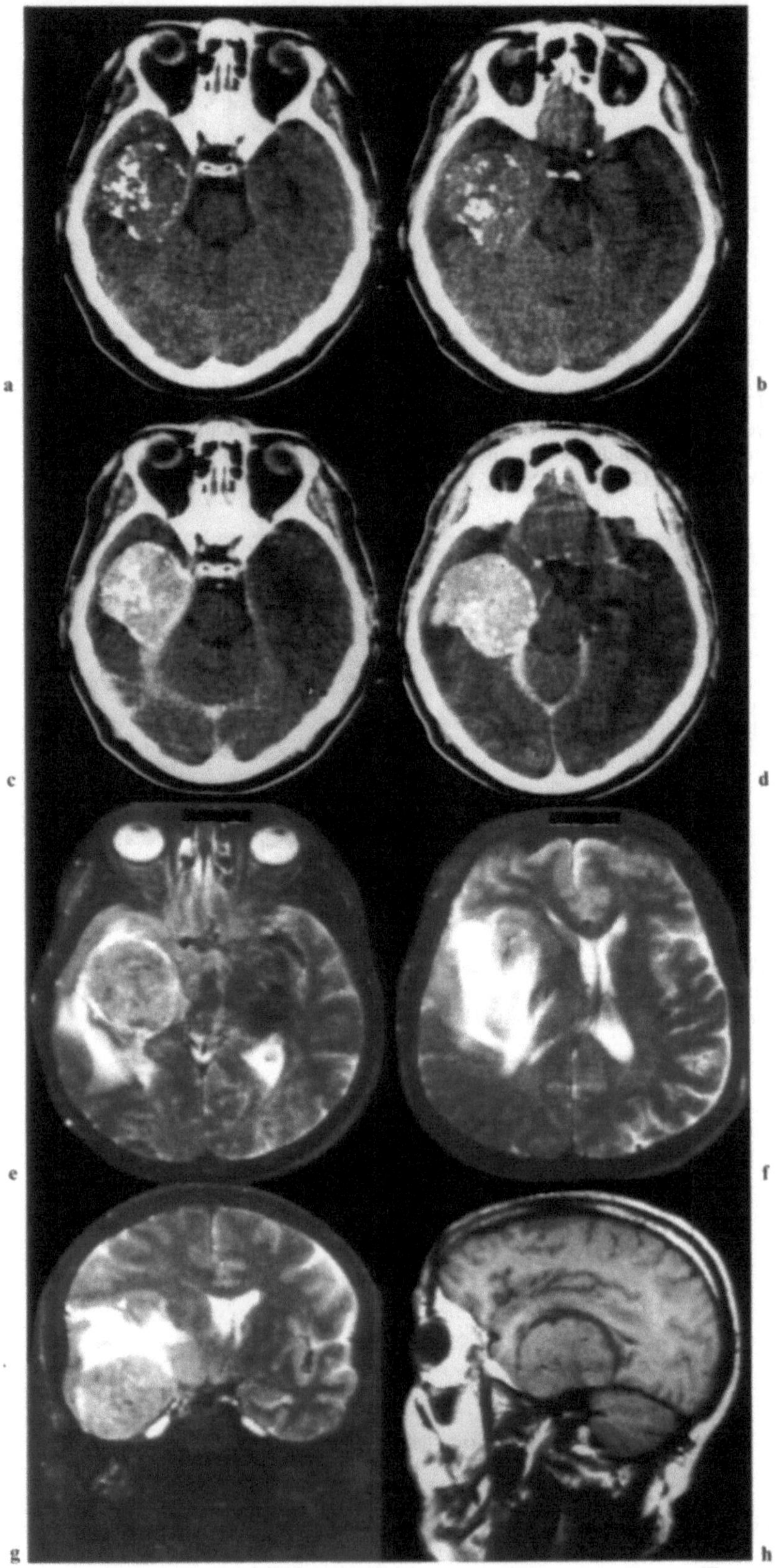
a
b
c
d
e
f
g
h

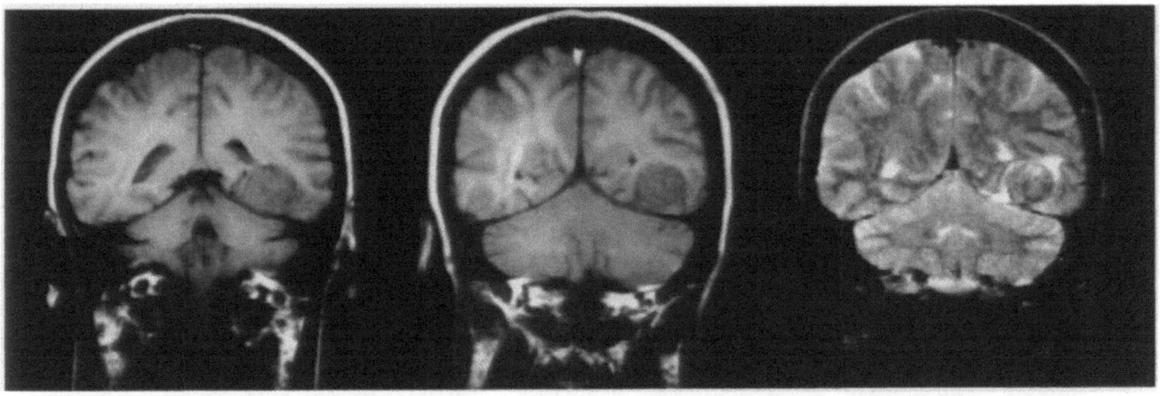

Fig. D 2.62. Tentorial meningioma occupying the right supratentorial space in a 46-year-old woman with headaches as her only symptom. MR *left* and *center* SE 500/30, *right* SE 2500/120, all coronal. The T1-weighted images (*left* and *center*) demonstrate a hemispheric tumor that appears contiguous to the tentorium. The T2-weighted sequence (*right*) discloses a thin rim of hyperintense edema

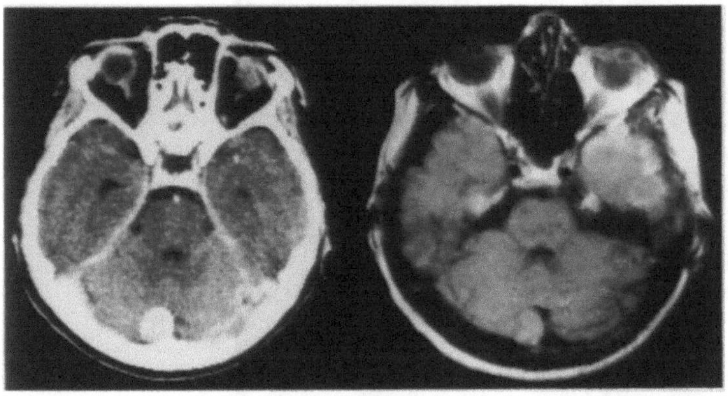

Fig. D 2.63. Infratentorial meningioma at the confluence of the sinuses on the left side in a 58-year-old woman with intractable headaches. Postcontrast CT *left*. MR *right* SE 2500/30. The tumor is displayed with higher contrast on the enhanced CT scan than on the unenhanced MR image

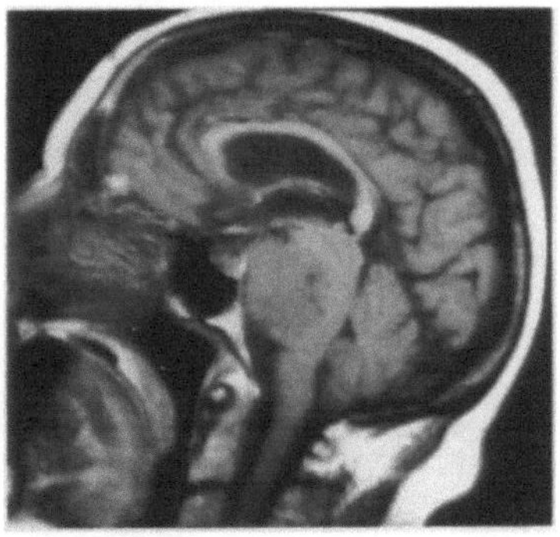

Fig. D 2.64. Tentorial meningioma lying partly anterior to the brainstem in a 69-year-old woman with slowly progressive left-sided hemiparesis, trigeminal neuropathy, and diplopia. MR: SE 500/30 sagittal. The tumor, appearing isointense to brain on the T1-weighted sequence, is compressing and displacing the pons posteriorly

Fig. D 2.61 a–h. Left temporal meningioma arising partly from the tentorium. The 56-year-old woman presented with a history of cerebral seizures for 6 months, headache, subtle right-sided hemiparesis, and mild dysphasia. CT: **a, b** precontrast, **c, d** postcontrast. MR: **e** SE 2500/120, **f** SE 2500/120, **g** SE 2500/120 coronal, **h** SE 500/30 parasagittal. Plain CT shows a slightly hyperdense tumor with calcifications. The lesion enhances markedly with contrast medium. The T2-weighted image at the basal level (**e**) shows a slightly hyperintense tumor with a nonhomogeneous signal pattern. Scan **f** further demonstrates peritumoral edema, which gives a very intense signal. The tumor is isointense to brain on the T1-weighted image (**h**) and well delineated. Its relation to the temporal base is apparent

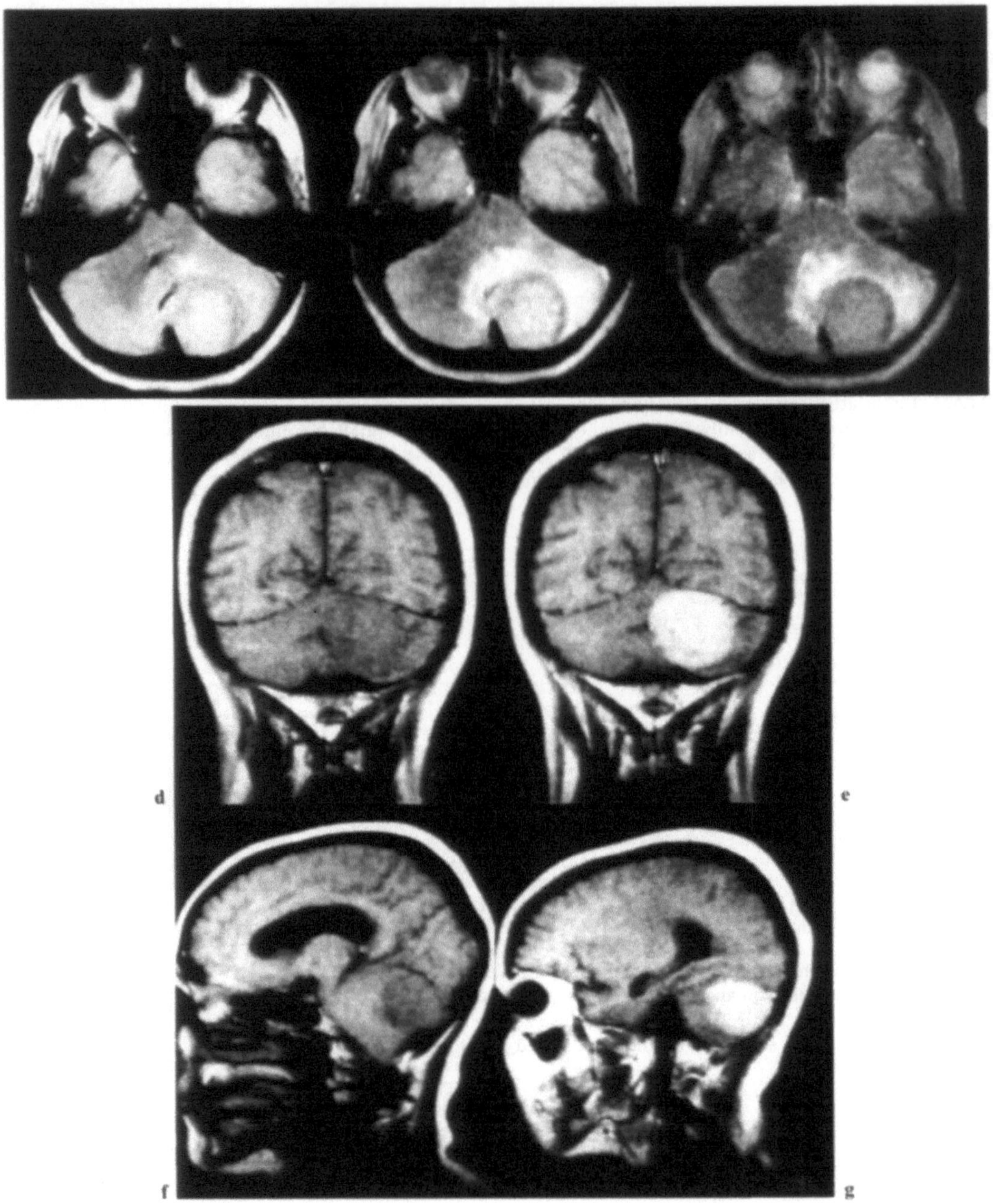

a–c d e f g

Fig. D 2.65 a–g. Tentorial meningioma in a 58-year-old woman with a history of intermittent crises of increased intracranial pressure for 2 years and mild disturbance of equilibrium. MR: **a** SE 1600/30, **b** SE 1600/90, **c** SE 1600/180, **d** SE 400/35 coronal, **e** SE 400/35 post Gd-DTPA coronal, **f** SE 400/35 parasagittal, **g** SE 400/35 post Gd-DTPA parasagittal. The T2-weighted image (**c**) affords the best contrast between the spherical tumor and the surrounding, hyperintense edema. The lesion enhances markedly with Gd-DTPA (**e, g**). Its relation to the tentorium and its infratentorial growth are apparent

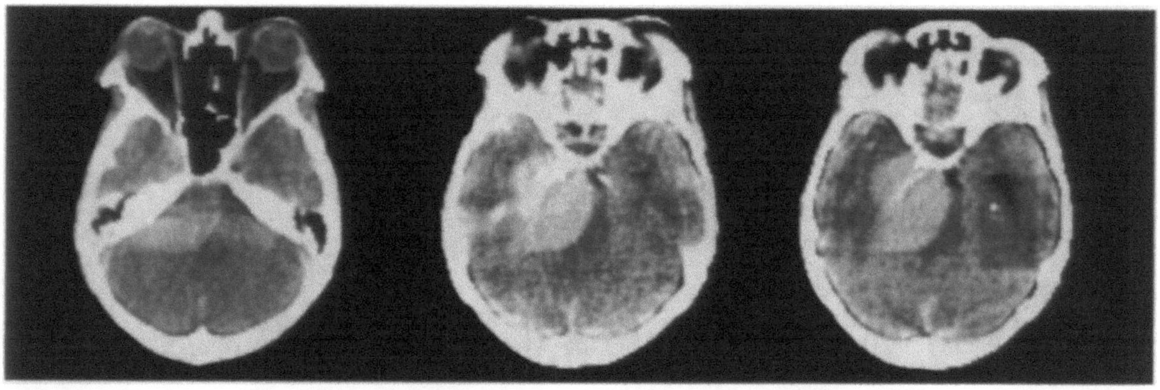

Fig. D 2.66. Very large meningioma in the left cerebellopontine angle with extension toward the clivus, dorsum sellae, and middle fossa in a 55-year-old woman. The brainstem is displaced far to the right and is greatly compressed. Postcontrast CT

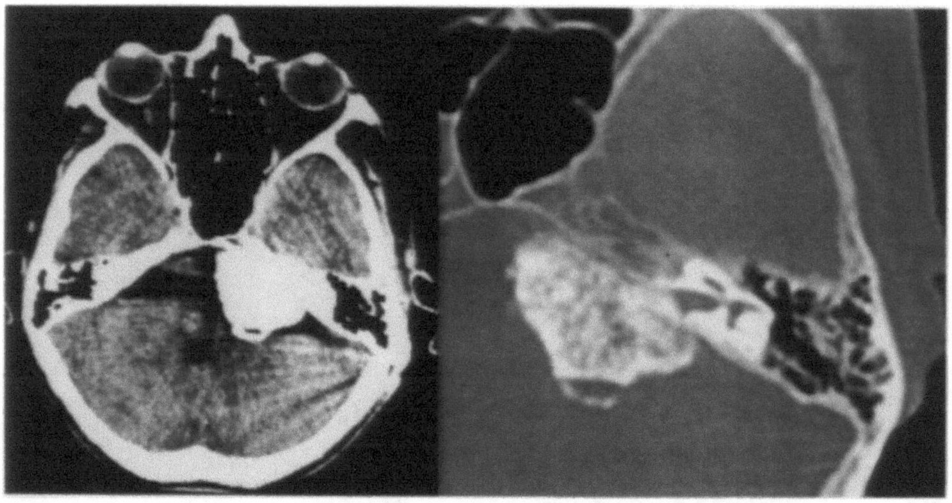

Fig. D 2.67. Completely calcified meningioma in the right cerebellopontine angle of an 80-year-old woman with retrocochlear hearing loss. CT scan at *left* is noncontrast! *Right* bony window

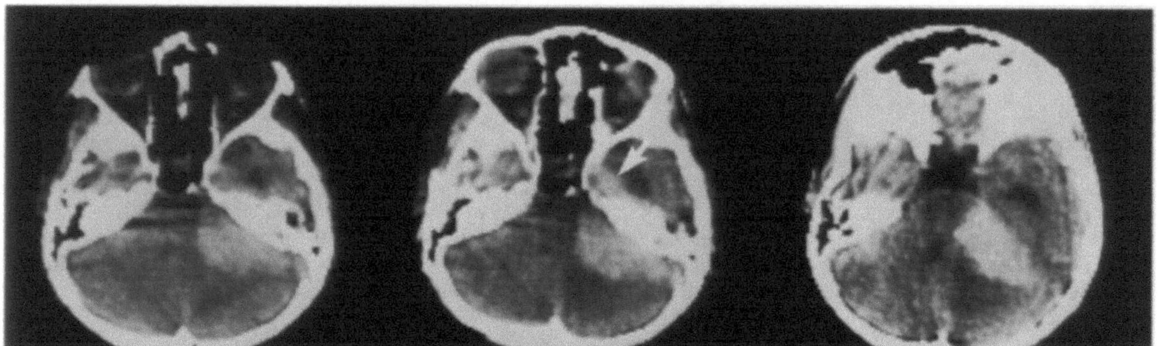

Fig. D 2.68. Meningioma with en-plaque features in the right cerebellopontine angle of a 50-year-old woman. The sharp, diagonal demarcation of the tumor by the tentorium and the border of the petrous pyramid establishes the infratentorial location of the mass. A small nubbin of tumor projects into the middle fossa (*arrow*). Postcontrast CT

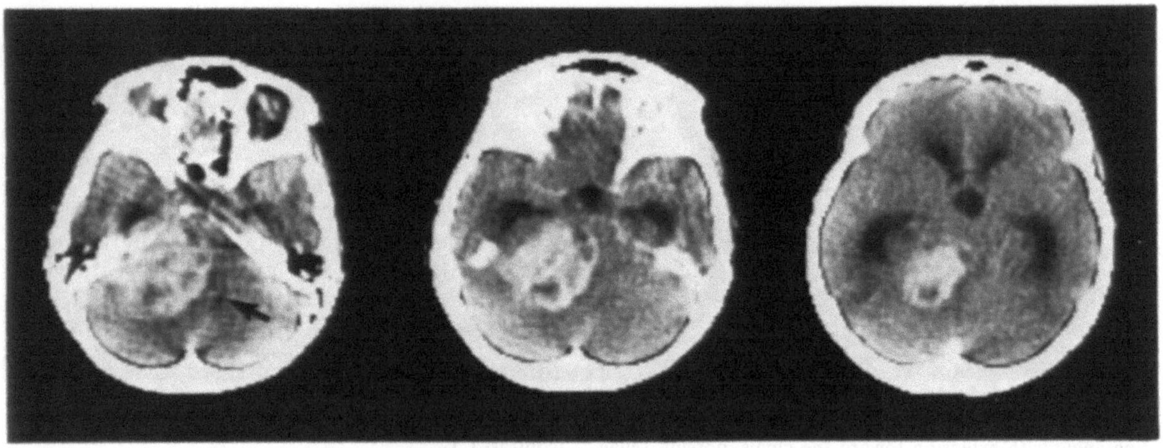

Fig. D 2.69. Large meningioma in the left cerebellopontine angle with foci of regressive change in a 50-year-old woman. There is compression and displacement of the aqueduct and fourth ventricle (*arrow*) causing obstructive hydrocephalus. Postcontrast CT

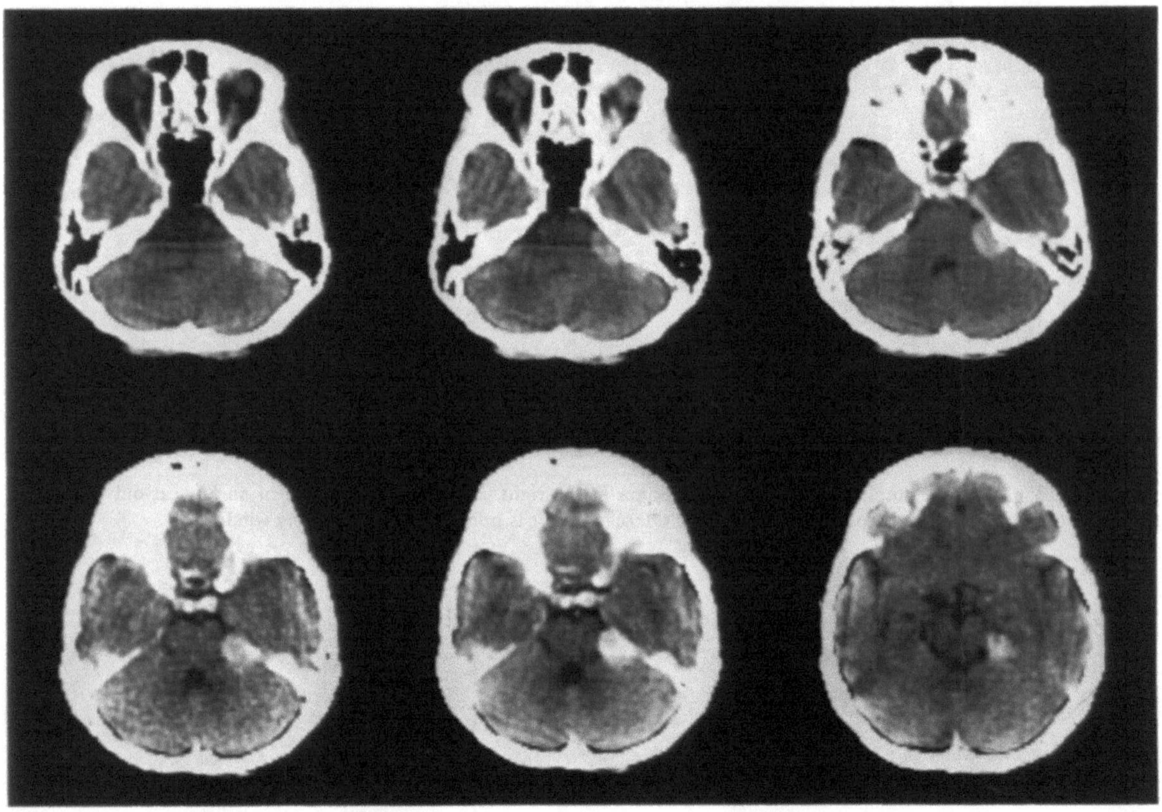

Fig. D 2.70. Small meningioma in the right cerebellopontine angle of a 53-year-old woman. The lesion is clearly visible on the noncontrast scans (*left*) and shows marked contrast enhancement (*center* and *right*). Note amputation of the ambient cistern by the upward-projecting tumor. The marked hyperdensity of the lesion on plain scans would not be consistent with acoustic neurinoma

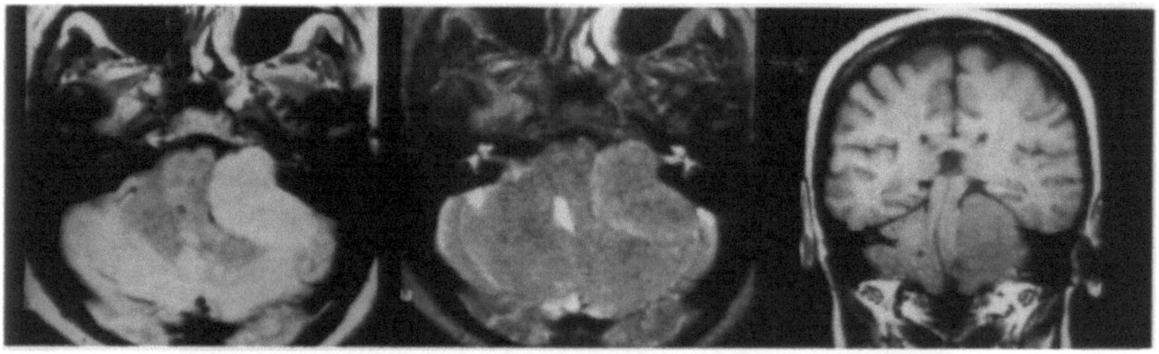

Fig. D 2.71. Large meningioma of the right cerebellopontine angle in a 45-year-old woman with a 6-month progressive history of tinnitus and hypoacusis on the right side and ataxia. MR: *left* SE 1500/30, *center* SE 2500/120, *right* SE 500/30 coronal. The tumor, slightly hyperintense on the proton-density image (*left*), is compressing and displacing the brainstem and cerebellum. The tumor is isointense on the T1-weighted image

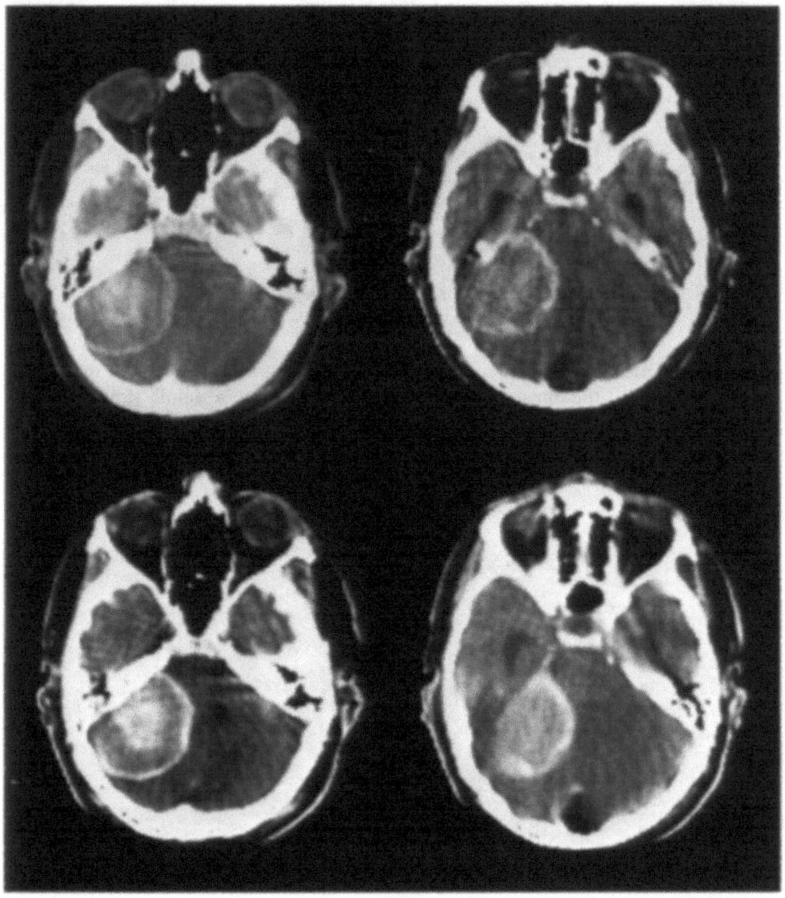

Fig. D 2.72. Infratentorial meningioma along the border of the left pyramid in a 65-year-old man. The CT appearance is not characteristic of meningioma, the bull's-eye pattern resulting from asbestos-like calcifications at the center and periphery of the mass. Note the straight, oblique demarcation of the tumor at higher levels by the tentorium. *Upper* scans are precontrast, *lower* scans postcontrast. The tumor shows minimal enhancement

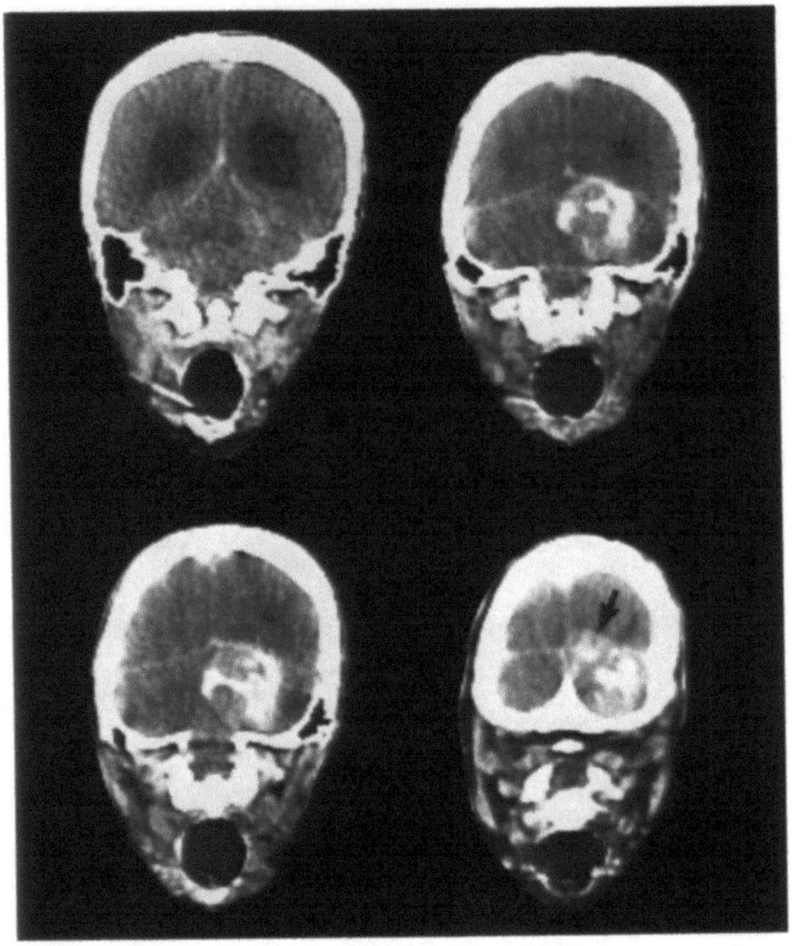

Fig. D 2.73. Partially calcified subtentorial meningioma in a 59-year-old man. The coronal scans at the most posterior level demonstrate a small supratentorial component (*arrow*). Marked obstructive hydrocephalus is present. Postcontrast CT

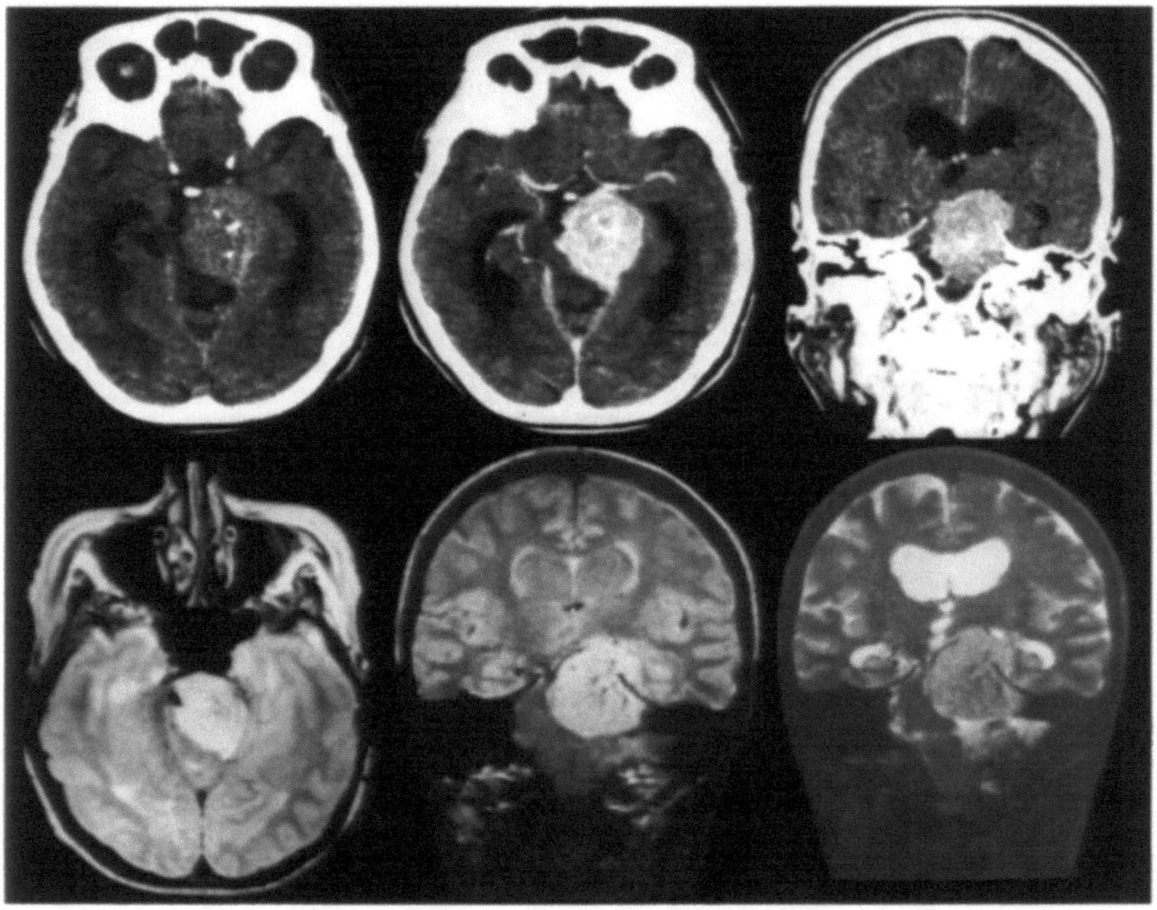

a–c

d–f

Fig. D 2.74 a–f. Supra- and infratentorial meningioma on the right side in a 61-year-old woman with a 2-year history of progressive right-sided hemiparesis. CT: **a** precontrast, **b** postcontrast, **c** postcontrast coronal. MR: **d** SE 3000/30, **e** SE 3000/30 coronal, **f** SE 3000/90 coronal. Plain CT demonstrates flecks of calcification in a slightly hyperdense mass. The predominantly infratentorial tumor enhances brightly (**b, c**) on postcontrast scans. The lesion is slightly hyperintense on proton-density MR sequences (**d, e**), the calcium deposits producing a signal void. The T2-weighted image demonstrates the relation of the tumor to the tentorium

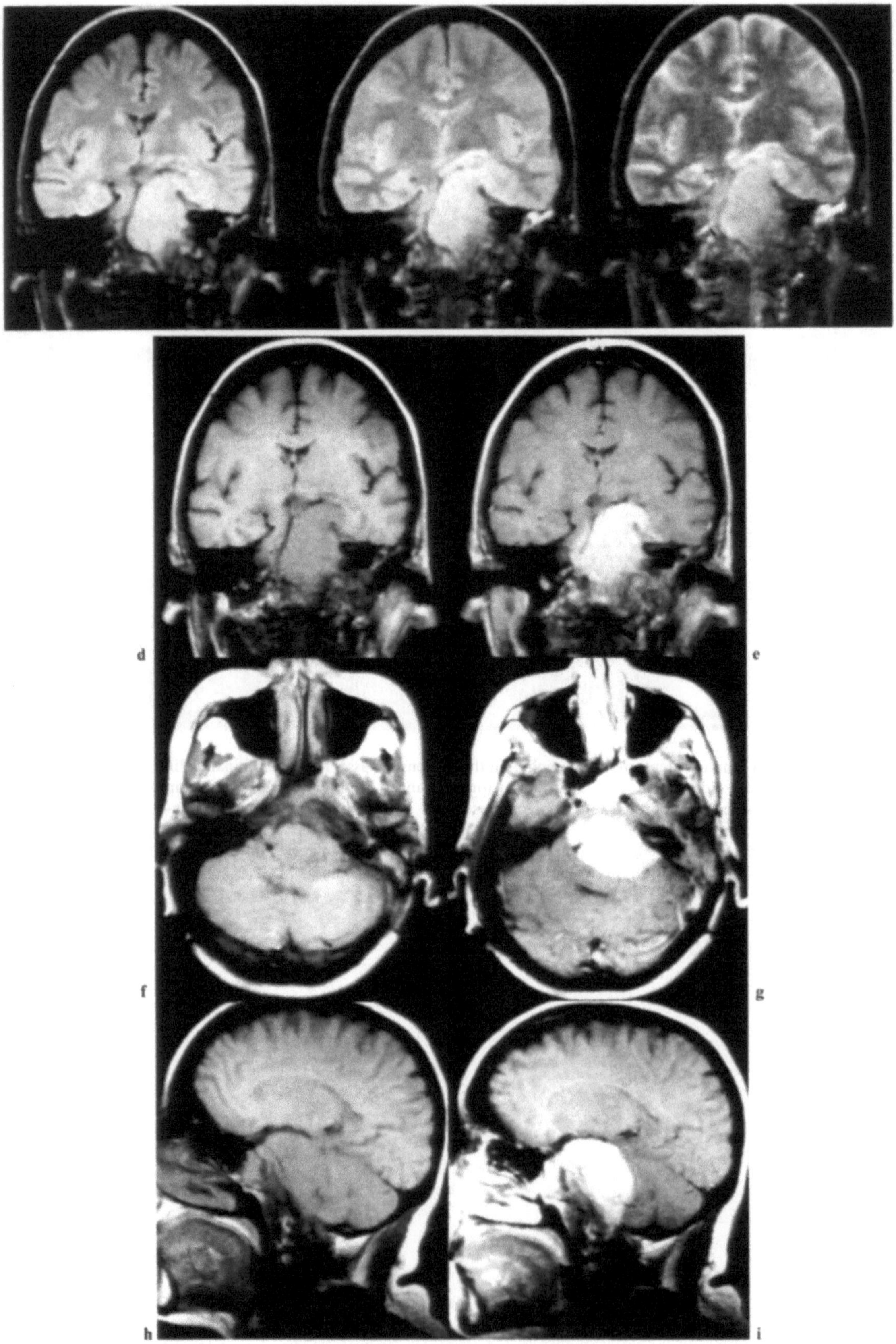
a–c
d
e
f
g
h
i

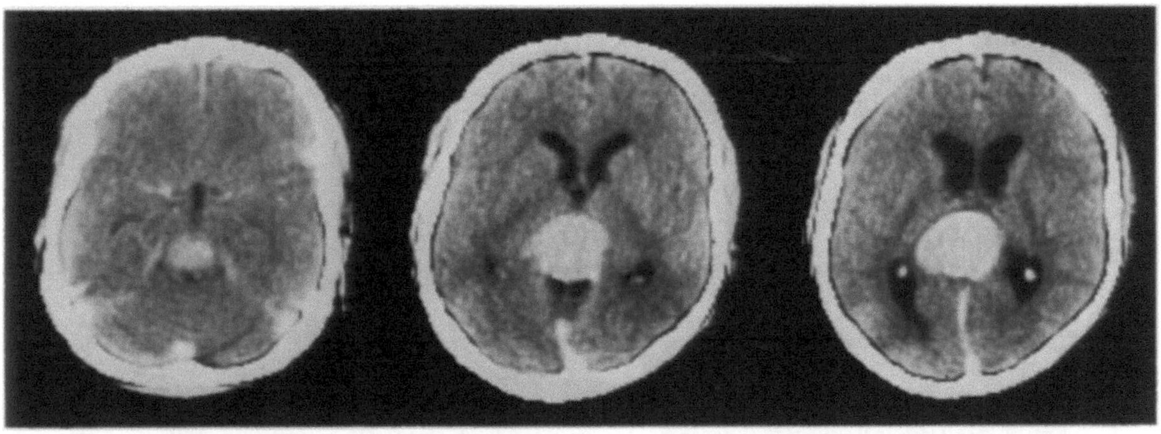

Fig. D 2.76. Meningioma occupying the tentorial incisure in a 44-year-old man. The relations of the basal part of the tumor to the tentorial margin on both sides are more consistent with meningioma than with a pineal neoplasm. Scans reveal stippled calcifications in the tumor (*left*) and homogeneous contrast enhancement. The ventricles are dilated by obstruction to CSF flow in the region of the aqueduct. Postcontrast CT

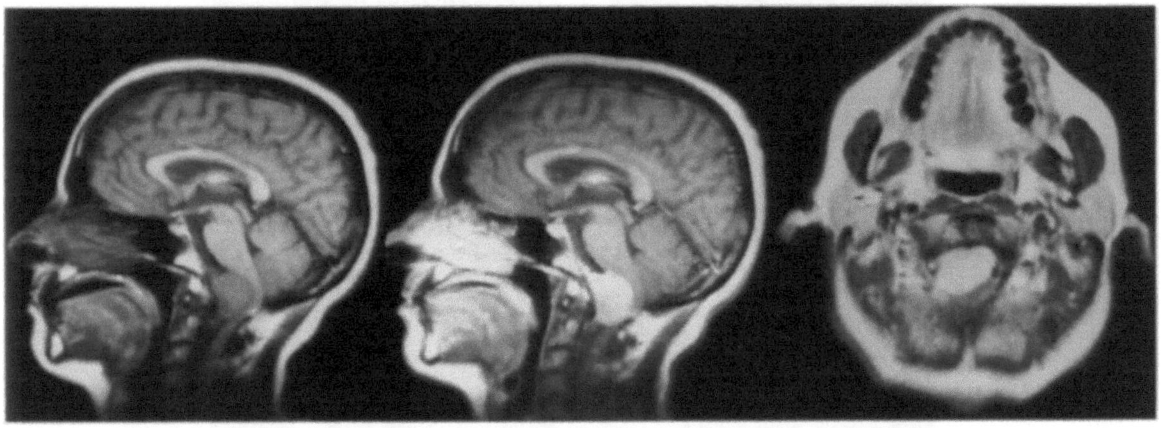

Fig. D 2.77. Meningioma at the craniocervical junction in a 43-year-old woman with a history of progressive tetraparesis in previous years. MR *left* SE 500/30 sagittal, *center* SE 500/30 sagittal post Gd-DTPA, *right* SE 500/30 axial post Gd-DTPA. The intensely enhancing tumor (*center*) is causing severe compression of the medulla oblongata and spinal cord

Fig. D 2.75a–i. Recurrent meningioma of the right petroclival area in a 51-year-old woman with headache, mild left-sided hemiparesis, peripheral facial paresis on the right side, right-sided trigeminal hypoesthesia, and complete hearing loss in the right ear. MR: **a** SE 1600/30, **b** SE 1600/90, **c** SE 1600/150, **d** SE 400/30, **e** SE 400/30 post Gd-DTPA (all coronal); **f** SE 400/30, **g** SE 400/30 post Gd-DTPA (both axial); **h** SE 400/30, **i** SE 400/30 post Gd-DTPA (both parasagittal). The gadolinium-enhanced T1-weighted parasagittal image demonstrates the hyperintense tumor riding broadly on the clivus in the area of the cerebellopontine angle. The mass is causing marked compression of the brainstem and cerebellum

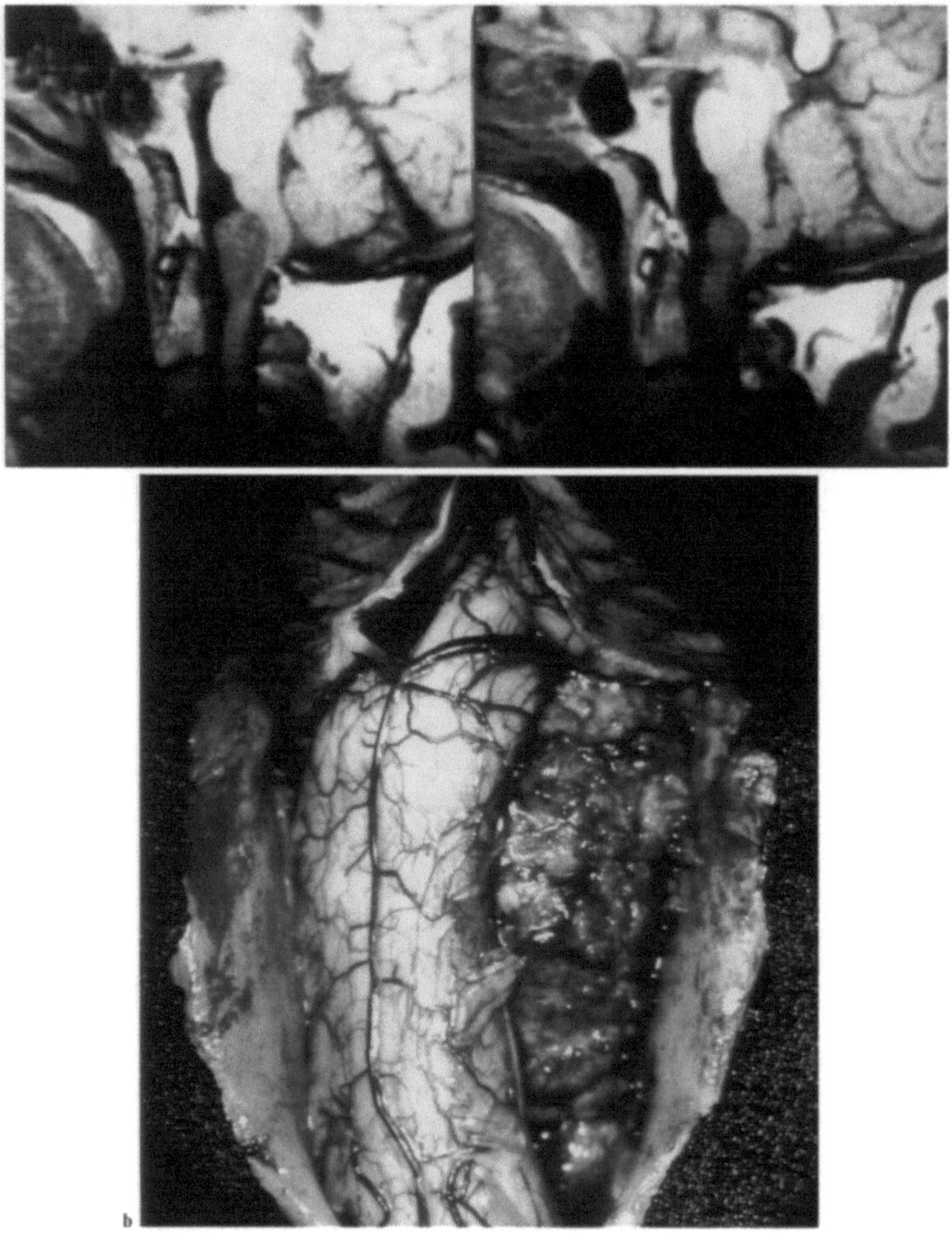

Fig. D 2.78 a, b. Meningioma of the craniocervical junction, chiefly involving the right side. The 64-year-old man presented with a 1-year history of progressive, incomplete tetraparesis and sensory symptoms of a transverse cord lesion. **a** MR, SE 500/30 sagittal. T1 weighting displays the tumor as a hypointense mass extending to C1/C2. **b** Appearance of the lesion at operation

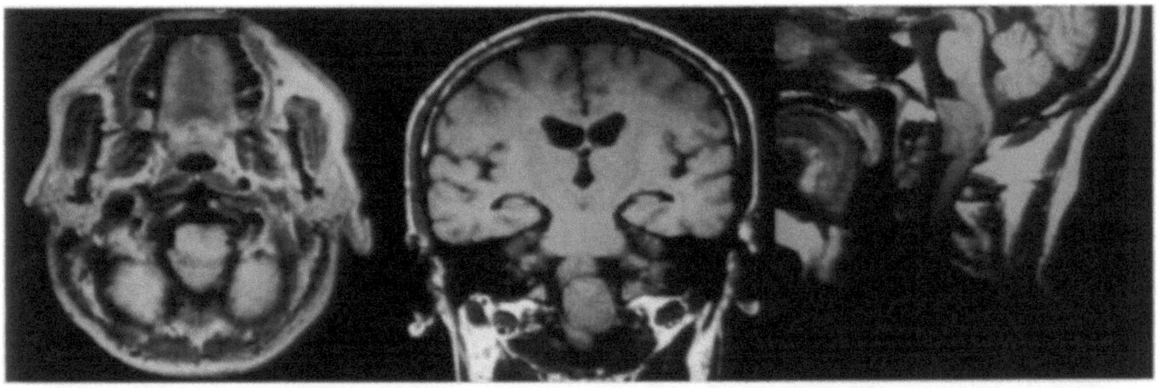

Fig. D 2.79. Meningioma at the craniocervical junction in a 41-year-old woman with a 9-month history of progressive tetraparesis and occipital headaches. MR: *left* SE 3000/30, *center* SE 700/30 coronal, *right* SE 500/30 sagittal. The lesion appears isointense to brain on the T1-weighted sequences (*center* and *right*). The tumor is severely compressing the brainstem from the right side on the coronal view (*center*) and from the anterior side on the sagittal view (*right*)

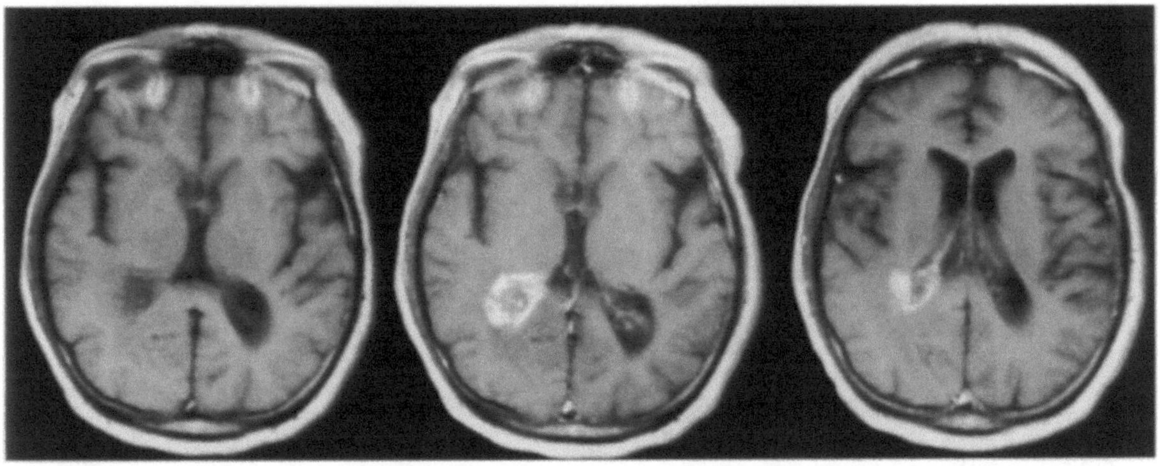

Fig. D 2.80. Atypical choroid plexus meningioma in the area of the left trigone in a 45-year-old man with a 5-month history of headaches. Neurologic exam was negative. MR: *left* SE 400/30, *center* SE 400/30 post Gd-DTPA, *right* SE 400/30 post Gd-DTPA. The region of the left occipital horn enhances intensely with Gd-DTPA. The focus of lower signal at the center of the mass represents the calcified choroid plexus

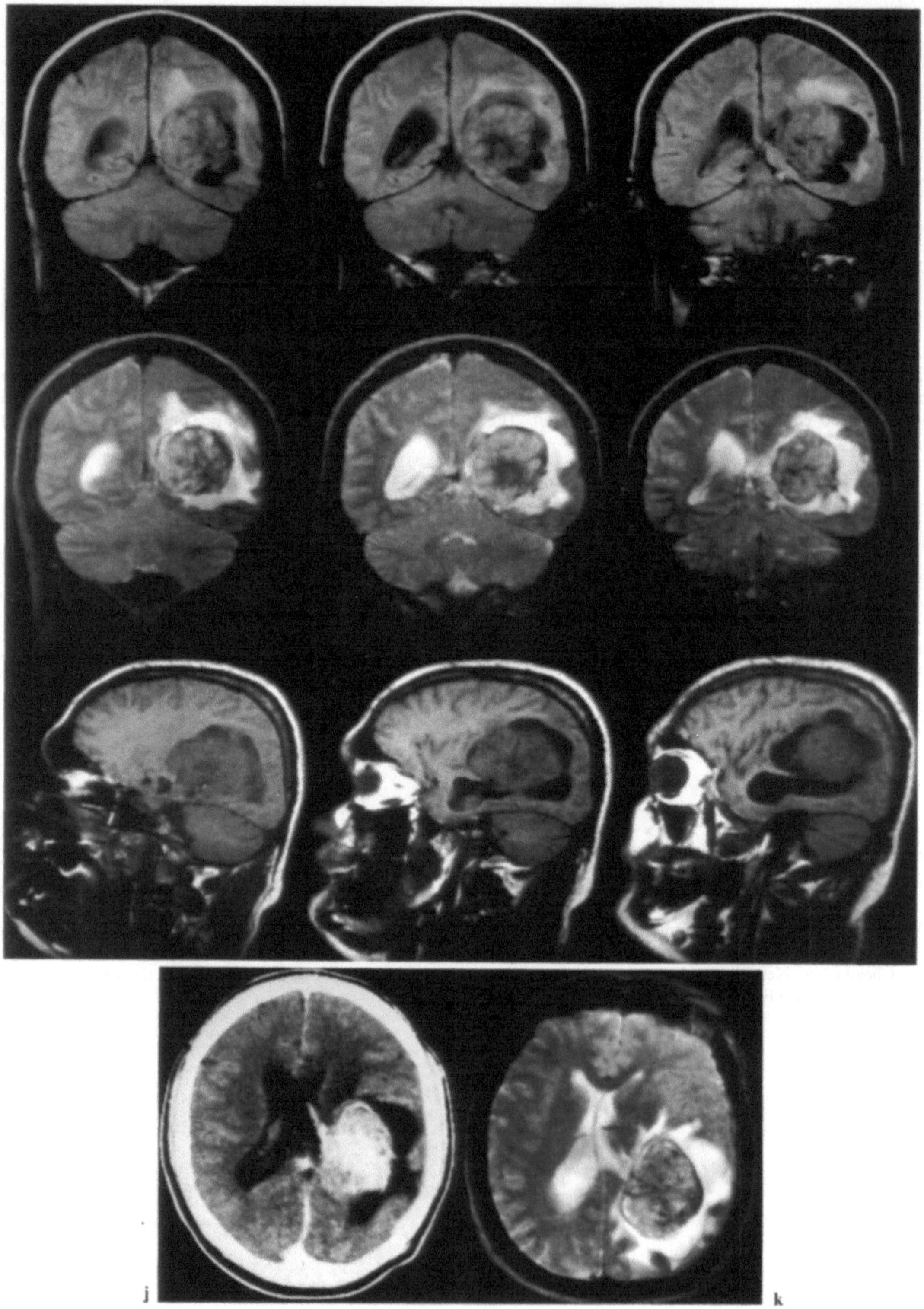

Fig. D 2.81 a–k. Large meningioma of the right occipital horn and trigone region in a 44-year-old man with a history of headaches for 6 months, lassitude of sudden onset, and altered mental status. MR: **a–c** SE 2500/30, **d–f** SE 2500/120 (all coronal), **g–i** SE 500/30 parasagittal, **k** SE 2500/120. CT: **j** postcontrast. T2-weighted sequences (**d–f, k**) demonstrate a sharply delineated, predominantly isointense lesion with a nonhomogeneous signal pattern. The surrounding edema is hyperintense

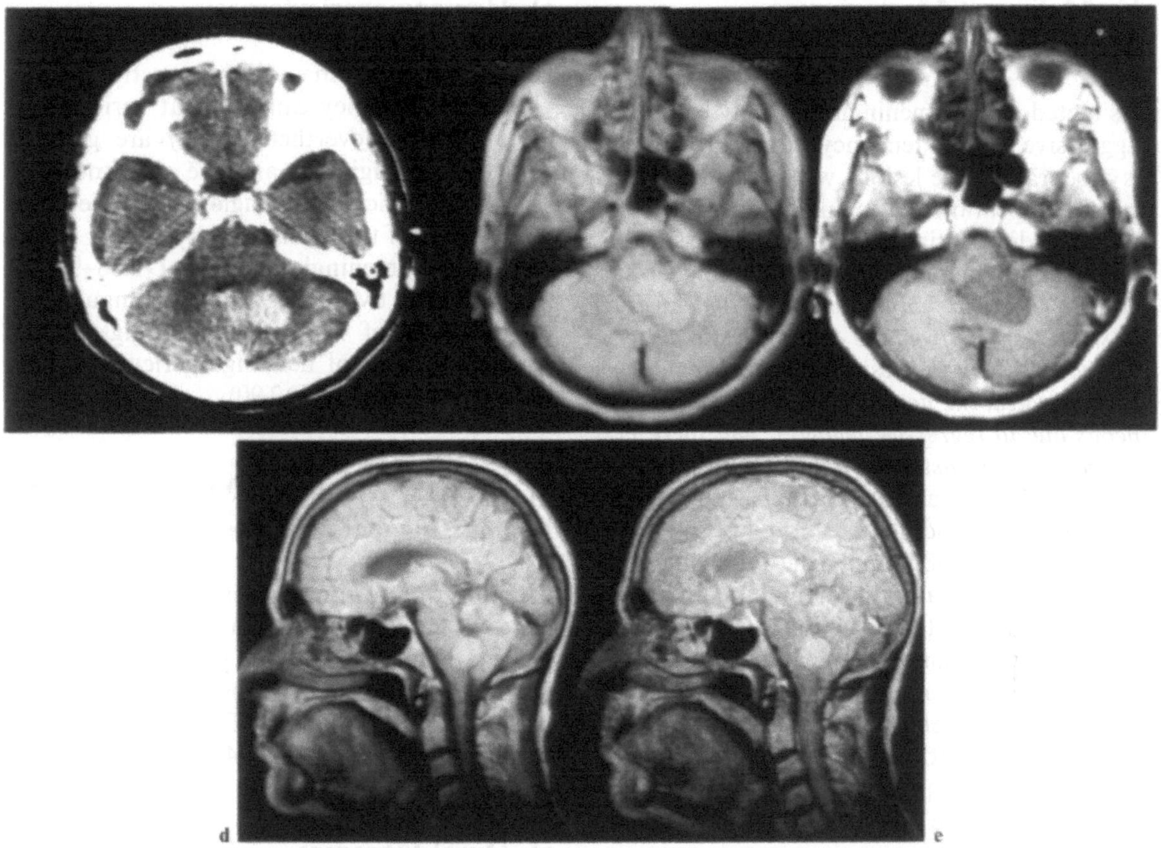

Fig. D 2.82 a–e. Meningioma in the lateral recess of the fourth ventricle in a 69-year-old woman with bilateral facial paresis and ataxia of stance and gait. CT: **a** postcontrast. MR: **b** SE 1600/35, **c** SE 400/35, **e** SE 1600/70; **d, e** sagittal. The tumor shows marked contrast enhancement on CT. T1-weighted MR (**c**) shows a hypointense mass completely filling the fourth ventricle. T2 weighting (**e**) demonstrates a hyperintense mass between the brainstem and cerebellum

b) Malignant Meningiomas, Meningeal Sarcomas

As stated earlier, meningiomas may exhibit an aggressive growth tendency. If the growth rate is moderate, these lesions will present the typical CT appearance of meningiomas. But if the tumor dedifferentiates further, it is classified as a malignant meningioma or "meningeal sarcoma." *The CT features of these tumors differ in some respects from the characteristic pattern: The borders of the lesion appear irregular or even serrated, the density pattern is nonhomogeneous due to regressive changes, and there may be patchy contrast enhancement* (Figs. D2.83–87). Vassilouthis and Ambrose (1979) have reported similar findings.

New et al. (1982) apply the following criteria to the CT diagnosis of malignant meningioma: significant destruction of bone, irregular tumor margins, significant necrosis, little or no calcification, and fungoid spread of the tumor over the hemisphere. Shapir et al. (1983) describe an additional CT sign of malignant meningioma: the presence of a pathologic vein coursing from the margin of the tumor toward the midline.

A histologic diagnosis cannot be made with CT unless scans are able to demonstrate the site of tumor origin from the meninges (see Fig. D2.83).

c) Hemangiopericytomas

Hemangiopericytomas differ from true meningiomas in that they can occur at various sites in the body. Nevertheless, they are grouped with the meningiomas and are also known as "hemangiopericytic meningiomas." Indeed, the CT features of these tumors very closely resemble those of meningioma (Figs. D2.88–90, 92, 93), and the two types are indistinguishable on the basis of CT or MR findings. A few congenital cases of hemangiopericytoma have been described (Fig. D2.90).

d) Primary Meningeal Melanomas and Leptomeningeal Melanosis

Circumscribed primary meningeal melanomas have the same CT presentation as intracranial metastatic melanomas (see pp. 442–448).

Leptomeningeal melanosis without mass effect is not detectable by CT, as our own observations indicate (Fig. D2.94).

e) Dural Fibromas

In rare cases fibromas can arise from dural tissue. These lesions are indistinguishable from meningiomas on the CT scan (Fig. D2.91).

Fig. D2.83. Malignant meningioma of the left temporoparietal region in a 59-year-old woman. The tumor appears heterogeneous and shows patchy contrast enhancement. The knobbly appearance of the medial surface of the tumor is reminiscent of meningioma. Grade II–III perifocal edema is present. Midline structures are greatly displaced, and the contralateral ventricle is dilated (postcontrast CT). *Below:* Transverse brain section on the same plane as the CT scans (myelin sheath stain) shows the knob of tumor growth on the meninges with invasion of the white matter

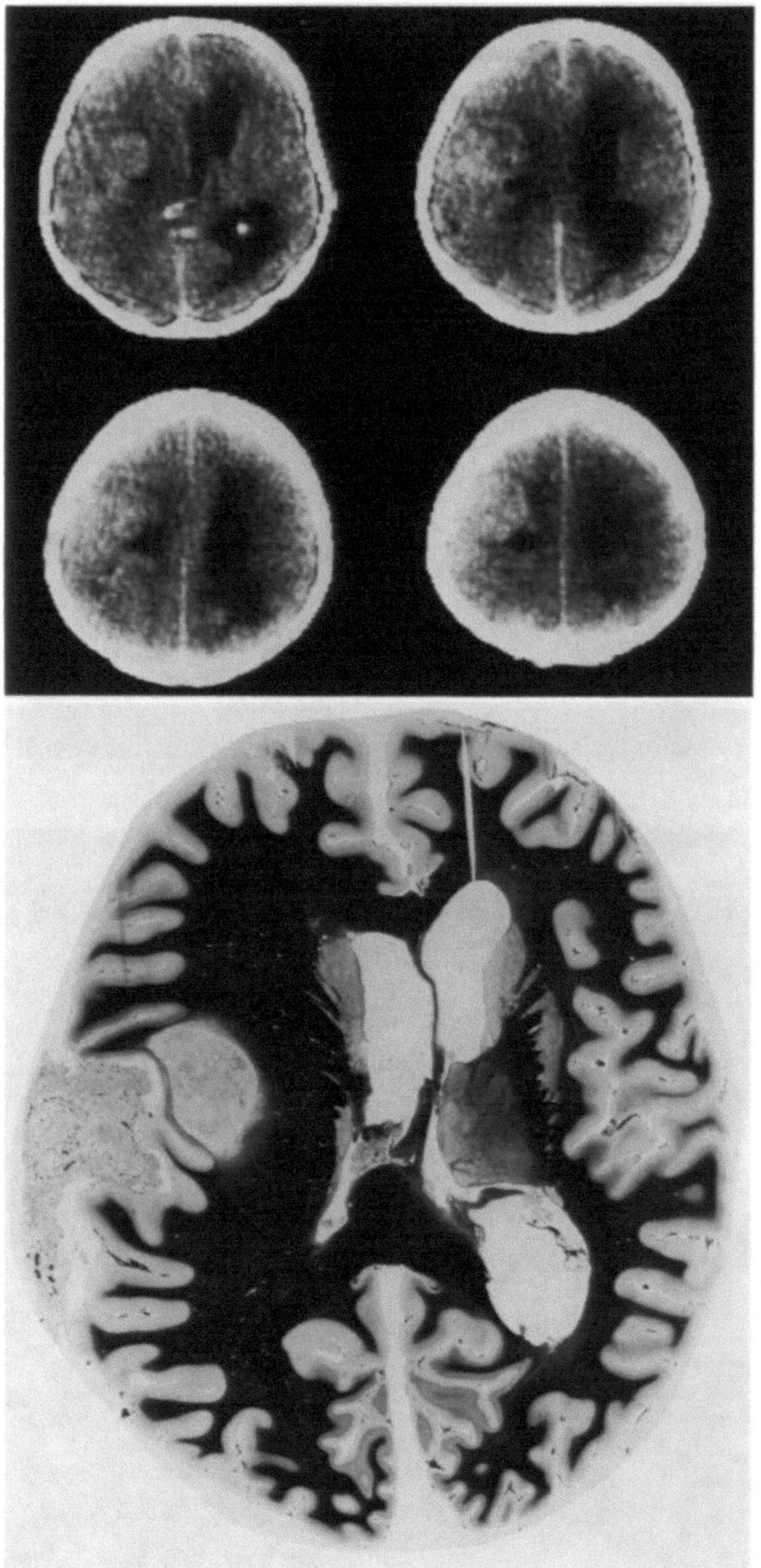

D2.84 ▶

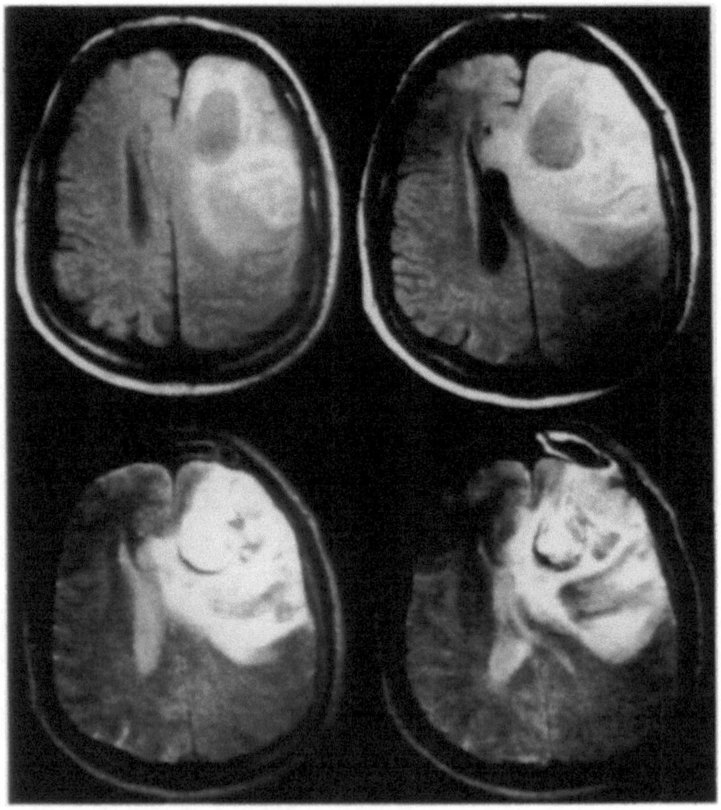

D2.85
▼

a–c

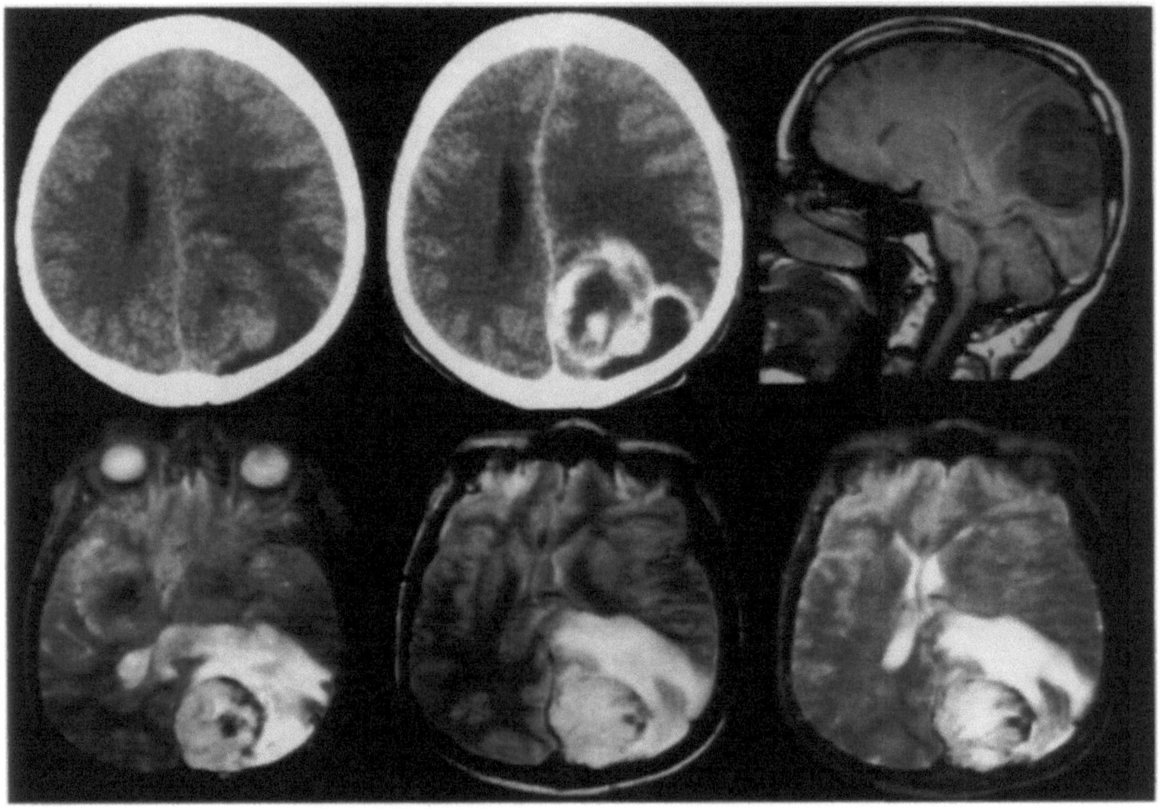

d–f

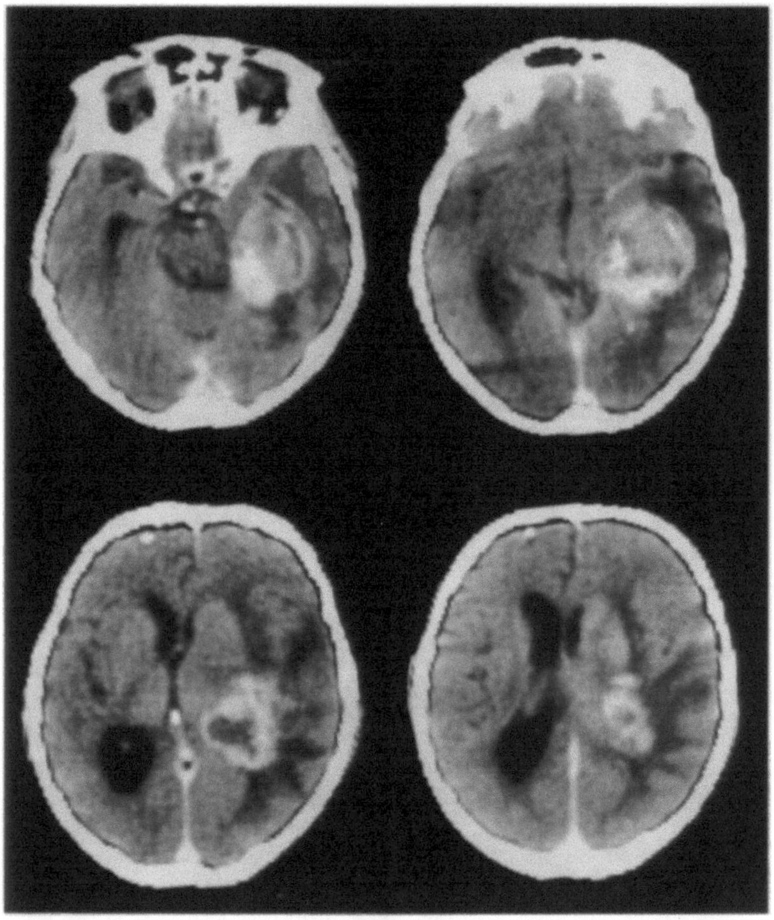

Fig. D 2.86. Malignant meningioma of the right temporobasal region arising from the tentorium in a 60-year-old man. CT findings are atypical and include numerous hypodense areas of regressive change within the lesion. Perifocal edema is marked, and there is moderate shift of midline structures. The brainstem is compressed in the tentorial incisure, and there is obstruction to CSF flow causing contralateral ventricular dilatation. CT findings do not permit a definitive diagnosis of meningioma. Postcontrast scans

Fig. D 2.84. Malignant meningioma in a 52-year-old man with a history of headache, seizures with an olfactory aura, and mild alteration in mental status in previous weeks. MR: *top* SE 2000/30, *bottom* SE 2000/120. Proton-density weighting reveals a hyperintense lesion with a central hypointense area and extreme mass effect (*top*). More structural details are appreciated on the T2-weighted sequences (*bottom*), although the margin between tumor and edema is poorly resolved

Fig. D 2.85 a–f. Recurrence of malignant meningioma in the right occipital region of a 59-year-old woman with headache, altered mental status, and left homonymous hemianopia. CT: **a** precontrast, **b** postcontrast. MR: **c** SE 700/30 parasagittal, **d** SE 3000/90, **e** SE 3000/30, **f** SE 3000/90. A garland pattern of enhancement is observed on postcontrast CT. The entire lesion appears hypointense and clearly delineated on the T1-weighted image (**c**). The signal pattern becomes nonhomogeneous and predominantly hyperintense on the proton-density image (**e**), peritumoral edema giving a bright signal. The T2-weighted images (**d, f**) display the edema clearly and show the mass compressing the right occipital horn and displacing the ventricular system toward the left

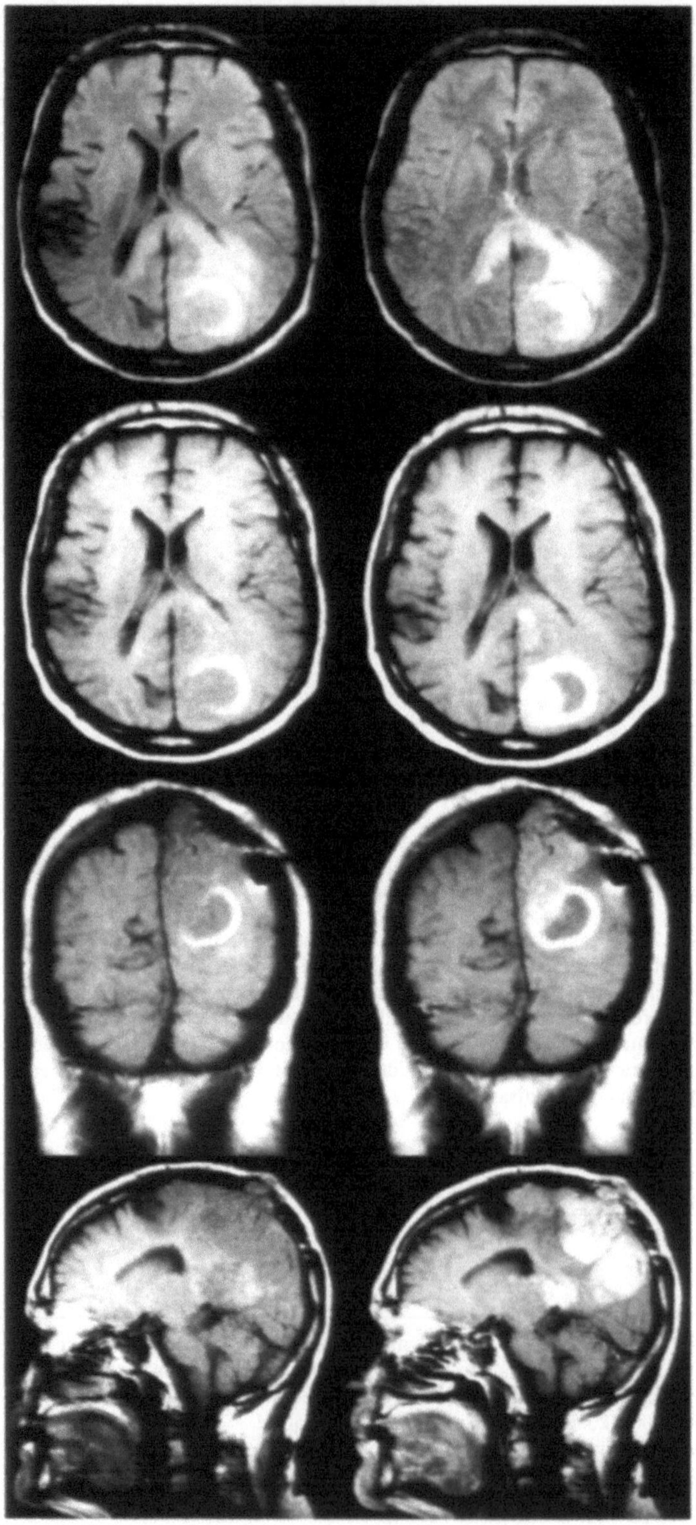

Fig. D 2.87 a–h. Recurrence of a mid- to posterior-third meningosarcoma on the right side with intratumoral hemorrhage in a 62-year-old man with left hemianopia and left-sided hemiparesis. MR: **a** SE 1600/35, **b** SE 1600/70, **c** SE 400/30, **d** SE 400/30 post Gd-DTPA, **e** SE 400/30 coronal, **f** SE 400/30 post Gd-DTPA coronal, **g** SE 400/30 sagittal, **h** SE 400/30 post Gd-DTPA sagittal. The intratumoral hemorrhage appears on the proton-density and T2-weighted images (**a, b**) as a laterally sited crescent of high signal intensity; edema is additionally visible on image **b**. The post-Gd-DTPA sequences (**d, f, h**) show enhancement of the solid, paramedian tumor component and capsule; the hemorrhage persists as a nonenhancing area of low signal intensity

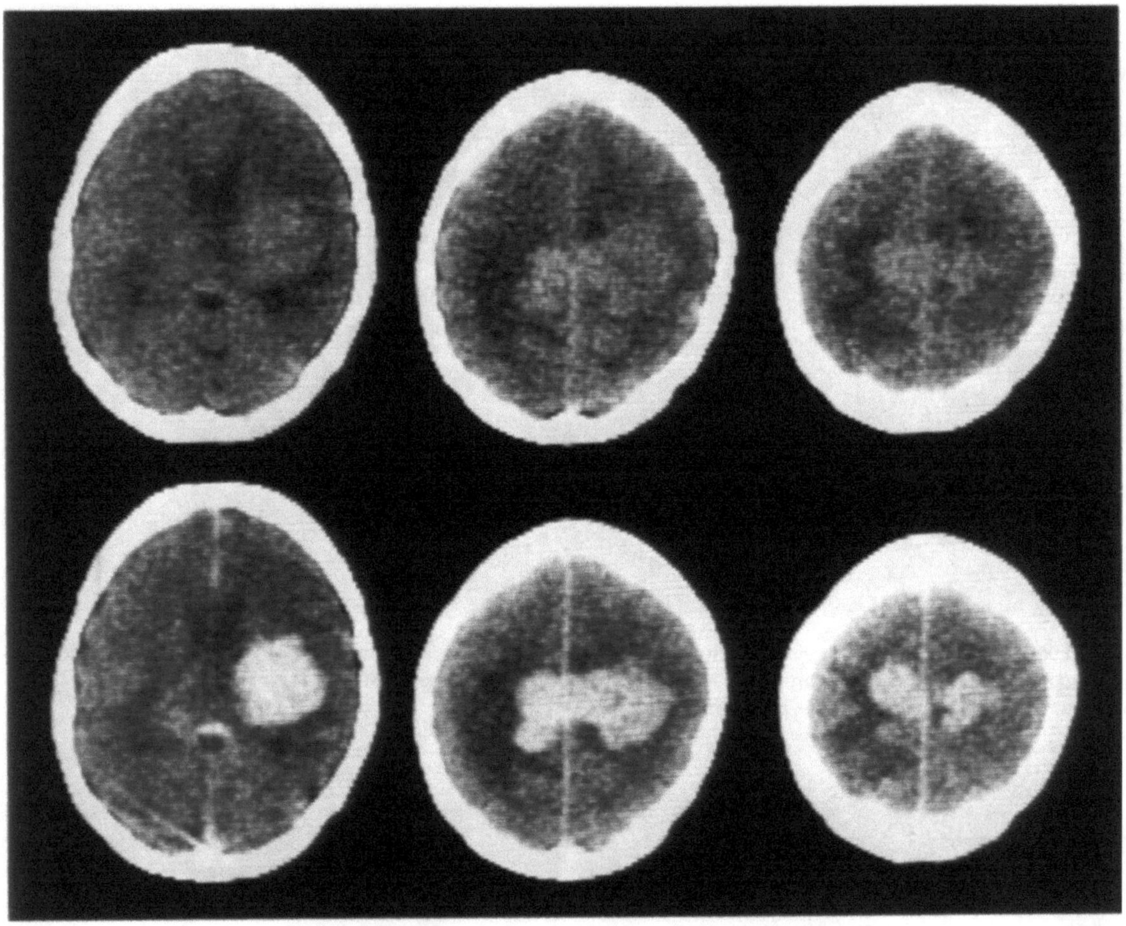

Fig. D 2.88. Hemangiopericytic meningioma with bilateral extension arising from the falx in a 49-year-old woman. The lesion is minimally hyperdense on the noncontrast CT scans (*top*) and on postcontrast scans shows the intense, homogeneous enhancement characteristic of meningiomas (*bottom*)

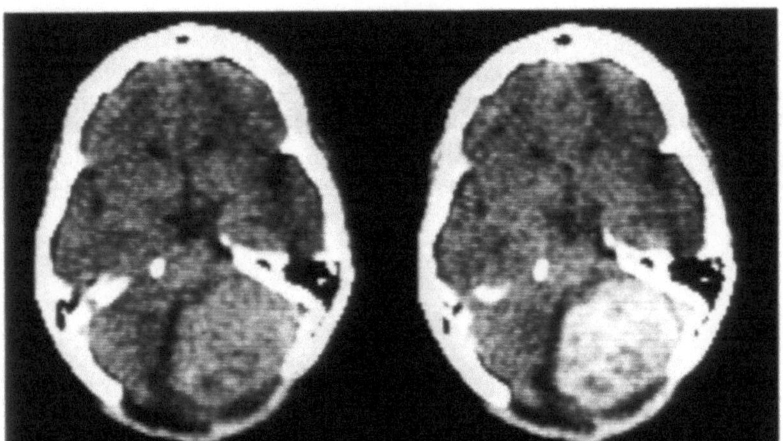

Fig. D 2.89. Large recurrence of hemangiopericytoma in the right posterior fossa. The tumor is clearly visible on the plain CT scan (*left*) by virtue of its increased density. Contrast enhancement is largely homogeneous (*right*). These CT findings are characteristic of meningioma

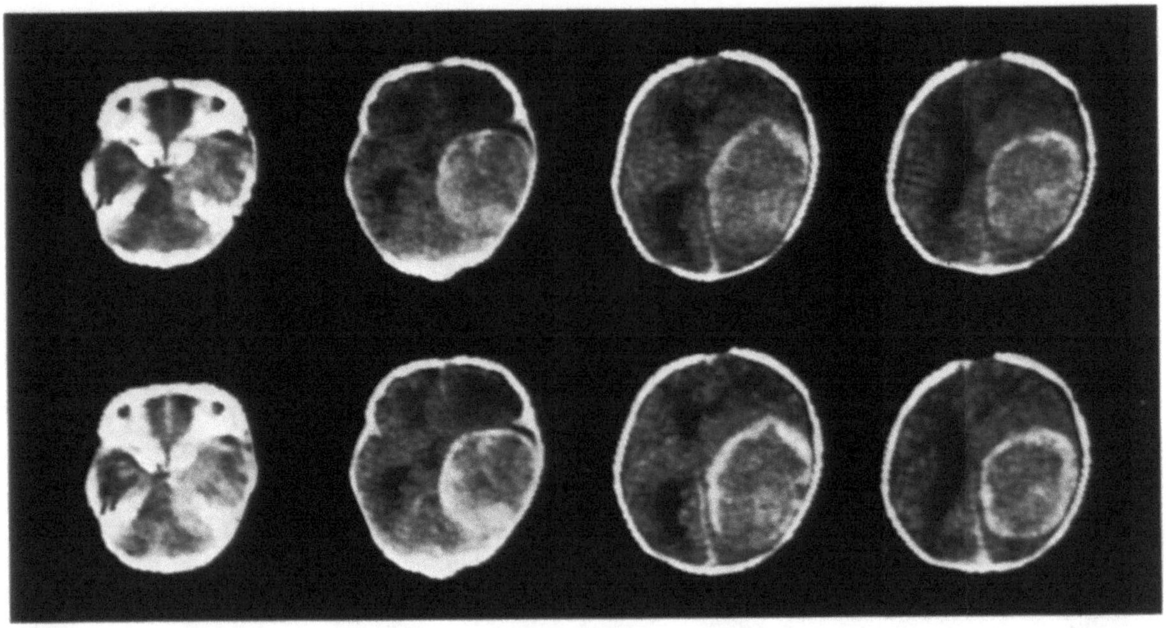

Fig. D 2.90. Congenital hemangiopericytoma in a 13-day-old infant. The tumor occupies large portions of the right cerebral hemisphere. The lesion presents a bull's-eye pattern with weak enhancement mostly at the periphery. *Top* precontrast CT, *bottom* postcontrast

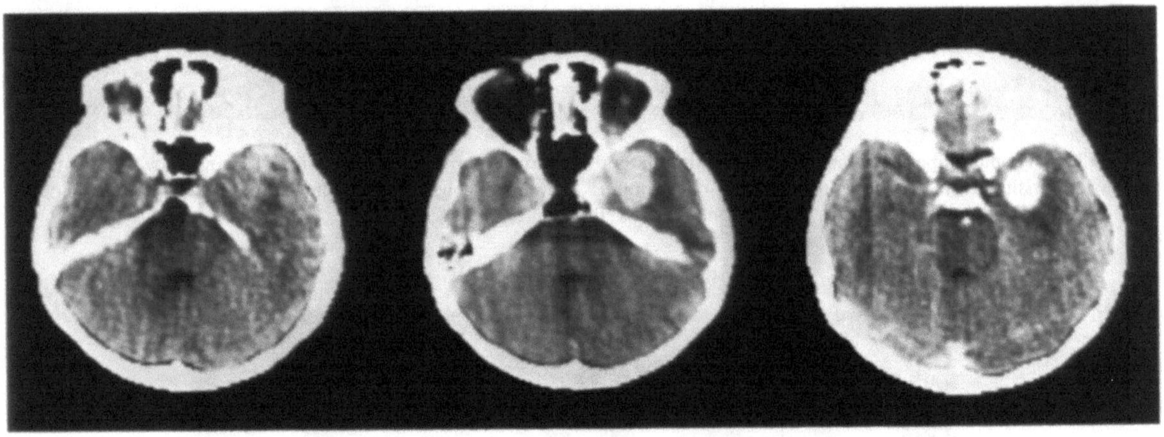

Fig. D 2.91. Dural fibroma in the right parasellar area of the middle fossa and below the temporal pole in a 62-year-old woman. CT findings are characteristic of meningioma. *Left* precontrast CT, *center* and *right* postcontrast

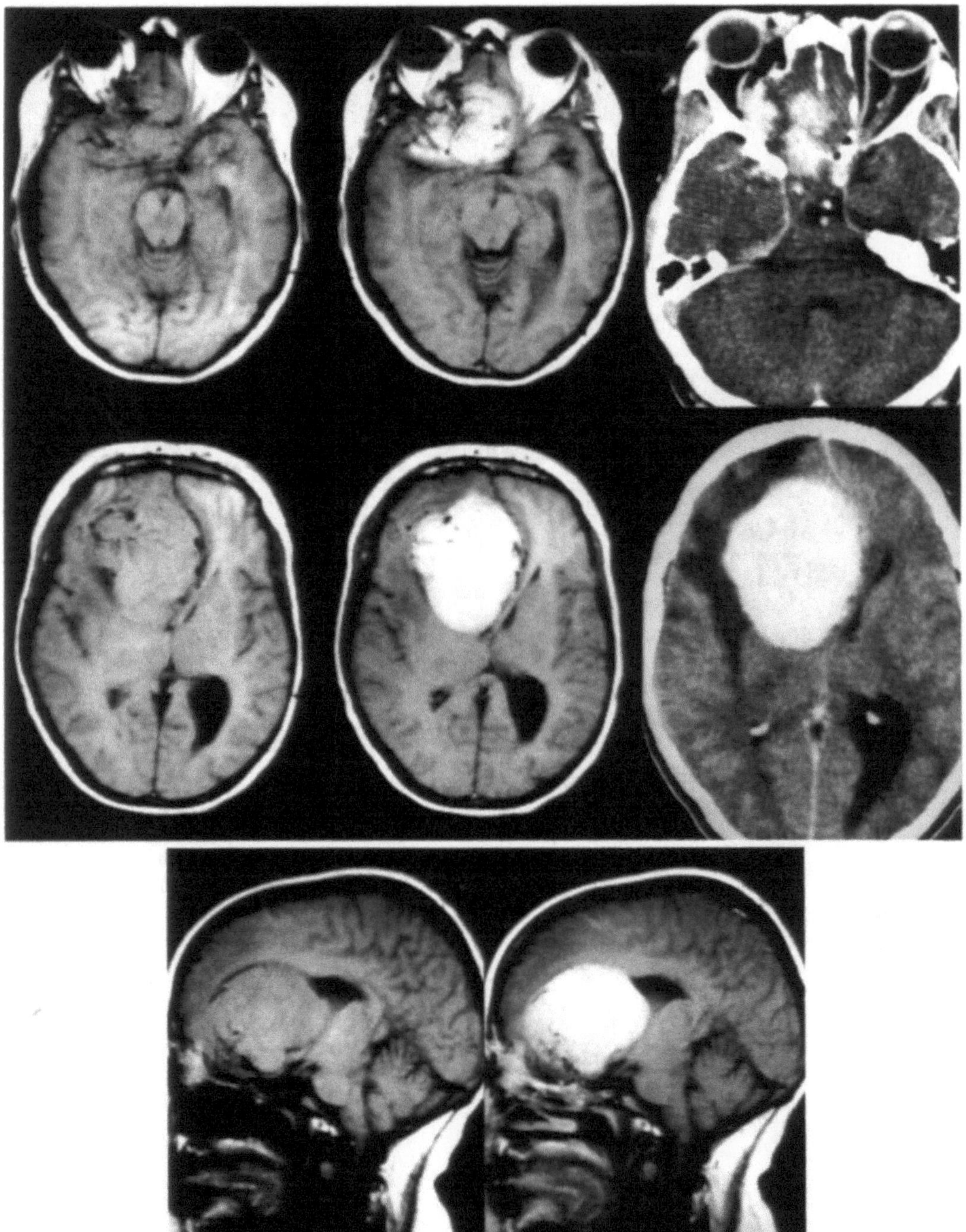

a–c

d–f

g h

Fig. D 2.92 a–h. Fist-size hemangiopericytoma of the left frontal region with destruction of the bony skull base in a 28-year-old woman with a 6-month history of frontal headaches. Patient presented with anosmia, bilateral papilledema, and bitemporal hemianopia. Postcontrast CT: **c, f.** MR: **a** SE 400/30, **b** SE 400/30 post Gd-DTPA, **d** SE 400/30, **e** SE 400/30 post Gd-DTPA, **g** SE 400/30, **h** SE 400/30 post Gd-DTPA parasagittal. CT reveals extensive destruction of the skull base with infiltration of the sphenoid sinus and ethmoid cells (**c**). The tumor enhances very brightly on the postcontrast scan (**f**). The lesion also shows intense enhancement with Gd-DTPA (**e, h**). The displaced pericallous artery and the tumor vessels appear as signal voids

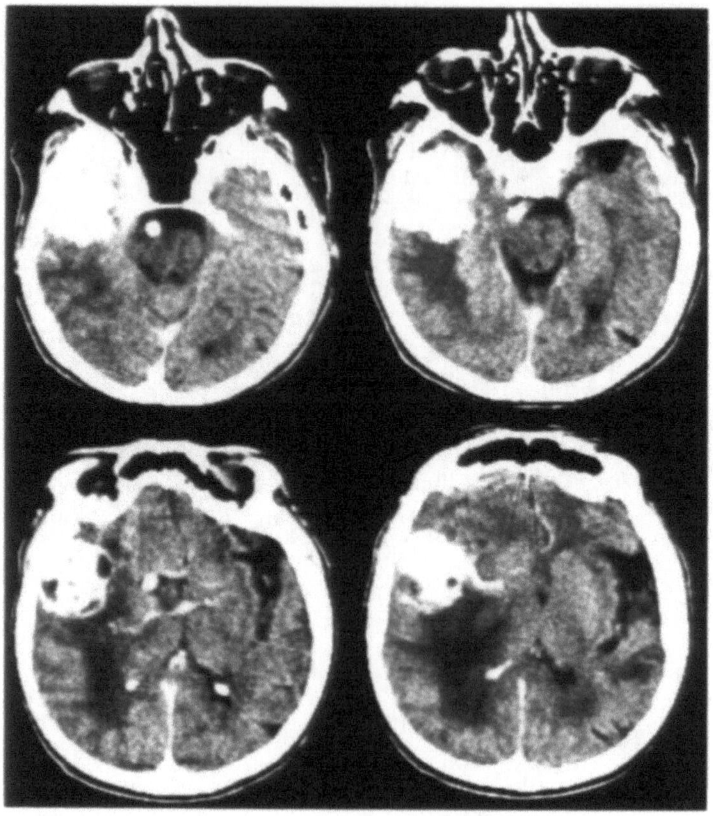

Fig. D2.93. Hemangiopericytoma of the left temporal region in a 72-year-old woman with increasing headaches and two episodes of syncope. She presented with mimic facial paralysis on the right side and mild dysphasia. Postcontrast CT scans show very dense enhancement of the tumor, which contains small cystic components. The entire left hemisphere is involved by edema

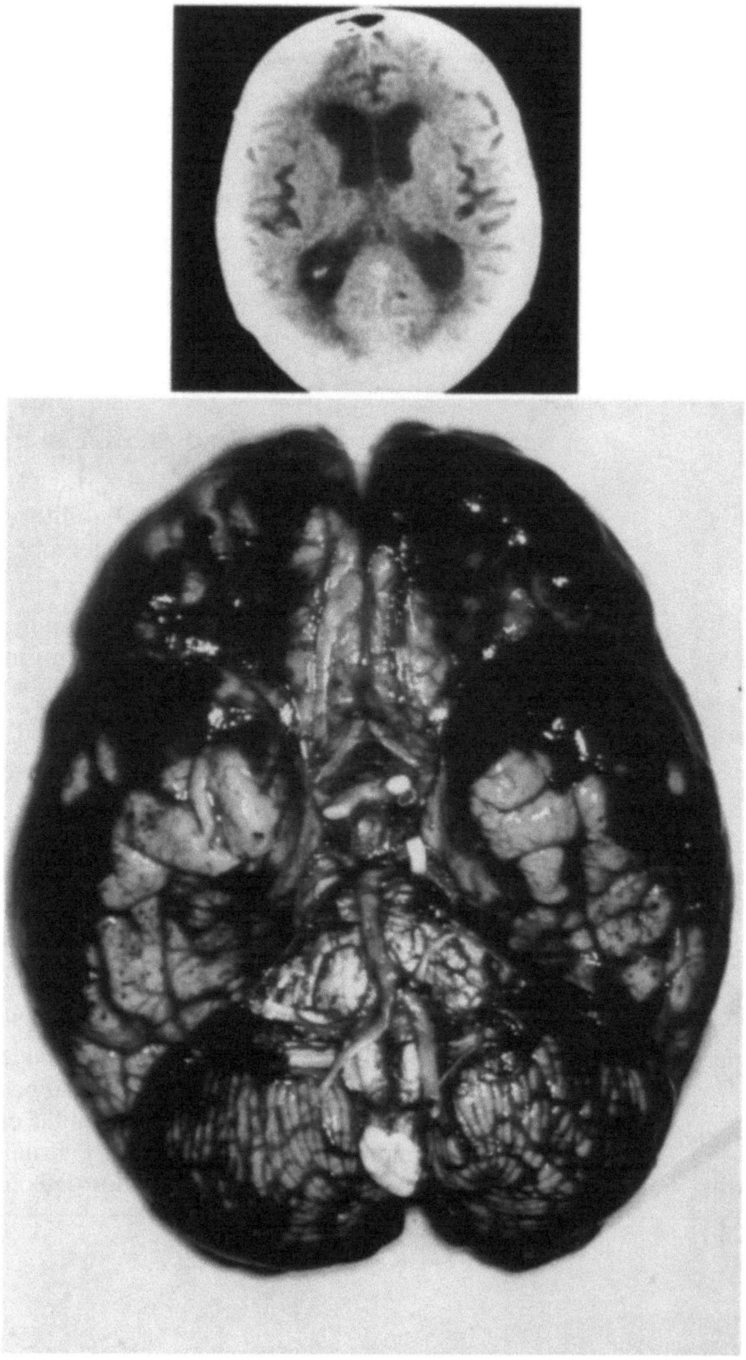

Fig. D 2.94. Primary melanomatous leptomeningeosis in a 58-year-old man with generalized seizures and altered mental status; no headaches, meningism, or cranial neuropathies. Contrast-enhanced CT (*top*) shows signs of cerebral atrophy with expansion of the internal and external CSF spaces. Photo of the necropsy specimen (*bottom*) shows the base and convexity covered with dark melanomatous masses that were not visible on the CT scan

3. Neurinomas

Incidence	5%–8% of all brain tumors
Age predilection	35–60 years
Sex predilection	2:1 female preponderance
Typical sites	1. Arising from statoacoustic nerve in cerebellopontine angle 2. Arising from trigeminal nerve at base of middle fossa
Main clinical features	Site 1: hearing loss, vestibular disorders, later trigeminal hypoesthesia Site 2: pain and sensory disturbances in distribution of trigeminal nerve
Skull radiograph	Site 1: frequent widening of internal auditory canal Site 2: well-defined bone defect at trigeminal impression of petrous pyramid
Angiography	Displacement of blood vessels by tumor, faint tumor staining due to increased supply by normal vessels, slight blush
Other contrast studies	Even small tumors can be demonstrated by cisternography
CT	
Noncontrast scan	Tumors are very often isodense and so usually not directly visualized; indirect signs only when neurinoma large enough to displace or obliterate fourth ventricle or expand or obliterate pontocerebellar cistern
Contrast enhancement	Always pronounced, mostly homogeneous
Postcontrast appearance	Solid tumor nodule in cerebellopontine angle or at medial base of middle fossa. Perifocal edema with larger tumors. Tumors smaller than 0.5 cm (especially intracanalicular lesions) are poorly visualized and usually require air cisternography for detection

MR	
Noncontrast scan	Tumor hypo- to isointense on T1-weighted sequences and poorly demarcated from surrounding brain. Tumor gives higher signal on T2-weighted images, but borders may still be poorly defined
Gadolinium enhancement	Very intense
Post Gd-DTPA appearance	Marked signal increase even in intracanalicular portion of acoustic neurinoma

Differential diagnosis

Site 1	Site 2
Meningioma	Meningioma
Metastasis	Pilocytic astrocytoma
Ependymoma	Gangliocytoma
Glomus tumor	Giant aneurysm
Angioblastoma	
Aneurysm	
Ectatic basilar artery	
Choroid plexus papilloma	
Cerebellar sarcoma	
Abscess	

Reports in the literature place the incidence of intracranial neurinomas at 3%–8% of all brain tumors. The incidence in our series was 6.6% (565 tumors). Most patients are between 35 and 60 years of age, although some cases occur in adolescence. Females are affected about twice as often as males. Neurinomas are histologically benign (grade I).

Typical Sites

a) Acoustic Neurinomas

These tumors originate from the *statoacoustic nerve*, and most lie in the cerebellopontine angle. Tumor growth begins in the auditory canal, usually on the vestibular nerve, and the tumor expands the canal as it enlarges. The lesions vary greatly in size. They do not infiltrate adjacent structures, but their expansive growth can distort the brainstem and displace the cerebellar hemisphere.

Neurinomas vary in consistency from firm to soft, depending on the presence and degree of regressive changes. Cystic components are rare, although arachnoid cysts of varying size may form on the surface of the lesion.

The facial nerve may be displaced, thinned, and stretched as it crosses the tumor capsule. In some cases the nerve cannot be separated from the tumor itself.

Bilateral acoustic neurinomas are known and may represent a forme fruste of von Recklinghausen's neurofibromatosis. The tumors may also occur in conjunction with meningiomas (see Figs. D3.20, 21).

The main clinical manifestation of acoustic neurinoma is unilateral hearing loss, which may be partial or complete. This may be associated with a vestibular disturbance. With larger tumors, otoneurologic disorders may be accompanied by purely neurologic symptoms (facial or trigeminal neuropathies) and by evidence of cerebellar dysfunction. Hydrocephalic headache and papilledema may occur with tumors large enough to obstruct CSF flow.

b) Trigeminal Neurinomas

Neurinomas arising from the *trigeminal nerve* are far less common than acoustic neurinomas. They lie anterior to or within Meckel's cave, causing neuralgia (constant pain!) and paresthesias in the distribution of the trigeminal nerve.

Involvement of other cranial nerves (caudal group) is extremely rare and produces corresponding neuropathic symptoms.

Additional Diagnostic Procedures

Standard skull radiographs and special views may demonstrate expansion of the internal auditory canal by acoustic neurinoma (40%–80% of cases according to the literature, see Canigiani 1978). Films may additionally show erosion of the pyramidal apex (Figs. D 3.1, 3.5). Secondary signs of intracranial hypertension are seen only with very large tumors.

With trigeminal neurinoma, radiographs will often show a clearly defined bone defect at the trigeminal impression of the petrous pyramid.

Serial cerebral angiograms in acoustic neurinoma will demonstrate displacement of the anterior inferior cerebellar artery, and faint tumor staining may be evident.

Other contrast studies include pneumoencephalography and especially cisternography with positive contrast media. Positive cisternography can detect even small tumors that are confined to the internal auditory canal (Wende and Nakayama 1978) (Fig. D 3.10).

a) Acoustic Neurinomas

Computed Tomography
(Figs. D 3.1–10, 20)

Noncontrast Scan
The tumor tissue is *predominantly isodense and so is not directly visualized.* In our series 61% of 190 acoustic neurinomas were isodense on the unenhanced scan. Minimal degrees of hypo- or hyperdensity may be noted in some cases. Some isodense tumors are detected from the presence of perifocal edema. *Cystic components* outside the tumor also may be visualized (Fig. D 3.3). A major indirect sign of tumor is *displacement of the fourth ventricle* (60% of cases, see Fig. D 3.8). *Nonvisualization of the fourth ventricle* with correctly executed CT is another indirect sign of tumor (17% of cases in our series), as is *dilatation or unilateral absence of the pontocerebellar cistern.* Very large tumors may elevate and twist the ipsilateral temporal horn and compress the brainstem (Figs. D 3.14–16).

CT scanning with a large window width will reveal *expansion of the internal auditory canal* and other changes in the bony pyramid when the scan is performed on the appropriate plane (Figs. D 3.1, 2).

Postcontrast Scan
Almost all neurinomas undergo *rapid contrast enhancement* that is maximal at only 2 min after injection and fades thereafter.

Most neurinomas are visible only on the postcontrast CT scan. Enhancement is intense, averaging 21 HU in our series. Of 194 neurinomas evaluated by postcontrast CT, 173 (89.2%) enhanced, the great majority homogeneously. Only necrotic or cystic components failed to enhance, causing a distinctive ring pattern to appear in some cases (Fig. D 3.4). Very large acoustic neurinomas always contain foci of regressive change that are easily recognized on the CT scan (Figs. D 3.4, 5, 9).

Tumor size is a key factor determining CT detectability. *Acoustic neurinomas less than 0.5 cm in diameter are rarely detected on axial CT scans.*

The extent of the tumor and its relation to the tentorium are appreciated better on craniocaudal projections than on axial views.

Acoustic neurinomas too small to be detected on plain CT or CT enhanced with iodinated contrast media can be made visible on CT scans by the intrathecal injection of Amipaque or Solutrast M. The contrast medium enters the basal cisterns, and the tumor is outlined by a filling defect at the acoustic pore.

Combined Use of Computed Tomography and Pneumocisternography

The combined use of CT and pneumocisternography, first described by Sortland in 1978, has proved to be a major advance in the diagnostic imaging of small acoustic neurinomas. This technique provides optimum visualization of the pontocerebellar cistern and internal auditory canal, making it possible to detect even very small intracanalicular growths. Kricheff et al. (1979) and Wende (1980) reported similar results (Figs. D 3.7, 10).

Examination Technique. CT is performed before and after i.v. contrast injection to exclude a large mass lesion in the cerebellopontine angle. If the scans are negative, lumbar puncture is performed with the patient in the sitting position. The head is inclined toward the unaffected side, and 5–6 ml of air is injected through the lumbar needle at a fairly rapid rate. In this position the air will enter the affected pontocerebellar cistern and internal auditory canal. The patient is then placed on his side and moved into the CT scanner, which must allow thin-slice scanning (5 mm maximum) with a high-resolution matrix (e.g., 320×320). The patient's head is rotated about 45° so that the air-filled pontocerebellar cistern and internal auditory canal are uppermost. With proper slice selection, the cerebellopontine angle will be visualized on the CT scan. The contralateral cerebellopontine angle region can be examined next by turning the patient to the opposite side. Intracanalicular acoustic neurinomas, even those with extracanalicular extension, can be demonstrated with great clarity (Fig. D 3.10).

The foregoing method is simple and provides a rich source of diagnostic information. Moreover, it is safe in cases where no contraindications exist to lumbar puncture. Mild headache is reported by some patients and is the only known side effect.

b) Trigeminal Neurinomas

Computed Tomography

Most trigeminal neurinomas in our series showed very intense, homogeneous contrast enhancement on CT scans. The tumors occur at the medial base of the middle fossa and are in contact with the brainstem (see Figs. D 3.18, E 15). Coronal projections may be useful.

Magnetic Resonance Imaging
(Figs. D 3.6, 11–16, 20–22)

Noncontrast Scan

MR is the optimum modality for evaluating the cerebellopontine angle region. It yields a primary subtraction image in which bony structures appear as voids and the seventh and eighth cranial nerve bundles and their divisions are delineated. Images are free of artifacts, and the plane selection capability of MR allows the cranial nerves to be examined in their entirety.

Acoustic neurinoma appears hypo- to isointense on the T1-weighted image and is poorly differentiated from surrounding brain. The tumor is markedly hyperintense to brain on T2-weighted sequences (Figs. D 3.6, 11–16).

Post-Gadolinium Scan

Owing to the very intense enhancement of *acoustic neurinomas* with Gd-DTPA, even the smallest intracanalicular tumors can be detected with confidence. The boundary between tumor and brain is particularly well defined on heavily T2-weighted images (Figs. D 3.6, 11–14, 16). The high sensitivity of gadolinium-enhanced images makes MR the modality of choice for the detection of intracanalicular acoustic neurinomas. MR and CT are roughly equivalent in their ability to detect larger acoustic neurinomas.

Because *trigeminal neurinomas* are often difficult to recognize on the CT scan, MR is the preferred modality for these tumors owing to the absence of bone artifact and the strong gadolinium enhancement of the lesion.

Differential Diagnosis

The differential diagnosis of *acoustic neurinomas* should include meningiomas, metastases, and less common lesions such as glomus tumors, angioblastomas, ependymomas, aneurysms, desmoplastic medulloblastomas, choroid plexus papillomas, epidermoids, lipomas, and abscesses.

Some *meningiomas* may appear isodense on plain scans, but they are rarely found in the cerebellopontine angle region. Their enhancement characteristics are similar to those of neurinomas, so differentiation must usually rely on clinical findings. The otorhinolaryngologic examination is especially helpful in this regard. Calcifications and erosive changes in the petrous apex are more consistent with meningioma. This diagnosis is also suggested by a tumor that is broadly contiguous to the tentorium and is separated from it by a sharp border, although acoustic neurinomas also can become quite extensive. **MR** can differentiate meningioma from acoustic neurinoma by the shape of the meningioma and its lack of extension into the internal acoustic meatus.

Of particular importance are large, sometimes fusiform *aneurysms of the basilar artery* that project into the cerebellopontine angle. Often these lesions can be diagnosed on postcontrast CT scans, and distinguished from acoustic neurinoma, by their very intense enhancement and by their tortuosity (see Fig. F82).

Epidermoid cysts of the cerebellopontine angle pose no problems of differential diagnosis because of their very low density on the CT scan, equal to that of CSF (see Figs. D6.44, 45).

In rare cases *lipomas* may occur in the cerebellopontine angle region and produce the same clinical symptoms as acoustic neurinomas. Again, densitometry will serve to identify the specific tumor type.

The main lesions to be differentiated from *trigeminal neurinoma* are meningiomas of Meckel's cave and large pilocytic astrocytomas, which also show marked contrast enhancement. Temporobasal gangliocytomas usually contain calcifications, which are never present in trigeminal neurinomas. Giant aneurysms of the carotid artery and posterior cerebral artery may have the same location as trigeminal neurinomas, but their profound contrast enhancement serves to make their identity clear. Thrombosed aneurysms are surrounded by a densely enhancing ring representing the aneurysm capsule (see Fig. F81).

The criteria employed in MR for the differentiation of metastases, medulloblastomas, aneurysms, epidermoids, and lipomas are discussed under the appropriate headings.

c) Neurofibromatosis (von Recklinghausen's Disease)

Von Recklinghausen in 1882 described a condition characterized by the development of multiple fibrous tumors of the skin. Since then a great many reports have been published which have expanded our knowledge of neurofibromatosis (Canale and Bebin 1972). The disease is one of three groups of tumors that are known to have a familial or hereditary occurrence, the other two being tuberous sclerosis (Bourneville-Pringle disease, subependymal giant cell astrocytoma) and angiomatosis of the CNS (hemangioblastoma, von Hippel-Lindau disease). Van der Hoeve (1933) coined the term "phacomatoses" for these disease entities. Zülch (1986) prefers the term "hamartoblastosis."

Today three forms of neurofibromatosis are recognized on the basis of their distinctive clinical and pathologic features (Rubinstein 1972):

1. A *peripheral form* with numerous nerve sheath tumors arising from peripheral and subcutaneous nerves and with multiple café au lait spots on the skin.
2. A *central form* with multiple intracranial and intraspinal tumors that may arise from the brain or its coverings, from the cranial nerves, and from spinal nerve roots.
3. A *visceral form* with various neurogenic tumors involving the viscera and autonomic nervous system. This form may be associated with other tumors of the neural crest such as peripheral neuroblastomas, adrenal ganglioneuromas, and pheochromocytomas.

Here we are concerned exclusively with the *central form* of neurofibromatosis. Schaltenbrand (1933) and many authors after him have described the tumors and combinations of tumor types that may occur in this form.

Besides bilateral acoustic neurinomas, the disease may be associated with multiple meningiomas, which sometimes are heavily calcified. It appears that the choroid plexus may also be involved. Often the bilateral acoustic neurinomas are the only signs of the disease, although neurinomas of the spinal roots are also observed.

There is a significant incidence of *gliomas* in the central form of neurofibromatosis, most notably:

1. *Pilocytic astrocytomas* on the midline (optic nerve, optic chiasm, hypothalamus, third ventricle, pons, medulla oblongata, spinal cord; see Fig. D 1.123)
2. *Ependymomas*, which occur mostly in the spinal canal (Zülch 1956)

The disease usually appears in the third decade of life but is also common in adolescence. Males and females appear to be affected about equally. The reported incidence is 0.5% of intracranial tumors (central type, Glowacki 1963). Rodriguez and Berthrong (1966) reported the following incidence data for the different types of neoplasia in cases of central neurofibromatosis:

Bilateral acoustic nerve tumors	82%
Unilateral acoustic nerve tumors	18%
Multiple meningiomas (42% having a combined intracranial and intraspinal location)	54%
Strictly intraspinal tumors	4%
Gliomas	45%

In a review of 3007 patients with brain tumors who underwent treatment over a 36-year period at the Neurosurgical Clinic of the Free University of Berlin, it was found that 12 patients had the central form of neurofibromatosis (0.4%). Four of these had bilateral acoustic neurinomas, while eight had bilateral acoustic neurinomas combined with multiple meningiomas and less frequently with gliomas. Neurofibromatosis was diagnosed in three other patients as well, but the tumor combinations were atypical (Öztürk et al. 1987):

- Anaplastic astrocytoma occurring a short time after removal of a large neurofibroma from the left brachial plexus
- Pilocytic astrocytoma of the cerebrum occurring after removal of a spinal neurofibroma
- Ingrowth of a large cervical neurofibroma into the posterior fossa plus numerous cutaneous tumors

The clinical picture of the central form is characterized by hearing loss, which is usually bilateral, and by the location and size of coexisting tumors. Central or spinal deficits are observed accordingly.

Computed Tomography

Contrast medium is necessary for the detection of acoustic neurinomas. Meningiomas, on the other hand, are generally easy to detect on noncontrast scans, especially when calcifications are present (Fig. D 3.20). Spinal tumors with associated bone destruction (enlargement of the intervertebral foramen) are also detectable with CT, especially when their location is cervical (Fig. D 3.20).

Magnetic Resonance Imaging

MR is a valuable adjunct to the detection of acoustic neurinomas, meningiomas, and gliomas in neurofibromatosis owing largely to its capability for arbitrary plane selection. However, the full potential of MR is utilized only in gadolinium-enhanced sequences (Figs. D 3.21 and 22). There is no alternative to MR in the detection of tumors at the craniospinal junction. The MR image enables the surgeon to plan the operation effectively and to select the sequence of procedures that will be of greatest benefit to the patient.

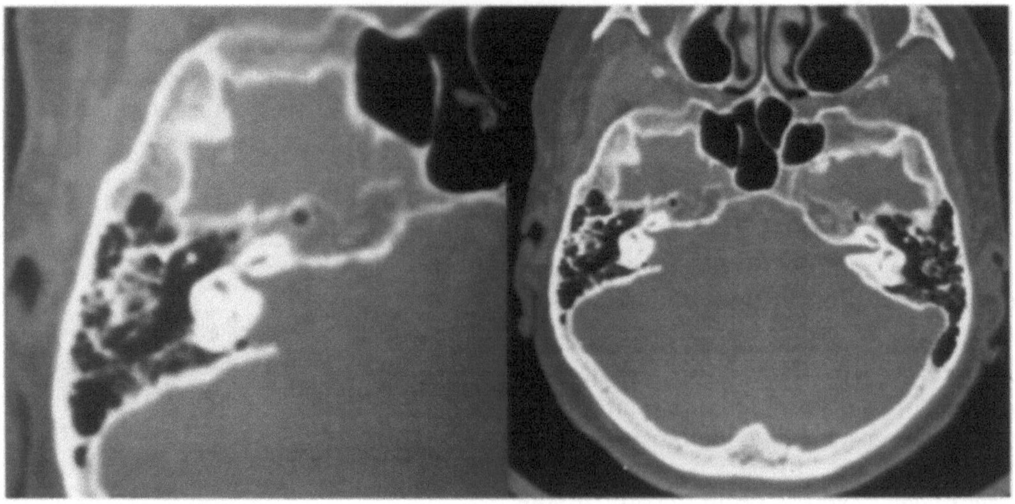

Fig. D 3.1. Acoustic neurinoma of the left side in a 64-year-old man with a 10-year history of hearing disturbances and tinnitus. CT reveals destruction of the left pyramid as far as the labyrinth. The right internal auditory canal appears normal

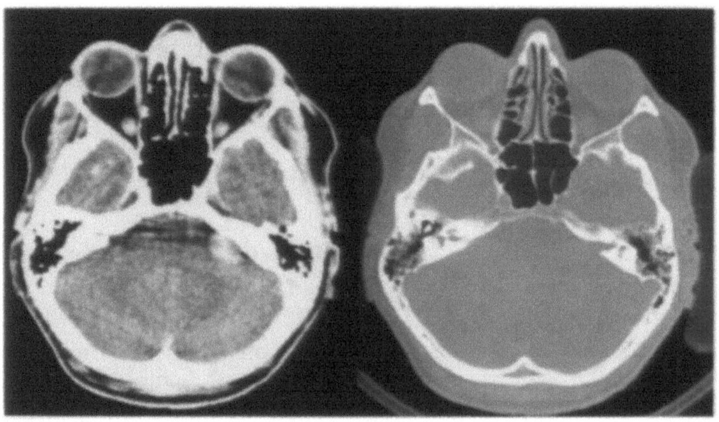

Fig. D 3.2. Acoustic neurinoma of the right side in a 50-year-old man with a 3-year history of progressive hearing loss and tinnitus in the right ear. CT: *left* postcontrast, *right* bony window. The right internal auditory canal is markedly expanded. The contrast scan shows circumscribed enhancement of a tumor extending out of the internal auditory canal

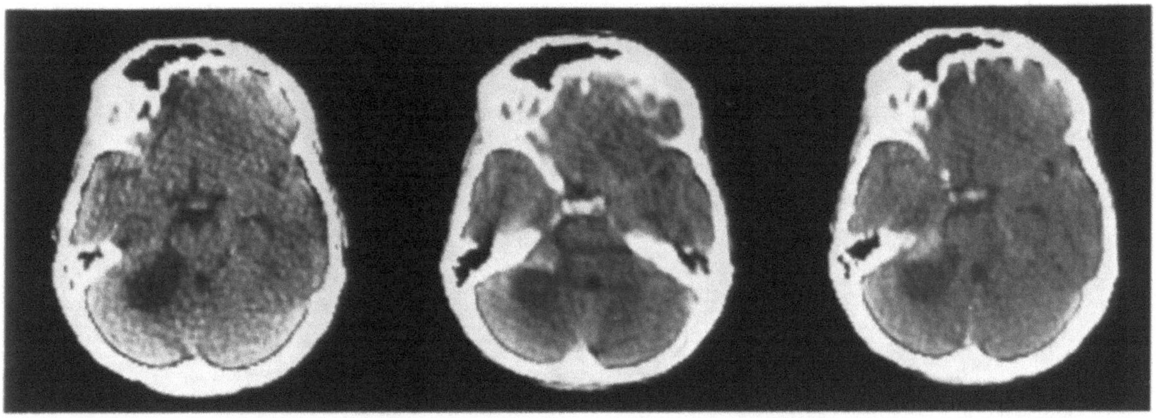

Fig. D 3.3. Acoustic neurinoma of the left side surrounded by a large cyst in a 47-year-old woman. The cyst permits detection of the tumor on the precontrast scan (*left*). The solid tumor component is depicted better on the postcontrast scans (*center* and *right*)

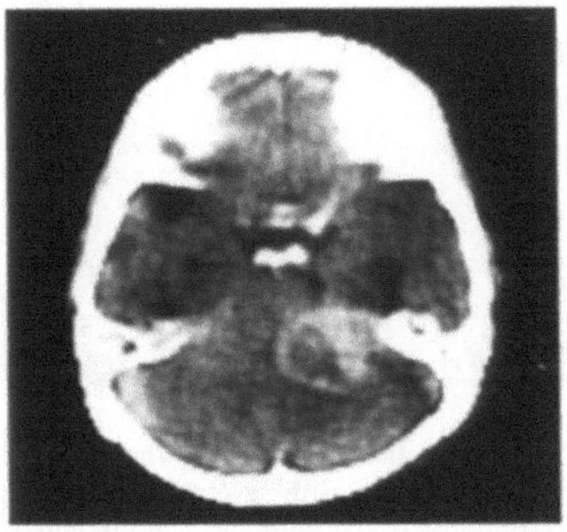

Fig. D 3.4. Acoustic neurinoma of the right side with central necrosis and ring enhancement in a 69-year-old woman

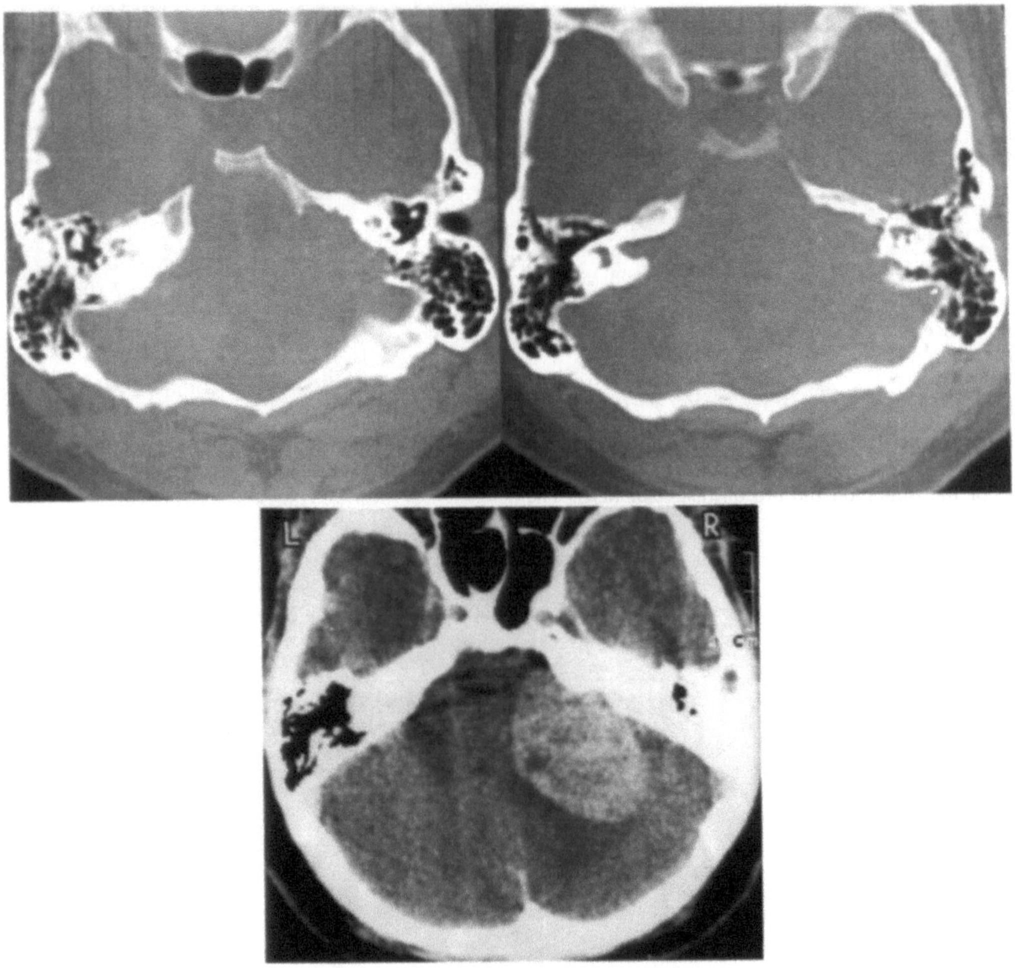

Fig. D3.5. Acoustic neurinoma of the right side in a 50-year-old woman with several years of progressive hearing loss in the right ear. She presented with hypoesthesia in the distribution of the second and third trigeminal nerve divisions, increasing ataxia, and headache. CT: *top* precontrast, *bottom* postcontrast. Scans show extensive destruction of the right pyramid; the internal auditory canal is no longer discernible. Contrast enhancement discloses a large acoustic neurinoma extending as far as the tentorium and greatly displacing the brainstem

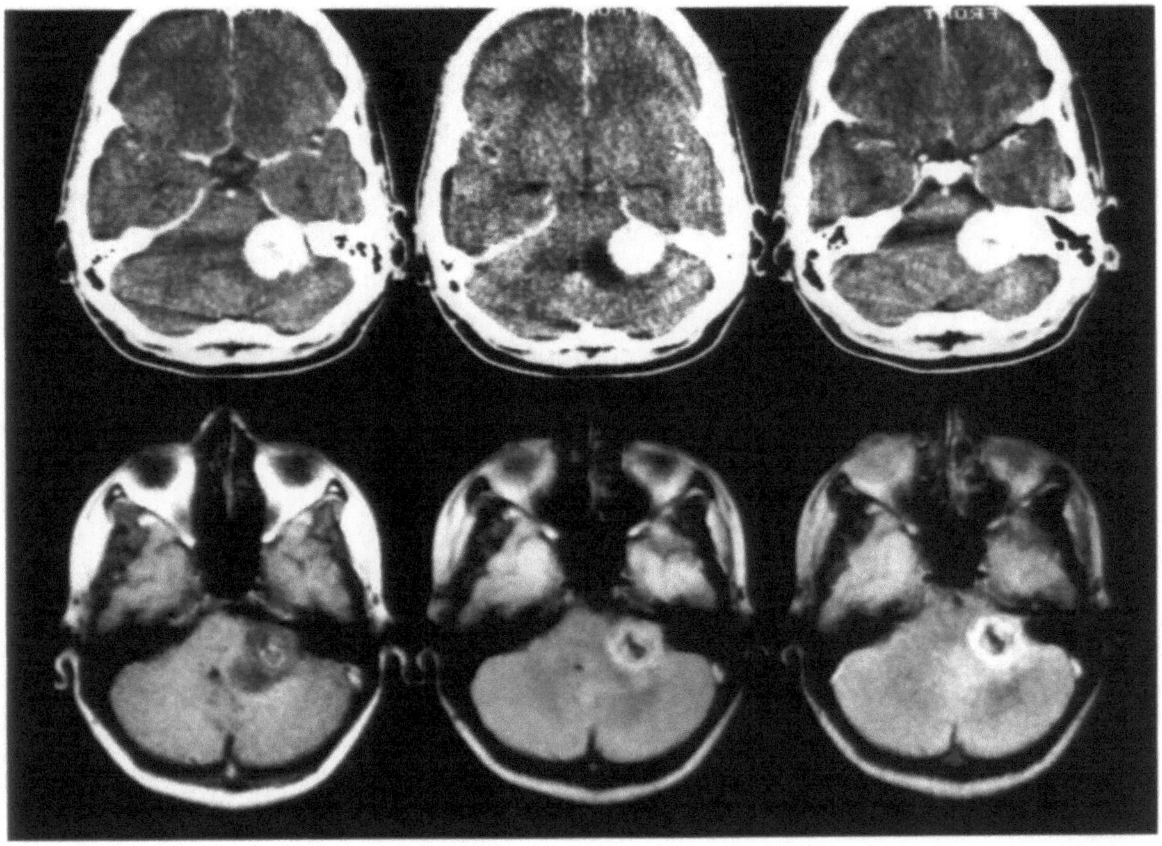

a–c

d–f

Fig. D 3.6 a–f. Acoustic neurinoma of the right side in a 33-year-old woman with a history of hearing loss in the right ear for 16 years, tinnitus for 1 year, and numbness of the right corner of the mouth and right side of the tongue for 15 months. CT: **a–c** postcontrast. MR: **d** SE 400/35, **e** SE 1600/35, **f** SE 1600/70. CT demonstrates a large, densely enhancing acoustic neurinoma on the right side. Moderate edema is apparent medial to the tumor. MR reveals necrotic breakdown at the core of the tumor, which is displacing the fourth ventricle. The tumor extends to the brainstem

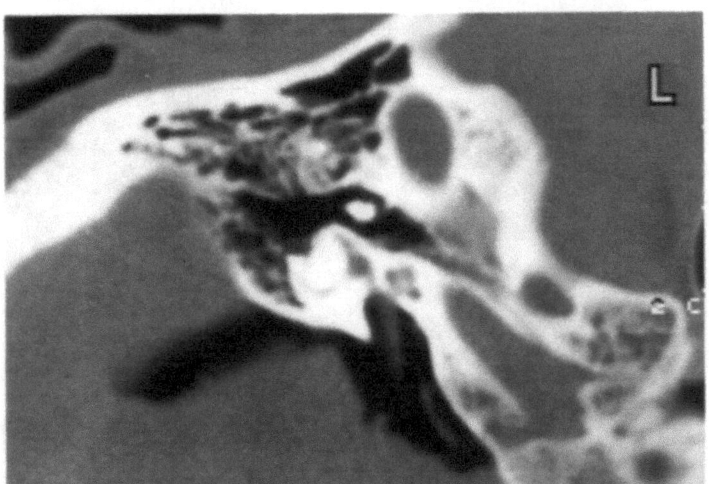

Fig. D 3.7. CT after insufflation of air into the pontocerebellar cistern and internal auditory canal. Findings are normal. The facial nerve and statoacoustic nerve are clearly visualized

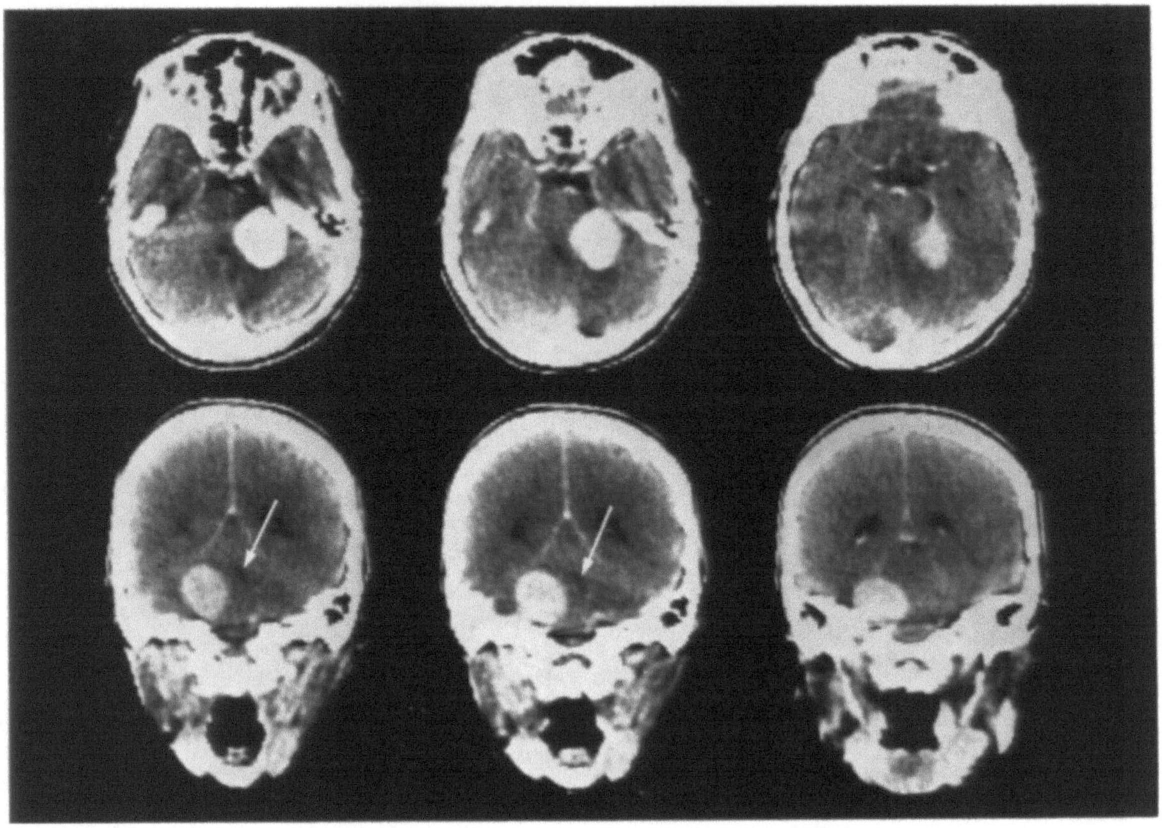

Fig. D 3.8. Comparison of axial and coronal postcontrast CT scans of a right-sided acoustic neurinoma in a 39-year-old woman. The coronal scans clearly demonstrate the displaced and distorted aqueduct and fourth ventricle (*arrows*). The tumor extends below the tentorium

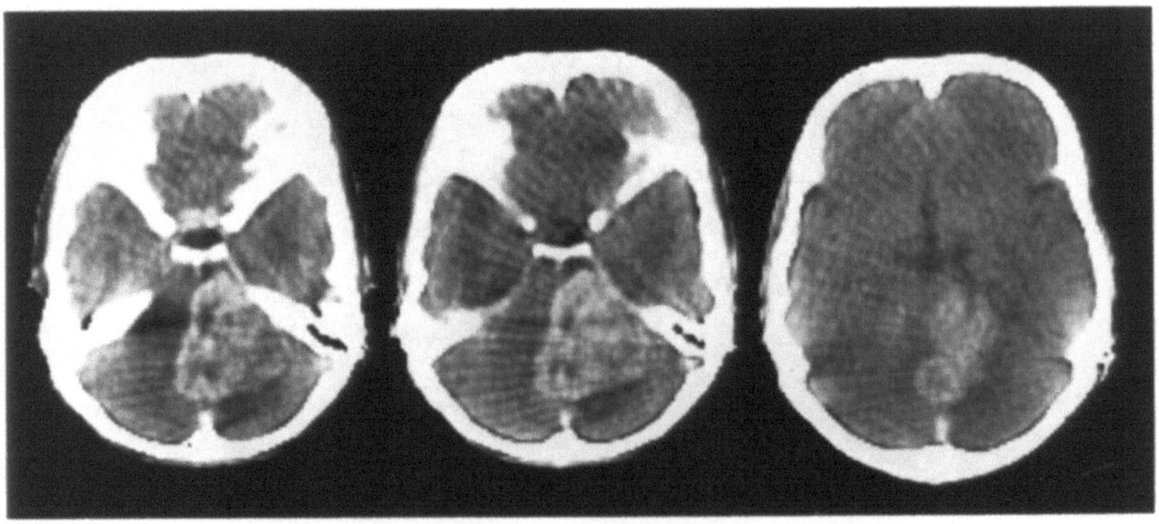

Fig. D 3.9. Very large acoustic neurinoma with extensive regressive changes in a 37-year-old woman. The tumor extends from the foramen magnum to the tentorium and superior vermis. Artifacts emanate from a shunt previously implanted on the right side (all CT scans are contrast-enhanced)

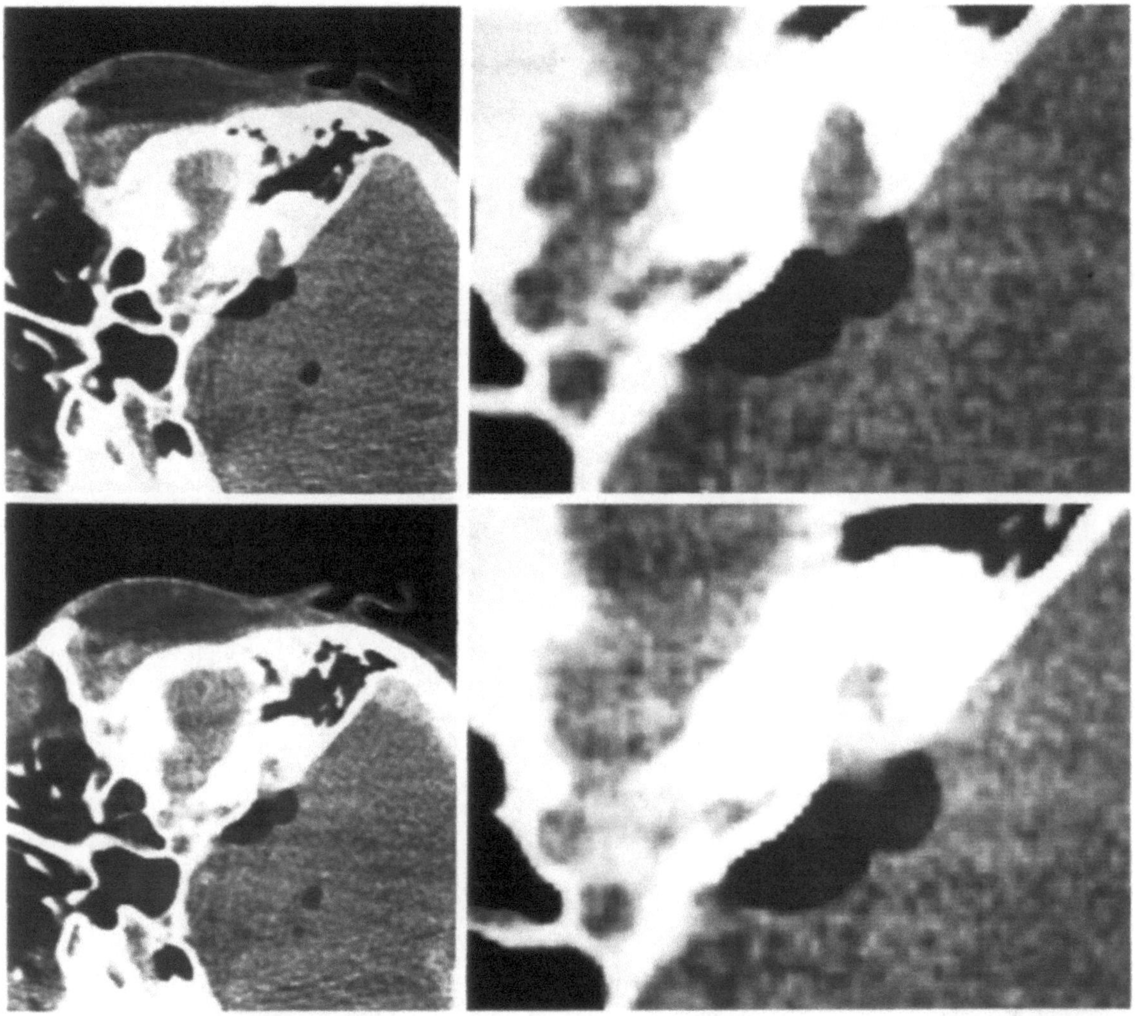

a a′

b b′

Fig. D 3.10 a, b. Combined CT-pneumocisternographic evaluation of a predominantly intracanalicular acoustic neurinoma. The tumor completely fills the right internal auditory canal and has a small extracanalicular extension clearly visible in the air-filled pontocerebellar cistern. **a′** and **b′** are detail views of 5-mm slices; **b** and **b′** are contrast-enhanced

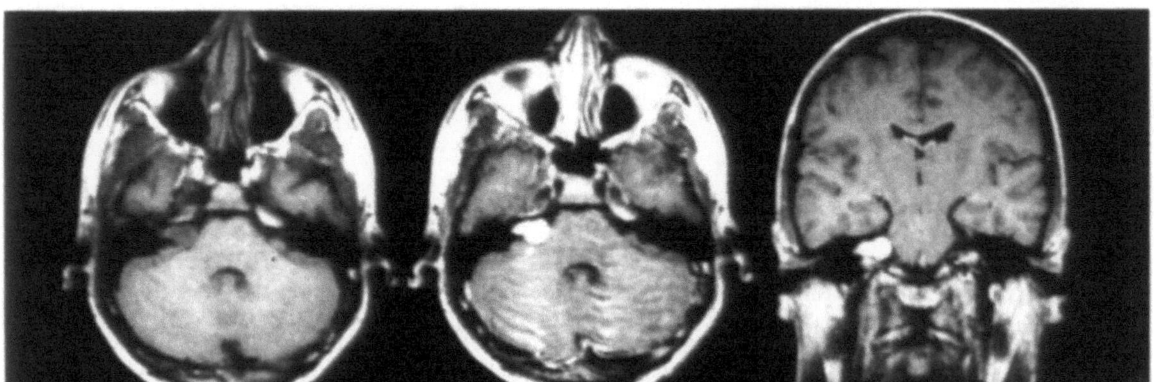

Fig. D 3.11. Acoustic neurinoma of the left side in a 20-year-old man with decreased hearing and tinnitus in the left ear and vestibular hypoexcitability. MR: *left* SE 400/30, *center* SE 400/30 post Gd-DTPA, *right* SE 400/30 post Gd-DTPA coronal. Scans demonstrate a hyperintense tumor projecting into the pontocerebellar cistern on the left side

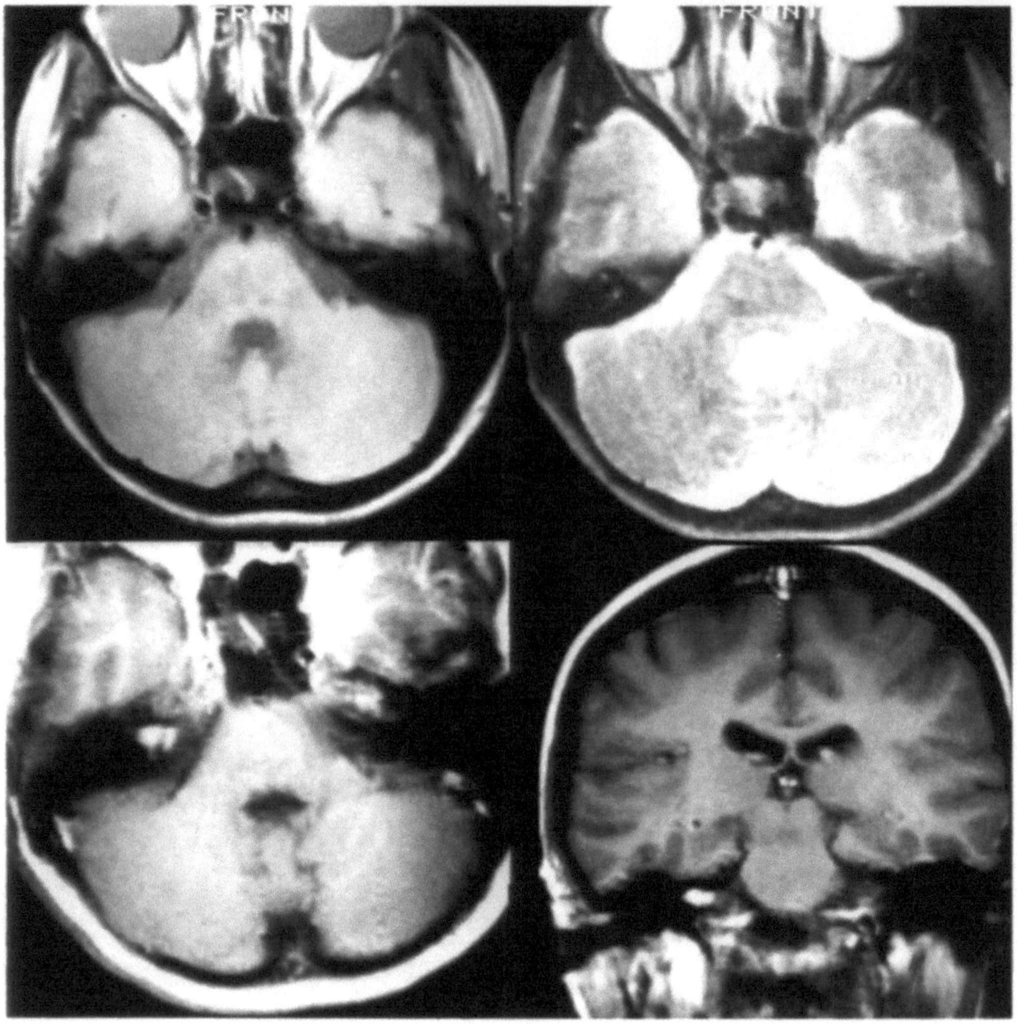

a b c d

Fig. D 3.12 a–d. Small intracanalicular acoustic neurinoma of the left side in a 42-year-old woman with progressive labyrinthine hearing loss in the left ear. MR: **a** SE 1600/30, **b** SE 1600/120, **c** SE 400/30 post Gd-DTPA, **d** SE 400/30 post Gd-DTPA coronal. The unenhanced proton-density and T2-weighted images (**a**, **b**) give no clear evidence of a tumor. However, the small intracanalicular tumor is displayed with high signal intensity on the post-Gd-DTPA images (**c**, **d**)

Fig. D 3.13 a–e. Acoustic neurinoma of the right side in a 60-year-old woman with a 1-year history of decreased hearing in the right ear. MR: **a** SE 400/30, **b** SE 400/30 post Gd-DTPA, axial; **c** SE 400/30 post Gd-DTPA coronal; **d** SE 400/30, **e** SE 400/30 post Gd-DTPA, parasagittal. The acoustic neurinoma appears hypointense on the plain images and enhances markedly with Gd-DTPA. The tumor extends to the brainstem

Fig. D 3.14 a–d. Acoustic neurinoma of the right side in a 59-year-old man with a 6-month history of vertigo, headache, and hypoacusis in the right ear; mild evidence of ataxia was found on examination. MR, SE 400/30: **a** axial, **b** axial post Gd-DTPA, **c** coronal, **d** coronal post Gd-DTPA. The postcontrast images show a large, brightly enhancing, right-sided acoustic neurinoma indenting and displacing the brainstem. The fourth ventricle is also displaced

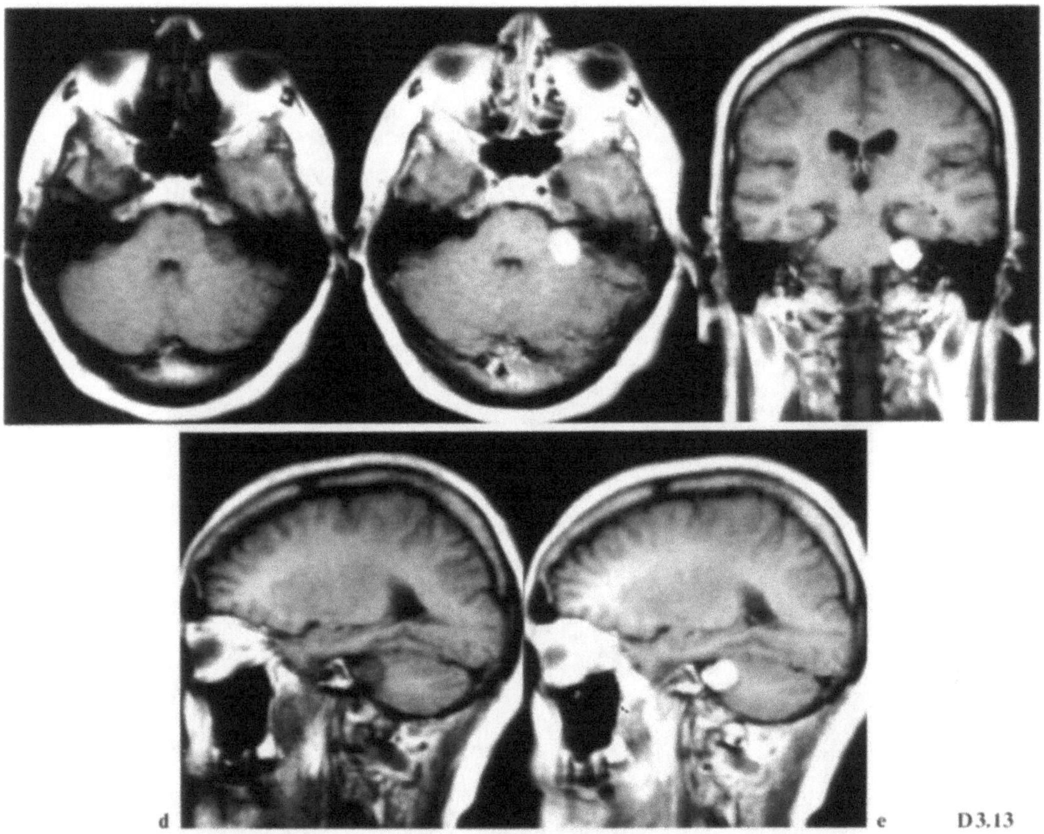

a–c

d e D3.13

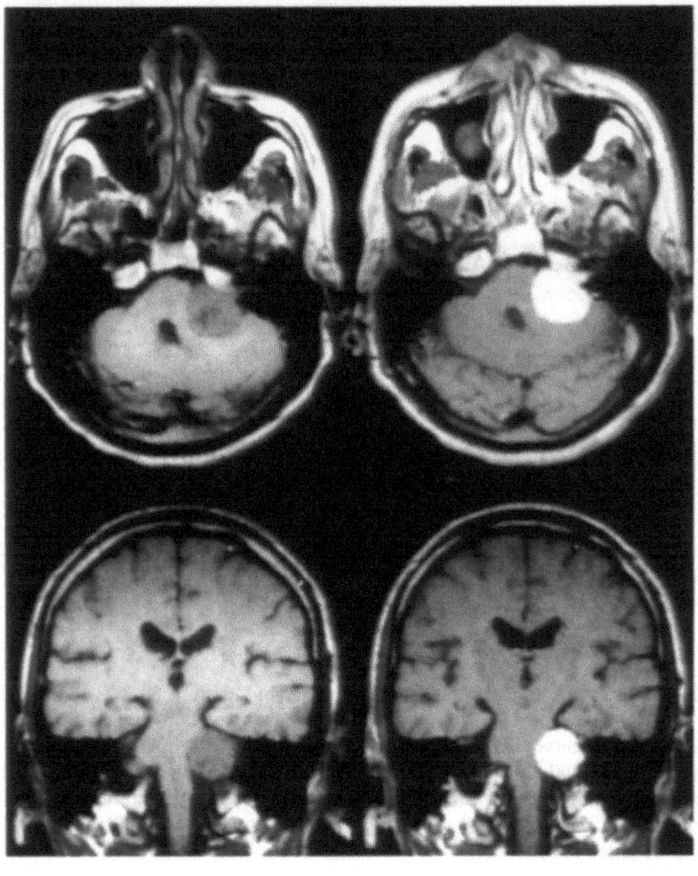

a b

c d D3.14

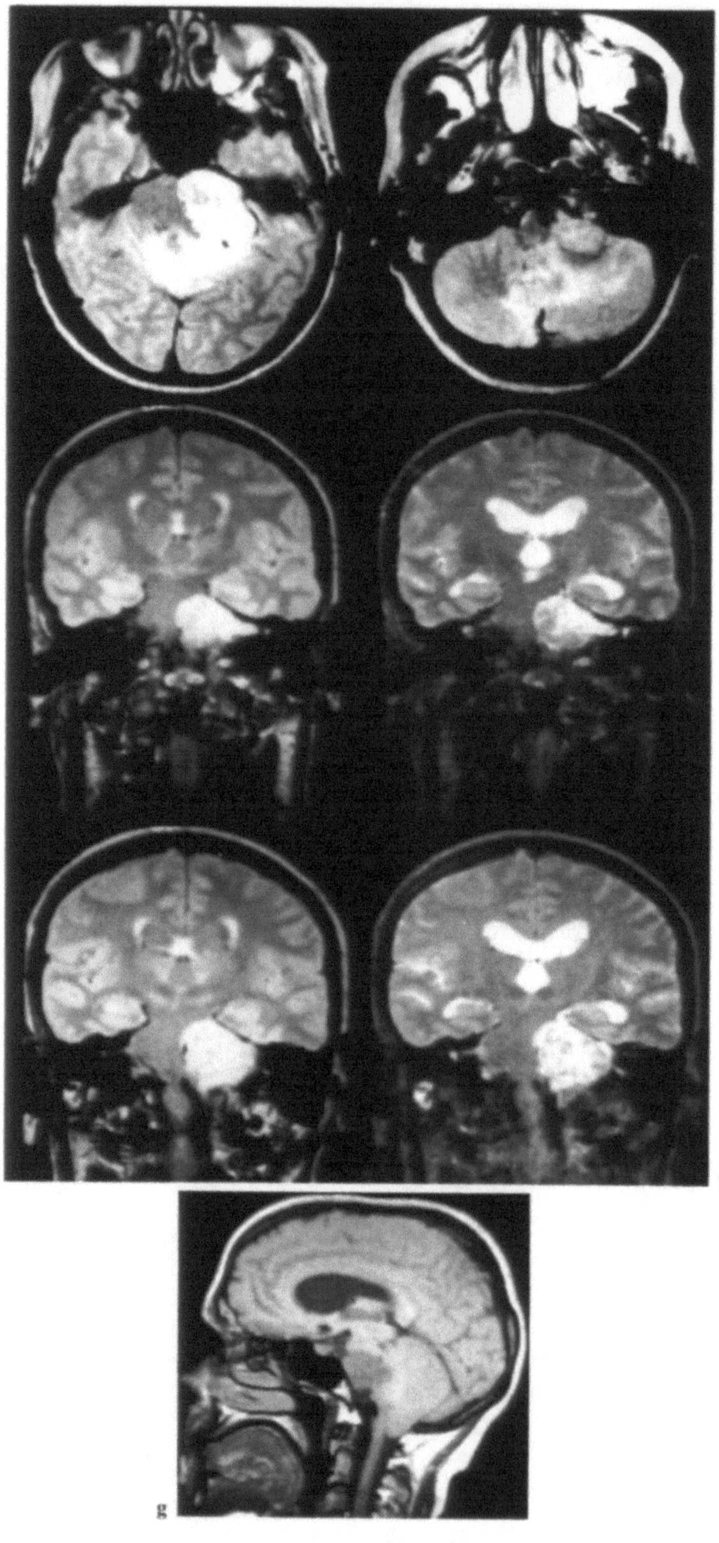

a b c d e f g

Fig. D3.15a–g. Acoustic neurinoma of the right side in a 50-year-old man with right-sided hearing loss and cranial neuropathies involving the fifth and seventh nerves. MR: **a, b** SE 3000/30 axial, **c, e** SE 3000/30 coronal, **d, f** SE 3000/90 coronal, **g** SE 700/30 parasagittal. The T1-weighted image (**g**) demonstrates a low-signal tumor compressing the brainstem. The tumor and perifocal edema give higher signals on the proton-density and T2-weighted images

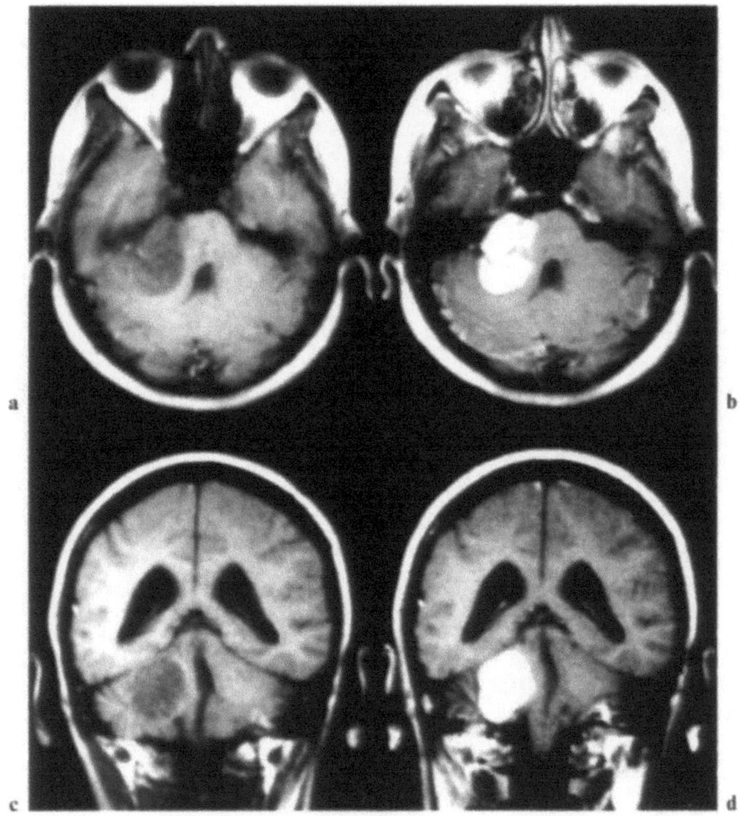

Fig. D3.16a–d. Acoustic neurinoma of the left side in a 50-year-old woman with a 2-year history of left-sided hearing loss, tinnitus, and attacks of vertigo. MR: **a, c** SE 400/30 without Gd-DTPA; **b, d** SE 400/30 post Gd-DTPA. Post-contrast images show a large, brightly enhancing acoustic neurinoma on the left side indenting and displacing the brainstem and fourth ventricle

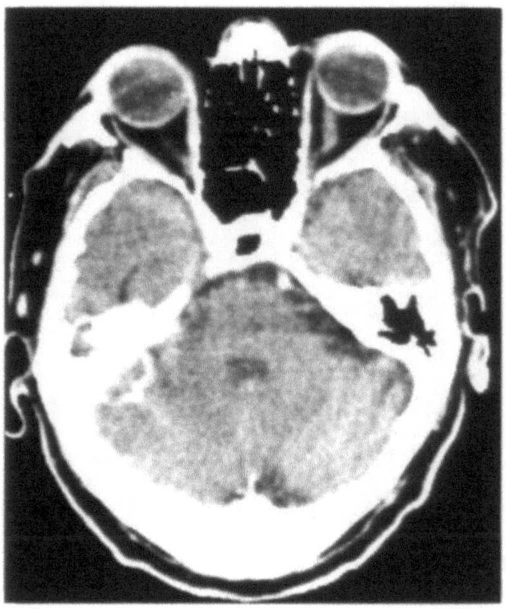

Fig. D3.17. Cholesteatoma of the left side in a 60-year-old man with a history of "chronic ear problems." Postcontrast CT demonstrates a peripherally enhancing mass lesion in the left cerebellopontine angle, representing the penetration of a clinically known cholesteatoma into the cranial cavity

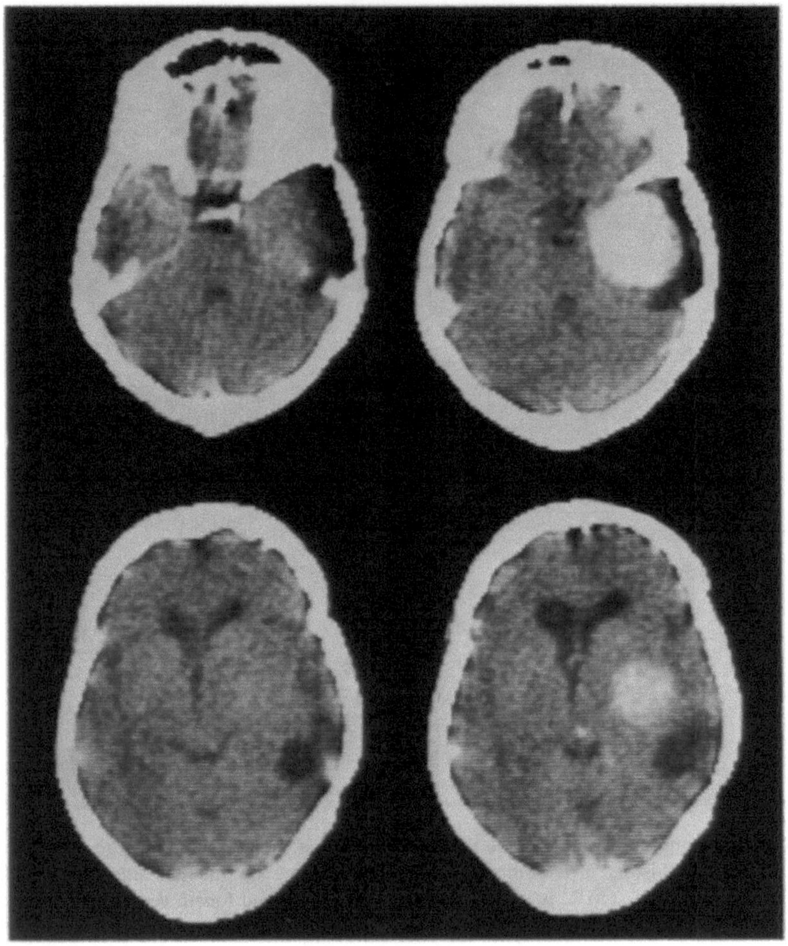

Fig. D3.18. Large recurrence of a right-sided trigeminal neurinoma in a 65-year-old woman. Solid tumor tissue is isodense on the plain CT scans (*left*) and shows intense, uniform enhancement with contrast medium (*right*)

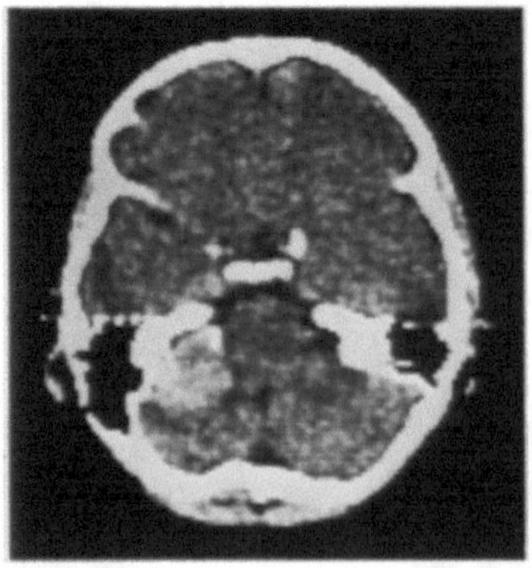

Fig. D3.19. Neurinoma of the left vagus nerve in a 14-year-old boy. The tumor occurs at a somewhat lower level than acoustic neurinoma; otherwise its CT appearance is similar

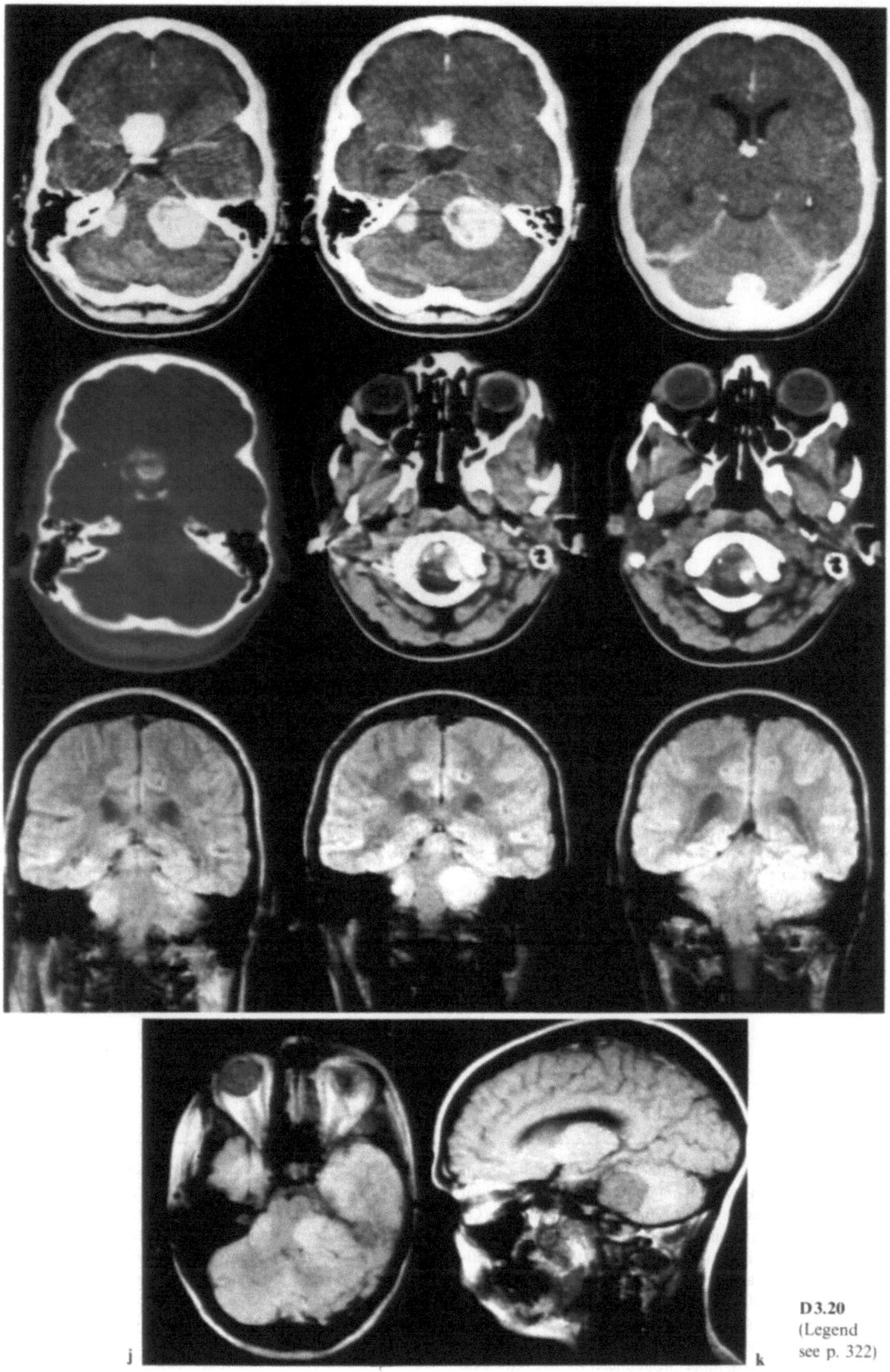

a–c

d–f

g–i

j

k

D 3.20
(Legend see p. 322)

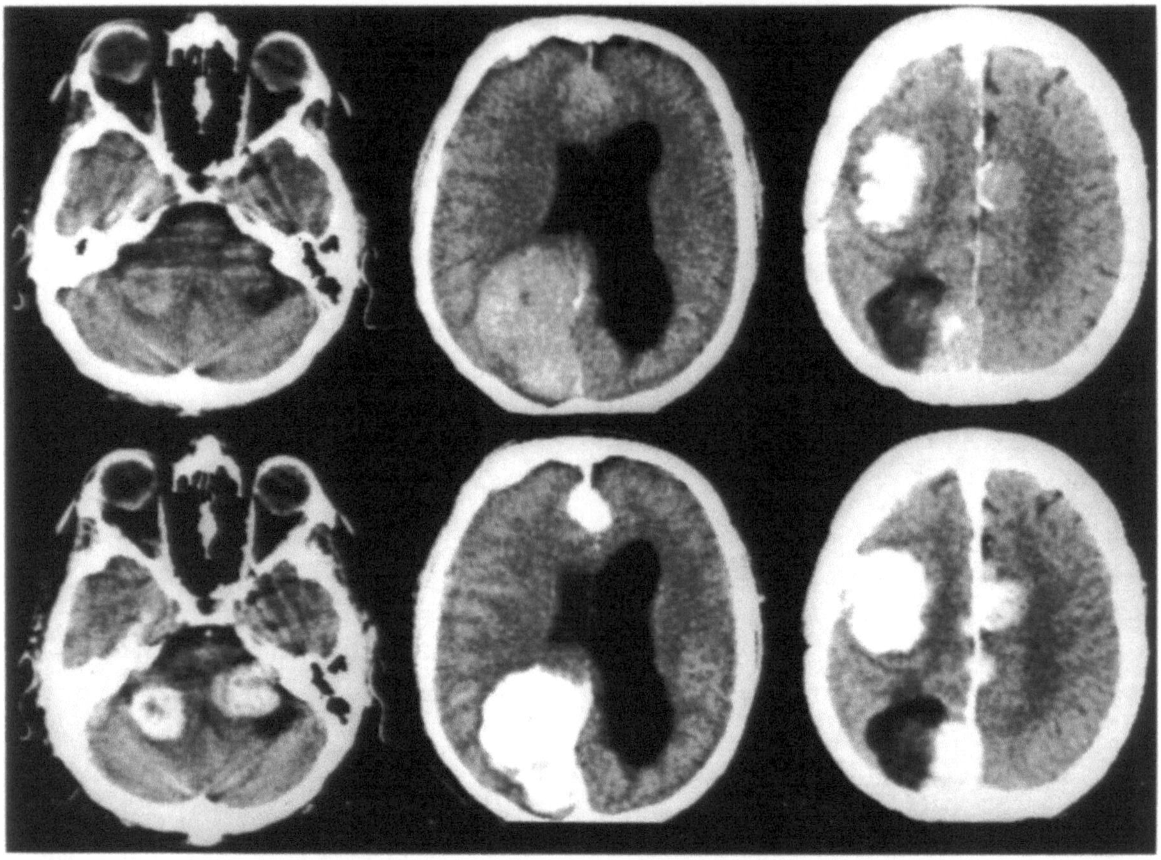

a–c

d–f

Fig. D 3.21 a–n. Von Recklinghausen's disease with bilateral acoustic neurinomas and multiple meningiomas in a 43-year-old woman with hearing loss since 10 years of age and focal seizures with late generalization since 13 years of age. Patient underwent removal of a right occipital meningioma at age 19. Seizures began to recur at age 32, and a neurofibroma was removed from the right side of the neck at age 39. Patient presented at age 43 with increased intracranial pressure and refractory seizures, left homonymous hemianopia, bilateral anacusis, and ataxia of gait and stance on the left side. CT: **a, b** precontrast, **c–f** postcontrast. MR: **g** SE 800/35, **h** SE 800/35 post Gd-DTPA, **i** SE 800/35, **j** SE 800/35 post Gd-DTPA, **k, l** SE 400/30 post Gd-DTPA coronal, **m, n** SE 400/30 post Gd-DTPA parasagittal. The acoustic neurinomas are poorly delineated on the plain CT scans but enhance markedly after contrast injection (**d**). The supratentorial meningiomas are partly cystic and appear moderately hyperdense on the plain scans. These lesions, too, show marked contrast enhancement. The T1-weighted MR sequences (**g, i**) show a combination of hypointense (acoustic neurinomas) and isointense lesions (meningiomas). Both tumor types enhance brightly with Gd-DTPA

◄

Fig. D 3.20 a–k (see p. 321). Von Recklinghausen's disease in a 20-year-old woman with meningiomas at the tuberculum sellae, at the confluence of the sinuses, and at the C1/C2 level of the spinal cord; bilateral acoustic neurinomas, more pronounced on the right side; known intrathoracic neurifibroma. Patient had a 4-year history of recurring crises of increased intracranial pressure and grand mal seizures, and a 6-month history of gait ataxia, vertigo, visual acuity loss in the right eye, diplopia, bilateral nystagmus in the direction of gaze, and hypoacusis, more pronounced on the right side than the left. CT: **a, b, c, e, f** postcontrast, **d** bony window. MR: **g–i** SE 1600/35 coronal, **j** SE 1600/35 axial, **k** SE 400/35 parasagittal. Meningiomas and neurinomas enhance well on postcontrast CT. Partially calcified meningioma on the tuberculum sellae. The tumors are poorly delineated on the unenhanced MR images, appearing hypointense on the T1-weighted sequence (**k**). The tumors are slightly hyperintense to surrounding brain on the proton-density images (**g–j**)

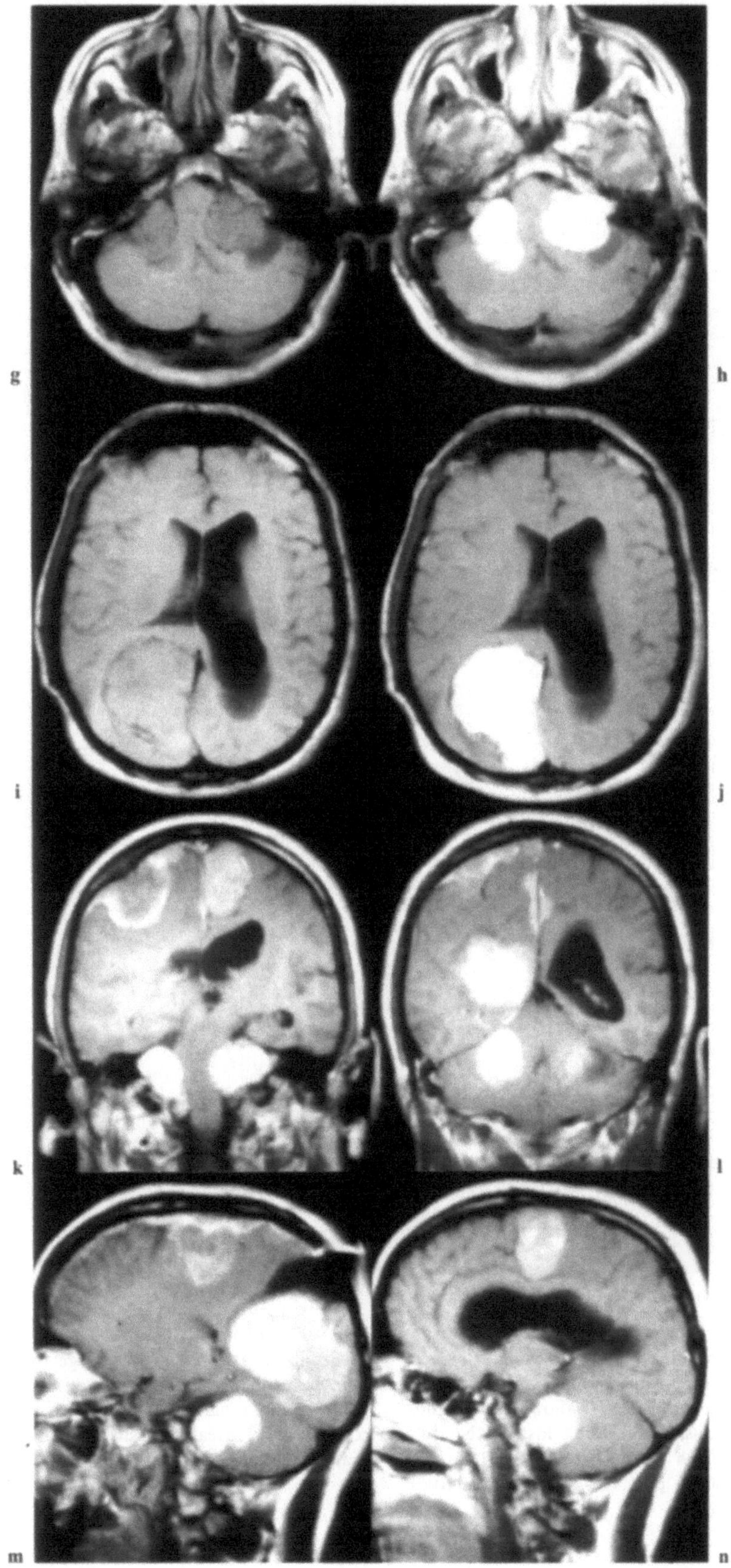
g
h
i
j
k
l
m
n

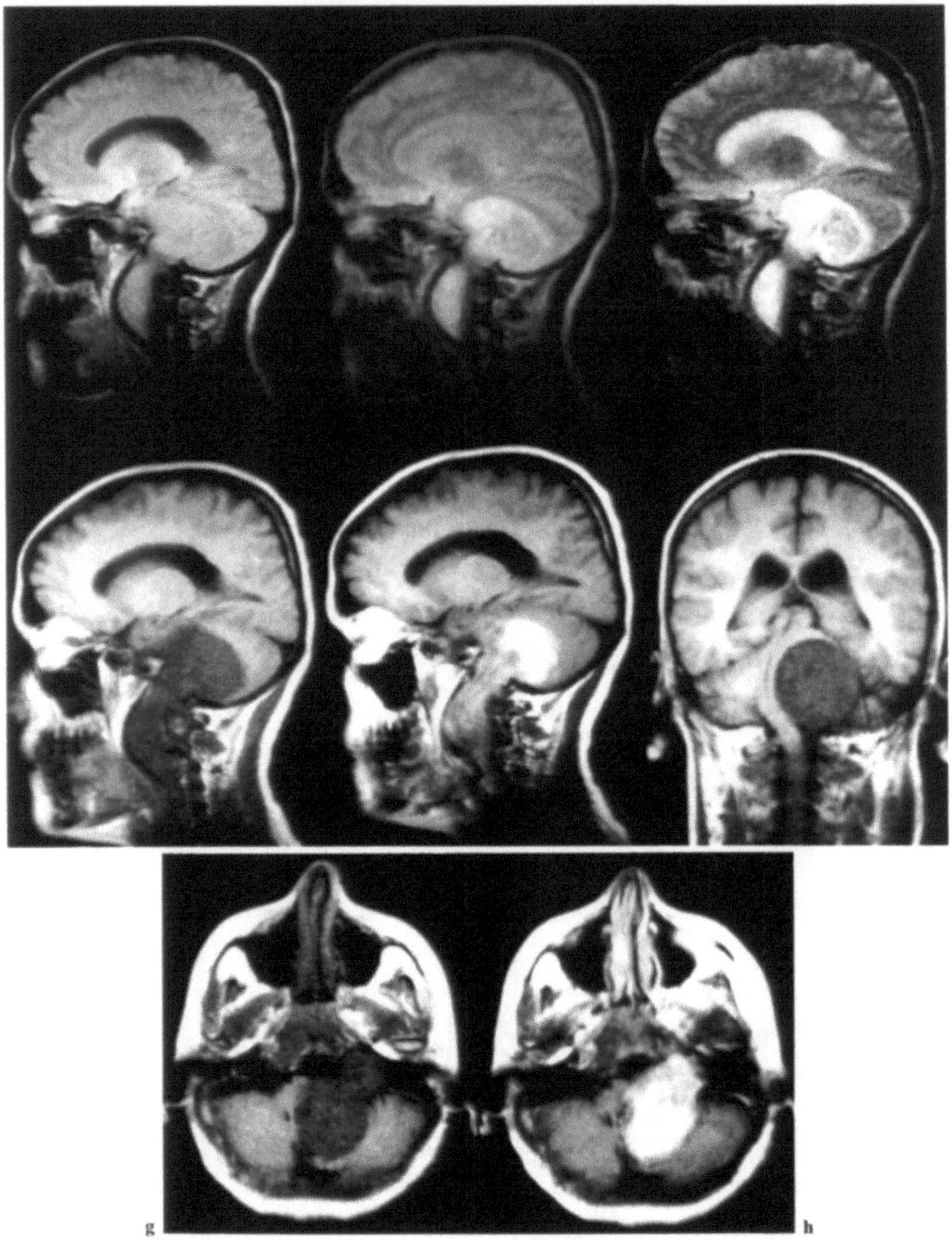

a–c

d–f

g

h

Fig. D3.22a–h. Von Recklinghausen's disease with a giant neurofibroma of the posterior fossa and caudal splanchnocranial spread in a 20-year-old woman with a painless swelling on the right side of the neck, swallowing difficulties, horizontal gaze nystagmus, and hearing loss in the right ear. MR: **a** SE 1600/30, **b** SE 1600/90, **c** SE 1600/150, **d** SE 400/30, **e** SE 400/30 post Gd-DTPA (all sagittal); **f** SE 400/30 coronal; **g** SE 400/30, **h** SE 400/30 post Gd-DTPA (both axial). The very large tumor is markedly hypointense to surrounding brain on the T1-weighted images (**d, f, g**) and enhances brightly with Gd-DTPA (**e, h**). The coronal view reveals massive lateral displacement of the brainstem by the mass

4. Pituitary Adenomas

Incidence	8%–12% of all brain tumors
Age predilection	25–60 years
Sex predilection	Roughly equal distribution
Typical site	Sellar region
Main clinical features	Hormonal disorders (hormone excess: acromegaly, hyperprolactinemia, Cushing's syndrome; pituitary insufficiency); visual (chiasmal) disturbances
Skull X-ray	Primary sellar changes
Angiography	Suprasellar extension elevates horizontal limb of anterior cerebral artery; parasellar extension displaces carotid siphon. Angiography may be omitted if lesion adequately demonstrated by MR
Special examinations	Endocrinologic function studies
CT	
Noncontrast scan	Tumors frequently hyperdense, less commonly isodense; mixed density may result from cyst formation producing low-density areas at pentagon or sellar entrance
Contrast enhancement	Generally positive in solid parts of tumor
Postcontrast appearance	Smooth-bordered tumor at sellar entrance or above sella, occasionally with para- or retrosellar extension. Cysts clearly delineated. Purely intrasellar lesions generally not demonstrated on routine scans
MR	
Noncontrast scan	T1-weighted images: tumors slightly hypointense to normal pituitary, cysts markedly hypointense with well-defined borders, intratumoral hemorrhage hyperintense. T2-weighted images: tumor slightly hyperintense, cystic, necrotic, and hemorrhagic components markedly hyperintense
Gadolinium enhancement	Moderate
Post Gd-DTPA appearance	Mild enhancement
Differential diagnosis	
Suprasellar meningioma Craniopharyngioma Pilocytic astrocytoma Aneurysm Empty sella	Less frequently: metastases, chordoma, ectopic pinealoma, malignant lymphoma, epipharyngeal tumors, histiocytosis X

Pituitary adenomas are extra-axial tumors derived from the anterior lobe of the pituitary gland. Zülch (1986) states that these tumors comprise 6.6% of all intracranial neoplasms; Olivecrona (1967) reports 8.6%. The incidence was 10% in our series of 3750 tumors. With advances in the endocrinologic diagnosis of pituitary microadenomas, the incidence in recent years has risen to 12.4% of 8514 intracranial tumors.

Pituitary adenomas are most common during middle age. However, the peak incidence, put at between 35 and 55 years by Zülch, is manifesting a downward trend owing to the more frequent detection of microadenomas.

Men and women are affected about equally, although microprolactinomas show a marked predilection for females.

Sites, Classification

Pituitary adenomas are divided into microadenomas and macroadenomas, a diameter of 10 mm being the cutoff point between the micro and macro forms. All originate within the sella turcica and subsequently expand in the suprasellar, parasellar, retrosellar, and/or subfrontal directions. Adenomas expanding toward the skull base may extend laterally into the cavernous sinus and downward into the sphenoid sinus. Large adenomas may expand in all directions simultaneously, and this behavior is especially common in recurrent growths. Seeding via the CSF is a rare complication.

Very large pituitary adenomas with extension to the foramen of Monro can incite obstructive hydrocephalus.

Pituitary adenomas were formerly classified by light microscopic criteria as eosinophil, basophil, chromophobe, or mixed type. The preferred classification today is based on *endocrinologic criteria* and characterizes tumors as functioning (hormone-secreting) or nonfunctioning (non-hormone-secreting) as established by immunohistochemical tests or cell culture studies.

Main Clinical Features

Pure intrasellar growths can stimulate excessive hormone production resulting in acromegaly, hyperprolactinemia (amenorrhea-galactorrhea syndrome), or Cushing's syndrome. These and functioning tumors can exert pressure on the anterior lobe of the pituitary resulting in anterior lobe insufficiency with secondary hypogonadism, hypothyroidism, and adrenocortical insufficiency. Chiasmal disturbances occur only if there is suprasellar extension sufficient to impinge on the undersurface of the optic chiasm. Bitemporal hemianopia is observed in about half of cases. Rare parasellar extension can irritate the ocular motor nerves, especially the third cranial, causing diplopia.

Headache may result from obstruction of the foramen of Monro or intratumoral hemorrhage. Frontal headache is common in acromegaly.

Additional Diagnostic Procedures

Plain skull X-rays continue to be a mainstay in the initial diagnostic workup of pituitary adenoma. The great majority of microadenomas can be detected on plain skull films or conventional tomographic surveys of the sella by a double outline, unilateral excavation, or slight bowing of the sellar floor. However, an undistorted sella of normal size on these studies does not necessarily exclude microadenoma. Conventional tomography may be omitted in some cases owing to the superiority of CT in the detection of these lesions (see below). Often diagnosis must rely upon special hormonal studies, especially in patients with Cushing's disease.

Only adenomas exceeding 8 mm in diameter cause enlargement of the sella turcica, thinning of the floor, and decalcification of the dorsum sellae, which may subsequently evert and contribute to enlargement of the sellar entrance.

Angiographic findings in large adenomas with suprasellar extension include elevation of the horizontal segment of the anterior cerebral artery. The carotid siphon may be opened or laterally displaced, especially with parasellar extension.

A normal vascular pattern on angiograms does not exclude a supra- or parasellar neoplasm, however, since the tumor may lack a capsule and fail to displace vessels as it grows. Angiography traditionally has been indicated whenever parasellar growth is suspected. However, these criteria are no longer considered valid owing to the vascular imaging capabilities of MR.

Computed Tomography

(Figs. D4.1–11, 13, 16, 18, 21, 24, 26, 31)

Noncontrast Scan

Pituitary macroadenomas generally appear as well-defined rounded or oval lesions that are hyperdense (65.8%) or isodense (17.5%) to brain and fill all or part of the chiasmatic cistern. A small percentage of adenomas (12.5%) acquire mixed densities due to the presence of cystic or older hemorrhagic components (Figs. D4.5, 7, 8, 10, 11). Cysts also may develop outside the tumor itself (Fig. D4.18). Calcifications are very rare, occurring in less than 1% of cases. Only adenomas that have undergone extensive cystic transformation appear hypodense (4.2%), except for pituitary microadenomas, which generally present a lower density than normal intrasellar pituitary tissue. The attenuation values of solid tumor tissue average 35–50 HU. Higher values suggest intratumoral hemorrhage, especially in patients who report headache and visual disturbance of sudden onset (Figs. D4.7, 8). This complication, which may be associated with ocular motor nerve palsies and severe endocrine disturbances, is quite rare (1% incidence in our series). CT is also useful for the detection of postoperative hemorrhage.

Contrast Enhancement

More than 95% of pituitary adenomas enhance densely in their solid portions with intravenous contrast. The enhancement is usually homogeneous and ranges from 12 to 34 HU (average 16 HU) immediately after the contrast injection, depending on the dose administered. The enhancement fades rapidly.

Postcontrast Findings

Pituitary adenoma with suprasellar extension usually appears as a well-defined area of high density within the chiasmatic cistern (Figs. D4.1–4, 6, 9–11, 13, 18, 24). In many cases the tumor configuration can be accurately assessed only on the contrast-enhanced scan. Parasellar, retrosellar, and subfrontal extensions are displayed with much greater clarity and indeed may not be visualized on the nonenhanced scan. Today the coronal and sagittal CT views are utilized routinely in selecting the route of surgical approach. Cysts, older hemorrhages, and other foci of regressive change within the tumor do not enhance and appear as well-defined areas of low density (Figs. D4.5, 10). Larger vessels such as the internal carotid artery and basilar artery usually appear on axial sections as circumscribed, rounded structures that enhance densely at the tumor margin (Fig. D4.5). Long segments of these vessels are portrayed on coronal sections, which may demonstrate the division of the internal carotid into the anterior and middle cerebral arteries. Enhancement in the cavernous sinus can simulate parasellar extension of tumor.

Tumor extending from the sella toward the sphenoid is detected by the presence of enhancing tissue in spaces that are normally air-filled.

Functioning *microadenomas* are detectable by endocrinologic studies but cannot be demonstrated with CT unless they are larger than 5 mm. These lesions can be visualized, however, using special reconstructions of thin (2-mm) CT sections.

Empty sella represents an intrasellar herniation of the opticochiasmatic cistern into the radiographically enlarged sella turcica. It appears on the CT scan as an area of CSF density occupying the sella (Fig. D4.26). An empty sella in older patients may not signify disease and may represent a physiologic involution of the pituitary with depression of the diaphragma sellae (30% of persons over 40 years of age).

The *pituitary stalk* is visible in the posterior part of the sellar entrance.

Coexisting intrasellar herniation of the opticochiasmatic cistern is present in approximately 20% of patients with microadenoma.

Magnetic Resonance Imaging

(Figs. C16, D4.12–29)

Normal Anatomy

MR can provide optimum visualization of sellar anatomy on both the coronal and sagittal projections. T1-weighted sequences using a thin-slice technique (2–3 mm) are most suitable. The infundibulum, optic chiasm, and other adjacent structures are displayed with exceptional clarity owing to the low signal intensity of CSF in the surrounding cisterns. The anterior lobe of the pituitary gives a moderate, homogeneous signal intensity on the T1-weighted image, matching that of the white matter. The posterior lobe of the pituitary is displayed as a hyperintense structure in most cases. The 1- to 1.5-mm-thick infundibulum always contrasts well with the surrounding CSF. The bony structures of the sphenoid sinus (midsagittal scan) cannot be identified due to the absence of signal from bone. The dorsum sellae and clinoid processes give an intense signal due to the presence of fat marrow.

Noncontrast Scan

Microadenomas appear slightly hypointense to normal brain parenchyma on the T1-weighted scan. Morphologically, there is asymmetric expansion of the gland contour with contralateral displacement of the infundibulum. With very small microadenomas (Cushing's disease), the sensitivity of MR is comparable to that of CT (Figs. D4.22–24, 26). Little additional information is gained by obtaining T2-weighted sequences.

Macroadenomas likewise appear hypointense to brain and normal pituitary tissue on the T1-weighted image. In many cases normal pituitary tissue can no longer be recognized when the tumor becomes very large. The T2-weighted image shows a slight hyperintensity that does not contribute significantly to diagnosis.

Anatomic structures surrounding or traversing the tumor, such as the optic chiasm, carotid artery, and cavernous sinus, are displayed with great clarity. It is easy to determine whether these structures are displaced or enveloped by tumor. The low-signal CSF clearly outlines the tumor boundaries relative to surrounding structures, especially the optic chiasm, which gives a slightly higher signal intensity than the tumor (Figs. D4.20–23, 25).

Cysts appear hypointense on T1-weighted sequences and hyperintense on T2-weighted sequences, as do areas of necrosis. Intratumoral hemorrhage can be identified by its high signal intensity on both T1- and T2-weighted sequences (Figs. D4.14, 23).

Post-Gadolinium Scan

Pituitary adenomas enhance with Gd-DTPA, but in general this does not provide significant additional information.

Differential Diagnosis

1. Suprasellar Meningioma. This tumor and pituitary adenoma have the same densities, enhancement kinetics, and sites of occurrence on the CT scan (see Fig. D2.45). Differentiation is possible, however, by noting bone changes typical of meningioma on the plain skull radiograph and by obtaining an additional view on the sagittal plane. Meningioma is not associated with primary sellar enlargement or with endocrine abnormalities (see drawings in Fig. D4.30).

The midsagittal MR image is excellent for establishing the topographic relations of the tumor.

2. Aneurysms. Large aneurysms of the ophthalmic artery and circle of Willis can mimic pituitary adenoma. However, the contrast enhancement of these lesions is extremely dense (see Figs. F74, 75). It is not unusual to find crescent- or ring-shaped calcifications in the aneurysm wall, which are visible on the noncontrast CT scan and should direct suspicion toward a vascular lesion (see Figs. F74, 76). Findings of this kind are an urgent indication for carotid angiography. Generally these large aneurysms do not bleed and tend to produce the manifestations of a space-occupying lesion, most notably visual disturbances.

These aneurysms appear on MR images as areas of signal void. This serves to distinguish them from other types of lesion.

3. Craniopharyngiomas. Craniopharyngioma is not always distinguishable from pituitary adenoma on the CT scan. This is especially true of uncalcified, cystic midline tumors that show peripheral enhancement (Figs. D6.12, 13, 22). A presumptive diagnosis of craniopharyngioma is justified in patients under 25 years of age who develop diabetes insipidus in the setting of a hormonal deficiency (see also drawings in Fig. D4.30). A Rathke's pouch cyst presents simply as an intrasellar cyst (Fig. D6.23). Its contents give a high signal on T1-weighted MR images, serving to distinguish it from the low-signal cyst in pituitary adenoma.

4. Pilocytic Astrocytoma. Pilocytic astrocytomas of the chiasmal/hypothalamic region (older terms: optic glioma, spongioblastoma of hypothalamus, infundibuloma) are distinguished on CT by their irregular configuration, the encasement of one or both optic nerves by tumor, or hypothalamic extension. Calcifications are almost as common as in craniopharyngiomas and are extremely rare in adenomas. Density patterns on plain and enhanced CT scans may be indistinguishable from adenoma.

Again, MR is very useful for establishing the topographic relations of the tumor.

5. Ectopic Pinealoma, Germinoma. The CT features of these neoplasms can closely resemble adenoma, although sagittal and coronal scans will generally show that the tumor lies above the pituitary in proximity to the infundibulum (see Fig. D 1.217). Children and adolescents are most commonly affected. As with other rare tumors of this region, biopsy is necessary to establish a histologic diagnosis. Diabetes insipidus was present in our patients.

MR is superior to CT in evaluating the topography of the disease.

6. Other Tumors of the Sellar Region. *Metastases* are extremely rare in the pituitary and more commonly arise from the skull base or paranasal sinuses. Like other, primary malignancies of this region (*adenoid cystic carcinoma, esthesioneuroblastoma,* etc.), metastases cause destructive changes that are detectable on X-ray films and CT scans.

Our series includes several *chordomas* of this region, which contain numerous flecks of calcification and enhance with contrast medium (see Fig. E 13 a, b). CT findings differ markedly from those of adenoma.

We were unable to distinguish a *malignant lymphoma* of the sellar region from a pituitary adenoma. The same is true of *histiocytosis X*, which may develop anywhere in the hypothalamic-pituitary system (see Figs. D 1.201–203).

One of our patients, a 50-year-old woman, had a *choristoma* (tumor arising from the posterior lobe of the pituitary) which appeared on CT as a large, smooth-bordered mass in the sellar region and could be distinguished from pituitary adenoma only by its vast suprasellar extension (Fig. D 4.31).

Zülch (1986) notes the occurrence of *gangliocytomas* in the sellar region as well.

7. Empty Sella. The high signal intensity of CSF on heavily T2-weighted MR sequences differentiates the empty sella from other conditions with absolute confidence. An intrasellar cyst (e.g., Rathke's pouch cyst) gives a less intense signal than CSF (Figs. D 4.27–29, D 6.23, 24).

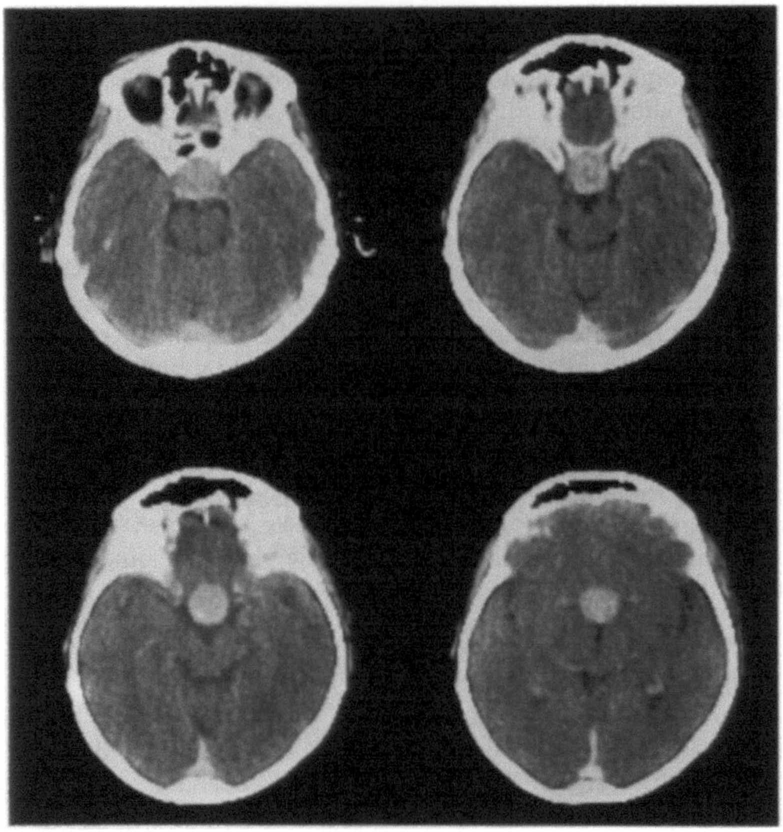

Fig. D4.1. Pituitary adenoma with symmetric intra- and suprasellar growth in a 50-year-old man with bitemporal hemianopia. Postcontrast CT

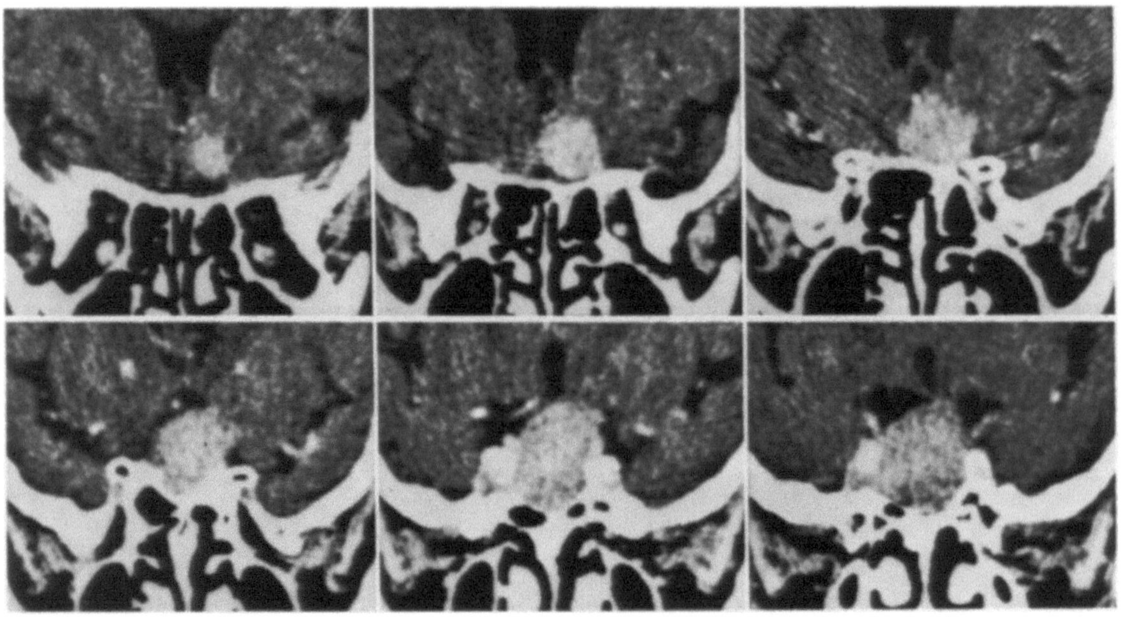

Fig. D4.2. Asymmetric pituitary adenoma with intra- and suprasellar extension in a 71-year-old woman. Enhanced coronal CT

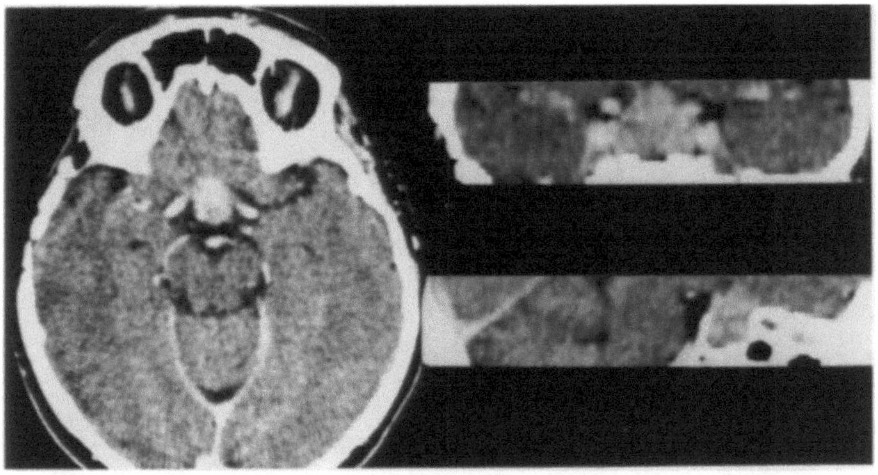

Fig. D 4.3. Pituitary adenoma in a 58-year-old woman who underwent two pituitary operations. Patient was left with residual visual acuity loss and was receiving hormone replacement therapy. She developed a clinically asymptomatic recurrence. The postcontrast axial CT scan and the coronal and sagittal reconstructions demonstrate an intensely enhancing tumor

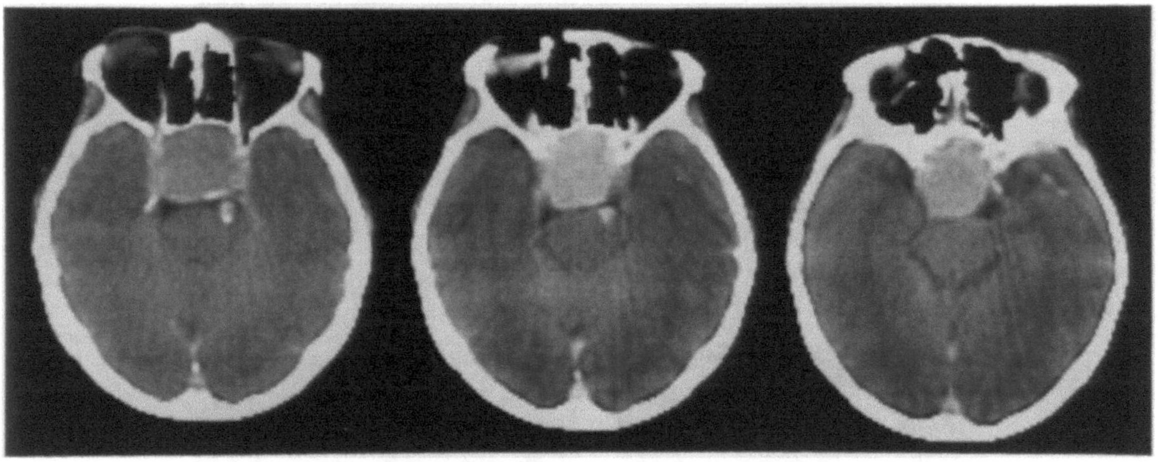

Fig. D 4.4. Large pituitary adenoma projecting into the sphenoid sinus, with complete destruction of the dorsum sellae. Postcontrast CT

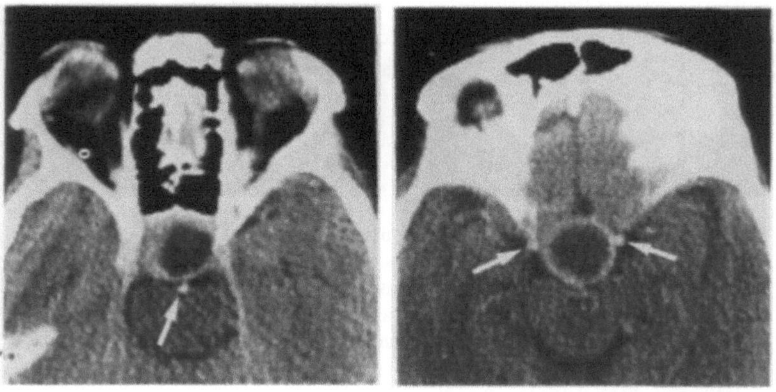

Fig. D 4.5. Cystic pituitary adenoma in a 70-year-old woman with chiasmal disturbances. Ring enhancement is seen in solid parts of the tumor. The large arteries in contact with the tumor capsule, cut at right angles by the scan, show very dense enhancement (right and left internal carotid arteries, basilar artery, *arrows*). An old hemorrhage was found in the adenoma at operation

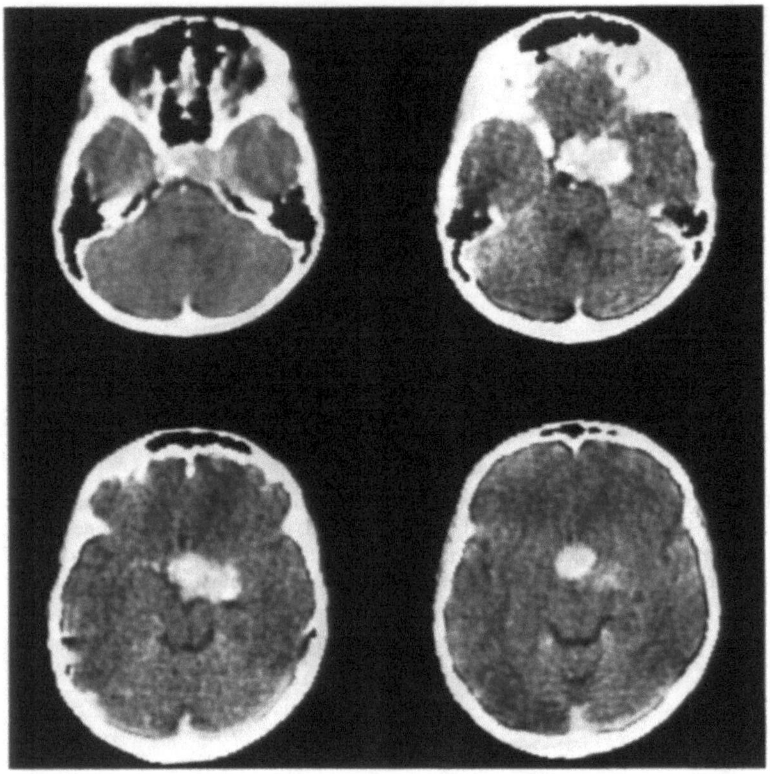

Fig. D 4.6. Pituitary adenoma with intrasellar, suprasellar, and right parasellar extension in a 43-year-old woman. Postcontrast CT

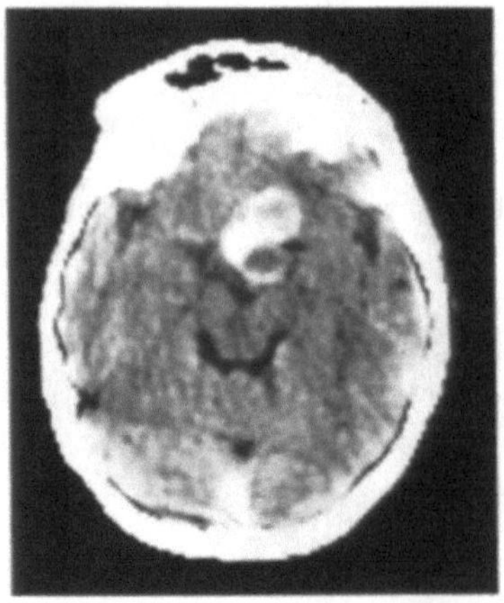

4.7

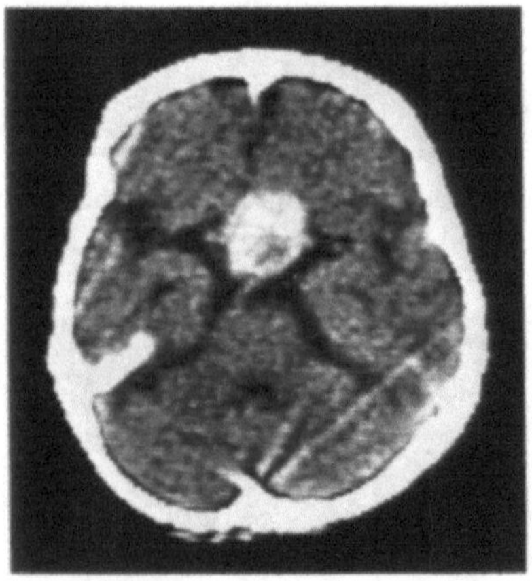

4.8

Fig. D 4.7. Pituitary adenoma with subfrontal extension and hemorrhagic components in a 38-year-old woman with right-sided amaurosis and partial oculomotor paresis of acute onset. The tumor contained very dense foci (70–80 HU) on the noncontrast scan, which were identified as fresh hemorrhages at operation. Behind them was an area of older hemorrhage that resembled a cyst. Postcontrast CT

Fig. D 4.8. Massive hemorrhage into a pituitary adenoma in a 69-year-old man with bilateral amaurosis of acute onset. The density values in the tumor are consistent with freshly clotted blood

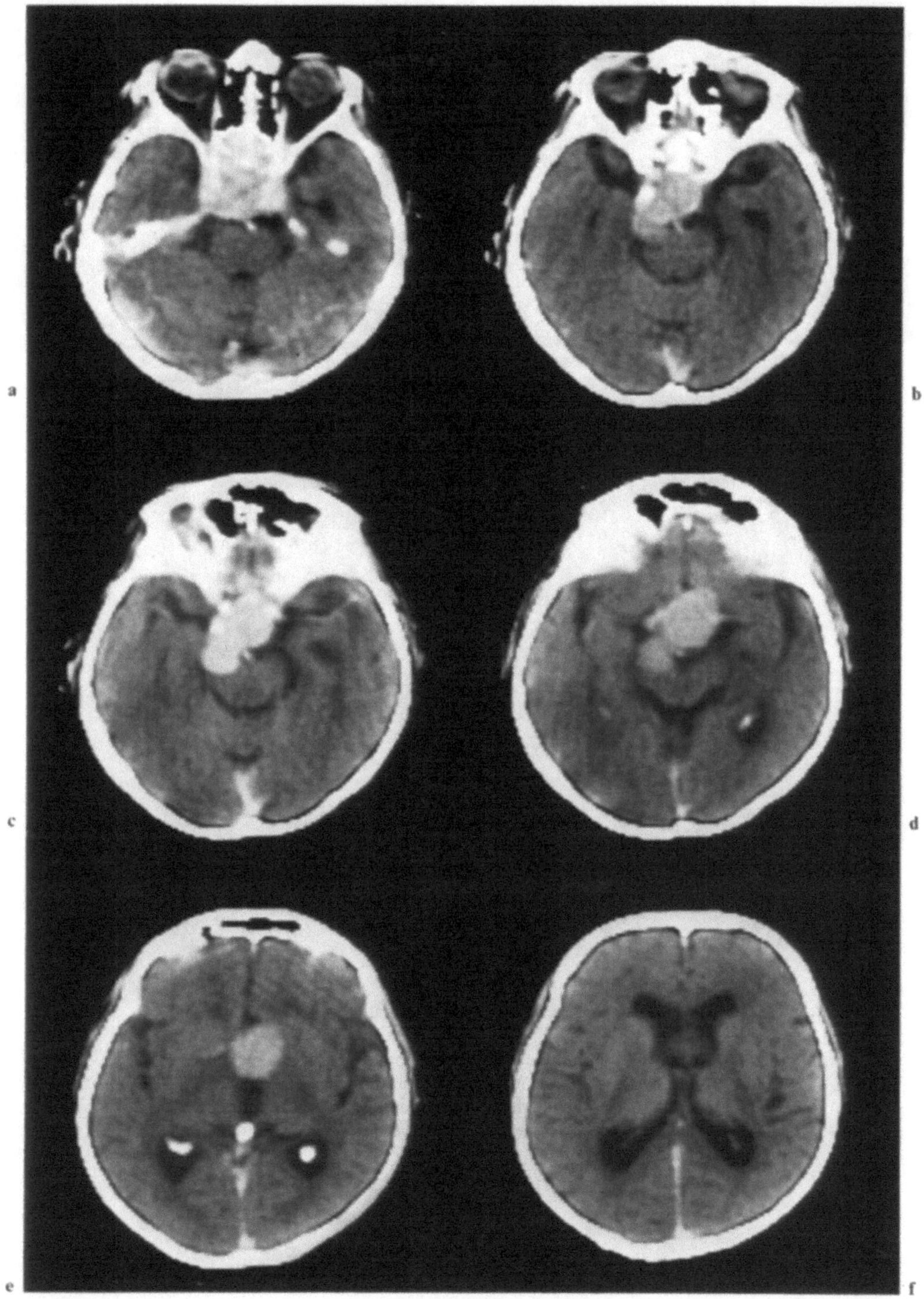

Fig. D 4.9 a–f. Large pituitary adenoma in a 71-year-old man. The tumor has invaded the sphenoid sinus (**a**). A small retrosellar extension projects toward the left cerebral peduncle (**b, c, d**). There is a very high suprasellar extension encroaching on the foramen of Monro (**e, f**). Postcontrast CT

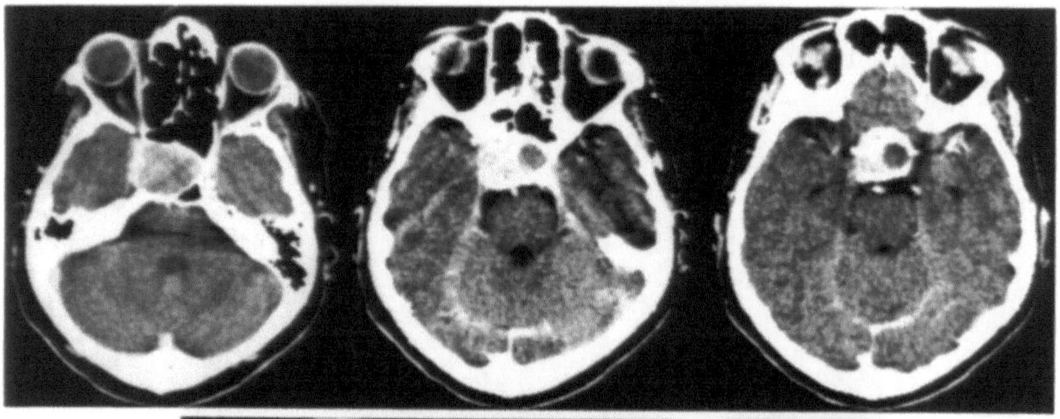

a–c

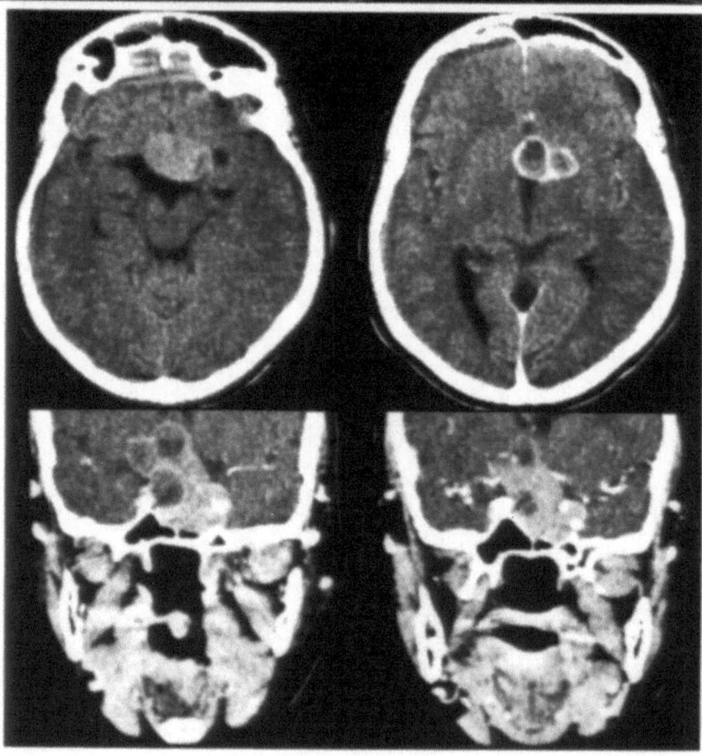

d e f g

Fig. D 4.10 a–g. Chromophobe pituitary adenoma with para- and suprasellar extension, cystic components, and intratumoral hemorrhage in a 42-year-old woman with hemorrhage-related amaurosis. Postcontrast CT: **f, g** coronal. Scan **c** shows the cyst clearly as a hypodense area in the intensely enhancing tumor

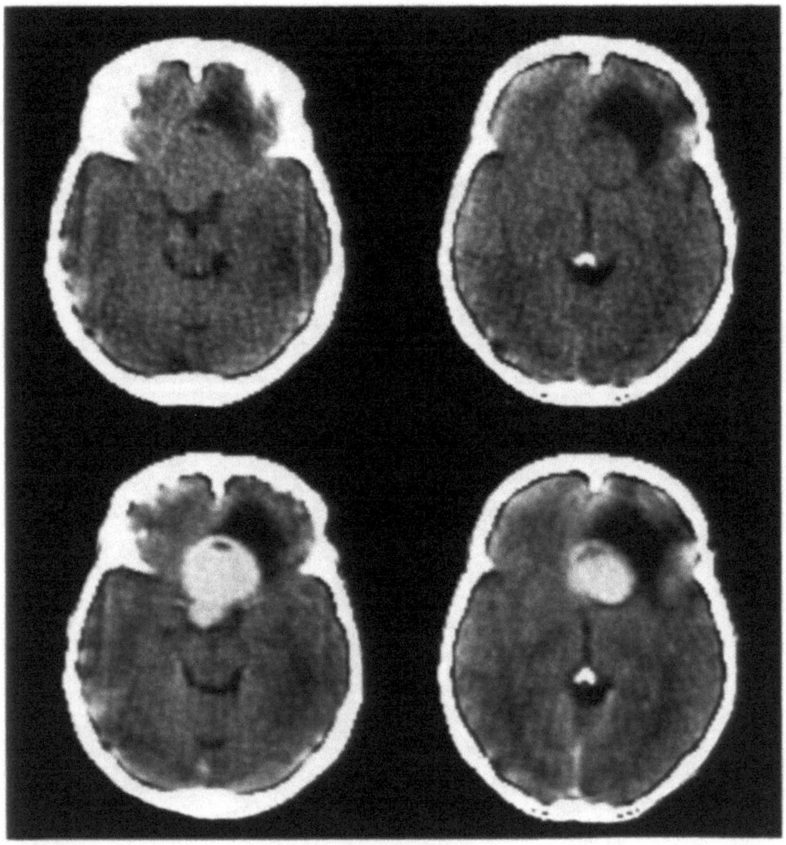

Fig. D4.11. Large supra- and retrosellar recurrence of pituitary adenoma with an adjacent cyst in the right frontal lobe of a 35-year-old woman. The tumor is isodense on the plain CT scans (*top*), and its solid portions enhance intensely and almost homogeneously on the postcontrast scans (*bottom*)

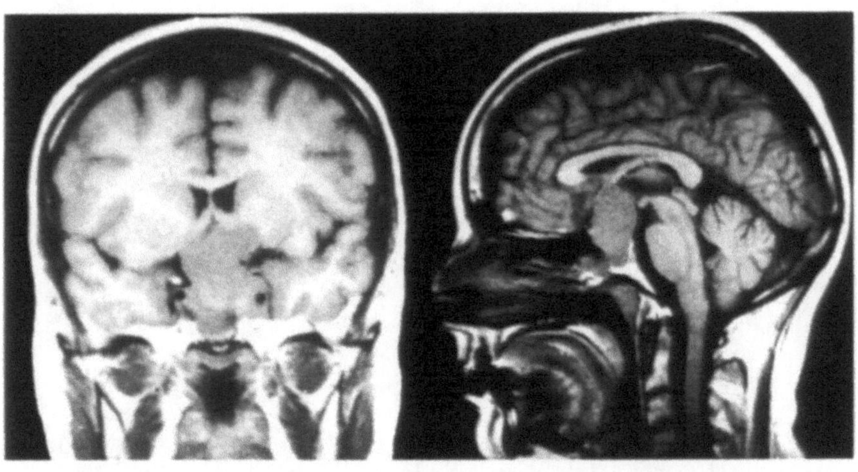

Fig. D4.12. Large intra- and suprasellar pituitary adenoma in a 40-year-old woman with secondary amenorrhea. MR: *left* SE 500/30 coronal, *right* SE 500/30 sagittal. The T1-weighted images show a hypointense tumor adjacent to the third ventricle extending to the foramen of Monro

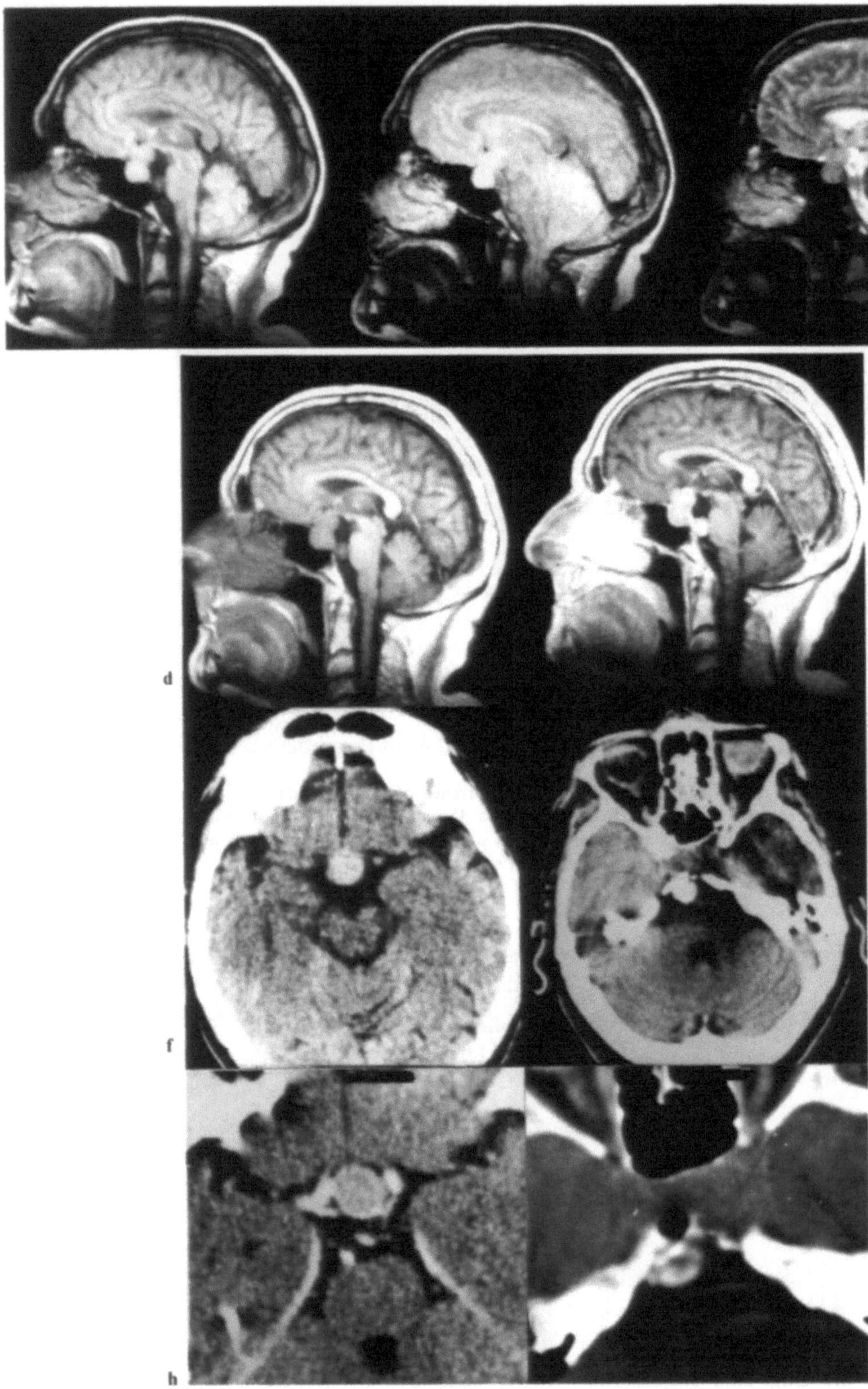

a–c d e f g h i

Fig. D 4.13 a–i. Intra- and suprasellar pituitary adenoma in a 75-year-old man. MR: **a** SE 1600/30, **b** SE 1600/90, **c** SE 1600/180, **d** SE 200/16 post Gd-DTPA, all images sagittal. CT: **f, g, i** precontrast, **h** postcontrast. The intra- and suprasellar components are hyperintense on the proton-density image (**a**). Image **c** shows evidence of a second lesion of almost equal signal intensity between the clivus and pons (calcified basilar artery aneurysm, requires differentiation from calcified clivus meningioma). Both lesions enhance with Gd-DTPA (**e**). The tumor appears hyperdense on the plain CT scans. The lesion near the clivus presents a very high density in the magnified view (**i**)

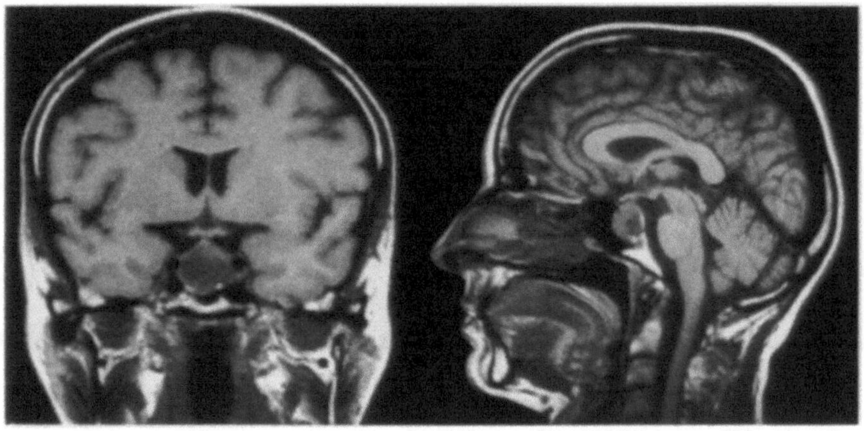

Fig. D 4.14. Intrasellar pituitary adenoma with a cyst in a 51-year-old woman with secondary amenorrhea and hyperprolactinemia. MR: *left* SE 500/30 coronal, *right* SE 500/30 sagittal. The cyst is somewhat more hypointense than the tumor tissue on the T1-weighted sequences

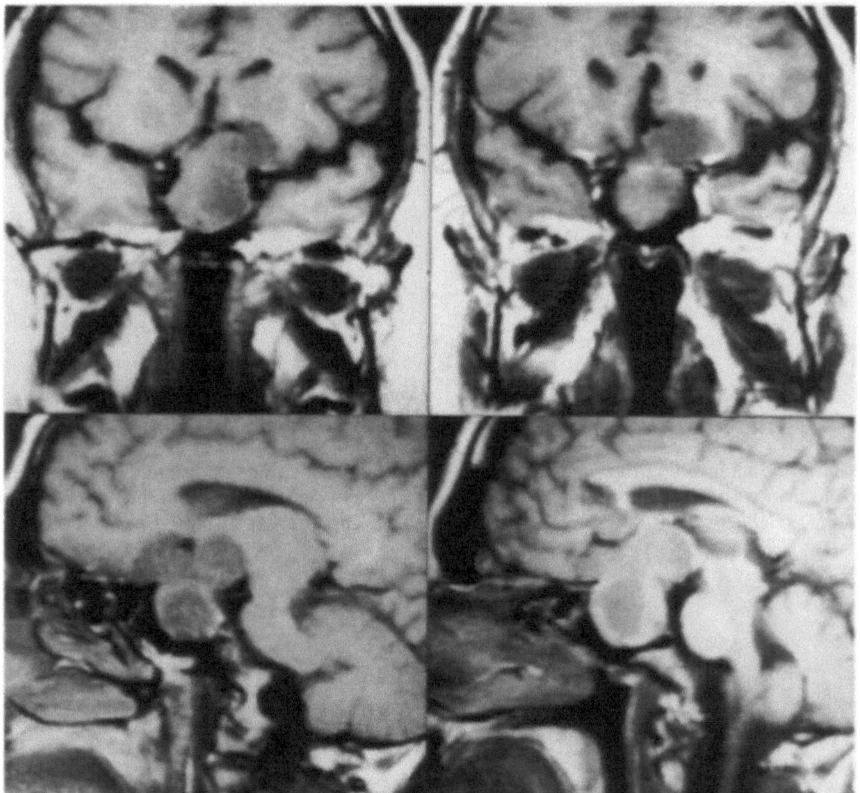

Fig. D 4.15. Large, functioning pituitary adenoma with intrasellar, suprasellar, retrosellar, and subfrontal extension in a 50-year-old man with chiasmal disturbances. MR: *top* SE 700/30 coronal, *bottom* SE 700/30 sagittal. The T1-weighted images demonstrate a mixed-intensity tumor. The sagittal image shows the subfrontal extension compressing the ventricles from below

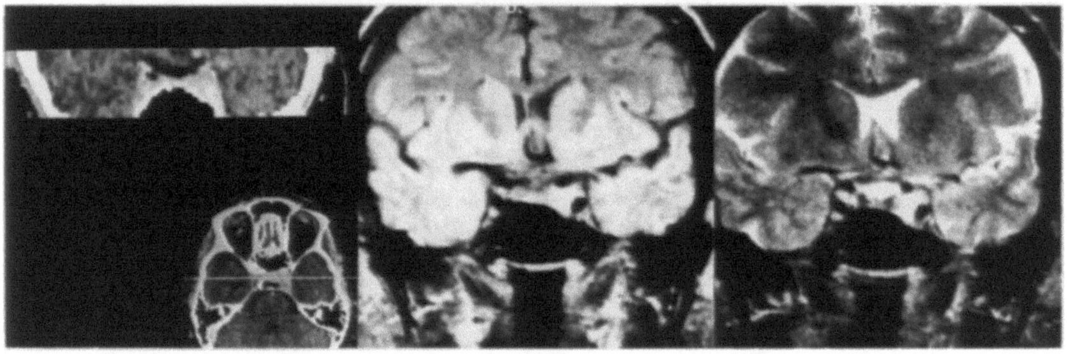

Fig. D4.16. Parasellar and extraglandular pituitary adenoma in a 41-year-old woman with acromegaly. Postcontrast CT: *left* coronal reconstruction. MR: *center* SE 2500/35, *right* SE 2500/120. The right parasellar tumor is isointense to the pituitary on the T2-weighted image and is clearly demarcated from it (*right*)

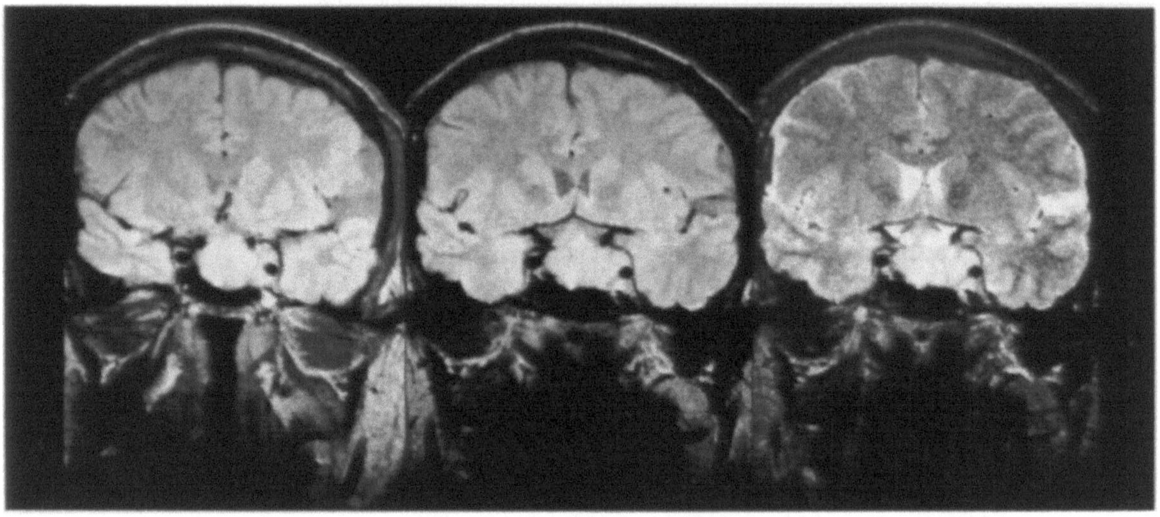

Fig. D4.17. Pituitary adenoma invading the right cavernous sinus in a 43-year-old man with florid acromegaly. MR: *left* and *center* SE 3000/35, *right* SE 3000/90, all coronal. The proton-density and T2-weighted images display the carotid artery as a signal void within the tumor-infiltrated cavernous sinus. The artery is displaced basolaterally

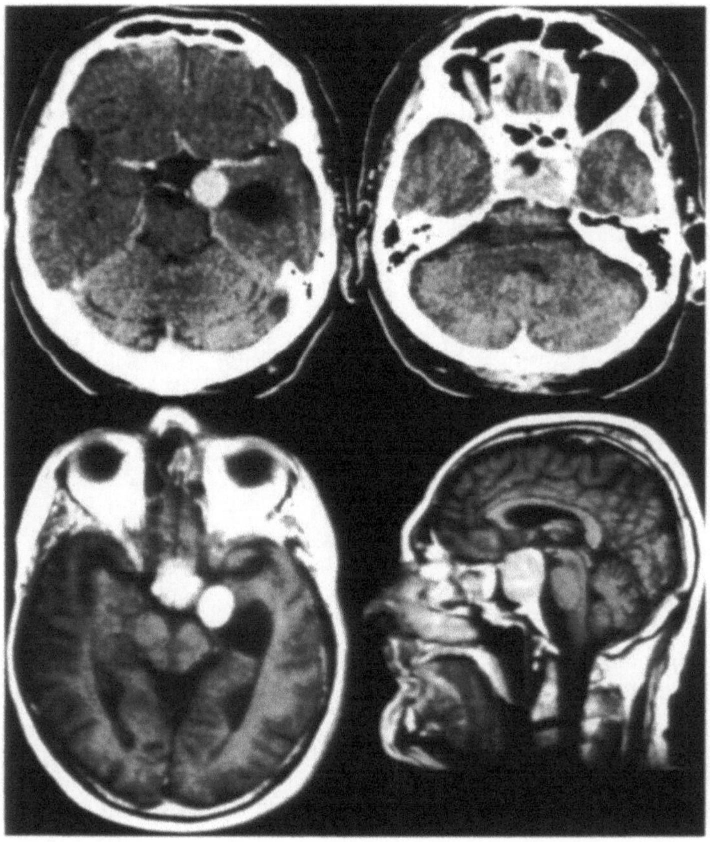

a b c d

Fig. D4.18a–d. Intra- and right parasellar pituitary adenoma with a temporal cyst in a 73-year-old man with subjective visual disturbances and pronounced altered mental status. CT: **a, b** postcontrast. MR: **c** SE 400/30 post Gd-DTPA, **d** SE 400/30 sagittal post Gd-DTPA. The signal characteristics of the intra- and parasellar tumor components differ markedly on the T1-weighted image (**c**). Suprasellar extension is apparent on the sagittal view (**d**)

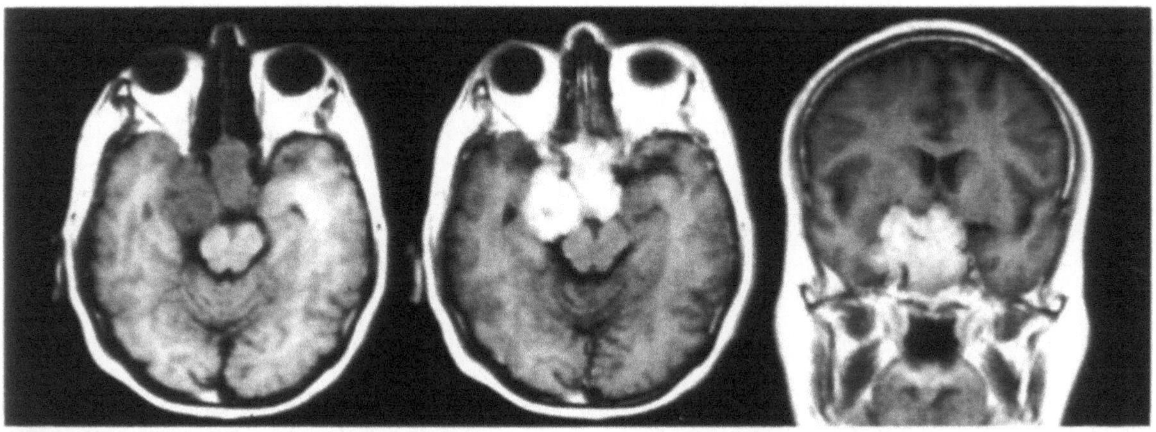

Fig. D4.19. Eosinophil pituitary adenoma with invasion of the sphenoid sinus and destruction of the clivus. The 40-year-old man presented with a 2-year history of discharge of CSF via the nose, impotence, bitemporal hemianopia, and bilateral visual acuity loss. MR *left* SE 400/30, *center* SE 400/30 post Gd-DTPA, *right* SE 400/30 post Gd-DTPA coronal. The lesion enhances intensely on the post-Gd-DTPA T1-weighted scans

a–c

d–f

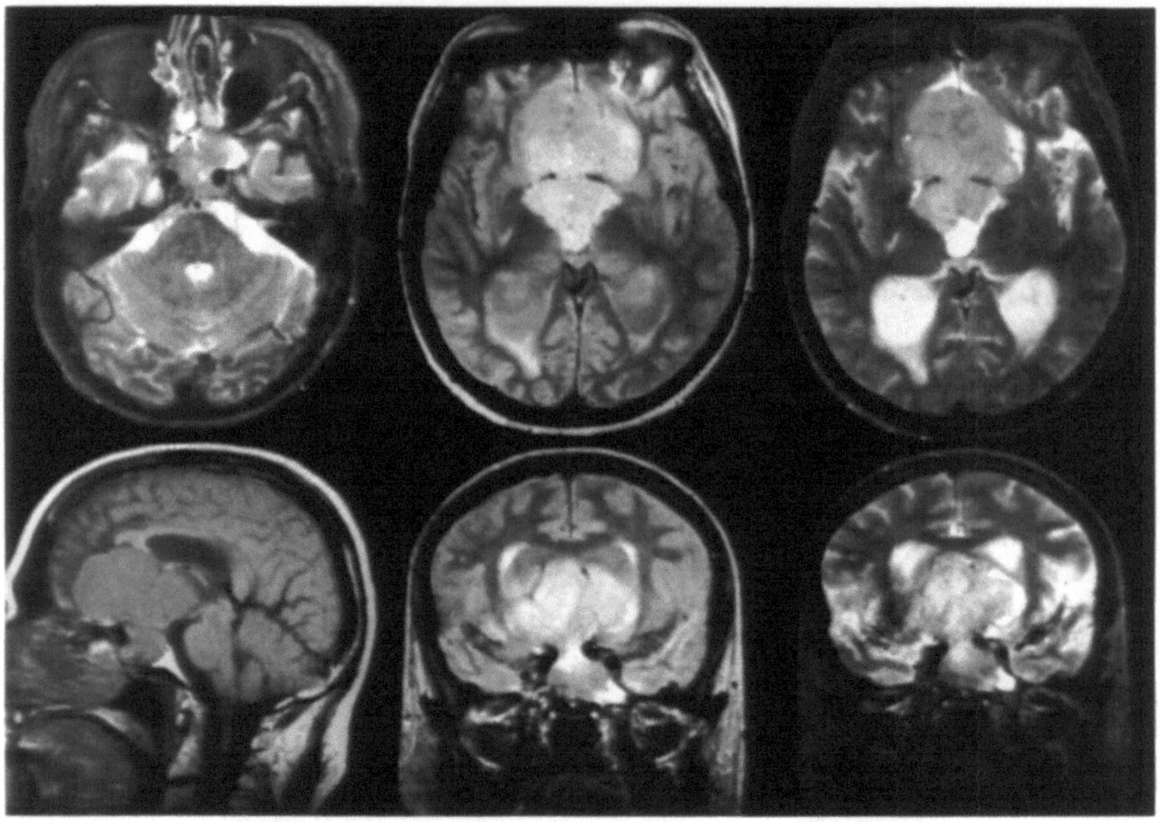

Fig. D 4.20 a–f. Giant pituitary adenoma with intrasellar, suprasellar, parasellar, retrosellar, and subfrontal extension in an 82-year-old man with increasing bitemporal hemianopia and subtle alteration in mental status consistent with a frontal brain lesion. MR: **a** SE 3000/90, **b** SE 3000/30, **c** SE 3000/90, **d** SE 700/30 sagittal, **e** SE 3000/30 coronal, **f** SE 3000/90 coronal. The T2-weighted images demonstrate a thin, bright rim of edema surrounding a massive, slightly hyperintense tumor (**c**). The suprasellar and subfrontal extensions appear homogeneous and nearly isointense to brain on the T1-weighted image (**d**)

Fig. D 4.21 a–h. Recurrent pituitary adenoma in a 53-year-old man with acromegaly and diabetes mellitus. CT: **a, b** noncontrast. MR: **c** SE 400/30, **d** SE 400/30 post Gd-DTPA, **e** SE 400/30 sagittal, **f** SE 400/30 sagittal post Gd-DTPA, **g** SE 400/30 coronal, **h** SE 400/30 coronal post Gd-DTPA. CT reveals a partially hypodense tumor with bone destruction affecting mainly the right side of the clivus; extension to the sphenoid sinus and ethmoid cells is apparent. On MR the carotid artery presents as a signal void within the tumor and cavernous sinus (**d, h**)

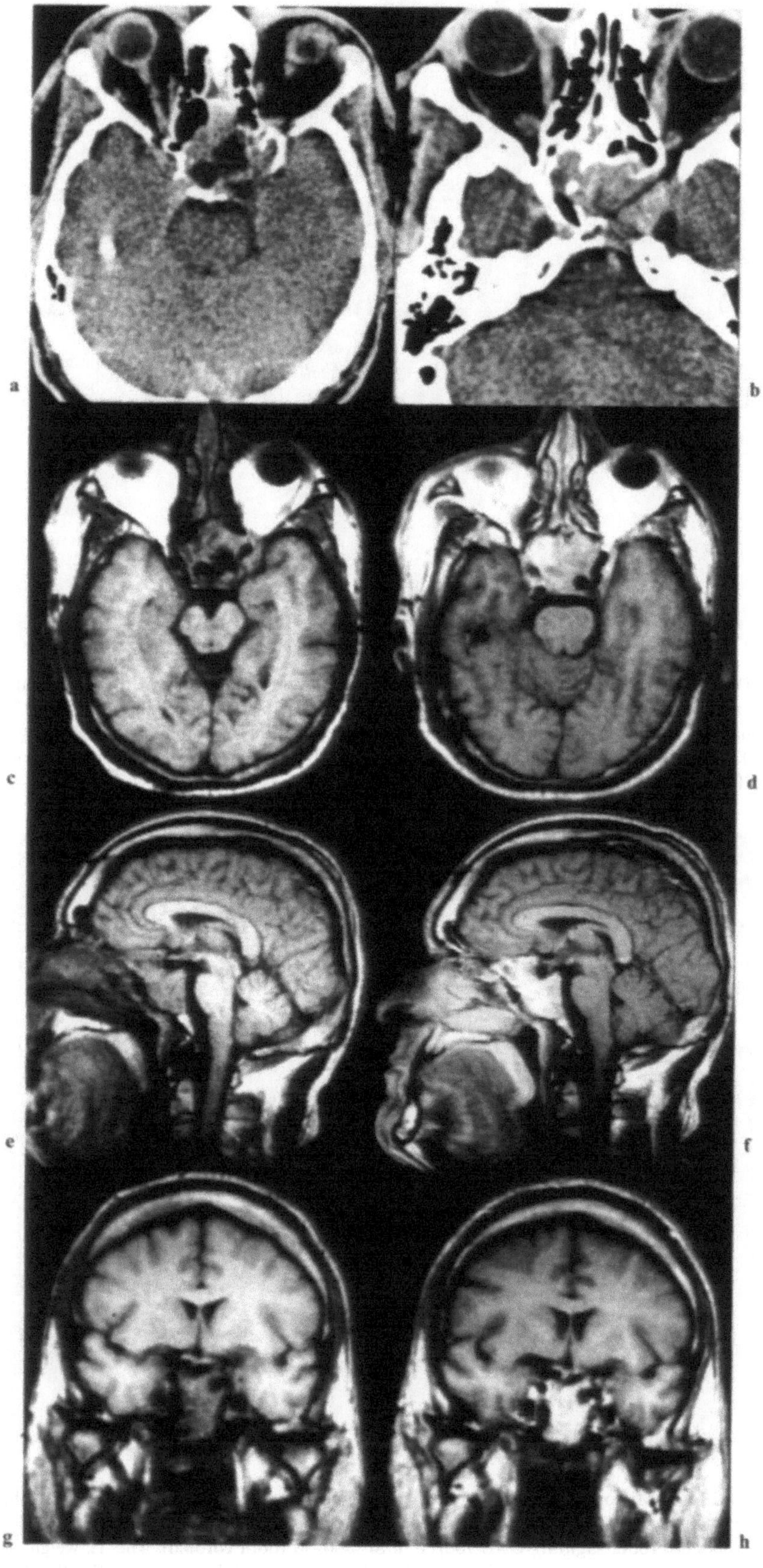
a
b
c
d
e
f
g
h

a b c d

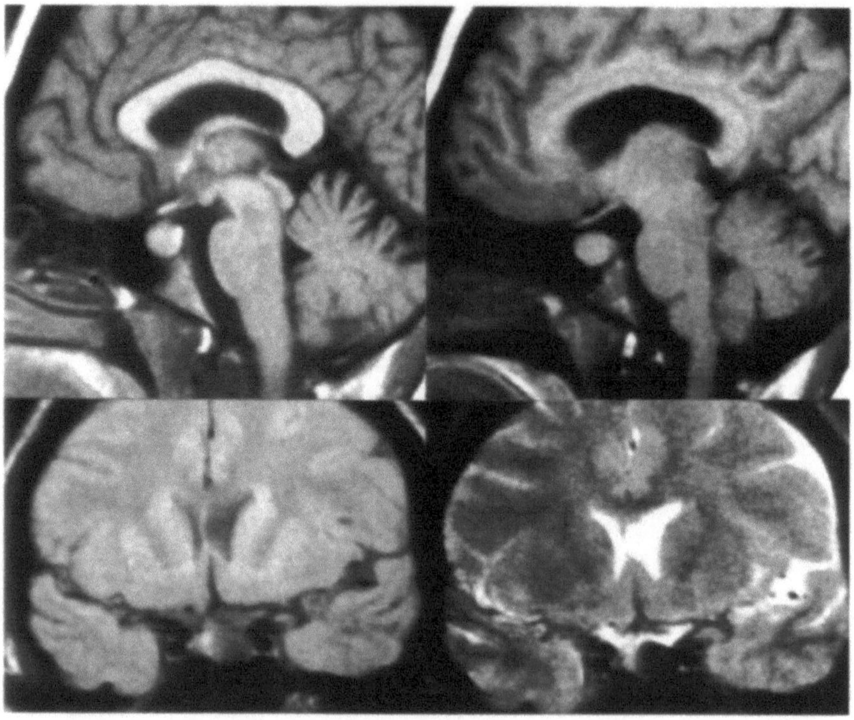

Fig. D 4.22 a–d. Intrasellar pituitary adenoma in a 41-year-old woman with acromegaly. MR: **a** SE 400/17 sagittal, **b** SE 400/17 parasagittal, **c** SE 2500/35 coronal, **d** SE 2500/120 coronal. The tumor is hypointense and poorly defined on the sagittal T1-weighted images (**a, b**). T2 weighting clearly demarcates the low-signal tumor relative to the hyperintense CSF (**d**)

a b c d

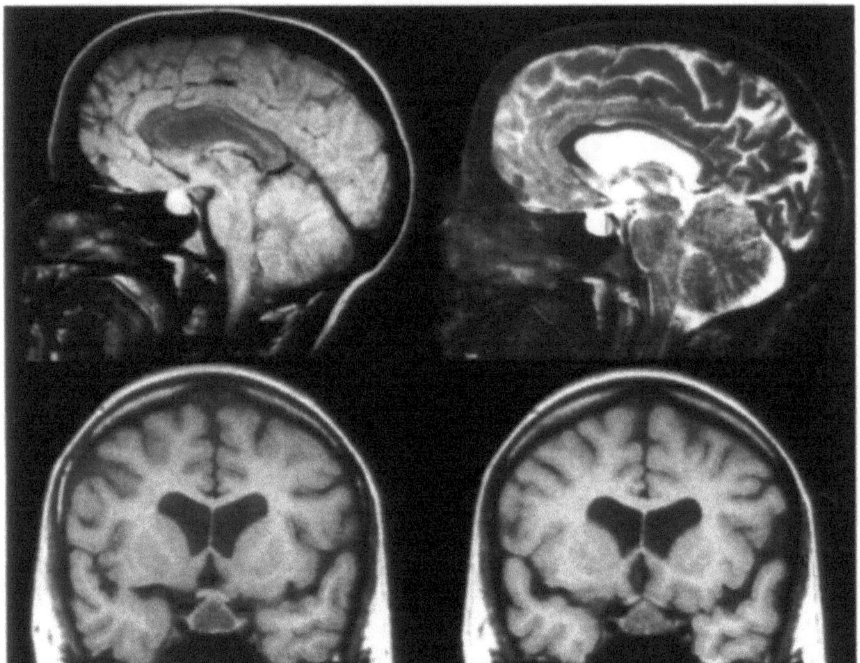

Fig. D 4.23 a–d. Microprolactinoma with an old hemorrhagic component in a 28-year-old woman with hyperprolactinemic amenorrhea and sellar enlargement. MR: **a** SE 2500/35, **b** SE 2500/120 (both sagittal), **c** SE 700/30, **d** SE 700/30 (both coronal). The T2-weighted image (**b**) demonstrates the fluid level of the old intratumoral hemorrhage. On the T1-weighted images (**c, d**) the hemorrhage appears encapsulated and gives a higher signal than the hypointense pituitary tumor

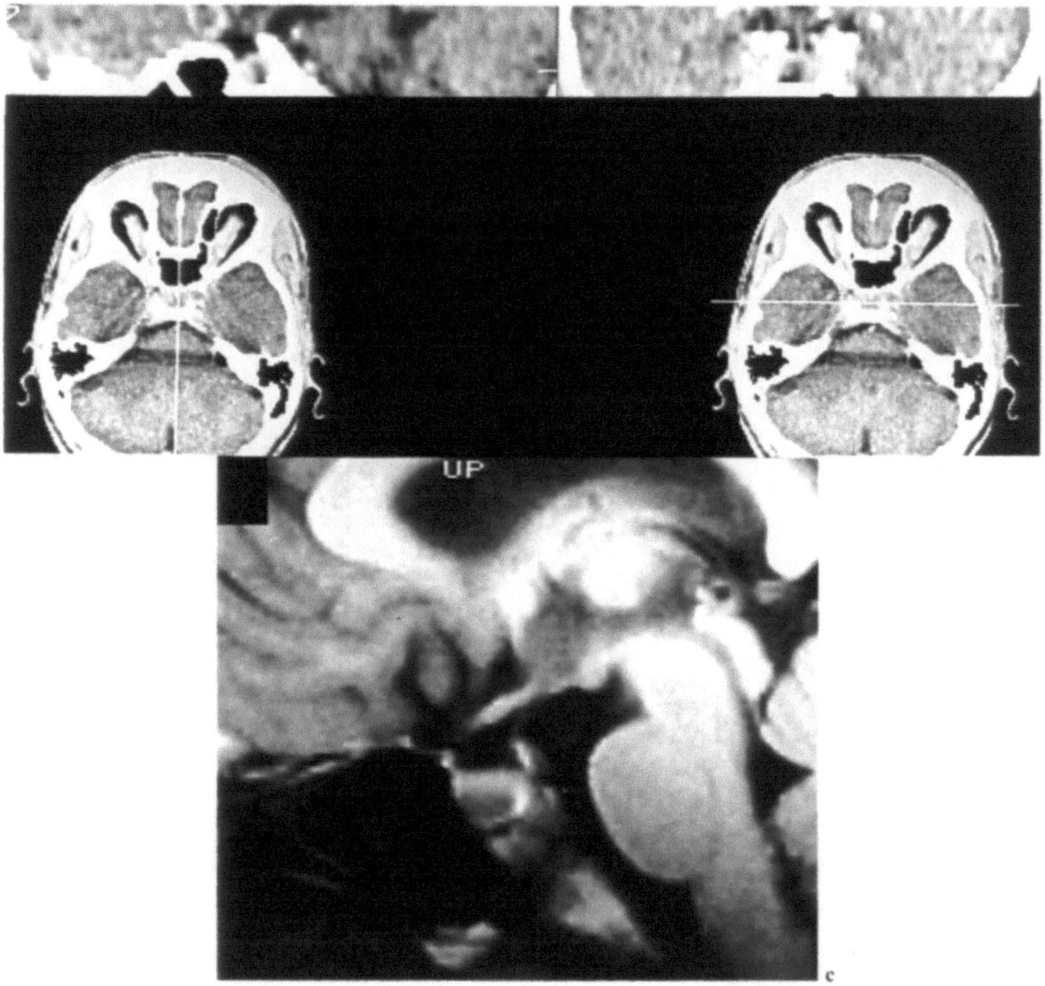

a b c

Fig. D 4.24 a–c. Mediobasal microadenoma 5–6 mm in diameter in an 18-year-old male with central (hypothalamic-pituitary) Cushing's syndrome. CT: **a, b** postcontrast in sagittal and coronal reconstructions. MR: **c** SE 600/15 sagittal. The adenoma presents on MR as a hypointense area that contrasts with the overlying isointense anterior lobe tissue and the hyperintense posterior lobe tissue behind it. Similarly, postcontrast CT scans on the sagittal and coronal planes show a hypodense lesion displacing the infundibulum slightly toward the right side

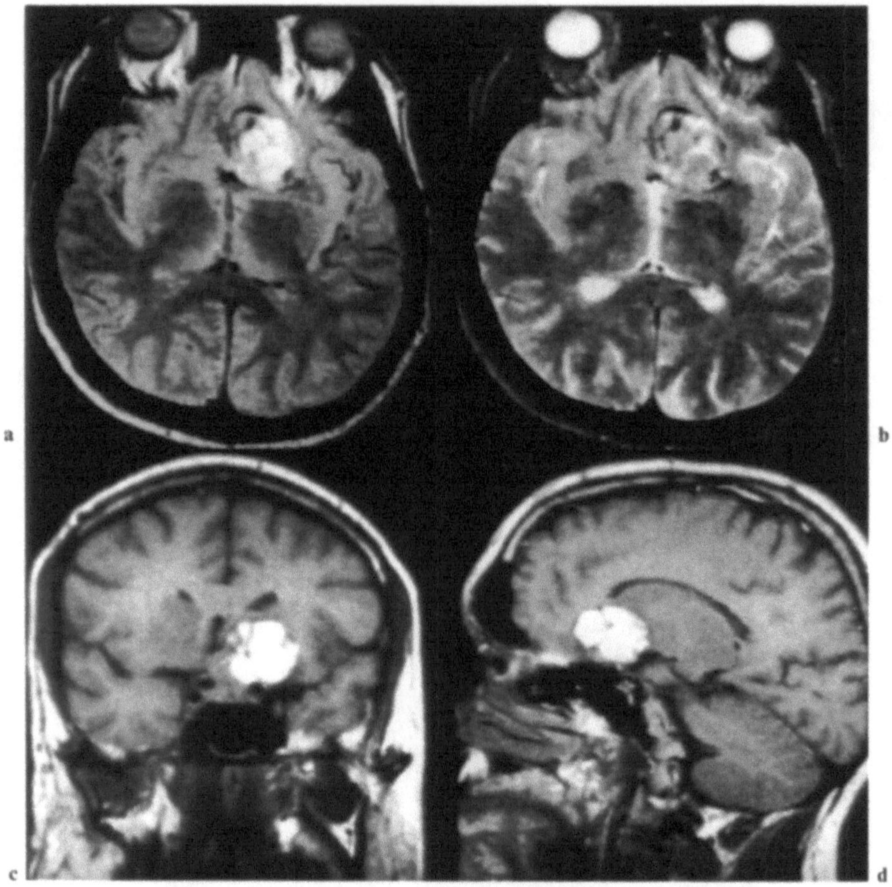

Fig. D 4.25 a–d. Pituitary adenoma with extra- and parasellar extension in a 37-year-old man with a history of headaches for 1 year, altered mental status, and mild visual impairment in the right eye. MR: **a** SE 3000/30, **b** SE 3000/90, **c** SE 700/30 coronal, **d** SE 500/30 sagittal. The tumor shows mixed signal characteristics on the proton-density and T2-weighted sequences (**a**, **b**). It appears markedly hyperintense on the T1-weighted image!

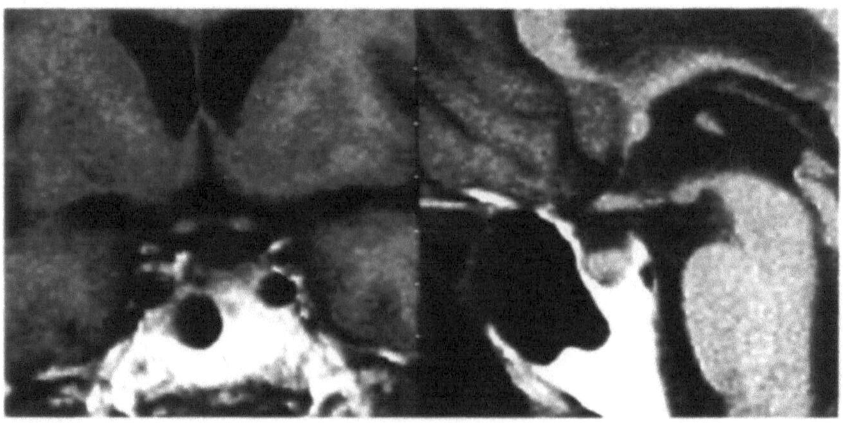

Fig. D 4.26. Microadenoma 4 mm in diameter in a 51-year-old woman with Cushing's disease. MR *left* SE 600/15 coronal, *right* SE 600/15 sagittal. The left paramedian microadenoma is displayed as a hypointense area on the coronal scan. It appears as a basal hypointensity on the sagittal image (*right*) (4-mm slice thickness with intermediate sections)

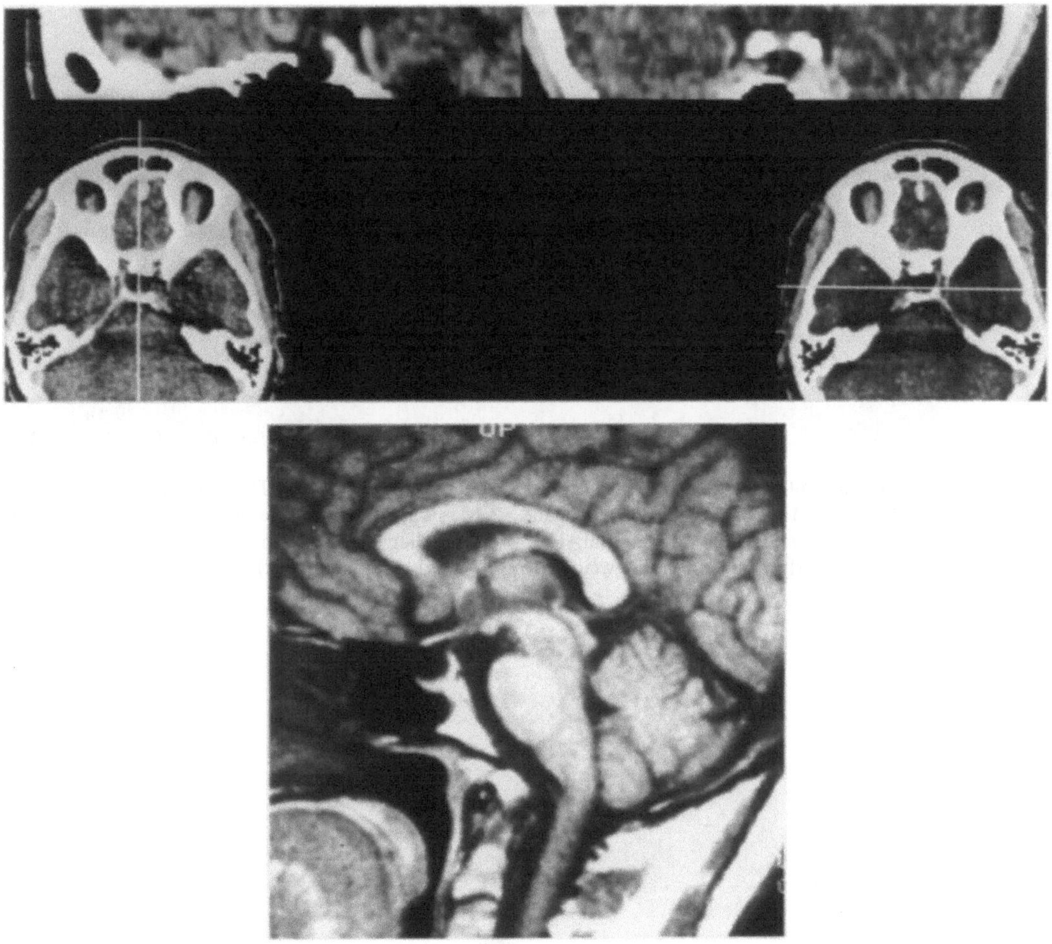

Fig. D 4.27. Empty sella discovered incidentally in a 39-year-old asymptomatic male. CT at *top* with sagittal and coronal reconstructions. MR *bottom* SE 400/17. The sellar region gives virtually no signal on the T1-weighted image

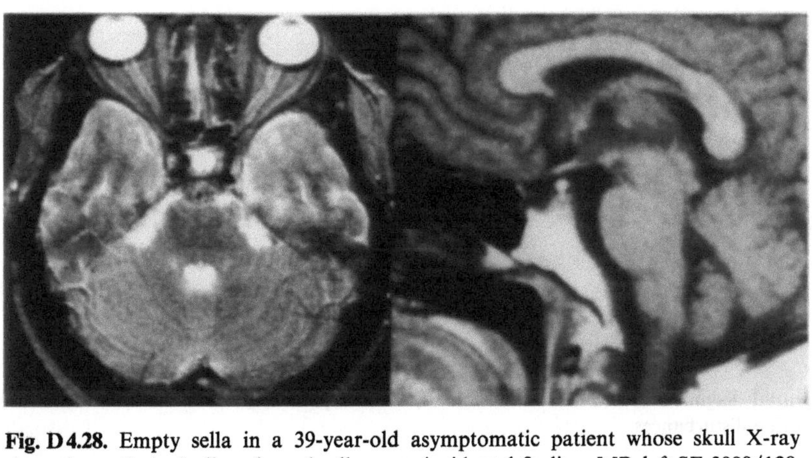

Fig. D 4.28. Empty sella in a 39-year-old asymptomatic patient whose skull X-ray showed a pathologically enlarged sella as an incidental finding. MR *left* SE 3000/120, *right* SE 400/17. The sella gives a low signal on the T1-weighted image (*right*) and appears isointense to CSF on the T2-weighted image (*left*)

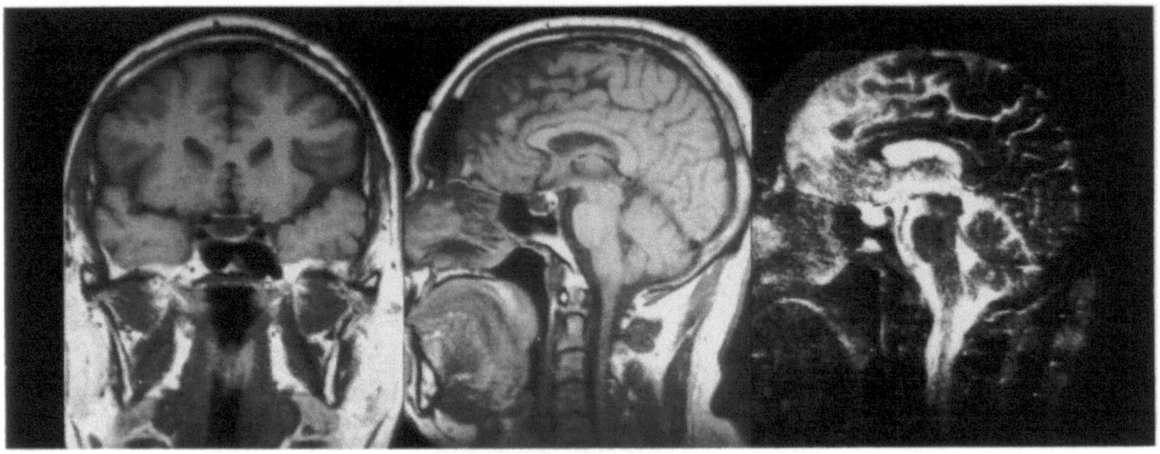

Fig. D 4.29. Empty sella in a 49-year-old man with accompanying hypoprolactinemia. MR *left* SE 400/30 coronal, *center* SE 400/30 sagittal, *right* SE 2200/210 sagittal. The empty, hypointense sella is clearly visible on the T1-weighted images (*left* and *center*). The pituitary appears as a hyperintense peripheral structure on the sagittal view (*center*). The entire sellar region is as hyperintense as CSF on the heavily T2-weighted image (*right*)

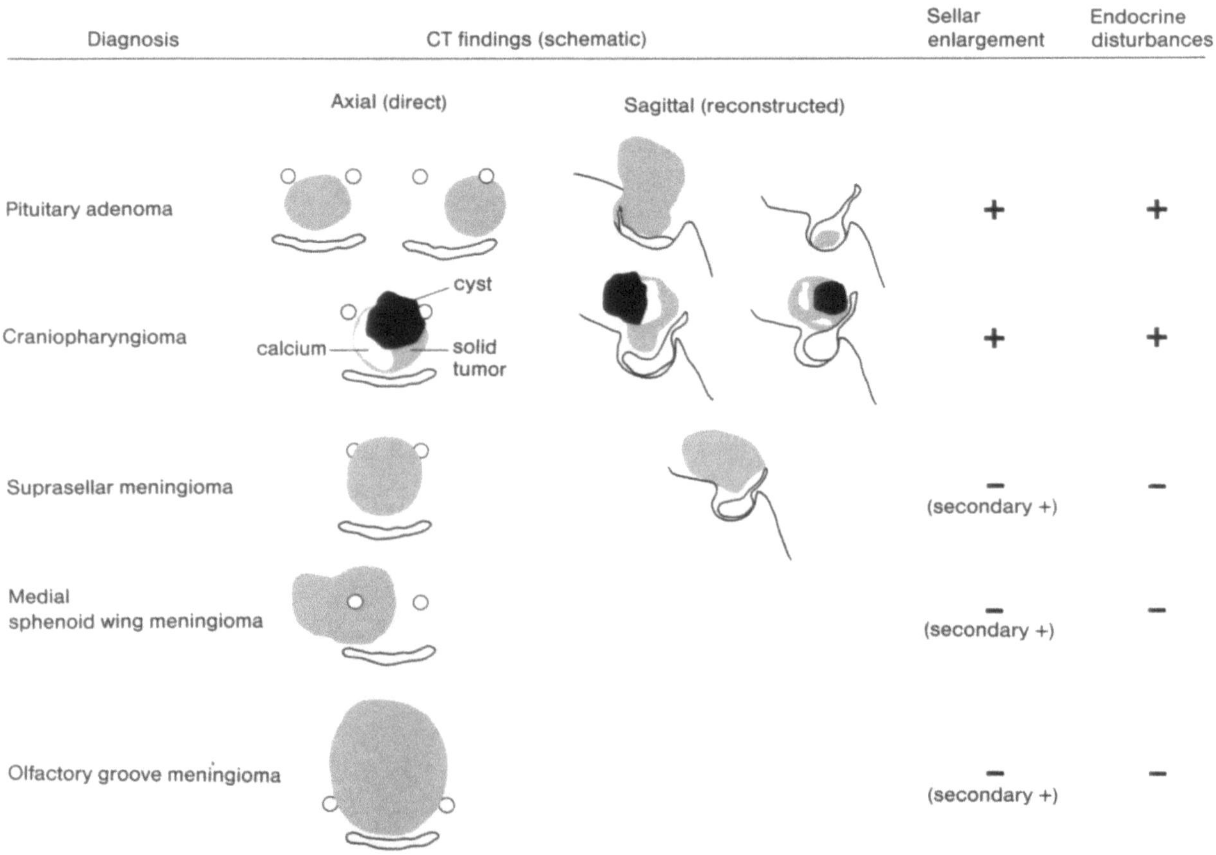

Fig. D 4.30. Differential diagnosis of the most common supra- and parasellar tumors on the basis of CT findings, sellar changes, and endocrine disturbances

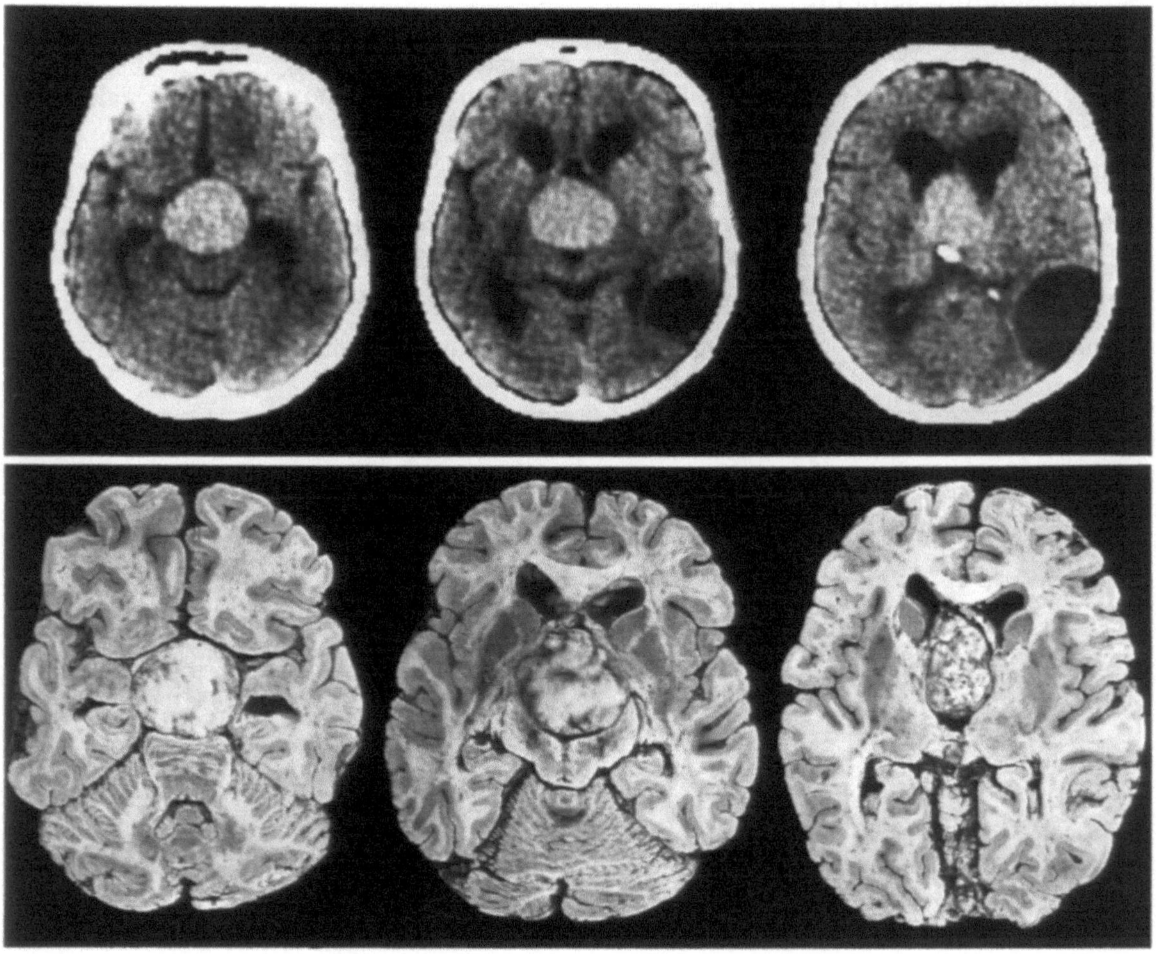

a

b

Fig. D 4.31 a, b. Choristoma of the posterior lobe of the pituitary in a 58-year-old man. CT reveals a large suprasellar mass that is slightly hyperdense on the plain scan. Enhanced scans demonstrate bilateral obstruction of the foramina of Monro (**a**). An arachnoid cyst in the right posterior temporal region is an incidental finding. Postcontrast CT. Note the anatomic correspondence in the brain sections obtained at the levels of the CT scans

5. Hemangioblastomas

Incidence	1%–2% of all brain tumors (most common cerebellar tumor in adults)
Age predilection	30–60 years
Sex predilection	Preponderance of males
Typical site	Cerebellum
Main clinical features	Signs and symptoms of cerebellar dysfunction
Angiography	Densely enhancing tumor nodule, often combined with an avascular space
CT	
Noncontrast scan	Hypodense area very common
Contrast enhancement	Marked in solid tumor nodule
Postcontrast appearance	Cyst with or without mural tumor nodule; ring enhancement occasionally observed; solid tumor with no cystic component may also be seen
MR	
Noncontrast scan	Cyst and solid tumor nodule hypointense on T1-weighted sequences. Both structures homogeneous and hyperintense on T2-weighted sequences
Gadolinium enhancement	Markedly positive in solid tumor nodule
Post Gd-DTPA appearance	Cyst gives low signal on T1-weighted images and is readily distinguished from hyperintense nodule. Enhancement identical in tumors with ringlike configuration. CT and MR appearances very similar. Midsagittal projection best for establishing topographic relationships
Differential diagnosis	
Tumor with large cyst:	Pilocytic astrocytoma Arachnoid cyst "Simple cyst" Enlarged fourth ventricle secondary to obstruction of foramina of Magendie and Luschka
Ringlike tumor with central cyst:	Pilocytic astrocytoma Metastasis Abscess Monstrocellular sarcoma
Solid tumor nodule:	Metastasis Meningioma Acoustic neurinoma Aneurysm/angioma Malignant lymphoma

Hemangioblastoma (synonyms: angioblastoma, hemangioendothelioma, Lindau's tumor) is a grade I tumor derived from the blood vessels. Zülch (1986) reports an incidence of 1.3%, Cushing (1932) 1.2%, and Olivecrona (1967) 2.3%. The prevalence in our series was 1.3%.

Hemangioblastoma is the most common cerebellar tumor in adults, occurring chiefly between 30 and 60 years of age. It is rare in children. Males are affected preferentially by a 2:1 ratio. Occurrence in multiple generations is not uncommon, and inheritance is considered to be established for cases where choroid tumors coexist with tumors of the cerebellum (von Hippel-Lindau disease). Multiplicity of hemangioblastomas is occasionally observed. Cysts in the pancreas and kidneys are not unusual and are regarded as a component of von Hippel-Lindau disease.

Typical Sites, Main Clinical Features

Hemangioblastomas grow almost exclusively in the cerebellum, often in association with a large cyst. They occur rarely in the spinal cord and are extremely rare in the cerebrum. Cerebellar symptoms therefore predominate.

Additional Diagnostic Procedures

The solid part of the tumor shows dense opacification on cerebral angiograms. A large cyst appears as an avascular space. Other adjunctive studies do not aid in the diagnosis of hemangioblastoma.

Computed Tomography (Figs. D 5.1–3)

Noncontrast Scan

In the great majority of cases (73%), plain CT scans demonstrate the tumor as a smooth-bordered hypodensity in the posterior fossa (Fig. D 5.1, 2). The low-density area represents the cystic component, which has a mean density of 20–22 HU. In one case we measured only 12 HU. It is claimed in the literature that 75%–90% of hemangioblastomas possess a cystic component (Ganti et al. 1982; Heiss and Albert 1982).

The solid tumor tissue may have the same density as the surrounding cerebellar tissue, or its density may be slightly higher or lower. Consequently an angioblastoma without a cystic component may escape detection on nonenhanced CT scans.

Contrast Enhancement

Enhancement occurs only in solid tumor components and is very pronounced (averaging 15–20 HU). Because of its vascular nature, the tumor enhances densely and very rapidly after intravenous contrast injection, and washout is also rapid.

Postcontrast Appearance

The solid tumor component is demonstrated with contrast medium in slightly more than half of cases. One pattern that may occur is a *small peripheral tumor nodule with a large cyst* (Fig. D 5.1, 3). Recognition of this pattern can be difficult if the nodule is in direct contact with bone (Fig. D 5.1). A second pattern is a *peripherally enhancing tumor with a central cyst* (Fig. D 5.2). Finally, contrast medium may reveal a *large, solid tumor nodule* that shows almost homogeneous enhancement.

Mild perifocal edema is seen in only a small percentage of angioblastomas and occurs exclusively around noncystic tumors.

Magnetic Resonance Imaging
(Figs. D 5.4–11)

The MR appearance of hemangioblastomas is often very similar to their appearance on CT (see Figs. D 5.4–6).

The cyst and possibly the tumor nodule give a low signal on T1-weighted sequences without contrast medium. The cystic component in particular gives an intense signal on T2-weighted sequences, but it may not be possible to detect a solid nodule (Figs. D 5.7, 10). Gadolinium enhancement of the T1-weighted image provides good separation of the intense tumor nodule from the low-signal cyst. In one case we observed faint ring enhancement of the entire cyst wall and a brightly enhancing tumor nodule on the post Gd-DTPA image (Fig. D 5.6).

MR is especially useful for evaluating the relation of the tumor to the brainstem (Fig. D 5.10). The midsagittal projection is best for this purpose. The situation is more difficult to interpret when intratumoral hemorrhage is present. Large feeding and draining vessels, which may resemble an AV malformation, are occasionally noted on the MR image (Fig. D5.11).

Coronal and midsagittal images can demonstrate concomitant cerebellar and spinal involvement, which is not too unusual (Fig. D5.11).

Differential Diagnosis

The presence of a *large cyst* should arouse suspicion of pilocytic astrocytoma, although that tumor occurs mainly in children. Calcifications favor a diagnosis of pilocytic astrocytoma. Faint contrast enhancement of the entire cyst wall is extremely rare in hemangioblastoma and is far more typical of pilocytic astrocytoma.

An arachnoid cyst can almost always be distinguished from an angioblastomatous cyst by densitometry. The contents of the arachnoid cyst have the same density as CSF, while the attenuation values in angioblastomatous cysts tend to be significantly higher (see above).

It is not possible to differentiate between a "simple cyst" (see Fig. F53) and an angioblastoma presenting as a solitary cyst, since the xanthochromic fluid in a simple cyst also may have slightly higher density values than CSF.

Severe enlargement of the fourth ventricle secondary to obstruction of the foramina of Magendie and Luschka with concomitant narrowing of the aqueduct can simulate a midline angioblastomatous cyst, as can an epidermoid of the fourth ventricle. Density values in both conditions are comparable to those of CSF, and this can serve to distinguish them from angioblastoma. In addition, epidermoid cysts usually present a maplike surface structure.

A *ring-shaped tumor* with a central cyst should again raise suspicion of pilocytic astrocytoma. In some cases CT findings may not allow positive differentiation.

Cerebellar metastases and abscesses may occasionally resemble angioblastoma. Differentiation in these cases relies mainly on the history and clinical findings.

Monstrocellular sarcomas of the cerebellum may be indistinguishable from angioblastomas on the CT scan when a ringlike tumor configuration is observed.

A *solid tumor nodule* may be found in a great many tumors and vascular lesions including metastasis, meningioma, acoustic neurinoma, giant aneurysm, cerebellar angioma, and malignant lymphoma. Differentiation relies on the history, clinical data, otorhinolaryngologic findings, plain skull radiographs, and vertebral angiography.

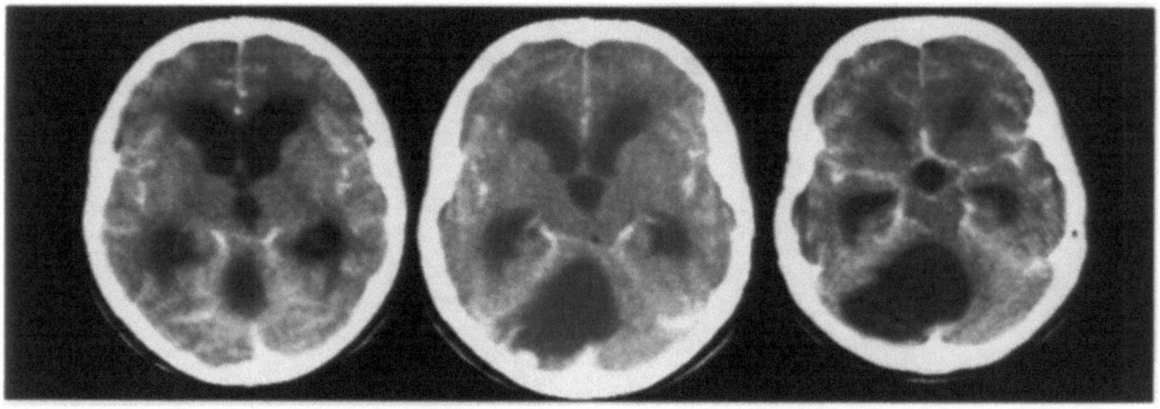

Fig. D5.1. Hemangioblastoma of the left cerebellar hemisphere in a patient with a 4-month history of increasing symptoms of raised intracranial pressure and ataxia. Postcontrast CT demonstrates a solid tumor nodule near the calvarium with a large cyst and associated obstructive hydrocephalus

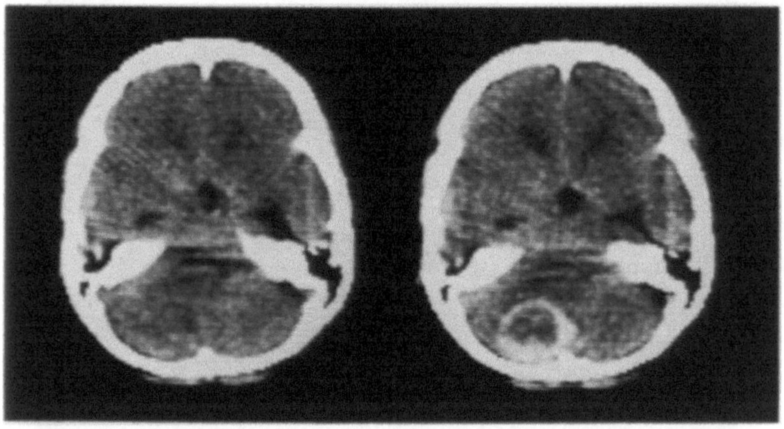

Fig. D5.2. Angioblastoma of the left cerebellar hemisphere with no evidence of a cyst in a 38-year-old woman. The lesion appears isodense on the plain CT scan (*left*) and shows intense ring enhancement on the postcontrast scan (*right*), arousing suspicion of a vascular lesion

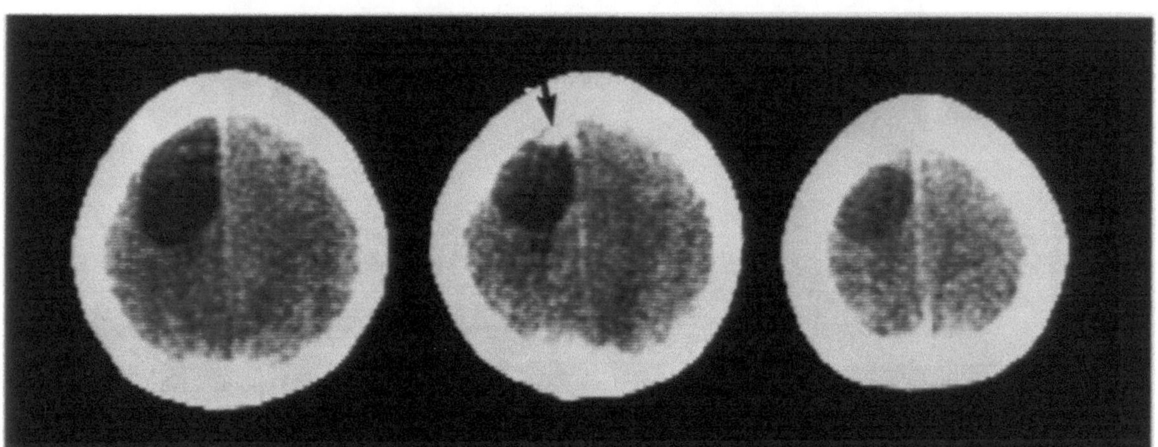

Fig. D5.3. Cerebral angioblastoma in a 70-year-old man with focal seizures. Postcontrast CT scans demonstrate a large hypodense lesion with peripheral, nodular enhancement (*arrow* indicates solid tumor nodule). This location is highly unusual for angioblastoma

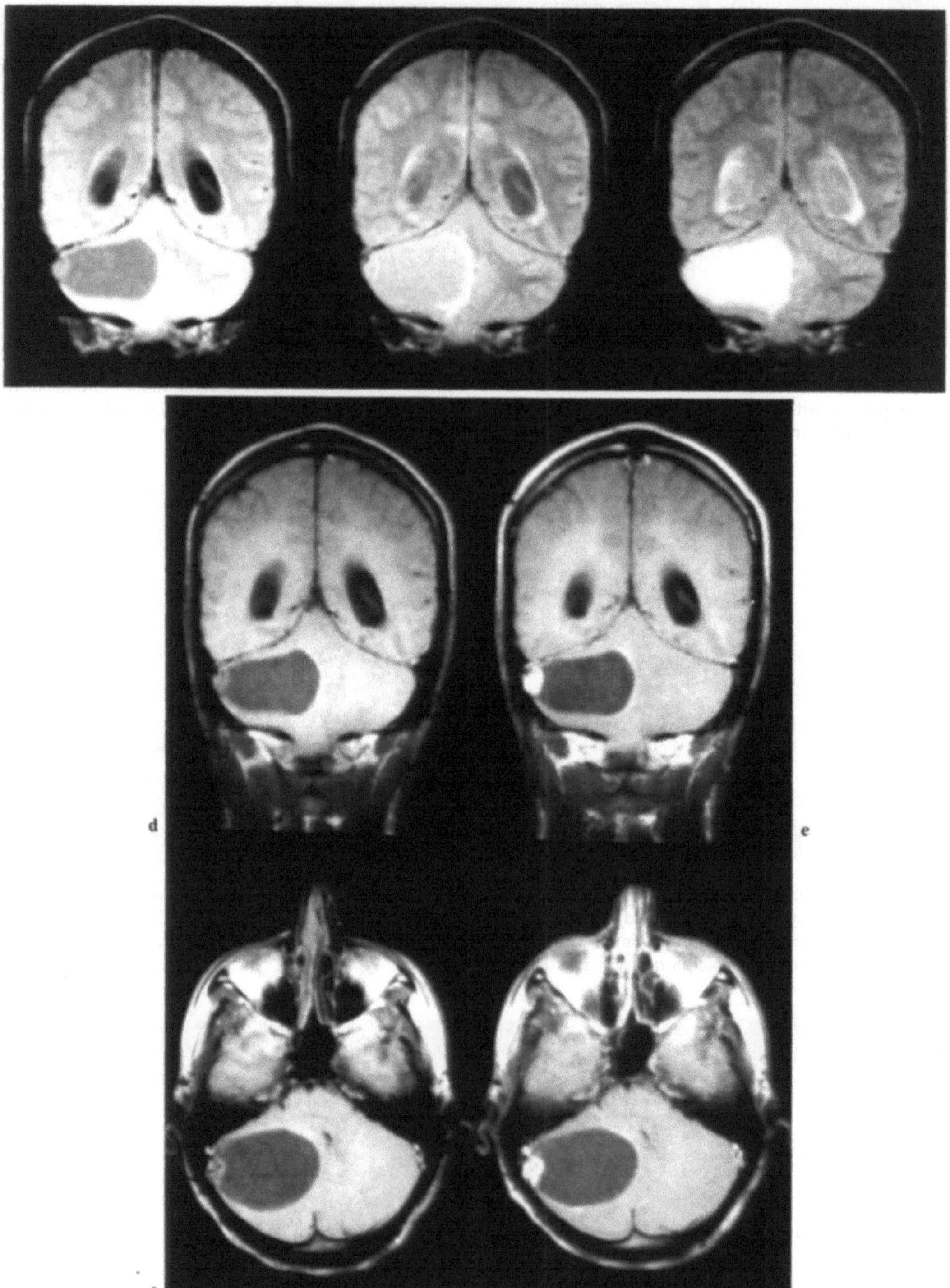

a–c d e f g

Fig. D 5.4 a–g. Hemangioblastoma of the left cerebellar hemisphere with a lateral, solid tumor nodule and large cyst in a 19-year-old man with a 6-week history of increased intracranial pressure, left abducens paresis, ataxia, and latent right hemiparesis. MR: **a** SE 1600/30, **b** SE 1600/60, **c** SE 1600/90, **d** SE 400/30, **e** SE 400/30 post Gd-DTPA, all coronal; **f** SE 400/30, **g** SE 400/30 post Gd-DTPA, both axial. The lateral tumor nodule and cyst are well discriminated on the proton-density image (**a**). The T2-weighted image (**c**) displays only the hyperintense cyst. The solid component enhances markedly with Gd-DTPA (**e, g**)

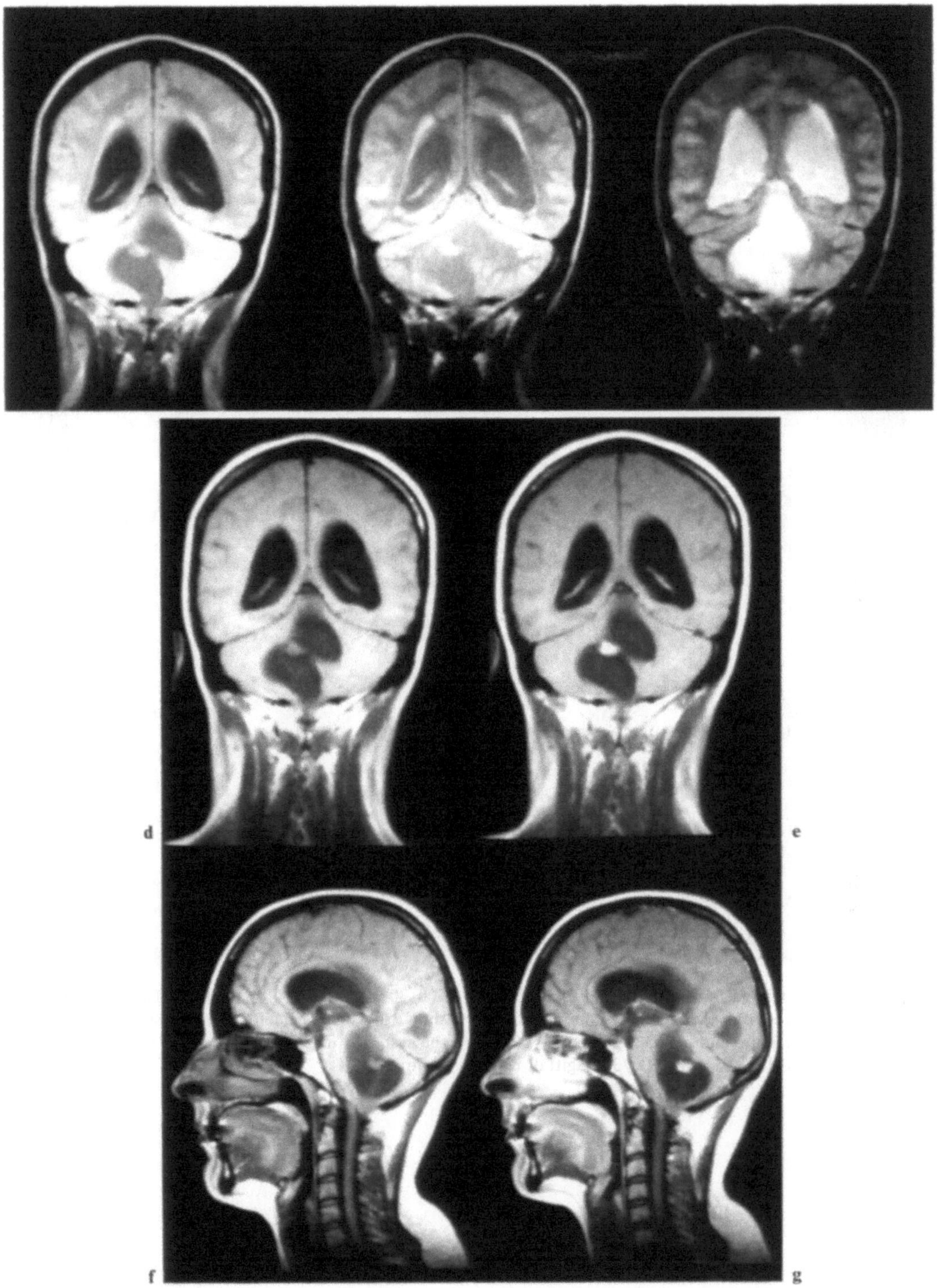

a–c d e f g

Fig. D5.5a–g. Hemangioblastoma with a solid tumor nodule and two cysts in a 17-year-old male with a history of headaches for 3 months, left-sided dysdiadochokinesia, and ataxic stance. MR: **a** SE 1600/30, **b** SE 1600/60, **c** SE 1600/120, **d** SE 400/30, **e** SE 400/30 post Gd-DTPA, all coronal; **f** SE 400/30, **g** SE 400/30 post Gd-DTPA, both sagittal. The proton-density image (**a**) shows the solid tumor nodule flanked by two paramedian cysts. The cysts appear bright on the T2-weighted image (**c**), but the solid tumor is not visualized. The nodule enhances markedly with Gd-DTPA (**e, g**). There is equivocal evidence of a coexisting angioblastoma of the frontobasal cerebrum and a cystic lesion in the occipital lobe

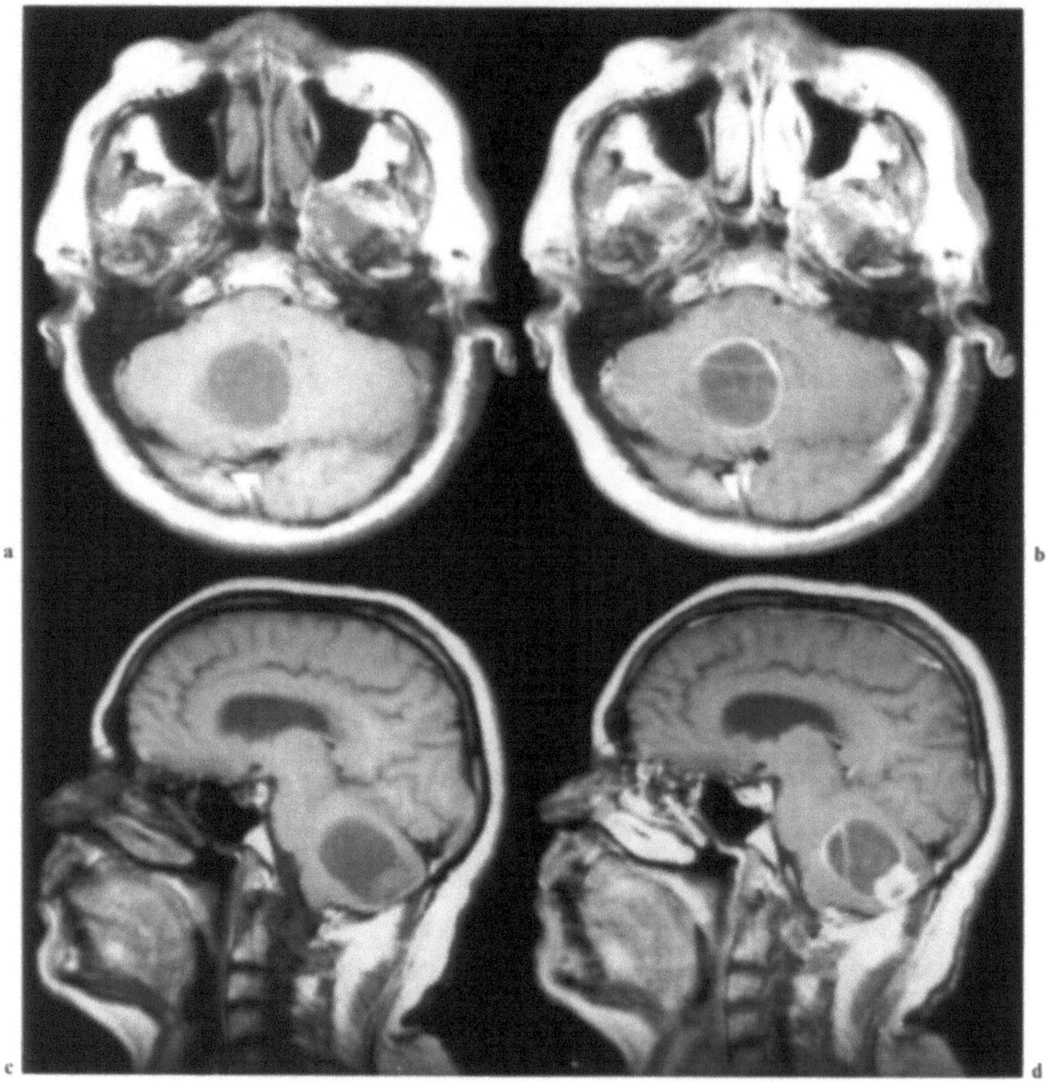

Fig. D 5.6 a–d. Hemangioblastoma of the left cerebellar hemisphere in a 20-year-old man with symptoms of increased intracranial pressure and ataxia. MR: **a** SE 500/30, **b** SE 500/30 post Gd-DTPA, **c** SE 500/30 sagittal, **d** SE 500/30 post Gd-DTPA sagittal. The postcontrast images show ring enhancement of the cyst wall, a septum within the cyst, and marked enhancement of the large, solid tumor component

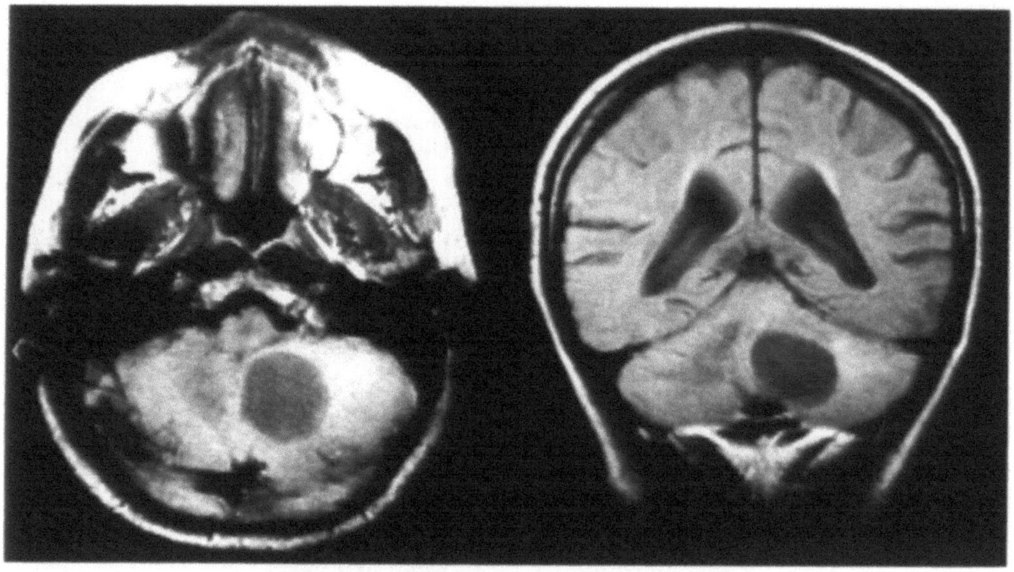

Fig. D5.7. Cystic angioblastoma of the right cerebellar hemisphere in a 73-year-old woman with a 3-month history of progressive ataxia and vertigo. MR: *left* SE 2000/35 axial, *right* SE 2000/35 coronal. The T1-weighted images reveal an entirely cystic mass that is markedly hypointense to the surrounding cerebellum. Hydrocephalus is present

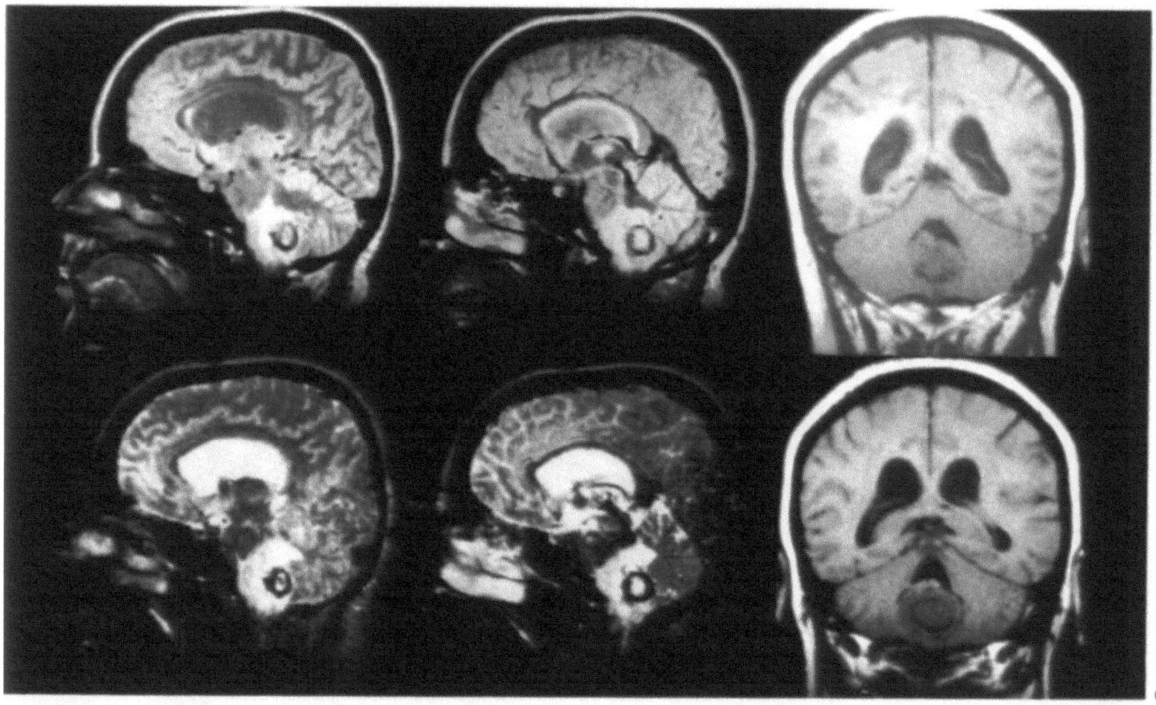

a–c

d–f

Fig. D5.8a–f. Large, predominantly solid hemangioblastoma of the cerebellar vermis in a 44-year-old woman with a 6-week history of ataxia and scanning speech. MR: **a, b** SE 2500/30 sagittal, **c** SE 500/30 coronal, **d, e** SE 2500/120 sagittal, **f** SE 500/30 coronal. The midsagittal and parasagittal proton-density images (**a, b**) demonstrate a solid tumor nodule isointense to the cerebellum and surrounded by a hypodense ring, which sharply delineates the mass. T2-weighted images additionally demonstrate edema of the cerebellar hemispheres (**d, e**)

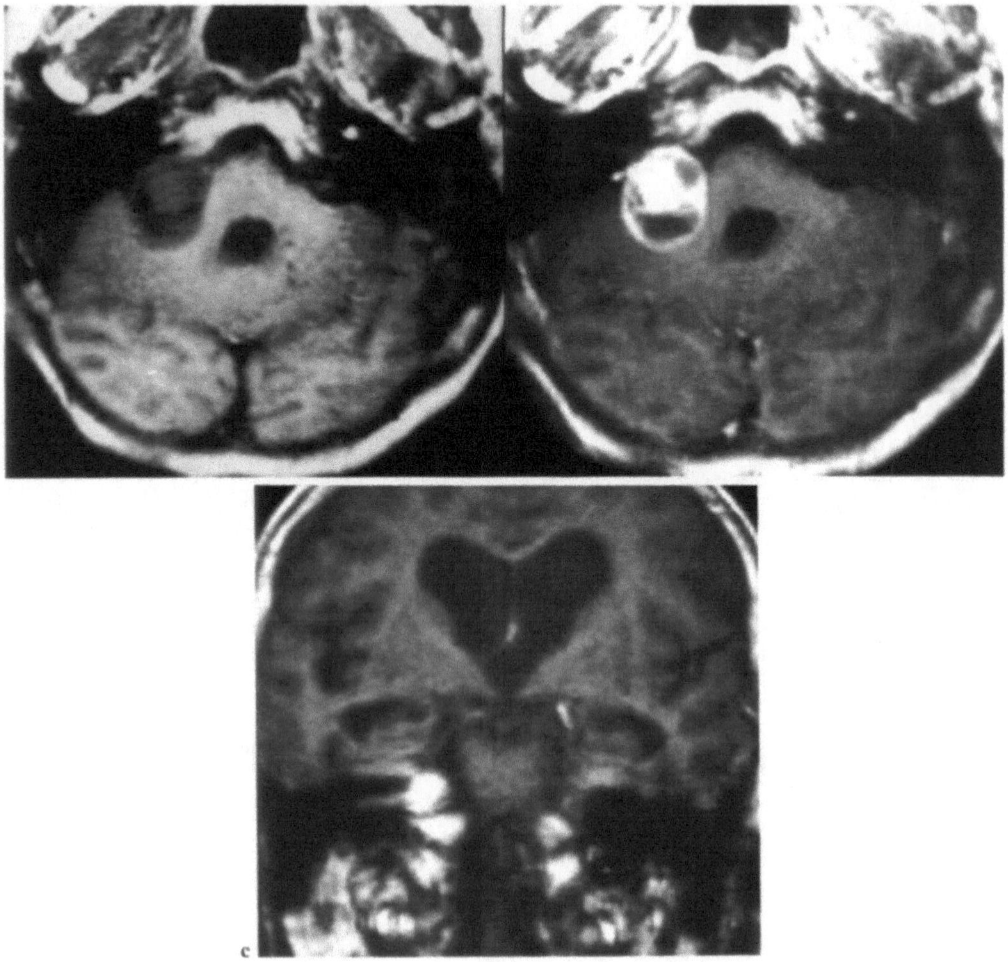

Fig. D5.9a–c. Hemangioblastoma in the left cerebellopontine angle in a 60-year-old man with progressive hearing impairment. MR: **a** SE 400/30, **b** SE 400/30 post Gd-DTPA, **c** SE 400/30 coronal. The very intense, solid tumor nodule and low-signal cyst are clearly discriminated on the post-Gd-DTPA T1-weighted image (**b**)

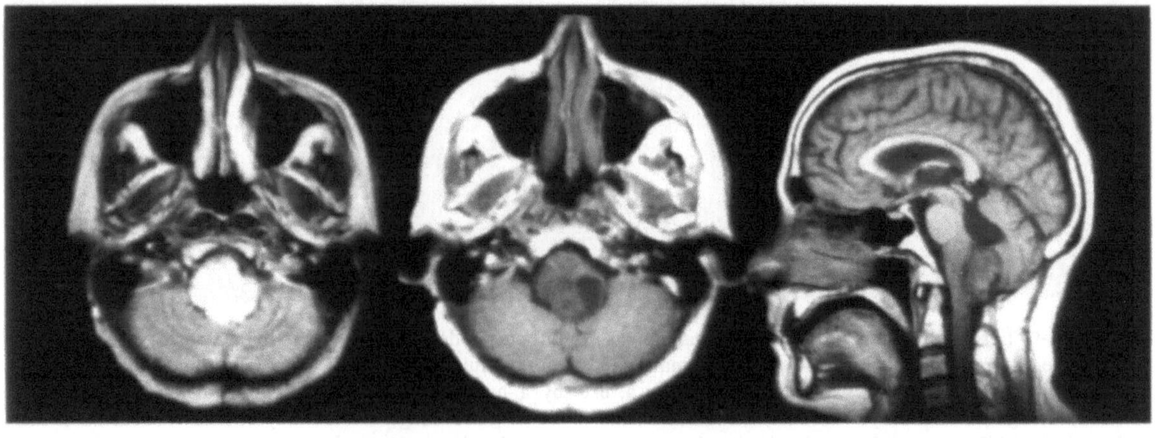

Fig. D5.10. Cystic angioblastoma of the brainstem in a 41-year-old man with increasing intracranial pressure, gait disturbance, somnolence, diplopia in all directions of gaze, and latent right hemiparesis. MR: *left* SE 1600/70, *center* SE 400/30, *right* SE 400/30 sagittal. The entire brainstem appears hyperintense on the T2-weighted image (*left*), while the T1-weighted image displays multiple cysts as rounded areas of low signal intensity (*center*). The midsagittal scan demonstrates the location of the tumor and shows associated compression of the brainstem and cerebellum; the fourth ventricle is enlarged

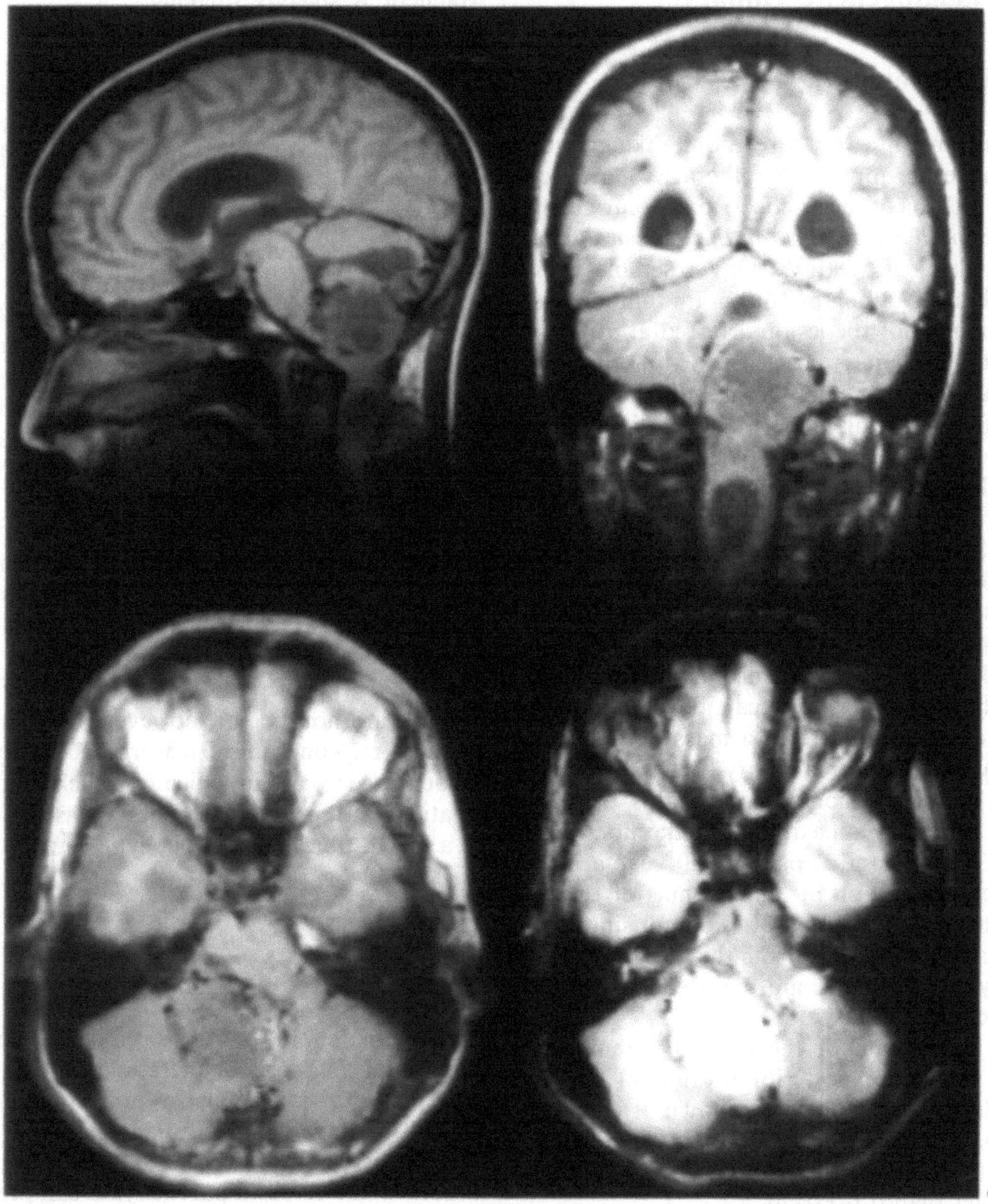

a b c d

Fig. D5.11 a–d. Cerebellar and spinal hemangioblastoma at the C3 level in a 20-year-old man with increasing ataxia and tetraparesis. MR: **a** SE 400/30 sagittal, **b** SE 400/30 coronal, **c** SE 400/30 axial, **d** SE 1600/90 axial. The images demonstrate two separate components of the richly vascularized tumor. The large mass with its cystic core and vascularized periphery (low-signal areas) is demonstrated on all images. The small nodule in the right cerebellar hemisphere is clearly visible only on the T2-weighted image (**d**). The spinal extension gives a low signal and appears as a predominantly cystic lesion on the T1-weighted sequences

6. Dysontogenetic Tumors

a) Hamartomas

Hamartomas are very rare glioma-like growths that have no apparent proliferative tendency, cause little or no mass effect, and occur chiefly in the *mediobasal part of the temporal lobe.* Their histologic features may resemble those of all known autochthonous brain tumors, with development of the lesion arrested at a particular stage. There is no clear dividing line that separates hamartomas from gangliocytomas. Patients harboring these malformations commonly experience cerebral seizures while still in childhood or adolescence. Seizures tend to be of the complex focal type (psychomotor) and often are refractory to medical treatment. The neurologic examination is generally unrewarding, but EEG frequently demonstrates a temporal focus.

Other sites of occurrence are known: Hypothalamic hamartomas can develop on the tuber cinereum and form a mass between the pituitary stalk and mamillary bodies. The hallmark of these lesions is precocious puberty, which generally appears during the first years of life. Diebler and Ponsot (1983) gave a more detailed description of hamartomas of the tuber cinereum in a large series comprising their own patients and cases from the literature. Various types of seizures are reported in addition to precocious puberty.

A hamartoma of the tuber cinereum appears within the posterior portion of the interpeduncular cistern (also known as the pentagon). The tumor can attain a diameter of more than 2 cm, although many are nodules no larger than 0.7–1.0 cm.

Computed Tomography
(Figs. D6.1, 3, 5)

Temporal lobe hamartomas are easily detected on nonenhanced CT owing to the frequent presence of calcifications and cysts (Fig. D6.1, 3). In our experience these lesions rarely show significant contrast enhancement.

Magnetic Resonance Imaging
(Figs. D6.2–4, 6, 7)

The T1-weighted image shows a nonspecific isointense mass lesion. T2 weighting demonstrates hyperintense zones in the mediobasal part of the temporal lobe. Venous hamartial elements, if present, produce a hypointense focus within the high-intensity zone (Fig. D6.4). Comparisons of tumor extent on CT and MR may well reveal a greater extent on MR owing to the superiority of that modality in demonstrating gliotic tissue reaction (Fig. D6.3). MR is also superior for detecting temporal mediobasal hamartomas owing to the absence of bone artifact and the capacity for arbitrary plane selection.

The midsagittal MR scan is excellent for detecting *hamartomas of the tuber cinereum*, especially if the lesion extends into the cistern. Hamartomas at this location are predominantly isointense and do not enhance with Gd-DTPA (Diebler and Ponsot 1983). These findings are nonspecific, however, and diagnosis must rely on clinical features. Recently we encountered a case in which one such lesion in a patient with precocious puberty was found to be a mixed fibrillary and pilocytic astrocytoma (Fig. D6.8).

Differential Diagnosis

Hamartoma should always be included in the differential diagnosis of the adolescent patient with temporal lobe epilepsy and corresponding CT findings. The CT diagnosis is at best presumptive, however, because other lesions or tumors of the cerebral parenchyma can present the same features.

The main tumors requiring differentiation from hamartoma are *pilocytic astrocytomas* (cysts) and *oligodendrogliomas* and *gangliocytomas* (calcifications). Transitional forms also may occur (see Fig. D6.5). The intratumoral hemorrhage that we observed in one hamartoma underscores the dysontogenetic character of the lesion. This cannot, however, be considered typical.

b) Cavernous Hemangiomas

Cavernous hemangiomas (synonym: cavernoma) are very rare dysontogenetic tumors that can occur anywhere in the brain. The cerebral hemispheres are most commonly affected. The orbital region is another frequent site (see Chap. G). Less common sites are the lateral ventricles, fourth ventricle, basal ganglia, cerebellopontine angle, brainstem, and cerebellar hemispheres. Cavernous hemangiomas occasionally arise from the dura mater, especially that lining the floor of the middle fossa (Mori et al. 1980). Signs and symptoms vary widely according to the site of the lesion. Seizures characterize involvement of the cerebral hemispheres, while basal cavernous hemangiomas tend to produce cranial nerve palsies (especially of the second and third nerves). Intratumoral hemorrhage is also observed. The tumors are most common in adolescents and young adults, although some are detected in infancy (congenital). The lesion is known to possess some growth potential despite its dysontogenetic character.

Computed Tomography
(Figs. D6.9, 10)

Most cavernous hemangiomas show increased density on the plain CT scan, and calcifications are not uncommon (Fig. D6.9). Often the lesion enhances intensely with intravenous contrast and in that respect can resemble meningioma. This is especially true of lesions occurring in the middle fossa. Lesions typically appear spherical or lobulated and are sharply demarcated from adjacent brain. It is virtually impossible to make a specific diagnosis from CT findings alone. The very intense enhancement is consistent with a heavily vascularized lesion but is insufficient to distinguish the tumor from meningioma.

In our experience a presumptive diagnosis of cavernous hemangioma is justified when the lesion is entirely intracerebral, since we have not observed other tumors of similar appearance occurring within the brain parenchyma (Figs. D6.9, 11).

Magnetic Resonance Imaging
(Fig. D6.11)

To date, examiners have had very little experience with the MR appearance of cavernous hemangiomas. As Fig. D6.11 illustrates, the tumor produces a very high signal even on T1-weighted sequences. In the case depicted there was no hemorrhagic component in the mass that might have accounted for the high signal intensity. T2 weighting did not alter the signal pattern significantly, and the lesion did not enhance further with Gd-DTPA.

With other cavernous hemangiomas, T1-weighted images have demonstrated signal intensities comparable to those of the cerebral gray matter.

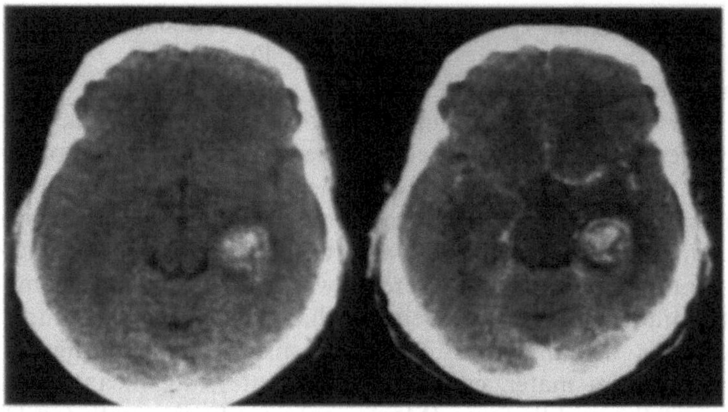

Fig. D6.1. Hamartoma in the posteromedial portion of the right temporal lobe. The 36-year-old man presented with a history of mild seizures since adolescence and late generalized seizures. Plain CT (*left*) demonstrates a mixed-density lesion with calcified elements. Ring enhancement of the tumor capsule is noted on the postcontrast scan (*right*)

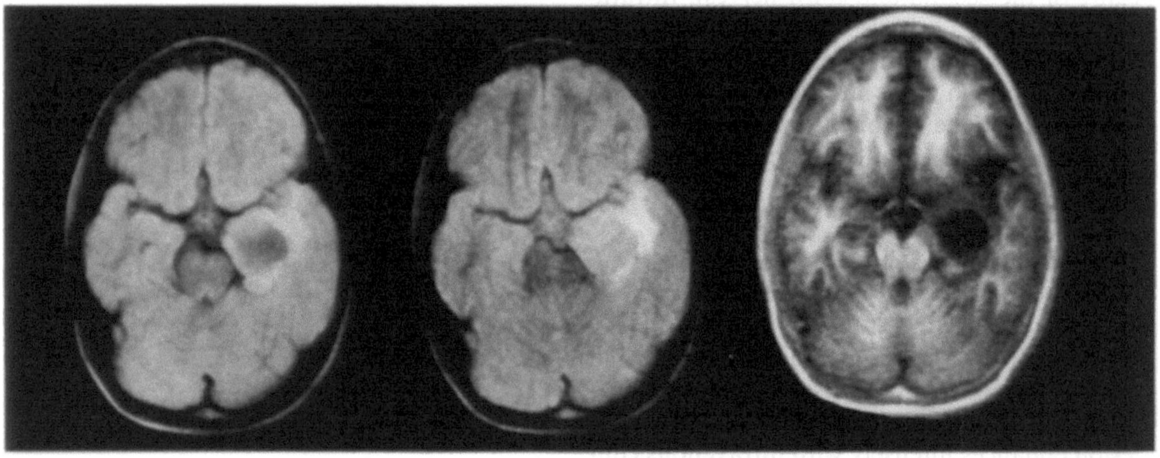

Fig. D6.2. Right mediobasal hamartoma in an 8-year-old girl who experienced nodding spasms at 10 months of age, followed later by psychomotor seizures. MR: *left* SE 1600/35, *center* SE 1600/70, *right* IR 1500/400/35. The proton-density image (*left*) discloses a low-signal area in the mediobasal portion of the right temporal lobe. The T2-weighted image (*center*) shows a peripheral, fingerlike area of increased signal intensity and edema. The IR sequence (*right*) reveals a sharply defined area of signal void. The images at *left* and *center* show slight evidence of brainstem compression

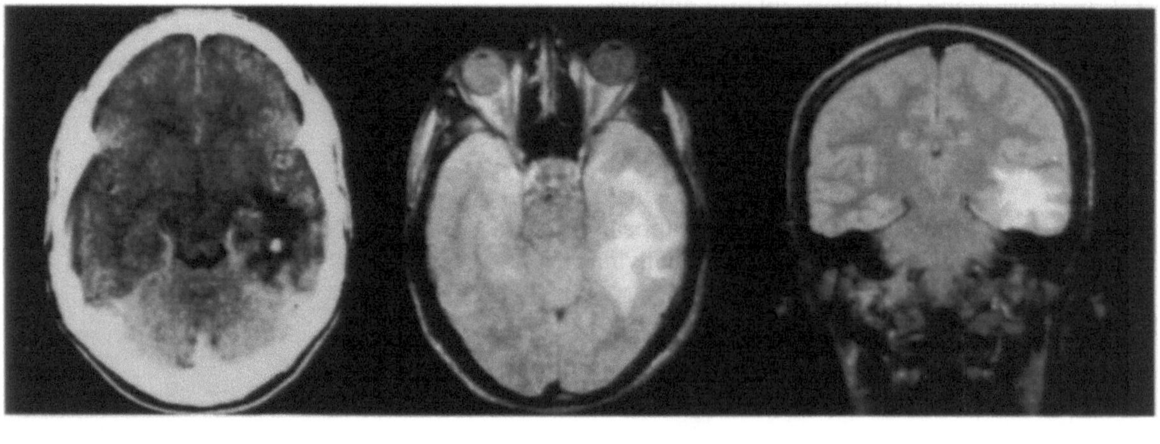

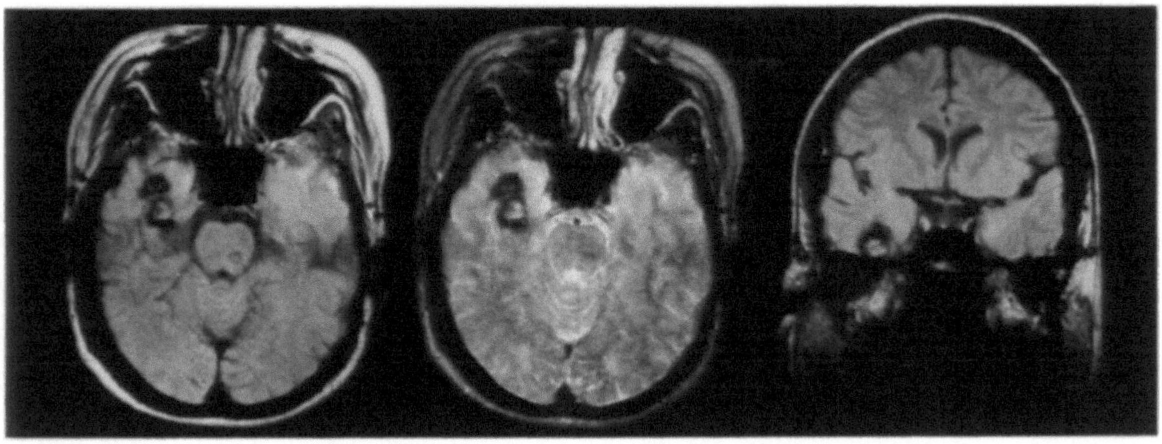

Fig. D 6.4. Hamartoma in the mediobasal portion of the left temporal lobe in a 28-year-old man with a 1-year history of refractory temporal lobe seizures. MR: *left* SE 2500/30, *center* SE 2500/120, *right* SE 2500/30 coronal. The proton-density image (*left* and *right*) and T2-weighted image (*center*) demonstrate a hyperintense lesion surrounded by areas of low signal intensity

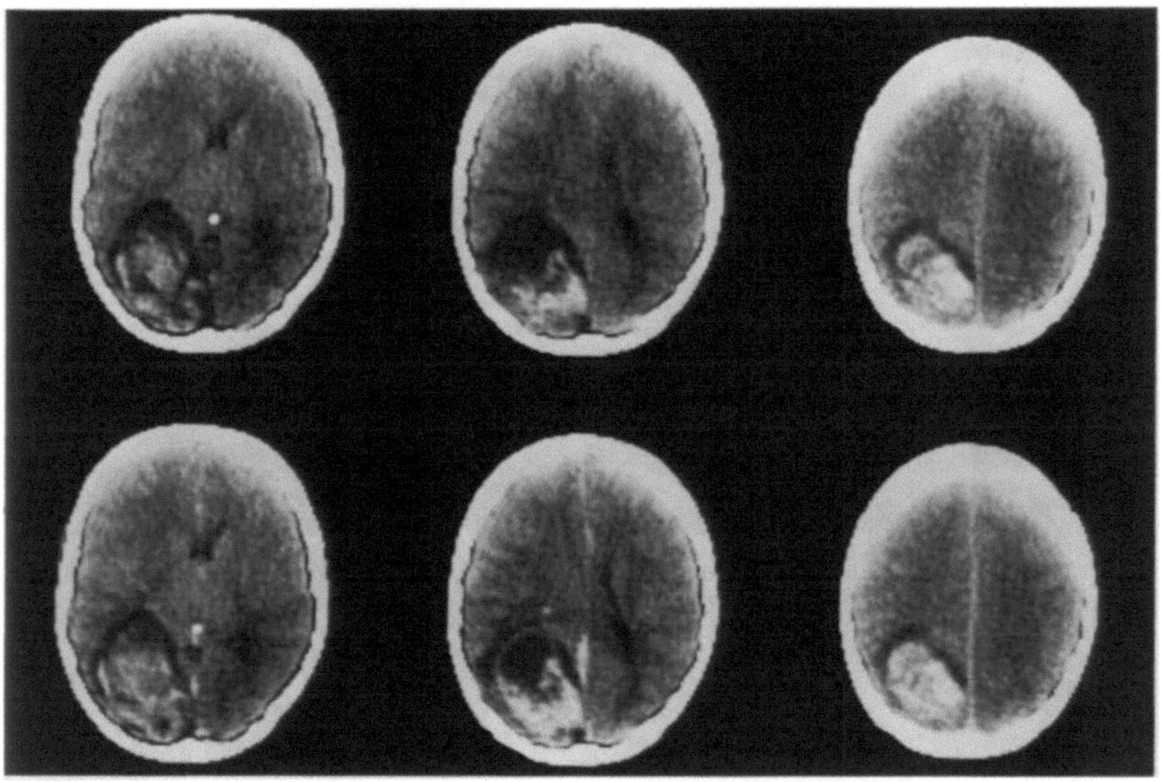

Fig. D 6.5. Combination of hamartoma and oligodendroglioma with a hemorrhagic component in the left occipital lobe of a 17-year-old girl with a history of seizures in previous years. The plain CT scans (*top*) show a clearly delineated lesion containing areas of varying density. The attenuation values in the higher slices are consistent with clotted blood. The contrast-enhanced scans (*bottom*) show a marked density increase in the primarily isodense areas of the lesion with faint capsular enhancement (*center* scan). CT findings were consistent with a combined solid and cystic tumor with a fresh hemorrhagic component, confirmed at operation

Fig. D 6.3. Right mediobasal hamartoma in a 30-year-old man with late epilepsy; neurologic exam was negative. CT: *left* postcontrast. MR: *center* SE 1600/70 axial, *right* SE 1600/70 coronal. CT demonstrates a hypodense lesion with central specks of calcification. The T2-weighted images show a hyperintense lesion of greater extent than on the CT scan

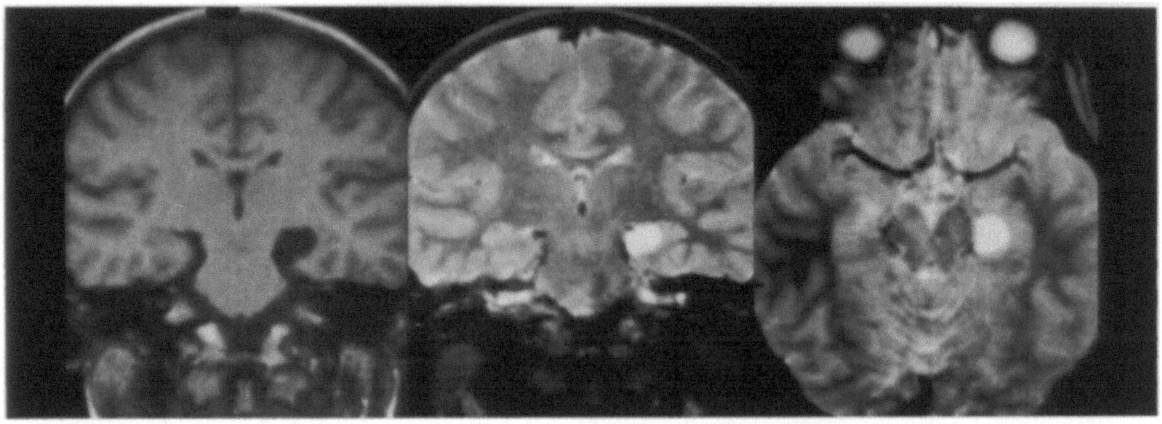

Fig. D6.6. Hamartoma on the right hippocampal uncus in a 12-year-old girl with an 8-month history of psychomotor seizures. MR: *left* SE 500/30 coronal, *center* SE 3000/90 coronal, *right* SE 3600/90 axial. The T1-weighted image shows a hypointense tumor whose signal density progressively increases with T2 weighting

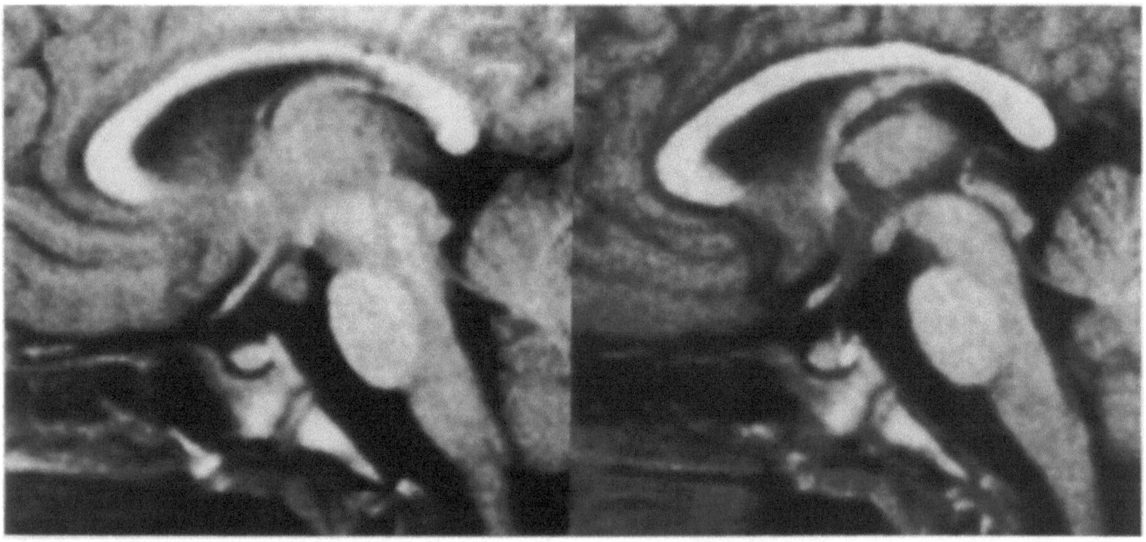

Fig. D6.7. Hamartoma arising from the floor of the third ventricle, confirmed at operation. The 4-year-old boy was admitted with precocious puberty and elevation of luteinizing hormone. MR: SE 400/17 sagittal, parasagittal. The T1-weighted images demonstrate a clearly defined tumor isointense to brain

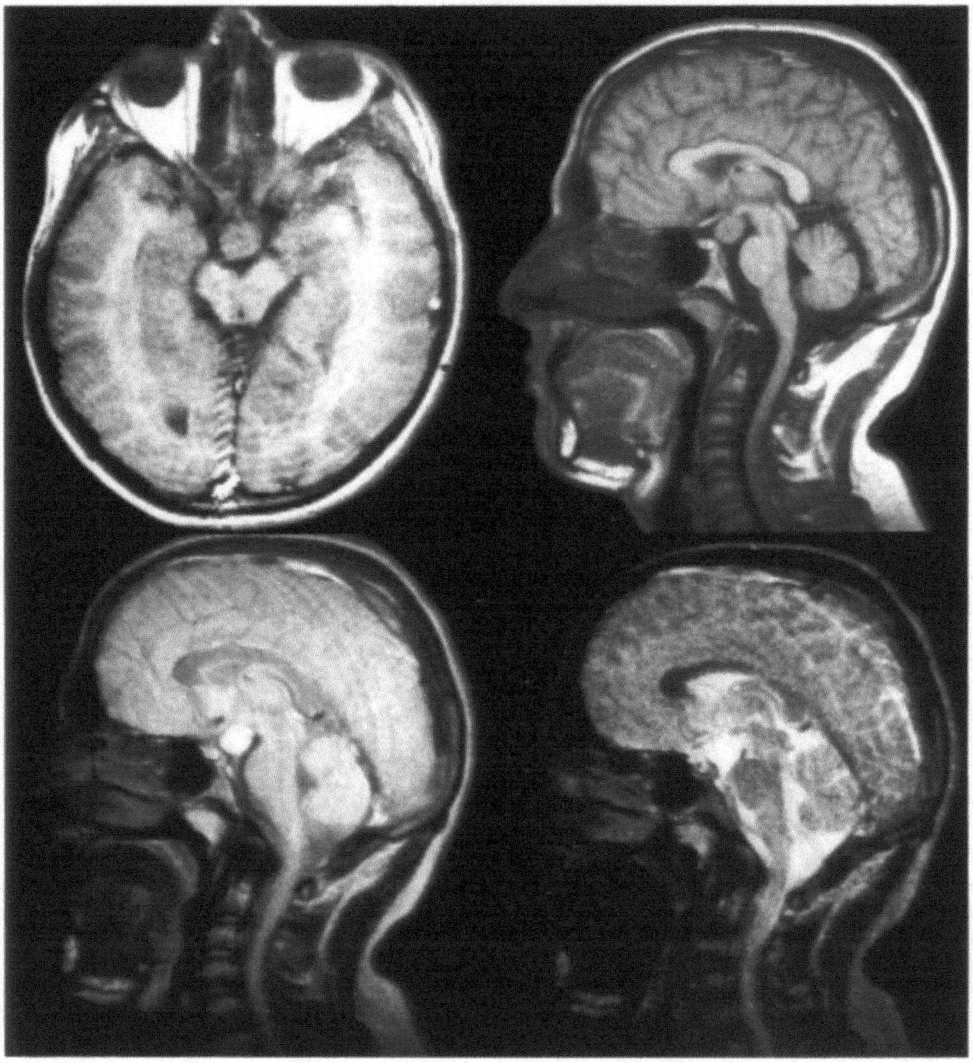

a b c d

Fig. D 6.8 a–d. Mixed fibrillary and pilocytic astrocytoma between the hypothalamus and tuber cinereum, confirmed at operation, in a 10-year-old boy with precocious puberty. MR: **a, b** SE 400/30 axial, sagittal; **c** SE 1600/60 sagittal; **d** SE 1600/150 sagittal. The tumor is isointense to surrounding brain on the T1-weighted sequences (**a, b**). The T2-weighted sequences (**c, d**) show a marked signal increase, the tumor displaying the same intensity as CSF in the late echo (**d**)

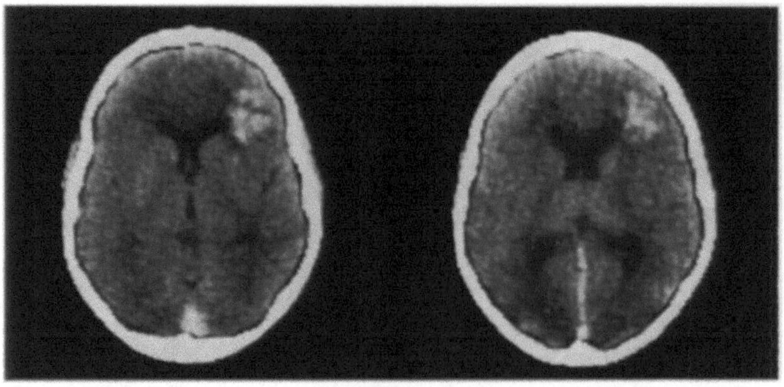

Fig. D 6.9. Cavernous hemangioma of the right frontotemporal region in a 14-year-old girl with cerebral seizures. CT defines the lesion as an irregular area containing patchy hyperdensities (calcifications). Contrast enhancement is minimal

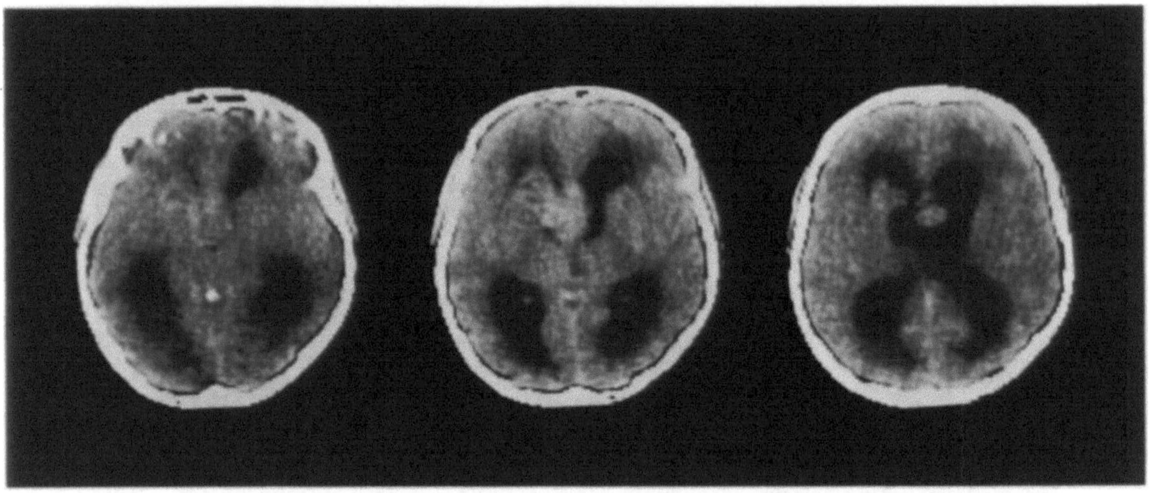

Fig. D 6.10. Cavernoma at the left foramen of Monro with extension to the left frontal horn in a 17-year-old girl with headache and papilledema. There is obstructive hydrocephalus with periventricular lucency. Plain CT scans show an irregular configuration with hyperdense areas. This pattern changes little on the contrast-enhanced scans

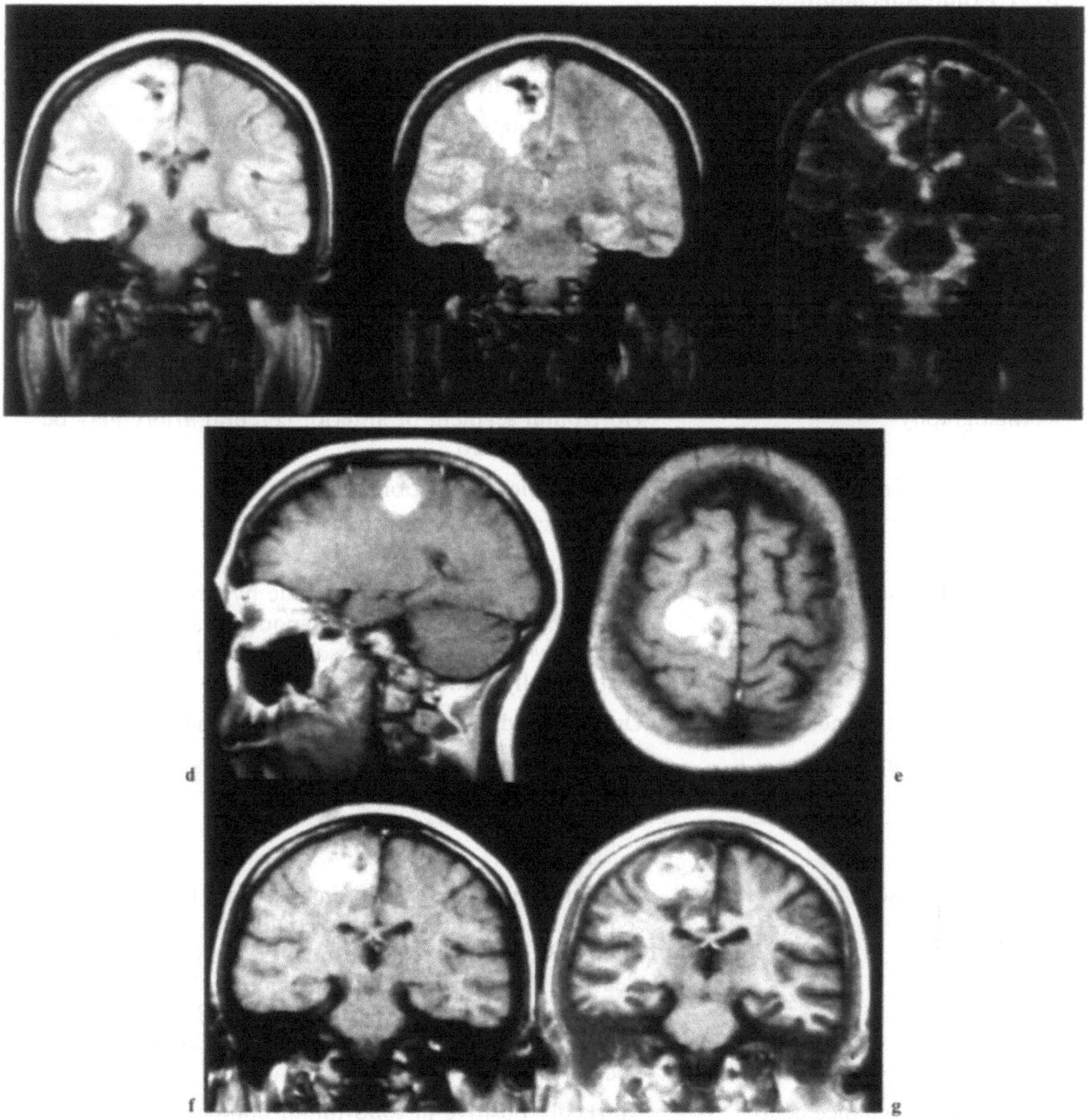

a–c d e f g

Fig. D6.11 a–g. Cavernoma of the left central region in a 51-year-old woman with focal and generalized seizures and hemiparesis predominantly affecting the right leg. MR: **a** SE 1600/30, **b** SE 1600/90, **c** SE 1600/120, **a–c** coronal; **d–f** SE 400/35 post Gd-DTPA sagittal, axial, coronal; **g** IR 1500/400/35 post Gd-DTPA. Tumor and edema give a bright signal on the T2-weighted image (**c**) and are separated by a thin ring of low intensity. Heavily vascularized areas appear as signal voids. The gadolinium-enhanced T1-weighted sequences show a marked rise of signal intensity partially affecting the blood vessels

c) Craniopharyngiomas

Incidence	2%–4% of all brain tumors
Age predilection	All age groups, peak incidence at 10 years
Sex predilection	Preponderance of males
Typical site	Suprasellar region
Main clinical features	Visual disturbances, signs of increased intracranial pressure; pituitary insufficiency; in children, growth retardation and delayed puberty, occasionally adiposogenital dystrophy; diabetes insipidus not uncommon
Skull X-ray	Suprasellar calcifications, primary sellar changes
Angiography	Horizontal segment of anterior cerebral artery may be deflected upward
Special examinations	Endocrinologic function studies
CT	
Noncontrast scan	Appearance variable, may include hyperdensities caused by calcifications and hypodense areas representing cystic components; solid, uncalcified tumor parts usually isodense
Contrast enhancement	Only in solid, uncalcified tumor components
Postcontrast appearance	Suprasellar tumor nodules, sometimes associated with cysts and calcifications
MR	
Noncontrast scan	Appearance variable. Hypointense on T1-weighted sequences. Protein-rich cystic contents typically give high signal on T1-weighted images (distinguishes them clearly from cysts in pituitary adenomas). Solid tumor parts and cysts both hyperintense on T2-weighted sequences and not clearly differentiated; calcifications poorly displayed
Gadolinium enhancement	Markedly positive in solid tumor components
Post Gd-DTPA appearance	Improved visualization of solid tumor components

Differential diagnosis

Pituitary adenoma
Pilocytic astrocytoma
Gangliocytoma
Meningioma
Carotid artery aneurysm
Chordoma
Epipharyngeal carcinoma

Craniopharyngioma is derived from the craniopharyngeal duct. Its development may be intrasellar, suprasellar, or a combination of both. It is the second most common tumor of the sellar region after pituitary adenoma. Incidence is reported to range from 2% to 4% in the literature, and the prevalence in our series was 1.9%. This grade I tumor may have a solid, soft consistency, may include firm, calcified components, or may contain cysts. The cysts often contain a thick, brownish fluid resembling motor oil, and they can attain a huge size.

Main Clinical Features

By inhibiting the secretion of growth hormone, these tumors in children and adolescents cause pituitary dwarfism with delayed puberty. Adiposogenital dystrophy is occasionally seen. Many patients develop a diabetes insipidus that may terminate in antidiabetes.

Suprasellar extension of the tumor causes visual acuity loss and visual field defects, and growths obstructing the foramen of Monro can increase the intracranial pressure. These symptoms may be reversible following complete removal of the tumor.

Additional Diagnostic Procedures

Flecks of calcification in the suprasellar region are the most characteristic finding on skull X-rays. Very large calcific foci may also be seen. In contrast to pituitary adenoma, primary sellar changes are frequently absent. Increased intracranial pressure in children may be manifested by separation of the cranial sutures and increased digital impressions.

Upward deflection of the horizontal segment of the anterior cerebral artery may be noted on cerebral angiograms. Tumor staining does not occur.

Endocrinologic function studies can be performed to evaluate for hormonal deficits.

Computed Tomography
(Figs. D6.12–15, 19, 22)

Noncontrast Scan
The CT findings of craniopharyngioma vary widely due to the diverse combinations of solid, cystic, and calcified elements that may exist in the tumor (Figs. 6.12–15). Some 80% of craniopharyngiomas are hyperdense or present a mixed density. Purely hypodense areas represent larger cystic components (Figs. D6.12, 13, 22) with attenuation values approximating those of CSF. Other craniopharyngiomatous cysts have absorption values only slightly less than those of normal brain. Ambrose (1974) described one craniopharyngioma containing a multilocular cyst with negative EMI numbers, but we were unable to duplicate this finding in our own series.

The *calcifications* in craniopharyngioma vary in size and shape, ranging from small, punctate foci to chestnut-size, well-defined masses of very high density (Figs. D6.14, 15). The solid tumor components are usually isodense or slightly hypodense (Fig. D6.15). Purely solid tumors, then, can be detected only on the basis of indirect signs on the nonenhanced CT scan.

Postcontrast Scan
Approximately two-thirds of craniopharyngiomas enhance with contrast medium, the average degree of enhancement being 12–14 HU.

Only the solid, uncalcified parts of the tumor enhance. The mixture of solid tumor nodules, calcifications, and cysts frequently produces a bizarre pattern, especially in recurrent growths (Fig. D6.15). Ring enhancement is occasionally seen around cysts (Figs. D6.13, 22). Cysts that are minimally hypodense are defined with greater clarity on postcontrast scans.

Equivocal findings, such as a cystic tumor with a very thin capsule, can be clarified by repeating the CT examination after the intrathecal administration of contrast medium (Fig. D6.22).

Magnetic Resonance Imaging
(Figs. D6.15–21)

As on CT, craniopharyngiomas present a diversity of MR patterns owing to their variegated composition.

The capacity for arbitrary plane selection allows for precise anatomic localization of midline craniopharyngiomas on midsagittal and coronal views, especially if the lesion has para- and suprasellar extension. A distinctive feature of MR is its very hyperintense portrayal of cystic contents on T1-weighted sequences, consistent with the appearance of protein-rich and crystalline substances. MR thus allows positive differentiation between the protein-rich craniopharyngiomatous cysts on the T1-weighted image and the cysts of pituitary adenoma, which give a low signal.

Small flecks of calcification often are poorly displayed on MR images. Consequently that feature is not available as a criterion for histologic classification.

The solid parts of the tumor, which often appear isointense on the noncontrast T1-weighted image, enhance well with Gd-DTPA. This makes it easier to recognize smaller calcifications as foci of signal void. *Cysts* do not enhance on the post-Gd-DTPA T1 image, and it is more difficult to separate cyst from solid tumor.

Differential Diagnosis

Calcifications are the main CT criterion for differentiating craniopharyngioma from pituitary adenoma, as they are observed in only about 1% of the latter. In some cases, however, the CT appearances of craniopharyngioma and pituitary adenoma may be identical.

In the presence of cysts, MR can aid differential diagnosis by demonstrating the higher signal intensity of the protein-rich fluid in craniopharyngiomatous cysts on the T1-weighted image. Differentiation from other suprasellar mass lesions is discussed in the section on pituitary adenomas (Sect. D4).

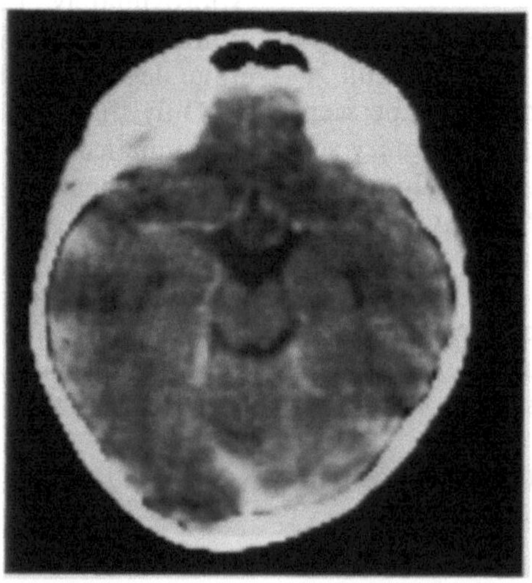

Fig. D6.12. Cystic craniopharyngioma in an 11-year-old boy with growth retardation and hormonal deficits. The postcontrast CT scan demonstrates a spherical mass with faint peripheral enhancement inside the pentagon. The density of the tumor cyst is appreciably greater than that of CSF

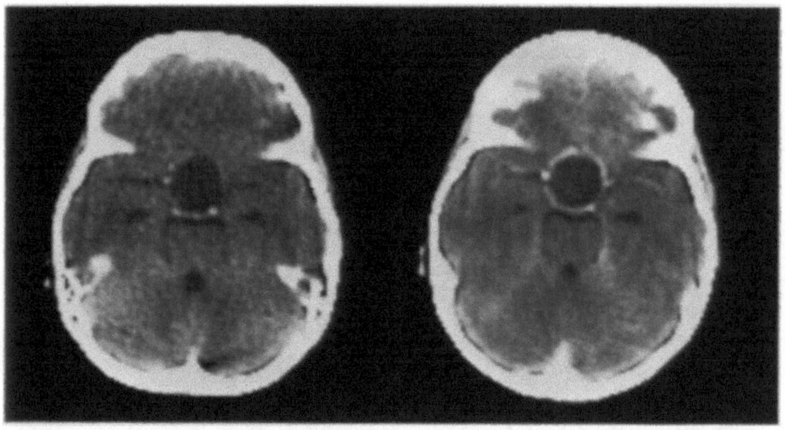

Fig. D 6.13. Large cystic craniopharyngioma completely filling the chiasmatic cistern in a 12-year-old girl with rapidly progressive loss of visual acuity. *Left* noncontrast scan; *right* contrast scan showing ring enhancement of solid tumor portions. A similar pattern might be seen in pituitary adenoma with a cystic or older hemorrhagic component. The patient's age is an essential criterion for differential diagnosis!

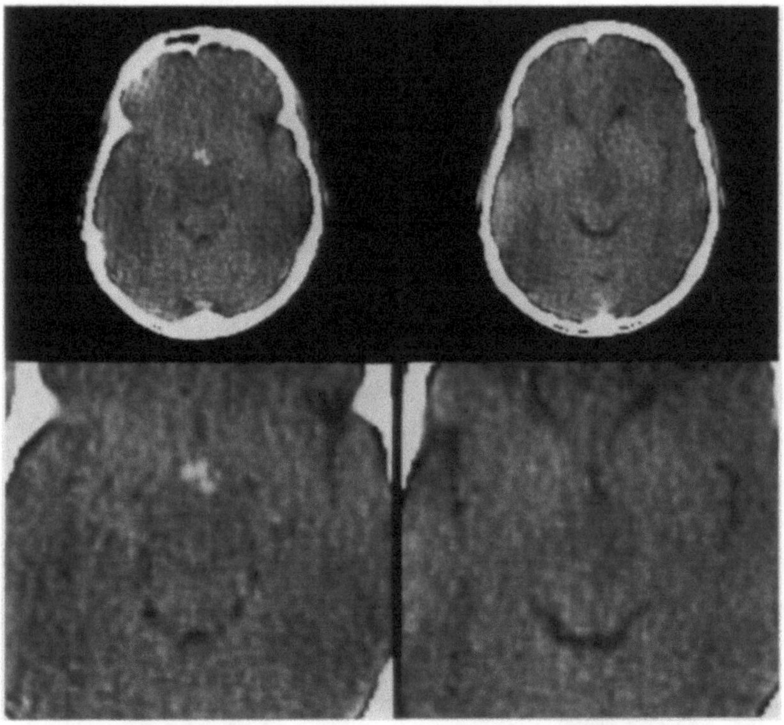

Fig. D 6.14. Large, solid craniopharyngioma with a small peripheral calcification in a 50-year-old man. The tumor completely fills the chiasmatic and prepontine cisterns. The lesion appears slightly hypodense on the noncontrast CT scans. Contrast medium was withheld because of allergy

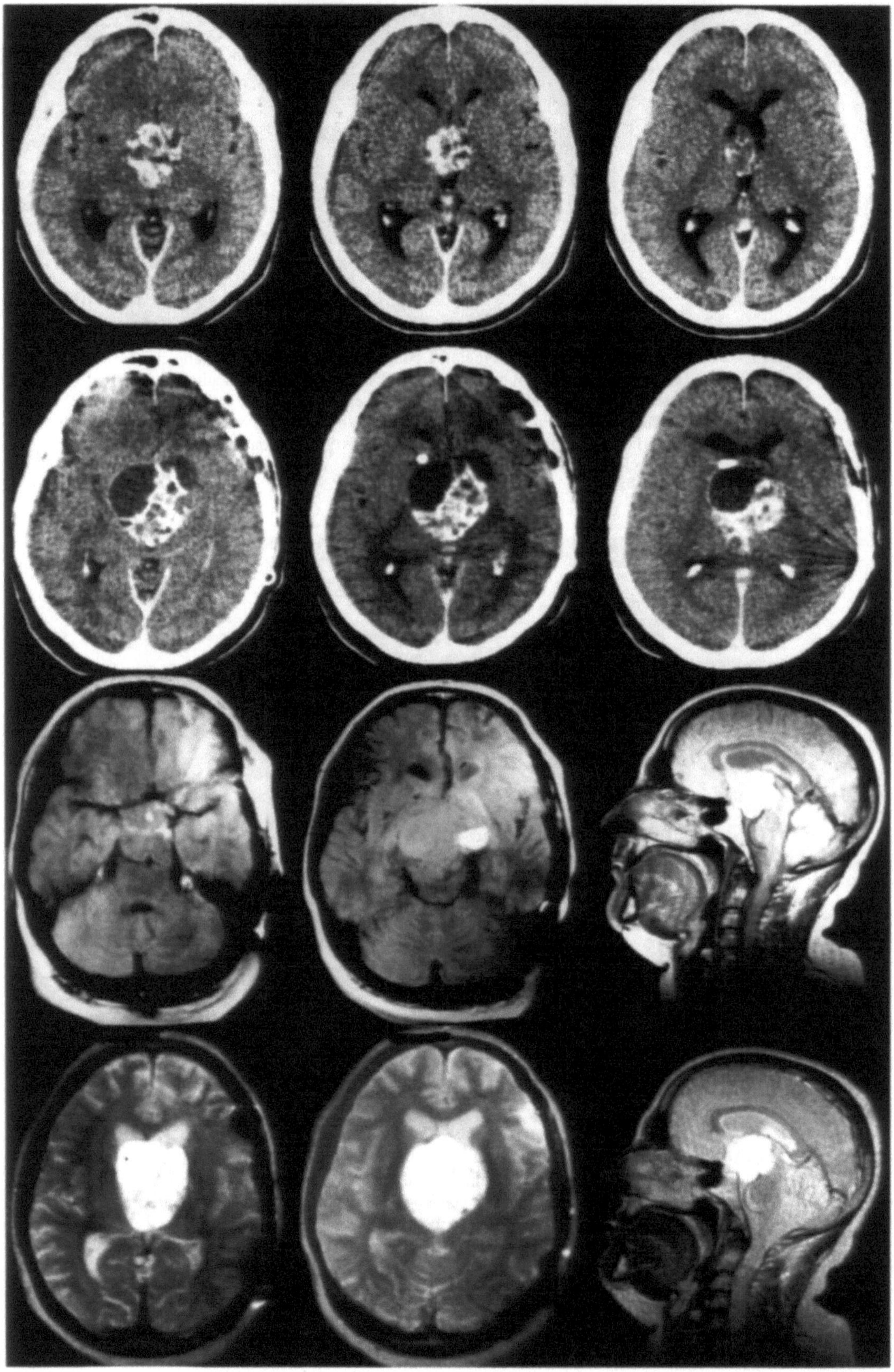

a–c

d–f

g–i

j–l

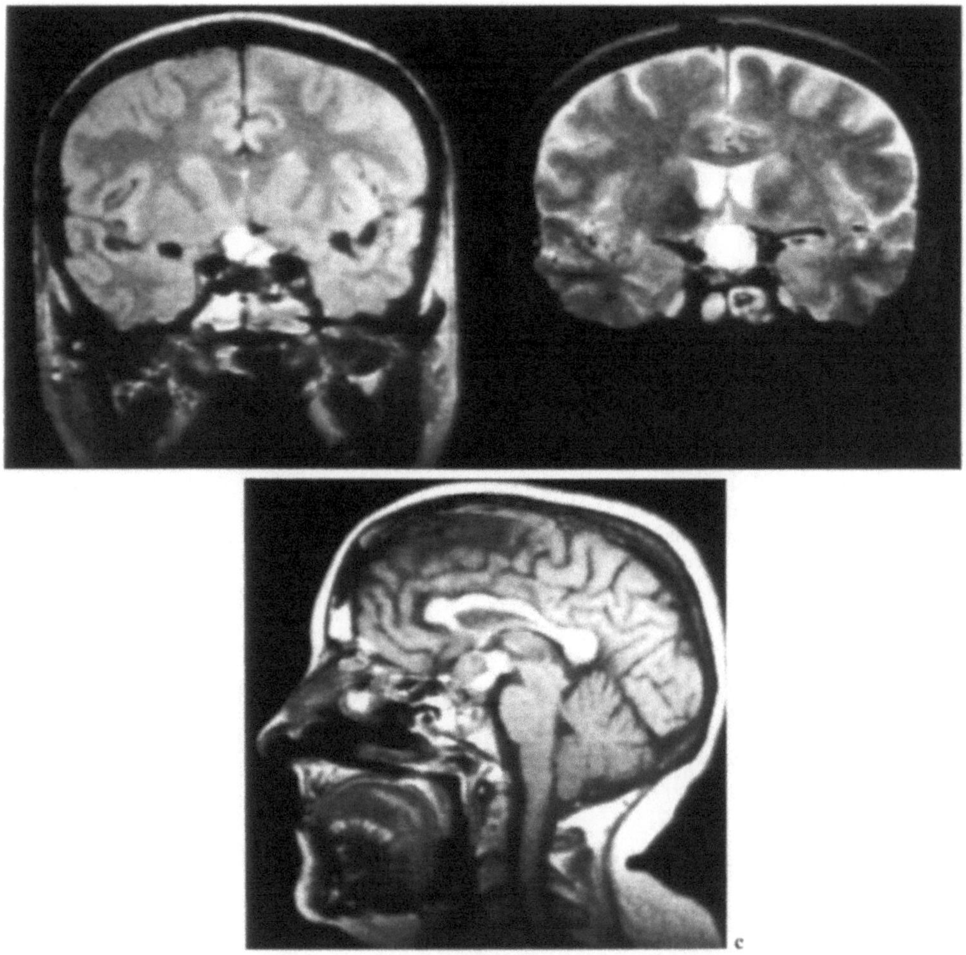

a b c

Fig. D6.16a–c. Craniopharyngioma in a 59-year-old woman with chiasmal disturbances and adynamia. MR: **a** SE 3000/30, **b** SE 3000/90, both coronal; **c** SE 300/30 sagittal. The cysts appear very hyperintense on the proton-density and T2-weighted images. On the sagittal section (**c**) the tumor is seen to contain two areas of different signal intensity representing solid tumor components and cyst

Fig. D6.15a–l. Extensive craniopharyngioma with solid components, cysts, and calcifications in a 58-year-old woman known for 3 years to have an intracranial tumor. She presented clinically with chiasmal disturbances, altered mental status, and marked obesity. CT: **a–f** postcontrast. MR: **g, h** SE 2000/40, **i** SE 2000/35, **j, k** SE 2000/110, **l** SE 2000/70. The protein-rich cystic fluid gives a very high signal on the proton-density and T2-weighted sequences. The calcifications appear only as faint signal voids

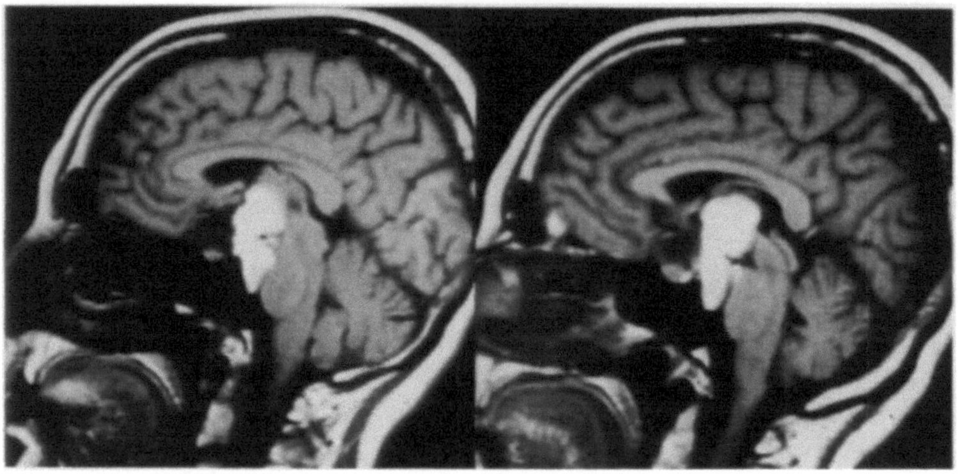

Fig. D6.17. Craniopharyngioma in a 53-year-old woman with mild chiasmal disturbances, diabetes insipidus, and hyperprolactinemia. The SE 600/17 sagittal images demonstrate extension of tumor from the sphenoid sinus to the third ventricle and prepontine region. The anterior, sellar, and suprasellar tumor components give a low signal. The posterior component is hyperintense owing to the protein-rich cystic fluid

a b c d

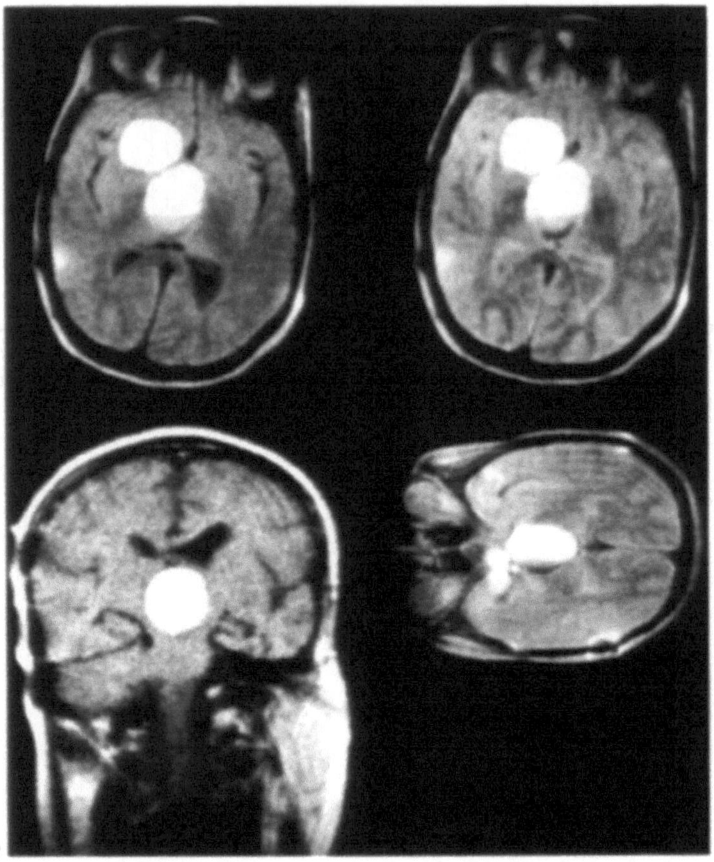

Fig. D6.18a–d. Craniopharyngioma in a 21-year-old man with bilateral amaurosis and hemiparesis predominantly affecting the right leg. MR: **a** SE 1600/35, **b** SE 1600/70, **c** SE 400/45 coronal, **d** SE 1600/70. The cyst is equally hyperintense on the proton-density and T2-weighted sequences; a fluid level is visible in the supra- and left parasellar portion. The cyst is also hyperintense on the T1-weighted image (**c**) and displays considerable suprasellar extension. Image **d** shows the change in the fluid level with the head turned 90°

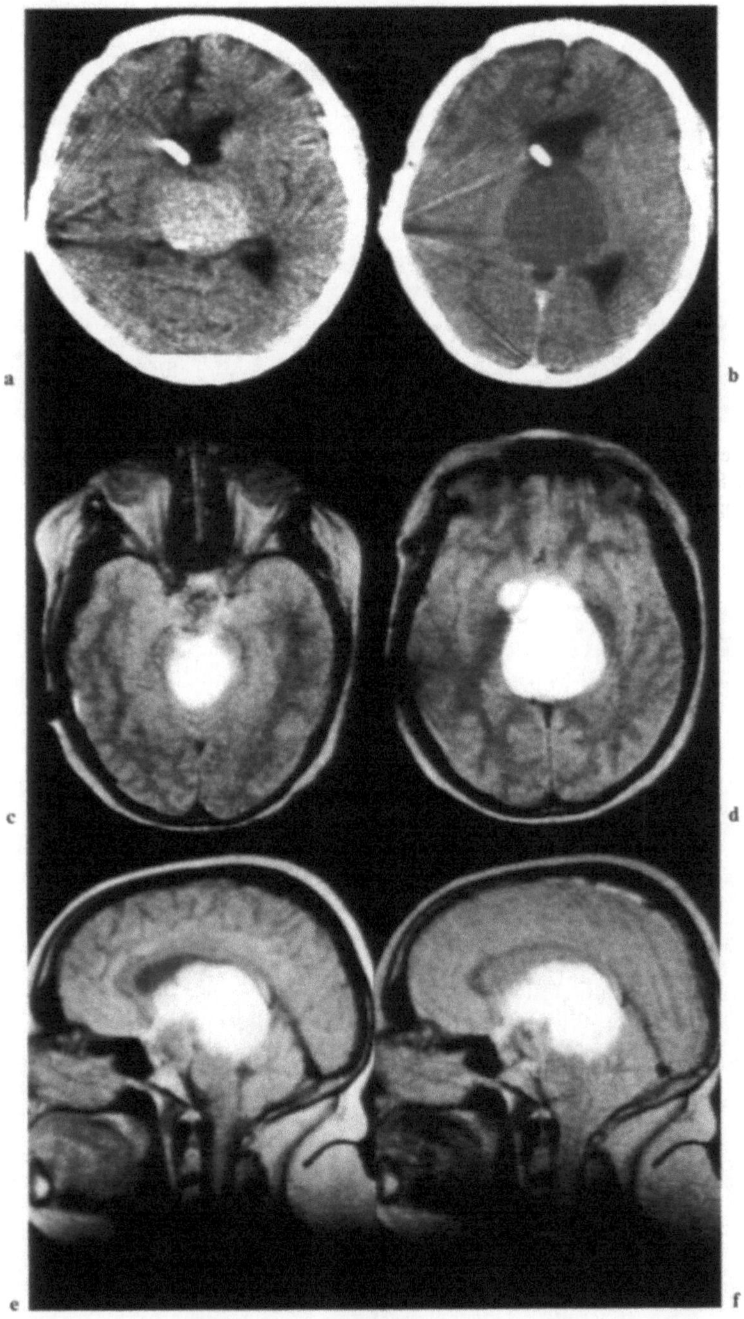

Fig. D 6.19 a–f. Recurrence of craniopharyngioma in a 19-year-old woman. Following initial surgery at age 11, the patient had developed bilateral visual acuity loss, gaze paresis toward the right, trigeminal hypoesthesia, latent right-sided hemiparesis, and overt features of Cushing's syndrome. CT: **a, b.** MR: **c, d** SE 1600/70, **e** SE 1600/35 sagittal, **f** SE 1600/70 sagittal. Plain CT shows hyperdense cystic contents (ventricular catheter appears in the left frontal area). Two days later, following aspiration of the cyst, a marked decrease in density is observed. MR demonstrates the hyperintense cystic fluid

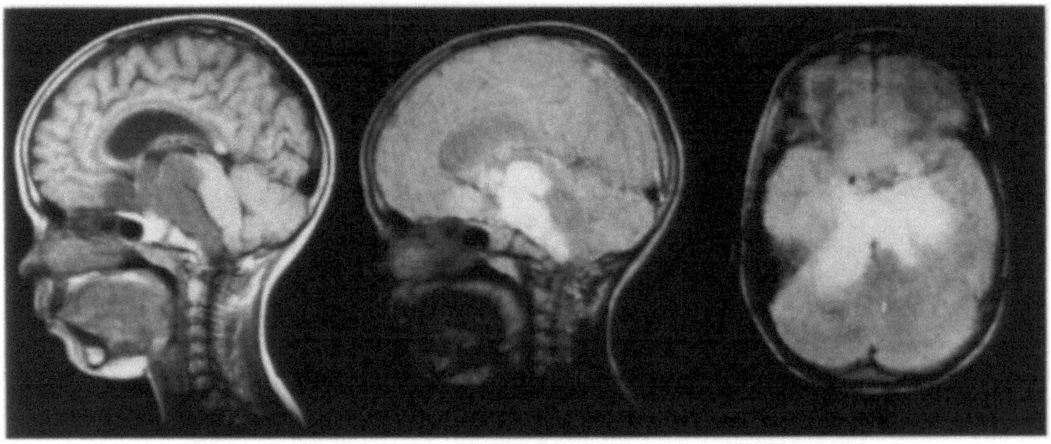

Fig. D 6.20. Recurrence of craniopharyngioma in a 7-year-old boy with bilateral visual acuity loss and optic nerve atrophy. MR: *left* SE 400/35, *center* and *right* SE 1600/70. The tumor gives a low signal on the T1-weighted image (*left*) and appears more intense on the T2-weighted image

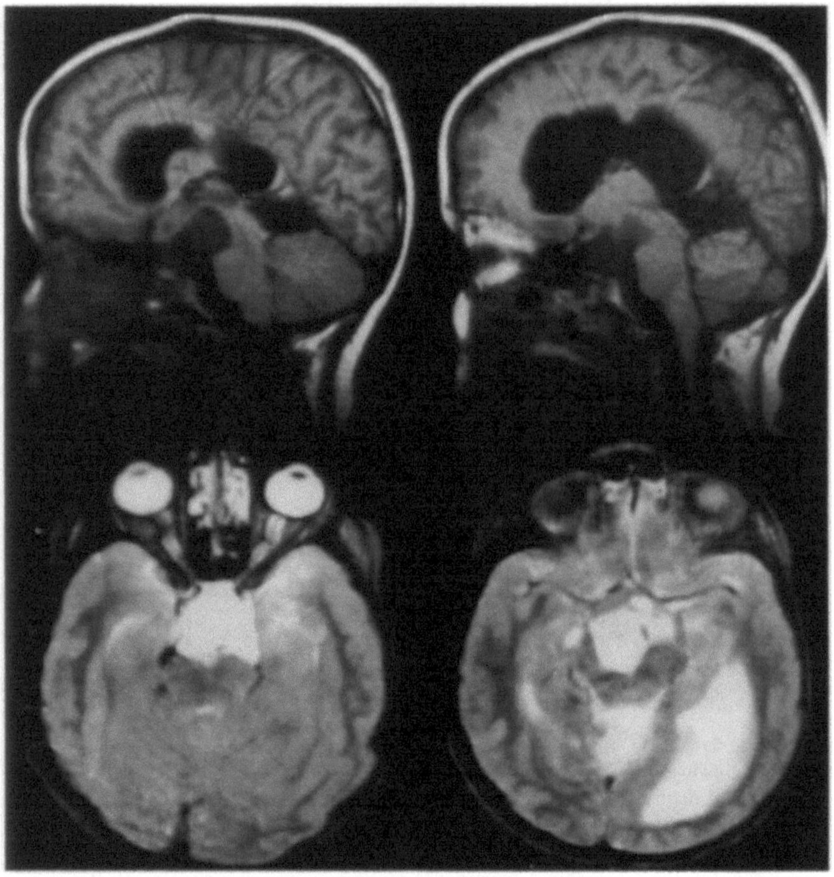

Fig. D 6.21. Craniopharyngioma in an 8-year-old boy with developmental retardation. MR: *top* SE 500/30, *bottom* SE 3000/90. The T1-weighted images show hypointense tumor components extending from the sella to the third ventricle. The tumor appears hyperintense on the T2-weighted images (*bottom*). Hydrocephalus is apparent

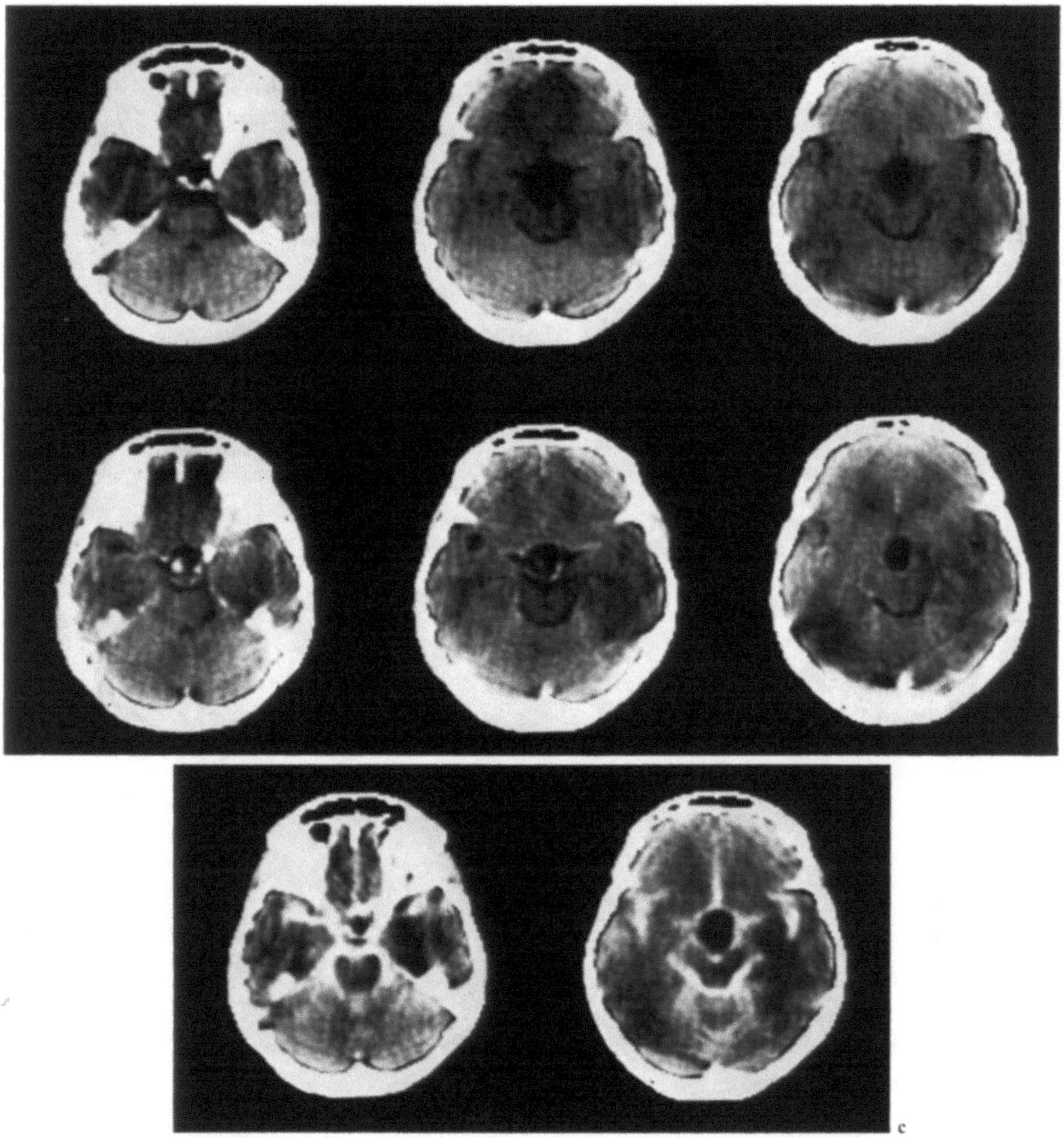

Fig. D 6.22 a–c. Cystic craniopharyngioma in a 45-year-old woman with visual disturbances (bilateral enlargement of the blind spot). Noncontrast CT scans demonstrate a large hypodensity (18–25 HU) in the region of the chiasmatic cistern (**a**). Postcontrast scans show thin peripheral rim enhancement (**b**). Combined metrizamide cisternography and CT demonstrates lack of communication between the cyst and the other CSF spaces (**c**)

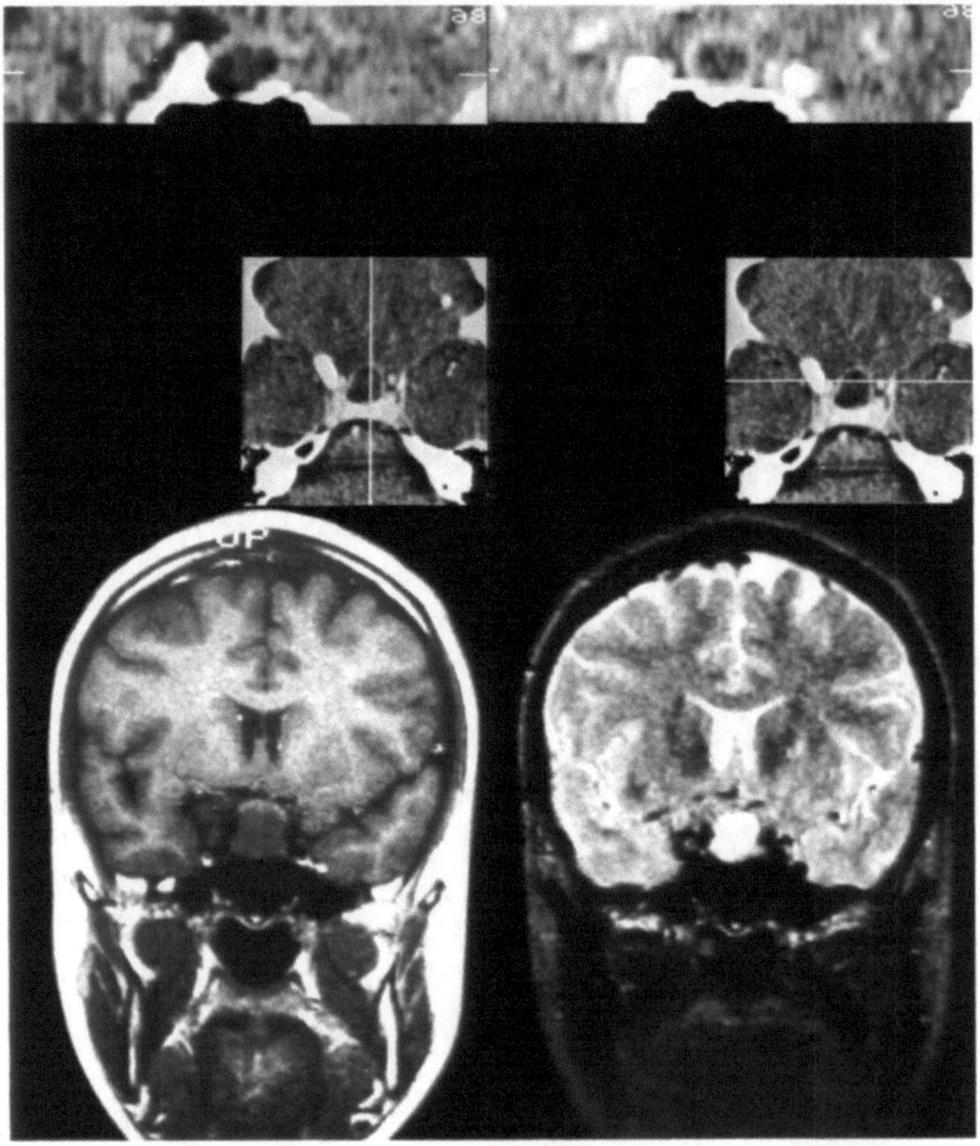

Fig. D 6.23 a–f. Rathke's pouch cyst in a 29-year-old woman with secondary amenorrhea and diabetes insipidus. CT: **a, b** reconstructions of **c** and **d**, all noncontrast. MR: **e** SE 300/17, **f** SE 2500/120, both coronal. The cyst is displayed most clearly on the T2-weighted image, where it appears hyperintense

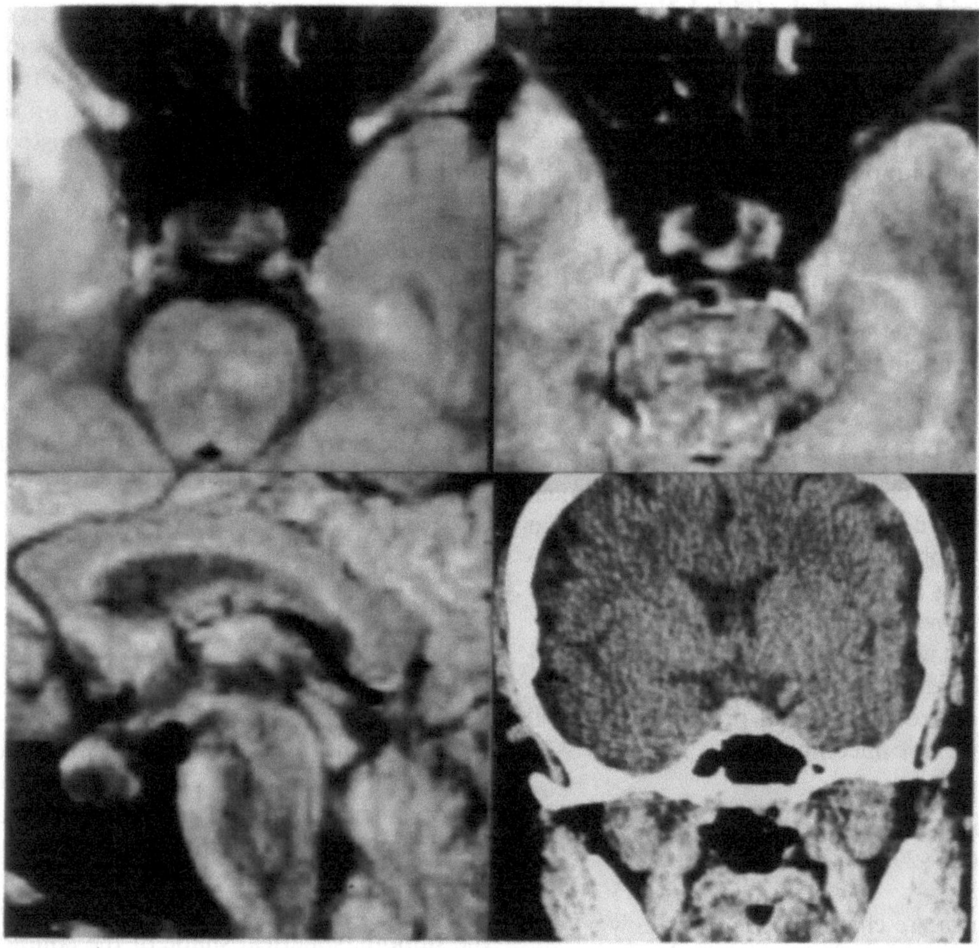

Fig. D 6.24 a–d. Primary sellar cyst with no evidence of tumor. MR: **a** SE 2500/30 axial, **b** SE 2500/120 axial, **c** SE 2500/30 sagittal. CT: **d** noncontrast, coronal

d) Colloid Cysts of the Third Ventricle

These cysts (synonyms: foramen of Monro cysts, ependymal cysts, paraphyseal cysts, neuroepithelial cysts) arise from the tela choroidea of the choroid plexus at the site where the lateral ventricle joins the roof of the third ventricle.

These relatively rare dysontogenetic "tumors" comprised 0.48% of the intracranial tumors in our series. The cyst sac is lined by mucus-producing epithelium. The cyst contents are yellowish-green and have a gelatinous consistency.

Colloid cysts range from a few millimeters in diameter to cherry-size in cases where clinical symptoms are pronounced. The cyst acts like a ball valve, obstructing the foramen of Monro and causing a hydrocephalus that affects only the lateral ventricles.

Patients with this malformation suffer intermittent headaches and show increasing symptoms of raised intracranial pressure. Syncopal attacks are not uncommon.

Computed Tomography
(Figs. D6.25–29)

CT findings are characteristic and allow a confident prediction of the histologic diagnosis. Colloid cysts appear on the axial CT scan as rounded, smooth-bordered foci in the anterior part of the third ventricle between the foramina of Monro. In some 80% of cases the lesion is markedly hyperdense on the noncontrast scan. Attenuation values may reach 60 HU, consistent with a fresh hemorrhage or calcification (Figs. D6.25, 26, 28). However, the high density of the colloid is mainly attributable to its high electrolyte content (Isherwood et al. 1977), and a high protein content may also play a role. Some colloid cysts are isodense and therefore are very difficult to detect with CT (Figs. D6.27, 29). The possibility of a colloid cyst should always be considered when both lateral ventricles are dilated and the third ventricle appears normal. Occasionally, intermediate slices are necessary to demonstrate the malformation since routine sections may fail to traverse the cyst completely.

It is our experience that colloid cysts do not enhance with contrast medium. Enhancement may be simulated by superposition of the adjacent choroid plexus or by imaging on slightly different planes for the pre- and postcontrast studies.

Magnetic Resonance Imaging
(Fig. D6.28)

MR is advantageous in detecting colloid cysts that are small or isodense and would require contiguous scanning with CT. These lesions are displayed clearly on the midsagittal MR image.

Colloid cysts appear hyperintense on the T1-weighted image. MR can demonstrate internal lamination of the cyst, resulting in a higher signal intensity at the periphery of the lesion than at the center.

Differential Diagnosis

It is unusual for lesions other than colloid cysts to occur in the anterior part of the third ventricle. Choroid plexus papillomas occur there rarely, and meningiomas are rarer still. Both these tumors enhance significantly with contrast medium, and both rarely exhibit the smooth, spherical shape of the colloid cyst.

e) Endodermal Cysts

Endodermal cysts are ectopic, intrameningeal malformations whose epithelial lining resembles that of the alimentary tract. They almost invariably occur in the spinal canal. We observed one endodermal cyst in the posterior fossa that presented as a smooth-bordered, nonenhancing midline hyperdensity located near the cranial vault (Fig. D6.30a). Meningioma was considered in the differential diagnosis but was excluded because the lesion did not enhance. At operation a large cyst containing dark, viscous fluid resembling motor oil was found between the cerebellar hemispheres extending the length of the vermis (Fig. D6.30b).

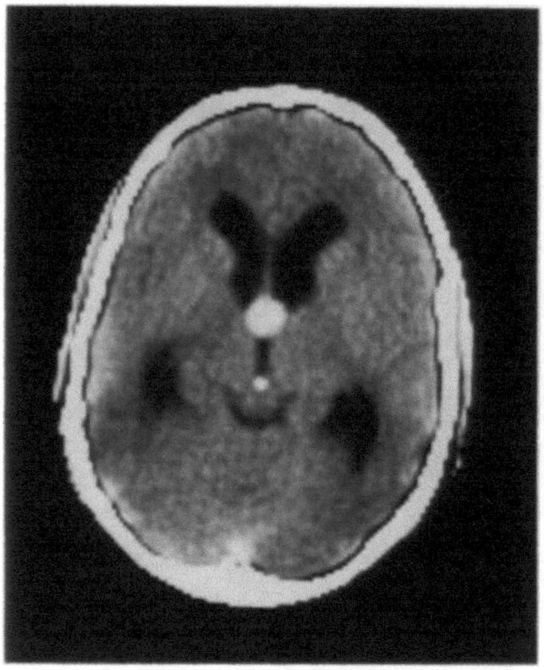

Fig. D 6.25. Colloid cyst of the third ventricle with hydrocephalus caused by bilateral obstruction of the foramina of Monro in a 17-year-old male with intermittent headache. The circular cyst always occupies the anterior part of the third ventricle, where it acts as a ball valve to obstruct both lateral ventricles. The cyst appears very dense (64 HU) on the plain CT scan and does not enhance with contrast medium

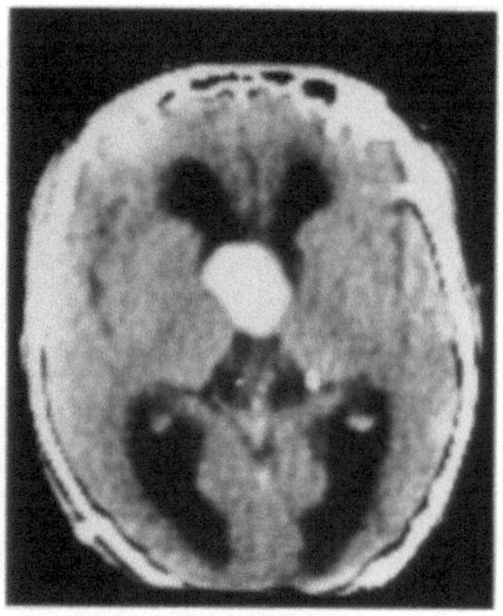

Fig. D 6.26. Colloid cyst of the third ventricle with obstructive hydrocephalus in a 52-year-old man with gait disturbance. The cyst appears extremely dense (100 HU) on the noncontrast CT scan. A friable, cheesy mass was found at operation

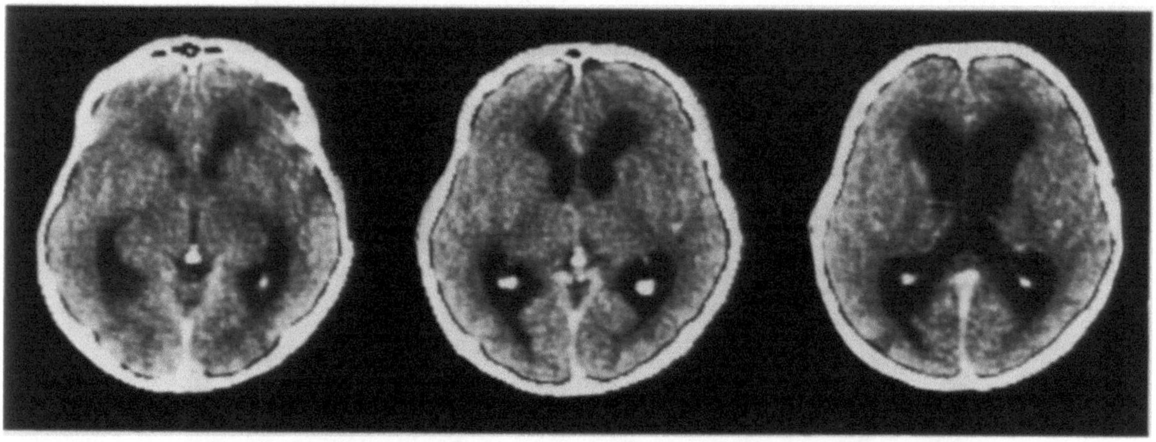

Fig. D 6.27. Isodense colloid cyst of the third ventricle in a 43-year-old man with signs of increased intracranial pressure. The hemispheric defect between the frontal horns (*center*) is consistent with this type of cyst. The site of the lesion is further evidenced by the normal size of the third ventricle posterior to the cyst (*left*). There is severe hydrocephalus secondary to obstruction of both foramina of Monro

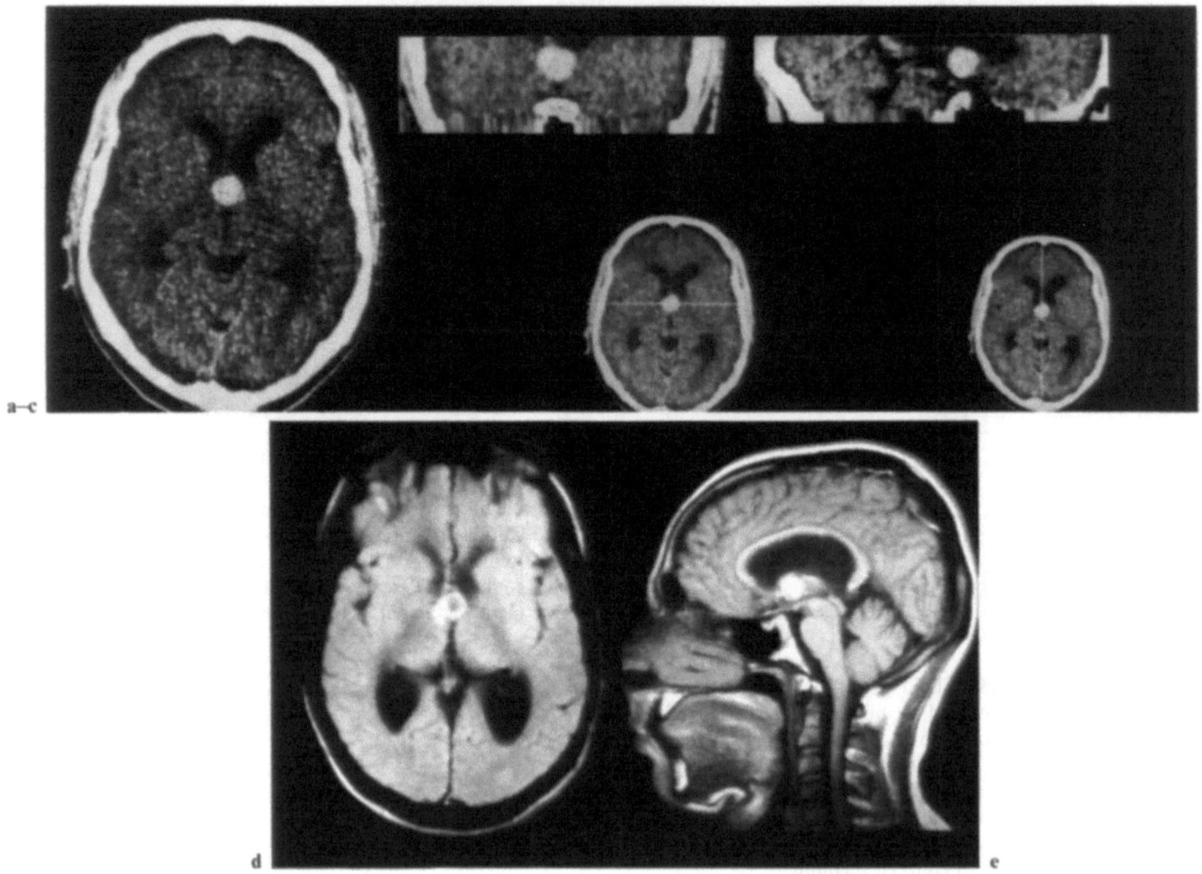

Fig. D 6.28 a–e. Colloid cyst in a 45-year-old woman with intermittent increased intracranial pressure and memory impairment. CT: **a** noncontrast, **b** coronal reconstruction, **c** sagittal reconstruction. MR: **d, e** SE 400/30 axial, sagittal. CT shows a hyperdense, rounded structure lodged in the anterior part of the third ventricle. MR shows a hyperintense, spherical tumor with a hypointense core

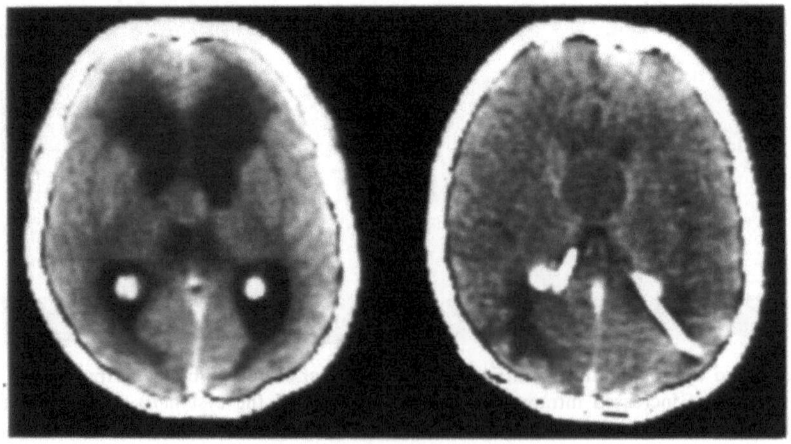

Fig. D 6.29. Colloid cyst of the third ventricle in a 60-year-old woman with increased intracranial pressure. Four years after shunt implantation she developed failure of short-term memory accompanied by adynamia and anisocoria. Plain CT scan (*left*) shows a nearly isodense cyst with associated hydrocephalus. Postcontrast CT 4 years later (*right*) demonstrates marked enlargement of the cyst with ring enhancement of the capsule. Ventricular catheters are visible in both occipital horns

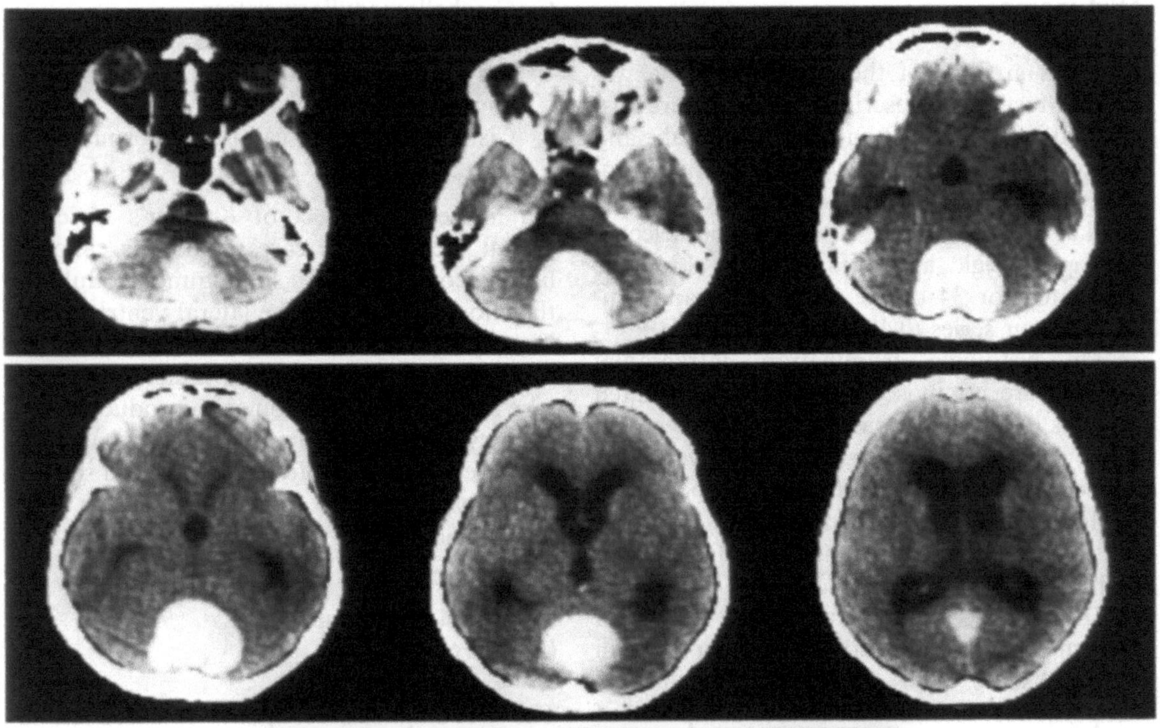
a

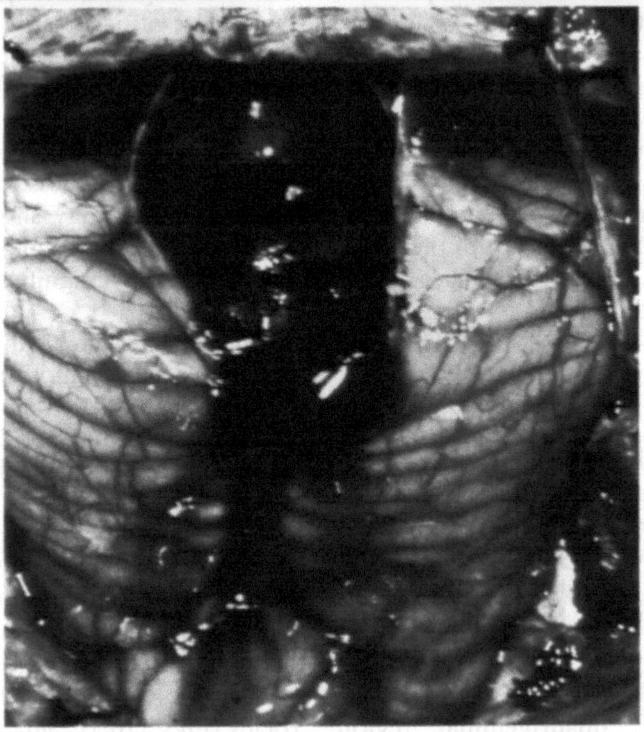
b

Fig. D6.30. a Endodermal cyst on the posterior fossa midline in a 29-year-old woman with cerebellar symptoms. The lesion appears as a well-defined area of extremely high density (96 HU). It does not enhance with contrast medium. The fact that a dermal sinus on the occipital midline had been resected several years previously suggested the dysontogenetic nature of the lesion. Meningioma was excluded due to the extreme density of the lesion and the fact that meningiomas do not calcify in such a homogeneous fashion. **b** A large cystic cavity filled with a dark brown, oily fluid was exposed at operation

f) Lipomas

Lipomas are one of the rare intracranial tumors. Most cases described to date were discovered incidentally at autopsy. Vonderahe and Niemer (1944) found only 4 intracranial lipomas in 5000 postmortem examinations, while Budka (1974) found 9 cases in 1956 selected neuropathologic autopsies (0.46%). Lipomas accounted for 34 of the 8516 intracranial tumors in our series (0.40%).

On histologic examination, intracranial lipomas are composed of fully differentiated fat cells, often accompanied by other types of tissue such as blood vessels, connective tissue, and occasionally muscle fibers. The periphery of the tumor is apt to contain areas of fibrosis, calcifications, and even plaque-like foci of ossification.

Intracranial lipomas are ectopic lesions of dysontogenetic origin and are not neoplasms in the strict sense. Willis (1953) describes them as "superfluous tumorlike structures composed of an incongruous mixture of tissues." They are related to teratoid and teratomatous lesions and participate in general organ growth without manifesting the autonomous growth patterns of, say, ventricular wall tumors in tuberous sclerosis or neurofibromas. Thus, clinical progression in patients with intracranial lipomas is due not so much to growth of the lesion as to the effects of regressive changes in the lipoma on surrounding tissues.

Typical Sites

The most common site of occurrence is the region of the corpus callosum, which is involved in 28%–50% of cases. The next most frequent sites are the tuber cinereum and the quadrigeminal plate. Krainer (1935) identified the sites of predilection for these rare intracranial tumors on the basis of his own observations and a review of the literature:

1. Ambient cistern, quadrigeminal region (junction of colliculus and brachium)
2. Chiasmatic cistern and infundibulum
3. Interpeduncular cistern
4. Cistern of sylvian fossa
5. Lateral pontine cistern (cerebellopontine angle)
6. Cerebellomedullary cistern
7. Tela choroidea of lateral ventricles and third ventricle, choroid plexus, velum triangulare
8. Cistern of corpus callosum (corpus callosum lipomas)

An interesting aspect of Krainer's review is that it includes five cases of corpus callosum lipoma coexisting with small tumor nodules on the choroid plexus of the lateral ventricles (see Figs. D6.37, 38).

Reports in the literature indicate that it is rare for intracranial lipomas to produce neurologic symptoms. Lipomas of the corpus callosum are usually manifested by cerebral seizures and less commonly by hemiparesis or other neurologic disturbances.

Computed Tomography
(Figs. D6.31–42)

The CT diagnosis of lipoma is based on the typical site of occurrence and especially on the attenuation characteristics of the tumor. Fatty tissue has attenuation values of approximately −100 HU, and these are typical of lipoma. It should be noted, however, that smaller tumor nodules occupying less than the thickness of a whole CT slice may show higher attenuation values as a result of volume averaging. Density does not increase significantly with intravenous contrast.

Plaque-like calcifications at the periphery of large corpus callosum lipomas are visible on plain skull X-rays and may be diagnostic. These calcifications are displayed most clearly on coronal sections (Fig. D6.39b). We have not observed calcifications in lipomas at other sites. Corpus callosum lipoma is commonly associated with partial or complete aplasia of the corpus callosum, resulting in a separation of the lateral ventricles (Figs. D6.38, 39a). Multiple lipomas may occur and are most likely to involve the choroid plexus of the lateral ventricles (Figs. D6.37, 38).

Magnetic Resonance Imaging
(Fig. D 6.43)

Lipomas have characteristically short T1 and T2 values on MR images. Even on T1-weighted sequences the tumor appears hyperintense and well-defined. The tumor gives a very high signal on heavily T2-weighted scans. Lipomas of the corpus callosum (the most common site of involvement) are displayed exceptionally well on midsagittal images. The high sensitivity of MR permits the detection of very small bits of aberrant fatty tissue anywhere in the CSF pathways.

MR is inferior to CT in its ability to detect calcifications.

Differential Diagnosis

Dermoid cysts and teratomas may have CT density values comparable to those of lipoma. Unlike epidermoid cysts, which usually are isodense to CSF and are easy to differentiate, dermoid cysts and teratomas are very rare, and experience with these lesions is meager. Nevertheless, four definite sites of predilection are known: the third ventricle, with the tumor arising from the pineal body; the ambient cistern; the fourth ventricle; and the cribriform plate with extension into the frontal and temporal white matter. To the best of our knowledge, there have been no verified reports of lipomas occurring at the last two sites. The nonhomogeneity of the hypodense cystic contents of dermoids and teratomas is an additional aid to the CT diagnosis of these lesions. Histograms indicate a homogeneous density pattern in lipoma only if the tumor is at least 25–30 mm in diameter. The variation is greater in smaller lipomas due to the partial volume effect; the standard deviation is similar to that in dermoid cysts.

Lipomas in the region of the ambient cistern are generally much smaller than dermoid cysts at that location. The characteristic plaques of calcifications in lipomas of the corpus callosum are sufficient to distinguish those lesions from dermoid cysts of the third ventricle.

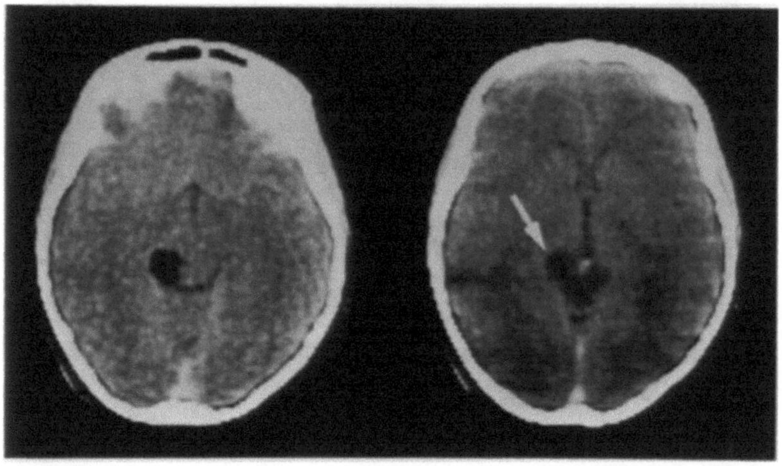

Fig. D 6.31. Lipoma in the left ambient cistern of a 9-year-old boy with brainstem seizures. CT demonstrates a very low density mass (–48 to –52 HU) the size of a hazelnut

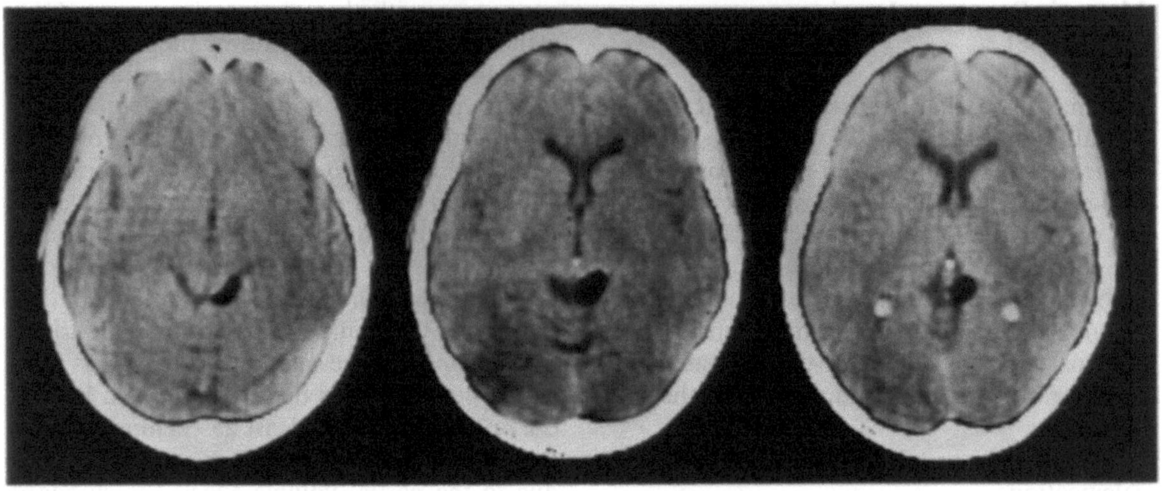

Fig. D 6.32. Lipoma in the region of the right ambient cistern and quadrigeminal plate in a 36-year-old woman with a 2-year history of headache and a single seizure episode. The mean density of the lesion is −72 to −88 HU, consistent with lipoma. The diagnosis was confirmed at operation

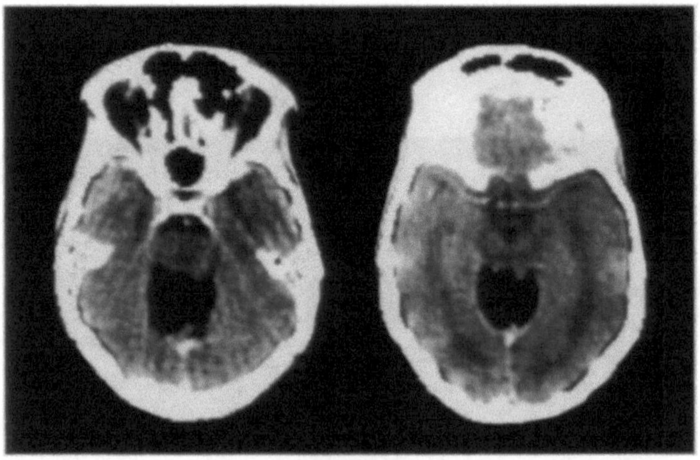

Fig. D 6.33. Large lipoma at the center of the superior vermis and its cistern in a 40-year-old man with papilledema of 2 diopters. Postcontrast CT

Fig. D 6.34. Lipoma of the quadrigeminal plate in a 67-year-old man with pronounced hydrocephalus secondary to tumor obstruction of CSF flow in the aqueduct. Mean tumor density is −70 HU

Fig. D 6.35. Lipoma in the cistern of the velum interpositum in a 43-year-old woman. Mean tumor density is −40 HU. Incidental finding

Fig. D 6.36. Lipoma in the region of the chiasmatic cistern, probably on the infundibulum, in a 12-year-old boy evaluated for increasingly aggressive behavior. Density −42 HU

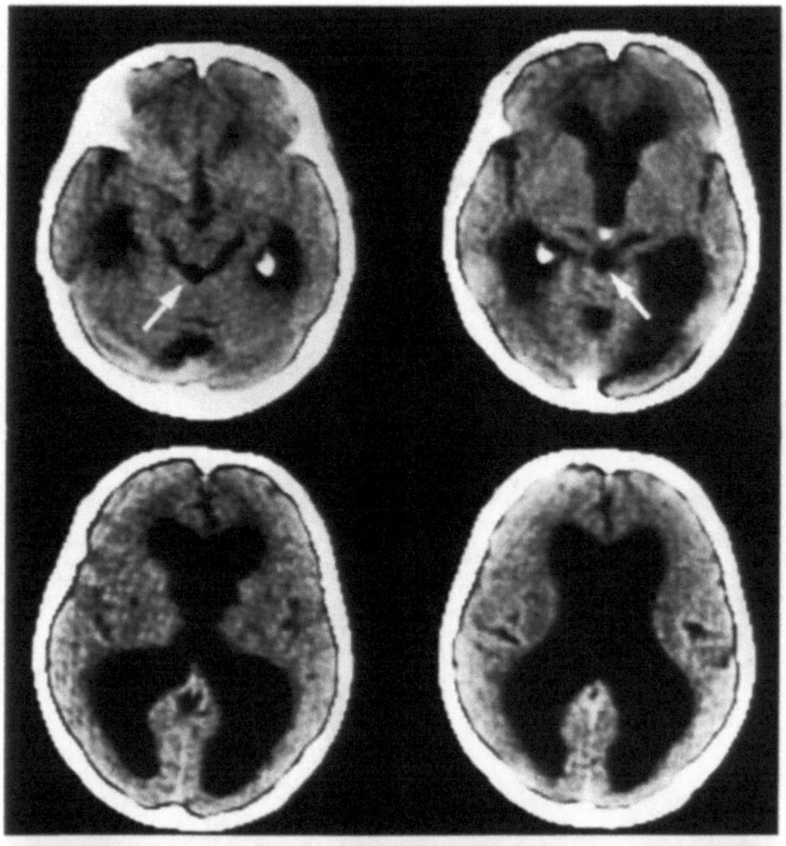

D 6.34

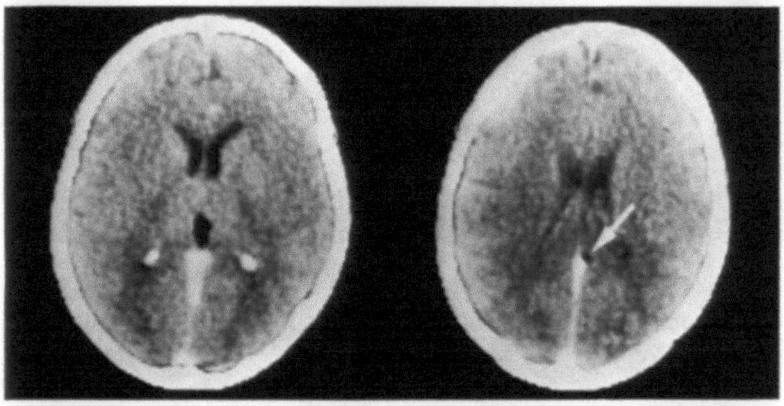

D 6.35

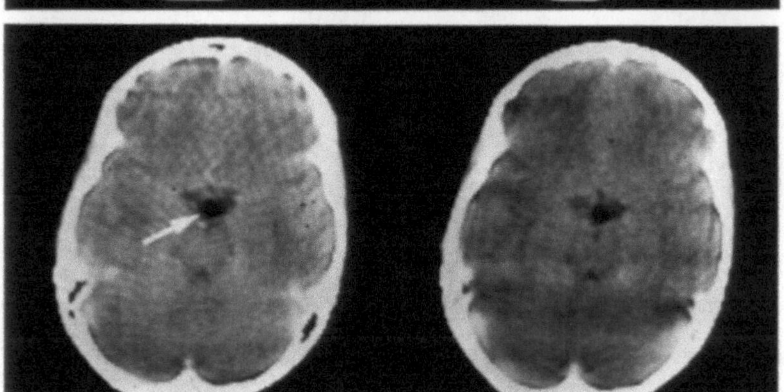

D 6.36

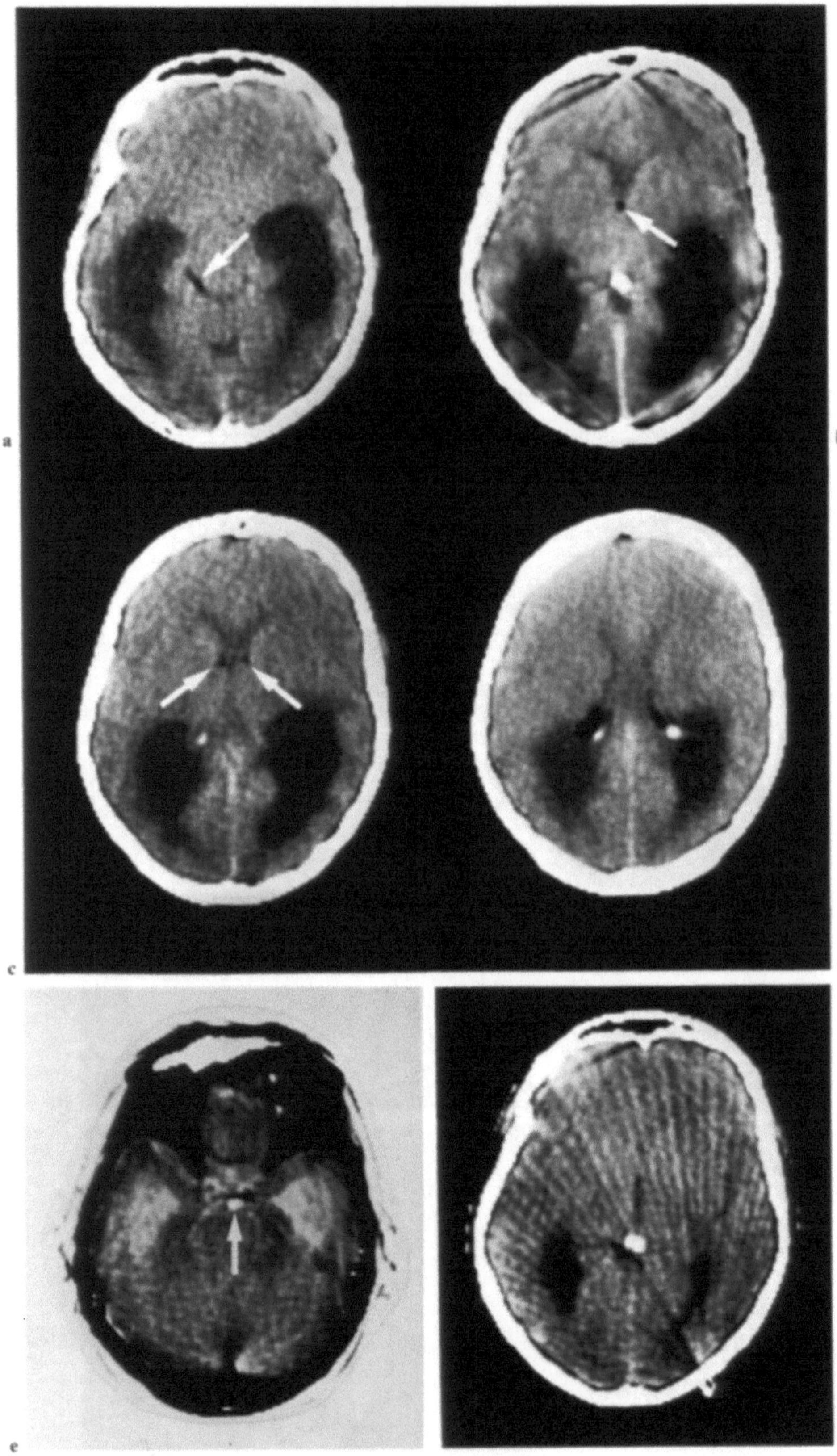

a b c d e f

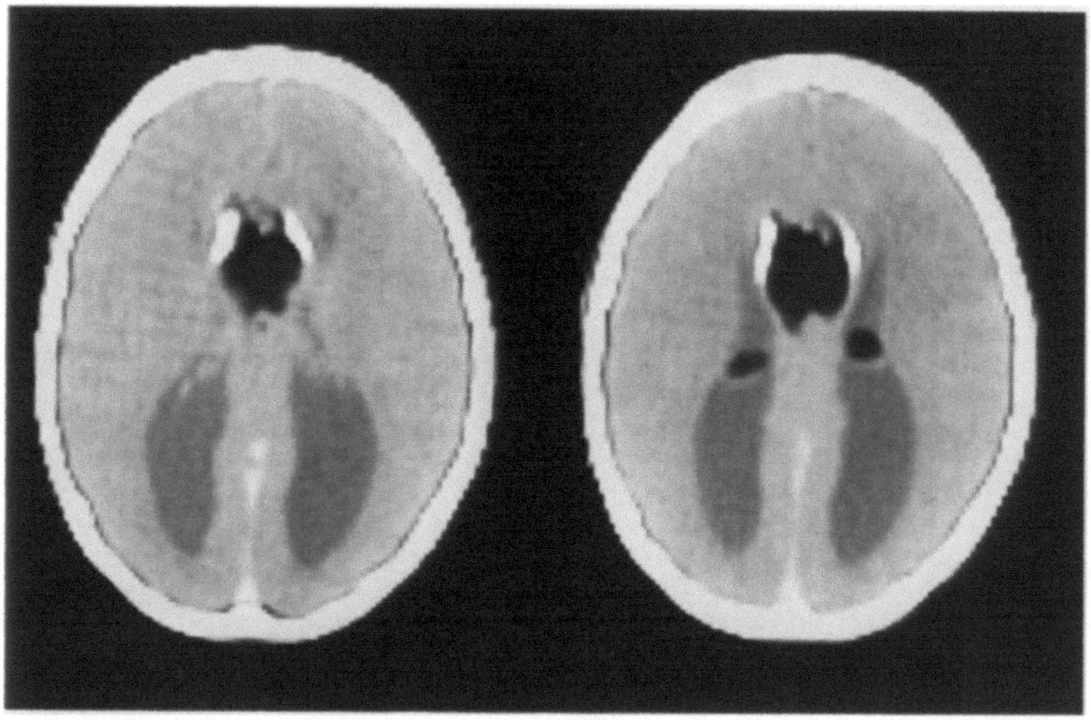

Fig. D 6.38. Lipomas on the choroid plexus of both lateral ventricles with a coexisting lipoma of the corpus callosum, which presents typical shell-like calcifications at its interface with adjacent brain. The 21-year-old woman presented with a 2-year history of psychomotor seizures and a 3-month history of paroxysmal headaches (referrable to obstructed CSF flow in the occipital horns). Density values in the lipomas range from −33 HU in the left choroid plexus to −67 HU in the right choroid plexus and −106 HU in the corpus callosum

Fig. D 6.37 a–f. Multiple intracranial lipomas in a 60-year-old man with profoundly altered mental status, decreased vision, vertigo, and micturation difficulties. **a** Small lipoma on the left side of the ambient cistern (*arrow*). **b** Small lipoma in the anterior part of the third ventricle (*arrow*). **c** Small lipomas on the choroid plexus of the lateral ventricles near the foramina of Monro (*arrows*). **d** Lipomas on the glomus of the choroid plexus in the lateral ventricles, obstructing both occipital horns and causing severe hydrocephalus and periventricular lucency. **e** Small lipoma in the interpeduncular fossa (*arrow*). The negative of the CT image is shown to demonstrate the lipoma more clearly. **f** Marked regression of ventricular dilatation is noted 6 weeks after a drainage procedure (artifacts are from the metal parts of the shunt). Density values in the different lipomas range from −15 to −52 HU

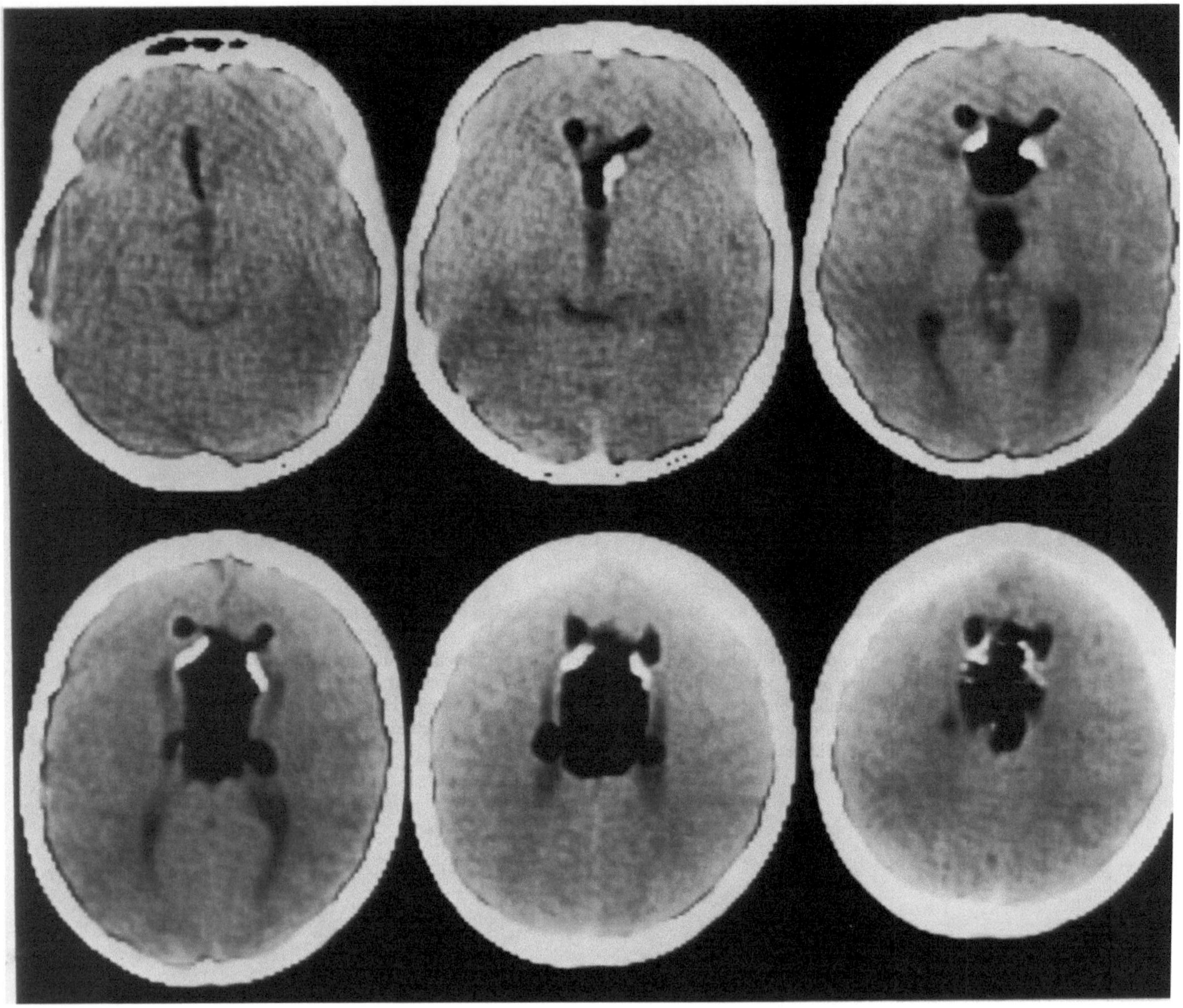

a

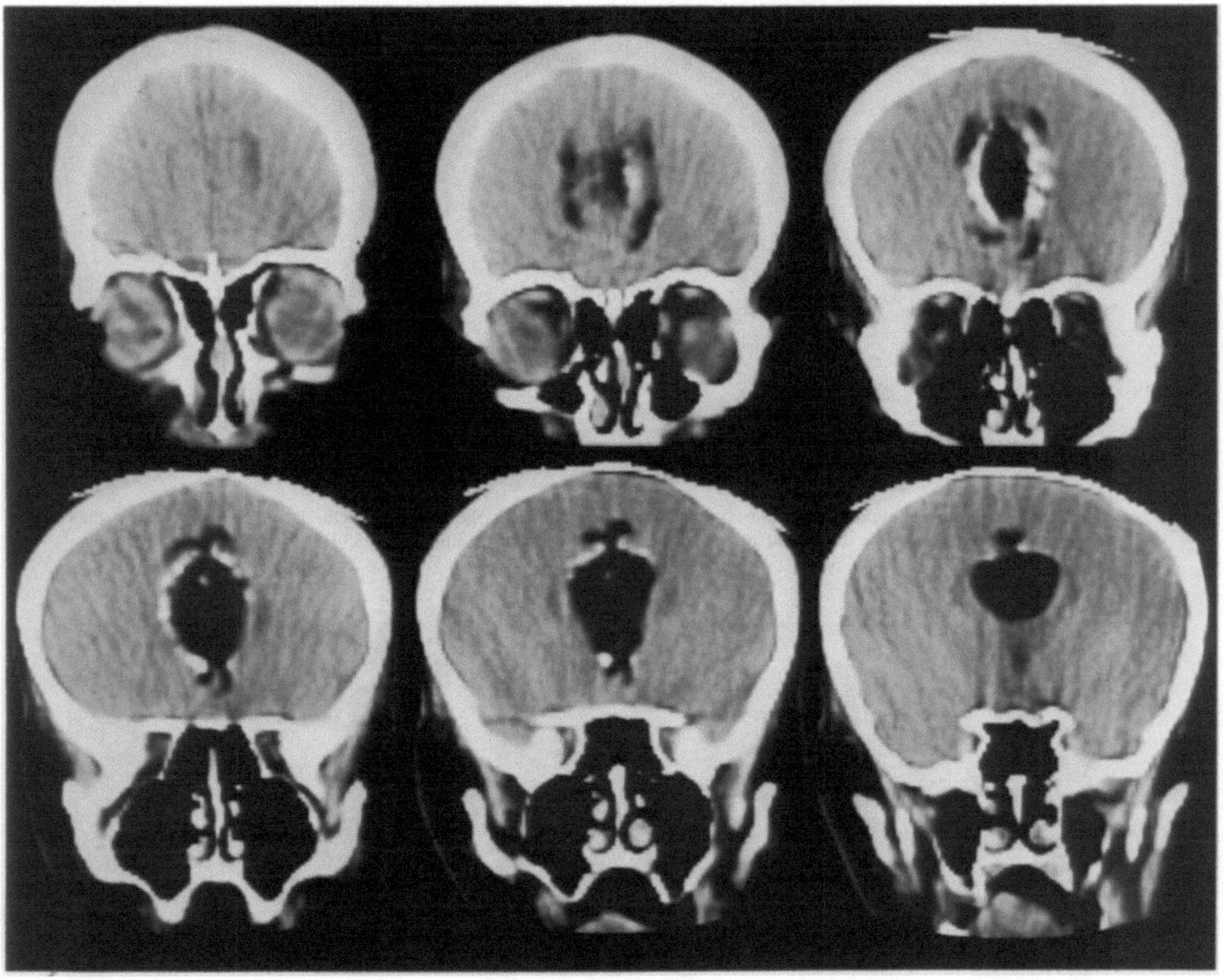

b

Fig. D 6.39 a, b. Atypical corpus callosum lipoma in a 22-year-old woman with cerebral seizures. **a** Axial CT scans demonstrate a large lipoma replacing almost the entire corpus callosum (aplasia) with small calcium plaques at the tumor border and multiple smaller, coexisting lipomas in the lateral ventricle adjacent to the main tumor. **b** The plaque-like calcifications are displayed more clearly on coronal scans. In most cases these calcifications can be detected on standard skull X-rays

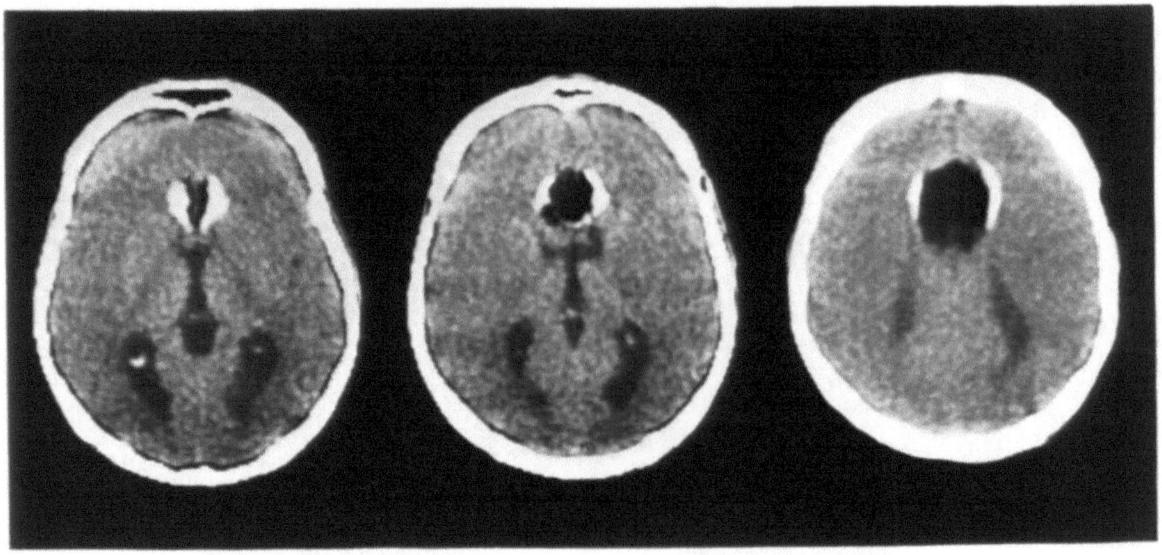

Fig. D 6.40. Corpus callosum lipoma in a 20-year-old man with cerebral seizures. Note the typical plaque-like calcifications at the periphery of the fatty tumor. Density at the center of the lipoma is −55 HU

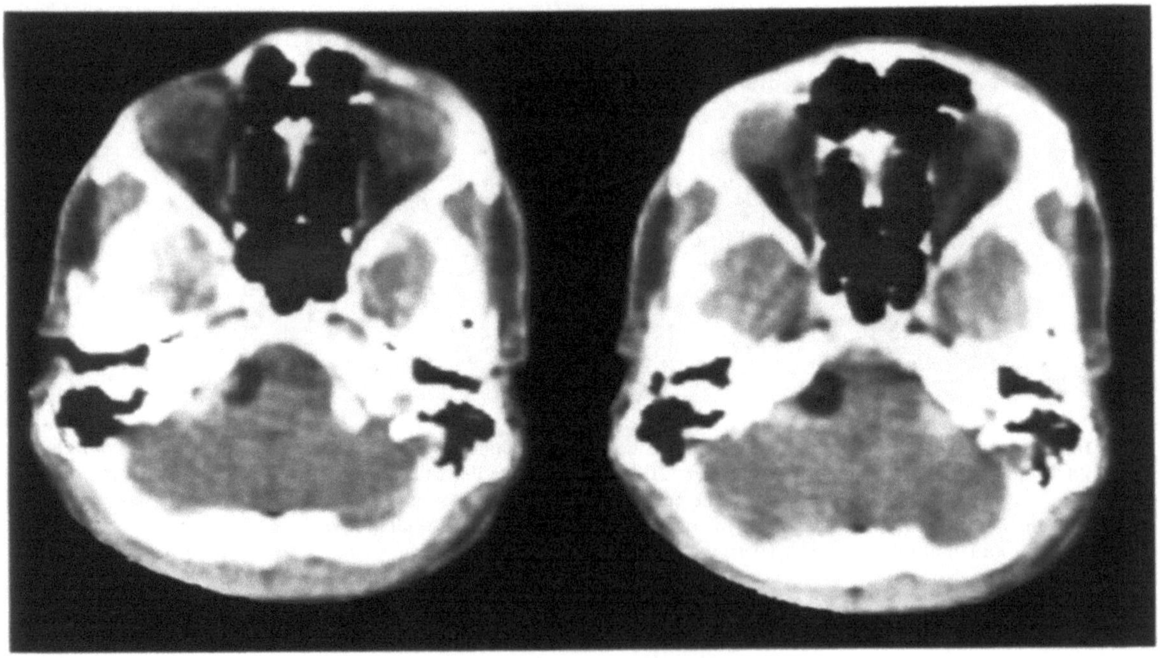

Fig. D 6.41. Small lipoma at the left pyramidal apex in an 18-year-old male with symptoms of a cerebellopontine angle mass. Mean density is −55 HU

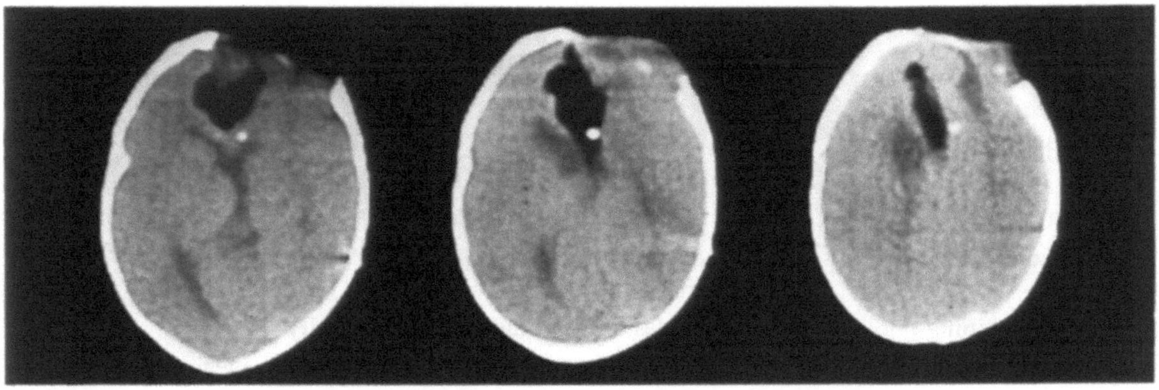

Fig. D 6.42. Large lobulated lipoma (mean density −117 to −125 HU) between the frontal lobes (arising from the anterior corpus callosum?) in a child who previously underwent removal of a right frontal encephalocele

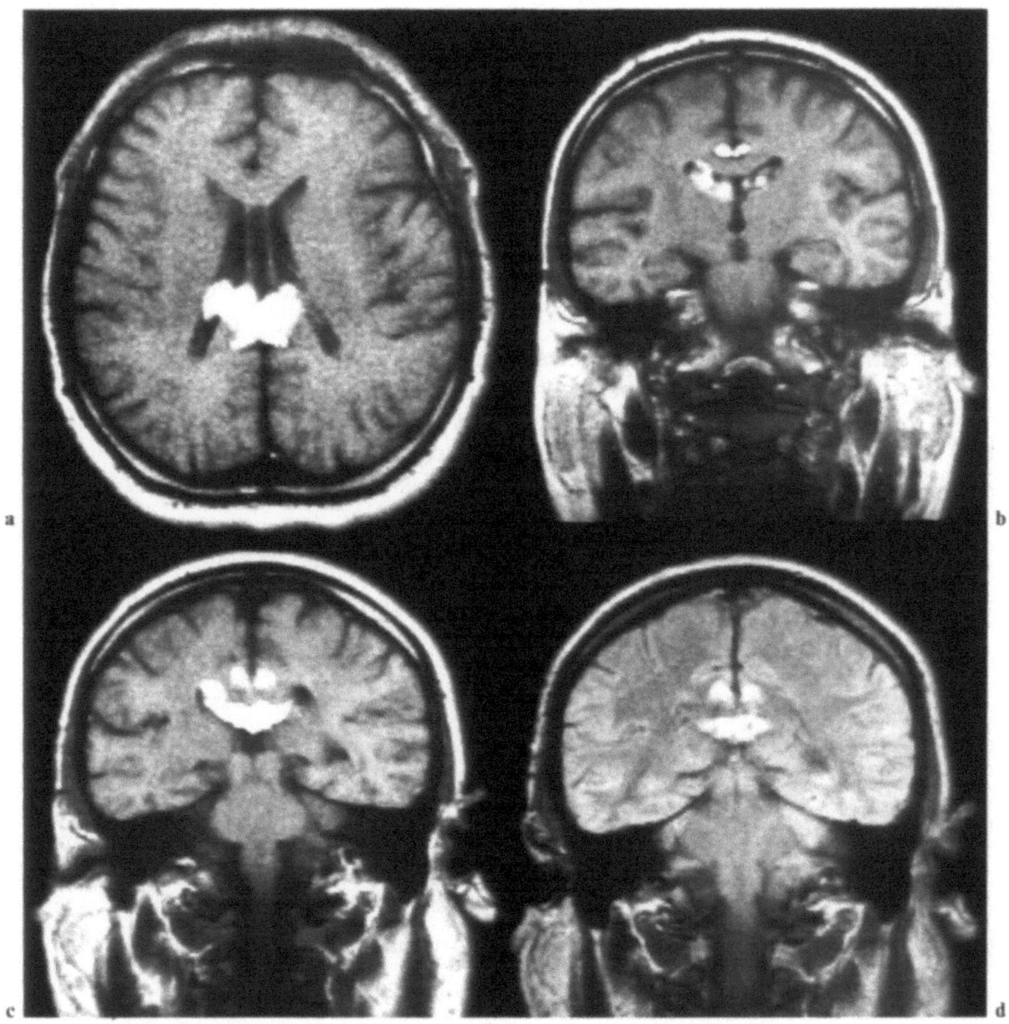

Fig. D 6.43 a–d. Corpus callosum lipoma in the region of the posterior callosal cistern with associated aplasia of the corpus callosum, detected incidentally in a 54-year-old man with Parkinson's disease. Patient experienced no headaches or seizures. MR: **a** SE 400/35, **b–d** SE 400/35 coronal. Because of its fat content, the tumor gives a bright signal on the T1-weighted image

g) Epidermoids, Dermoids, Teratomas

Incidence:	
Epidermoids	0.6%–1.5%
Dermoids	0.1%
Teratomas	0.3% of all brain tumors
Age predilection	Second to fourth decades; teratomas also occur in small children
Sex predilection	Males and females affected equally
Typical sites	Epidermoids: cerebellopontine angle, parapontine area, lateral ventricle, fourth ventricle, third ventricle, corpus callosum, chiasmal region, quadrigeminal region, sylvian fissure, cranial diploe Dermoids: parapituitary region, anterior fossa closure lines, region of third ventricle and pineal body, ambient cistern, posterior fossa midline Teratomas: pineal region, third ventricle, sellar region, lateral ventricle
Main clinical features	Signs of increased intracranial pressure, local symptoms, "aseptic meningitis"
Skull X-ray	Erosion of cranial bone adjacent to tumor
Angiography	Vascular displacement
CT	
Noncontrast scan	Epidermoids: hypodense area, isodense to CSF, with peripheral hyperdense foci (calcifications) Dermoids: very hypodense area, isodense to fat, often with peripheral calcifications Teratomas: same as dermoids, or unevenly scattered areas of varying density
Contrast enhancement	Positive in teratomas of high malignancy
Postcontrast appearance	No significant change in epidermoids or dermoids, heterogeneous pattern in malignant teratomas
MR	
Noncontrast scan	Epidermoids: usually have long relaxation times on T1-weighted images (hypointense) and T2-weighted images (hyperintense) Dermoids: variable relaxation times; fatty components have shorter T1 times (hyperintense) and longer T2 times
Gadolinium enhancement	Positive in highly malignant teratomas
Post Gd-DTPA appearance	No significant change; unknown for teratomas

Differential diagnosis

Epidermoids:	Arachnoid cyst Other cysts Cysticercosis Old hemorrhagic cavity Gumma
Dermoids and teratomas:	Lipoma

Epidermoids, dermoids, and teratomas are rare dysontogenetic tumors for which Zülch (1986) reports an incidence of 1.8% (in 9000 tumors). Both sexes are affected equally. The incidence in our series was only 1.5%. The prognostic classification is grade I.

Epidermoids (epidermoid cysts, pearly tumors, cholesteatomas) account for approximately three-fourths of these dysontogenetic lesions. Epidermoids and dermoids are diagnosed chiefly in the middle decades, while teratomas may be diagnosed in childhood.

Epidermoids are composed of epidermis, connective tissue, and an aggregation of horny scales arranged in lamellae and enclosed within a thin membrane. This is responsible for the tumor's transparency and mother-of-pearl sheen. *Dermoid cysts* may contain saponified fatty tissue, epidermis, skin appendages with hair follicles, hair, sebaceous glands, and sweat glands.

Teratomas likewise contain epidermis and skin appendages in addition to bone, cartilage, endodermal tissue, and other organic tissue structures.

The *typical sites* of occurrence are as listed in the box above. Clinical manifestations include signs of increased intracranial pressure and local symptoms, as well as "aseptic meningitis" incited by the entry of epidermal plaques or fat into the CSF.

Additional Diagnostic Procedures

Plain skull X-rays are of value only in epidermoids that arise from the diploe. Dermoids in the anterior fossa cause erosive bone change along the closure lines. Teratomas may be evidenced by large intracranial calcifications or even tooth formation.

Computed Tomography

(Figs. D6.44, 45, 47–50, 52–64; E 17)

Noncontrast Scan

All three of these dysontogenetic tumors have predominantly low, cystlike attenuation values. Small calcifications are occasionally seen at the periphery of the mass (Figs. D6.44, 45).

Densitometry is of major value and in *epidermoids* will show values approximating those of CSF (+2 to +10 HU). Consequently, epidermoids will tend to have the same gray level as CSF on analog images, although the standard deviation is usually higher in epidermoids than in CSF.

Our experience is consistent with the results of Fawcitt and Isherwood (1977) and New and Scott (1975). However, Gyldensted and Karle (1977) reported on three suprasellar epidermoids and Braun et al. (1977) on three epidermoids in the posterior fossa that appeared isodense or even hyperdense on plain CT scans. Some of these lesions enhanced, raising the possibility of confusion with meningioma. It is unclear from these publications whether the lesions were in fact epidermoid cysts. One tumor is described as a "black mass" (cf. case in Fig. D6.30).

Dermoid cysts have mean densities in the negative range of the Hounsfield scale because of their high fat content. Mean values as low as −1000 HU may be registered depending on the degree of saponification. Dermoids therefore tend to appear darker than CSF on the CT scan (Figs. D6.56–59, 61). The standard deviation is often very high due to the varying densities of the cyst components, and may exceed 20 HU.

The CT features of *teratomas* are much more variable. Again, components with negative densities predominate, and the pattern may be identical to that of a dermoid cyst (Fig. D6.63). However, certain other components in teratomas may have high density values, so that measurements at different sites in the tumor will show a greater range of variation than in dermoids. The different components of this dysontogenetic tumor can be visualized by changing the window level while viewing the CT image (Fig. D6.62).

Postcontrast Scan

We observed no measurable contrast enhancement in any of the epidermoids or dermoids in our series. Only malignant teratomas show significant enhancement, which may assume bizarre patterns (Fig. D6.64).

The CT examination may be repeated with intrathecal metrizamide to help identify other cystic lesions, especially epidermoids of the ambient cistern (Fig. D6.49).

Magnetic Resonance Imaging

(Figs. C3; D 1.222, D 6.44–46, 50, 51, 54, 59, 60, 65; E 17)

Because these dysontogenetic tumors frequently occur near the skull base or in the posterior fossa, MR is advantageous in that it can provide an artifact-free image. This is especially useful in the detection of small lesions. The major disadvantage of MR is the poor visualization of calcium deposits. Dermoids and epidermoids often appear isointense to CSF on T2-weighted sequences. MR can clearly demonstrate the laminar arrangement of epidermal plaques within epidermoid cysts.

Rarely, epidermoids give a high signal intensity on the T1-weighted sequence. These tumors appear increasingly hyperintense as T2 weighting is increased. Epidermoids and dermoids do not enhance with Gd-DTPA.

Differential Diagnosis

1. Epidermoid Cysts. Arachnoid cysts located near the calvarium produce a characteristic thinning and bulging of the cranial wall. However, an arachnoid cyst in the quadrigeminal region may be indistinguishable from an epidermoid due to its identical attenuation values and absence of other changes. The same applies to an arachnoid cyst of the cisterna magna. An irregular configuration would favor a diagnosis of epidermoid, whereas arachnoid cysts always present a round or oval contour.

A solitary *hydatid cyst*, an old *hemorrhagic cavity*, or a *gumma* may contain hypodense areas (same density as CSF) in addition to peripheral calcifications, creating a very strong resemblance to an epidermoid cyst. A lesion confined to the brain parenchyma and having no contact with the CSF is probably not an epidermoid.

2. Dermoid Cysts and Teratomas. Given the extremely low densities of these lesions, lipoma is the only other tumor that need be considered in the differential diagnosis. Only one location poses a problem in this regard: the ambient cistern, which can be a site for lipomas as well as dermoids (see Fig. D6.49).

Malignant teratomas in young children lack the very low-density components that are seen in benign tumor forms. Other malignant childhood tumors, such as germinomas, should be considered in the differential diagnosis.

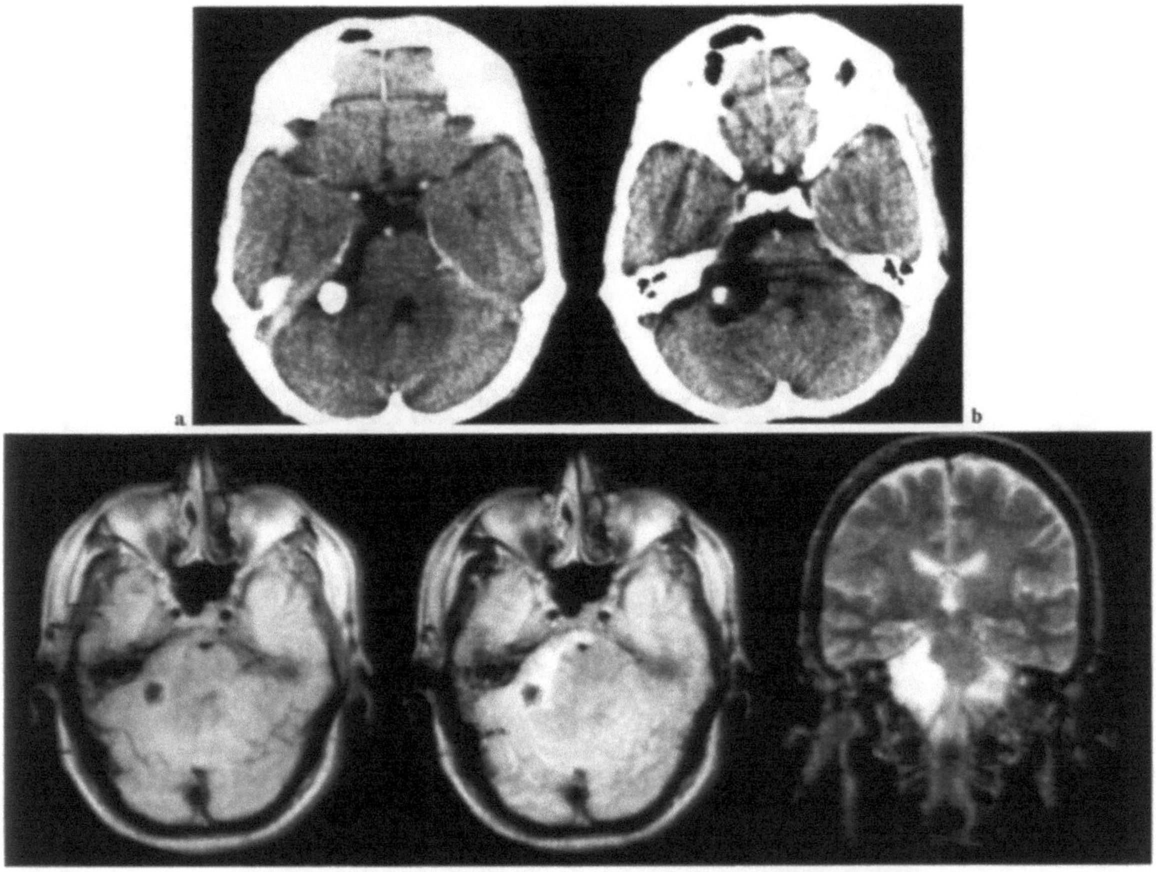

a b c–e

Fig. D 6.44 a–e. Epidermoid cyst in the left cerebellopontine angle of a 51-year-old man with headache, vertigo, unsteady gait, tinnitus, and left-sided hypoacusis. CT: **a, b** noncontrast. MR: **c** SE 1600/35, **d** SE 1600/70, **e** SE 1600/180 coronal. The epidermoid is markedly hypodense on the CT scan (**b**) and contains calcifications (**a**). The tumor is not delineated on the proton-density or T2-weighted images (**c, d**), and the calcification presents as a signal void. On the heavily T2-weighted coronal image (**e**), the tumor is nearly isointense to CSF. Torsion of the brainstem is apparent

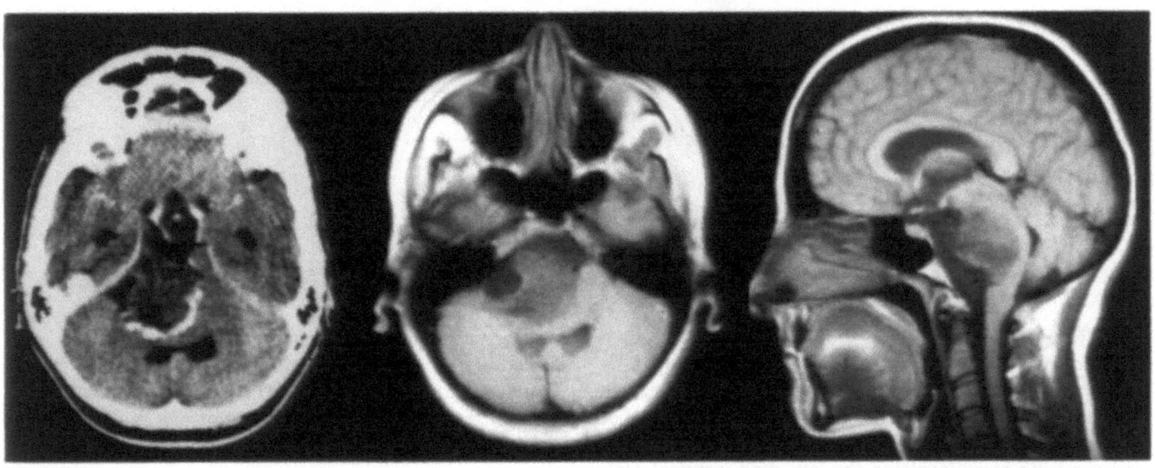

Fig. D 6.45. Prepontine epidermoid cyst in a 47-year-old woman with attacks of vertigo, left abducens paresis, decreased hearing, dysarthria, and dysphagia. CT: *left* contrast-enhanced. MR: *center* and *right* SE 400/30 axial and sagittal. On CT the cyst extends from the prepontine area to the left cerebellar hemisphere and shows peripheral plaque-like calcification. The T1-weighted sequences (*center* and *right*) show a mixed-intensity lesion that is predominantly hypointense. The sagittal view reveals marked brainstem compression. The calcification is not visualized

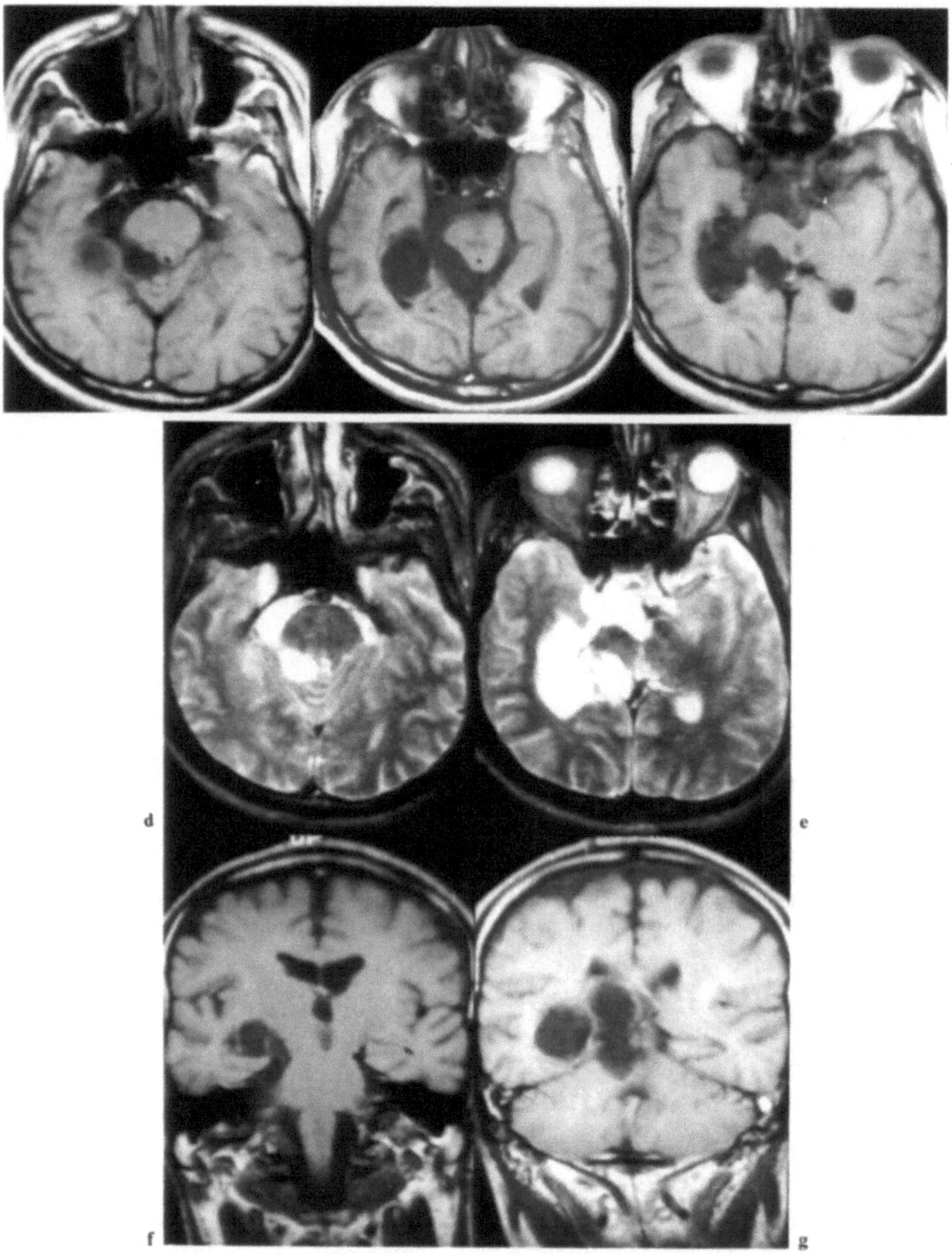

a–c d e f g

Fig. D 6.46 a–g. Epidermoid of the posterior fossa in a 47-year-old man with a 6-month history of right hemiparesis, profoundly altered mental status and temporal lobe seizures. MR: **a–c** SE 700/30, **d, e** SE 3000/90, **f, g** SE 700/30 coronal. The T1-weighted images (**a–c, f, g**) show a hypointense retro- and perisellar mass involving the left quadrigeminal plate region and compressing the brainstem from the left side. The tumor is virtually indistinguishable from CSF by its signal pattern on the T1- and T2-weighted sequences. The coronal sections (**f, g**) show the tumor extending along the brainstem and past the tentorium

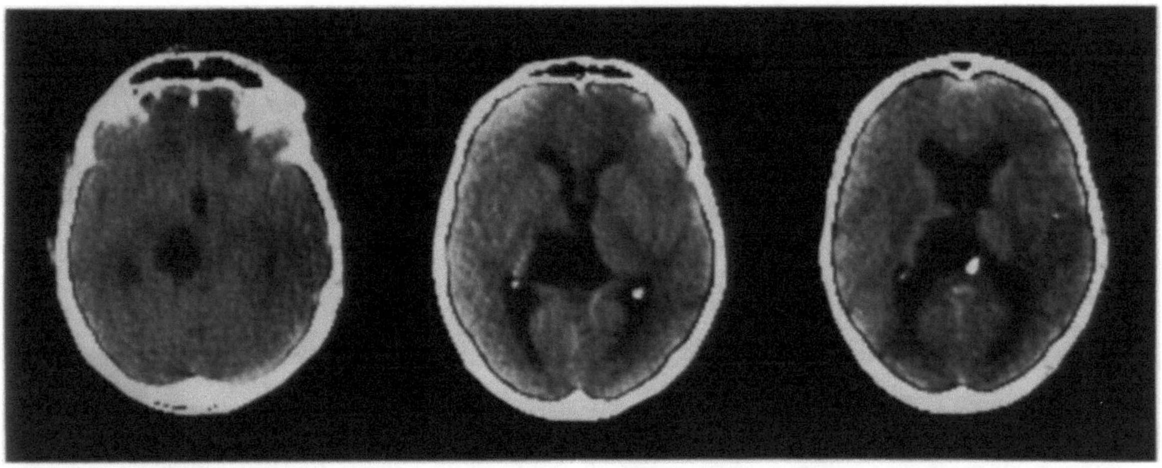

Fig. D 6.47. Large epidermoid cyst, isodense to CSF (9.8 HU), of the quadrigeminal region, thalamus, and left cerebral peduncle in a 47-year-old man with slowly progressive right-sided hemiparesis. The scan on the *right* shows a fine membranous partition between the left occipital horn and the epidermoid cyst; this feature was crucial in forming a diagnosis. Incipient hydrocephalus is present

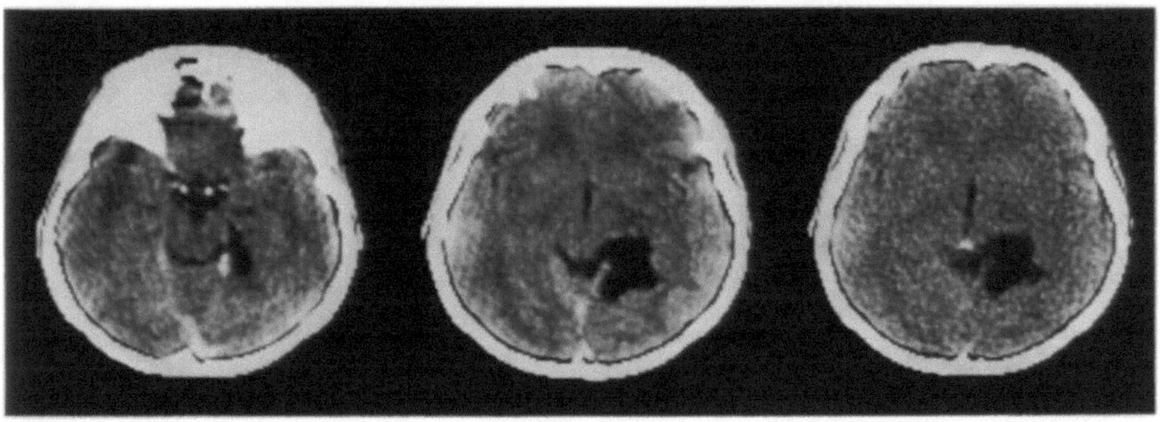

Fig. D 6.48. Epidermoid cyst in the right ambient cistern with extension into the right occipital lobe and right cerebral peduncle in a 34-year-old woman with intermittent hemiparesis on the left side. Multiple sclerosis had been incorrectly diagnosed several years earlier. The lesion is isodense to CSF

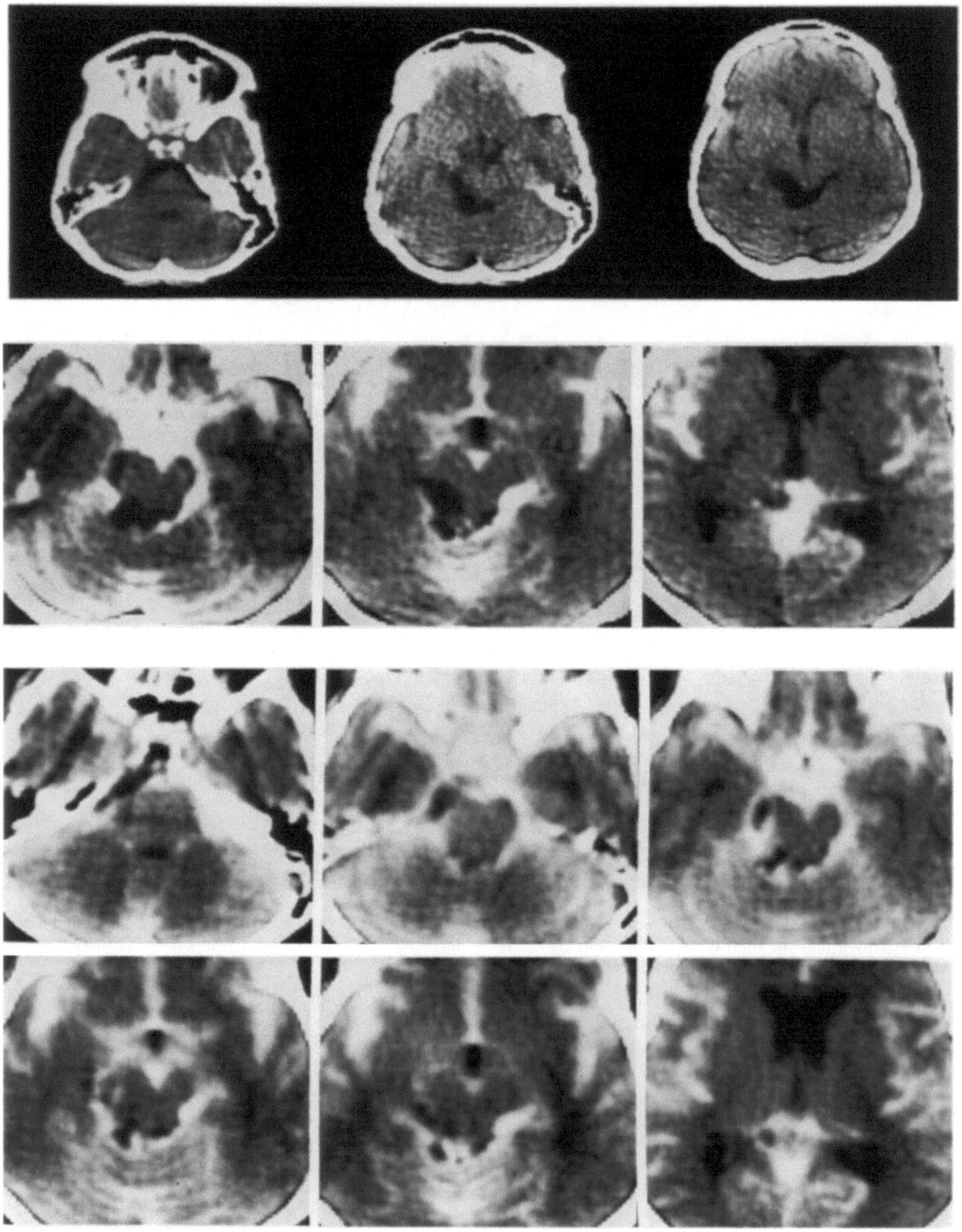

a

b

c

Fig. D 6.49 a–c. Small epidermoid in the ambient cistern, predominantly on the left side, in a 49-year-old woman with cranial nerve dysfunction and psychomotor seizures. **a** Plain CT scan shows apparent dilatation of the ambient cistern on the left side. **b** Repeat CT examination 3 h after intrathecal metrizamide identifies the dilatation as a mass lesion isodense to CSF. Diagnosis: epidermoid cyst. **c** Entry of contrast medium into the epidermoid cyst 6 h after postinjection

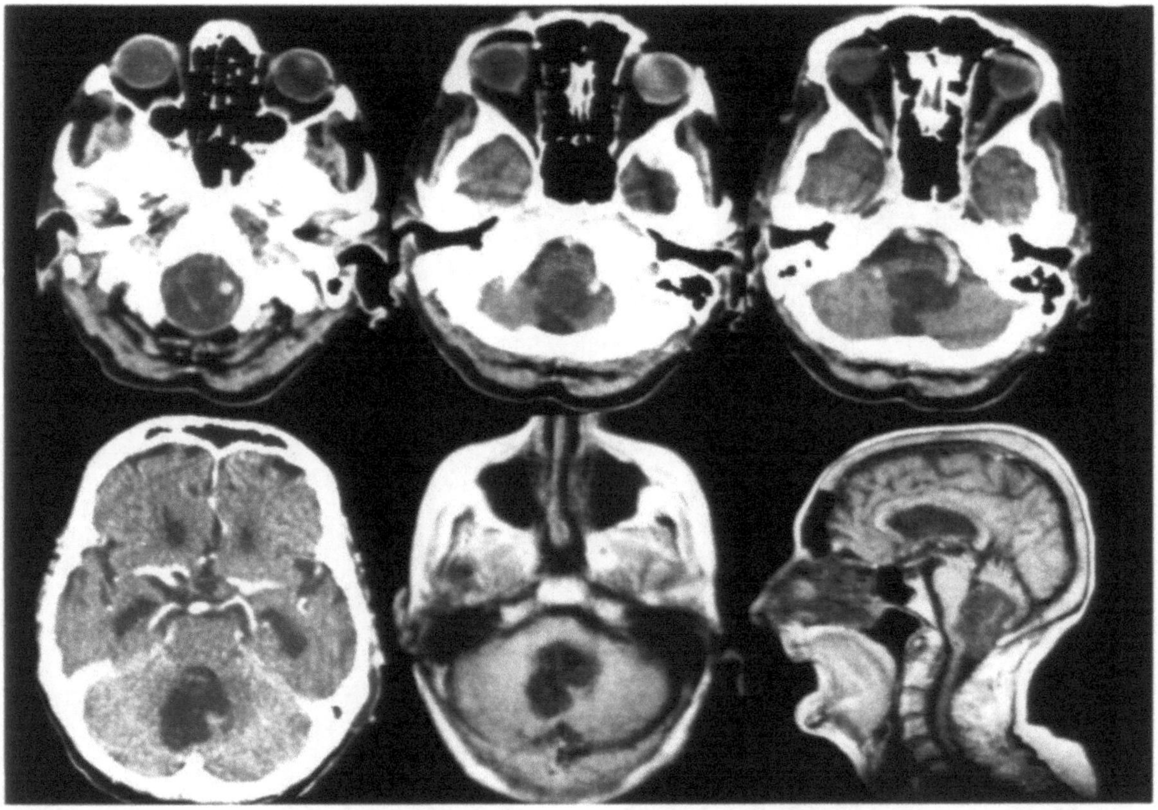

a–c

d–f

Fig. D 6.50 a–f. Epidermoid cyst extending downward from the cerebellum through the foramen magnum in a 74-year-old woman with syncopal episodes and ataxia of gait and stance. CT: **a–d**. MR: **e** SE 400/30 axial, coronal. CT reveals a hypodense tumor with calcification of the basilar and vertebral arteries. The sagittal T1-weighted image (**f**) shows a mass of low signal intensity extending far through the foramen magnum while compressing and displacing the cerebellum upward. The brainstem is compressed by a small anterior projection of tumor

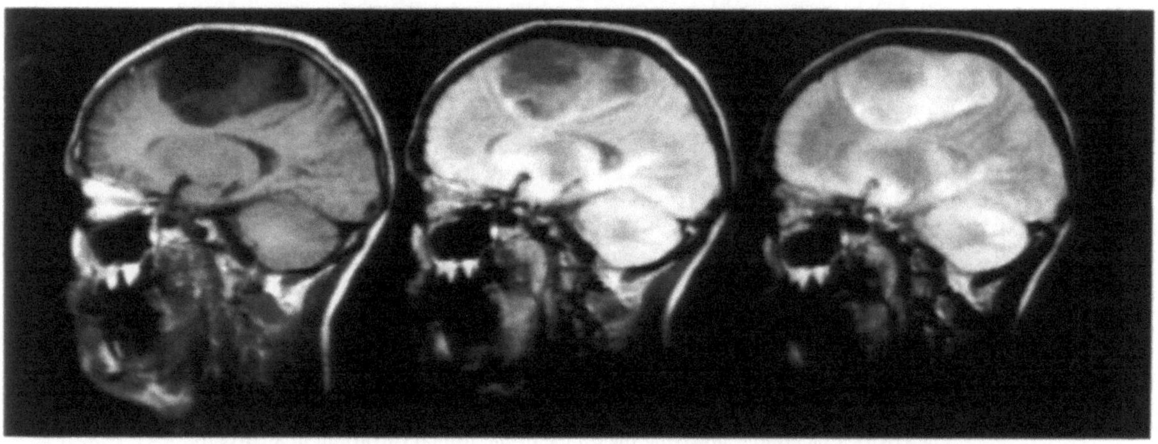

Fig. D 6.51. Epidermoid cyst involving frontal, precentral, and parietal regions of the cerebrum in a 32-year-old man with focal seizures and progressive hemiparesis predominantly affecting the left leg. MR: *left* SE 1600/30, *center* SE 1600/60, *right* SE 1600/120, all sagittal. The proton-density image (*left*) demonstrates a hypointense tumor, which acquires a clumped, mixed-density appearance as T2 weighting is increased (*center* and *right*)

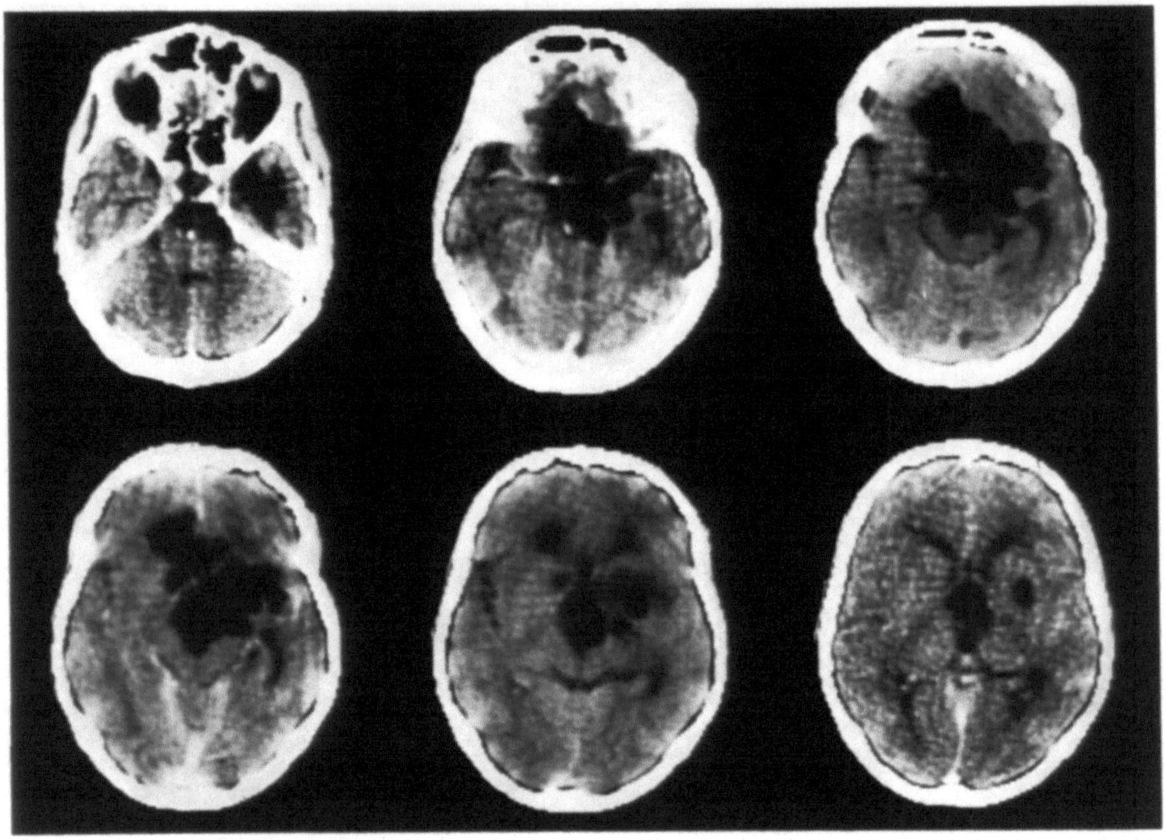

Fig. D 6.52. Very large epidermoid cyst with maplike boundaries at the base of the middle fossa in a 35-year-old man. The tumor extends to the interpeduncular cistern, the prepontine area, the subtemporal and subfrontal regions, and into the third ventricle from below

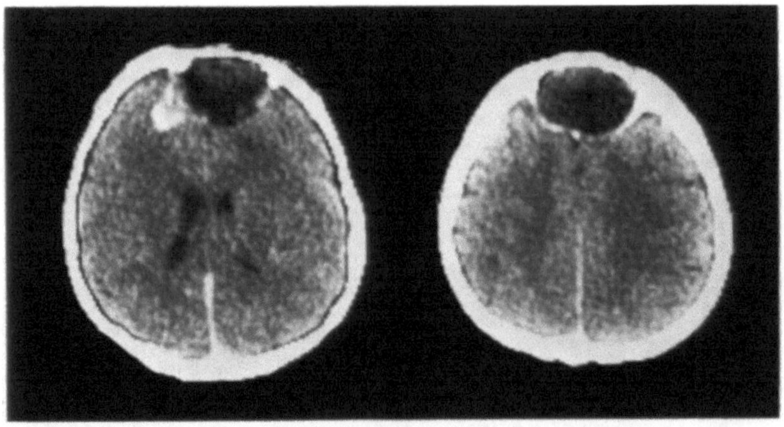

Fig. D 6.53. Epidermoid involving the diploe of the frontal calvarium in a 53-year-old man. The dysontogenetic tumor is predominantly hypodense and is largely demarcated from normal brain by a membrane of calcific density. The epidermoid is bordered on the left by an area of increased density, which enhanced with contrast medium. This area proved to be granulation tissue

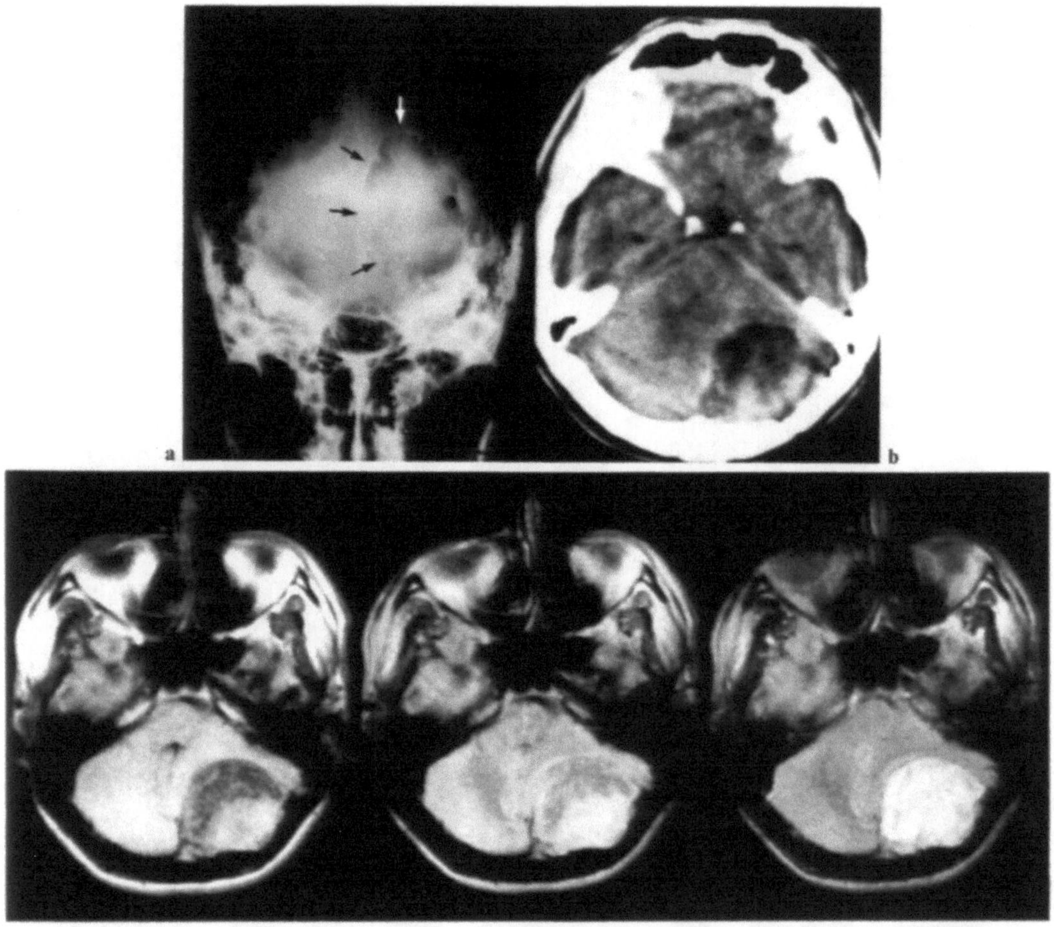

Fig. D 6.54 a–e. Extradural epidermoid cyst of the right posterior fossa in a 40-year-old man with headache, unsteady gait, and palpable bossing of the occiput. **a** Plain skull X-rays indicate marked destructive bone change (*arrows*). CT: **b** noncontrast. MR: **c** SE 400/35, **d** SE 1600/35, **e** SE 1600/70. CT shows a mixed iso- and hypodense tumor with associated thinning of the calvarium. T1-weighted MR (**c**) demonstrates a cup-shaped (extradural!) hypointense mass that shows increased signal at the calvarium, appearing isointense to the cerebellum. T2 weighting (**e**) brings out the tumor with greater definition

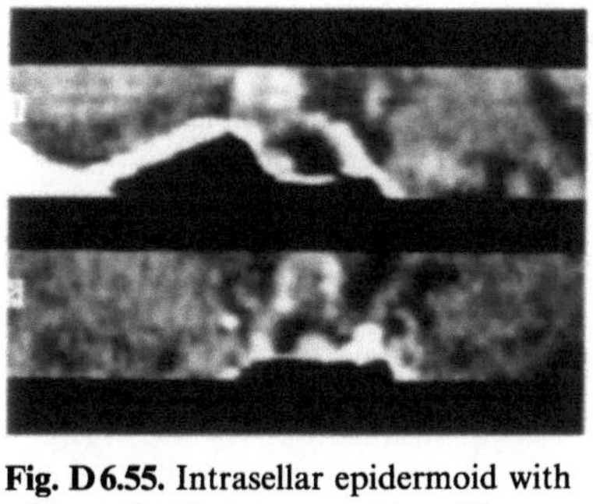

Fig. D 6.55. Intrasellar epidermoid with a hemorrhagic component in a 33-year-old man with diabetes insipidus and impotence. Noncontrast CT: *top* sagittal, *bottom* coronal reconstruction

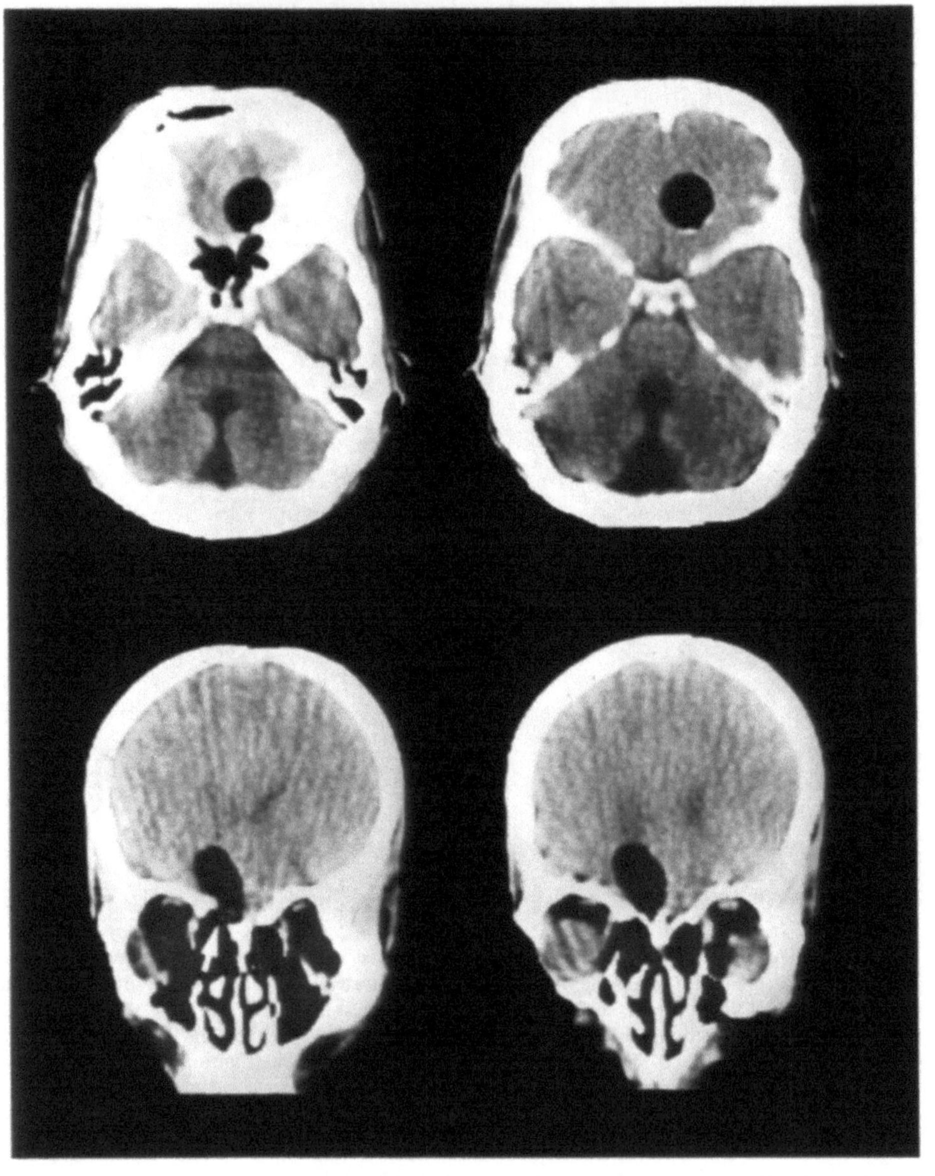

Fig. D 6.56. Dermoid cyst of the right frontal region. The coronal scan shows the dermoid cyst arising from the cribriform plate, where the bone is thinned and deepened (*arrow*). Mean density of the lesion is −68 HU. Faint calcifications are visible on the cyst wall (*upper right*). Aplasia of the cerebellar vermis is present as an incidental finding

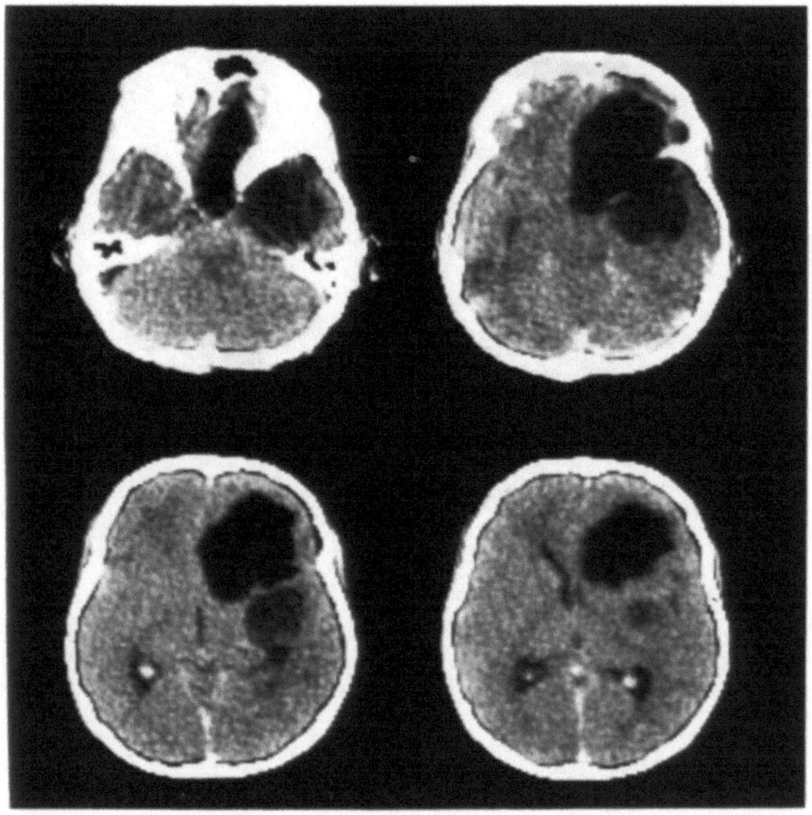

Fig. D 6.57. Dermoid cyst of the right frontal region arising from the sellar fossa, coexisting with an epidermoid cyst of the right temporal region, in a 20-year-old man with severe headache and papilledema. The lesions are separated from each other by the sylvian fissure and its vessels. Mean densities range from −3 HU in the dermoid to +6 HU in the epidermoid

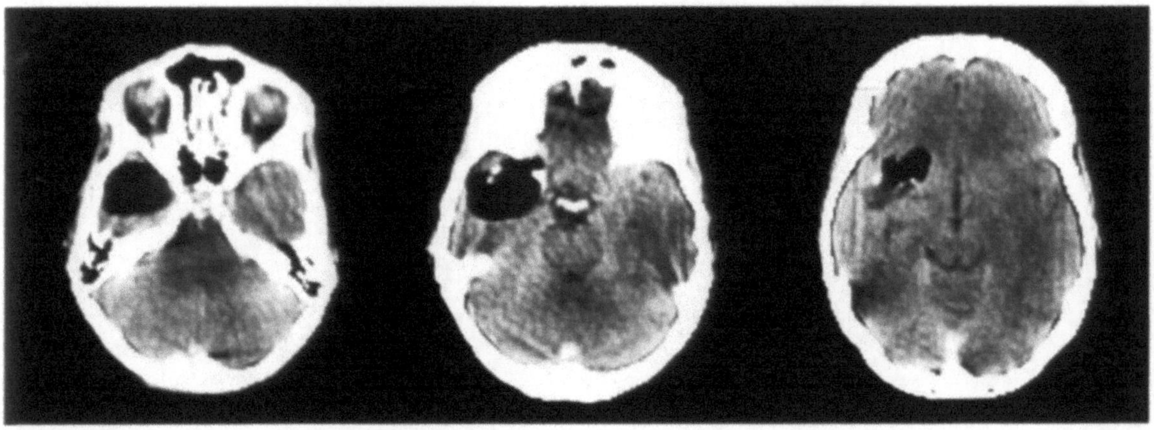

Fig. D 6.58. Dermoid cyst at the base of the middle fossa on the left side with a bone defect in the medial sphenoid wing (*center*). Faint calcification is visible at the margin of the dermoid cyst, which has a mean density of −66 HU (33-year-old woman)

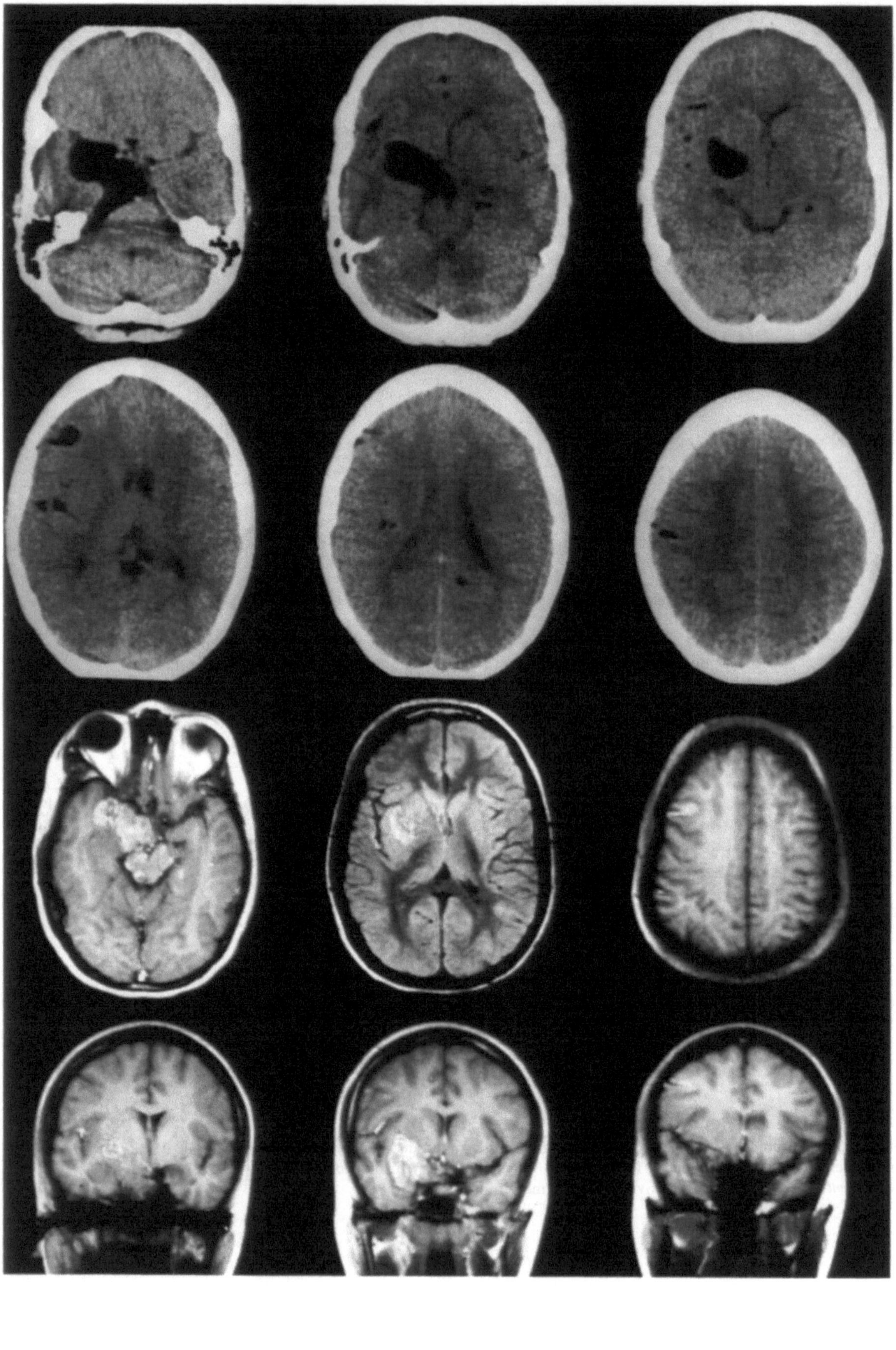

a–c

d–f

g–i

j–l

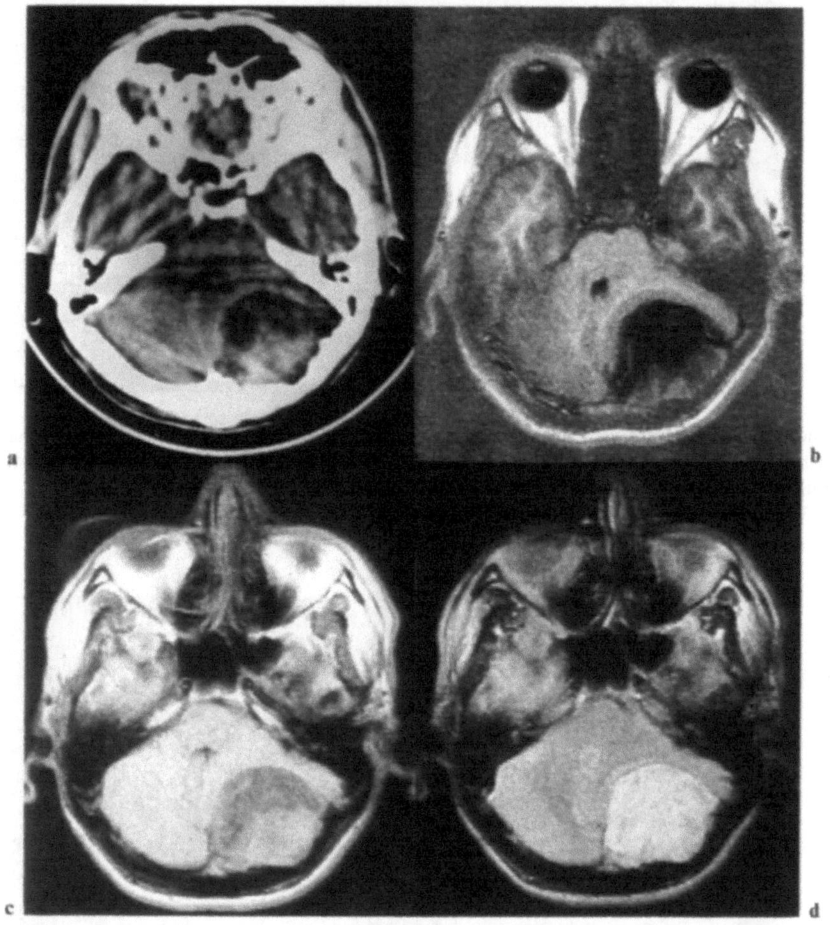

Fig. D 6.60 a–d. Epidermoid in the posterior fossa of a 31-year-old man with a 3-month history of headaches and attacks of vertigo. Postcontrast CT: **a**. MR: **b** IR 1500/400/35, **c** SE 400/35, **d** SE 1600/70. Postcontrast CT (**a**) demonstrates a predominantly hypodense, clearly delineated mass in the right half of the posterior fossa with thinning of the contiguous skull. The lesion shows peripheral ring enhancement and is displacing the fourth ventricle. T1-weighted MR (**b, c**) defines the lesion as an area of decreased signal intensity. The solid tumor component on the T1-weighted SE image (**c**) matches the enhancing area on the CT scan. The lesion gives a much brighter signal on the T2-weighted image (**d**), but its components cannot be differentiated

Fig. D 6.59 a–l. Temporobasal dermoid extending past the tentorium to the prepontine area with multiple additional foci in a 19-year-old woman with a 1-year history of temporal lobe epilepsy. CT: **a–f** noncontrast. MR: **g** SE 400/30, **h** SE 1600/35, **i** SE 310/14, **j** SE 310/14, **k** SE 400/30, **l** SE 310/14, **j–l** coronal. CT shows multiple circumscribed areas of very low density, representing dermoids. These lesions appear hyperintense on the T1-weighted sequences. Brainstem compression is apparent on the axial scan (**g**)

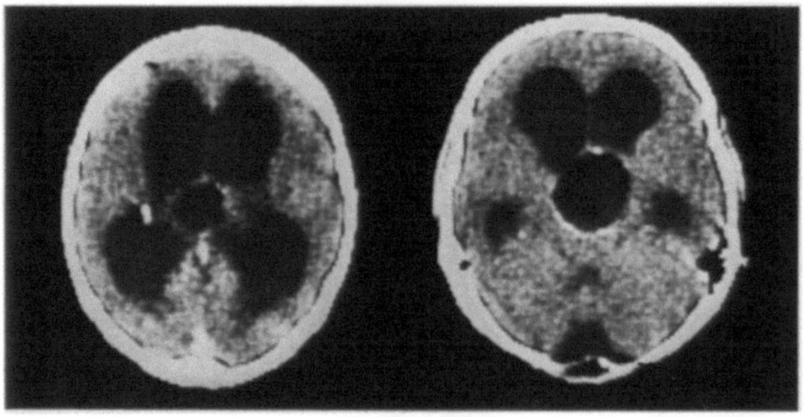

Fig. D 6.61. Dermoid cyst in the third ventricle of a 32-year-old man with a history of visual disturbances, incorrectly diagnosed as multiple sclerosis. The mean density in the dermoid cyst is −35 HU. Plaque-like calcifications are visible on the cyst capsule. Severe hydrocephalus is present. The bright spot in the left lateral ventricle represents the tip of a Torkildsen drainage catheter

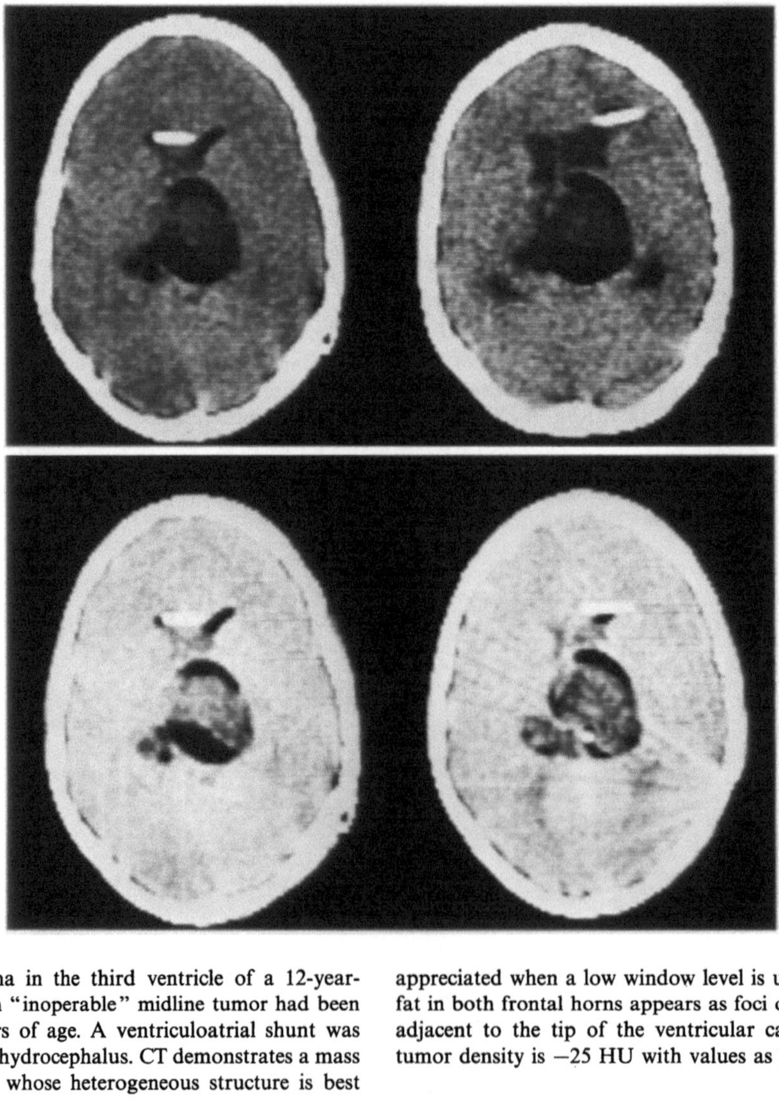

Fig. D 6.62. Teratoma in the third ventricle of a 12-year-old boy in whom an "inoperable" midline tumor had been diagnosed at 8 years of age. A ventriculoatrial shunt was inserted for relief of hydrocephalus. CT demonstrates a mass of very low density whose heterogeneous structure is best appreciated when a low window level is used (*bottom*). Free fat in both frontal horns appears as foci of very low density adjacent to the tip of the ventricular catheter. The mean tumor density is −25 HU with values as low as −54 HU

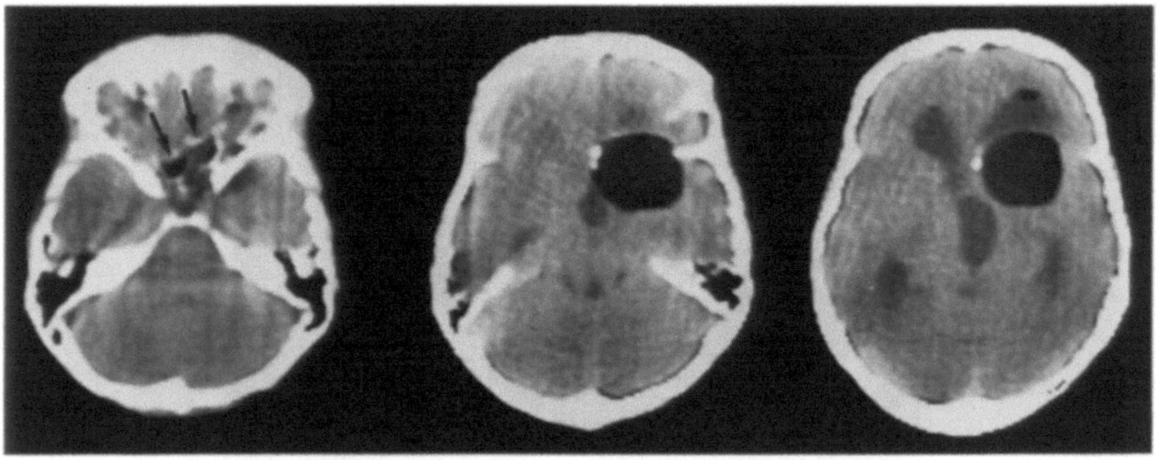

Fig. D 6.63. Dermoid cyst with a teratomatous component in a 34-year-old woman with intermittent left-sided hemiparesis. The presumptive clinical diagnosis was multiple sclerosis. CT reveals a cyst with extremely low density values (−71 to −77 HU at the center) and calcifications in its medial wall. The basal slice shows excavations in the planum sphenoidale (*arrows*), indicating the site of tumor origin. There is free fat in both frontal horns, especially on the right side. A large dermoid cyst was exposed at operation. Its medial wall contained a firm component that was identified as a teratoma

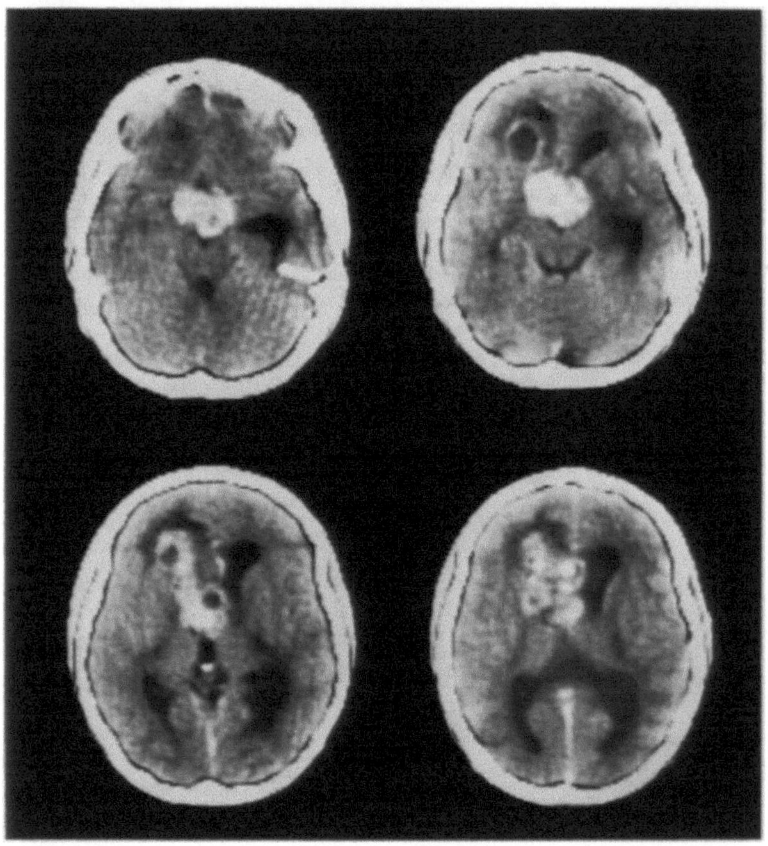

Fig. D 6.64. Malignant teratoma in a 9-year-old boy. From its origin in the sellar region, the tumor has extended through the hypothalamus to reach the left lateral ventricle and left basal ganglia. Contrast enhancement is extremely nonhomogeneous. Mild perifocal edema is apparent. There is internal hydrocephalus secondary to obstruction of the foramen of Monro. CT findings are not specific enough to provide a histologic diagnosis

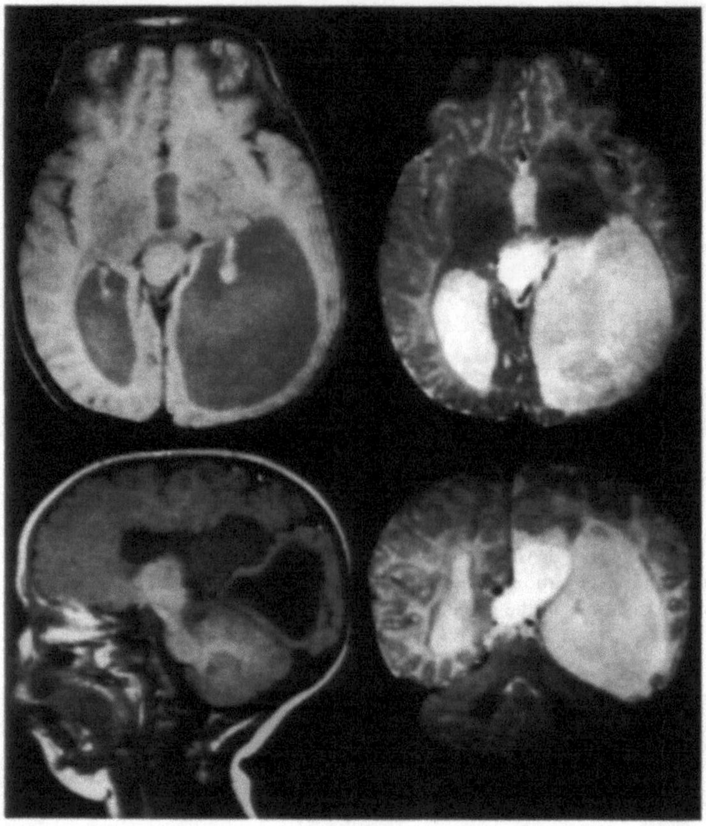

Fig. D 6.65 a–d. Mature teratoma in the region of the quadrigeminal plate, trigone, and right parietal region with expansion of the right inferior and occipital horns in a 7-month-old infant with cranial enlargement. MR: **a** SE 3000/30, **b** SE 3000/90, **c** SE 500/30 sagittal, **d** SE 3000/90. The proton-density and T1-weighted images (**a**, **c**) show an isointense tumor with slightly hyperintense elements. The tumor gives a very bright signal on the T2-weighted sequences

h) Primitive Neuroectodermal Tumors of the CNS (PNET)

PNET is a collective term applied to rare, poorly differentiated tumors of the CNS. It is not always possible to assign these tumors to a specific histologic category such as medulloepithelioma, ependymoblastoma, central neuroblastoma, polar spongioblastoma, pinealoma, or medulloblastoma. PNETs are most aptly defined, then, as malignant neuroepithelial cerebral neoplasms occurring predominantly in children. As there is no evidence for neuronal or glial differentiation, these tumors are classified as "primitive" and "neuroectodermal" (Hart and Earle 1973; Kosnick et al. 1978).

There are no clear histologic or immunohistologic criteria by which PNETs can be differentiated from medulloblastomas. This can be done only by establishing the site of occurrence. Among the PNETs, only desmoplastic medulloblastoma with frequent astroglial differentiation, detectable by the GFAP reaction, merits recognition as a separate tumor entity.

CT demonstrates these primitive tumors as predominantly hypodense mass lesions with variable patterns of contrast enhancement (Fig. D6.67a, b).

To date, only one PNET in our series has been demonstrated with **MR** (Fig. D6.66).

There are no CT or MR criteria that are specific for these neoplasms. PNET should be considered in the differential diagnosis of pediatric tumors that are difficult to categorize.

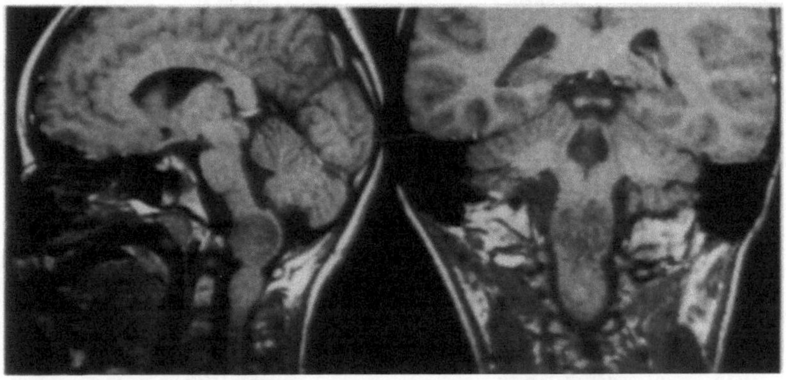

Fig. D6.66. Primitive neuroectodermal tumor (PNET) in a 9-year-old child with tetraparesis, bilateral dysfunction of the lower cranial nerves, and swallowing difficulties. MR: *left* SE 500/30 sagittal, *right* SE 500/30 coronal. The tumor presents a globular or dumbbell shape and is expanding the medulla and upper cervical cord. Its borders appear relatively well defined. The upper part is predominantly hypointense to normal brain while the lower part is nearly isointense to brain on the T1-weighted images. Histologic examination identified the apical portion as a ganglioglioma and the caudal portion as a PNET

31. 1. 1984

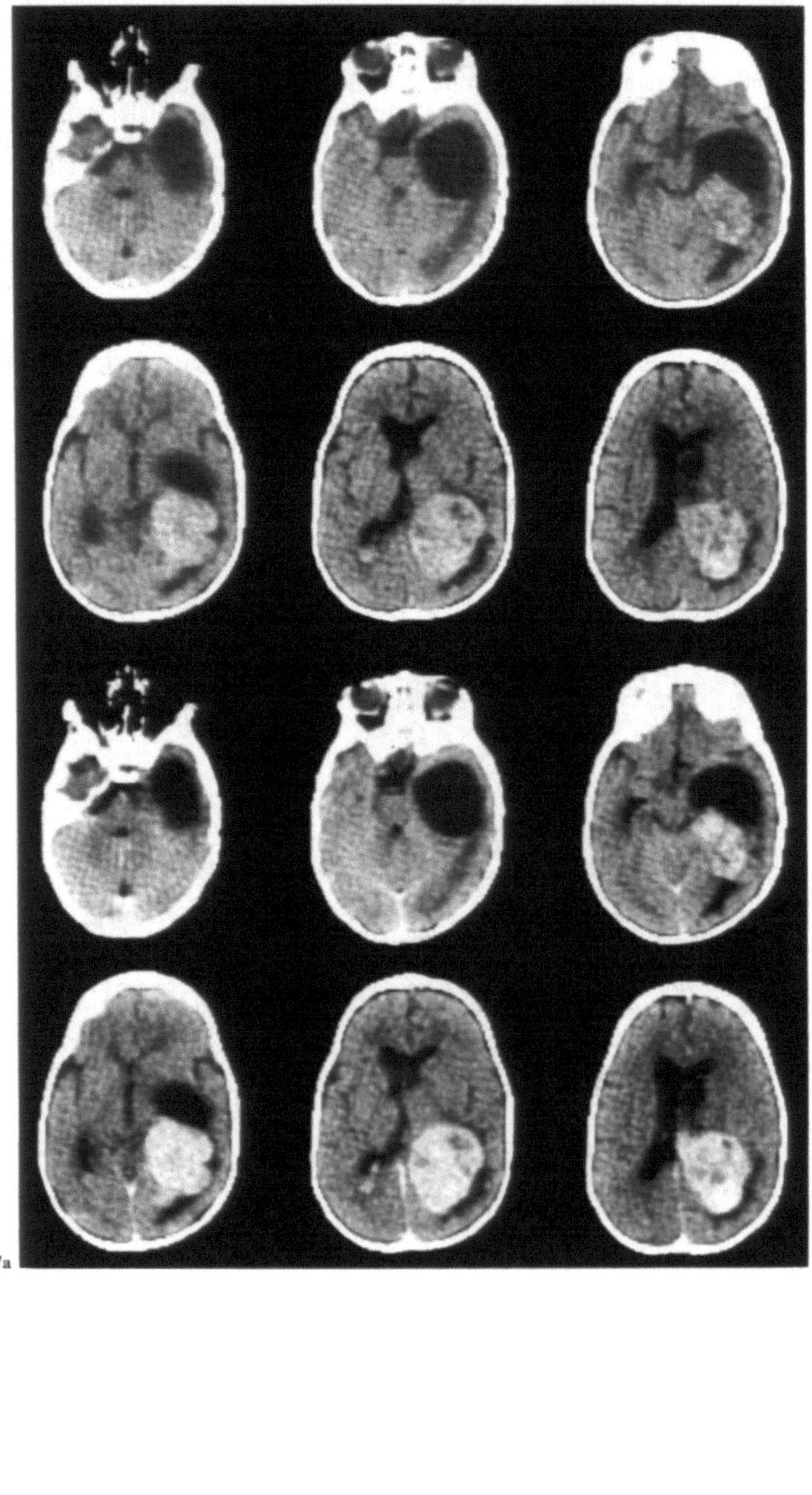

D6.67a

2.5.1984

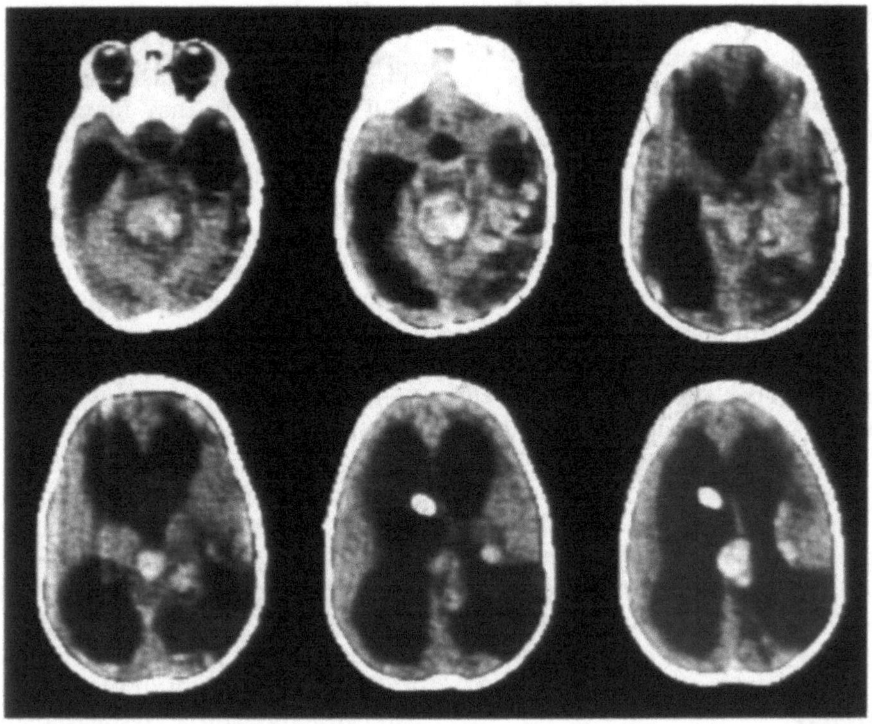

b

Fig. D 6.67 a, b. Primitive neuroectodermal tumor in a 6-month-old boy with fever, vomiting, and weight loss. Pre- and postcontrast CT scans taken on January 31, 1984 (**a**) demonstrate a large, relatively smooth-bordered hyperdensity in the right trigone region. The right temporal horn is dilated, and midline structures are shifted to the left. The tumor enhances markedly with contrast. At operation 10 days later the tumor was grossly removed in toto, and an Ommaya reservoir was inserted for intrathecal methotrexate therapy. Postcontrast CT scans taken on May 2, 1984 (**b**) reveal marked internal hydrocephalus with tumor seeding in the region of the pons, pineal, and right hemisphere. The Ommaya reservoir is visible

7. Intracranial Tumors of Skeletal Origin

Intracranial tumors of skeletal origin include osteomas, chondromas, and chordomas.

a) Osteomas

Osteomas can occur in all parts of the cranial skeleton, to which they are solidly attached (see also Chap. E). They appear on CT as well-defined areas of ossific density contiguous to the cranial vault or base (Figs. D 7.1–3). Osteomas can be readily diagnosed on the plain skull X-ray. The main lesion requiring differentiation from osteoma is calcified meningioma. Generally this can be accomplished by selecting a sufficiently wide bone window.

b) Chondromas

Chondromas are extremely rare in the intracranial cavity. They are very dense tumors that contain numerous calcifications scattered throughout the mass and resembling bony trabeculae (Figs. D 7.4, 5). Solid, uncalcified tumor tissue enhances with contrast medium. Chondromas arise from the dura, chiefly in the falx region, and also from the skull base, where they are most commonly found about the foramen lacerum and at the apex of the petrous pyramid (Zülch 1986).

The malignant form of these bone tumors is known as **osteosarcoma** or **osteochondrosarcoma** (Figs. D 7.6, 7). The CT appearance of the malignancies does not differ significantly from that of the benign forms. On MR the less intense soft-tissue tumor component is clearly demarcated from the compressed and displaced brain tissue and from the soft tissues of the splanchnocranium by a clear, hypointense border on T1-weighted sequences.

c) Chordomas

Intracranial chordomas invariably occur at the skull base, where they may involve the sub- and parasellar region or the clivus (see also Chap. E). Extension toward the nasopharynx, optic chiasm, or suprasellar region is possible as a result of destructive tumor growth. Tumors that penetrate the clivus may spread to involve the lower brainstem and medulla oblongata. The consistency of the tumor ranges from soft and gelatinous to hard like cartilage. Some tumors contain many small hemorrhagic foci, and large calcifications are occasionally seen. Chordomas accounted for 0.38% of the intracranial tumors in our series. The peak incidence is in the 3rd and 4th decades of life, and the sexes are affected about equally. The initial symptoms are headache and deficits involving the fifth to seventh cranial nerves and especially the sixth nerve (Krayenbühl and Yasargil 1975; Raffel et al. 1985). Intratumoral hemorrhage can cause dysarthria, dysphasia, and unsteadiness of gait. The average length of survival is 6 years.

Noncontrast **CT** demonstrates chordomas as slightly hyperdense areas containing flecks of calcification (Figs. D 7.8, 9). The uncalcified parts of the tumor usually show marked contrast enhancement. The relations of clivus chordomas to the skull base are not always appreciated on the axial scan, and reconstructed images are helpful in establishing the diagnosis. Destructive changes are displayed best on scans taken with a bone window setting (Fig. D 7.9, see also Fig. E 13 a, b).

Experience with **MR** indicates that this modality is an indispensable adjunct to CT, since midsagittal images demonstrate the relations of the tumor to hypothalamic structures and the brainstem with exceptional clarity (Figs. D 7.9, 10; see also Chap. E).

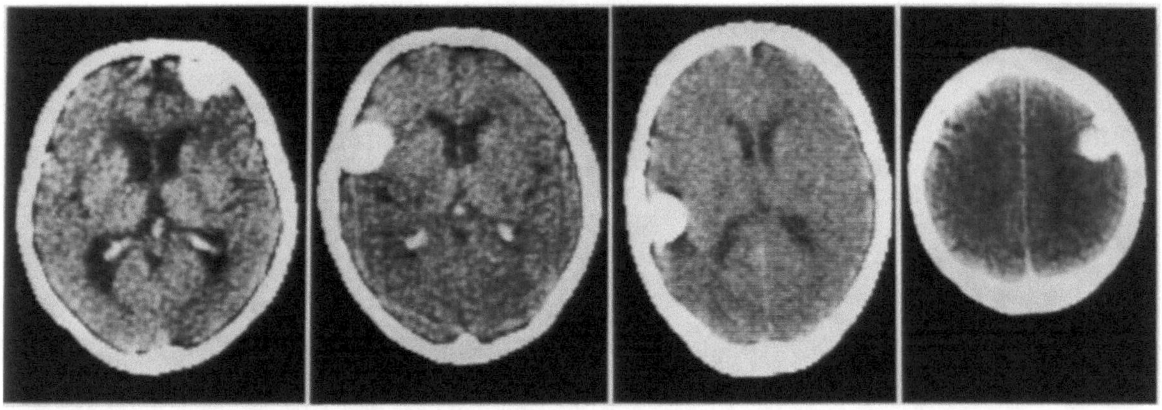

Fig. D 7.1. Four examples of intracranial osteomas occurring at various sites on the calvarium. The tumors are isodense to bone and are contiguous with the vault. Few of these tumors cause mass effect, and there is no perifocal edema

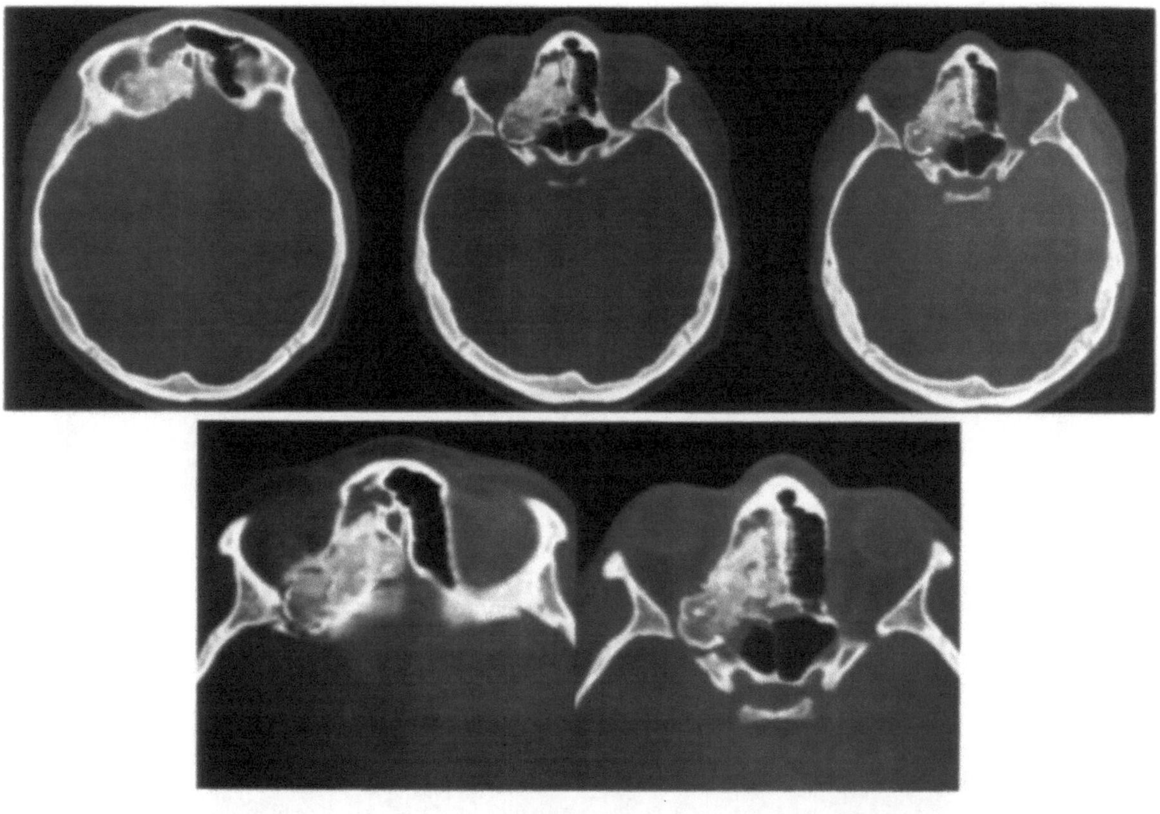

Fig. D 7.2. Osteoma of the left frontobasal region in a 17-year-old girl with decreasing vision in the left eye. CT with a bone window setting shows a clearly delineated osteoplastic tumor in the region of the left frontal sinus extending into the ethmoid cells. Tumor also protrudes into the left orbit behind the globe. The optic canal is no longer visualized

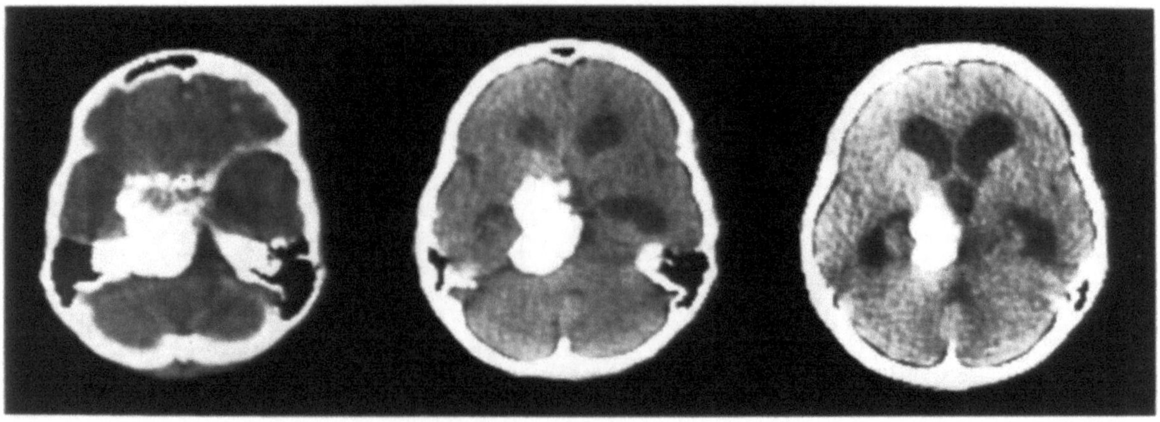

Fig. D 7.3. Very large osteoma at the base of the middle fossa with intracranial extension and obstructive hydrocephalus caused by blockage of the aqueduct in a 74-year-old woman

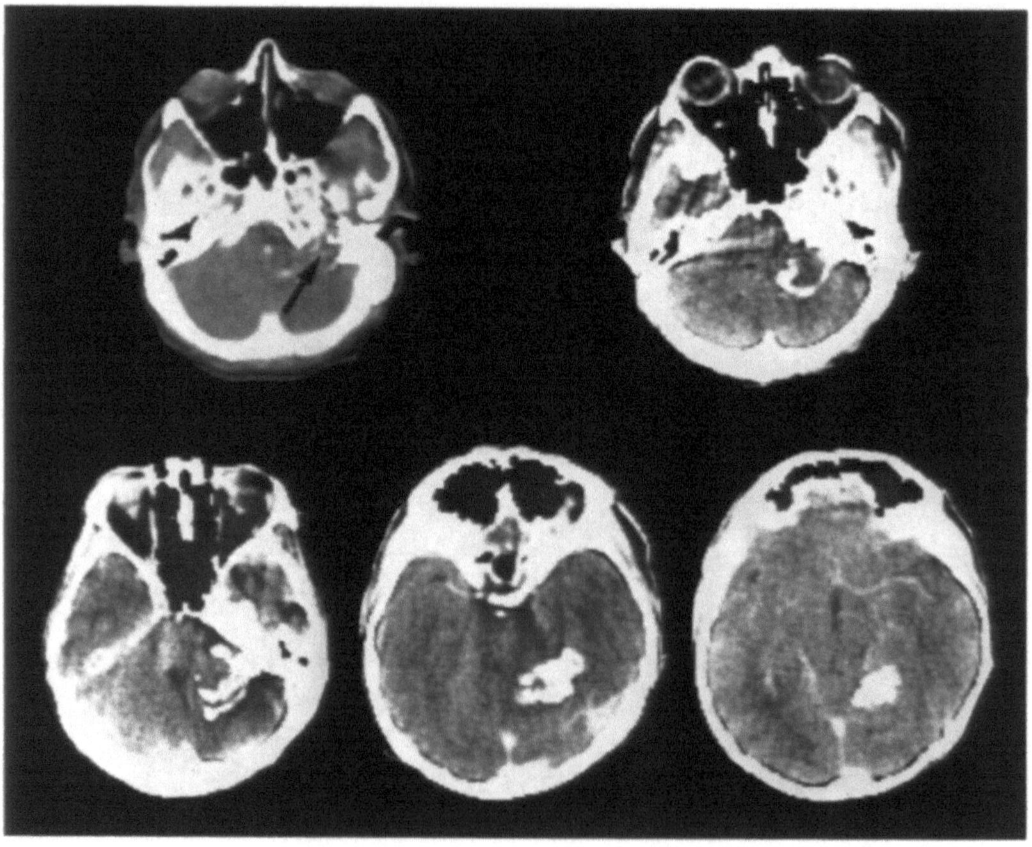

Fig. D 7.4. Large chondroma in the area of the right cerebellopontine angle and the right cerebellar hemisphere, extending as far as the tentorium, in a 28-year-old man. Postcontrast CT shows numerous, irregularly shaped calcifications

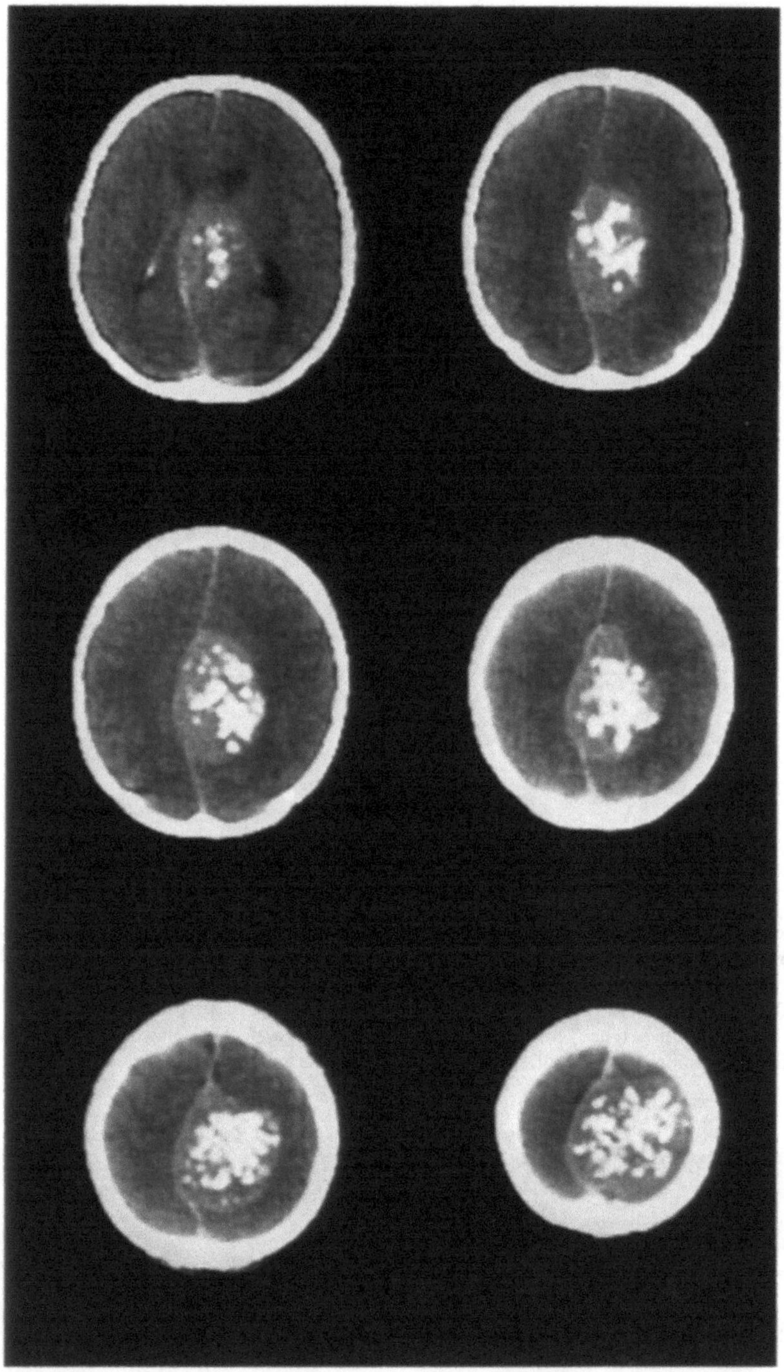

Fig. D 7.5. Chondroma adjacent to the falx at the middle third of the sagittal sinus in a 49-year-old man with focal and generalized seizures. The tumor contains many calcified flecks that resemble bony trabeculae and serve to distinguish the lesion from meningioma (see Fig. D 2.5). The solid, uncalcified parts of the tumor show minimal enhancement. The falx is markedly bowed toward the opposite side. Postcontrast CT with a 200 HU window width

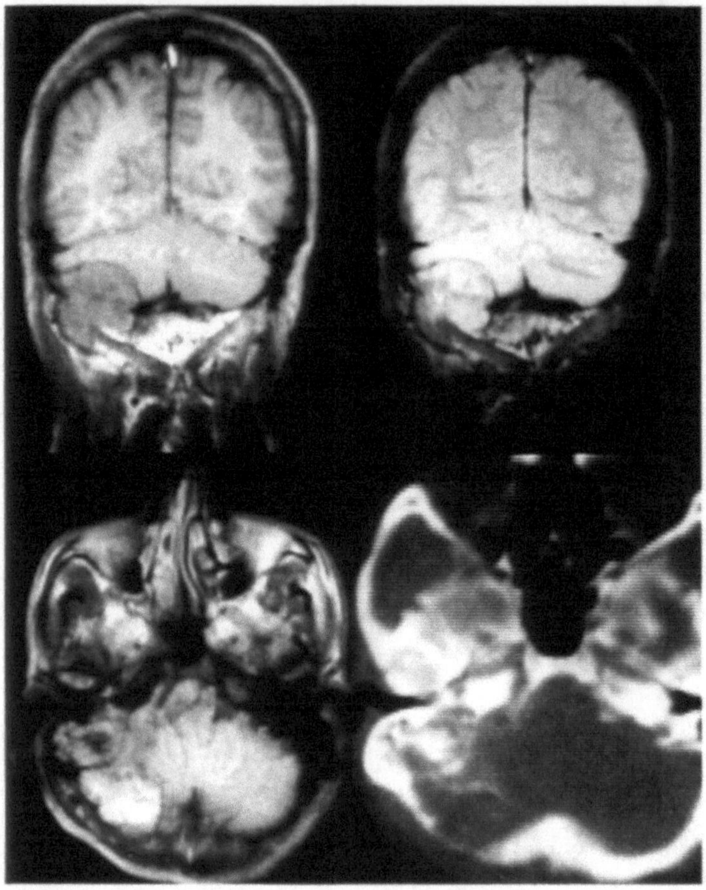

Fig. D7.6a–d. Osteosarcoma of the left lateral skull base in a 47-year-old man with an 8-year history of headache and 6-week history of left-sided hearing loss. MR: **a** SE 400/30, **b** SE 1600/35, both coronal; **c** SE 1600/35 axial. CT **d** noncontrast (bone window). The T1-weighted image (**a**) shows a hypointense tumor of the skull base with invasive intracranial growth. The left cerebellar hemisphere is compressed from below. The proton-density images (**b, c**) show a mixed isointense and hyperintense mass clearly demarcated from surrounding brain by a low-intensity border. CT (**d**) reveals ill-defined basal destruction of the petrous and occipital bones

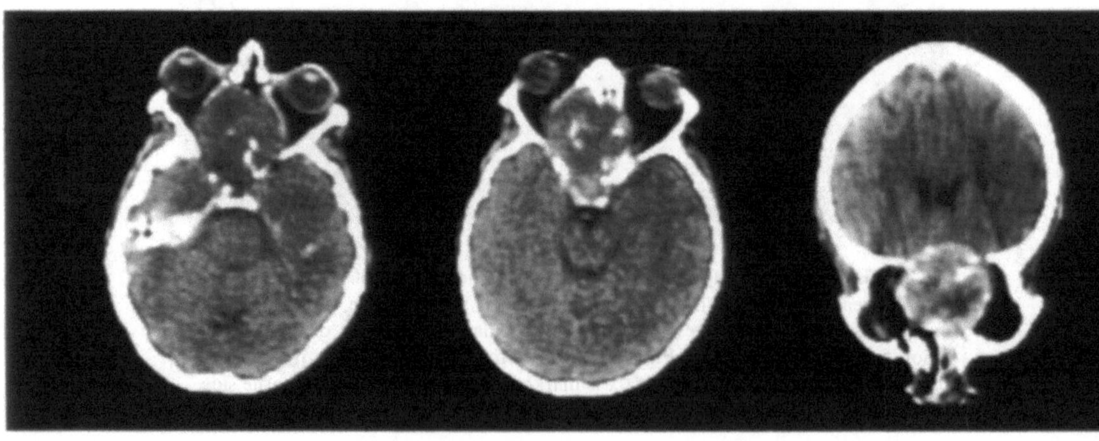

Fig. D7.7. Chondrosarcoma in a 63-year-old woman. Plain CT scans show the destructive tumor arising from the ethmoid cells

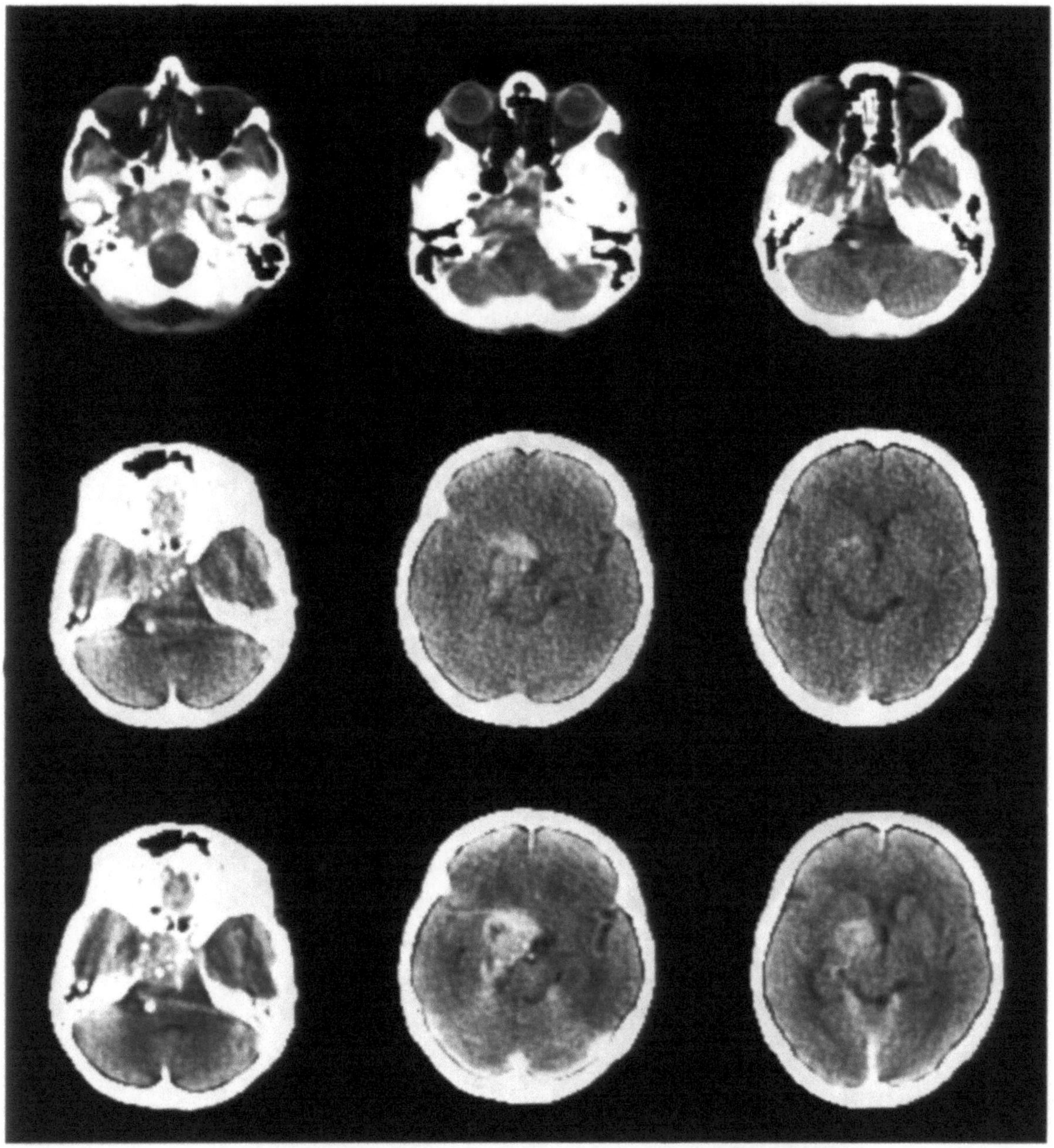

Fig. D 7.8. Clivus chordoma with extensive destruction of the bony skull base in a 58-year-old woman (*top*). The intracranial tumor extensions are hyperdense on the plain CT scans (*center*) and enhance markedly on the postcontrast scans (*bottom*). Small flecks of calcification are visible in the tumor

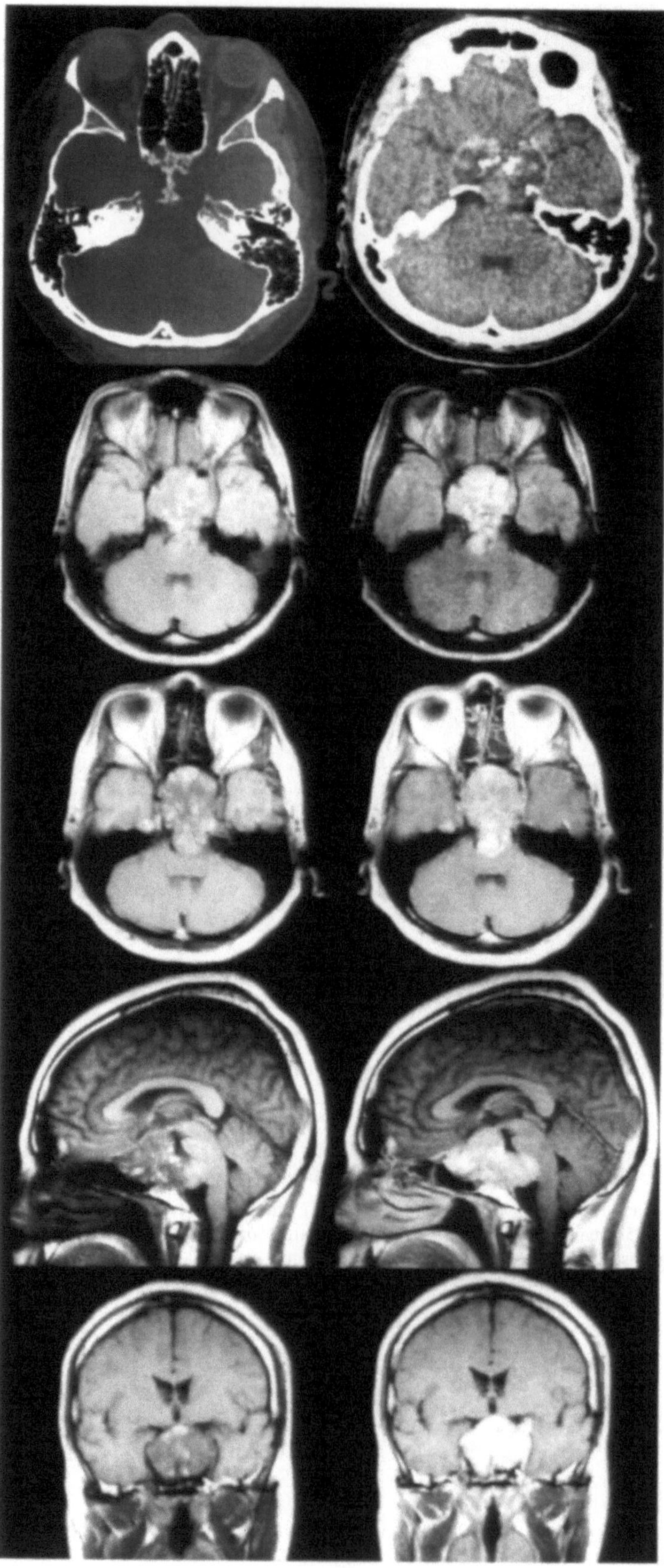

a b c d e f g h i j

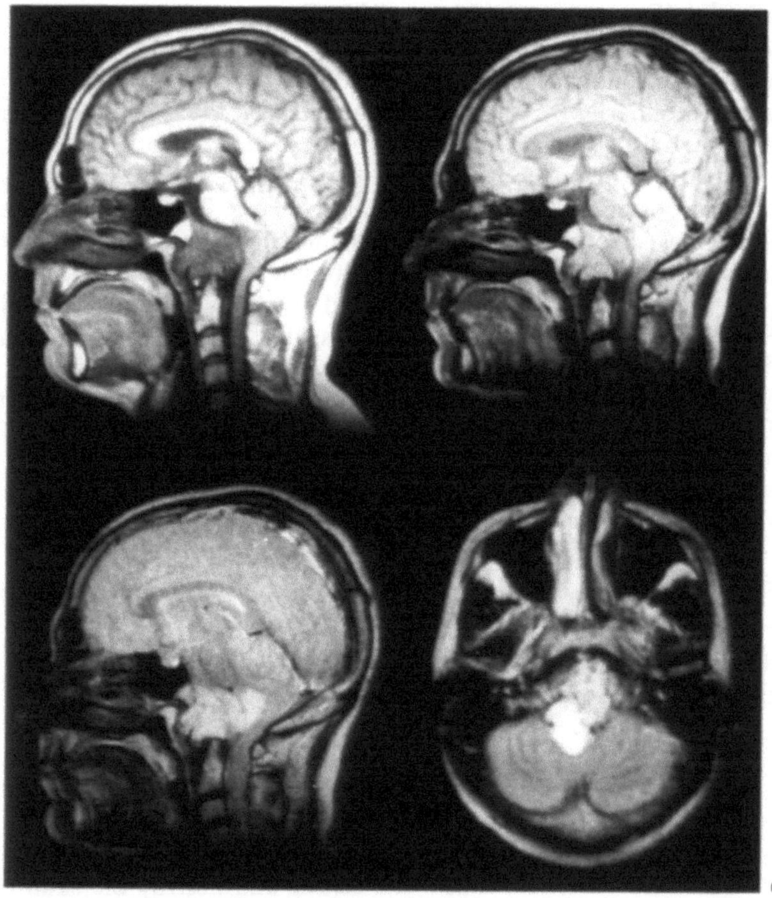

a b c d

Fig. D 7.10 a–d. Clivus chordoma in a 32-year-old man with a 6-month history of headache, tingling paresthesias in all extremities, marked tetraspasticity, paresis of the lower cranial nerves, and finally somnolence. MR: **a** SE 400/35, **b** SE 1600/35, **c** SE 1600/70, all sagittal; **d** SE 1600/70 axial. The tumor appears hypointense on the T1-weighted image (**a**), which shows destruction of the clivus and marked brainstem compression. The tumor give an increasingly intense signal on the proton-density and T2-weighted images

←

Fig. D 7.9 a–j. Clivus chordoma in a 44-year-old man with decreased vision in the right eye and no paresis. CT: **a** bone window, **b** noncontrast. MR: **c** SE 1600/35, **d** SE 1600/70, **e** SE 400/30, **f** SE 400/30 post Gd-DTPA, **g** SE 400/30 sagittal, **h** SE 400/30 sagittal post Gd-DTPA, **i** SE 400/30 coronal, **j** SE 400/30 coronal post Gd-DTPA. CT reveals destruction of the clivus with flecks of calcification in the suprasellar region. The proton-density MR image (**c**) demonstrates an isointense mass lesion whose signal intensity increases markedly on the T2-weighted image (**d**). The precontrast T1-weighted images (**e, g, i**) show a hypointense tumor with scattered foci of increased density, most likely punctate hemorrhages. Marked enhancement is seen after the injection of Gd-DTPA (**f, h, j**). Both the axial and sagittal views demonstrate clivus destruction, upward tumor extension to the third ventricle, and compression of the pons

8. Locally Invasive Tumors

Tumors of extracranial origin can gain access to the cranial cavity secondarily by way of the skull base. This process is always associated with erosion or destruction of portions of the bony skull base (see also Sect. E1). The following tumor types are most likely to invade the intracranial space by direct extension:

a) Cavernous hemangiomas (cavernomas) of the skull base
b) Paragangliomas (synonyms: chemodectomas, glomus jugulare tumors)
c) Angiofibromas
d) Paranasal sinus carcinomas
e) Adenoid cystic carcinomas (cylindromas)
f) Rhabdomyosarcomas
g) Esthesioneuroblastomas

All these tumors are relatively rare compared with primarily intracranial growths, i.e., invasion of the cranial cavity is the exception rather than the rule.

a) Cavernous Hemangiomas of the Skull Base

Cavernous hemangiomas of the skull base occur in the region of the carotid siphon, the base of the middle fossa, and the parasellar region. They can cause considerable expansion of bony structures, but the sclerotic tumor margins confirm the benign nature of the disease.

CT scans through the skull base demonstrate bone changes in addition to areas of increased density that show intense contrast enhancement (Fig. D 8.1), signifying a richly vascularized lesion. Nevertheless, it is unlikely that a specific diagnosis can be made from CT findings.

b) Paragangliomas

Tumors of the *glomus jugulare* and less frequently of the *glomus tympanicum* are called *paragangliomas* or *chemodectomas* (Helpap 1978). They are also referred to simply as *glomus tumors*. These tumors may spread along the jugular vein and invade the posterior fossa through the jugular foramen, producing signs and symptoms of a cerebellopontine angle mass if the tumor attains sufficient size. In most cases the diagnosis can be made from plain skull radiographs by noting characteristic bone changes (see Figs. E 10, 11).

CT demonstrates the soft tumor components, which are isodense or slightly hyperdense on the plain scan and enhance intensely with contrast, as well as erosive bone change (Fig. D 8.2). A specific diagnosis of tumor type can be made when typical bone changes are present.

c) Angiofibromas

Angiofibromas most commonly occur in the epipharynx of adolescents, from which they can invade and destroy the skull base. Differentiation from polyposis is difficult in the absence of destructive bone change. Dynamic **CT** shows marked contrast enhancement in the arterial phase, analogous to angiographic findings (see Table 9, p. 464). Both intra- and extracranial extension are possible.

MR can clearly distinguish the hypointense tumor tissue from the soft tissues of the retromaxillary space and from the brain, especially in the coronal view. The heavily vascularized tumor is seen to contain multiple oval or linear areas of signal void that represent larger intratumoral vessels and, like an AV malformation, can be recognized on the nonenhanced MR image (Fig. D 8.3).

d) Paranasal Sinus Carcinomas

Carcinomas of the paranasal sinuses can penetrate the skull base destructively to invade the cranial cavity or the orbit. In most cases the identity of the primary tumor is known, and CT is performed to evaluate for intracranial spread. Often this question cannot be resolved on axial scans alone, so it is recommended that coronal scans additionally be obtained (Figs. D 8.4, 5).

Contrast-enhanced **CT** is very helpful in defining the extent of the poorly to richly vascularized neoplasm (Fig. D 8.5). A tumor in the sphenoid sinus with associated destruction of the skull base and intracranial extension may represent a metastasis from a known or unknown primary, and this possibility should be considered in the differential diagnosis (Fig. D 8.6; see also Chap. E, Figs. E 23–26).

While CT provides a clear picture of skull base destruction caused by the sinus carcinoma, **MR** (especially with gadolinium enhancement) gives an accurate impression of the overall tumor extent, including the intracranial component, on the various planes of section (Fig. D 8.6).

e) Adenoid Cystic Carcinomas

Adenoid cystic carcinomas (formerly called cylindromas) can occur at either of two sites in the skull: nasopharyngeal tumors penetrate the skull base near the midline from below, showing a predilection for the region of the foramen ovale and gasserian ganglion, while tumors arising from the lacrimal gland invade the skull by way of the orbit (see Fig. G 23). Tumors of the first group cause local destruction of the skull base that is visible on X-rays, and there may be marked expansion of the foramen ovale. Cranial neuropathies, especially involving the trigeminal and oculomotor nerves, are the predominant clinical manifestations. **CT** will demonstrate any intracranial extensions, which appear sharply demarcated from brain. Diagnosis of tumor type relies mainly on radiologic signs and evidence of neurologic deficits.

f) Rhabdomyosarcomas

Rhabdomyosarcomas are malignant tumors of striated muscle that in rare cases penetrate the skull base, infiltrate the meninges, and attain a very large size within the cranial cavity (see Chap. E, Fig. E 20). These rare tumors are most commonly observed in children.

g) Esthesioneuroblastomas

Esthesioneuroblastomas (neuroblastomas of the olfactory nerve) arise in the olfactory nerve region and can invade the anterior fossa from the upper portions of the nasal cavity. The tumors are heavily vascularized and tend to grow slowly, although they infiltrate and destroy adjacent tissues and can even metastasize. Invasion of the orbit has been reported.

The **CT** findings of esthesioneuroblastoma are like those of other tumors that involve the anterior fossa by direct extension (Fig. D 8.7). **MR** provides a "subtraction image" of the soft-tissue tumor in the region of skull base destruction, and the true extent of the tumor is displayed to better advantage than with CT (see Fig. E 19).

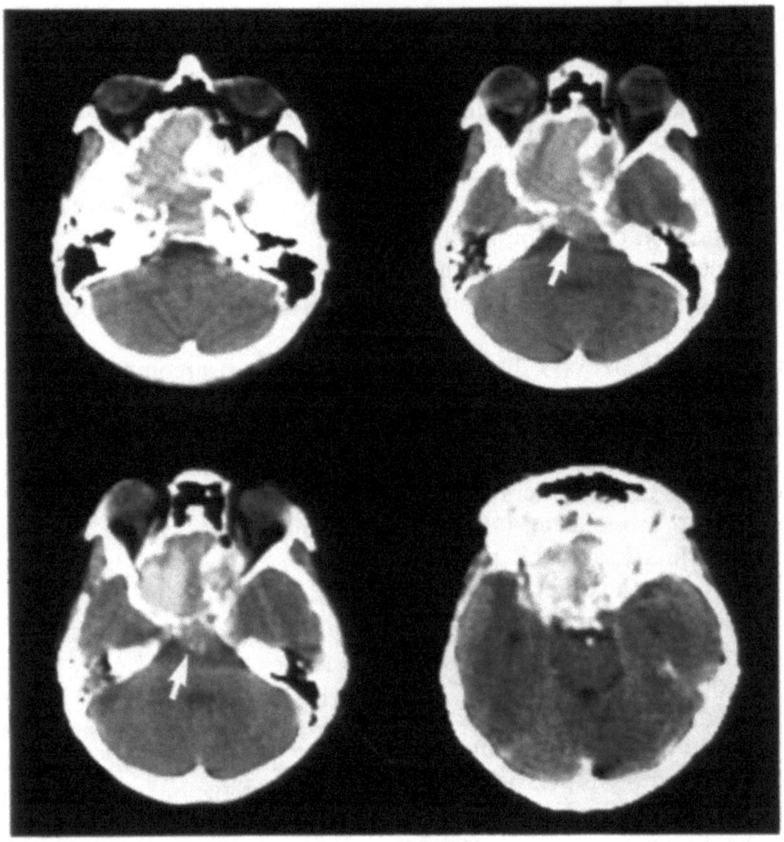

D8.1

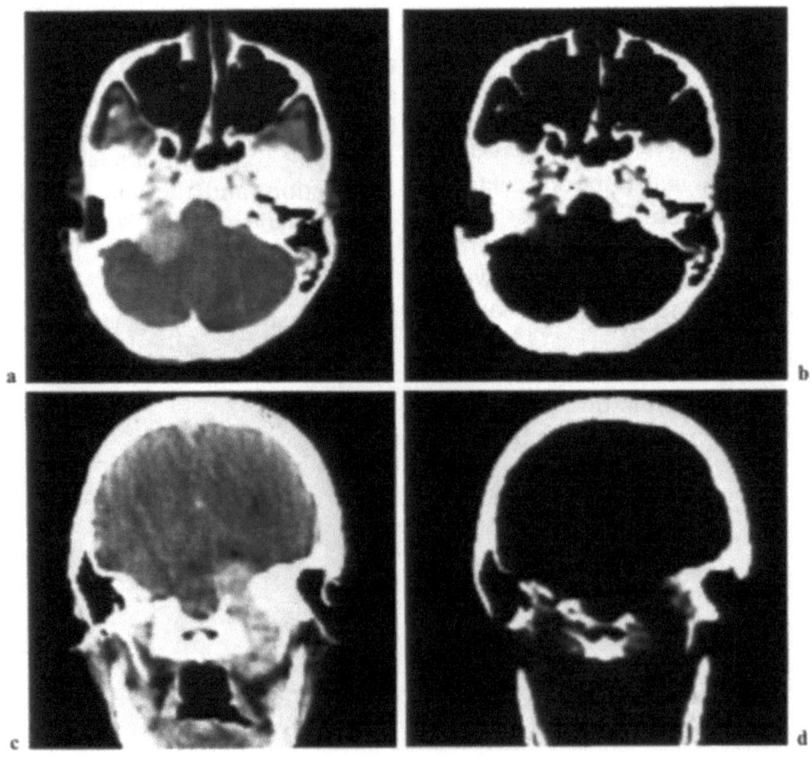

D8.2

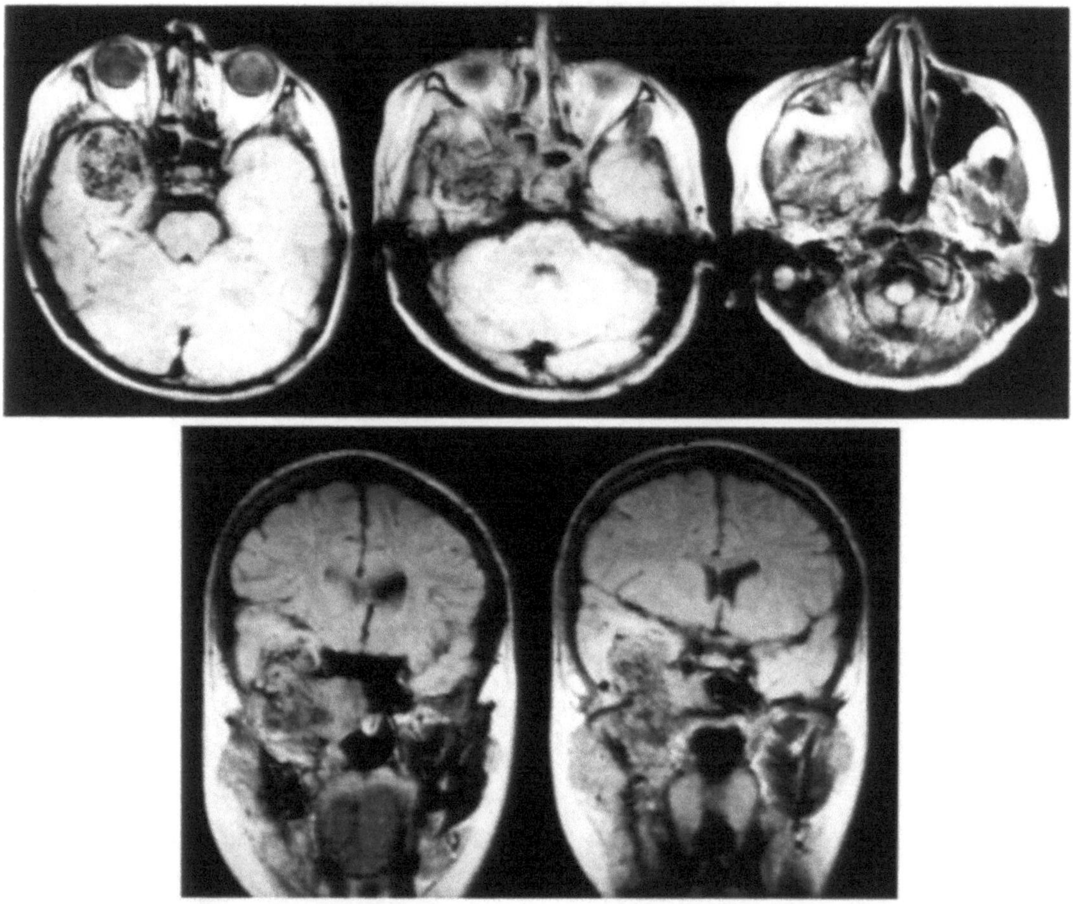

Fig. D8.3. Juvenile angiofibroma of the facial skeleton in a 16-year-old male with otorhinolaryngologic symptoms and negative neurologic exam. MR: *top* SE 1600/35 axial, *bottom* SE 1600/35 coronal. Images show a large tumor in the left retromaxillary space penetrating the middle fossa and extending toward the temporal lobe. The predominantly hypointense tumor contains garland-like areas of signal void which represent the larger intratumoral vessels and confirm the rich vascularity of the growth

◄

Fig. D8.1. Cavernous hemangioma originating from the sphenoid sinus in a 58-year-old woman. The tumor transgresses the boundaries of the sphenoid sinus and extends well into the cranial cavity, where growth is most pronounced along the clivus (*arrows*). The tumor enhances intensely with contrast medium (*bottom*). The sclerotic tumor margins indicate benignity

Fig. D8.2. **a** Glomus tumor in a 50-year-old woman. The tumor has invaded the intracranial space in the region of the left cerebellopontine angle and jugular foramen and is well defined by contrast enhancement. Destruction of the left petrous apex by the tumor is apparent (**b**). Coronal scans (**c, d**) define the full extent of the tumor from below the skull base into the cranial cavity. Characteristic destructive changes are appreciated better at the bone window setting (**b, d**)

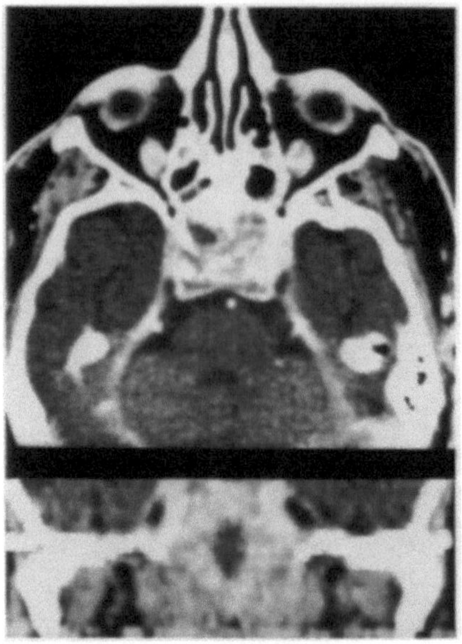

Fig. D8.4. Nasopharyngeal tumor in a 67-year-old man. CT: *top* axial, *bottom* coronal reconstruction (contrast-enhanced). Scans demonstrate a large tumor of the naso- and epipharynx with invasion of the sphenoid sinus and sellar cavity

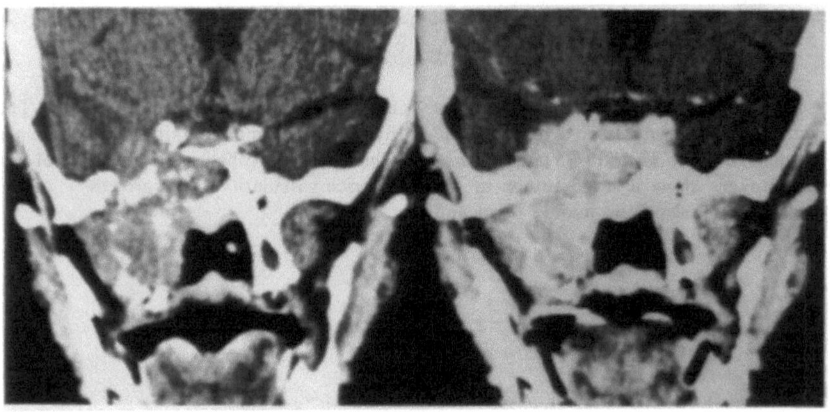

Fig. D8.5. Squamous cell carcinoma arising from the left maxillary sinus in a 73-year-old woman who underwent radiotherapy and endonasal biopsy. Neurologic exam revealed dysfunction of the sixth to eighth cranial nerves. CT: *left* coronal, noncontrast; *right* coronal, postcontrast. Scans show an extensive tumor of the left retromaxillary space with destruction of the pterygoid process and skull base. The tumor has invaded the sphenoid sinus and the temporal part of the cranial cavity. Contrast injection produces marked enhancement, which aids in delineating the tumor

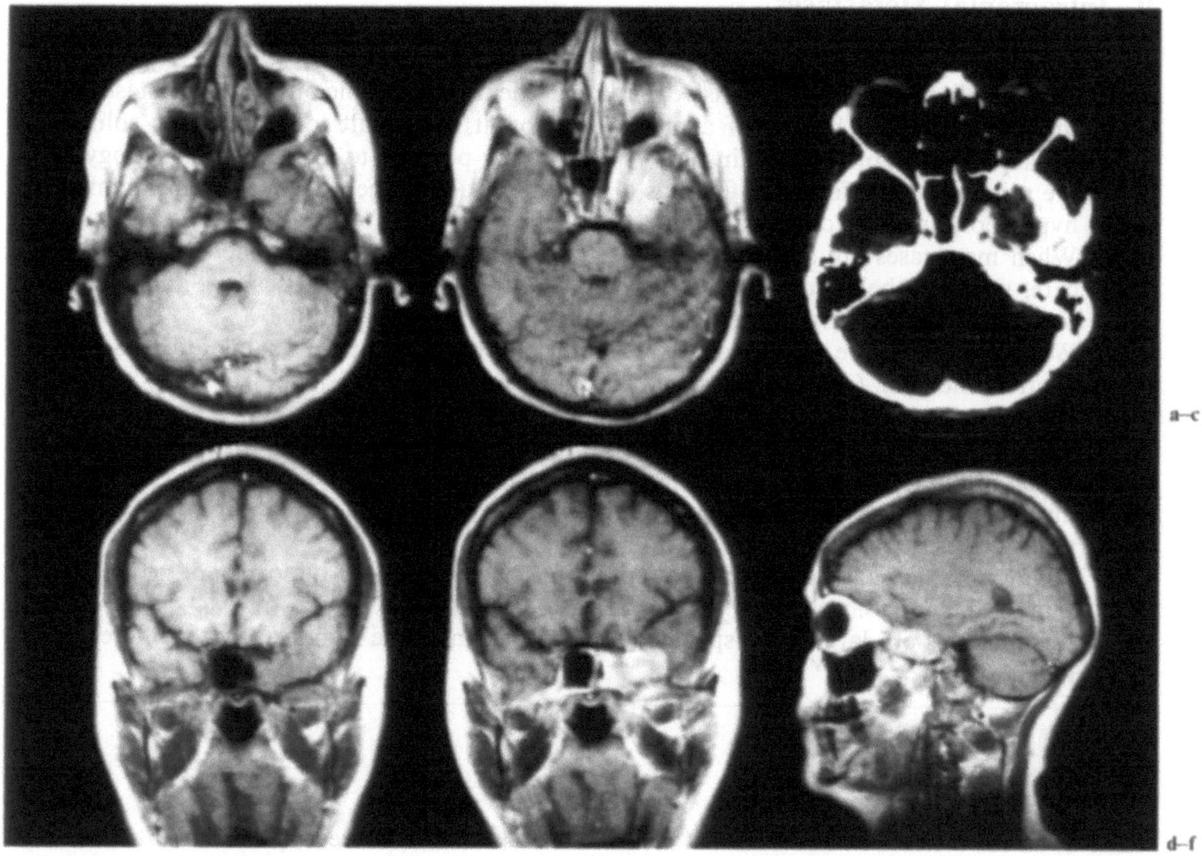

Fig. D 8.6 a–f. Metastasis from an unknown primary, probably small-cell bronchial carcinoma, in a 45-year-old woman with symptomatic trigeminal neuralgia on the right side and hypesthesia of the three trigeminal nerve divisions. MR: **a** SE 400/35, **b** SE 400/35 post Gd-DTPA, **d** SE 400/35 coronal, **e** SE 400/35 post Gd-DTPA coronal, **f** SE 400/35 post Gd-DTPA parasagittal. CT (**c** bone window) reveals pronounced hyperostosis of the skull base in addition to slight bone destruction. MR demonstrates involvement of the skull base, right sphenoid sinus, and right temporal lobe. The tumor enhances markedly with Gd-DTPA

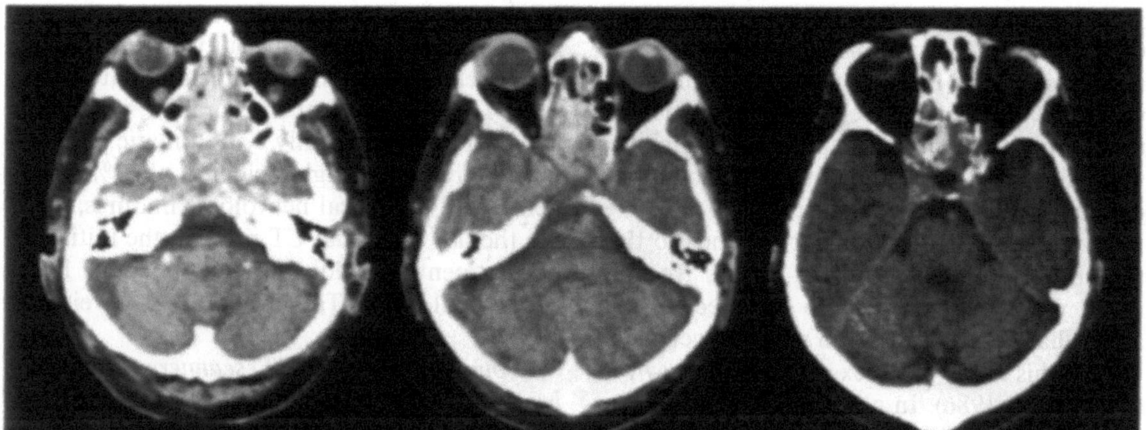

Fig. D 8.7. Esthesioneuroblastoma in a 59-year-old man with multiple cranial nerve dysfunctions. Postcontrast CT shows involvement of the ethmoid cells, sphenoid sinus, and right cranial cavity with destruction of the bony skull base. Contrast enhancement is mild

9. Intracranial Metastases

1. Very small tumors with extensive perifocal edema are suspicious for metastases. If the patient has no history of a primary tumor, it is difficult to differentiate solitary metastases from primary brain tumors. It is rarely possible to identify the histology of the primary tumor from CT findings (e.g., hemorrhage in metastases from melanomas, hypernephromas, or choriocarcinomas).
2. When metastases are suspected, the posterior fossa should be examined with utmost care, since cerebellar metastases frequently are isodense on CT scans. Similar close scrutiny should be given to the cortical portions of the parietal lobe.
3. When metastases are suspected, it is not sufficient to perform a CT examination without contrast medium. Contrast-enhanced CT alone will afford the same diagnostic yield as pre- and postcontrast studies combined.
4. The detection of a solitary tumor with CT by no means excludes multiple metastases.
5. When multiple intracranial mass lesions are detected, the differential diagnosis should include brain abscesses, multifocal glioblastomas, primary malignant lymphomas, and parasitic disease.
6. An intracranial mass lesion in a patient with a known primary tumor is not necessarily a brain metastasis.
7. MR findings are largely nonspecific and do not contribute significantly to differential diagnosis.

Reports on the incidence of intracranial metastases vary widely. Brain metastases were detected in 3.5% of the 4444 cases in the series of Olivecrona (Störtebecker 1954). Cushing (1932) reports an incidence of 3.2%, Zülch (1986) 3%–5%, while Henschen (1955) claims 37%–40%. Percy et al. (1972) reported 41% on the basis of necropsy statistics from large general hospitals. Cairncross et al. (1979) state that cerebral metastases occur in 12% of patients with systemic carcinoma. Rubinstein (1972) claims that 15%–25% of all intracranial tumors are metastases. The incidence in our own series was 13.8%. This relatively high figure is due to the fact that the participating CT facilities worked closely with numerous departments of oncology and internal medicine.

The age of predilection corresponds to that for primary malignancies and ranges from 40 to 70 years. Women tend to be affected at a somewhat younger age than men (55 versus 60 years); this is the only sex difference known to exist (Zülch 1986). In accordance with the frequency of the primary disease and the particular tendency of certain tumors to metastasize to the brain, the most common source of intracranial metastases is *bronchial carcinoma* (Jänisch et al. 1976), followed by *breast carcinoma, hypernephroma, gastrointestinal malignancies,* and *melanoma* (Henschen 1955; Bushe 1972).

Computed Tomography

(see also figures in Chaps. D8, E, G)

General Considerations

In recent years cranial CT has proved to be of major clinical value, especially in the staging of bronchial carcinoma and melanomatous disease. The detection of intracranial metastases in 94% of neurologically symptomatic patients, plus the relatively high incidence of 27% in patients with equivocal neurologic findings, justifies the use of cranial CT prior to the initiation of treatment (Ginaldi 1981; Hooper et al. 1984; Mintz et al. 1984; Tarver et al. 1984; Weisberg 1985).

Fourth-generation CT scanners can detect brain metastases as small as 1.5 mm in diameter with a certainty approaching 100%. The use of contrast medium is essential, especially in the posterior fossa, where artifacts from the bony skull base can obscure portions of the cerebellum. Small metastases, often without perifocal edema, are especially likely to be missed on the noncontrast scan. Contrast-enhanced CT alone can provide the same diagnostic accuracy as pre- and postcontrast CT (Butler and Kricheff 1978).

The CT findings in 338 patients of our series with intracranial metastases are summarized in Table 8. Breakdown by frequency of solitary versus multiple foci indicates that multiple metastases were found most often in patients with breast carcinoma (59.7%), followed by bronchial carcinoma (46.9%). Only 38% of the melanoma patients and only 27.3% of the patients with hypernephroma had multiple brain metastases.

Multiple metastases are easily missed in cases where clinical symptoms cause attention to be focused on a circumscribed portion of the cranial contents, such as the cerebellar region or supratentorial space. Hence, scans should always be performed from the foramen magnum to the apex of the skull if the potential of the CT technique is to be fully utilized. Multiple metastases can occur in any combination.

Despite the high resolution of modern CT scanners, the detection of a solitary tumor nodule does not exclude multiple metastases (Fig. D9.35). Thus, several larger metastases may be identified on the CT scan, but additional deposits may go undetected until necropsy. It can be difficult, of course, to correlate CT and postmortem findings due to the considerable time that may elapse between the CT examination and the patient's death and to the therapeutic interventions that may be undertaken during that period.

Noncontrast Scan

We observe *no consistent density pattern for intracranial metastases* on plain CT scans in our series. Increased attenuation values are the most common finding (33.8%; Fig. D9.39). Metastases of melanoma tend to show increased density on the noncontrast scan (Figs. 9.18, 19), making individual tumor nodules easy to detect. Many other brain metastases that form a solid tumor nodule are readily detected on plain CT scans, even when isodense, because of surrounding peritumoral edema (Fig. D9.29). Very high density values suggest intratumoral hemorrhage (Figs. 9.18, 40). Another one-third of intracranial metastases are mixed-density lesions whose inhomogeneity results from central necrosis (Figs. 9.2, 31, 33). Approximately one-sixth of intracranial metastases are isodense or hypodense on the nonenhanced scan.

Perifocal brain edema is unusually common with cerebral metastases (Fig. 9.28). This feature was present in 500 (87%) of 575 patients with brain metastases. Only glioblastomas had a higher association with peritumoral edema (91.7%). The edema surrounding metastases often spreads to involve large portions of a cerebral hemisphere, and we noted grade II or grade III edema in 57% of cases. An important fact of almost pathognomonic significance is that very small metastases can cause a disproportionately extensive edema that may

Table 8. CT findings in 338 patients with intracranial metastases

Diagnosis	*n*	Postcontrast appearance					
		Ring	Nodular	Ring + nodular	Hypo-density only	"Solitary"	Multiple
Bronchial carcinoma	113	48	31	30	4	60	53
Breast carcinoma	62	13	41	6	2	25	37
Malignant melanoma	34	3	21	8	2	21	13
Hypernephroma	22	8	10	4	–	16	6
Carcinoma of gastrointestinal tract	16	7	7	2	–	9	7
Other metastatic carcinomas[a]	91	14	40	33	4	43	48
Total	338	93	150	83	12	174	164
Percent	100	27.5	44.4	24.6	3.5	51.5	48.5

[a] Including 65 cases with an unknown primary.

involve the white matter of an entire cerebral hemisphere (Fig. D9.37).

Contrast Enhancement

Almost all brain metastases (94.4%) enhance markedly following the i.v. injection of contrast medium. In some of the negative cases in our series, intratumoral hemorrhage imparted maximal density to the lesion even on the noncontrast scan (Fig. 9.19). Other negative cases represented very small metastases that were suspected from the presence of extensive perifocal edema (Fig. D9.37).

Postcontrast Appearance

Metastases show *highly diverse patterns of enhancement* on the postcontrast CT scan. Enhancement may be of the *ring type, nodular, or combined ring and nodular* (see Table 8; Figs. D9.1, 13, 16, 33). The ring pattern signifies a more or less spherical tumor with a necrotic center, while the nodular pattern is characteristic of small metastases. The nature of the primary tumor cannot be established with certainty from the CT pattern, and a single patient may have multiple metastases that present different CT features. It should be kept in mind, however, that the CT pattern is chiefly a function of tumor size (small metastasis = solid tumor nodule, larger metastasis = ring pattern with central necrosis) (Fig. D9.16).

Nevertheless, there are features that tend to be more consistent with certain tumor types than others. Ring enhancement, for example, is seen in approximately 69% of patients with brain metastases of *bronchial carcinoma* (see Table 8; Figs. D9.1–3, 9, 10), whereas nodular enhancement predominates in metastases from *breast carcinoma* (66%; Figs. D9.12, 13, 16).

Deposits from *malignant melanoma* usually appear as solid tumor nodules that are hyperdense on plain CT scans (Figs. 9.18–21, 23–27), and hemorrhagic components are frequent (Potts et al. 1980; Weisberg 1985; Zülch 1986). Solid nodules were present in one-third of our patients with metastatic melanoma (Fig. D9.25), and some showed intratumoral hemorrhage (Fig. D9.19). Ring patterns are rarely seen in malignant melanoma (Fig. D9.23).

In metastases from *hypernephroma*, solid tumors and tumors with necrotic centers appear to be encountered with about equal frequency. A spherical tumor with a small necrotic core is typical (Figs. D9.28, 29).

Patterns also vary in metastases from *adenocarcinoma* of the gastrointestinal tract. In some cases we observed a garlandlike pattern otherwise found only in glioblastoma.

Metastases of *choriocarcinoma* usually present as an intracerebral mass hemorrhage. Differentiation from angiomatous or aneurysmal hemorrhage is not possible in patients having no history of a primary neoplasm.

Magnetic Resonance Imaging
(see also figures in Chaps. C 2, D 8, E)

Small metastases tend to appear isointense on nonenhanced T1-weighted images and are extremely difficult to detect. Both the metastasis and surrounding edema appear hyperintense on T2-weighted sequences. The metastasis enhances markedly on the post-Gd-DTPA T1-weighted scan, making it possible to separate the tumor from edema.

MR is more sensitive than any other modality and, unlike CT, can detect even the smallest intracranial metastases.

Differential Diagnosis

Multiple intracranial tumors discovered in a patient with a known primary tumor usually pose no problems of differential diagnosis. However, a solitary mass lesion in such cases may well represent a coexisting tumor of different origin, especially if a long period has elapsed between the two diseases.

Several diagnoses besides metastases should be considered in patients who have *multiple intracranial mass lesions* but no prior history of malignant disease: *multiple brain abscesses, multiple meningiomas, multifocal lymphomas, glioblastomas, tuberculomas,* and *parasitic infection.* When a metastatic tumor of the posterior fossa is suspected, hemangioblastoma (Lindau's tumor) should be included in the differential diagnosis (Zülch 1986).

One should also consider the possibility of *two different, coexisting brain tumors* when metastasis is suspected. A small, solitary intracranial mass with a necrotic center and/or extensive associated edema should always arouse suspicion of a metastatic deposit. No reliable CT or MR criteria have been established to distinguish solitary brain metastases from other tumors. Even a ring pattern can be difficult to distinguish from a brain abscess. Solitary metastases in the absence of a known primary tumor are most frequently misdiagnosed as an astrocytoma or glioblastoma.

Owing to its high sensitivity, MR detects very small metastases better than CT, especially when the lesions occur near the skull base, in the cerebellum, or in the brainstem, and especially when Gd-DTPA is administered. The clinical relevance of this fact will vary from one case to the next (Kazner et al. 1985; Kretzschmar et al. 1985).

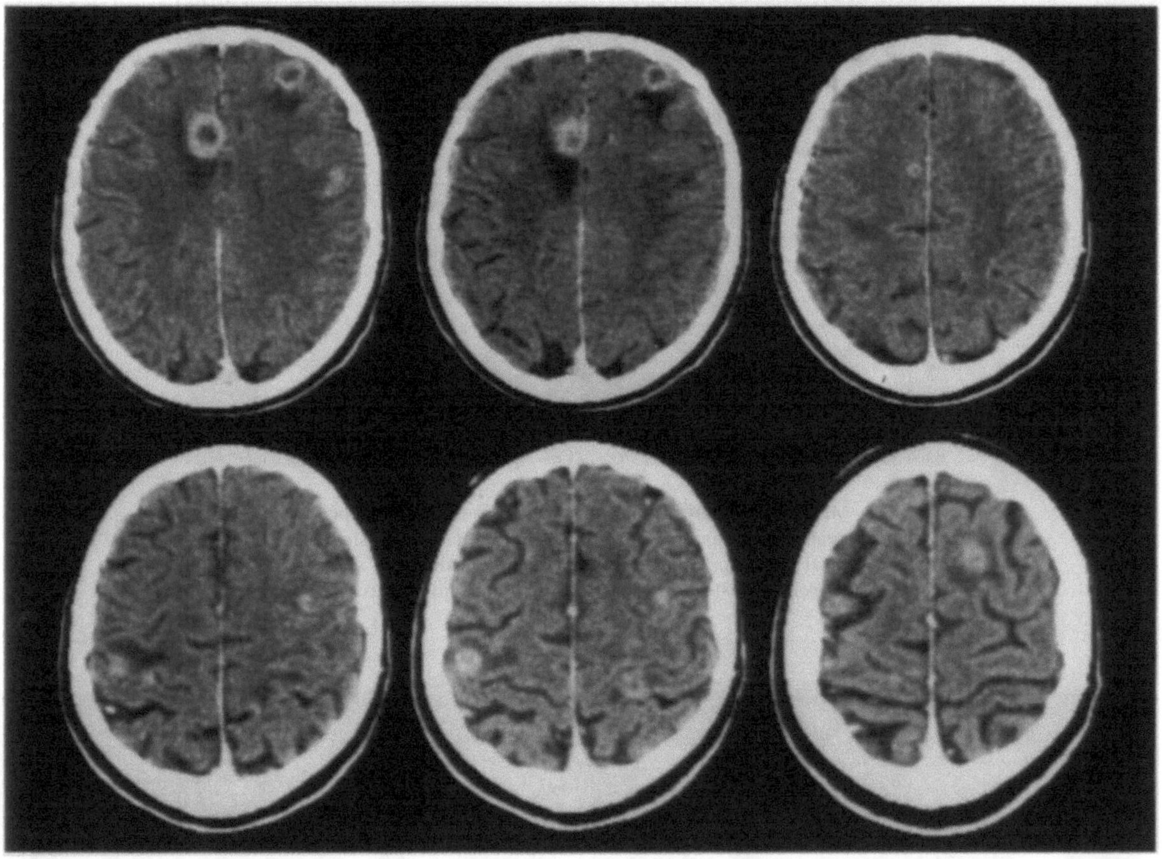

Fig. D 9.1. Multiple metastases of bronchial carcinoma in a 51-year-old man with several generalized seizures. Postcontrast CT shows multiple enhancing lesions over both hemispheres. Some of the lesions are solid, others have a necrotic center; all are associated with moderate edema

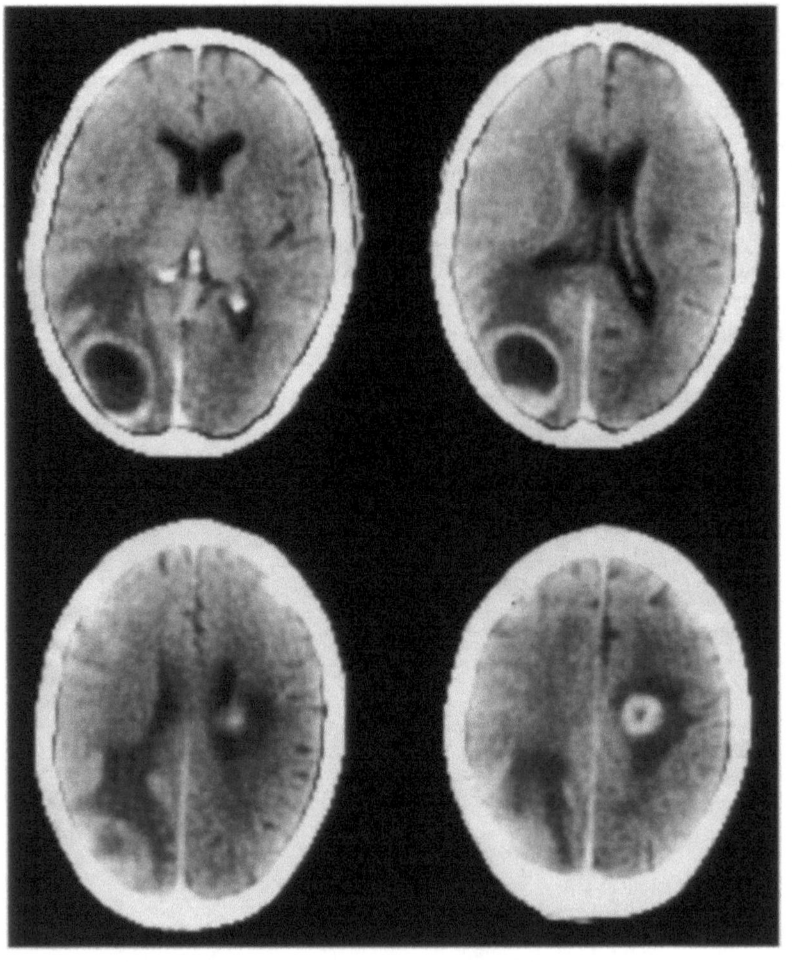

Fig. D9.2. Metastases of bronchial carcinoma in both cerebral hemispheres in a 60-year-old man. Both tumors show ring enhancement on postcontrast CT as a result of central necrosis. Even the smaller tumor on the right side has a necrotic center. Aside from metastases, this pattern is found only in cerebral abscesses

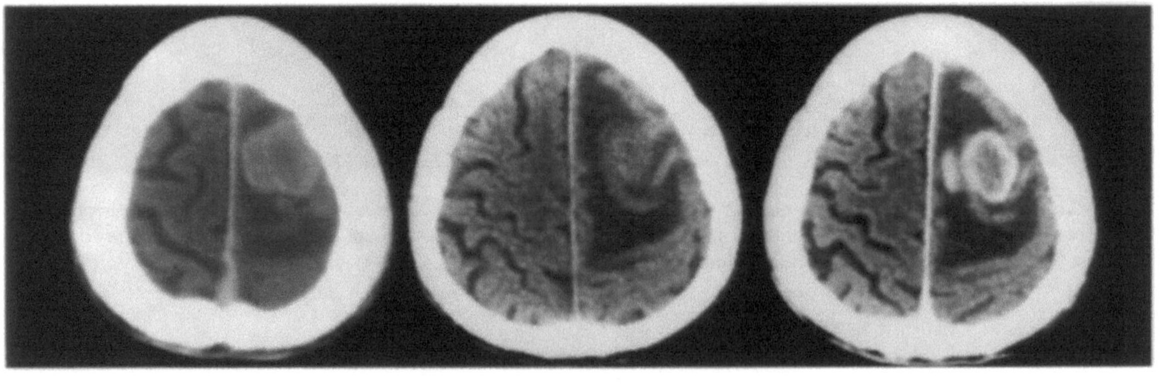

Fig. D9.3. Metastasis of bronchial carcinoma in the right frontal region of a 67-year-old man with jacksonian seizures. The postcontrast CT scan (*right*) shows marked enhancement of the tumor with central necrosis

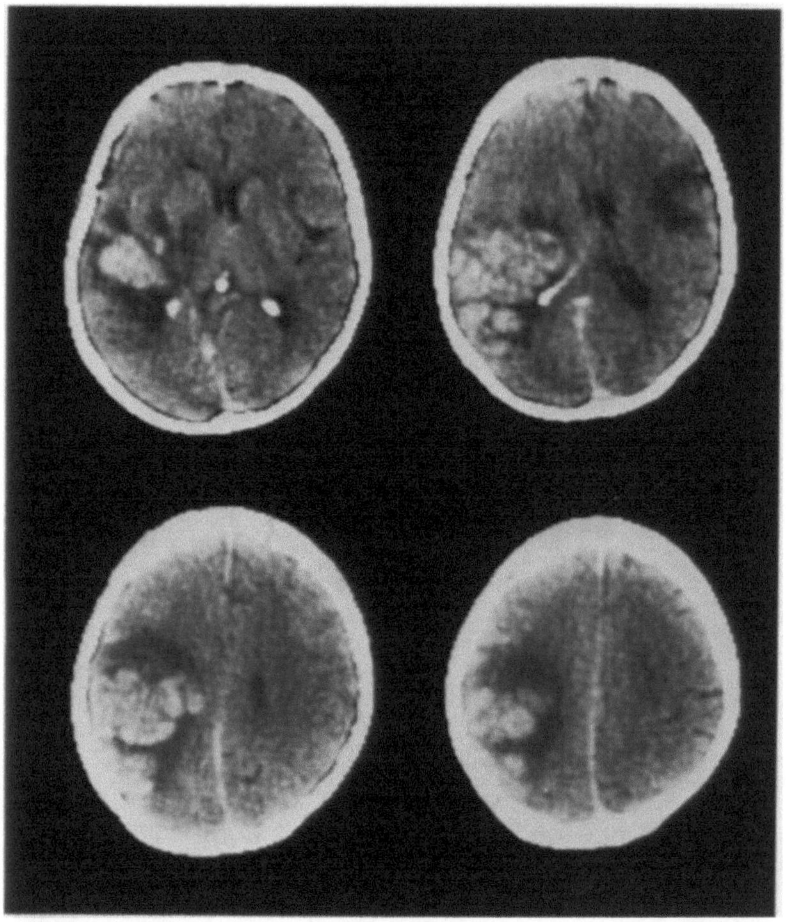

Fig. D9.4. Multiple metastases of bronchial carcinoma in a 68-year-old man. A collection of numerous hazelnut- to walnut-size tumor nodules occupy the central and posterior portions of the left cerebral hemisphere. An additional metastasis is noted at the junction of the frontal and temporal lobes (edema). Postcontrast CT

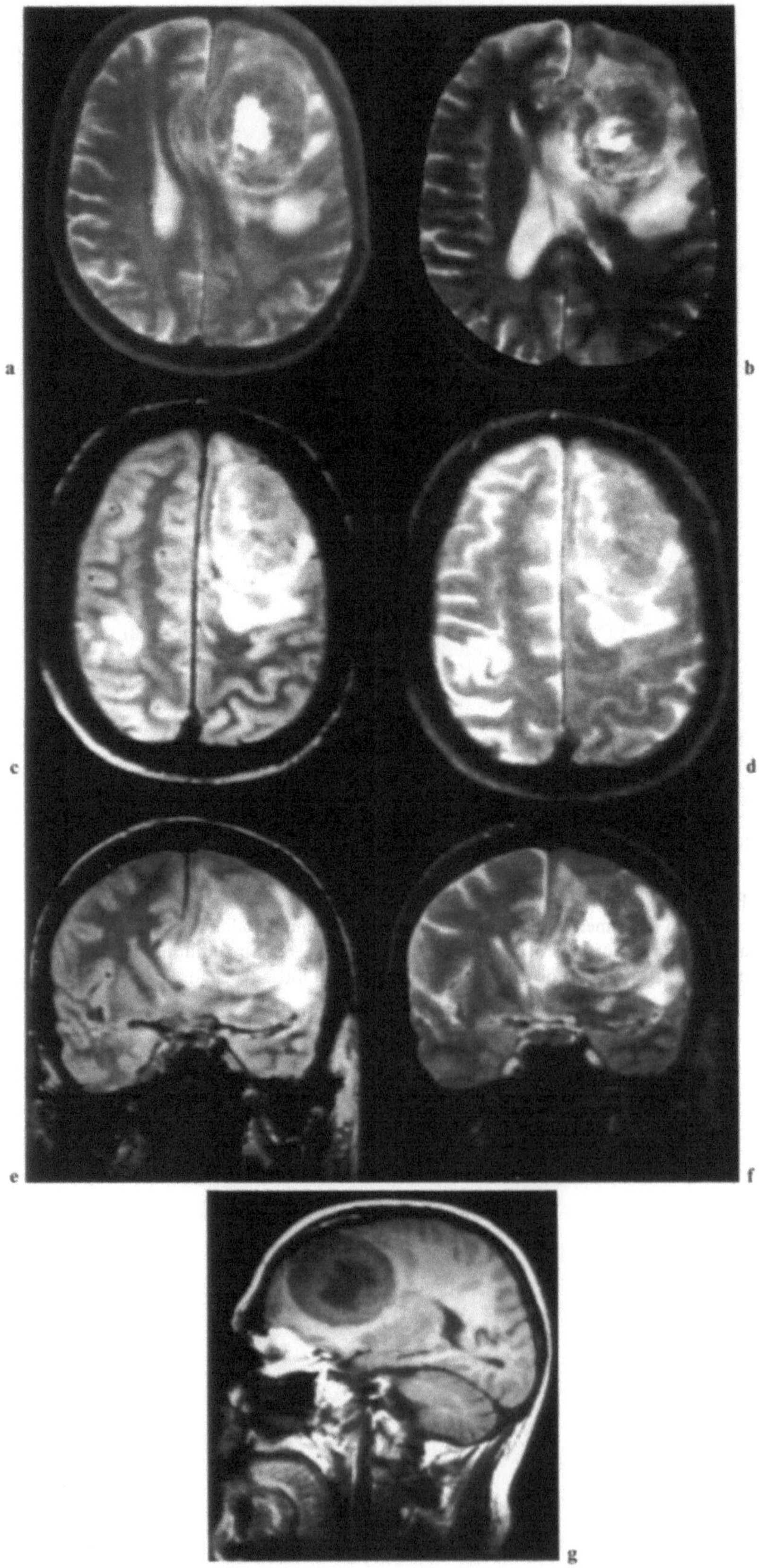
a
b
c
d
e
f
g

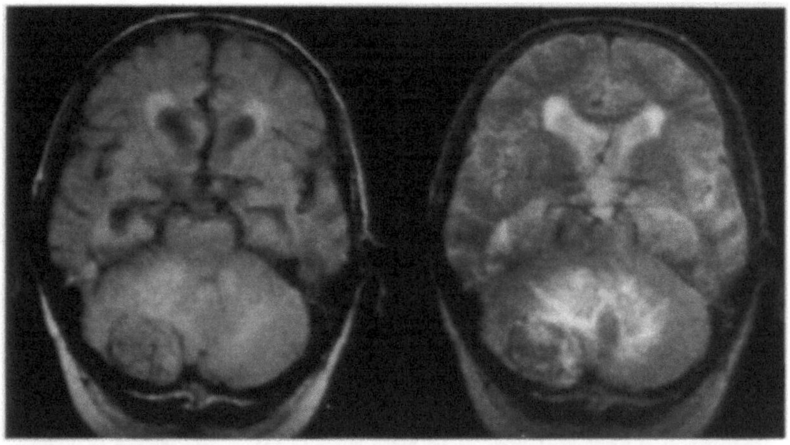

Fig. D 9.6. Metastasis from bronchial carcinoma in the left cerebellar hemisphere of a 71-year-old man with ataxia and altered mental status. MR *left* SE 2000/40, *right* SE 2000/110. The metastasis is sharply delineated on the proton-density image as an isointense mass. The T2-weighted image further discloses hyperintense edema in both cerebellar hemispheres

Fig. D 9.5 a–g. Metastasis of bronchial carcinoma in the right frontal region of a 61-year-old woman with altered mental status and mild left hemiparesis. MR: **a–d** SE 3000/90, **e** SE 3000/30 coronal, **f** SE 3000/90 coronal, **g** SE 700/30 sagittal. The T1-weighted scan (**g**) shows a hypointense, clearly delineated tumor with an even less intense center. The very bright perifocal edema on the T2-weighted images (**a–f**) clearly outlines the isointense tumor, whose cystic, necrotic core gives a very high signal

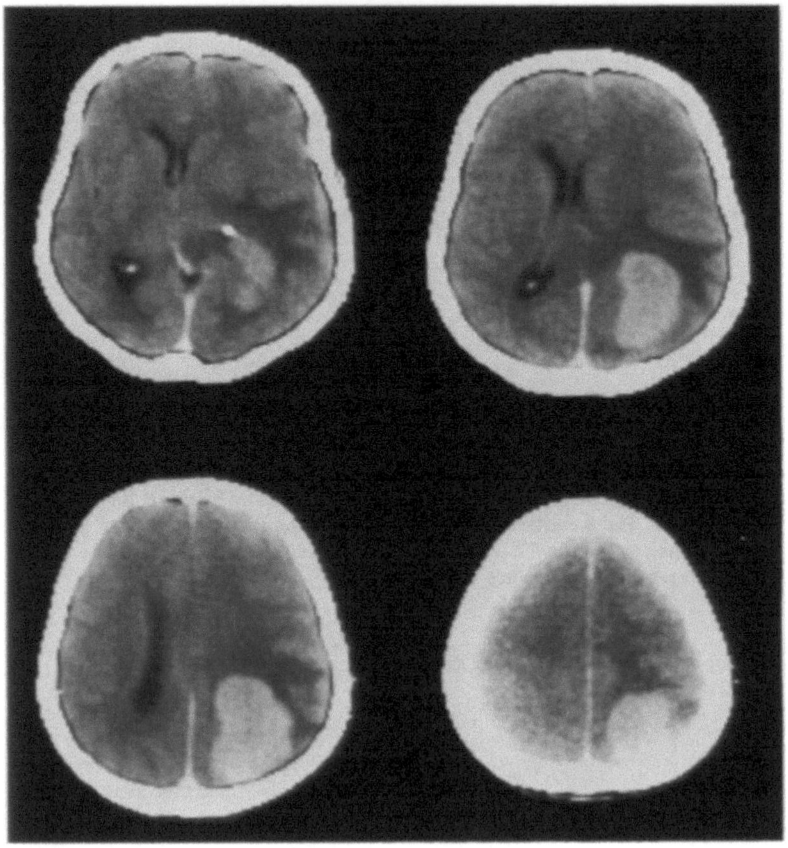

Fig. D9.7. Metastasis of bronchoalveolar adenocarcinoma in the right occipital-parietal region of a 55-year-old woman. The homogeneous enhancement of the cerebral metastasis resembles that of a meningioma or malignant lymphoma. Postcontrast CT

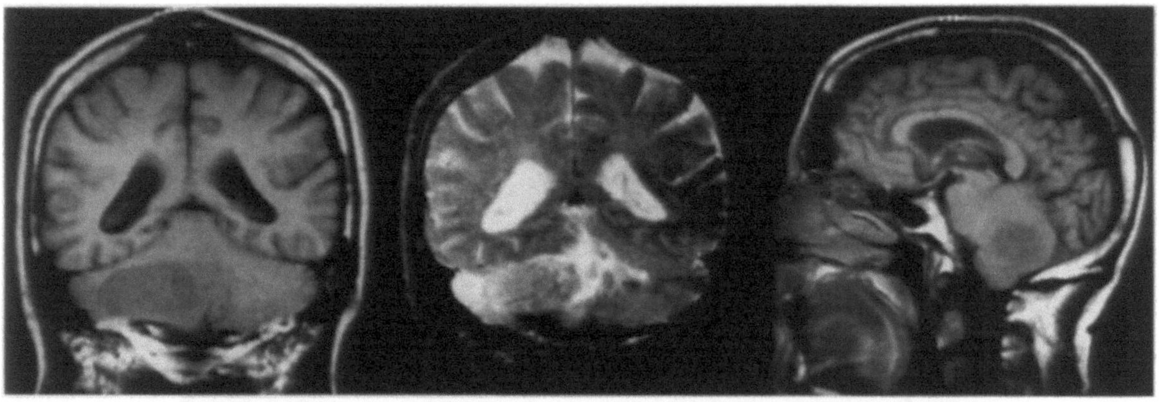

Fig. D 9.8. Metastatic bronchial carcinoma of the left cerebellar hemisphere in a 65-year-old man with symptoms of increased intracranial pressure for 1 month. MR *left* SE 500/30 coronal, *center* SE 2500/120 coronal, *right* SE 500/30 parasagittal. The tumor appears hypointense on the T1-weighted sequences (*left* and *right*), while perifocal edema appears very bright on the T2-weighted sequence (*center*)

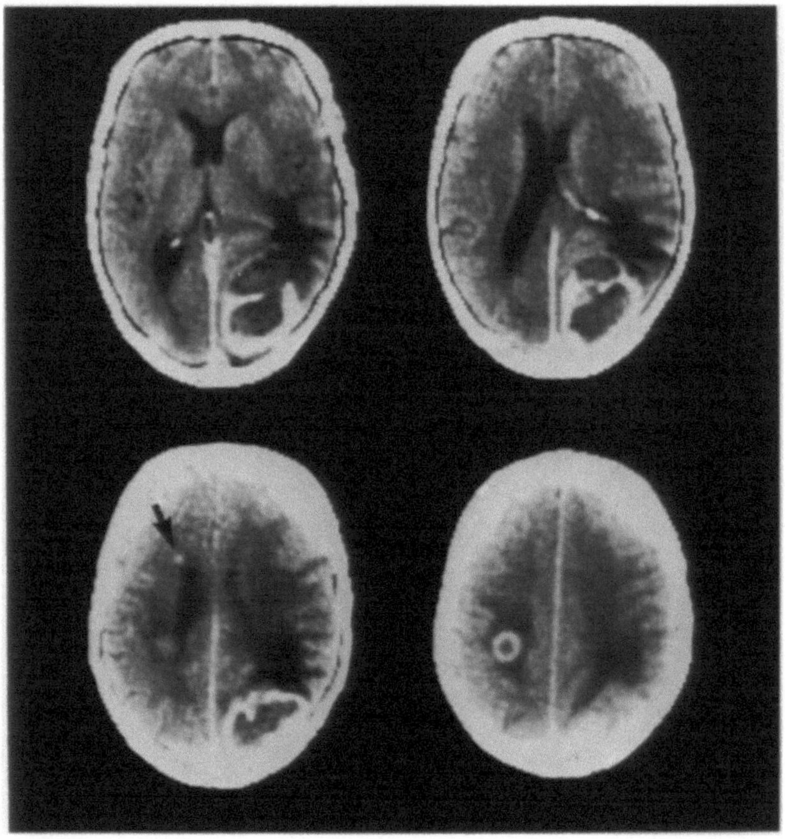

Fig. D 9.9. Multiple metastases of bronchial carcinoma in a 63-year-old man. The scan at *lower left* shows a 5-mm metastasis in the white matter of the left hemisphere close to the ventricle wall (*arrow*). Postcontrast CT

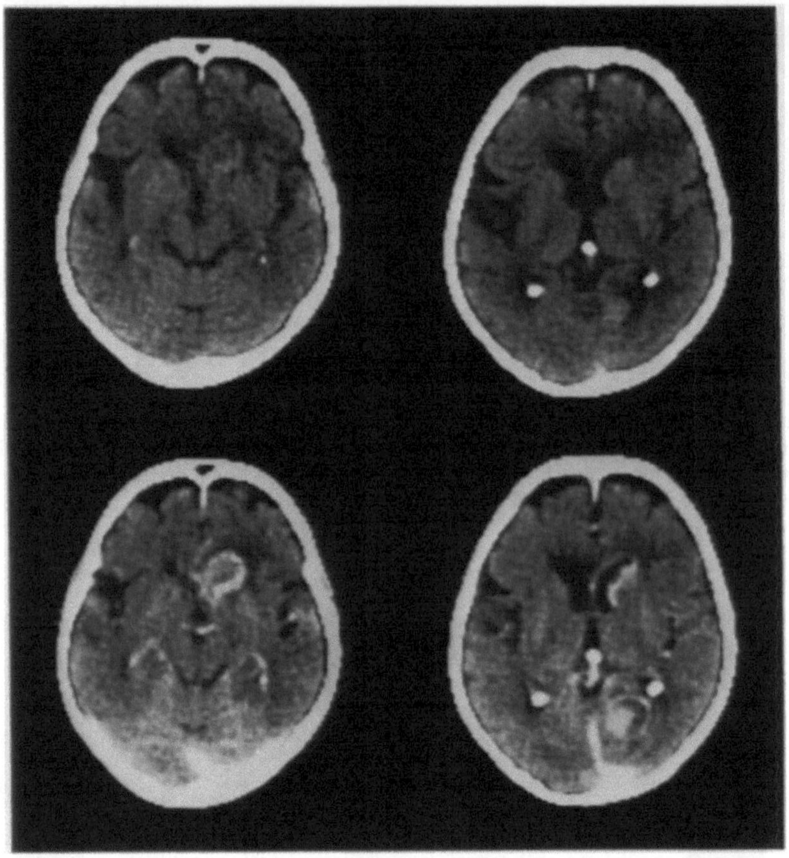

Fig. D9.10. Multiple metastases of bronchial carcinoma in a 68-year-old woman (*top* precontrast, *bottom* postcontrast). Scans demonstrate a metastasis in the right occipital region as well as an intraventricular metastatic growth in the right frontal horn with extension in the ventricle wall (*lower right*)

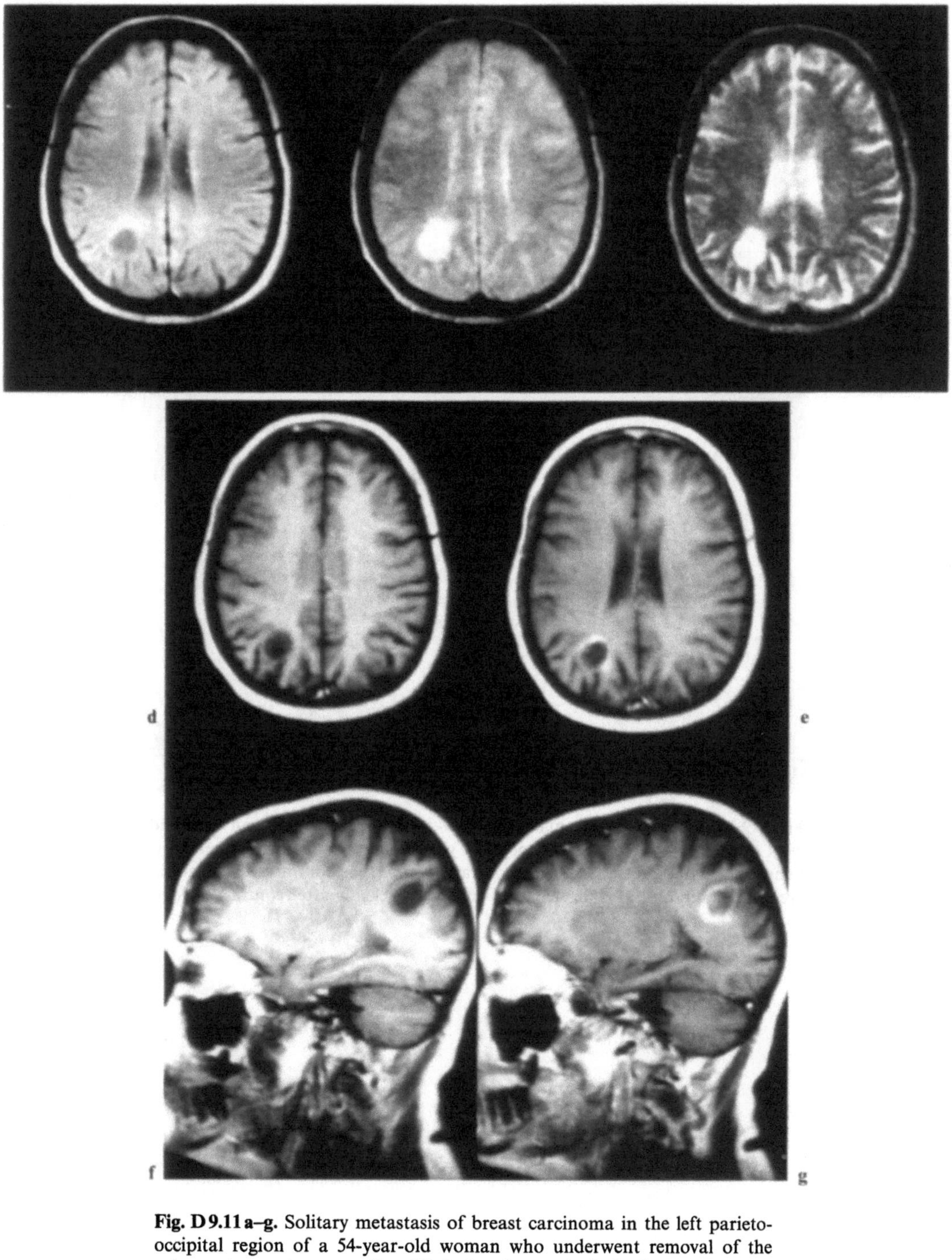

Fig. D9.11 a–g. Solitary metastasis of breast carcinoma in the left parieto-occipital region of a 54-year-old woman who underwent removal of the primary tumor 1 year earlier. Clinical and neurologic findings were unremarkable. MR: **a** SE 1600/30, **b** SE 1600/90, **c** SE 1600/210, **d** SE 400/30, **e** SE 400/30 post Gd-DTPA, **f** SE 400/30, **g** SE 400/30 post Gd-DTPA. The solitary metastasis gives a very intense signal as T2 weighting is increased (**c**). Ring enhancement is observed with Gd-DTPA (**e, g**)

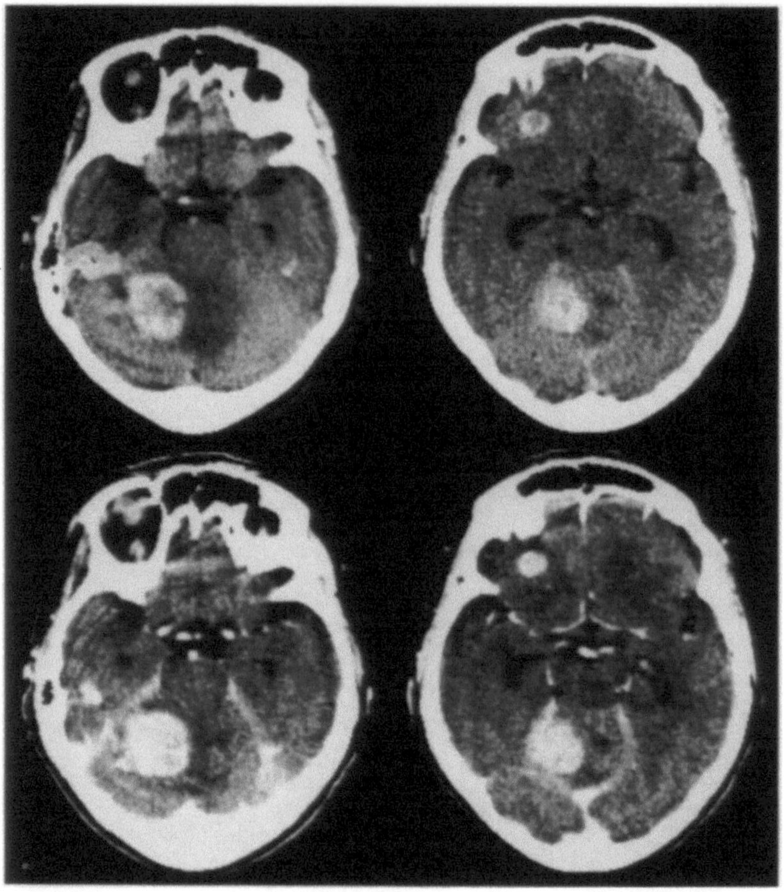

Fig. D9.12. Multiple intracranial metastases in a 40-year-old woman who underwent mastectomy for breast carcinoma 1 year earlier. The patient presented with nonspecific symptoms. CT *top* precontrast, *bottom* postcontrast. The metastases are visible even on the plain scan and enhance markedly after contrast injection

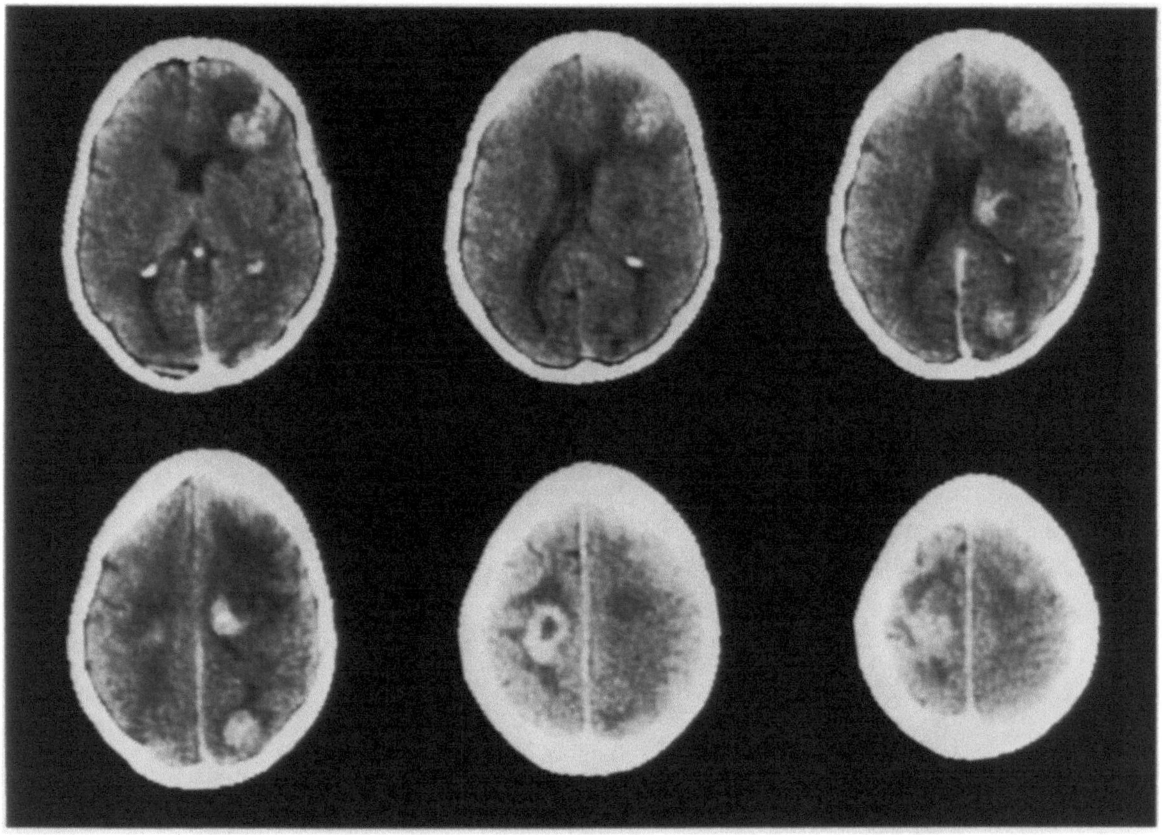

Fig. D9.13. Multiple metastases of breast carcinoma in a 53-year-old woman. Two of the four metastases show ring enhancement in at least one slice. The remaining two show largely homogeneous, nodular enhancement. Postcontrast CT

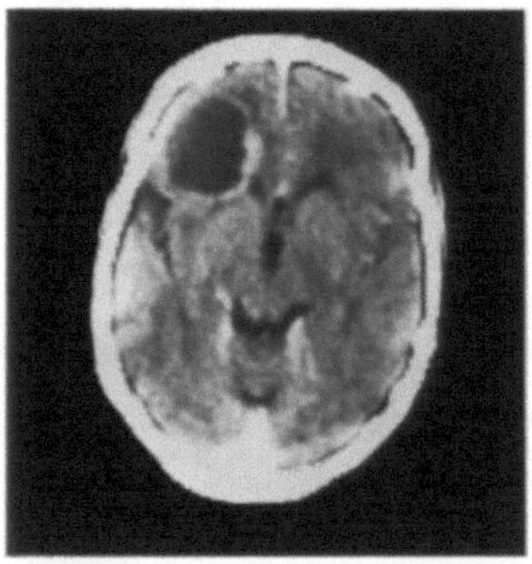

Fig. D9.14. Large solitary metastasis of breast carcinoma in the left frontal lobe of a 39-year-old woman. The thin peripheral tumor enhancement creates a ring pattern around a large necrotic core. This pattern is not typical of metastatic breast carcinoma. Postcontrast CT

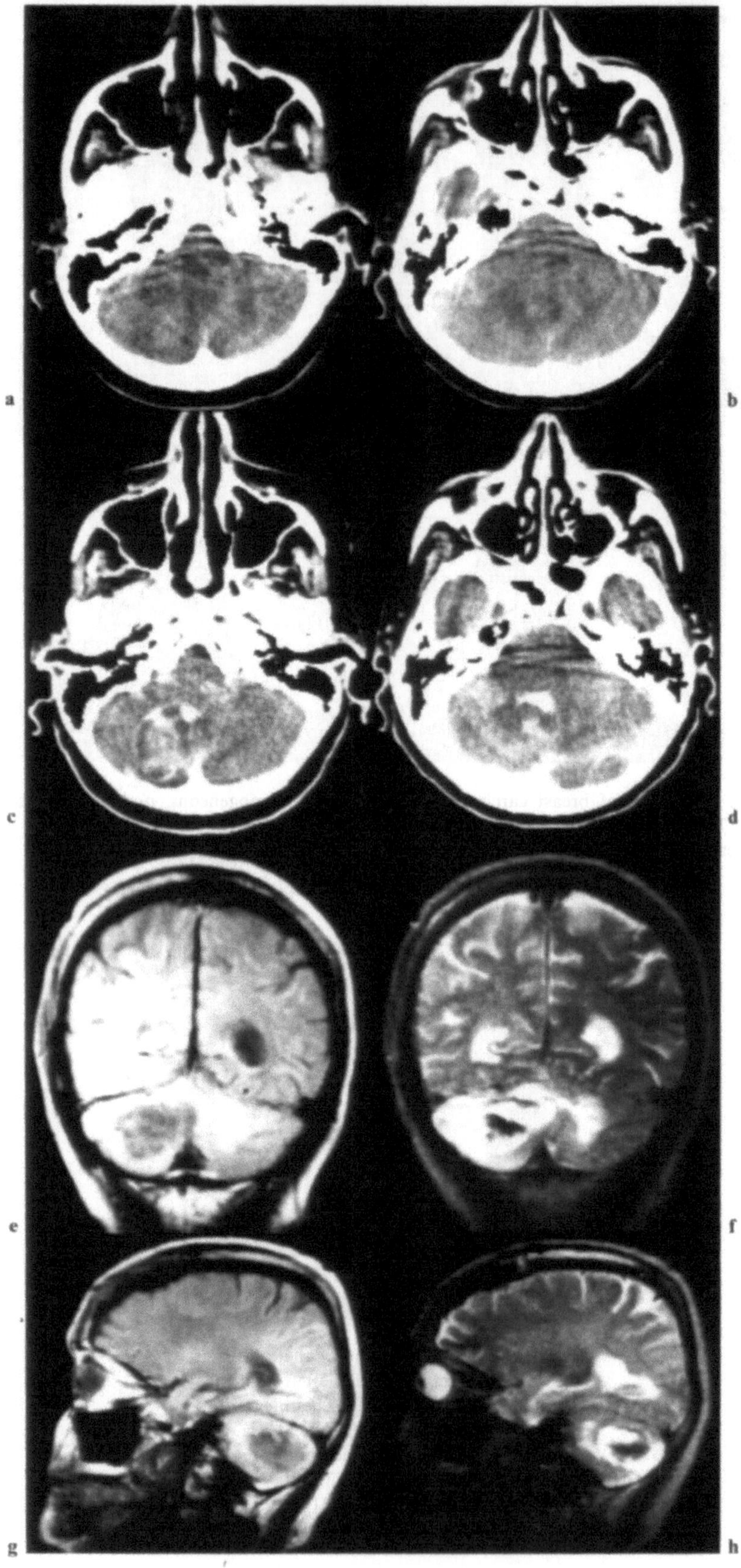
a
b
c
d
e
f
g
h

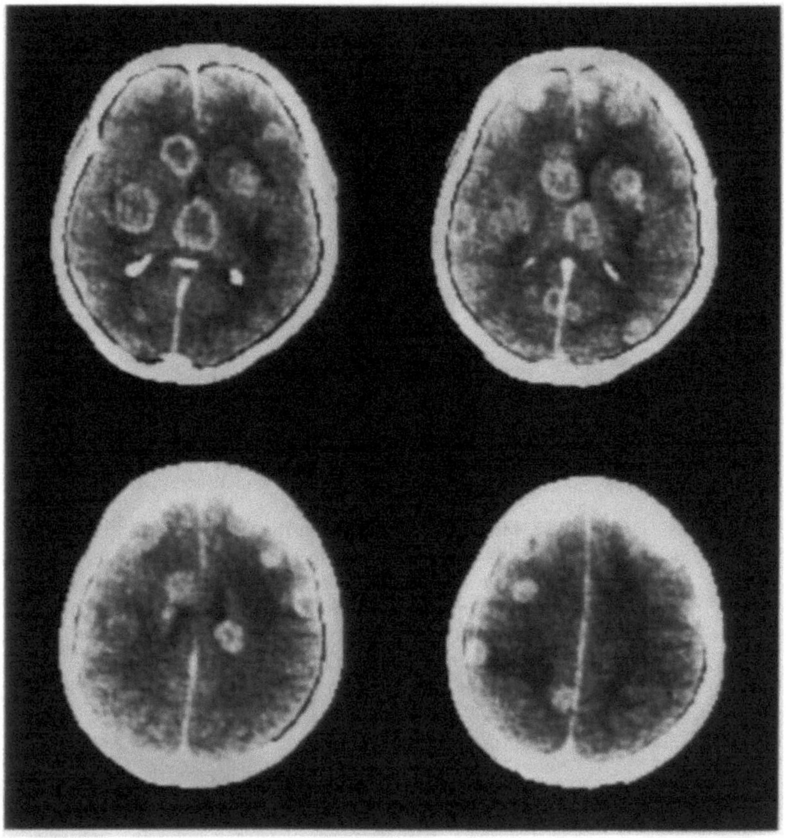

Fig. D 9.16. Multiple metastases permeating the cerebrum of a 44-year-old woman with breast carcinoma. The larger metastases show ring enhancement, while the smaller deposits appear as solid nodules. Postcontrast CT

◄

Fig. D 9.15 a–h. Metastatic breast carcinoma in the left cerebellar hemisphere of a 72-year-old woman with a 3-week history of ataxia and confusion. CT: **a, b** precontrast; **c, d** postcontrast. MR: **e** SE 2500/30, **f** SE 2500/120, both coronal; **g** SE 2500/30, **h** SE 2500/120, both parasagittal. Contrast-enhanced CT shows a well-defined tumor with patchy areas of degeneration. Proton-density MR (**e, g**) shows a predominantly hypointense mass with a nonhomogeneous signal pattern. The T2-weighted sequences (**f, h**) show a peripherally hyperintense tumor that contrasts poorly with the high-signal edema

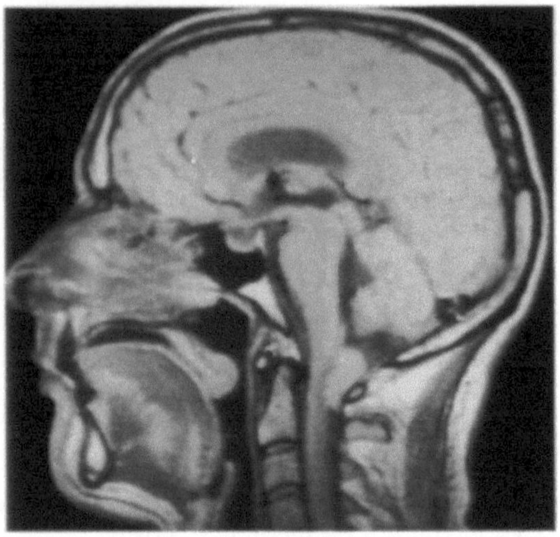

Fig. D 9.17. Metastatic melanoma at the craniocervical junction of a 44-year-old man who had two subarachnoid hemorrhages in the previous 3 months. Repeated cerebral angiograms failed to demonstrate pathology. Patient experienced severe paroxysmal headaches. MR: SE 1600/30. The proton-density image demonstrates a well-defined tumor impinging on the spinal cord from behind

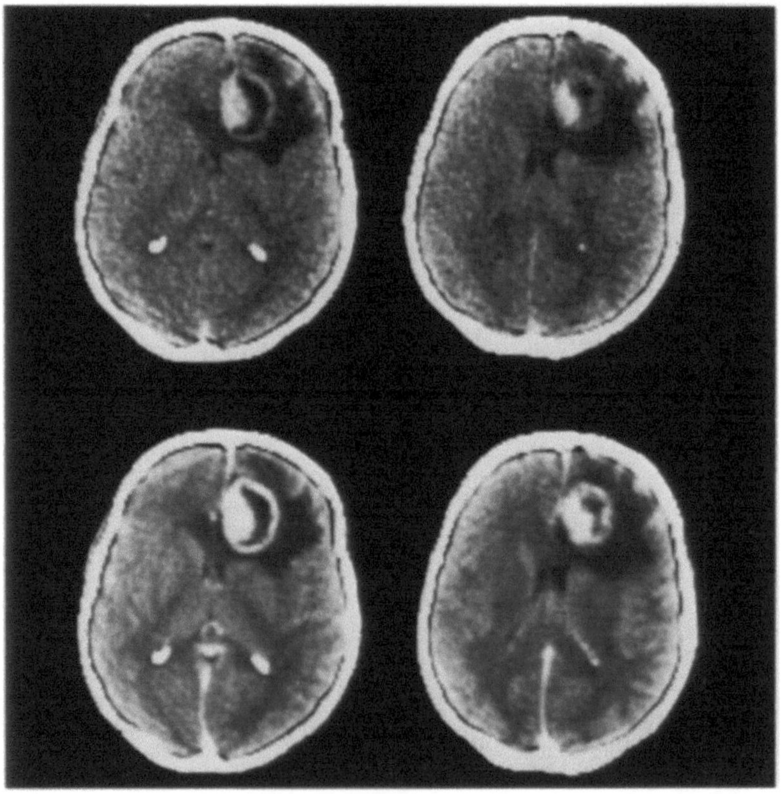

Fig. D 9.18. Metastasis of malignant melanoma in the right frontal lobe with typical frontal edema also extending to the left side. CT demonstrates a combination of ring and nodular patterns. The high density on the plain scans (*top*) is caused by intratumoral hemorrhage. The lesion enhances intensely on postcontrast scans (*bottom*)

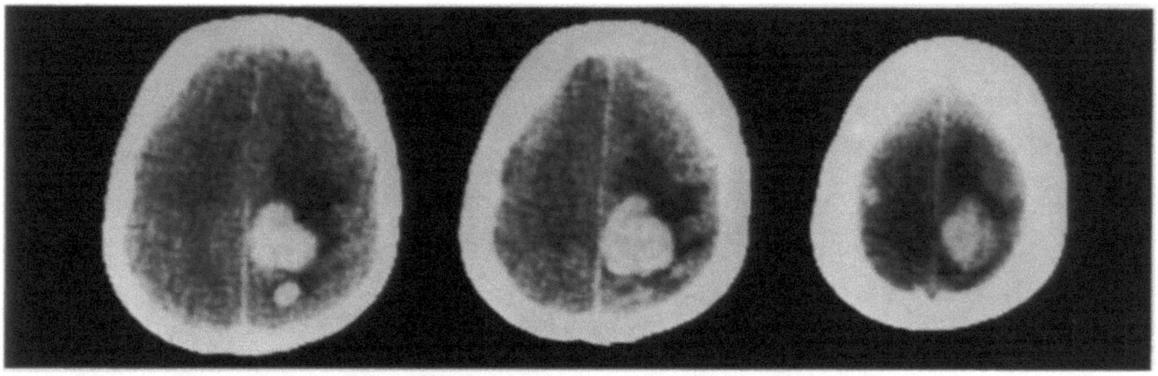

Fig. D9.19. Metastasis of malignant melanoma in the right parietal region with fresh hemorrhage in a 57-year-old man. The lesion does not enhance further with contrast medium due to the very dense attenuation of the clotted blood. Postcontrast CT

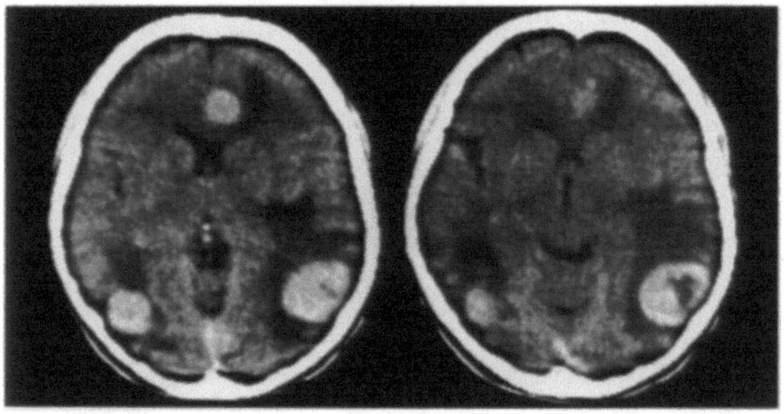

Fig. D9.20. Multiple brain metastasis from melanoma in a 43-year-old woman who underwent removal of a "mole" in the left inguinal area 10 years previously. Lymphadenectomy was performed 1 year later; after that she received no further therapy. Symptoms of increased intracranial pressure were evident for 5 weeks prior to CT examination. Scans demonstrate multiple cerebral metastases, some showing necrotic degeneration. Perifocal edema appears hypodense

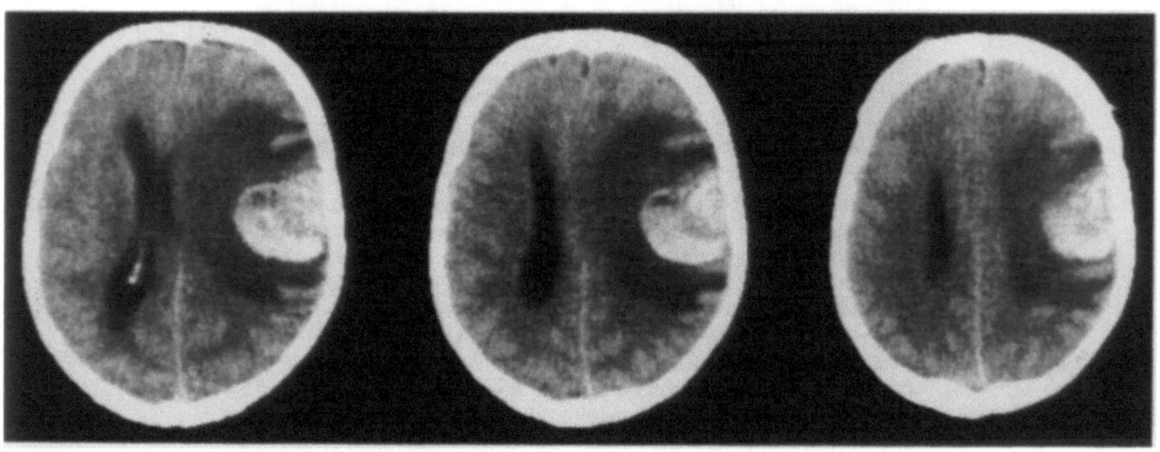

Fig. D9.21. Metastatic melanoma of the right frontoparietal region in a 47-year-old man with headache and progressive left hemiparesis. CT shows a smooth-bordered, predominantly hyperdense mass. The occipital parts of the tumor appear more dense than the other components (a "melanin lake" was found at operation). There is marked compression and displacement of midline structures and conspicuous perifocal edema

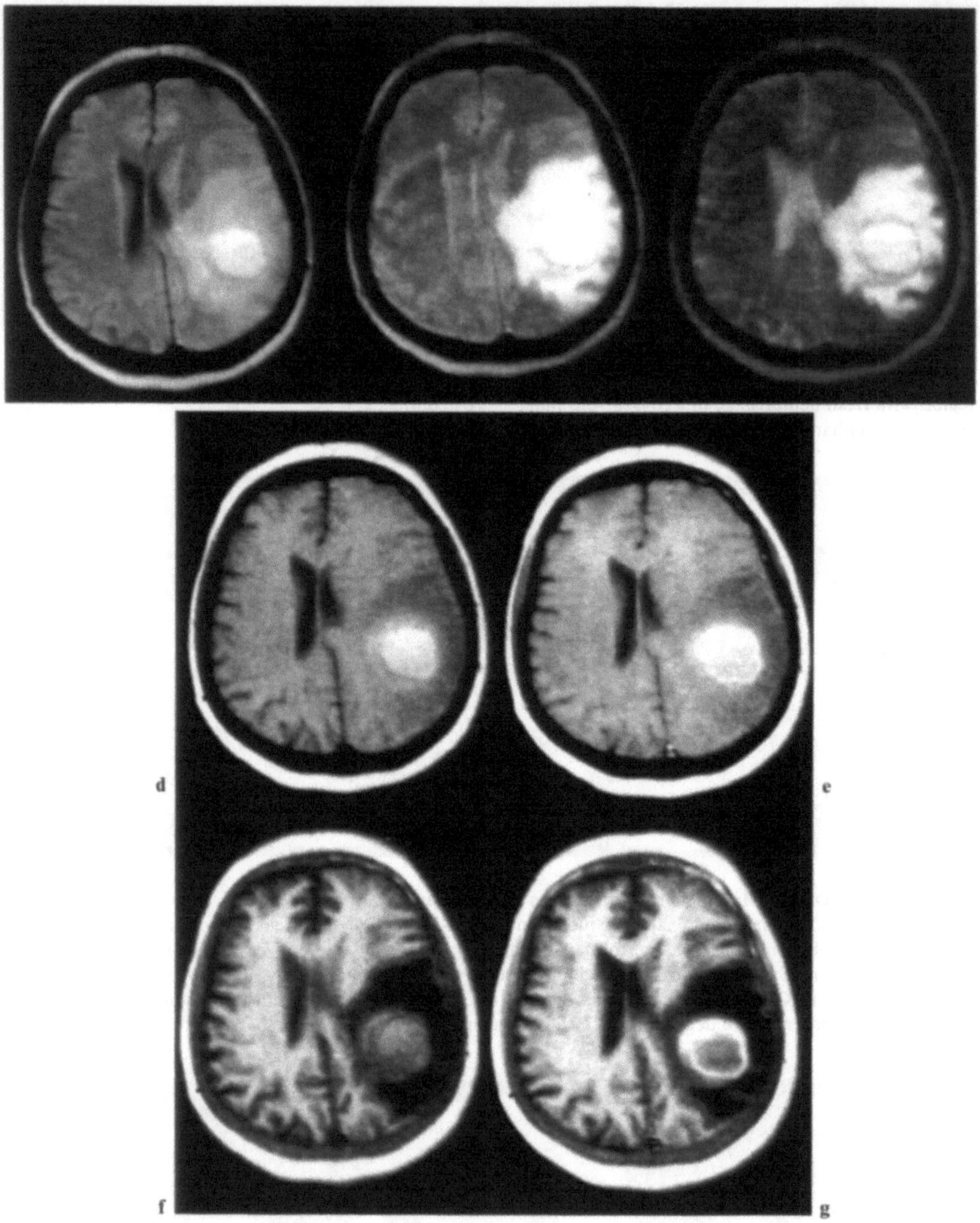

a–c d e f g

Fig. D 9.22 a–g. Metastatic melanoma of the right parietal region in a 50-year-old woman with a 3-week history of weakened grip in the left hand; headache, mild spastic left hemiparesis, loss of drive. MR: **a** SE 1600/30, **b** SE 1600/90, **c** SE 1600/180, **d** SE 400/35, **e** SE 400/35 post Gd-DTPA, **f** IR 1500/400/35, **g** IR 1500/400/35 post Gd-DTPA. The metastasis and perifocal edema give a high signal on the T2-weighted image (**c**) and are separated by a low-intensity ring around the tumor. Little enhancement is seen on the post-Gd-DTPA spin-echo sequence. The tumor is hypointense on the nonenhanced IR sequence, and surrounding edema gives a very low signal. Gadolinium produces ring enhancement of the tumor, whose central hypointensity indicates regressive change

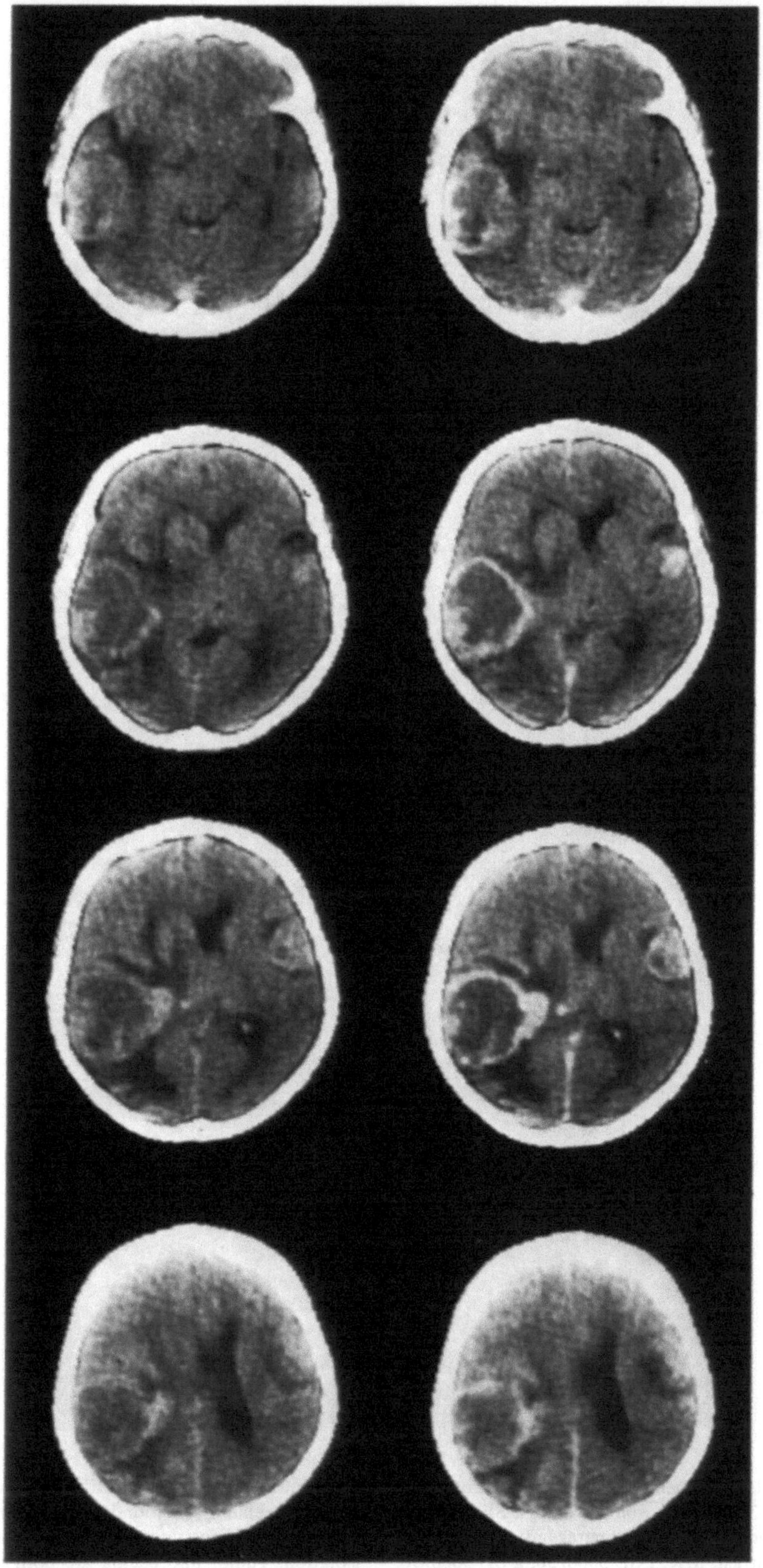

Fig. D 9.23. Multiple brain metastases from malignant melanoma in a 56-year-old woman. CT: *left* precontrast, *right* postcontrast. The tumor in the left hemisphere shows extensive central necrosis, unusual in metastatic melanoma

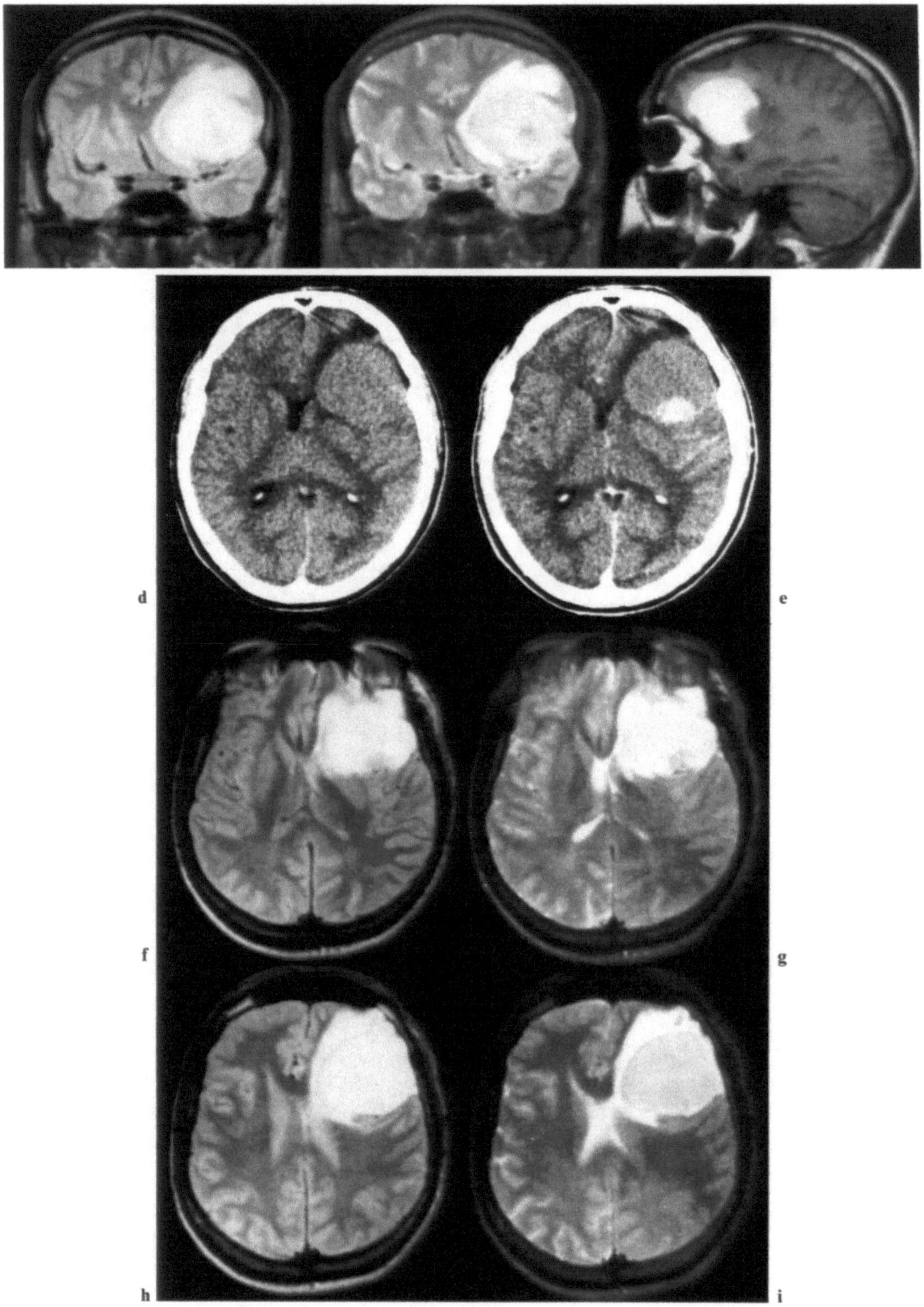

Fig. D 9.24 a–i. Metastatic melanoma in the right frontoprecental region of a 38-year-old woman. MR: **a** SE 3000/30, **b** SE 3000/90 coronal, **c** SE 500/30 parasagittal. CT: **d** precontrast, **e** postcontrast. MR: **f** SE 3000/30, **g** SE 3000/90, **h** SE 3000/30, **i** SE 3000/90. CT demonstrates an isodense mass with circumscribed contrast enhancement at its occipital pole (melanin cyst found at operation). The T1-weighted image (**c**) demonstrates the hypointense melanin cyst in isolation. Tumor and edema are both hyperintense on the T2-weighted images (**b, g, i**) but are easily separated

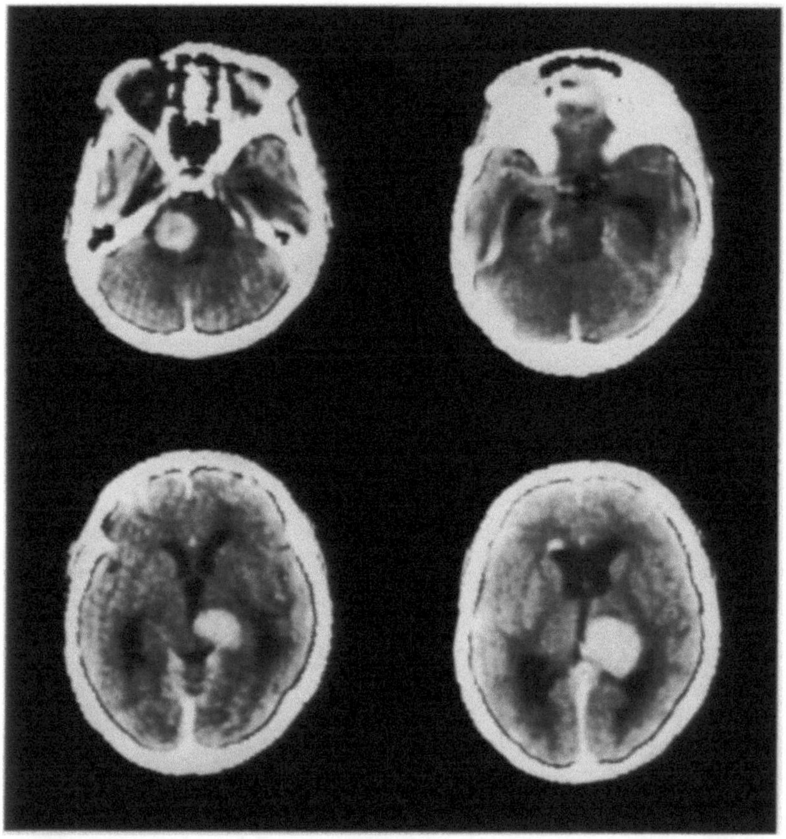

Fig. D9.25. Multiple metastases of malignant melanoma in a 36-year-old man. Postcontrast CT shows densely enhancing tumor nodules in the right thalamus, left cerebellopontine angle, and tip of the left frontal horn. The tumors appeared slightly hyperdense even on nonenhanced scans

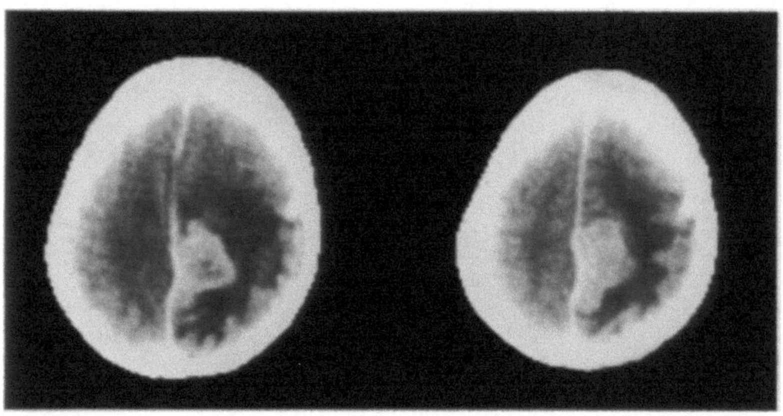

Fig. D9.26. Metastatic melanoma adjacent to the falx in a 52-year-old woman. A diagnosis of meningioma was considered because of the location and largely homogeneous enhancement of the tumor, but the history was more consistent with metastatic melanoma. Postcontrast CT

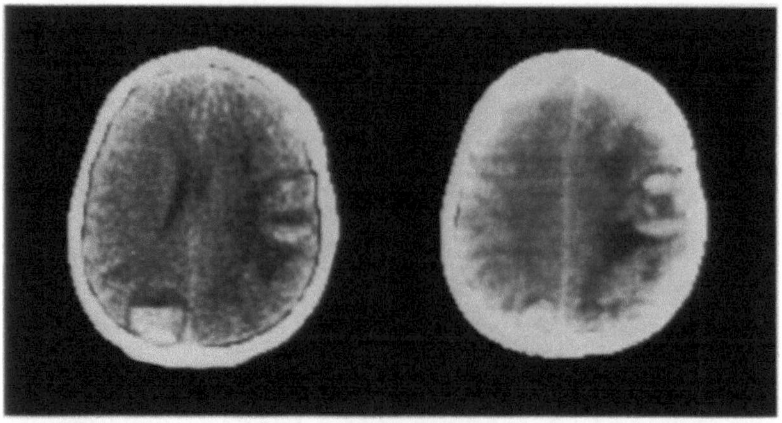

Fig. D9.27. Multiple metastases of melanoma in a 44-year-old man. The fluid level indicates a fairly recent intratumoral hemorrhage

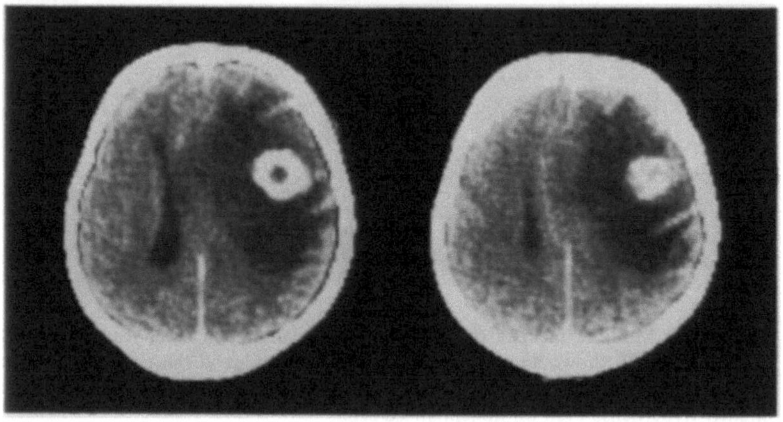

Fig. D9.28. Metastasis in the right precentral region of a 53-year-old man with hypernephroma. Postcontrast CT reveals a rounded tumor nodule with a small necrotic center and grade III perifocal edema with conspicuous mass effect

Fig. D9.29. Multiple brain metastases in a 59-year-old man with hypernephroma. CT: *left* precontrast, *right* postcontrast. The small tumor in the right frontal region enhances homogeneously, while the somewhat larger tumor in the left posterior temporal region shows central necrosis. Additional metastases near the calvarium in both occipital lobes are visible only on the enhanced scans (*arrows*). Bilateral edema of the occipital white matter suggested the presence of these tumors before contrast was administered

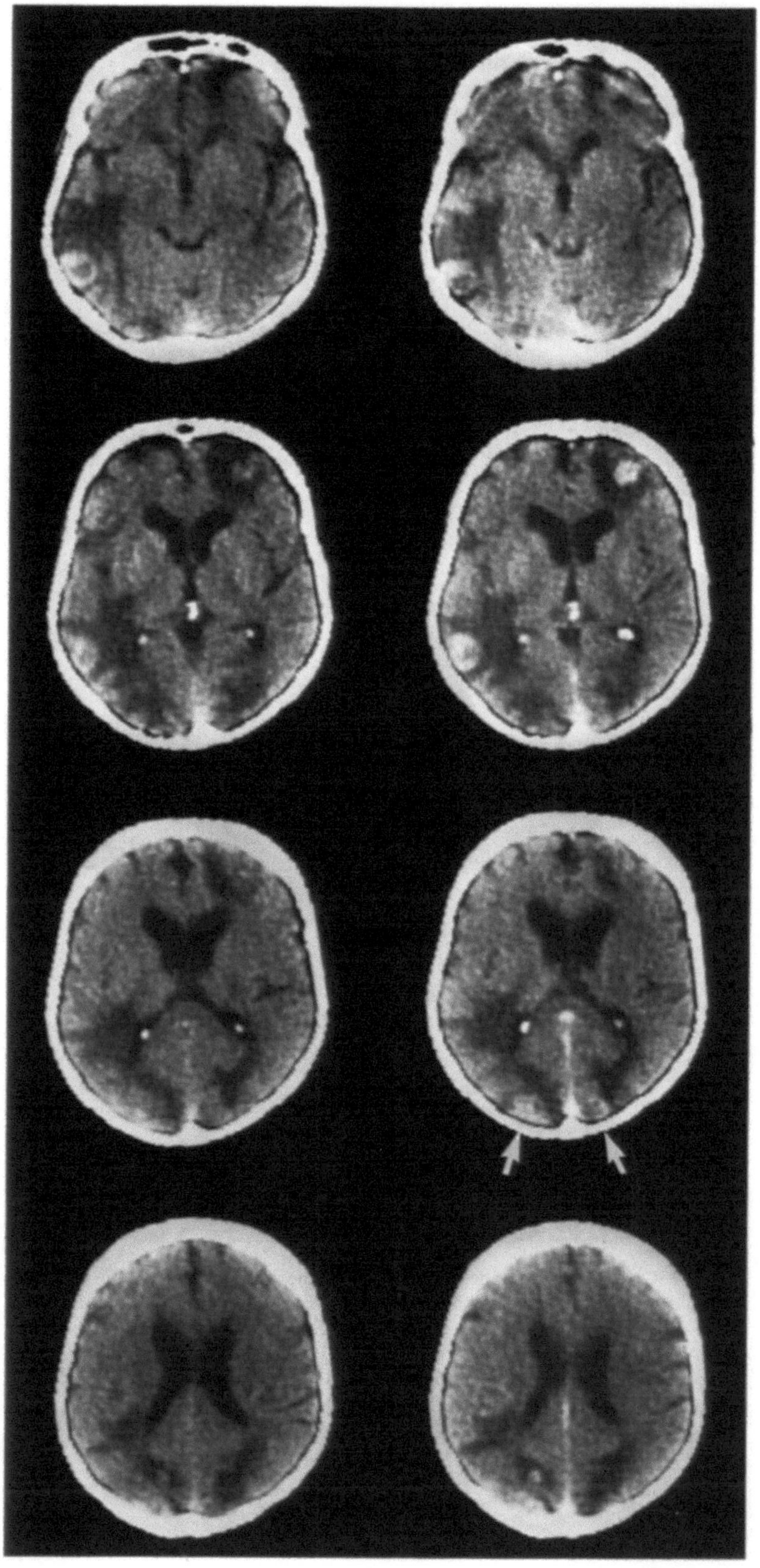

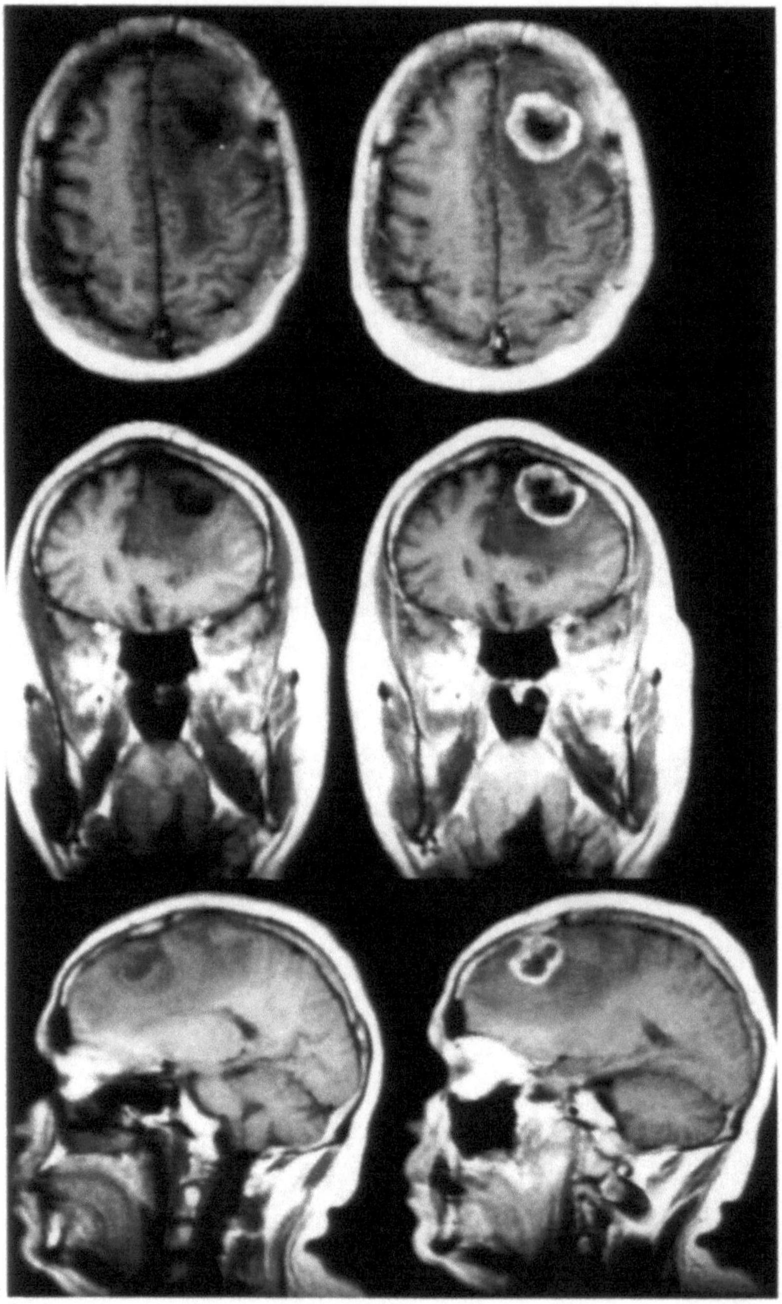

a b c d e f

Fig. D9.30a–f. Metastatic adenocarcinoma of the right frontal region in a 44-year-old man with latent left-sided hemiparesis and altered mental status. MR: **a** SE 400/30, **b** SE 400/30 post Gd-DTPA; **c** SE 400/30, **d** SE 400/30 post Gd-DTPA, both coronal; **e** SE 400/30, **f** SE 400/30 post Gd-DTPA, both sagittal. The tumor shows irregular ring enhancement after Gd-DTPA with a necrotic core. The peritumoral edema is hypointense

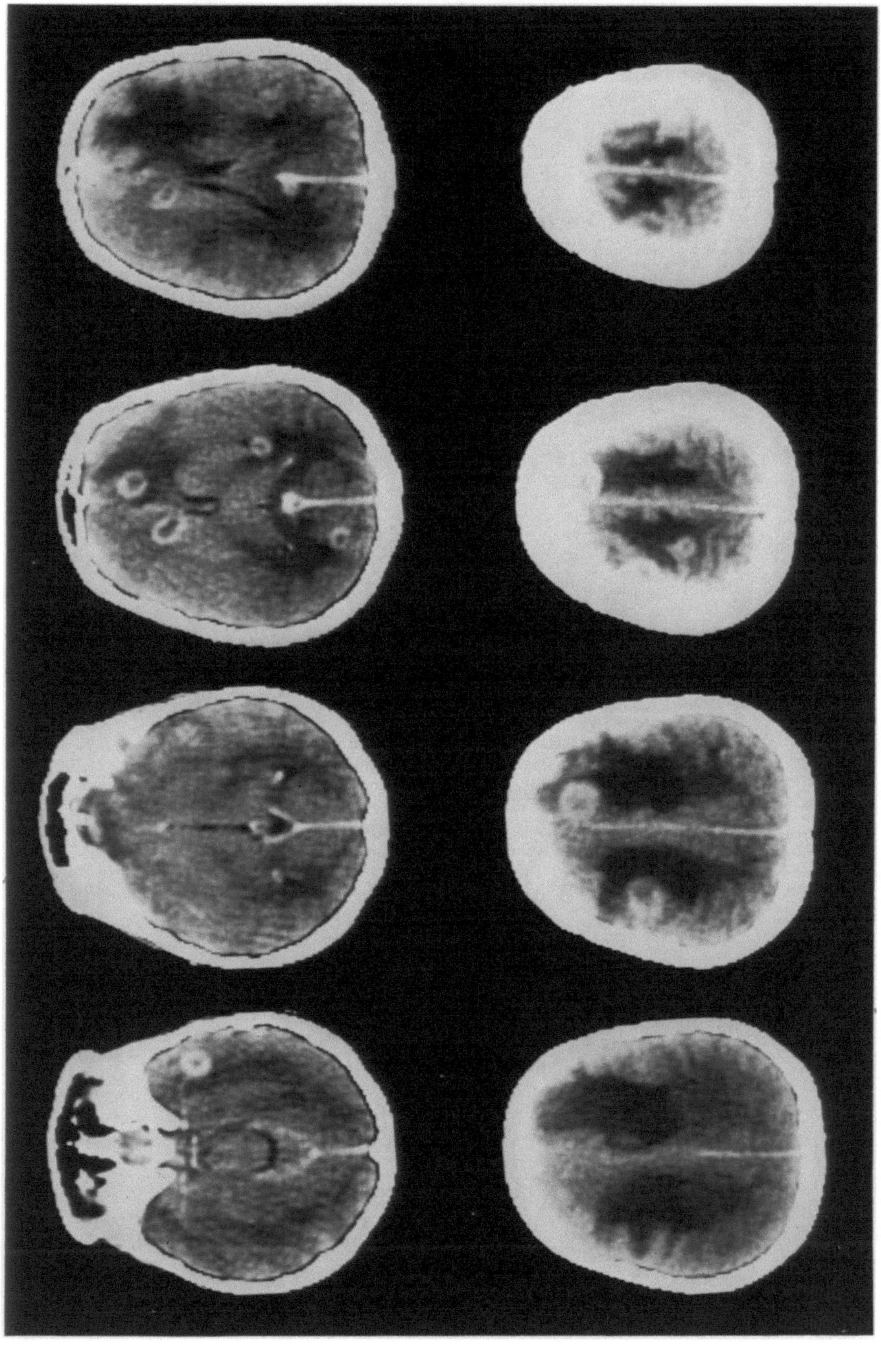

Fig. D 9.31. Multiple metastases of adenocarcinoma (unknown primary) in a 26-year-old woman. All nine metastases visible on the CT scans show central hypodensity consistent with necrotic change. Bilateral white-matter edema is especially pronounced in the centrum semiovale. Postcontrast CT

a b c d

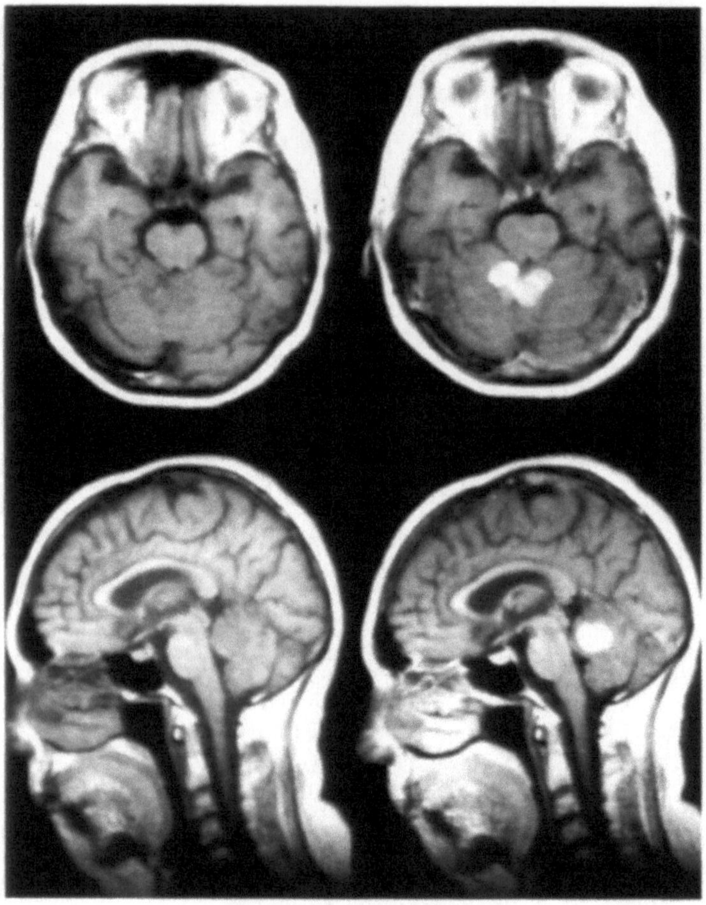

Fig. D 9.32 a–d. Solitary metastasis in the left cerebellar hemisphere of a 68-year-old woman with a 6-month history of vertigo and unsteady gait; mild truncal and stance staxia, bilateral dysdiadochokinesia. MR **a** SE 400/30, **b** SE 400/30 post Gd-DTPA, **c** SE 400/30, **d** SE 400/30 post Gd-DTPA. The tumor is nearly isointense and poorly delineated on the plain T1-weighted images. Intense, well-defined enhancement is seen on the post Gd-DTPA images

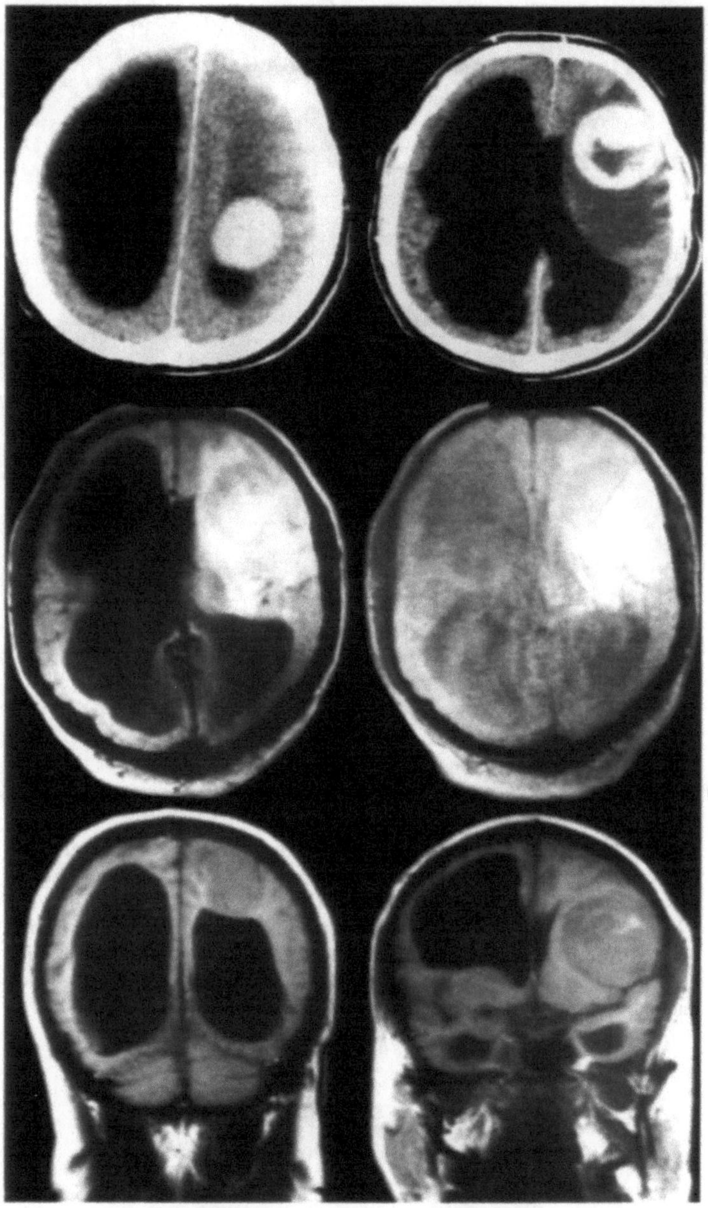
a b c d e f

Fig. D 9.33 a–f. Multiple metastases from an unknown primary in a 36-year-old man with a history of brain injury in early childhood. CT **a, b** postcontrast. MR **c** SE 2500/40, **d** SE 2500/90, **e, f** SE 500/30 coronal. CT reveals extreme dilatation of the ventricular system and two enhancing metastases in the right frontoparietal and parietal regions. There is conspicuous perifocal edema. The larger tumor appears isointense to brain on the T1-weighted images (**e, f**) and contains high-signal areas consistent with a small hemorrhage. The tumor and edema give equally high signals on the T2-weighted image (**d**) and are difficult to separate

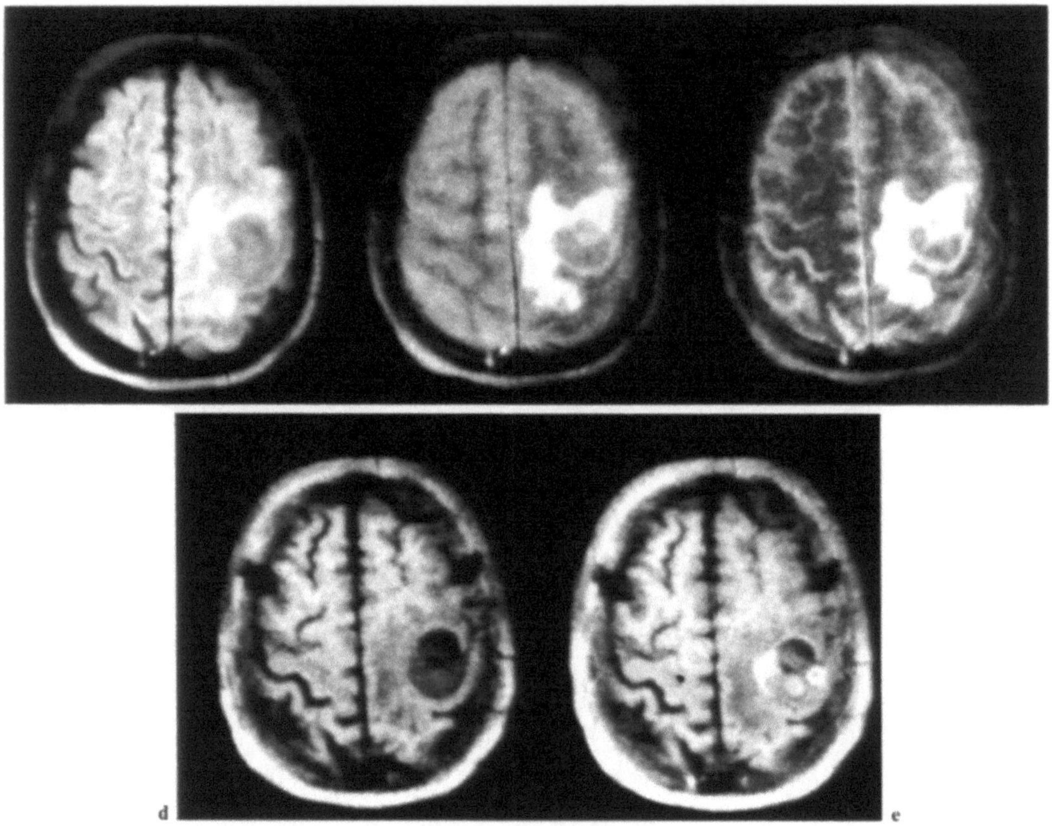

a–c d e

Fig. D 9.34 a–e. Solitary metastasis in the right centroparietal region of a 67-year-old man with spastic left hemiparesis and jacksonian seizures. MR: **a** SE 1600/30, **b** SE 1600/90, **c** SE 1600/150, **d** IR 1500/400/35, **e** IR 1500/400/35 post Gd-DTPA. The hypointense tumor is clearly distinguished from bright peritumoral edema on the T2-weighted sequences (**b, c**). The tumor appears very hypointense on the noncontrast IR sequence and shows spotty enhancement with Gd-DTPA

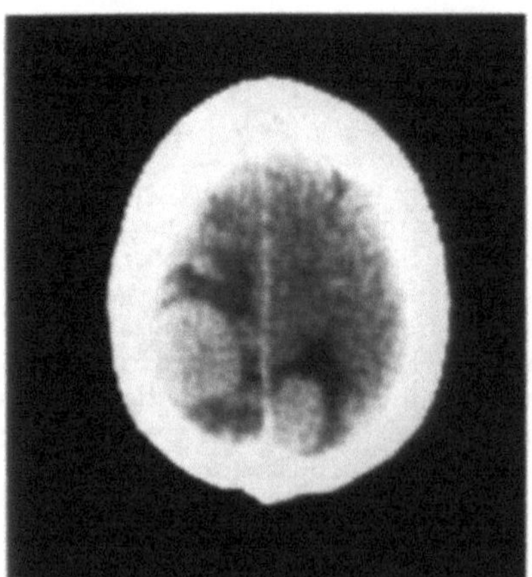

Fig. D 9.35. Multiple metastases of testicular teratoma appearing as solid tumor nodules in a 41-year-old man. Postcontrast CT

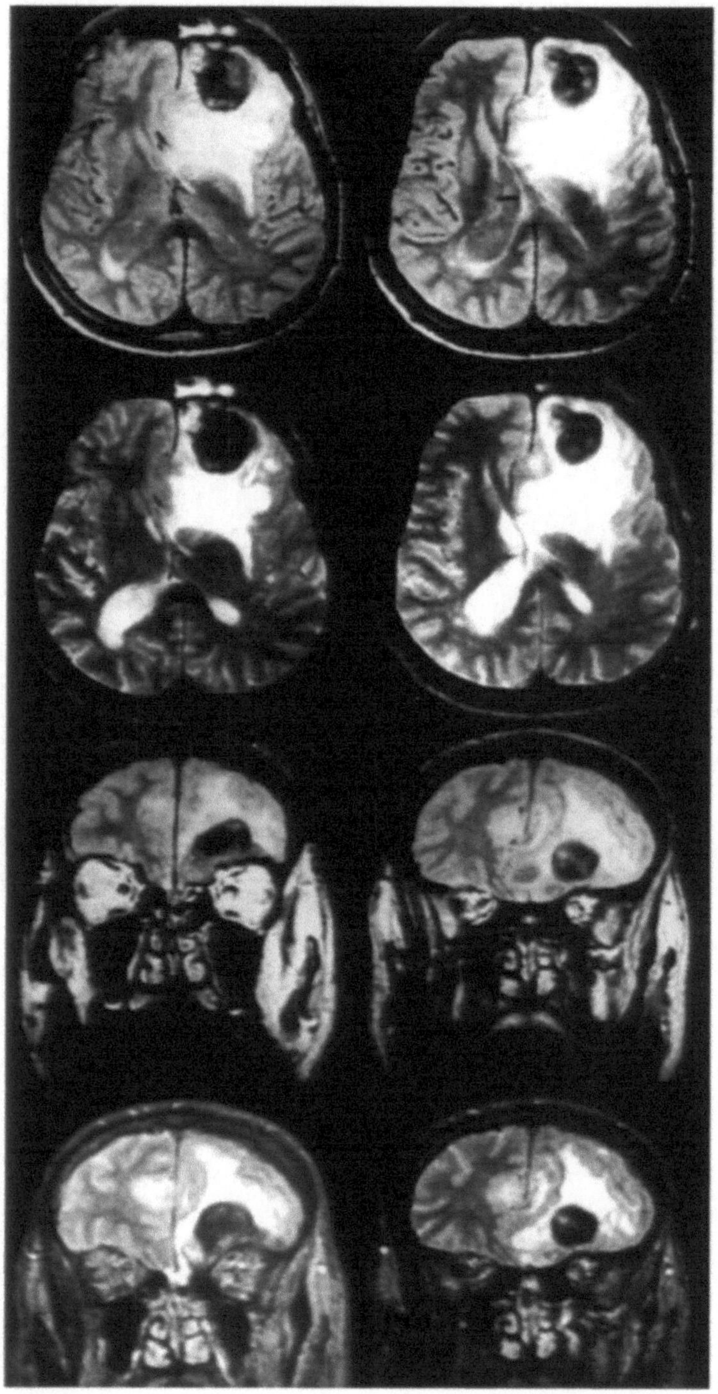

a b c d e f g h

Fig. D 9.36 a–h. Meningeal carcinomatosis from an unknown primary in a 60-year-old man with headache, progressive impairment of consciousness, and left hemiparesis. MR **a, b** SE 3000/30, **c, d** SE 3000/90, **e, f** SE 3000/30 coronal, **g, h** SE 3000/90 coronal. The solid tumor component gives a very low signal on the proton-density and T2-weighted sequences. The coronal view (**f**) additionally shows two less hypointense, circumscribed lesions medial to the original tumor. Edema is displayed as a sharply defined area of increased signal. There is mass effect with compression of the right frontal horn. Multiple metastases were found at operation

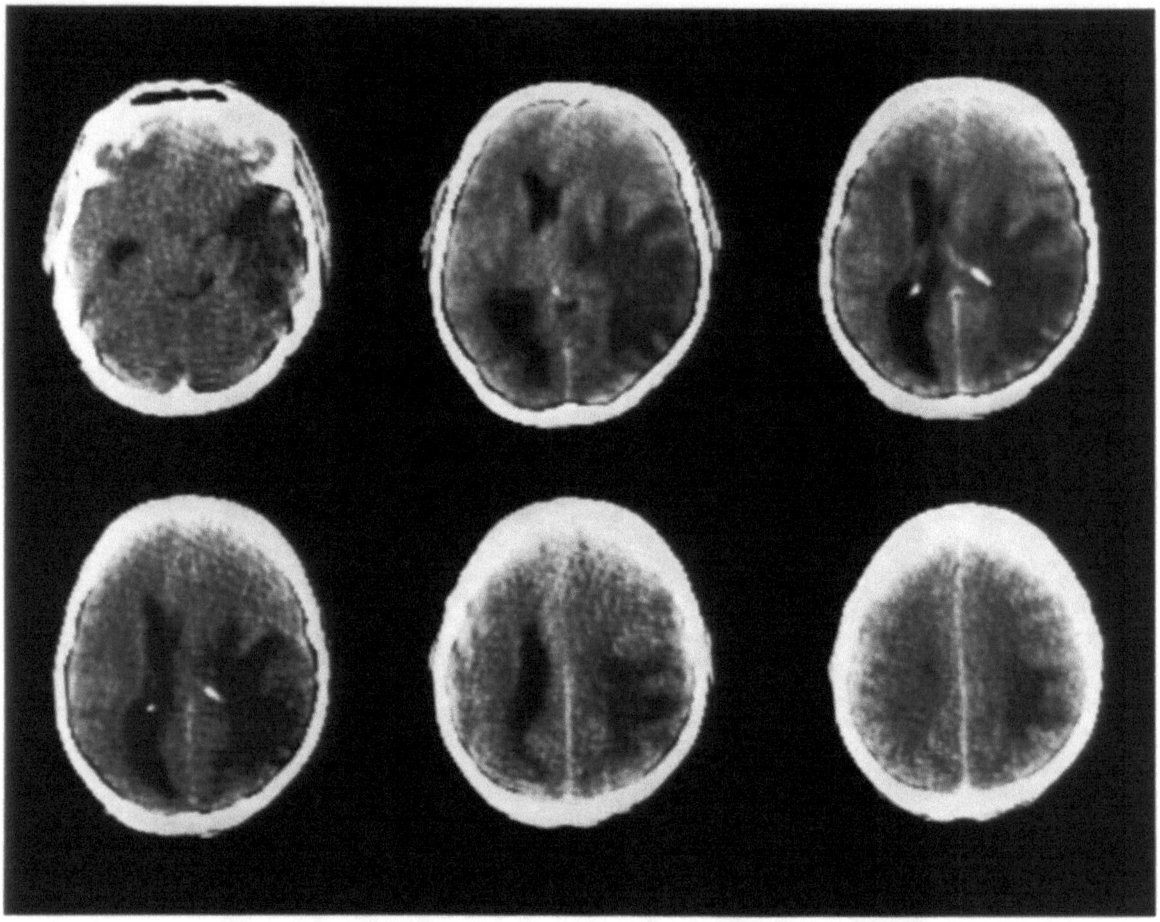

Fig. D 9.37. Metastatic squamous cell carcinoma of the right temporal region in a 40-year-old man. CT shows only a very extensive edematous zone with a typical fingerlike pattern following the course of the white matter. The actual tumor nodule is not visualized even with contrast medium

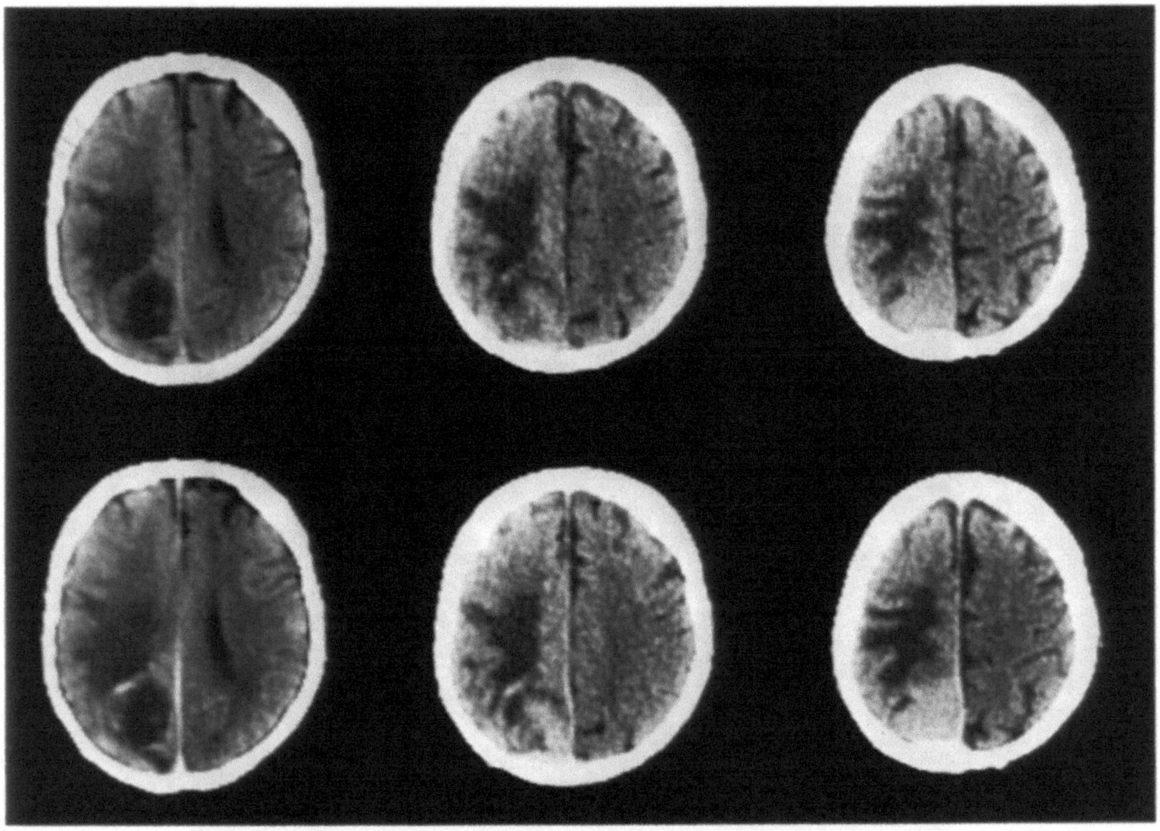

Fig. D 9.38. Osteoplastic metastasis of prostatic carcinoma in a 68-year-old man. At the time of the CT examination the primary tumor was unknown, so the most likely diagnosis was thought to be a meningioma at the dura-falcine angle with an adjacent cyst (*left* scans). The solid tumor tissue appears hyperdense even on the noncontrast scans (*top*), and the adjacent calvarium is markedly thickened (*right*). The tumor enhances moderately with contrast medium (*bottom*)

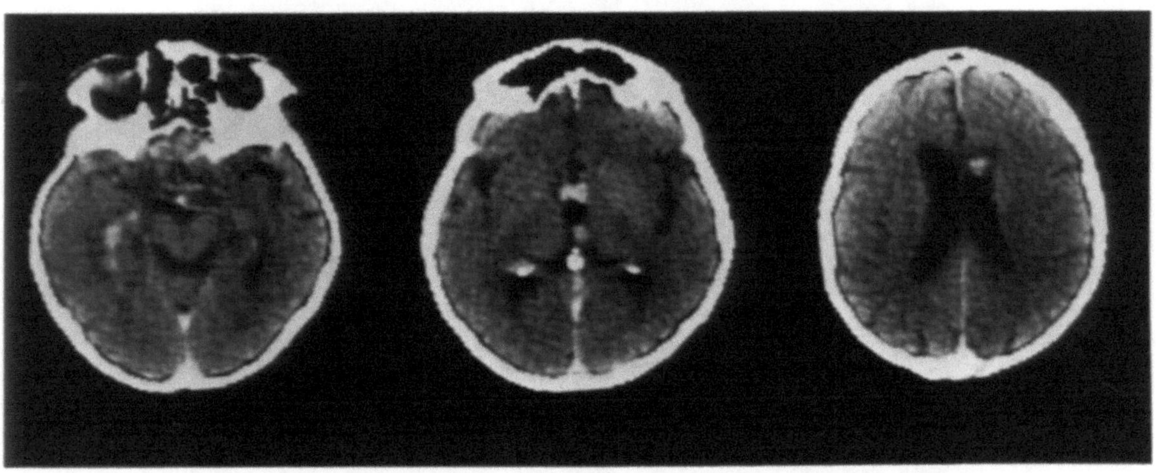

Fig. D 9.39. Multiple intraventricular metastases of seminoma in a 67-year-old man. The lesions occur in the left frontal horn, the third ventricle (two metastases), and in the region of the pars centralis of the right lateral ventricle. Postcontrast CT

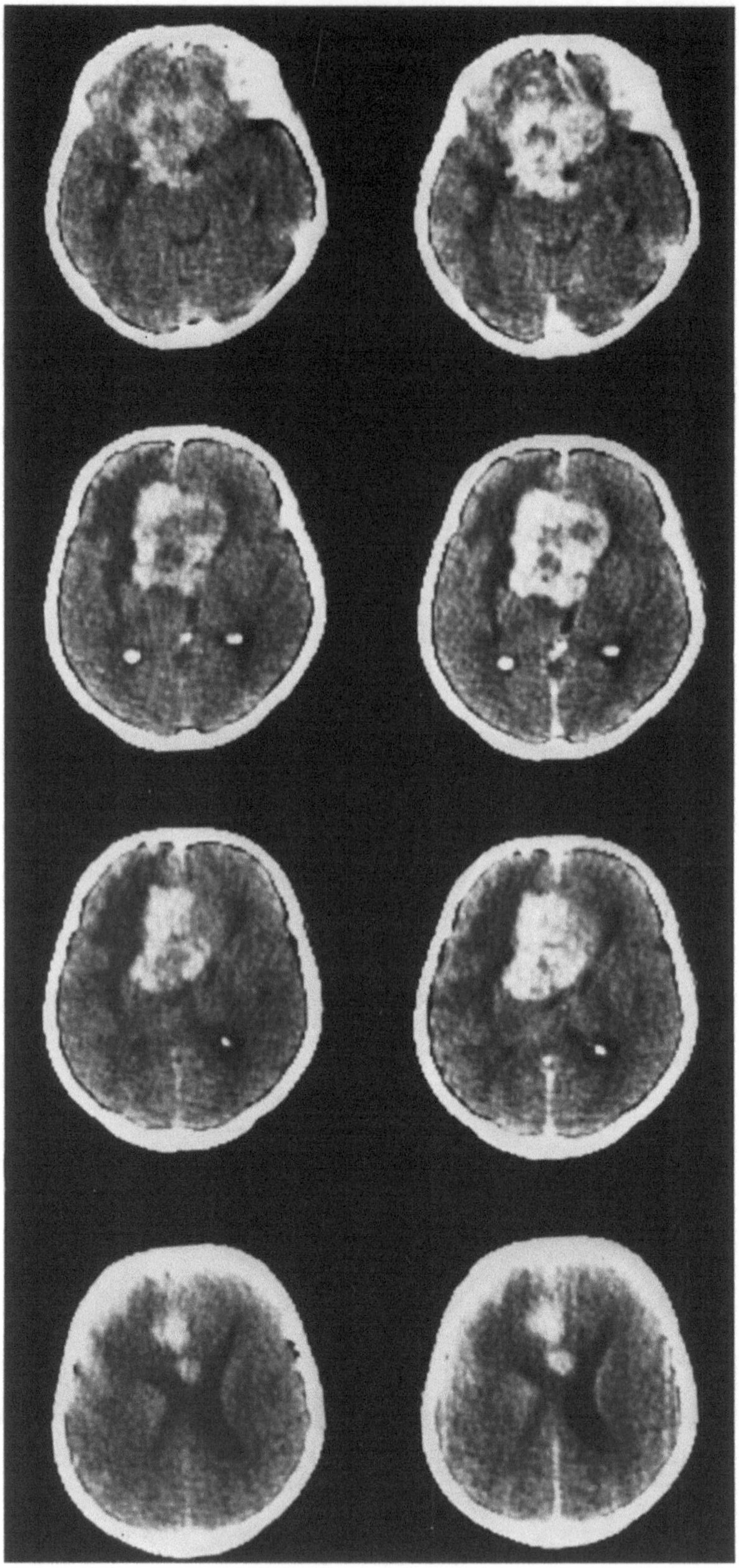

Fig. D 9.40. Very large bifrontal tumor metastatic to rectal carcinoma in a 64-year-old woman. There is evidence of extensive hemorrhage into the tumor, which shows further contrast enhancement in some slices. There is a typical funnel-shaped zone of edema in the left frontal region. The right frontal horn is grossly displaced by the tumor, which arises mainly from the left frontal lobe. *Left* precontrast, *right* postcontrast

E. CT and MR Imaging of Lesions of Skull Base and Cranial Vault

The importance of CT in examinations of the skull base, including its role in the planning of operative or radiation therapy, has long been recognized (Liliequist and Forsell 1976; Bradac et al. 1977 a, b; 1978 a, b; Hammerschlag et al. 1977; Caillé et al. 1977; Lohkamp et al. 1977; Huk and Schiefer 1978; Becker et al. 1978; Weinstein et al. 1978). In the present chapter we shall review the capabilities and limitations of this modality in the diagnosis of diseases involving the bony skull base and cranial vault. A more detailed discussion of specific tumor types may be found under the appropriate headings elsewhere in the book.

1. Skull Base

Examination Technique

Computed Tomography

Optimum visualization of the skull base with CT requires the use of contiguous slices no more than 4 mm thick. Overlapping slices about 1 mm thick should be used when examining very small anatomic structures like those in the petrous bone region. Contiguous slices are essential for multiplanar reformatting, especially on the sagittal and coronal planes.

Axial scans are oriented parallel to the orbitomeatal plane to allow for the physiologic slope of the skull base. Direct coronal projections also may be useful for demonstrating structures in the cerebellopontine angle, sella, and perisellar region. Bony as well as soft-tissue structures can be visualized with CT.

High-resolution thin-section CT provides additional information on bony changes (Fig. E1). This technique is used to evaluate the basal foramina, the cribriform plate, the superior and inferior orbital fissures, the infratemporal fossa, the middle ear structures including the ossicles, and the inner ear structures, especially the internal acoustic pore and the facial nerve canal.

Proper evaluation of the skull base anatomy and its variability requires a detailed knowledge of anatomy and embryology.

Asymmetries of the skull base not related to patient position are not always pathologic. This applies to the jugular foramen as well as to the size of the internal acoustic meatus, which may be considered pathologic only if comparison of both sides shows a disparity greater than 1.5 mm.

Dynamic CT makes it possible to evaluate the vascularization of tumors, especially tumors of the splanchnocranium that have infiltrated the skull base. This gives information helpful in making a differential diagnosis (Claussen et al. 1982). After the administration of intravenous contrast medium, one can employ a short scan time (< 5 s), short scan interval (<4 s), and high scan rate (>7 scans/min) to determine the time course of density changes. This can be quantitated by plotting time-density curves (Claussen and Lochner 1983).

Magnetic Resonance Imaging

In the skull base as elsewhere, the major advantage of MR is its capacity for variable image plane selection. However, it is necessary to limit the thickness of the image slice to a maximum of 5 mm, and this results in long imaging times compared with CT. Also, because of the weak or absent signal from cortical bone, the anatomic structures of the skull base are displayed with far less clarity than on the CT scan. Pathologic processes lead to marked signal changes on MR, and this makes MR su-

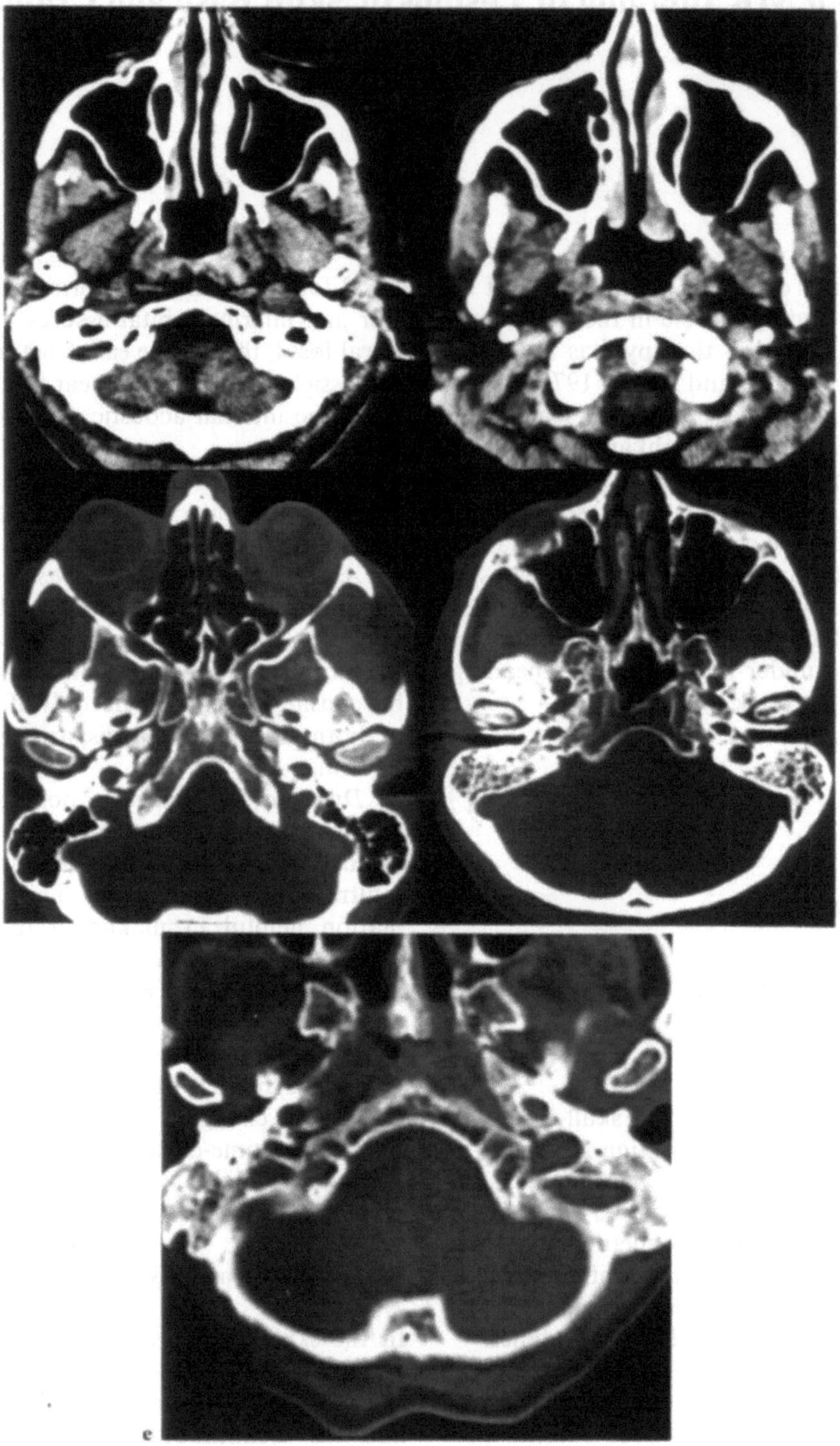

Fig. E1a–e. Normal appearance of the facial skeleton and skull base on high-resolution CT scans. **a, b** Normal window setting for the facial skeleton; **c–e** skull base imaged with a bone window setting

perior to CT in demonstrating the extent of a tumor and its infiltration of soft tissues, although the relation of the lesion to skull base anatomy is appreciated better on the CT scan.

Pathologic Findings

The types of pathology occurring in the skull base region may be grouped into several categories:

a) intracranial mass lesions that involve the skull base
b) primary lesions of the skull base or frontobasal region
c) primary extracranial tumors that infiltrate the skull base
d) metastases of the bony skull base

a) Intracranial Mass Lesions Involving the Skull Base

Intracranial lesions that involve the skull base include *perisellar meningiomas, pituitary adenomas* (which may invade the sphenoid sinus; see Chap. D4), *trigeminal neurinomas* (see Chap. D3 and Fig. E15), *acoustic neurinomas* (see Chap. D3), *cerebellopontine angle meningiomas, tuberculum sellae meningiomas, olfactory groove meningiomas, infraclinoid aneurysms, gliomas,* and *craniopharyngiomas* (see Chap. D6c). These lesions can produce the following changes in the skull base region:

- *Bone destruction*
- *Deformation of basal structures* (e.g., enlargement of sella and foramina)
- *Extension into adjacent cavities* (e.g., extension of sellar tumors into the sphenoid sinus)
- *Hyperostosis or sclerosis* (most common with meningiomas)

These four types of pathology in the skull base region may be encountered individually or in numerous combinations.

In some cases the bony changes are the only pathologic findings, so indirect signs may furnish the only evidence of an intracranial tumor on CT and MR images.

The differential diagnosis of skull base tumors characterized by sclerosis or hyperostosis of basal structures should include **osteoplastic meningiomas** in addition to other extra- or intracranial tumors. Osteoplastic meningiomas form a carpetlike growth on the bony skull base. CT demonstrates a localized, often extreme hyperostosis with thickening and increased density of the bone (Figs. E2–5). Intracranial extension cannot be demonstrated in many of these cases. MR displays the hyperostosis as an area of markedly reduced signal intensity (Fig. E2).

Meningiomas near the skull base can also produce destructive bone changes (Figs. E5, 6a). While the bone window setting clearly demonstrates osseous destruction of the skull base and pyramid by a cerebellopontine angle meningioma in both the axial and coronal projections, the contrast-enhanced scan with a soft-tissue window demonstrates the intracranial, infratentorial tumor in its entirety.

The tumor is clearly delineated on MR images and especially on T2-weighted sequences owing to its high signal intensity. Brainstem compression is appreciated better than on the CT scan. Often the hyperintense tumor cannot be distinguished from the equally intense perifocal edema unless Gd-DTPA is administered (Fig. E6b).

Large aneurysms near the skull base can also be a source of erosive or destructive bone change (Fig. E7).

The diagnosis of acoustic neurinomas is discussed in Chap. D3, the diagnosis of intrasellar tumors in Chap. D4.

b) Primary Lesions of the Skull Base or Frontobasal Region

Fibrous dysplasia is characterized by pronounced hyperostotic bone change with thickening of basal structures, especially the anterior and middle fossae, the bony orbits, and the lesser and greater sphenoid wings. This leads to compression and displacement of orbital structures and to narrowing of the basal foramina of the skull. CT usually shows a unilateral hyperostosis with the displacement of orbital structures (Fig. E8). Fibrous dysplasia requires differentiation from *ossifying fibroma* of bone, which occurs chiefly in the orbital and periorbital region.

Differential diagnosis should also include **von Recklinghausen's neurofibromatosis**, which is usually associated with partial or complete unilateral aplasia of the sphenoid bone. CT findings are very typical and consist in enlargement of the middle fossa by frontal displacement of the lesser and/or greater sphenoid wing, which may be hypoplastic or aplastic (Fig. E9). Coexisting soft-tissue tumors are occasionally detected in the face and orbit.

Glomus tumors are richly vascularized, locally destructive growths arising from the chemoreceptive glomerula of the ninth and tenth cranial nerves in the jugular fossa (glomus jugulare tumor) or from the glomerula of Jacobson's anastomosis at the promontory in the tympanic cavity (see also Chap. D 8). The glomus jugulare tumor may cause expansion of the jugular fossa with associated destruction of the bony membrane of the hypotympanum and carotid canal and invasion of the middle ear. This tumor also may extend intracranially as far as the fourth ventricle, with a potential for obstructive hydrocephalus. The glomus tympanicum tumors grow as space-occupying lesions in the tympanic cavity, frequently erode the promontory, destroy the tympanic membrane, and project into the external auditory canal. CT demonstrates sites of bone destruction (Figs. E10, 11) and a densely enhancing mass of soft-tissue attenuation. Involvement of atypical sites (e.g., the anterior skull base, sphenoid sinus, ethmoid cells, nasal cavity) by a tumor arising from the glomus pterygoideum is sometimes demonstrated (see Fig. E12).

Chordomas are composed of remnants of the embryonic notochord and occur in the skull base region, most commonly affecting the area of the dorsum sellae and clivus (see also Chap. D 7). Bone destruction is a common finding (Fig. E13a, b). Distant metastases are observed in 10% of cases. Chordomas appear on CT as slightly hyperdense masses with associated bone destruction. Flake-like calcifications are frequently seen in soft-tissue components. Most chordomas enhance moderately with intravenous contrast.

The sagittal MR image can more accurately depict the overall tumor extent in the skull base region and give a clearer impression of its relation to the retropharyngeal soft tissues and intracranial structures. Intracranial extension of the tumor, displacement and compression of the brainstem, and associated brainstem edema are appreciated better on the MR image than on the CT scan. CT findings are frequently degraded by artifacts emanating from the posterior fossa. Bone changes are appreciated only indirectly with MR (Treisch et al. 1986), and the inability to demonstrate calcifications in chordomas is a major drawback of that modality. The tumor enhancement seen on post Gd-DTPA images is comparable to that on contrast-enhanced CT (see Fig. D7.9).

The differential diagnosis of destructive lesions also includes **plasmocytoma**, the soft portions of which are more clearly visualized with MR than with CT. A plasmocytoma involving the clivus is indistinguishable from a chordoma on the basis of its MR signal characteristics (Fig. E14).

Cholesteatoma is a soft-tissue mass that grows slowly by expansion in the meso- or epitympanum, causing destruction of adjacent anatomic structures. It may transgress the boundaries of the middle ear, antrum, or mastoid and gain access to the middle fossa. Larger cholesteatomas that cause destruction of the petrous bone may spread into the cerebellopontine angle region and jugular fossa. Plain CT demonstrates the intracranial part of the tumor as a hypodense mass that shows ring enhancement of its capsule after intravenous contrast injection (see Fig. D3.17).

c) Primary Extracranial Tumors with Secondary Infiltration of the Skull Base
(see also Chap. D8)

The majority of these tumors arise in the splanchnocranium and infiltrate the skull base secondarily. The primary site may be in the paranasal sinuses, epipharynx, nasal cavity, external auditory canal, or parotid body. The following indirect signs on CT and MR may signify the presence of these tumors:

- Deformation or destruction of bone
- Obliteration of air-filled cavities in the facial skull
- Sclerosis of adjacent structures

A soft-tissue mass in the paranasal sinuses, nasal cavity, epipharynx, or retromaxillary space can be directly visualized with CT and MR. Both modalities can demonstrate intraorbital or intracranial tumor infiltration with associated skull base destruction. Contrast-enhanced CT can establish the degree of tumor vascularity and thus contribute to a pathologic diagnosis (see Tables 9, 10).

Benign tumors that secondarily cause bone destruction include **juvenile angiofibroma** (Fig. E 16, see also Fig. D 8.3).

Epidermoids and **dermoids** can also cause destructive changes in the bony skull base. Measured densities on CT scans are not always diagnostic (dermoids −50 to −100 HU, equivalent to fat), because the different tissue components can result in an overall density of about 0 HU, which is not suggestive of fat. Dermoids can be identified on MR images by the characteristically high signal intensity of fat on both T1- and T2-weighted sequences (Fig. E 17).

The malignant tumors that most commonly infiltrate the skull base from an extracranial source are the various grades of **carcinoma** (see Fig. G 29), **malignant lymphoma** (Fig. E 18), **adenoid cystic carcinoma**, **esthesioneuroblastoma** (Fig. E 19, see also Chap. D 8), **sarcoma** (including **rhabdomyosarcoma**, see Figs. E 20 and G 32), and **primary carcinoma of the external meatus** (Fig. E 21).

Mucoceles and **pyoceles** (see Figs. G 47, 48, 50–52) may develop as sequelae to sinusitis, traumatic fracture, or surgery. Obstruction of the excretory ducts with retention of secretions gives rise to a chronic expansive process that most commonly occurs in the frontal or ethmoid sinus and less frequently in the sphenoid or maxillary sinus. Mucocele formation leads to expansion of the sinus cavity with thinning and deflection of the adjacent bone. CT shows an expanded sinus filled with material of high or low density. Late cases usually present with foci of pressure erosion and bone destruction with a potential for intracranial involvement (Fig. E 22). Infection of the mucocele leads to a pyocele, which cannot be differentiated with CT or MR.

d) Bone Metastases of the Skull Base

Metastases are found in the skull base of many patients with primary carcinoma of the thyroid, breast, or lung (Figs. E 23–26). Foci of bone destruction are common and, when small, may be detectable only with CT. Sclerosis of adjacent bony structures is sometimes noted. Osteoplastic metastases may affect the skull base in patients with prostatic carcinoma (Fig. E 27). Histiocytosis X also may involve the skull base, especially the mastoid and paranasal sinuses, with soft tissue densities and osteolysis. In some patients with suspected cerebral metastasis, CT will reveal metastases in the bony skull base even when there are no definite clinical manifestations at the time of the examination.

Osteolytic processes cause detectable MR signal changes in the bone, but their relation to anatomic structures is demonstrated more clearly by high-resolution CT.

Conclusions

CT is excellent for examinations of the skull base, permitting the concurrent visualization of bone, brain parenchyma, and soft tissues of the splanchnocranium. High-resolution CT with a slice thickness less than 2 mm provides very high-quality images of the bony skull base and its foramina, and coronal scans may be taken to yield additional information.

MR is a useful adjunct to CT for certain lesions of the skull base. The extra- and intracranial extent of the soft-tissue component of the tumor is detected and delineated with greater accuracy than on the CT scan. What is more, the inflammatory response in the air-filled paranasal sinuses that may accompany a skull base tumor is readily distinguished from actual tumor infiltration on T2-weighted images by the higher signal intensity of the inflammatory change. CT lacks this capability.

Comparing high-resolution CT with conventional X-ray tomography, it is fair to say that CT at least equals the accuracy of X-ray tomography, and that most modern-day CT scanners surpass it.

Table 9. CT criteria for benign skull base tumors

	Site of predilection	Contrast enhancement	Calcification	Sclerosis, hyperostosis	Deformation, erosion	Osteolysis, destruction
Epidermoid, dermoid	Facial skeleton	−	+	+	+	+
Teratoma	Clivus	+	+	−	−	+
Chondroma	Clivus	+ − + +	−	−	+	+
Hamartoma	Sphenoid	0 − +	−	−	−	−
Juvenile angiofibroma	Paranasal sinuses, nasopharynx	+ +	−	−	+	+
Mucocele, pyocele	Paranasal sinuses	−	−	+	+	−
Chordoma	Clivus	+ − + +	+	−	+	+
Meningioma	Orbit, sphenoid	+ − + +	(+)	+	+	+
Osteoma	Base, vault	−	+	+	−	−
Paget's disease	Base, vault	+ +	(+)	(+)	+	+
Fibrous dysplasia	Paranasal sinuses, sphenoid, base	0 − +	−	+	+	−
Neurofibromatosis	Sphenoid, base, paranasal sinuses	0 − +	−	−	+	−

0 No enhancement; + enhancement by 30 HU or less; + + enhancement by more than 30 HU.

Table 10. CT criteria for malignant skull base tumors

	Site of predilection	Contrast enhancement	Calcification	Sclerosis, hyperostosis	Deformation, erosion	Osteolysis, destruction
Carcinoma	Nasopharynx, paranasal sinuses	0 − + +	−	−	−	+
Lymphoma	Paranasal sinuses, orbit	0 − +	−	−	−	+
Esthesio-neuroblastoma	Facial skeleton, base	+ +	−	−	−	+
Rhabdomyo-sarcoma	Parapharyngeal area, orbit	+	+	−	−	+
Fibrosarcoma	Sphenoid	+	−	−	−	+
Chondrosarcoma	Sphenoid, paranasal sinuses	−	+	−	−	+
Angiosarcoma	Paranasal sinuses	+ +	−	−	−	+
Osteosarcoma	Paranasal sinuses	+	+	+	−	+ +
Glomus tumor	Skull base	+ +	−	−	−	+
Plasmocytoma	Base, vault	0 − +	−	−	−	+
Malignant melanoma	Paranasal sinuses	+	−	−	−	+
Metastases	Base, vault	0 − + +	−	(+)	−	+

0 No enhancement; + enhancement by 30 HU or less; + + enhancement by more than 30 HU.

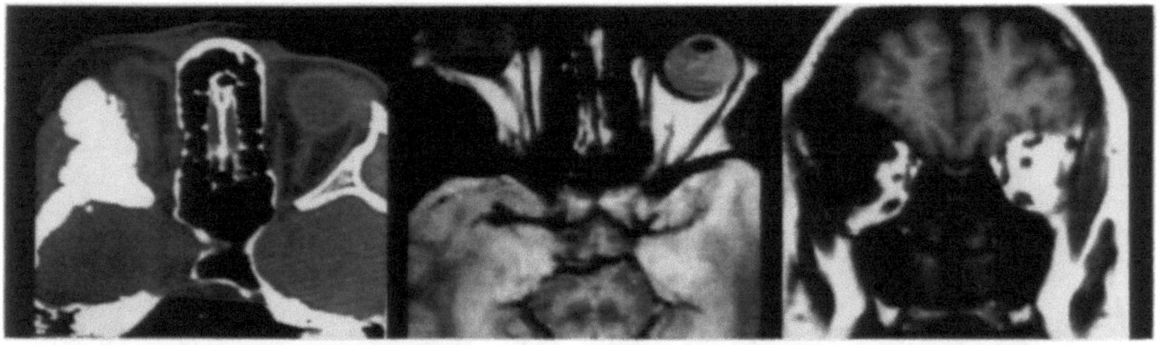

Fig. E2. Osteoplastic meningioma of the left sphenoid wing in a 49-year-old man. CT: *left*. MR: *center* SE 2500/30, *right* SE 500/30 coronal. CT shows osteoplastic change in the left sphenoid wing with displacement of the rectus lateralis muscle. The hyperplastic process appears hypointense on MR. The optic nerve and rectus lateralis stand out sharply against the hyperintense retrobulbar fat. Proptosis is present on the left side. The coronal image shows the extent of the hypointense lesion in the orbital roof area. There is marked constriction of the orbital funnel with displacement of the optic nerve and the lateral and superior rectus muscles

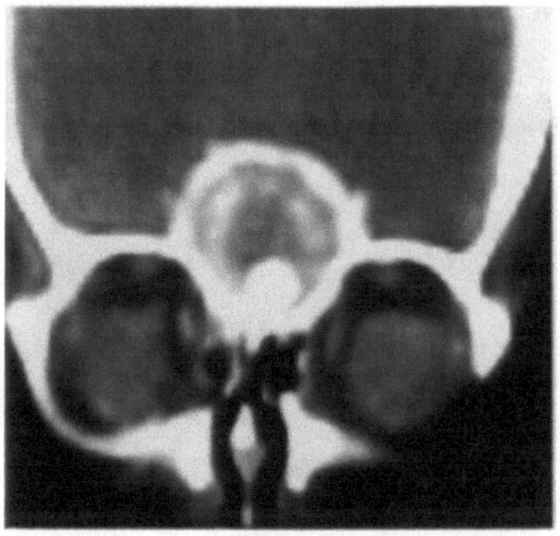

Fig. E3. Ossifying meningioma arising from the olfactory groove in a 36-year-old woman with olfactory disturbances. Coronal CT demonstrates an almost circular calcification above the olfactory groove. Mixed density is apparent within the lesion. The tumorous process has spread to involve the ethmoid cells

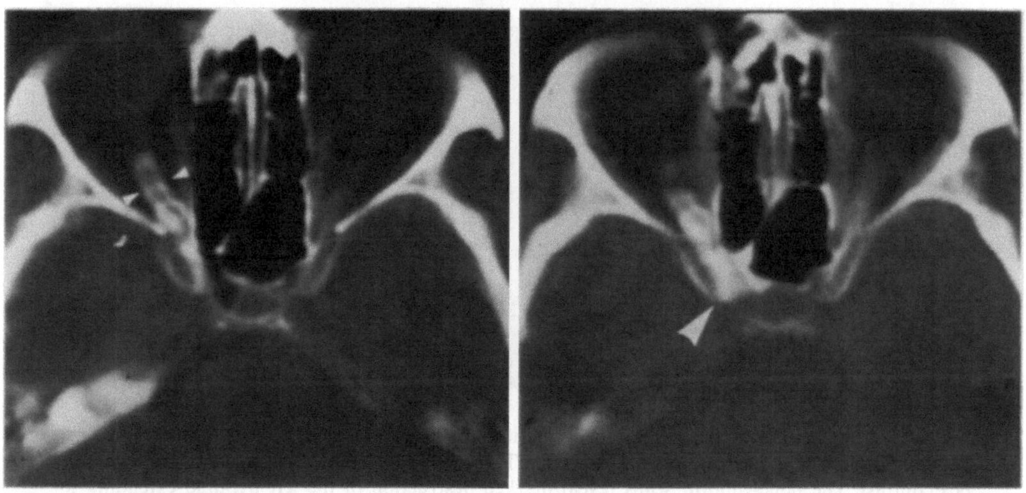

Fig. E4. Small meningioma of the left clinoid process with extension into the orbit. There is tumor-related hyperostosis (*large arrowhead*) at the level of the clinoid process and sphenoid sinus. A cuff of tumor envelops the optic nerve (*small arrowheads*) in the region of the optic sheath

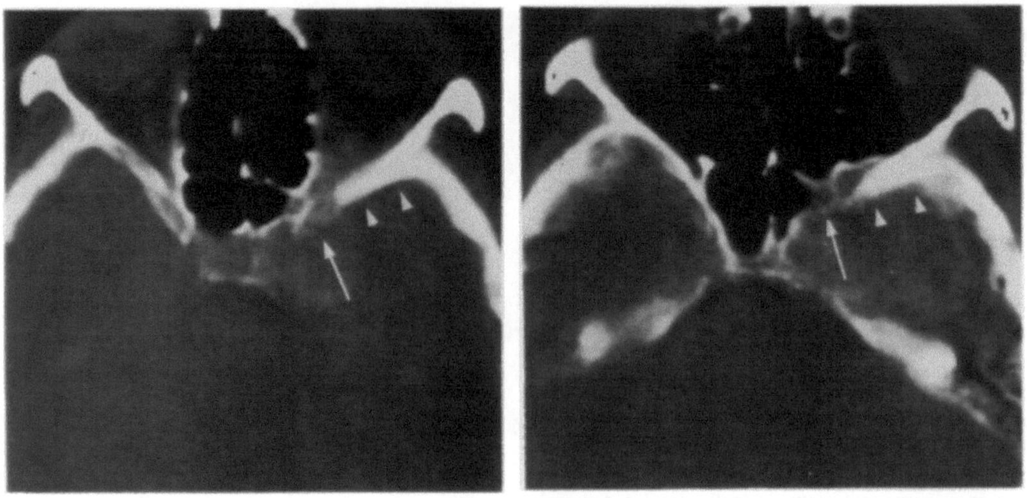

Fig. E5. Large parasellar meningioma on the right side. Visualization of bony structures shows erosion of the clinoid process and right orbital apex (*arrow*). There is bony hyperostosis of the lesser and greater sphenoid wings (*arrowheads*)

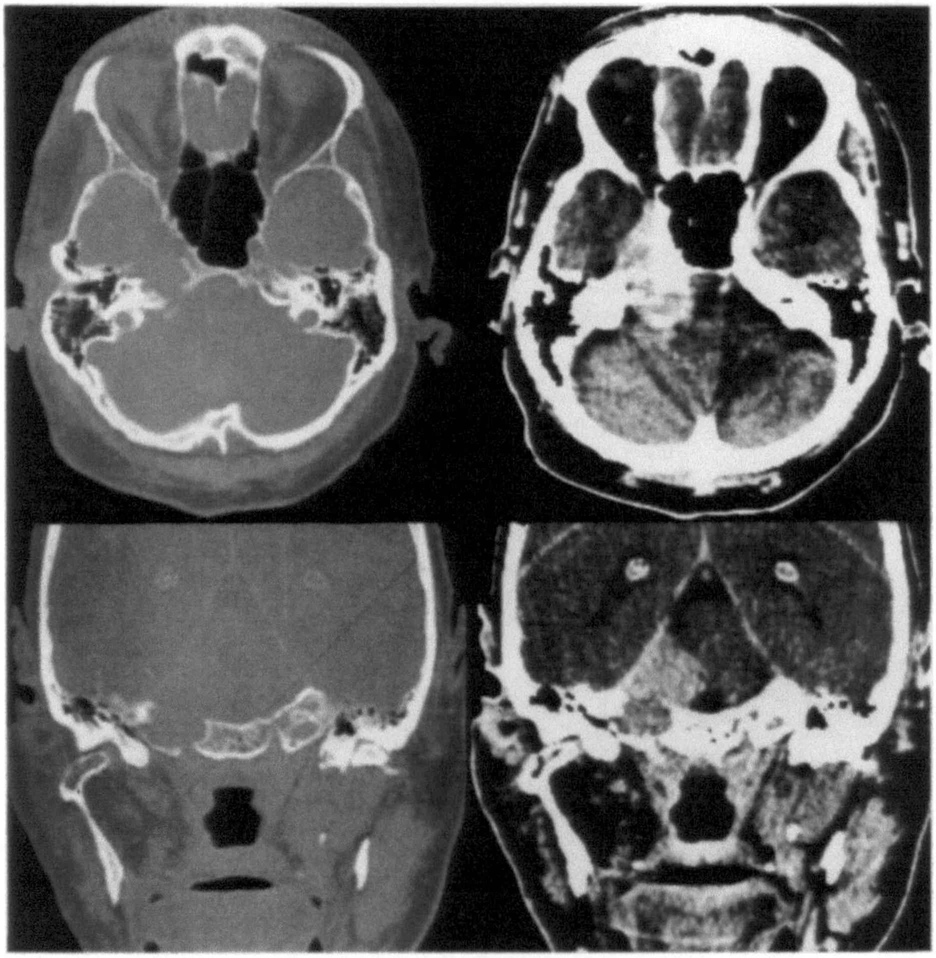

Fig. E6a. Meningioma of the left cerebellopontine angle with associated bone destruction in a 73-year-old man with hearing loss and ataxia. CT *left side* high-resolution precontrast; *right side* postcontrast. The bone-window scans reveal marked destruction of the left pyramid extending to the labyrinth (*upper left* axial, *lower left* coronal). The enhancing neoplasm extends into both the posterior and middle fossae and is bounded by the tentorial margin

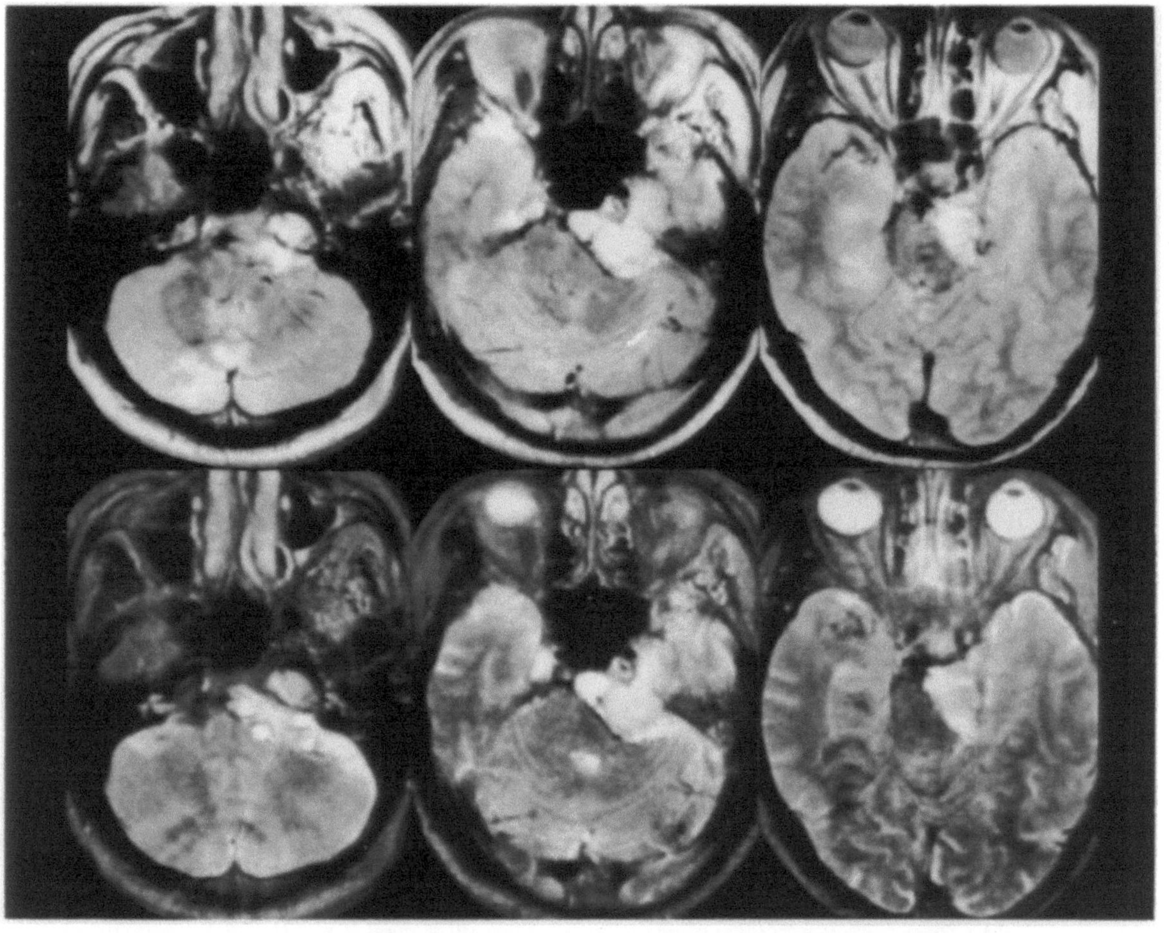

Fig. E6b. Meningioma in the right cerebellopontine angle in a 55-year-old man with isolated hyperesthesia in the distribution of the trigeminal nerve. MR: *top row* SE 3000/30, *bottom row* SE 3000/120. Images demonstrate an infratentorial growth extending to the temporobasal region and compressing the brainstem. The tumor gives a higher signal on the T2-weighted images (*bottom row*) and is more sharply delineated from the brainstem

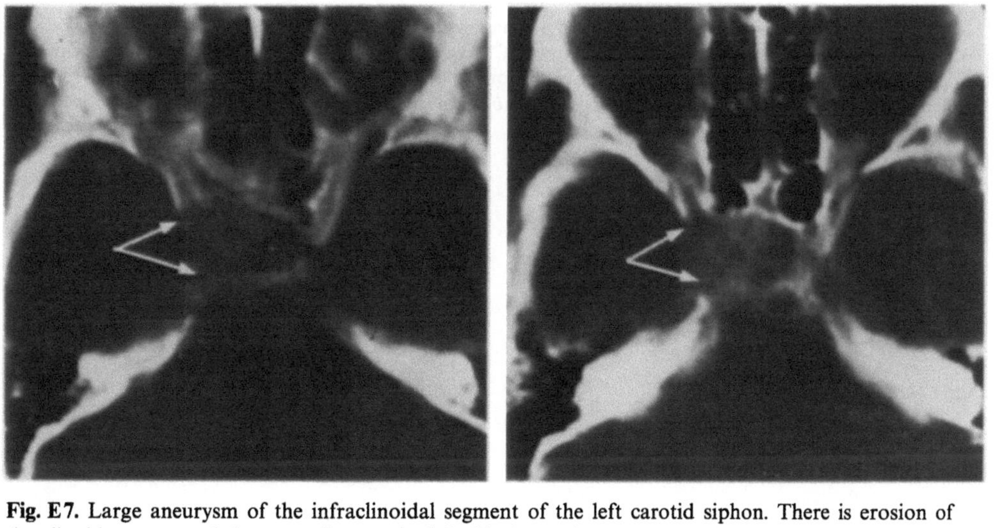

Fig. E7. Large aneurysm of the infraclinoidal segment of the left carotid siphon. There is erosion of the clinoid process and dorsum sellae on the left side (*arrows*)

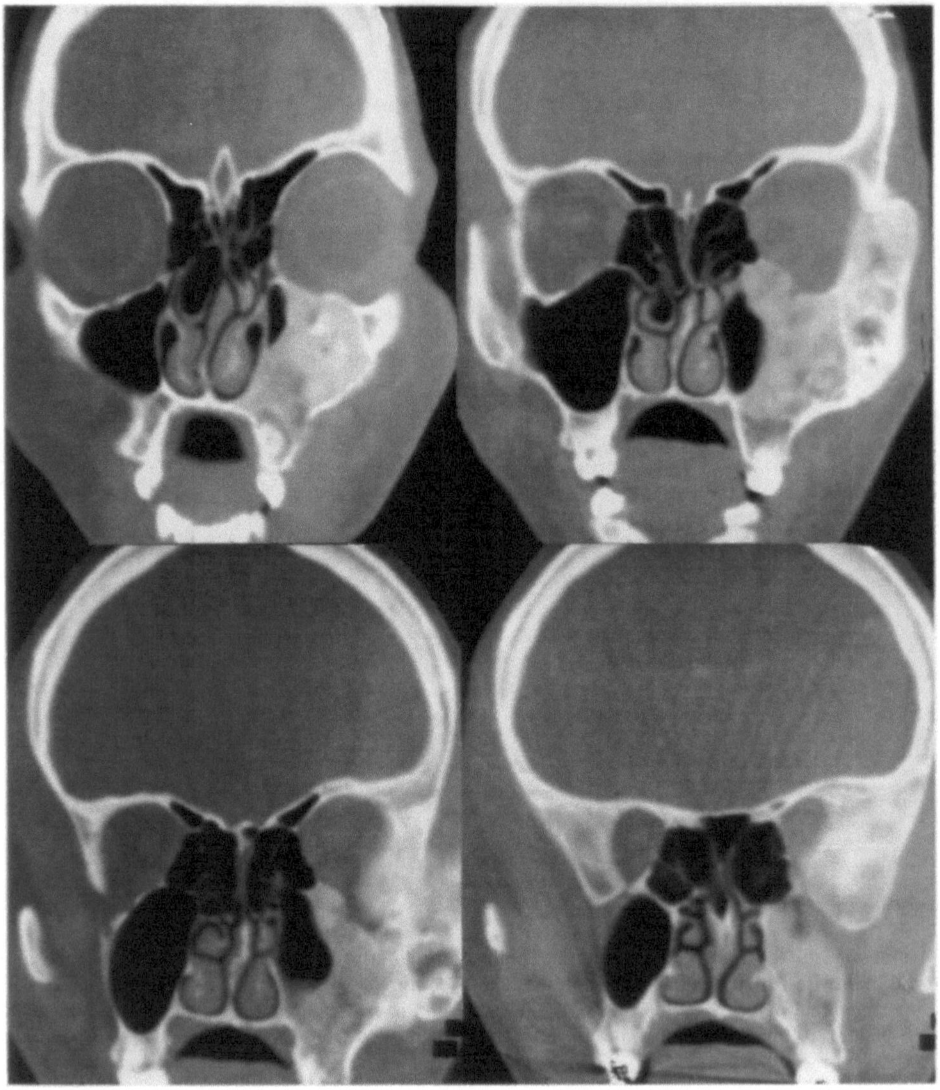

Fig. E8. Fibrous dysplasia in a 24-year-old woman with a 4-year history of swelling in the right half of the face with expansion of bone. Coronal CT (bone window) demonstrates a mass of calcific density in the right maxillary sinus with extension to the right zygoma and lower right portions of the cranial vault. The right orbital roof is also involved. Only the medial portion of the right maxillary sinus is still pneumatized

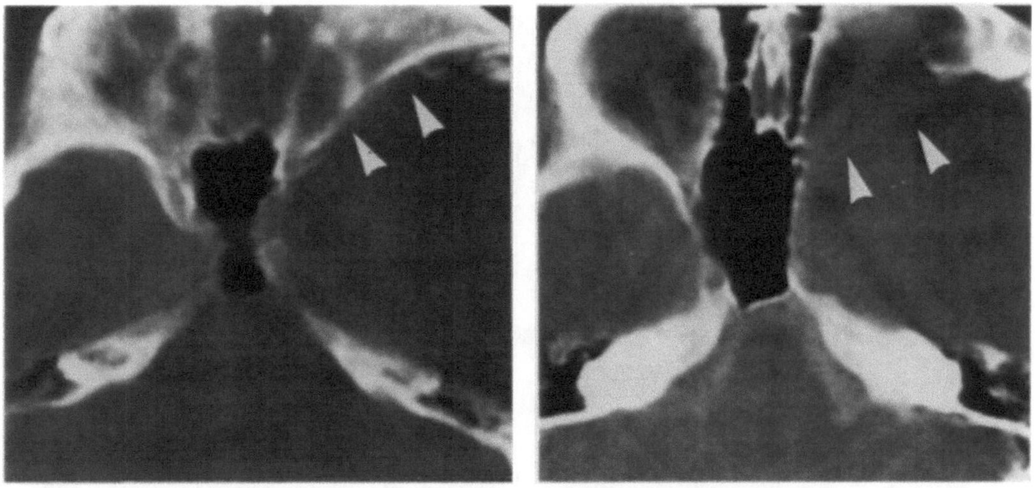

Fig. E9. Von Recklinghausen's neurofibromatosis. *Left:* The right middle fossa is enlarged by anterior displacement of the lesser sphenoid wing (*arrowheads*). *Right:* Aplasia of the greater sphenoid wing (*arrowheads*)

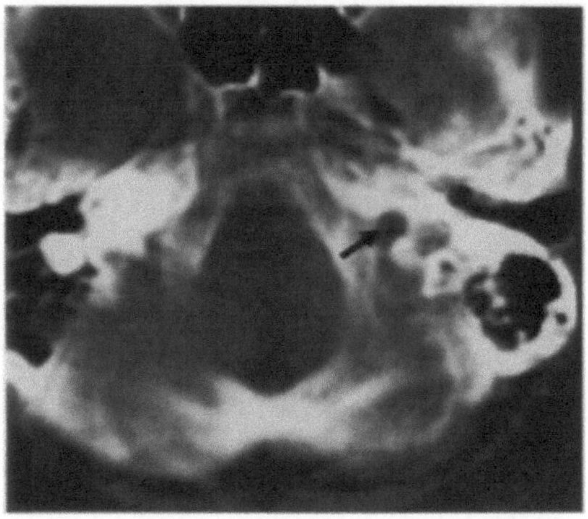

Fig. E10. Small glomus tumor at the right jugular foramen producing a conspicuous defect in the base of the pyramid (*arrow*). The destruction provides indirect evidence of the tumor

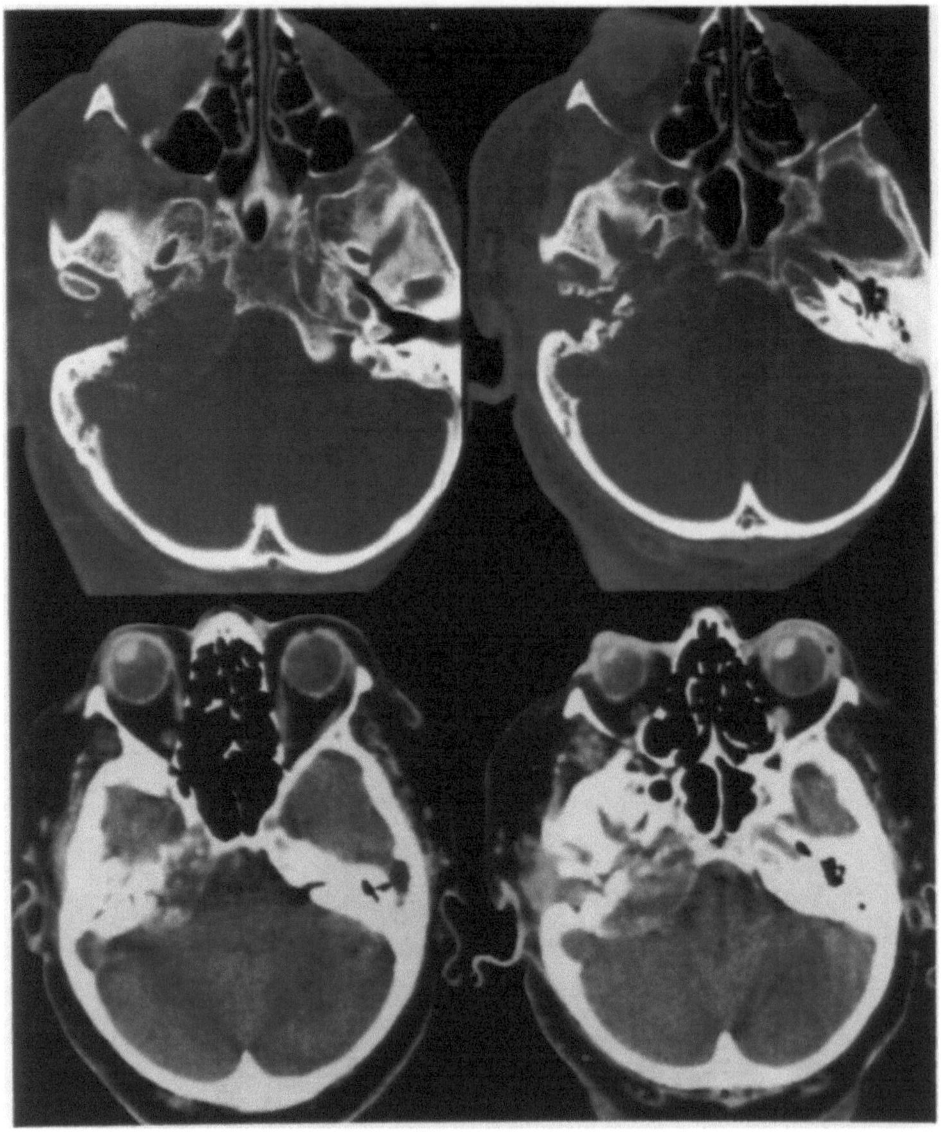

Fig. E11. Paraganglioma arising from the glomus jugulare in a 64-year-old woman with a 1-year history of progressive hearing loss and paresis of the fourth to twelfth cranial nerves. CT: *top* high-resolution scan, *bottom* soft-tissue window. The scans show complete destruction of the petrous bone and clivus on the left side and of adjacent skull base structures about the infratemporal fossa. The soft-tissue window (*bottom*) reveals tumor extension into the cerebellopontine angle with displacement of adjacent brain structures and additional soft components in the external ear canal

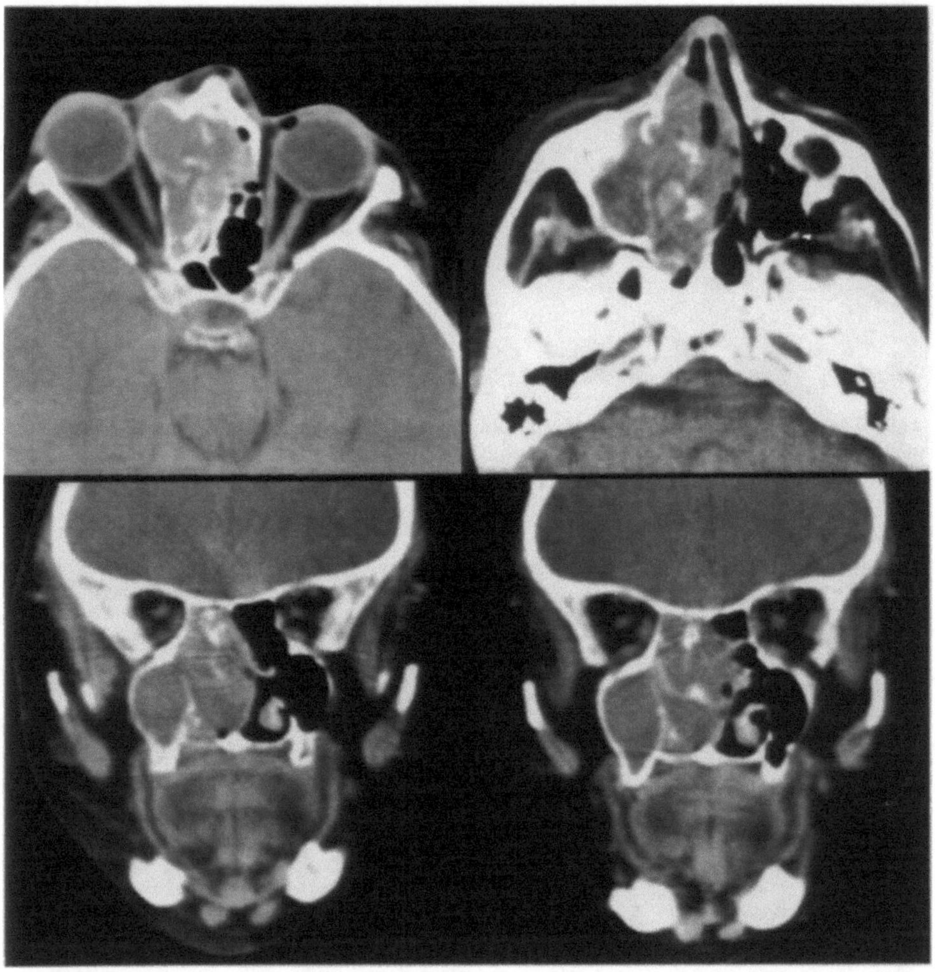

Fig. E12. Large tumor of the glomus pterygoideus involving the left maxillary sinus and ethmoid cells in a 40-year-old man with impaired nasal respiration and periodic epistaxis. CT: *top* axial, *bottom* coronal. Scans reveal a soft-tissue mass in the left maxillary sinus and left ethmoid cells with associated destruction of the medial antral wall and ethmoid structures. The tumor protrudes into the left orbit, causing proptosis. Bony structures of calcific density are visible in the tumor

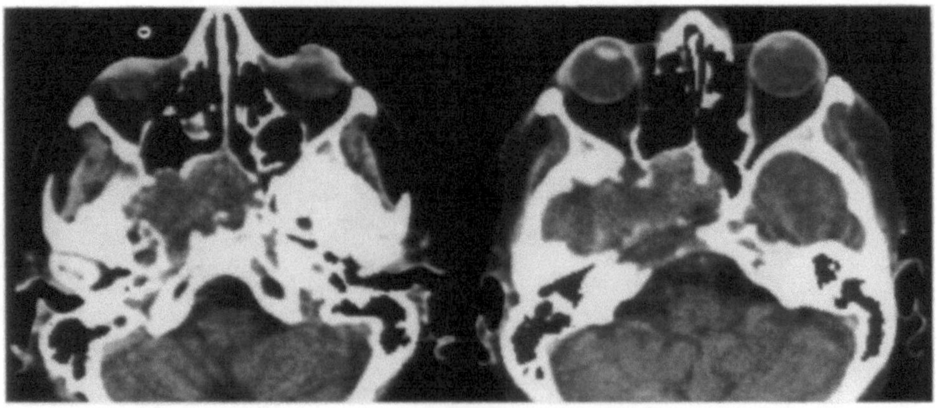

Fig. E13a. Parasellar chordoma in a 49-year-old woman. CT documents destruction of the sphenoid sinus and left pyramidal apex with extension into the middle fossa. Scattered calcifications are present in the tumor

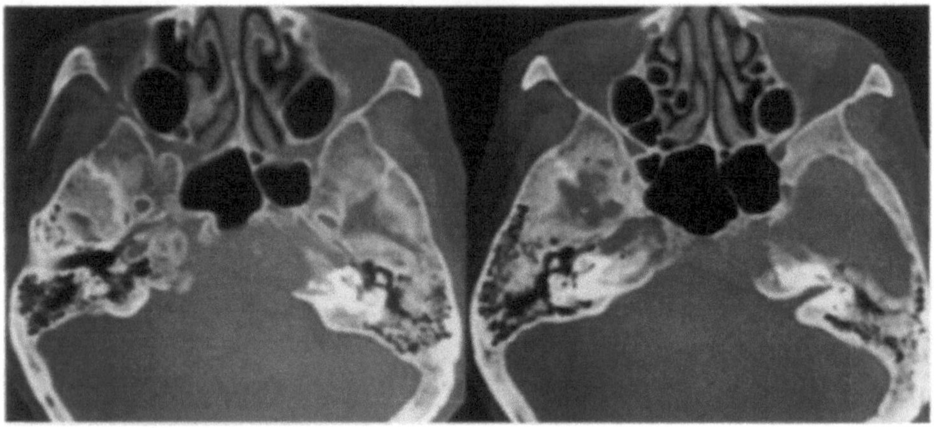

Fig. E13b. Clivus chordoma in a 42-year-old man. High-resolution CT shows pronounced destruction of the clivus and right pyramidal apex

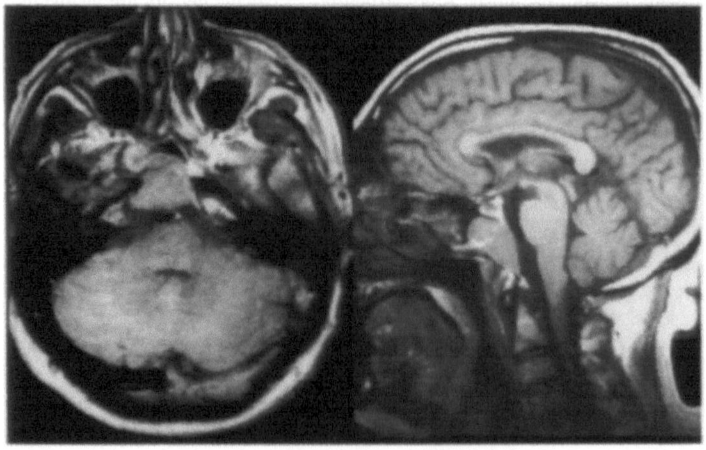

Fig. E14. Plasmocytoma of the clivus in a 62-year-old man with known generalized plasmocytoma. SE 500/30 sequences (*right* sagittal) demonstrate a clearly delineated tumor in the clivus region. Its signal intensity approximates that of brain tissue on the T1-weighted scans

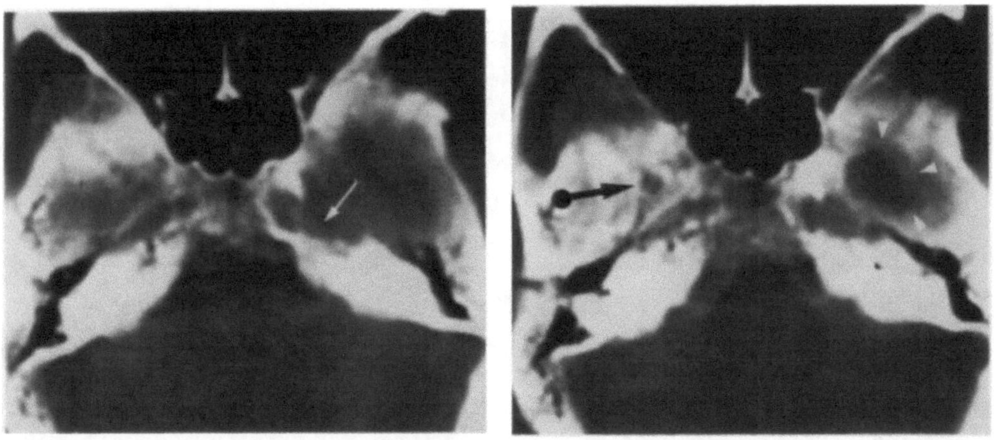

Fig. E 15. Trigeminal neurinoma on the right side. The *left* scan shows erosion of the anterior border of the pyramid. The *right* scan shows extreme expansion of the right foramen ovale (*white arrowheads*). Note the normal foramen ovale on the left side (*black arrow*)

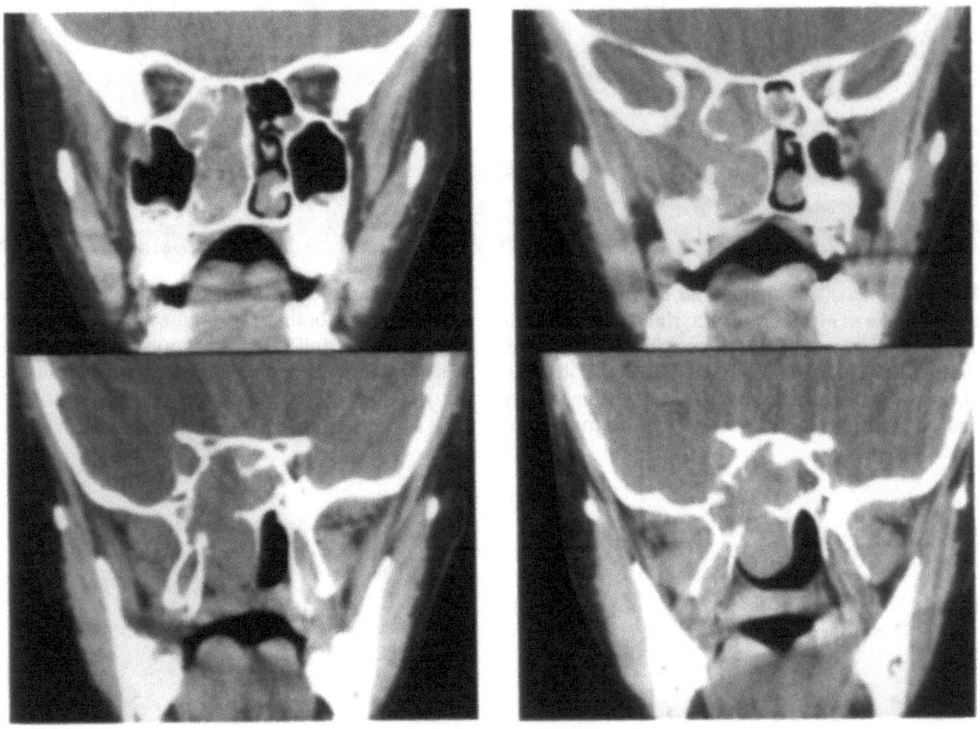

Fig. E 16. Juvenile angiofibroma in a 15-year-old male with recurrent epistaxis. Coronal CT demonstrates a large soft-tissue mass in the sphenoid sinus, left nasal cavity, and epipharynx with erosive bone changes and destruction of the lateral and caudal boundaries of the sphenoid sinus. The tumor has also eroded the superior portion of the pterygoid process

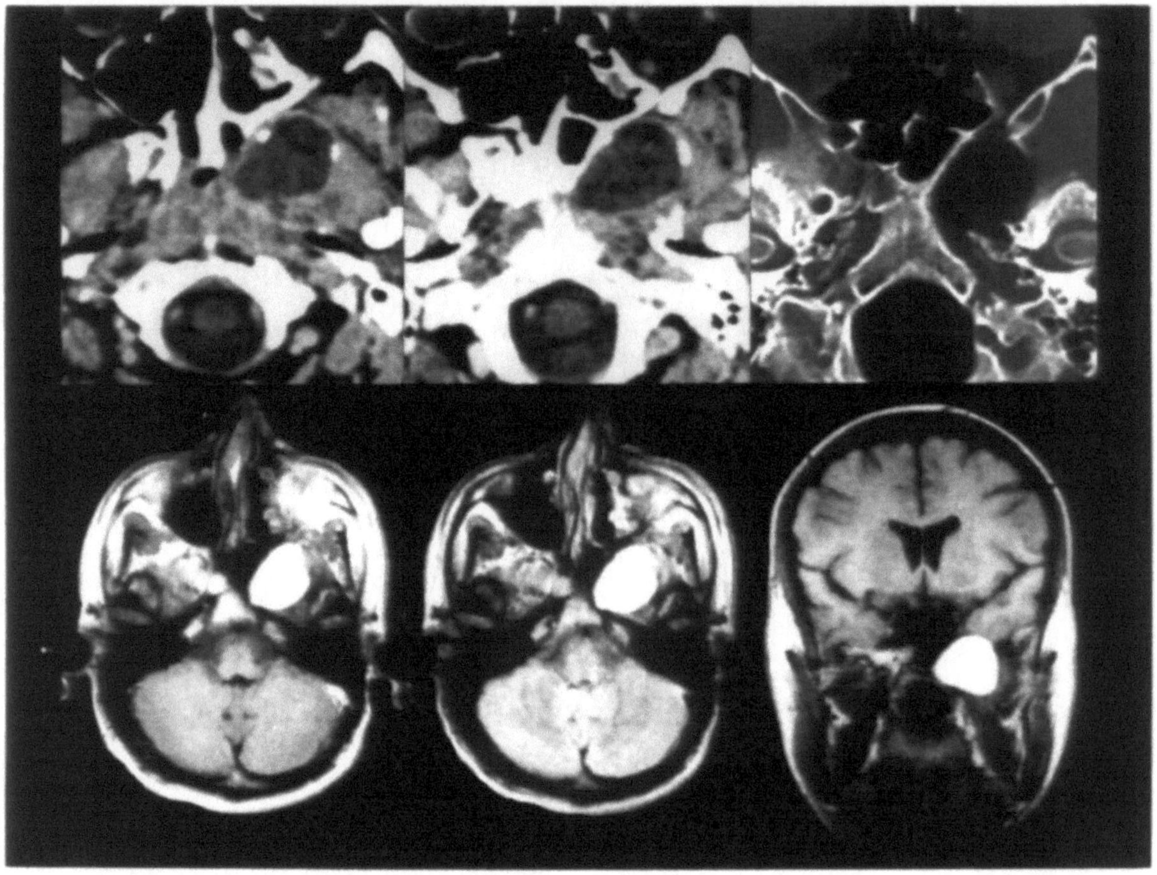

a–c

d–f

Fig. E17a–f. Retromaxillary epidermoid cyst in a 39-year-old man who underwent removal of a right-sided angiofibroma 25 years earlier. CT: **a, b** retromaxillary space, **c** skull base with bone window. MR: **d, e** SE 400/30; **f** SE 400/30 coronal. Scans demonstrate a retromaxillary mass lesion on the right side with associated destruction of the skull base but no infiltration of the ethmoid cells, sphenoid sinus, or brain. The tumor is hypodense on CT with plaque-like peripheral calcification. T1-weighted MR shows a smooth-bordered mass whose hyperintensity reflects the fatty consistency of the tumor

Fig. E18a–e. Malignant lymphoma of the sphenoid sinus and sella in a 75-year-old man with dysfunctions of the third to fifth cranial nerves on the left side. CT: **a** axial, **b** coronal. MR: **c** SE 700/30 axial, **d** SE 700/30 coronal, **e** SE 700/30 sagittal. A large soft-tissue mass presents in the region of the sphenoid sinus and sella, more prominent on the left side. CT shows associated destruction of the anterior clivus and adjacent skull-base structures. T1-weighted MR demonstrates a mixed-intensity lesion that is hypointense to brain parenchyma

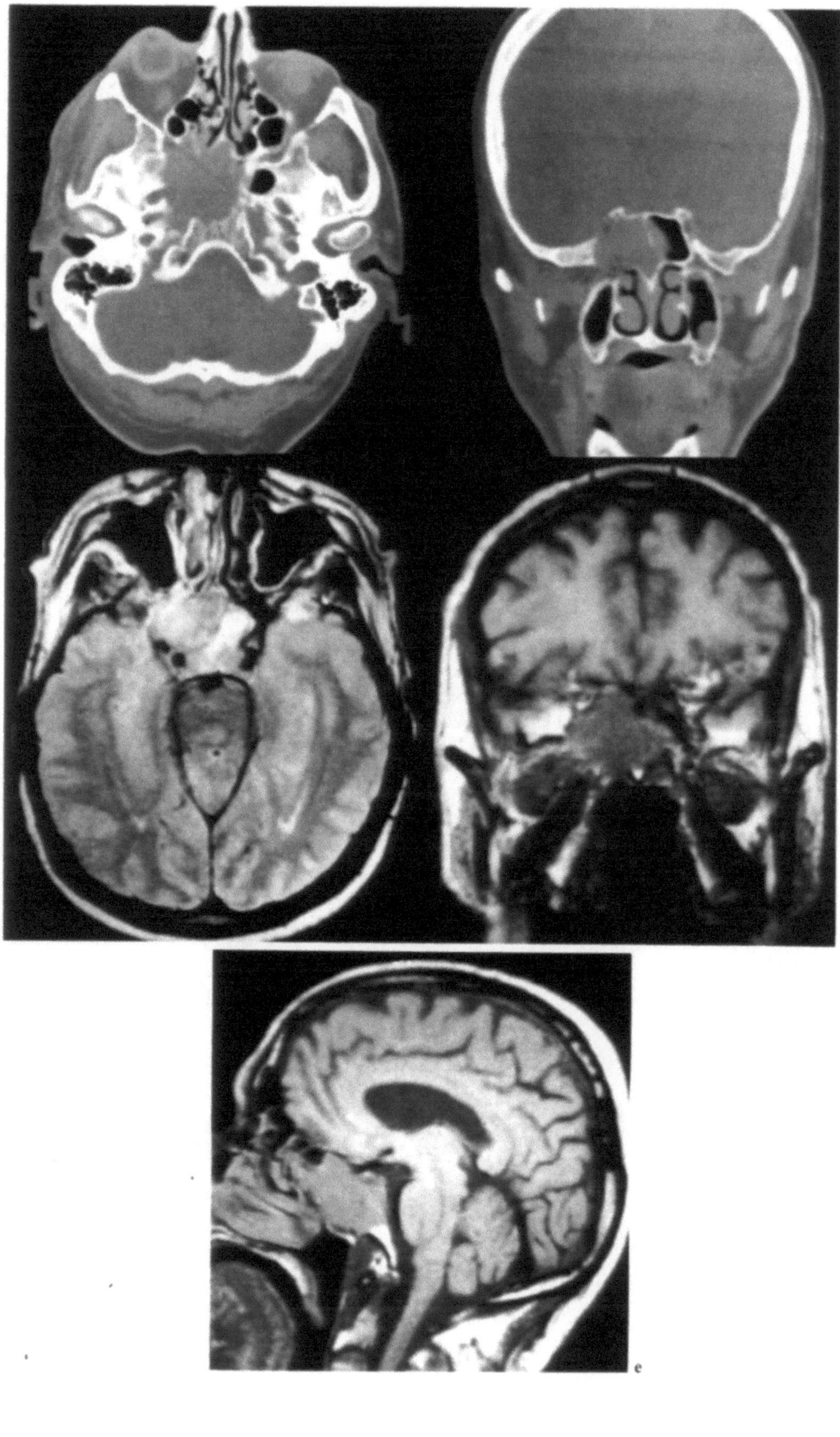

a b c d e

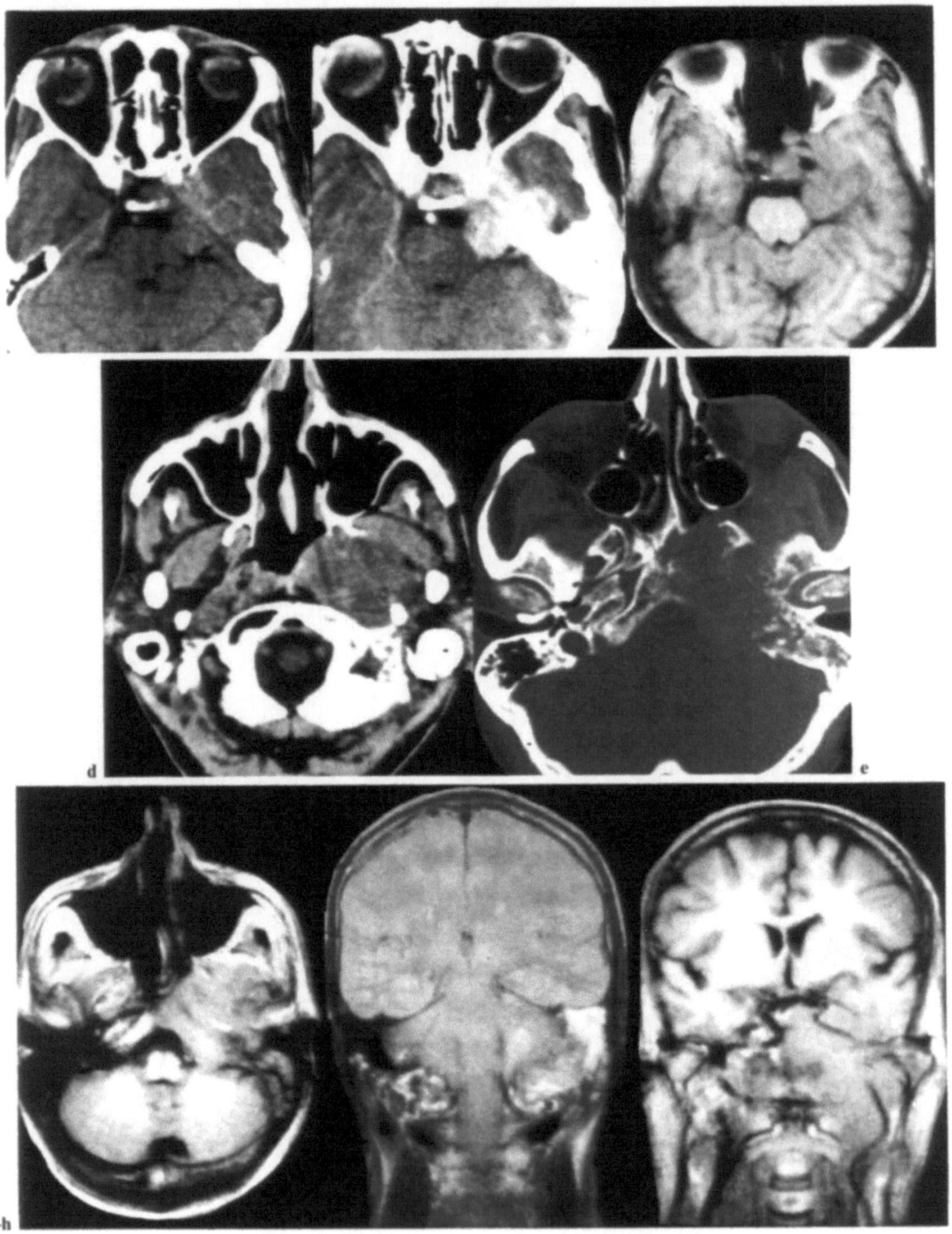

a–c

d

e

f–h

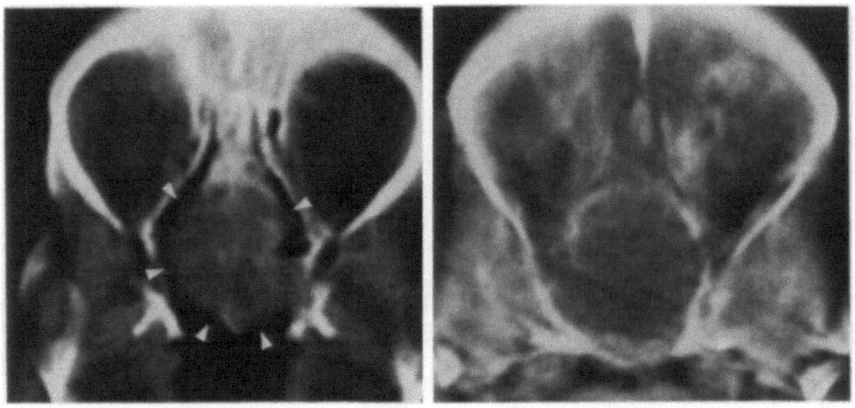

Fig. E 20. Rhabdomyosarcoma of the nasopharynx. *Left*: The nasopharynx is completely filled by tumor (*arrowheads*), and the vomer is destroyed. *Right*: infiltration of the anterior fossa by tumor

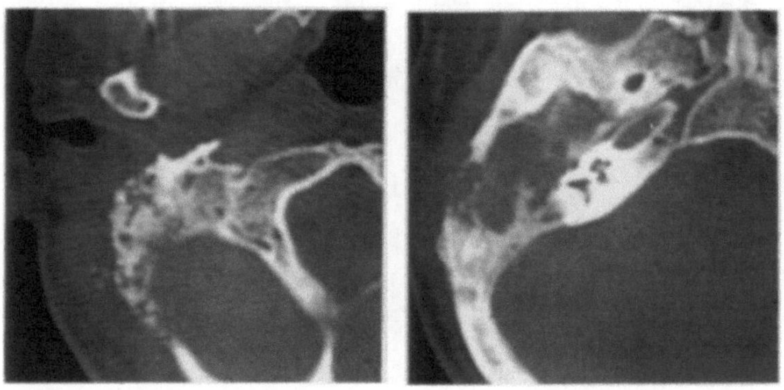

Fig. E 21. Squamous cell carcinoma of the left external auditory canal in a 79-year-old woman. CT with a bone window setting shows marked destructive changes in the left mastoid with extension to the pyramid

Fig. E 19 a–h. Esthesioneuroblastoma of the right retromaxillary space with destruction of the skull base and extension into the neurocranium in a 56-year-old man with right-sided cranial nerve dysfunctions. CT: **a** axial precontrast, **b** axial postcontrast, **d** facial skeleton, **e** skull base (bone window). MR: **c** SE 315/14 axial, **f** SE 315/14 axial, **g** SE 2000/70 coronal, **h** SE 315/14 coronal. CT demonstrates a large soft-tissue mass occupying the retromaxillary space and protruding into the nasopharynx (**d**). There is significant destruction of the right skull base and clivus (**e**). Postcontrast CT (**b**) shows a densely enhancing intracranial component extending into the posterior and middle fossae. T1-weighted images (**c, f, h**) demonstrate a soft-tissue mass arising from the facial skeleton and extending into the neurocranium. It is roughly isointense to brain. Part of the internal carotid artery is delineated within the tumor area (**h**). The cervical segment of the vessel (below the skull base) is displaced laterally by the tumor; the siphon portion is elevated and also displaced laterally. While CT shows only a soft-tissue density in the mastoid region (**b**), T2-weighted coronal MR (**g**) shows a hyperintense area in the right mastoid signifying an inflammatory response of the mastoid cells. This signal pattern is specific for inflammation and excludes tumor infiltration of the mastoid

a b c d

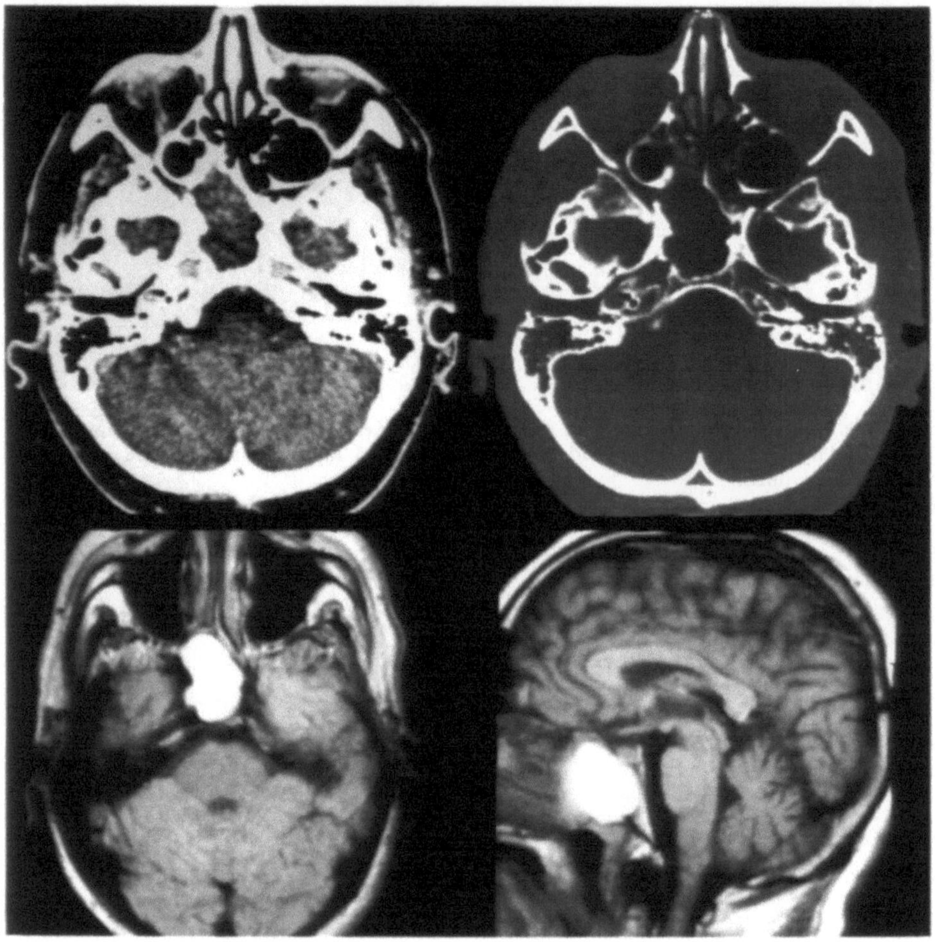

Fig. E22a–d. Mucocele of the sphenoid sinus in a 47-year-old man with radiographic opacity of the sphenoid sinus for 1 year and recurrent bouts of subfebrile temperatures. CT: **a, b** axial (**b** high-resolution). MR: **c** SE 400/35 axial, **d** SE 400/35 sagittal. CT demonstrates soft-tissue opacity of the sphenoid sinus. The bone-window scan (**b**) shows erosive bone change and expansion of the sphenoid sinus. The T1-weighted images show a hyperintense, smooth-bordered mass completely filling the sphenoid sinus. The signal pattern is consistent with fatty material. Mucocele was confirmed at operation

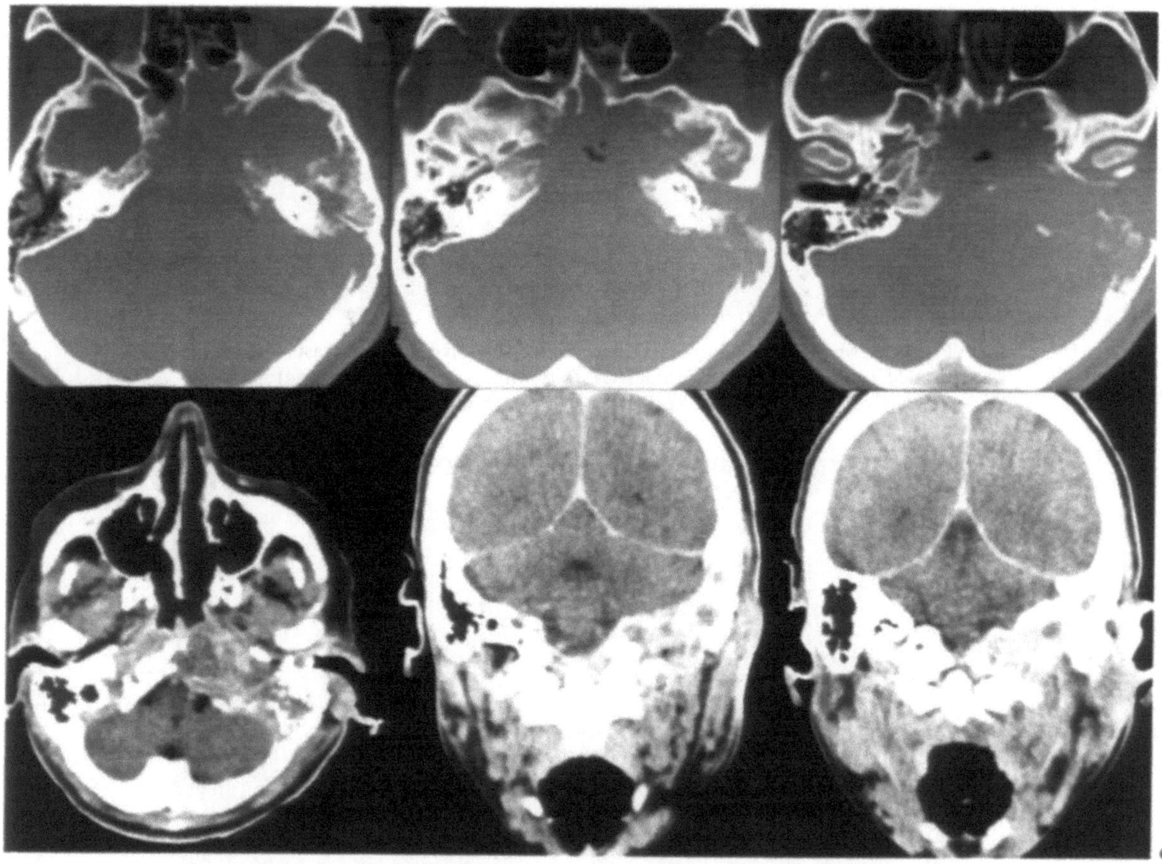

Fig. E 23 a–f. Metastasis from an unknown primary tumor in a 45-year-old woman with profound labyrinthine hearing loss on the right side. CT: **a–c** bone window setting, **d** axial, **e, f** coronal. The tumor has eroded through the skull base, destroying the right petrous bone and portions of the clivus on the right side. Some destruction of the cranial vault is also apparent. Postcontrast scans (**d–f**) define the tumor clearly despite its low enhancement. The lesion extends into the middle and posterior fossae and displaces the brainstem to the left

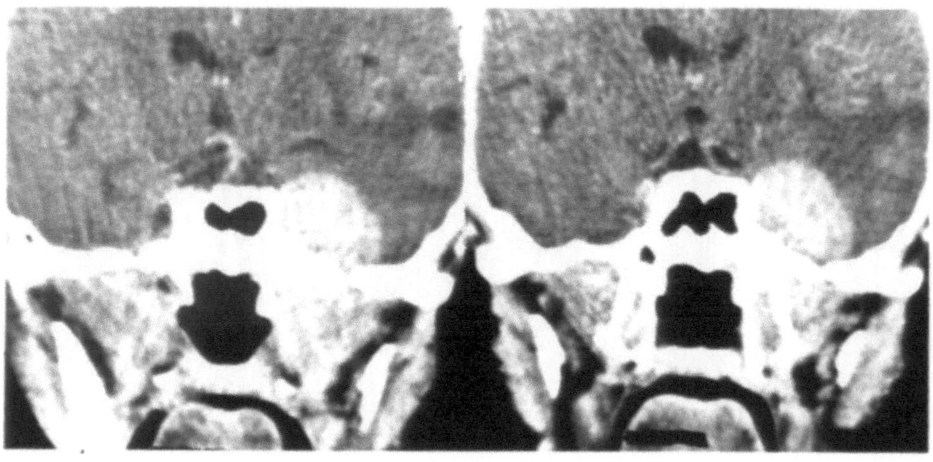

Fig. E 24. Metastatic carcinoma in a 64-year-old woman with breast cancer. Postcontrast coronal CT shows a clearly delineated densely enhancing tumor of the right parasellar region arising from the skull base and lateral sphenoid sinus wall. Differentiation from meningioma is required

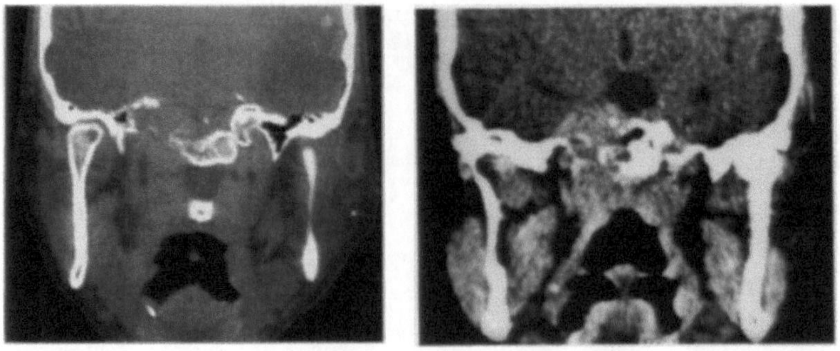

Fig. E25. Metastatis from an undifferentiated, invasive ductal breast carcinoma in a 55-year-old man (!). Coronal CT (*left* with bone window setting) shows a destructive tumor in the left skull base region with infiltration of the clivus

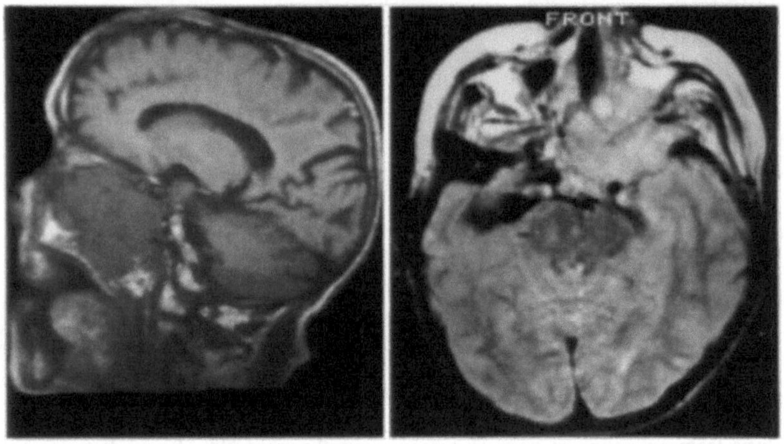

Fig. E26. Metastasis from an unknown primary (adenocarcinoma) in a 78-year-old man with local otorhinolaryngologic complaints. MR: *left* SE 500/30, *right* SE 3000/30. The tumor is hypointense to brain parenchyma on the T1-weighted image (*left*) and shows increased signal intensity on the proton-density sequence (*right*). The lesion completely fills the retromaxillary space and sphenoid sinus. Images also show infiltration of the sella and destruction of the skull base and sphenoid wing. The tumor extends to the right temporal lobe but does not infiltrate it; a sharp line of demarcation is seen between the tumor and temporal lobe

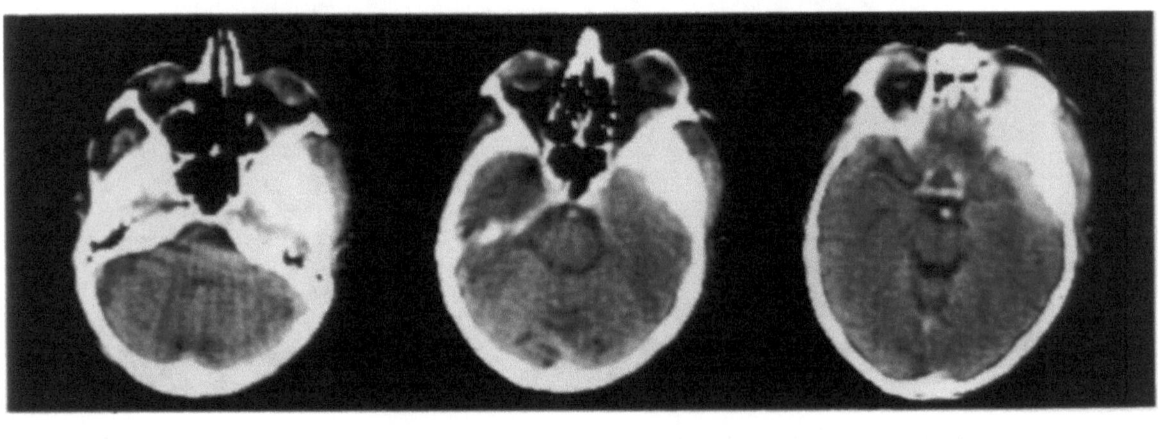

Fig. E27. Osteoplastic metastasis of prostatic carcinoma in a 76-year-old man with a soft swelling in the right temporal region. Postcontrast CT demonstrates marked thickening and increased density of the skull base, sphenoid, orbital roof, and temporal bone on the right side. The soft-tissue mass enhances densely and has both extra- and intracranial components

2. Cranial Vault

Plain skull X-rays continue to be the mainstay in the diagnosis of neoplastic disease of the cranial vault. CT serves only as an adjunct to conventional radiography and is especially useful for demonstrating coexisting soft-tissue components of the tumor. MR generally is not used for these investigations, because the bony structures of the outer and inner tables give almost no signal. The diploe, on the other hand, gives an intense signal due to its fat content, and so MR may have adjunctive value for certain diagnostic problems (e.g., plasmocytoma, epidermoid, or dermoid of the cranial vault) in cases where radiographic and CT findings are inconclusive.

The following tumors can cause bony changes in the cranial vault that are visible on the CT scan:

- Osteomas
- Paget's disease
- Hemangiomas of the cranial roof
- Aneurysmatic bone cysts
- Epidermoids and dermoids
- Meningiomas, including malignant forms
- Malignant lymphomas
- Plasmocytomas
- Metastases from carcinoma and other malignancies (e.g., neuroblastoma)

The skull is a common location for **osteomas**. Schwartz (1940) states that they account for approximately 1% of all cranial neoplasms. The majority develop in the frontal and ethmoid sinuses (see Fig. D 7.2), but some arise from the diploe of the cranial roof (see Chap. D 7, Fig. D 7.1). The superior border of the pyramid or petrous apex is also an occasional site of occurrence. Osteomas grow very slowly and rarely cause clinical symptoms. Many are detected incidentally. They are recognized on CT scans by their very high, uniform density which matches that of cortical bone. Osteoma may be difficult or impossible to distinguish from a heavily calcified meningioma.

Capillary and cavernous **hemangiomas of the cranial vault** produce characteristic radiologic changes. CT shows expansion of the cranial bone and depicts the trabecular internal structure of the vascular tumor (Fig. E 28).

Aneurysmatic bone cyst is a tumorlike lesion that most commonly affects the long bones (femur and tibia). Occurrence in flat bones is generally restricted to the spinal column. Aneurysmatic bone cysts in the cranial vault are rare and would represent either an "idiopathic" (primary aneurysmatic) bone cyst or a form developing in association with a benign or malignant bone tumor (secondary aneurysmatic bone cyst) (Freyschmidt 1980). Generally the diagnosis is established by plain X-rays. Conventional X-rays as well as CT scans demonstrate a thinning of the cortex, which is invested by a thin sheet of tense, calcified periosteum. The affected area is sharply demarcated from uninvolved bone, and the boundary is occasionally marked by a narrow sclerotic rim (Fig. E 29).

Epidermoids and **dermoids** likewise produce bone changes so characteristic that the plain skull X-ray is generally diagnostic. The lesion itself appears as a hypodense area on CT. Epidermoids arising in the diploe merit special mention. Dermoid cysts in the orbitotemporal region are associated with characteristic bone changes. These tumors arise from displaced embryonic ectodermal elements and tend to occur in the "closure lines" of the skull.

Meningiomas frequently cause changes in the cranial vault, including enostosis and thickening of the calvarium over the tumor. Some meningiomas grow mainly within the cranial vault, expanding and deforming the bone (see Fig. D 2.15). Usually there is an associated soft-tissue component that is clearly visualized with CT. Smaller meningiomas of the cranial vault cause a more circumscribed expansion (Fig. E 30). Again, an intracranial soft-tissue component is very often present.

Malignant meningiomas and **meningeal sarcomas** likewise can produce bone changes ranging from destruction of the bony architecture to expansion of the bone. Affected areas generally have lower attenuation values than normal bone.

Malignant lymphomas may originate in the cranial vault, causing destruction of the bony architecture and creating a soft-tissue mass that may extend to the scalp as well as intracranially, although it usually does not transgress the meninges (Fig. E 31).

A similar picture is seen with **plasmocytoma**, which destroys normal bone structures and on CT creates a lens-shaped soft-tissue mass interposed between the well-defined ends of the cranial defect (Fig. E32).

Metastatic carcinoma destroys normal bone and replaces it with tumor tissue. The osteolytic foci usually present ill-defined borders on X-ray and have a similar appearance on CT, which can also demonstrate the metastatic tumor itself (Figs. E33–35). Metastases in the cranium may be solitary, although multiple lesions are more common and may cause extensive bone destruction (Fig. E35). Osteolytic metastases in the cranial vault are most common in patients with bronchial carcinoma, hypernephroma, breast carcinoma, and thyroid carcinoma. Conventional radiography is superior to CT for the detection of multiple small metastases in the cranial vault. Plain skull X-rays in two projections furnish a diagnosis with considerably less time and effort than would be required for a CT examination.

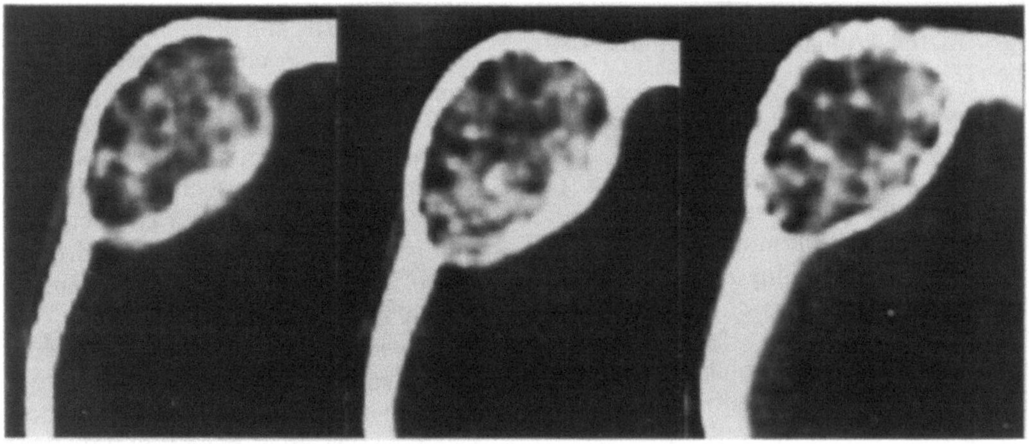

Fig. E28. Cavernous hemangioma of the cranial vault in a 15-year-old boy. CT shows fusiform expansion of the skull wall with minimal damage to the outer and inner tables. The vascular tumor presents the typical trabecular architecture of bone (magnified views with a window width of 400 HU)

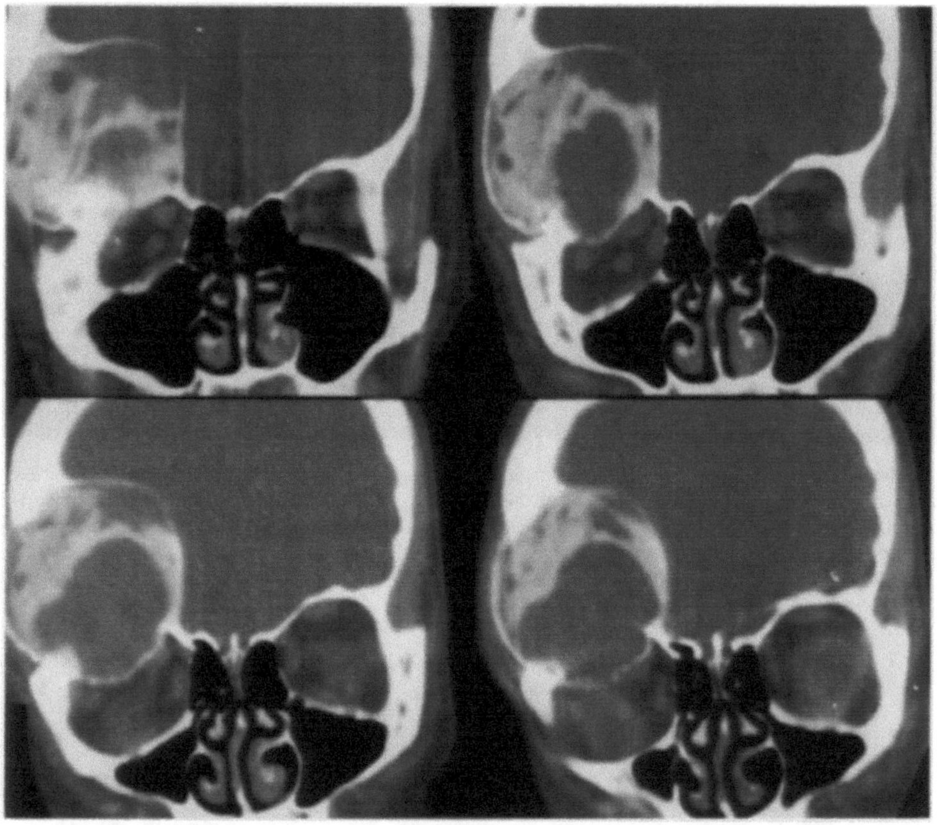

Fig. E29. Aneurysmatic bone cyst in a 26-year-old woman with a bulge in the region of the left temporal squama and left orbital roof. Coronal CT with a bone window reveals a pronounced structural change in the orbital boundaries. The orbital floor is displaced forward into the right maxillary sinus. The orbital roof is indented, and the external boundaries of the orbit appear enlarged. However, the orbital volume is diminished, resulting in proptosis. There is plaque-like hyperostosis with partial thinning of the cortex. The structure of the bone is irregular and rarefied, but there are no destructive changes sufficient to disrupt continuity

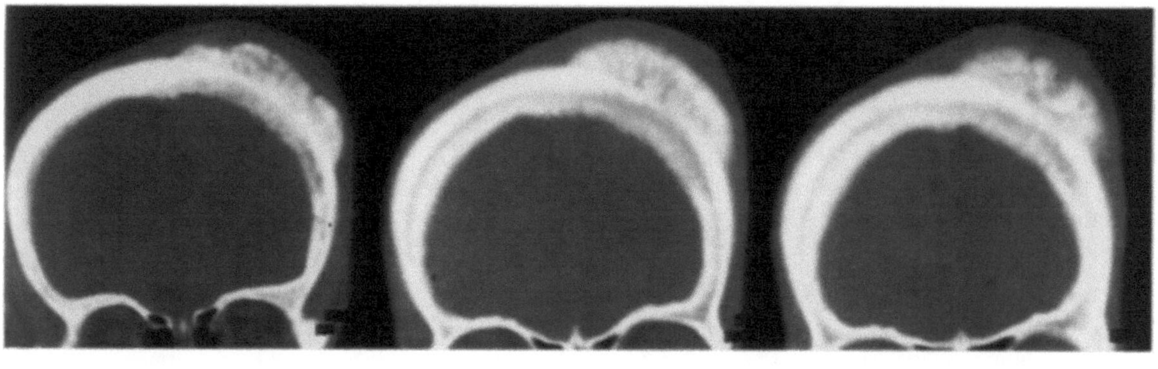

Fig. E30. Meningioma of the right parietal region in a 67-year-old man with headache and a noticeable bulge in the parietal cranium that had been present for several months. Coronal CT shows spicular expansion of the outer table of the skull in the right parietal area. The bone shows marked structural irregularities in the region of the inner table. The lesion proved to be a meningioma with intra- and extracranial extension

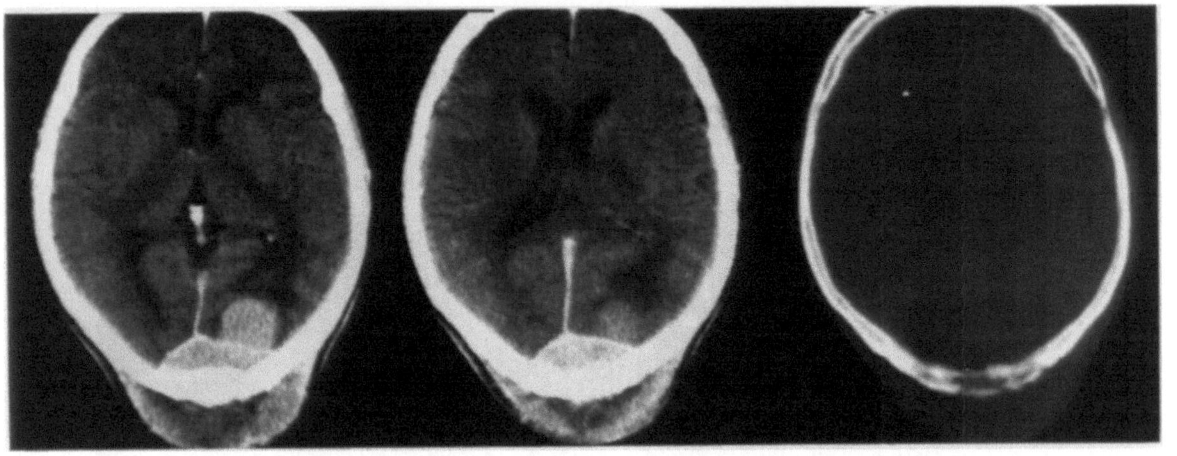

Fig. E31. Centroblastic non-Hodgkin's lymphoma in a 43-year-old man with no neurologic symptoms and a soft bulge on the occiput. Postcontrast CT: The scan at the bone-window setting (*right*) shows destruction of the occipital cranial vault. The scans at standard settings show bilateral tumor enhancement that is especially marked on the right side. An extracranial occipital mass of soft-tissue density is also visible. The low density in the right occipital area signifies peritumoral edema

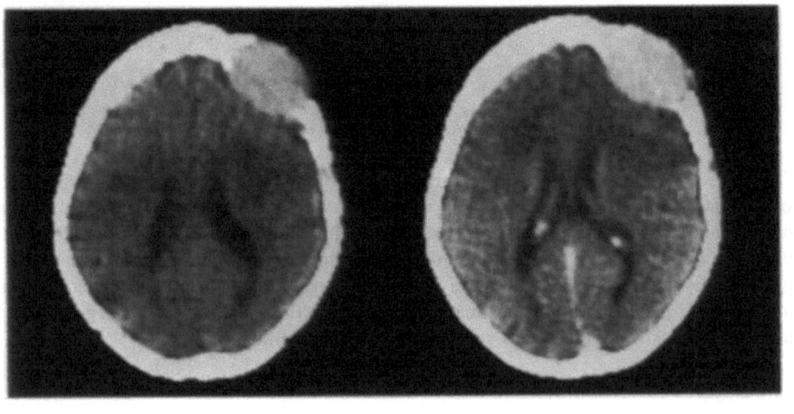

Fig. E32. Plasmocytoma of the cranial vault in a 64-year-old woman. The tumor has produced a sharply defined area of bone destruction in the region of the right frontal bone. The bone ends flank a spindle-shaped soft-tissue mass that shows marked contrast enhancement (*left* precontrast, *right* postcontrast)

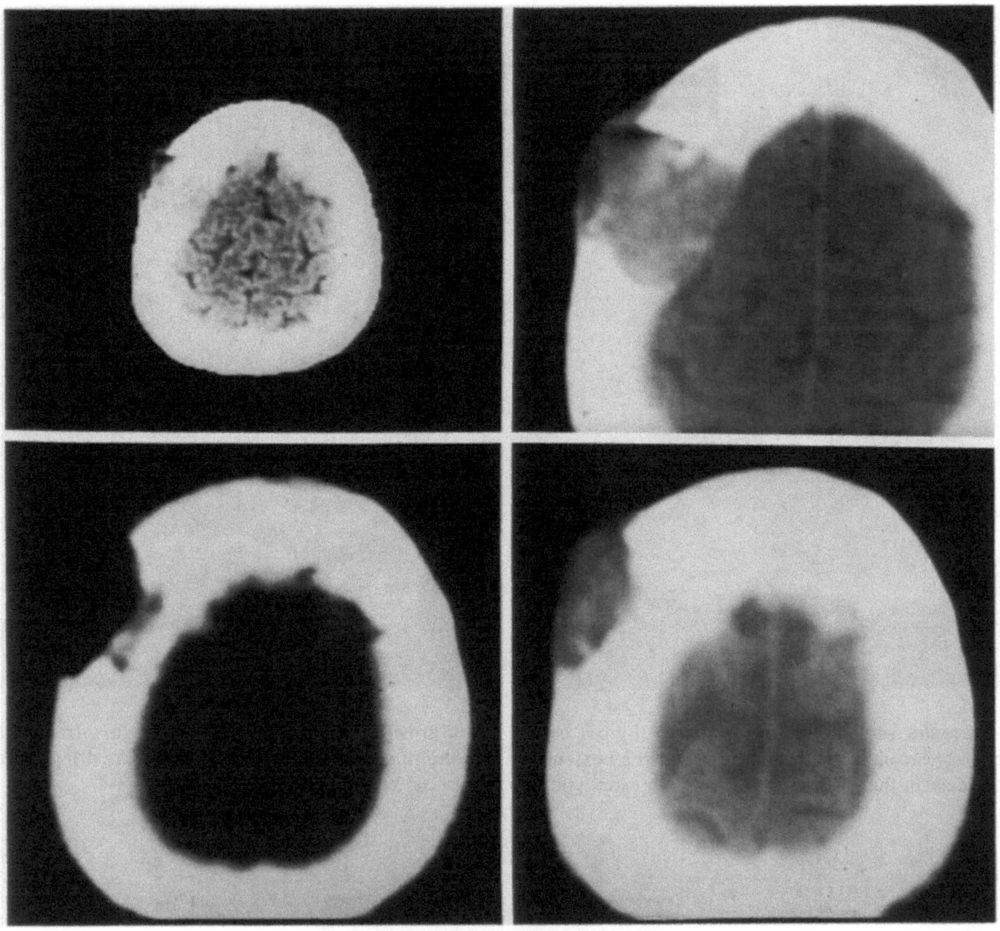

a b c d

Fig. E33. Metastatic carcinoma at the junction of the frontal and parietal bones on the left side. **a** Standard CT scan shows only a minor irregularity in the left frontoparietal contour of the skull. **b** Magnification of the same slice with a wider window (400 HU) reveals full-thickness permeation of the bone by metastatic tumor. **c** The next higher slice viewed with a bone window shows an ill-defined bony defect. **d** The soft-tissue window demonstrates extension of soft tumor tissue into the subcutaneous layer

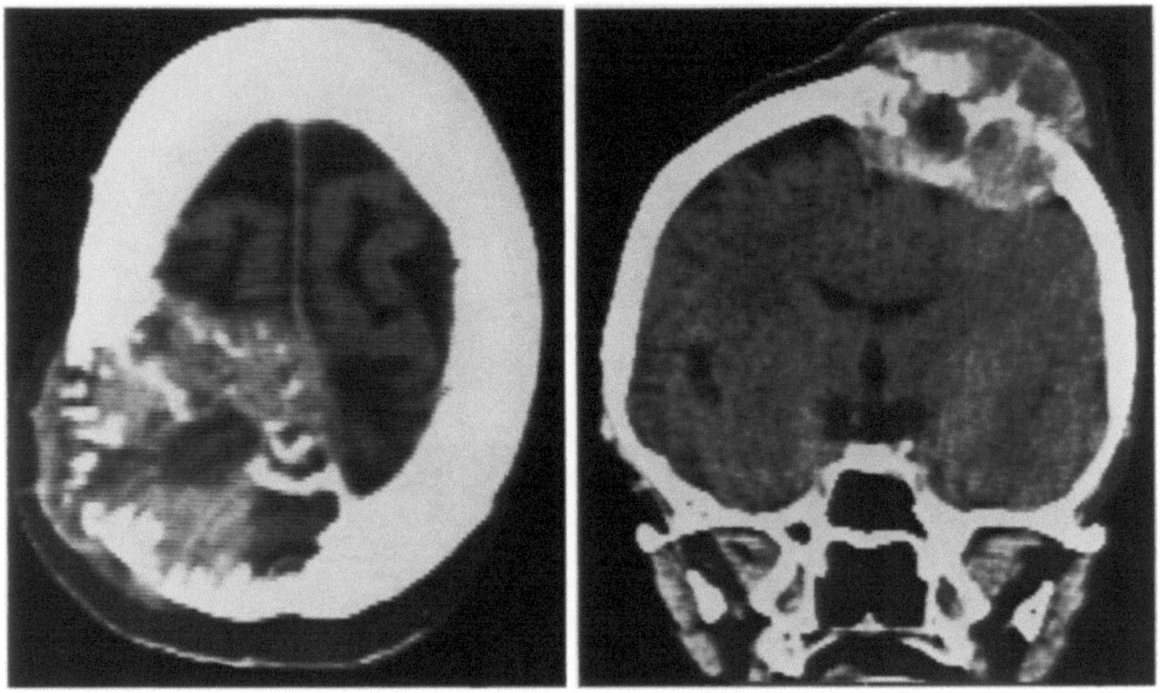

Fig. E34. Cranial vault tumor metastatic to thyroid carcinoma in a 62-year-old woman. Axial CT shows an extensive osteolytic focus in the left parietal region with exophytic tumor growth. The coronal scan shows the intracranial extent of the tumor, which is sharply demarcated from brain. The dura mater was intact at operation

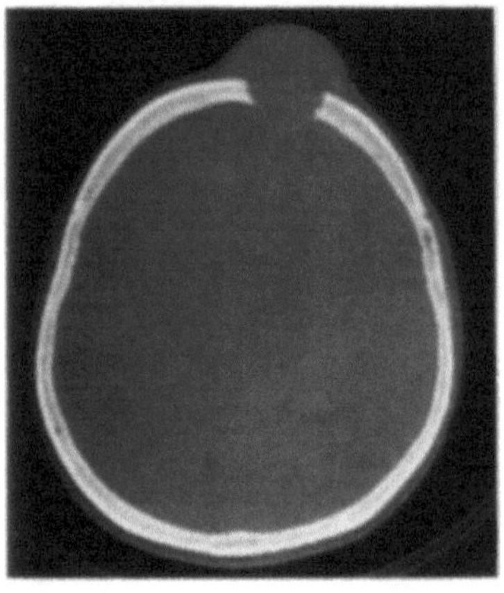

Fig. E35. Osteolytic metastasis of thyroid carcinoma in a 62-year-old woman with a soft-tissue bulge in the right frontal region adjacent to the midline. CT shows a conspicuous bone defect with a soft extracranial tumor component

F. CT and MR Imaging of Non-neoplastic Intracranial Masses

Many intracranial mass lesions of non-neoplastic origin present CT and MR features similar or identical to those of true neoplasms. In many cases a definitive diagnosis cannot be made from imaging findings alone, and misinterpretation is possible even when the history and clinical findings are considered. Yet an accurate preoperative diagnosis is an essential prerequisite for selecting candidates for a neurosurgical operation and planning the procedure. In some cases the full range of neuroradiologic techniques may have to be applied and evaluated in the context of clinical findings before the physician can accurately classify the disease and draw appropriate therapeutic conclusions.

The major non-neoplastic diseases that can produce an intracranial mass are listed in Table 11. The most important groups are *inflammatory diseases*, *granulomatous diseases*, and *cysts*, as these are most likely to mimic the features of an intracranial neoplasm.

Parasitic diseases with cerebral involvement are extremely rare at our latitudes but still should be considered in the differential diagnosis. Conditions that can mimic recurrent tumor growth include wall changes in the *surgical cavity* in the initial weeks following a tumor resection and *radionecrosis* developing in the aftermath of therapeutic irradiation.

Certain stages and presentations of *acute demyelinating diseases* can raise problems of differential diagnosis on CT and MR. Some cases resemble a neoplastic or metastatic process, while others resemble vascular disease.

CT and MR provide complementary information in the diagnosis of *acute and chronic intracranial hemorrhages* of any etiology. Acute hematoma is usually easy to recognize on CT, since the high density of the hemorrhage and the antecedent history almost always suggest the correct diagnosis. Chronic hematomas with isodense contents, especially when subdural, may have the CT presentation of an indeterminate mass lesion. Hematomas at this stage, however, are easily identified with MR.

Table 11. Non-neoplastic intracranial masses included in the differential diagnosis of brain tumors

1. **Inflammatory diseases**
   Brain abscess
   Subdural empyema, epidural abscess
   Meningoencephalitis
2. **Granulomatous diseases**
   Gummas
   Tuberculomas
   Granulomas in Boeck's disease
3. **Parasitic diseases**
   Cysticercosis
   Echinococcosis
4. **Brain diseases associated with AIDS**
5. **Cysts**
   Arachnoid cysts
   Dandy-Walker syndrome
   Other cysts
   Primary aqueduct stenosis, obstructions of the foramina of Luschka and Magendie
6. **Postoperative lesions**
   Radionecrosis
7. **Acute demyelinating diseases**
   Disseminated encephalomyelitis
   Diffuse sclerosis
8. **Intracranial hemorrhages**
   Spontaneous intracranial hemorrhages
   Old hemorrhages, chocolate cysts
   Chronic subdural hematoma
9. **Vascular malformations**
   Aneurysms
   Arteriovenous angiomas
   Sturge-Weber syndrome
   Basilar artery ectasia
10. **Cerebral infarction (arterial and venous)**
    Postinfarction edema with mass effect
    Cerebral infarction in the stage of disturbance of the blood-brain barrier
    Postinfarction hemorrhage with mass effect
    Cerebral venous or sinus thrombosis with edema and/or hemorrhage

Large *angiomas* and *aneurysms* likewise can mimic the appearance of a brain tumor. Specific CT criteria and the MR signal characteristics of thrombosis or flowing blood are helpful in these cases.

Enhancing *cerebral infarcts* examined in the stage of blood-brain barrier disruption and luxury perfusion pose a special diagnostic problem. Confusion with a brain tumor is not uncommon. Circumscribed cerebral venous thrombosis also may present as a space-occupying lesion.

In a special review of 7543 CT examinations which disclosed 1017 brain tumors we encountered such problems of differential diagnosis in 108 patients (Kazner et al. 1978). Disregarding cerebral mass hemorrhages, this meant that 10.6% of the cases were difficult to classify in terms of differential diagnosis. Although more recent data are not available, it is reasonable to assume that this percentage is not altered significantly by technical refinements in CT scanners or by adjunctive MR examination.

1. Inflammatory Lesions

a) Brain Abscesses

The high accuracy of **CT** in the detection and diagnosis of cerebral abscesses is widely acknowledged. Abscesses as small as 1 cm in diameter present a characteristic ring pattern with central liquefaction and a peripheral, densely enhancing capsule, perifocal edema, and mass effect, even when the lesions are multifocal (Figs. F 1–4).

MR imaging provides comparable specificity owing to the different relaxation times of the abscess contents, peripheral edema, and intervening capsule, which is roughly isointense to the parenchyma. Resolution of these features is further improved by the administration of Gd-DTPA. MR is superior to CT in demonstrating the spread of inflammation past the boundaries of the abscess along a needle track, into the ventricular system, or into the subarachnoid space. This potential complication of abscesses is evidenced by significantly shortened T1 and T2 relaxation times in the CSF and by increased signal intensity in the ependyma or meninges (Figs. F 5, 6).

However, both MR and CT have the same basic difficulties in assessing the age of the inflammatory lesion and in limiting the differential diagnosis. Animal experiments and clinical studies of cerebral abscesses have shown that CT can demonstrate an ill-defined area of decreased density with a central area of lower density due to incipient liquefaction on about the 4th day after the onset of infection. Contrast medium produces a faint ring of enhancement around the low-density core. This ring pattern can give the impression of a solid abscess capsule.

It takes 3–4 weeks for the lesion to progress through the granulation stage to encapsulation. The capsule itself appears as a hyperdense, strongly enhancing ring around a uniformly hypodense, necrotic center. As the abscess matures, there is a diminution of peripheral edema and mass effect (Figs. F 1–3, 5, 6). Although differences in cellularity, fiber content, vascularization, and blood-brain barrier breakdown lead to different time-density values of the ring patterns in the florid and mature abscess stages on contrast-enhanced scans, serial studies are required in order to make the confident evaluation necessary for planning operative treatment.

Measurements of CT densities and MR signal parameters are of little help in making a **differential diagnosis**. Unless the history and clinical manifestations suggest inflammatory disease, it is extremely difficult to distinguish a brain abscess from a centrally necrotic glioblastoma, especially in adults (Fig. F 1). Analyses of morphology, density, and enhancement kinetics contribute as little to differentiating the inflammatory lesion from a brain tumor (Mauersberger 1981) as do measurements of attenuation values of 19–23 HU in the necrotic center and increasingly prolonged T1 relaxation times as the core liquefies (Fig. F 5). Moreover, limitations of stage dependence apply equally to both types of lesion in terms of density or intensity characteristics, aggressiveness of growth, development of central necrosis, and the degree of perifocal brain edema. Even the reduction of ring enhancement or decrease in perifocal edema with corticosteroid therapy is not helpful for differential diagnosis.

The only criterion specific for brain abscess is gas formation within the ring-shaped lesion (Fig. F3).

In some cases angiography can provide a more confident diagnosis by demonstrating opacification of the abscess capsule or, if a tumor is present, of the pathologic vessels supplying the lesion.

Ring enhancement is seen not only in glioblastomas and anaplastic astrocytomas but also in cerebral metastases. Pilocytic astrocytoma should be considered in the differential diagnosis of a ring-enhancing lesion in the posterior fossa.

A *multilocular brain abscess* can also mimic the appearance of a glioblastoma or metastasis (Fig. F2).

Multifocal brain abscesses mainly require differentiation from cerebral metastases. Multifocal glioblastomas are occasionally observed. Finally, parasitic disease and especially *cysticercosis* should be considered whenever multiple brain lesions are encountered.

b) Subdural Empyemas and Epidural Abscesses

Intra-axial brain abscess and extra-axial empyema coexist in approximately 20% of cases (Moseley and Kendall 1984). Subdural empyemas and epidural abscesses are most common in childhood and adolescence, and most arise secondary to the spread of inflammation from the paranasal sinuses or from infected injuries of the upper eyelid. More of these lesions are subdural than epidural. Confinement of the collection to one hemisphere with ipsilateral demarcation by the interhemispheric fissure or falx serves to identify the lesion as subdural. Epidural lesions transgress the midline and separate the falx from the calvarium (Figs. F7–10).

The early stages of an extraparenchymal pus collection are difficult to recognize on **CT**. Frequently the diameter of the collection is small, it causes little mass effect, its contents are isodense, and the encapsulating meninges do not enhance. With passage of time the pus becomes decreasingly dense, almost CSF-like, and within 3 weeks there is a densely enhancing capsule composed of the dura and arachnoid (Figs. F8, 9). Subdural empyema appears in the interhemispheric fissure as a tubular or lens-shaped mass alongside the falx with peripheral contrast enhancement and perifocal edema in the affected cerebral hemisphere (Fig. F7).

MR is more sensitive in detecting the inflammatory focus, even in its early stages. Increased signal intensity can be demonstrated in the subdural or epidural space, especially on T2-weighted sequences. The probable source of the infection can also be identified owing to its identical signal characteristics (Fig. F10).

Subdural empyemas over the cerebral convexity may ultimately attain a very large size and become loculated (Fig. F8). Empyemas over the cerebellar hemispheres in the posterior fossa are easily missed on CT scans but not on the multiplanar images provided by MR (Fig. F4).

Differentiation of subdural empyemas and epidural abscesses from chronic extraparenchymal hematomas or hygromas presents no difficulties when proper attention is given to the history, clinical manifestations, and enhancement kinetics.

c) Meningoencephalitides

The acute stage of *purulent meningitis* can present on **CT** as a mass lesion with widening of the subarachnoid spaces, increased density of the CSF (over 20 HU), and a rim of meningeal enhancement. In the subacute and chronic stages of the inflammation, the subarachnoid spaces may become isodense to brain as a result of leptomeningeal vascularization, perivascular infiltrates, or fibrin deposition. They enhance intensely with contrast medium (Bilaniuk et al. 1978; Cockrill et al. 1978).

In most cases CT demonstrates only the effects of the bacterial inflammation, consisting of adhesions in the CSF spaces or hydrocephalus secondary to obstruction of CSF flow.

MR is superior to CT in its ability to delineate the full extent of disease. The inflammation alters the water content and water-binding capacity of the meninges, ependyma, CSF, and affected brain areas, increasing their signal intensity and giving an accurate impression of the structures that are involved.

Tuberculous meningitis also is generally associated with significant hydrocephalus due to obstruction of CSF drainage by the characteristic gelatinous exudate in the basal cisterns. Blood vessels may become affected in their course along the skull base, with a potential for cerebral infarction and venous thrombosis. The tuberculous tissue can be directly visualized with CT when the inflammation is severe. To date MR (without gadolinium enhancement) has been unable to demonstrate the thick gelatinous infiltrates, and hydrocephalus and lacunar infarction provide the only diagnostic clues to tuberculous meningitis on MR images (Schroth et al. 1987).

Encephalitis is a diffuse, unilateral or focal inflammatory disease of the brain parenchyma which produces a mass effect in the acute stage. This effect is caused by mononuclear or lymphoid cell infiltrates, necrosis, and inflammatory exudation. Accordingly, **CT** shows decreased density in the affected brain area while **MR** shows increased proton signal intensity and prolonged T1 and T2 relaxation times. MR appears to be more sensitive in establishing the degree and extent of disease. The chronic stage is marked by an intense, garlandlike pattern of enhancement within the encephalitic focus or a serpiginous pattern of cortical enhancement caused by vascular proliferation and congestion. Although the CNS responses to all forms of encephalitis, most of them viral in origin, are similar, differences are observed relating to the pathogen and the topography and severity of the involvement (Figs. F11, 12).

Herplex simplex encephalitis type I displays a characteristic pattern of involvement. The inflammatory process incites a hemorrhagic necrosis that invades the limbic system and is sharply demarcated from the lenticular nucleus along the external capsule. Extension to the fronto-orbital brain area, the genu of the corpus callosum, and to the parietal lobe is possible, and bilateral inflammation of the temporal lobes is seen in the majority of cases (Fig. F34).

CT displays herpes simplex encephalitis as an ill-defined area of decreased density. Changes appear as early as 3 days after the onset of disease, although the average latent period is 5 days. Increasing mass effect and garland enhancement of the cortical parenchyma due to blood-brain barrier breakdown are observed in the 2nd week of the disease. At the same time, petechial areas of hemorrhage appear as hyperdense zones within the inflamed tissue. Resolution of the encephalitis is associated first with demarcation of the necrotic tissue and then with the formation of a cystic defect of CSF density. Cerebral atrophy predominantly affecting the temporal lobes is a common sequela.

MR is more sensitive than CT in the diagnosis of herpes simplex encephalitis and provides a more effective basis for instituting virostatic therapy. It can detect the changes of the disease at an earlier stage and more accurately portrays the extent of disease, especially in bilateral cases, owing to the increased proton density and prolonged relaxation times of affected tissues. These signal changes coincide with the earliest clinical manifestations of the encephalitis, and their distribution allows a prompt, definitive diagnosis to be made (Schroth et al. 1987) (Figs. F13, 34).

While spread of the type I virus is mediated by the fifth cranial nerve branches and appears to be transmitted by the axons (Davis et al. 1978; Damasio and van Hoesen 1985), *herpes simplex encephalitis type II* is a rampant infection which causes a diffuse or disseminated inflammation of the brain parenchyma in neonates. The infection is believed to result from contamination during vaginal delivery. CT shows ill-defined areas of very low density scattered diffusely over both hemispheres and the brainstem or even over the cerebellum. These lesions enhance markedly with contrast medium. The rapidly progressive parenchymal destruction causes widespread cystic defect formation with calcium deposition that is most conspicuous in the subcortical tissues (Fig. F14).

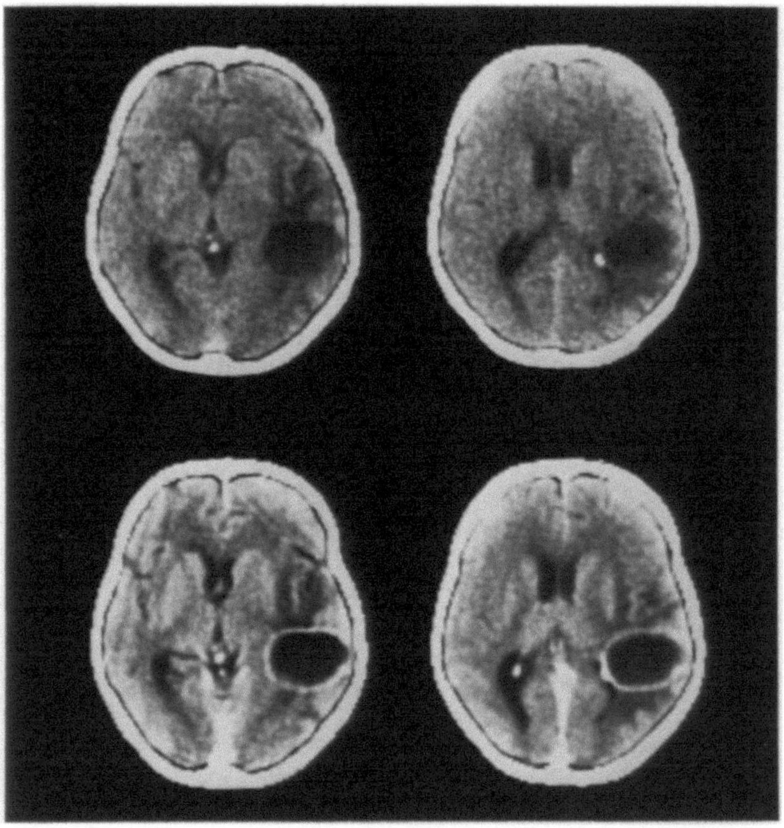

Fig. F1. Brain abscess in the right posterior temporal region of a 65-year-old woman. Plain CT scans (*top*) show a circumscribed area of decreased density with a fingerlike pattern of white matter edema. Postcontrast scans (*bottom*) show a narrow ring of enhancement outlining the abscess capsule. Differentiation is required from glioblastoma and metastasis

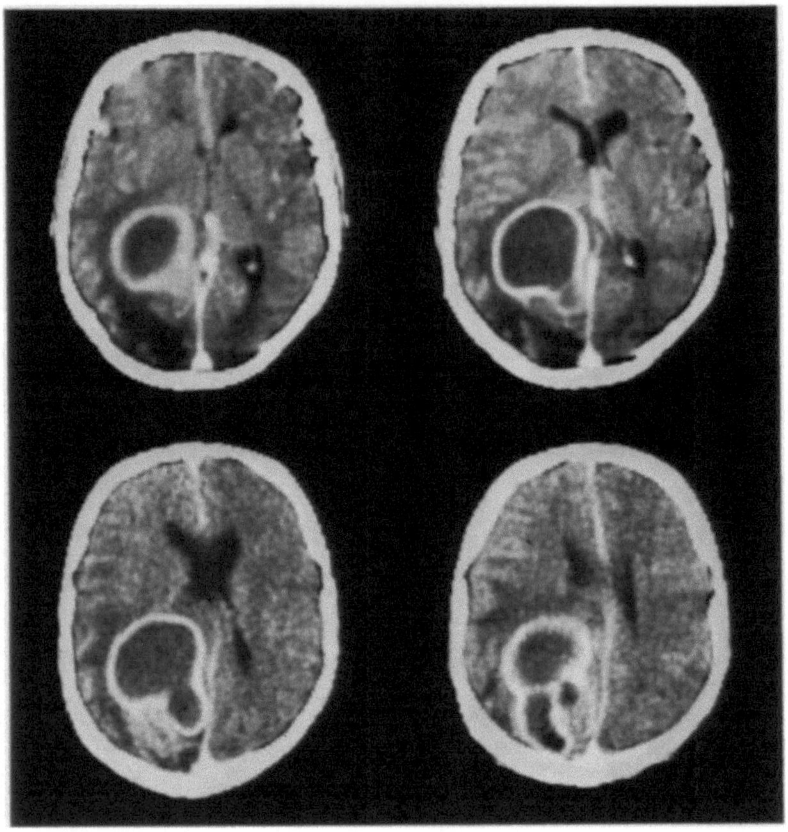

Fig. F2. Multilocular brain abscess in the left parieto-occipital region of a 14-year-old boy. Postcontrast CT

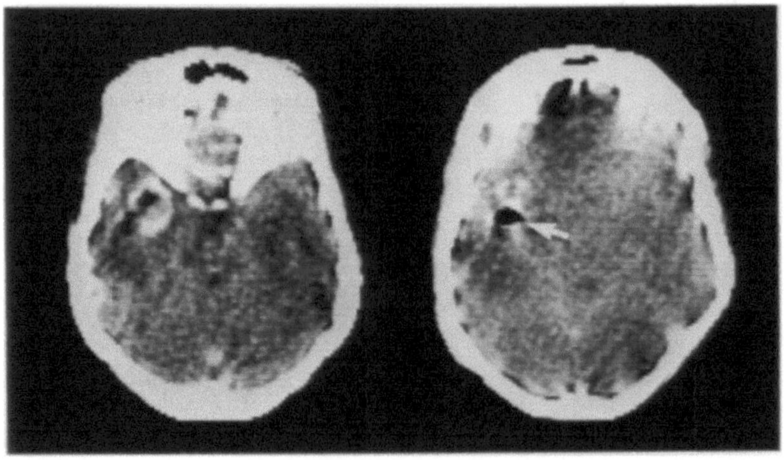

Fig. F3. Brain abscess with gas formation in the left temporal lobe of a 40-year-old woman with paranasal sinusitis. The extreme density gradient between the gas and abscess capsule produces an artifact due to "computer overswing" (*arrow*). Postcontrast CT

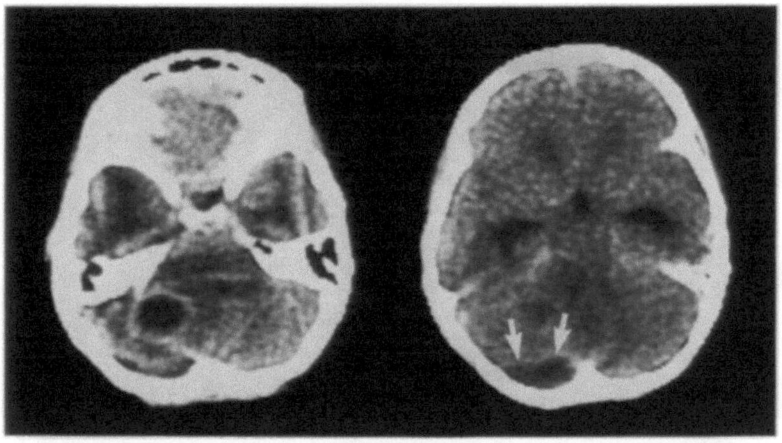

Fig. F4. Cerebellar abscess with ring enhancement and subdural empyema over the left cerebellar hemisphere in a 25-year-old woman, with enhancement in the visceral layer of the inflammatory lesion (*arrows*). There is pronounced edema of the cerebellar white matter

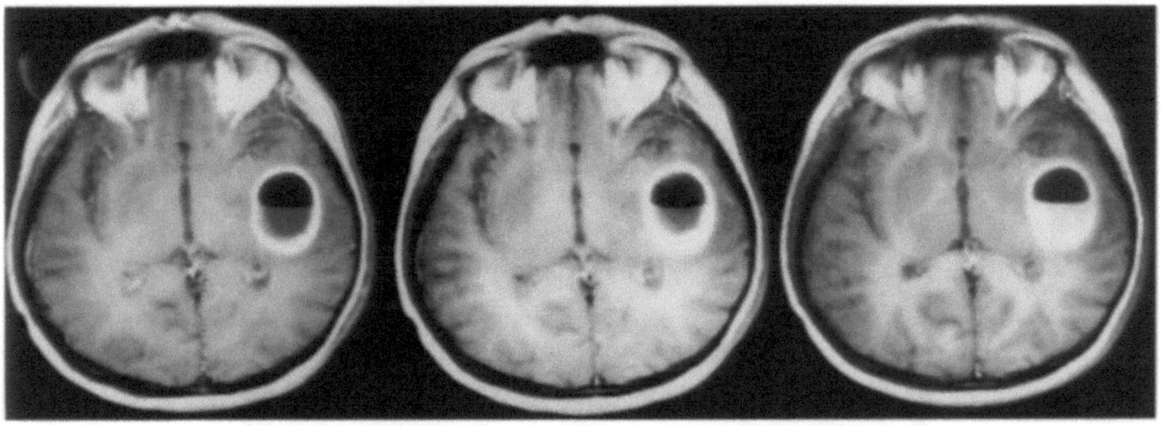

Fig. F5. Otogenic brain abscess in a 29-year-old woman who had her first generalized seizure following untreated otitis media. She presented with mild neurologic symptoms on the left side. SE 400/30 images were taken 10 min (*left*), 30 min (*center*), and 60 min (*right*) after the administration of Gd-DTPA. The serial images show increasing hyperintensity of the abscess capsule and especially of the abscess contents

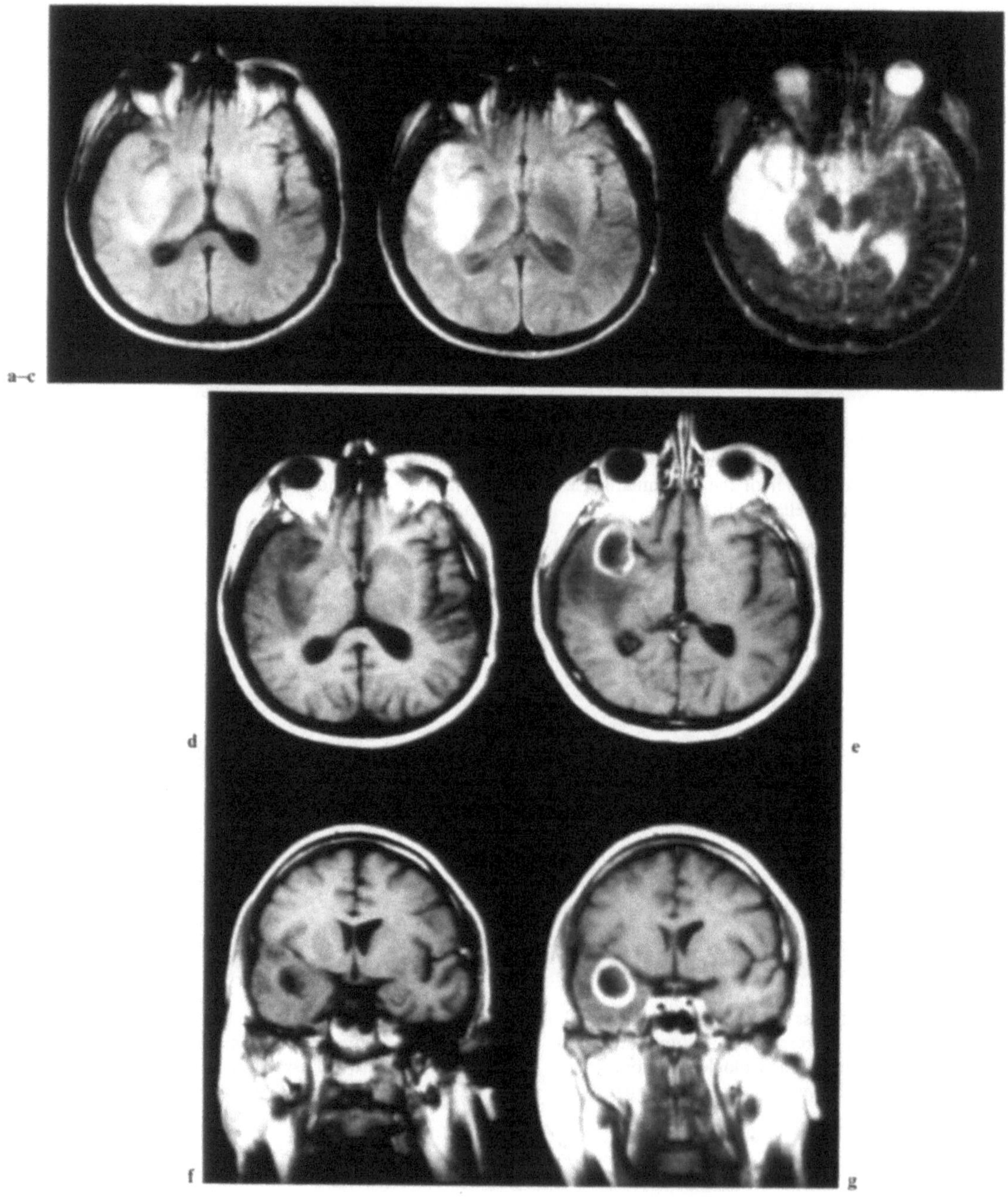

Fig. F6a–g. Brain abscess in the left temporal lobe of a 45-year-old man with a 2-month history of left temporal headache and left-sided proptosis. Neurologic exam disclosed partial ophthalmoplegia. MR: **a** SE 1600/30, **b** SE 1600/60, **c** SE 1600/210, **d** SE 400/30, **e** SE 400/30 post Gd-DTPA, **f** SE 400/30, **g** SE 400/30 post Gd-DTPA. There is conspicuous edema of the left hemisphere with a relatively well-defined abscess in the left temporal lobe (**c**). Ring enhancement clearly outlines the abscess on the post Gd-DTPA scans

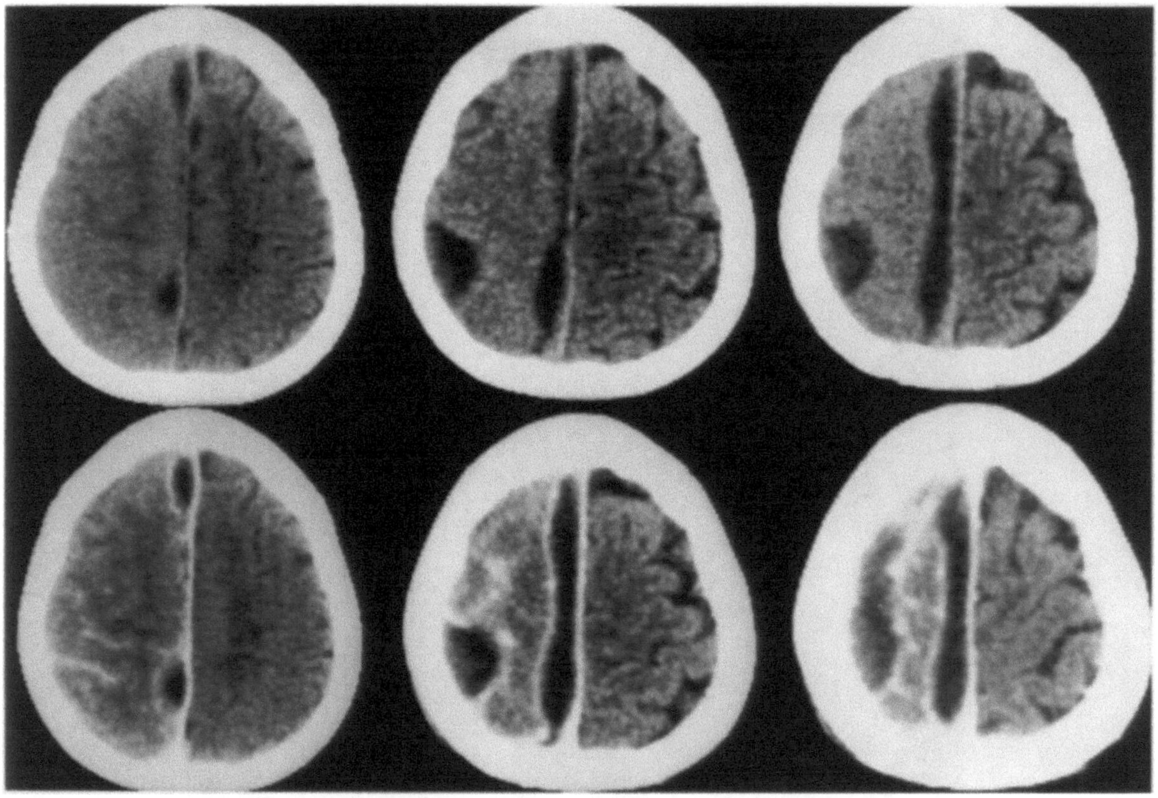

Fig. F7. Subdural empyema of the left interhemispheric fissure and left parietal region in a 9-year-old girl acutely ill with fever, impaired consciousness, and right hemiparesis. *Top* plain CT, *bottom* postcontrast CT. The space-occupying empyema is particularly well defined on the enhanced scans. Disturbance of the blood-brain barrier is apparent over the left hemisphere

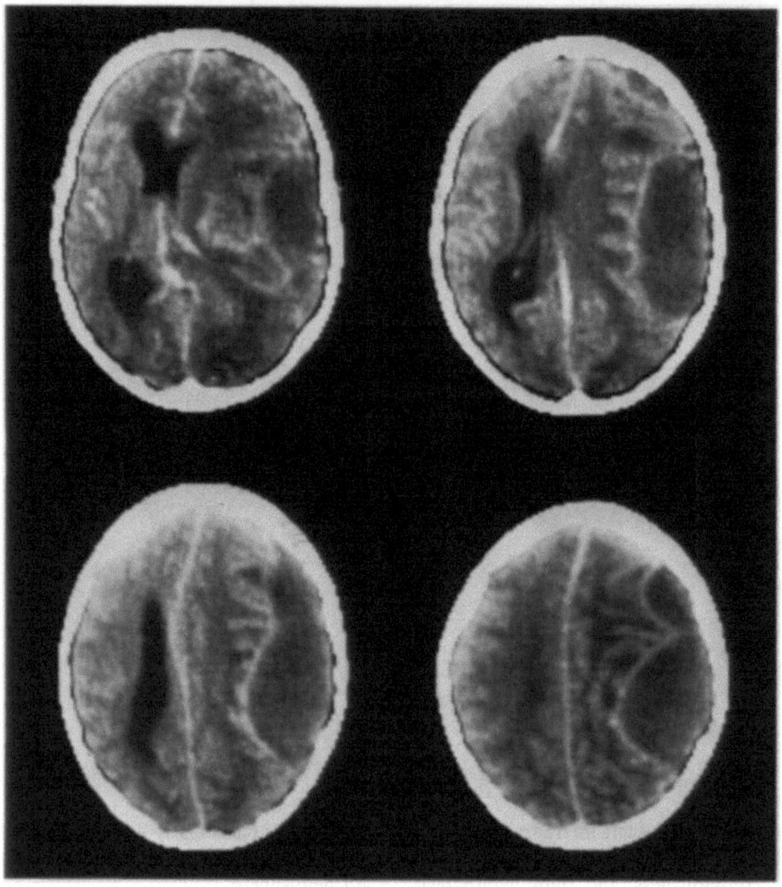

Fig. F8. Very extensive, loculated subdural empyema over the right cerebral hemisphere in a 12-year-old boy. The entire right hemisphere is involved by white matter edema. There is marked displacement of midline structures with enhancement in the visceral layer of the empyema capsule. Postcontrast CT

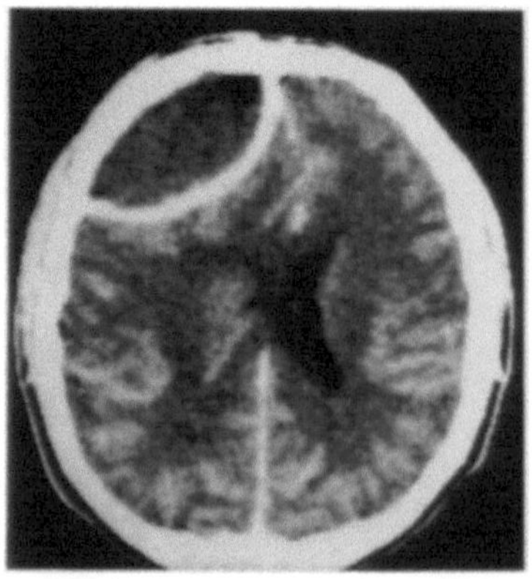

Fig. F9. Epidural abscess of the left frontal region in a 17-year-old male secondary to purulent sinusitis and an orbital abscess. Proptosis and severe headache developed 4 weeks after drainage of the abscesses. Neurologic findings were normal. Postcontrast CT demonstrates an epidural abscess with smooth borders, mass effect, and a strongly enhancing capsule

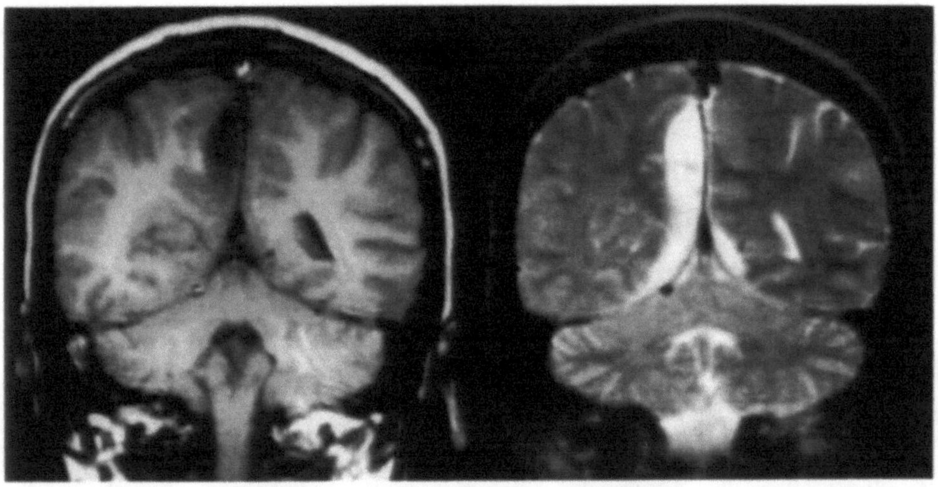

Fig. F10. Empyema along the falx in an 18-year-old male with sudden loss of consciousness following pansinusitis. MR: *left* SE 400/30, *right* SE 1600/120. The empyema appears hypointense on the T1-weighted image (*left*), but the full extension of the lesion to the tentorium is seen only on the T2-weighted sequence (*right*), where the empyema gives a bright signal

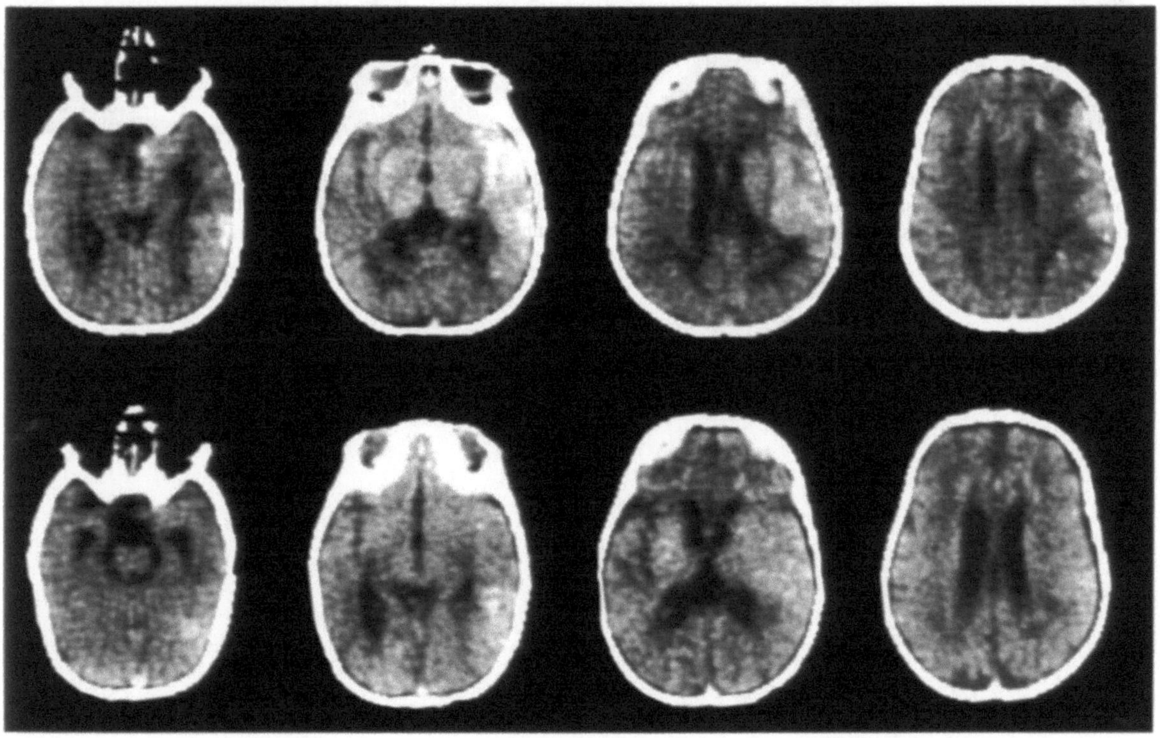

Fig. F11. Hemorrhagic encephalitis in an 8-month-old girl. The disease began 3 weeks earlier with dyspepsia followed by a generalized seizure and somnolence. Initial CT examination revealed hypodensity of the white matter, especially in the parietal region, in addition to a right temporal hemorrhage and incipient parenchymal necrosis. Reexamination 6 days later showed regression of the hemorrhagic encephalitis with increasing ventricular enlargement

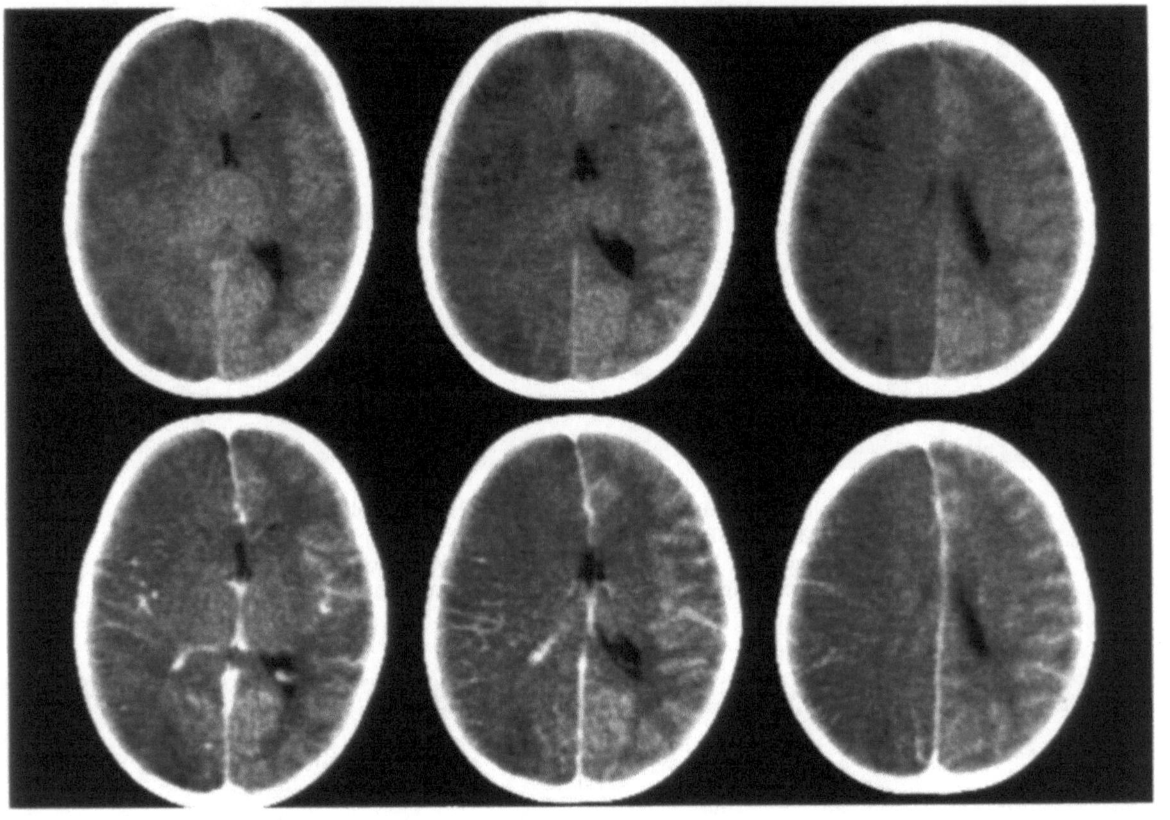

Fig. F12. Viral panencephalitis in a 2-year-old child with impairment of consciousness. *Top* plain CT, *bottom* post-contrast CT. Plain scans indicate low density over both hemispheres, especially on the left side, and compression of the lateral ventricles. Postcontrast scans demonstrate gyral enhancement

Fig. F13a–d. Confirmed herpes simplex encephalitis in a 60-year-old man with a history of lethargy and night sweats for 6 months, headache for 2 months, amaurosis fugax for 1 month, and acute left-sided hemiparesis and fever for 3 weeks. MR: **a** SE 1600/30, **b** SE 1600/70, **c** SE 400/30, **d** SE 1600/70. MR shows hyperintense lesions in the basal ganglia on both sides and in the right paraventricular area

Fig. F14. Status following herpes encephalitis in a 4-year-old boy. Postcontrast CT shows bilateral temporo-occipital and right frontoparietal parenchymal defects bounded sharply by the external capsule. Broad calcifications appear in the occipital lobes, and the CSF spaces are expanded

F 13

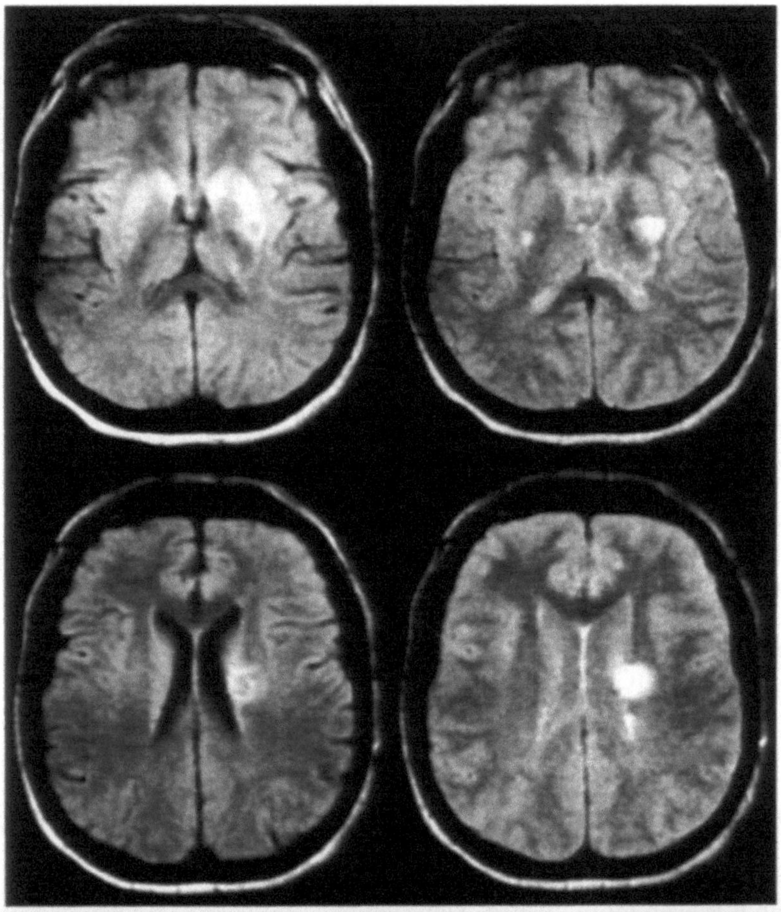

a b c d

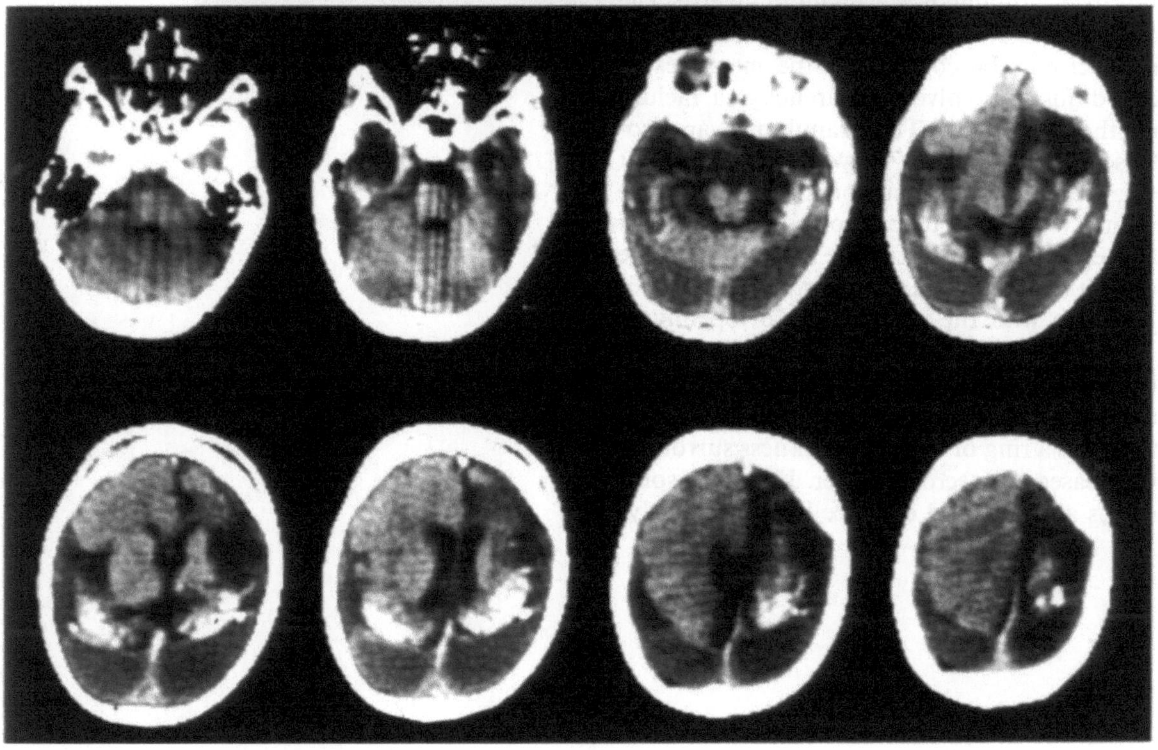

F 14

2. Granulomatous Lesions

a) Gummas

Gummas are so rare that there are no criteria for identifying specific forms or differentiating them from other types of lesion. In the absence of extracerebral involvement, histologic examination is necessary to establish a diagnosis.

The syphilitic granulation tissue of gummas has two types of presentation on **CT**. The most common involves a miliary, nodular seeding of deposits into the meninges and ependyma. These granulomas may be directly visualized on contrast-enhanced scans, or their presence may be inferred from hydrocephalus or cerebral infarction secondary to vascular infiltration. Large gummas of the cortex reportedly develop along the Virchow-Robin spaces from infiltrates in the subarachnoid space. They appear either as dense, enhancing nodules or as rings with necrotic centers (Godt et al. 1979) (Fig. F15).

b) Tuberculomas

Tuberculomas have basically the same **CT** appearance, although it is even more diverse. The miliary form consisting of small solid or ringlike foci may be confined to the meninges or may diffusely involve the parenchyma including the cerebellum. The granulomas are isodense on plain scans, show marked contrast enhancement, and are surrounded by extensive edema. With most tuberculomas of the cortex or deep periventricular white matter, the route of infiltration is apparent from the contact of the lesion with the leptomeninx or ependyma (Fig. F16). Less frequently, large granulomas develop from the coalescence of foci disseminated via the bloodstream. The predominant pattern is a ring of variable thickness surrounding a caseated, necrotic center. However, some lesions are solid and enhance homogeneously.

c) Granulomas in Sarcoidosis

Sarcoidosis of the CNS may present as a circumscribed, granulomatous meningitis with the development of conglomerate masses. These appear on **CT** as irregular, uniformly enhancing lesions (Fig. F17). Involvement may be diffuse and symmetrical or circumscribed. Some cases affect only one cistern or the sylvian fissure and adjacent parenchyma. A dense rim of edema surrounds the granulomas, which occur superficially in the cortex or in the periventricular region. In contrast to other types of granulomatous lesion, there is no central necrosis.

MR does not contribute to the differential diagnosis of the granulomas (Fig. F18). It demonstrates the granulomatous tissue as a circular or ringlike mass with prolonged T1 and T2 times that enhances with Gd-DTPA. Associated changes such as mass effect, hydrocephalus, or cerebral infarction are more easily demonstrated (Fig. F19).

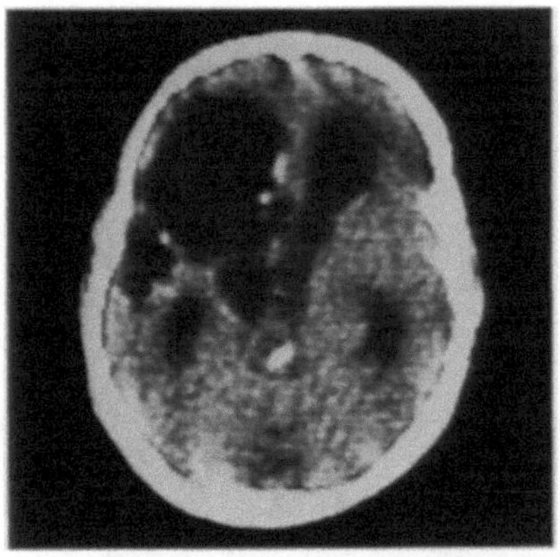

Fig. F15. Large gumma in the anterior portions of the left cerebral hemisphere in a 48-year-old man. The lesion presents as a clearly delineated zone of very low density with small peripheral calcifications. Confusion with an epidermoid cyst is possible

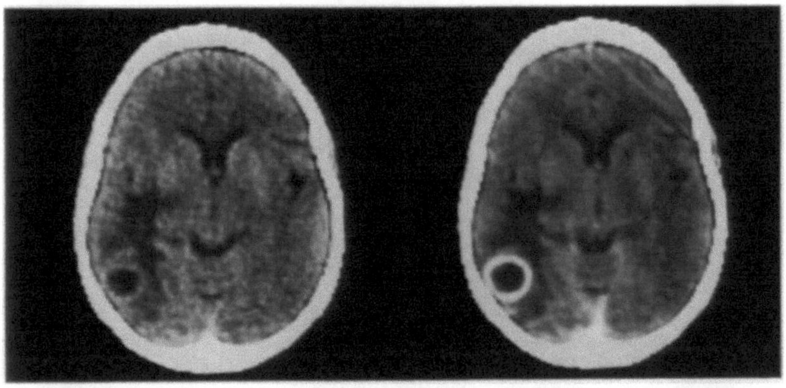

Fig. F16. Tuberculoma at the junction of the left temporal and occipital lobes with ring enhancement and extensive perifocal edema in a 66-year-old man. The lesion is indistinguishable from a brain abscess on CT. The patient had no known history of tuberculosis. *Left* plain scan, *right* postcontrast scan

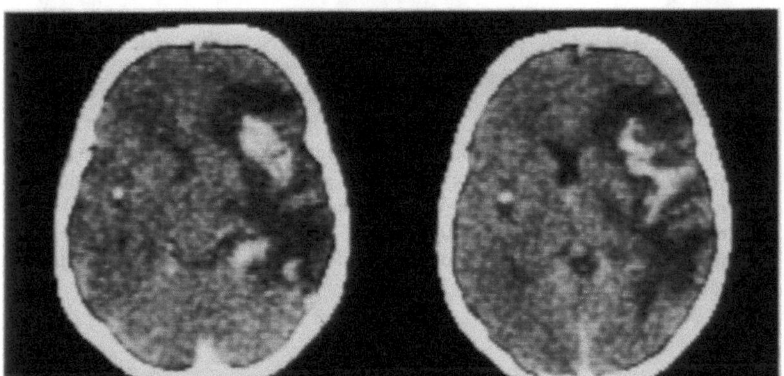

Fig. F17. Conglomerate sarcoid granulomas in the right frontotemporal region showing intense contrast enhancement and marked perifocal edema in an 8-year-old boy. The disease arises from the meninges in the sylvian fissure

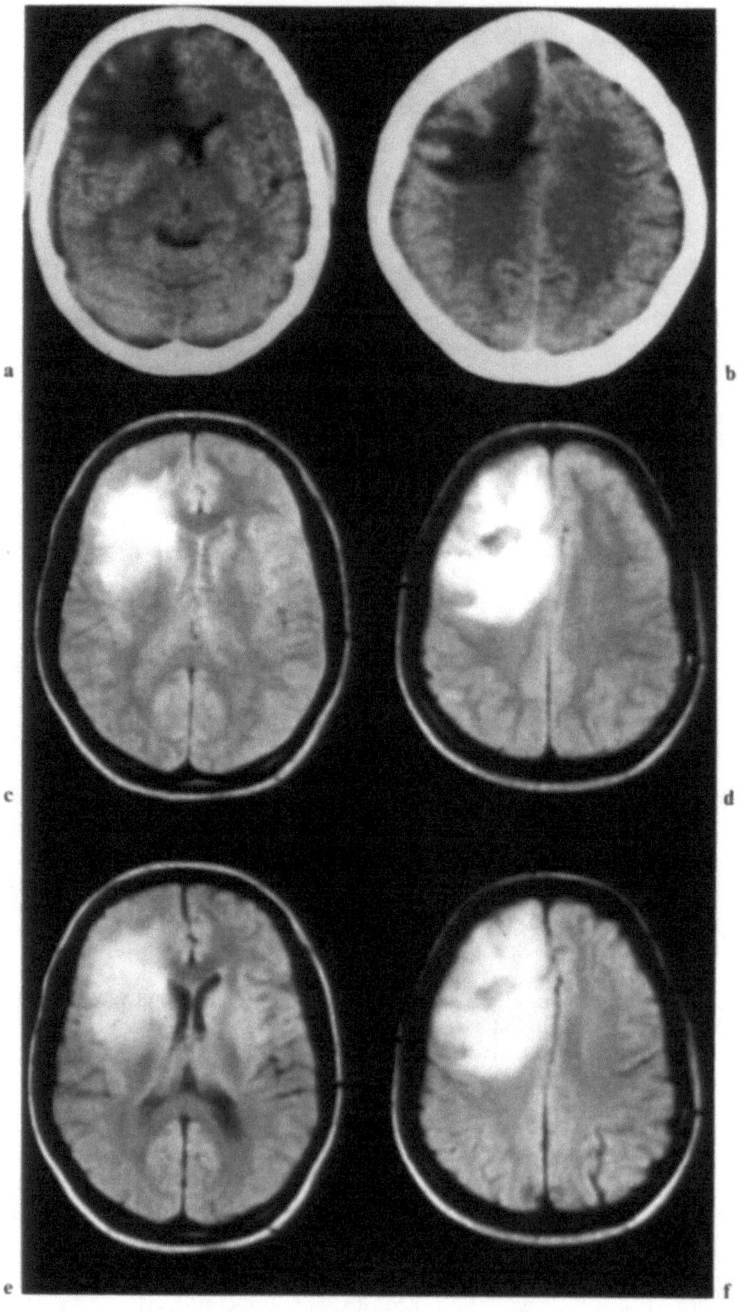

Fig. F18a–f. Tuberculoma in the left frontoprecentral region of a 25-year-old woman with a history of several generalized seizures in previous months. Neurologic findings were normal. CT: **a, b** noncontrast. MR: **c, d** SE 1600/70, **e, f** SE 1600/35. The circumscribed hyperintensity in the left frontoprecentral region with a low-signal center represents the tuberculoma and surrounding edema

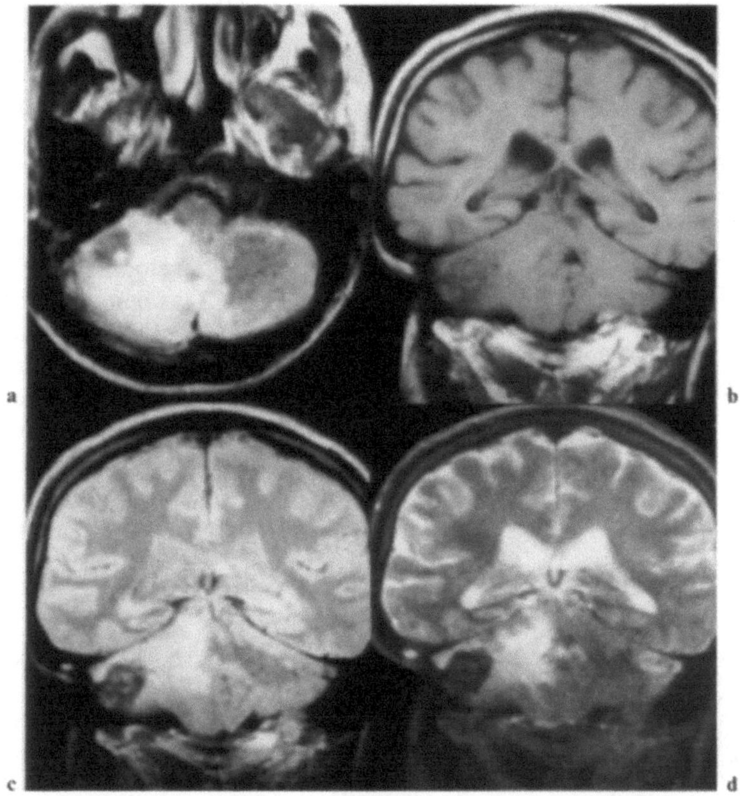

Fig. F 19a–d. Tuberculoma in the left cerebellar hemisphere of a 63-year-old man who sustained a gunshot injury of the left mastoid in 1943 ("chronic ear"). He presented with a 2-week history of vertigo and ataxia. MR: **a** SE 3000/30, **b** SE 700/30, **c** SE 3000/30, **d** SE 3000/90. There is marked edema of the left cerebellar hemisphere with displacement of the fourth ventricle toward the right side. A circumscribed lesion appears in the lateral part of the hemisphere

3. Parasitic Diseases

a) Cysticercosis

Though rare at our latitudes, parasitisms must be included in the differential diagnosis of intracranial cysts or non-neoplastic mass lesions (Figs. F20–25). Cysticercosis tends to produce a diffuse intraparenchymal involvement of the cerebral white matter (80% of cases). Cysticerci are rarely found in the ventricular system, subarachnoid spaces, ependyma, or meninges (Byrd et al. 1982).

Depending on the stage of the disease, **CT** demonstrates cysts of moderate size scattered diffusely in the brain parenchyma. The cyst contents are slightly hyperdense to CSF, and the larva appears as a circumscribed dense nodule on the cyst wall. The wall does not enhance with contrast medium. An inflammatory response leads to degeneration of the cyst with subsequent development of granulomas that appear on CT as densely enhancing nodules or rings. Final resolution is marked by the presence of scattered specks of calcification in the brain parenchyma. The parenchymatous form is characterized by the coexistence of different developmental stages of the parasite, the presence of cysticercus nodules in the cyst wall, and diffuse calcium deposits (Fig. F21).

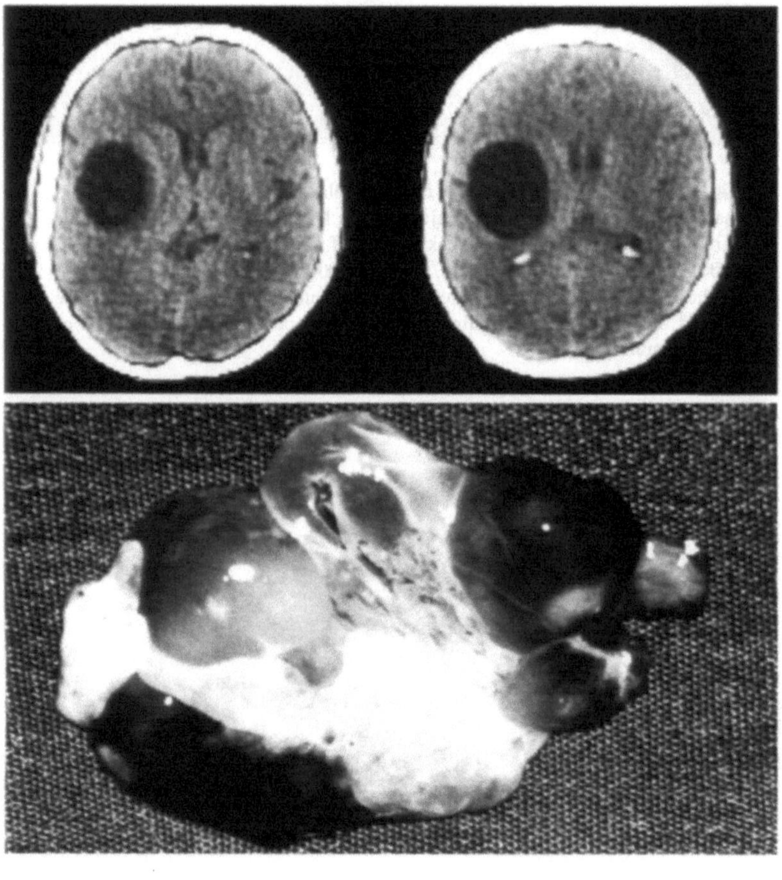

Fig. F20. CT reveals a cystic mass deep in the left cerebral hemisphere (*top*). The lesion was identified at operation as a cysticercus cyst (*bottom*)

On **MR**, the very intense appearance of the cysticercus nodule is diagnostic. The number of granulomas and the extent of perifocal edema are depicted more accurately on T2-weighted sequences. The disseminated calcifications appear as points of signal void in the parenchyma and are easily overlooked (Suss et al. 1986) (Figs. F22–25).

Intraventricular involvement with cysticercus cysts is seen in about 15% of patients (Zee et al. 1984). On CT scans the cyst contents are isodense to CSF, so detection of the cysts must rely on indirect signs: occlusion of the ventricular system or contrast enhancement of an associated ependymitis (Fig. F23). Noncalcified intraventricular cysts can be directly visualized only in ventriculographic studies using intrathecal contrast medium. This invasive contrast study can replace MR imaging.

Intraventricular cysts stand out clearly in the ambient CSF on proton-density MR images. T2-weighted images delineate the cyst wall and demonstrate associated periventricular reaction. Similar MR criteria can be used to identify subarachnoidal cysticercosis (Figs. F24, 25).

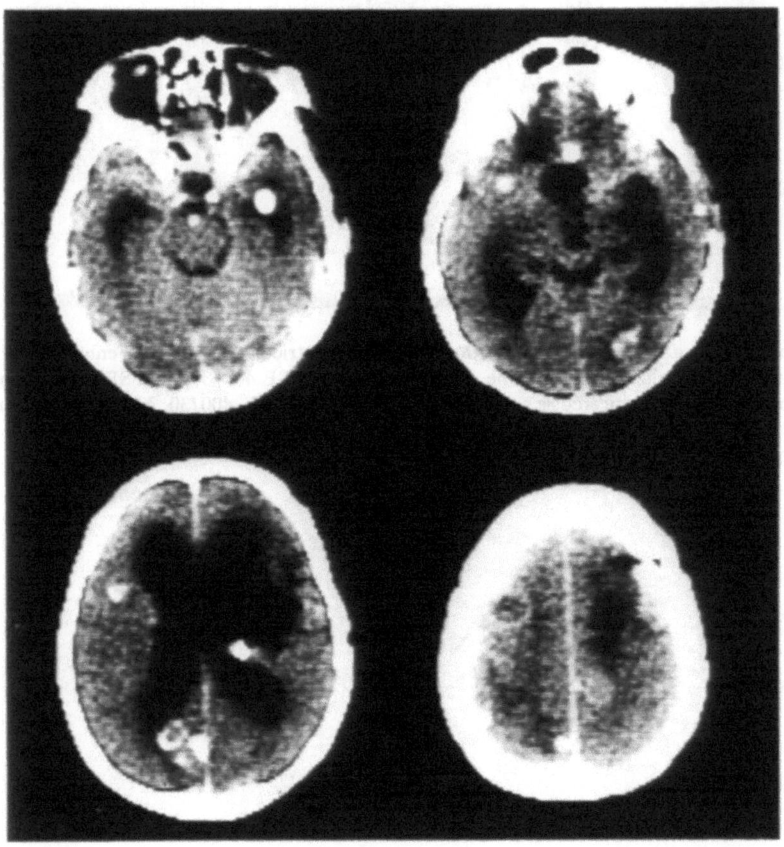

Fig. F21. Multiple cystic/solid lesions with calcifications or contrast enhancement in a 54-year-old man with cysticercosis (diagnosis previously established by burhole craniotomy in the right temporal area). Postcontrast CT

a–c

d–f

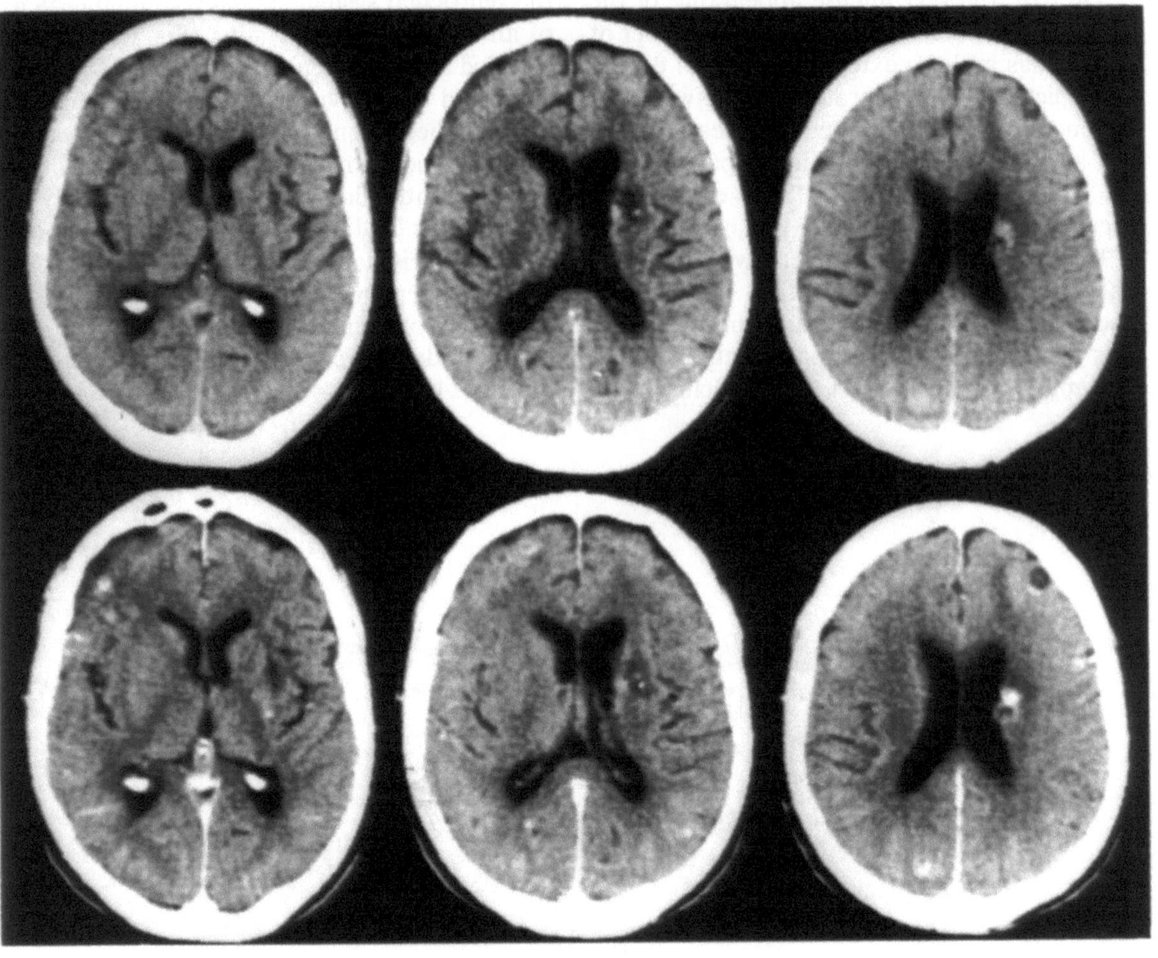

Fig. F22a–r. Cysticercosis in a 55-year-old man with a 6-year history of focal and generalized seizures. The patient had lived in India for some years. Cysticercosis was serologically confirmed. CT **a–c** precontrast, **d–f** postcontrast. Scans demonstrate multiple hyperdense foci in the cortex and paraventricular region that enhance with contrast medium. MR: **g–l** SE 400/30, **m–o** SE 1600/70, **p** SE 1600/35, **q** SE 1600/70, **r** SE 400/30. MR reveals more lesions than CT and defines them with greater clarity

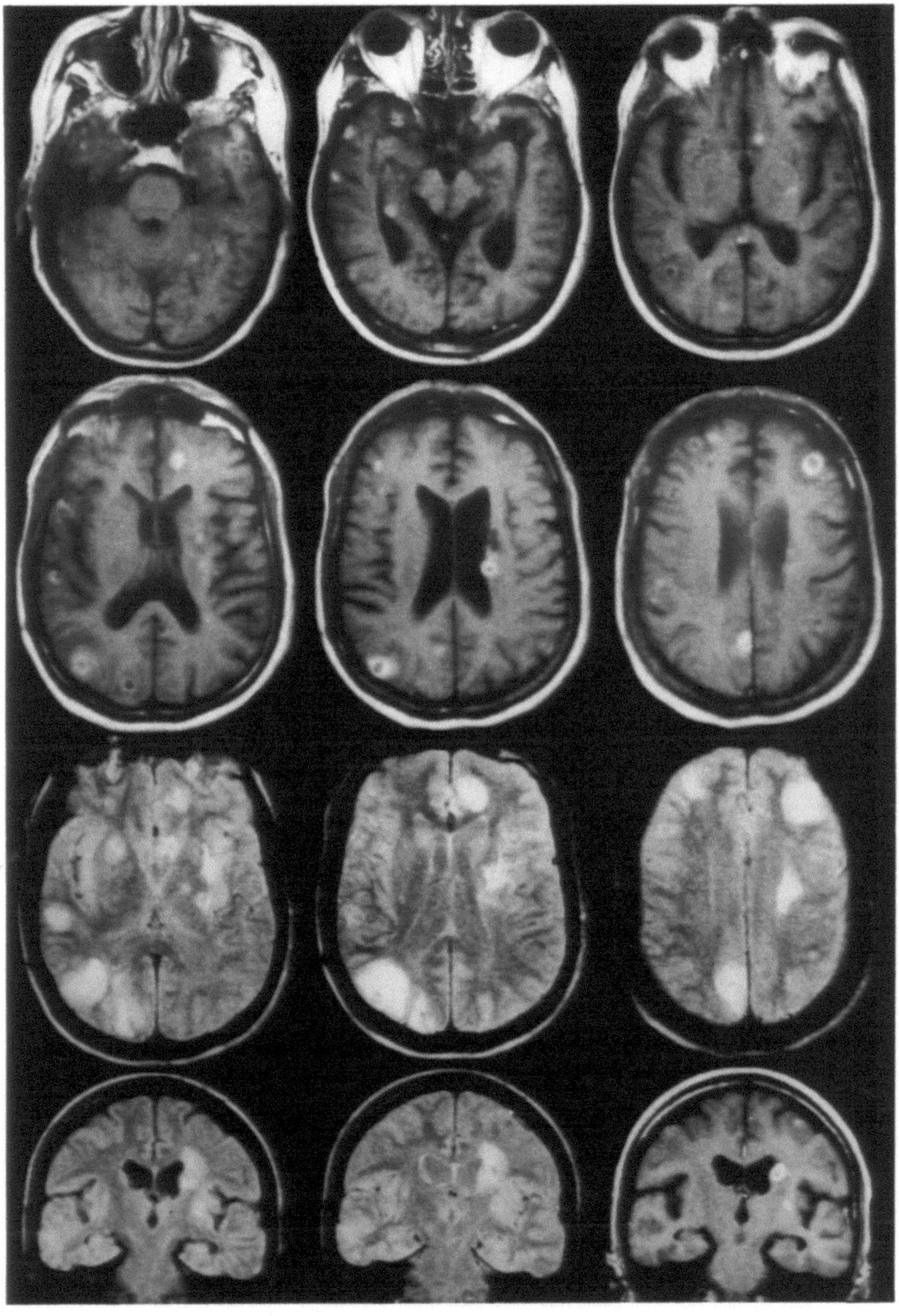

g–i

j–l

m–o

p–r

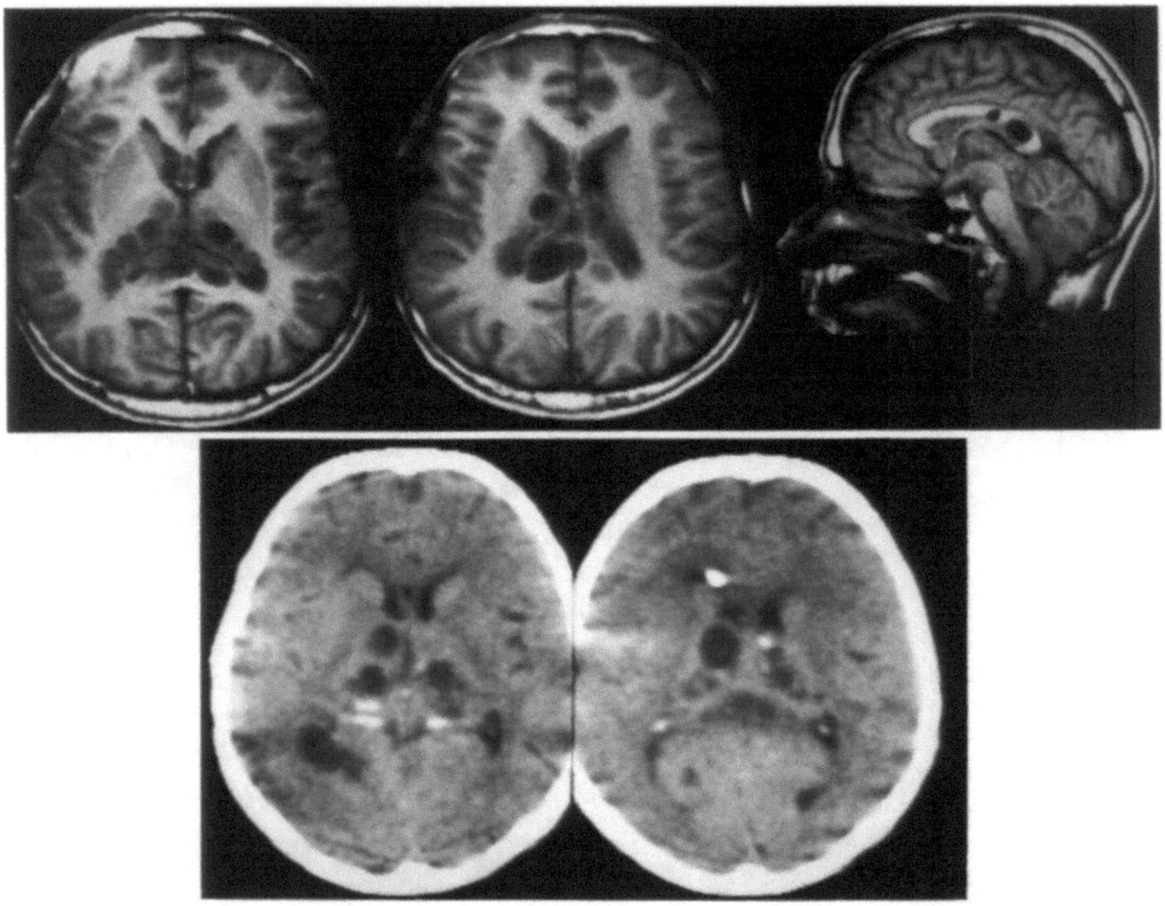

Fig. F23. Cysticercosis in a 16-year-old boy with headaches and generalized seizures. MR *top* SE 400/30. CT *bottom*. MR reveals a greater number of cystic lesions than CT but does not demonstrate the calcifications

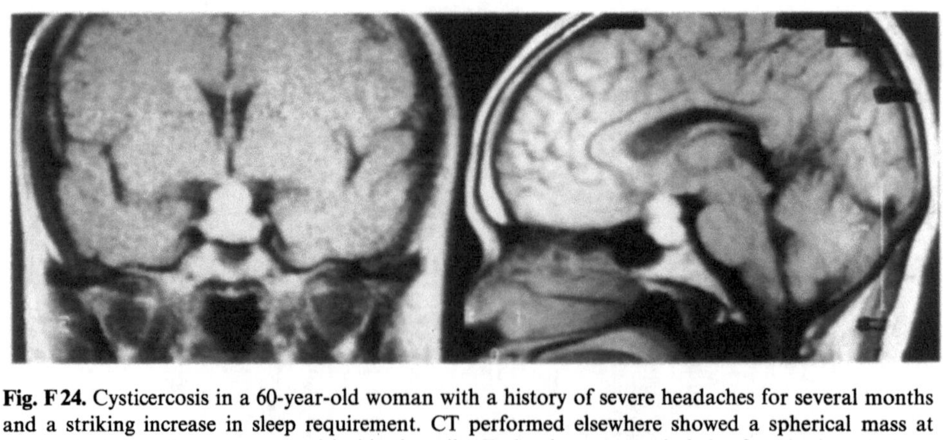

Fig. F24. Cysticercosis in a 60-year-old woman with a history of severe headaches for several months and a striking increase in sleep requirement. CT performed elsewhere showed a spherical mass at the level of the sellar entrance and inside the sella. Endocrine tests excluded a functioning pituitary tumor. MR: The T1-weighted images show a hyperintense, smooth-bordered mass in and above the sella. Operation disclosed a firm, yellowish, mucoid mass compressing and flattening the anterior lobe of the pituitary against the lateral sellar walls. Histology confirmed a cysticercus cyst

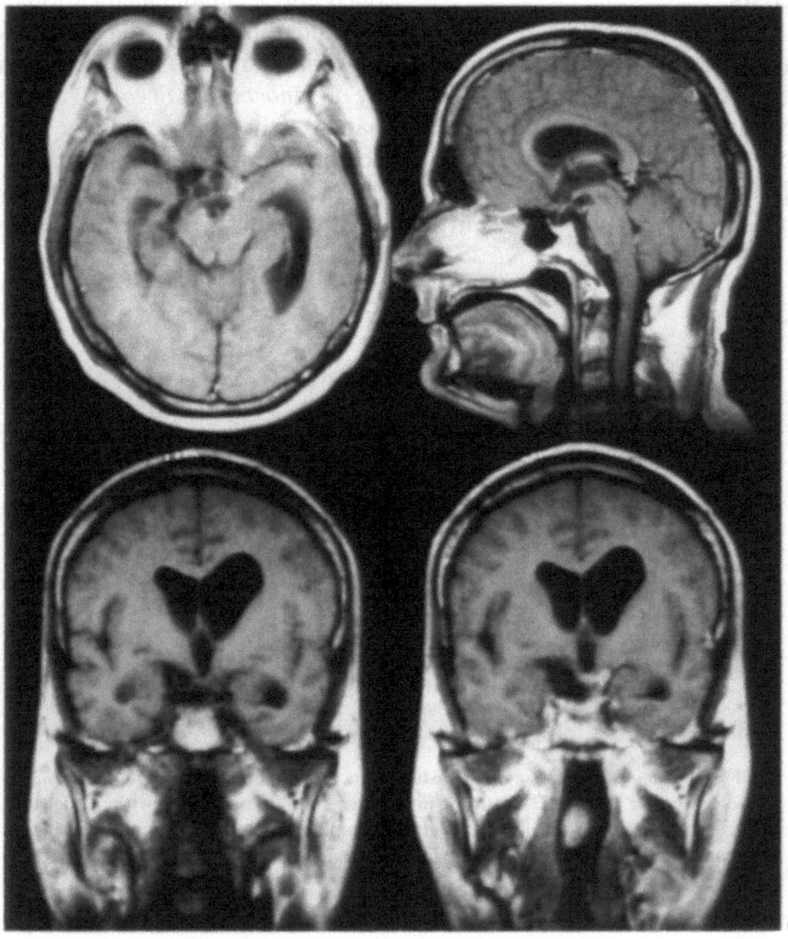

a b c d

Fig. F 25a–d. Cysticercosis in a 44-year-old woman with attacks of headache, visual disturbances, and paroxysmal weakness in both legs. CT disclosed an irregular multicystic lesion in the region of the opticochiasmatic cistern. MR: **a, c** SE 400/30 nonenhanced, **b, d** SE 400/30 post Gd-DTPA. MR demonstrates multiple cysts of varying size in the region of the opticochiasmatic cistern on all three image planes. Mild enhancement is seen around the cysts on the post-gadolinium scans

b) Echinococcosis

A large cyst characterizes echinococcal infection of the brain. The thin-walled, CSF-filled cyst does not enhance with intravenous contrast medium on CT. Surrounded by a narrow rim of inflammatory edema, the spherical cyst of *Echinococcus granulosus* causes little mass effect. Small calcifications in the cyst wall can aid differential diagnosis (McCorkell and Lewall 1985). In one case cerebral involvement by *Echinococcus alveolaris* was suspected in a patient who had a known history of hepatic echinococcosis. The CT appearance was not characteristic (Fig. F26), and only mild contrast enhancement was noted.

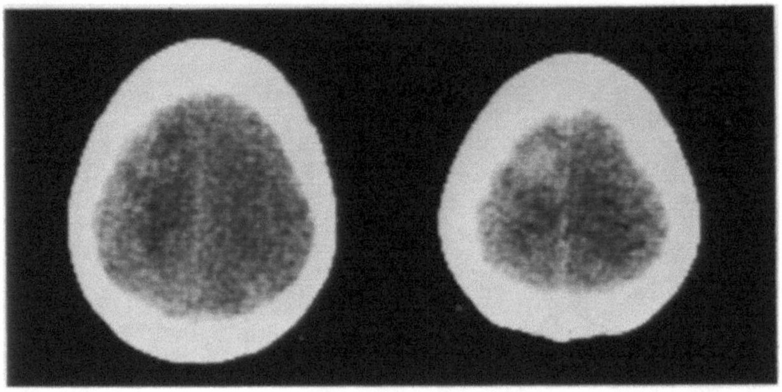

Fig. F26. *Echinococcus alveolaris* infestation in the left precentral region of a 43-year-old woman. Plain CT (*left*) demonstrates mild hypodensity with isodense zones. Postcontrast CT (*right*) shows minimal enhancement. A presumptive diagnosis was made on the basis of known echinococcosis in the liver and was later confirmed histologically

4. Brain Diseases Associated with AIDS

By the end of 1988 over 130000 cases of acquired immune deficiency syndrome (AIDS) had been reported to the World Health Organization. The magnitude of the problem is such that this single disease has strained the health facilities of many developing and developed countries alike.

Approximately 10% of AIDS patients initially present with neurologic symptoms (Levy RM et al. 1985). An additional 25%–30% of AIDS patients develop neurologic abnormalities during the course of their illness. Some 55%–95% of AIDS victims in whom autopsy is performed display pathologic evidence of central nervous system (CNS) disease. It is vital, therefore, that every radiologist become acquainted with the neurologic complications of AIDS.

Although AIDS was first described in June 1981, retrospective analysis suggests that cases may have existed as early as 1978. CDC criteria for diagnosis of AIDS are as follows: (1) demonstration of an opportunistic infection such as *Pneumocystis carinii* pneumonia or a disease such as Kaposi's sarcoma that suggests an underlying cellular immune deficit; (2) lack of another possible cause, such as the use of immunosuppressive drugs, that could explain the cellular immune deficiency.

Since the original description, the underlying organisms believed to be responsible for AIDS have been identified. They belong to a group of viruses known as retroviruses. Human T-cell lymphotrophic virus III (HTLV-III, Gallo et al. 1985), lymphadenopathy virus (LAV, Montagnier 1985), AIDS-associated retrovirus (ARV, Levy JA et al. 1984), and immunodeficiency-associated virus (IDAV, Barre-Sinoussi et al. 1983) represent separate but related viruses that most likely cause the immune deficit. Recently the terminology has been simplified, and all these viruses are now referred to as human immunodeficiency viruses (HIV). Transmission of the virus requires intimate contact. Specifically, there are no documented cases of transmission of these viruses from patient to health workers in the course of normal care.

Because the viruses can now be identified and tested for in blood, AIDS has been found to encompass certain conditions that also occur in patients who are not immunosuppressed. For example, histologically aggressive non-Hodgkin's lymphoma and disseminated histoplasmosis are manifestations of AIDS if they arise in a patient with a positive antibody test for HIV.

Although the putative viral agents have been isolated, AIDS is still primarily identified by a clinical syndrome. Outside the CNS, the most common opportunistic infections occurring in AIDS have protozoal and fungal causes. *Pneumocystis carinii* pneumonia is found in over 50% of patients. *Candida albicans* is the most common of the fungal infectious agents. Concurrent viral causes, especially cytomegalovirus (CMV), are also frequent. Causative bacterial agents include *Mycobacterium avium-intracellulare* and *Mycobacterium tuberculosis*. Pyogenic bacterial infections are unusual.

As in the rest of the body, involvement of the CNS in AIDS patients may be categorized as infectious or neoplastic. This review summarizes the neurologic manifestations of AIDS and the associated radiologic and MRI findings.

a) Infections

Nonviral Infections

Both nonviral and viral pathogens can attack the CNS in AIDS patients. Of the nonviral pathogens, *Cryptococcus neoformans* and *Toxoplasma gondii* are the most common (Levy RM et al. 1986). Although both organisms are frequently documented, they differ considerably in symptomatology, manifestations, and imaging appearance. Typically, *C. neoformans* leads to subacute meningitis with headache as the most common and occasionally the only symptom (Levy RM et al. 1985). Other findings with *C. neoformans* are fever, meningeal signs, confusion, seizures and, rarely, focal neurologic deficits (Kovacs et al. 1985). Pathologically, *C. neoformans* usually causes a granulomatous meningitis; the formation of cryptococcomas is much less common (Zuger et al. 1986). In most cases CT and MR are unrevealing, showing either normal findings or findings suggestive of early hydrocephalus. The basilar exudate typical of the fungal meningitides is rarely seen in AIDS patients with *C. neoformans* infection. The symptoms are often muted, perhaps because of the inability of AIDS patients to mount a significant cell-mediated immune response.

In contrast, toxoplasmosis, the other common nonviral infectious agent in AIDS, presents as a mass (Figs. F 27–31). Focal neurologic abnormalities, seizures, and deterioration of mental status are the most common clinical abnormalities (Anderson et al. 1983; Alonso et al. 1984; Wong et al. 1984). In addition, toxoplasmosis is more common in AIDS patients from tropical third-world countries than from developed countries, presumably due to the proportionately greater incidence of toxoplasmosis in the general population of those countries (Levy RM et al. 1986). Pathologically, toxoplasmosis produces necrotizing granulomas, usually with thin capsules (Moskowitz et al. 1984a). The parasites are often visible within the inflamed brain tissue and cause surrounding vasculitis, perivascular infiltrate, and peripheral astrocytosis.

Focal intraparenchymal lesions, such as toxoplasmosis, generally present as low-density areas on noncontrast **CT** (Post et al. 1983). These areas usually enhance in an irregular, nodular, or ring pattern after administration of contrast medium (Kelly et al. 1984) (Figs. F 27–29), although occasionally they do not enhance at all (Whelan et al. 1983). In these cases double-dose delayed scans may demonstrate enhancement (Whelan et al. 1983; Post et al. 1985). The lesions do not evolve as typical abscesses, and a clearly defined collagen capsule with a liquefied center is usually not present. The absence of a capsule is probably due to the muted immunologic response of the host (Post et al. 1983). Toxoplasmosis lesions are generally multiple and bilateral (Whelan et al. 1983). Involvement of the deep gray matter, especially the basal ganglia, occurs in 60%–90% of cases (Post et al. 1983; Snider et al. 1983; Levy RM et al. 1985).

In recent years **MR** has begun to supplant CT in the workup of AIDS patients with suspected masses (Figs. F 28–31). Because of its extreme sensitivity to altered water content and its lack of bony artifact, MR can demonstrate lesions not visible on CT scans (Fig. F 28). Lesions appear on T1-weighted images as ill-defined regions of low signal intensity. On T2-weighted images these regions are of medium to high intensity and are surrounded by the high signal intensity of edema. Irregularly enhancing lesions, often ringlike, are seen on T1-weighted images after the administration of Gd-DTPA.

The increased sensitivity of MR to toxoplasmosis lesions compared with CT allows therapy to be instituted earlier. Furthermore, even when CT is positive for such lesions, MR often demonstrates additional lesions that may be more accessible to biopsy (Fig. F 29). Finally, MR imaging, by demonstrating multiple lesions, may obviate the need for biopsy, since a trial of antitoxoplasmosis therapy is now advocated in such cases (Pitlik et al. 1983; Snider et al. 1983).

The response of toxoplasmosis lesions to therapy is often dramatic, with a visible decrease in the size of the lesions and surrounding edema in a few days. However, sequelae of the lesions, such as demyelination and gliosis, can result in permanent changes. Resolving lesions often remain low in density on CT scans, even after the injection of iodinated contrast medium. This low density on CT may help to differentiate active from inactive lesions. Foci of high signal intensity may persist on T2-weighted MR images, even after treatment.

Although several other nonviral pathogens can infect the CNS in patients with AIDS, they cannot be differentiated on the basis of imaging studies alone. These agents, which include *Candida albicans* and other fungi, mycobacteria, and rarely other bacteria, produce MR and CT changes that are often identical to those seen in the more common cryptococcosis and toxoplasmosis. Multiple microabscesses of the brain have been seen in both candidiasis and coccidiosis (Levy RM et al. 1985). In such cases CT scans are often unrevealing (Price et al. 1986), and the utility of MR imaging has not yet been determined. Aspergillus and mucormycosis abscesses also can occur in AIDS patients (Berger et al. 1984; Micozzi and Wetli 1985).

Mycobacteria infecting AIDS patients are represented by *Mycobacterium tuberculosis* and *Mycobacterium avium-intracellulare. Mycobacterium tuberculosis* has occurred most often in AIDS patients from tropical developing countries, especially Haiti. It chiefly affects populations in low socioeconomic strata, presumably because they have a higher rate of previous infection. Several AIDS patients, mostly Haitian, have been reported to have tuberculomas or tuberculous abscesses in the brain (Pitchenik et al. 1983; Pitlik et al. 1983; Fischl et al. 1985; Post et al. 1985). Again, these lesions closely resemble the prototype focal masses of toxoplasmosis. Tuberculous meningitis may also be present, although the typical thick, basilar, purulent exudate has not been reported, presumably due to the weakened defense system of the host.

Prior to the advent of AIDS, disseminated infection with *Mycobacterium avium-intracellulare* was considered a rare phenomenon, even in immunosuppressed patients. However, *Mycobacterium avium-intracellulare* has now been revealed to be a frequent pathogen in AIDS patients (Fauci 1985), although its involvement of the CNS is unusual. Probable granuloma formation has been noted in the brain of AIDS patients (Greene et al. 1982). This organism has been demonstrated at autopsy in the brain of an AIDS patient with encephalopathy (Snider et al. 1983). The remaining atypical mycobacterial infections occur in the rest of the body but have not yet been found in the CNS.

Pyogenic bacterial infections of the CNS are unusual in AIDS patients, probably because the primary deficit is one of cell-mediated rather than humoral immunity. Only one AIDS patient with *Escherichia coli* meningoencephalitis has been described (Berger et al. 1984). Another patient was found to have a mixed abscess composed of nocardia and salmonella (Holtz et al. 1985). Other bacterial pathogens occurring in AIDS are spirochetes and actinomycetes. Two cases of meningovascular syphilis have been reported in AIDS patients (Bredesen and Messing 1983; Berger et al. 1984). CT findings are normal in one; details of the other case are not available.

Viral Syndromes

Discovery of the HIV was soon followed by isolation of the nucleic acid of the viruses in the brain itself (Shaw et al. 1985). This isolation and the related evidence (Ho et al. 1985) suggest that the viruses may be directly involved in the pathogenesis of several of the acute and chronic neurologic syndromes associated with AIDS. By virtue of the neurotropism as well as the lymphotropism of these viruses, the CNS can suffer devastating consequences, not only from the opportunistic infections that typify AIDS in the rest of the body but also from the damage from the HIV themselves. If the viruses do have this capability, then the neural axis occupies a uniquely unfortunate niche in the body and possibly is affected by the most extensive range of AIDS-related abnormalities of any single organ system. The full effects of chronic HIV infection in the brain may not yet be apparent.

Viral syndromes can be divided into two categories: those which are clearly opportunistic, such as progressive multifocal leukoencephalopathy (Fig. F32), and those of which the cause is still in doubt. This latter group, more truly syndromes than specific disease entities, consists of subacute encephalopathy, recurrent or chronic aseptic meningitis, and subacute viral myelitis. Concerning the causative organism of the latter group of viral syndromes, most reports initially favored CMV as the prime suspect (Snider et al. 1983; Nielsen et al. 1984; Post et al. 1985, 1986; Levy RM et al. 1986). The typical "owl's eye" inclusion bodies of CMV have been documented in some of these syndromes. In others, positive immunohistochemical staining has been demonstrated (Nielsen et al. 1984; Wiley et al. 1986). However, several authors have disputed the hypothesis that CMV is the prime cause of CNS disease in AIDS, suggesting that CMV may often be a secondary opportunistic infection (Figs. F33, 35).

HIV have recently been proposed as the most likely primary pathogens (Ho et al. 1985; Kleihues et al. 1985; Levy JA et al. 1985). As mentioned earlier, HIV nucleic acids have been isolated in the brain of AIDS patients (Shaw et al. 1985). In addition, brain tissue cultures for HIV have proved positive in patients with AIDS-related dementia, even in patients in whom blood cultures were negative, making accidental contamination unlikely.

Syndromes Most Likely Due to HIV

The most common neurologic effect of AIDS is a subacute encephalopathy that is often attributed to HIV. It affects 22%–36% of all AIDS patients who have neurologic symptoms (Snider et al. 1983; Nielsen et al. 1984; Levy RM et al. 1985). Although the encephalopathy initially presents as mild confusion or loss of memory, it usually progresses to marked psychomotor retardation and dementia. Occasionally the symptoms are accompanied by focal findings or seizures. Coma and eventually death, usually due to intercurrent infection, can ensue. Pathologically, atrophy is prominent (Nielsen et al. 1984). Microglial nodules are present in the gray matter. White matter changes are typified by occasional microglial cells, perivascular infiltrates, focal vacuolation, and small, ill-defined foci of demyelination interspersed in a general pattern of myelin pallor (Price et al. 1986). White matter changes predominate in some patients, while in others the gray matter is much more extensively involved (Nielsen et al. 1984).

Radiologically, the encephalopathy is detected most consistently by **CT**, which shows only atrophy. Occasionally, diffuse low density is present in the white matter (Post et al. 1985). **MR** findings are similar to the CT findings. MR occasionally discloses areas of high signal intensity in the white matter on T2-weighted images. These lesions may be focal or coalesced and may involve much of the white matter. They may represent the pathologically demonstrated areas of demyelination.

HIV have recently been implicated in *subacute viral myelitis*. Postmortem cultures of the lumbar spinal cord in a patient with distal myelopathy and vacuolar degeneration grew HIV (Ho et al. 1985). Symptoms of this syndrome include leg weakness, incontinence, ataxia, and spasticity (Price et al. 1986). Histologic examination usually reveals a vacuolar myelopathy often associated with demyelination and primarily restricted to the lateral and posterior columns of the spinal cord, especially at the midthoracic level (Goldstick et al. 1985). This finding has been noted in 22%–50% of all patients with AIDS (Petito et al. 1985; Price et al. 1986). Since the spinal cord is grossly normal, myelography and adjunctive CT scanning have been normal. To date, pathologic findings in AIDS patients with subacute viral myelitis have not been correlated with MR findings. The cases we have encountered have shown normal findings on MR.

HIV have also been implicated in viral meningitis, with isolation of the virus in patients with AIDS or AIDS-related conditions (ARC) who present with unexplained chronic aseptic meningitis (Ho et al. 1985). In some cases recurrent or chronic aseptic meningitis precedes the initial diagnosis of AIDS. Symptoms are typified by headaches, fever, and meningeal signs. AIDS patients with *chronic aseptic meningitis* have normal CT and MR findings.

Opportunistic Viral Infections

Progressive multifocal leukoencephalopathy (PML) commonly affects patients with AIDS (Snider et al. 1983; Krupp et al. 1985; Levy RM et al. 1985). Symptoms are nonspecific and include headache, dementia, and focal deficits. The causative agent is a papovavirus, almost always the JC virus, which presumably becomes reactivated in immunosuppressed patients long after an asymptomatic childhood infection (Britton and Miller 1984). Histology demonstrates bizarre hypertrophic astrocytes and inclusion bodies within the oligodendrocytes. Because the JC virus attacks the myelin-producing oligodendrocytes, PML is manifested by demyelination and edema. **CT** demonstrates low-density areas in the white matter of the affected regions, typically in parieto-occipital distribution. However, approximately 10% of infections are entirely infratentorial, affecting the brainstem and/or cerebellum. Rarely, extension into the gray matter occurs. **MR** has proven superior in demonstrating the lesions. Because of its greater sensitivity to changes in water content, loss of the hydrophobic myelin, which results in increased local water content, appears as areas of high signal intensity on T2-weighted images (Fig. F32). But while MR is sensitive to the effects of the infection, MR findings are not specific. As previously noted, cases in which biopsy or autopsy did not show PML have shown MR findings consistent with encephalopathy.

Other viral encephalitides and myelitis. Although HIV have been implicated in many CNS diseases in AIDS patients, there is substantial evidence that CMV sometimes plays a role (Moskowitz et al. 1984a; Edwards et al. 1985; Wiley et al. 1986). Frank necrotic foci of acute encephalitis often demonstrate the typical inclusion bodies of CMV. The CT and MR appearances are identical to those of other mass lesions in AIDS. It is most likely that further work with AIDS will disclose many other viruses causing encephalitis. For example, Levy RM et al. (1985) report a probable case of *varicella zoster encephalitis* in which, though autopsy was not performed, the CSF was positive for varicella zoster cultures. This finding does not seem surprising in light of the known association between herpes zoster radiculitis and the later development of AIDS.

Because immunocompetent individuals occasionally acquire herpes simplex encephalitis, this disease by itself is not diagnostic of AIDS. However, although nearly all adult cases of herpes simplex encephalitis involve the herpes simplex virus I (HSV I), we have seen AIDS with *herpes simplex encephalitis* secondary to HSV II (Dix et al. 1985). MR scans of these AIDS patients disclose findings typical of HSV I encephalitis, unlike those reported in infants with HSV II encephalitis. The changes are often restricted to the temporal lobes, either unilaterally or bilaterally. MR imaging, as may be expected, is more sensitive. If changes are found in both temporal lobes, the specificity of MR increases because this appearance is almost pathognomonic for herpes simplex encephalitis (Fig. F34).

Ependymitis has been prominent in several AIDS patients, often as a near-terminal event. The distribution strikingly resembles that seen radiographically in congenital cytomegalic inclusion disease (Wiley et al. 1986). Cytomegalic cells are found in the periventricular areas (Post et al. 1986), and CMV has been grown from cultures of CSF (Edwards et al. 1985). Enhancing areas in the subependymal regions appear on contrast-enhanced CT scans, while MR images disclose areas of high signal intensity in periventricular distribution (Fig. F35). Irregular extension of the high intensity into the adjacent white matter may aid in differentiating this ependymitis from pure transependymal fluid flow typical of hydrocephalus, which generally appears as a smooth, thin band surrounding the ventricles.

Necrotizing myelitis, frequently severe and of rapid onset, is more unusual than subacute myelitis in AIDS patients. Two cases of necrotizing myelitis have been attributed to HSV II, either by means of positive cultures from the spinal cord or by immunohistochemistry (Britton et al. 1985; Dix et al. 1985). Myelography and CT scans showed negative findings in both cases. Another AIDS patient with ascending myelitis was considered at autopsy to have had CMV (Bagley et al. 1986). To our knowledge, MR imaging has not been performed in AIDS patients with suspected viral myelitis.

b) Neoplasms

Primary CNS Lymphoma

Before the advent of AIDS, primary CNS lymphoma was an unusual tumor, constituting less than 2% of all lymphomas. However, a high incidence of CNS lymphoma was known to occur in patients with immunodeficient states, whether congenital as in Wiskott-Aldrich syndrome, acquired as in Sjogren's syndrome, or iatrogenic as in patients who were organ transplant recipients (Letendre et al. 1982; Gill et al. 1985). It is not surprising, then, that CNS lymphoma has appeared in approximately 6.4% of all AIDS patients presenting with CNS disease (Levy RM et al. 1986). These patients usually exhibit symptoms consistent with focal masses, i.e., identical to those from other causes of intracerebral masses (Helle et al. 1984; Gill et al. 1985). The tumors appear histologically as high-grade lymphoma of either the immunoblastic sarcoma type or the small non-cleaved cell type (Gill et al. 1985; Ioachim et al. 1985; Levine et al. 1985) (roughly equivalent to the diffuse histiocytic lymphoma or diffuse undifferentiated lymphoma, respectively, of the Rappaport classification; Rosenberg et al. 1982). These are aggressive lesions, and the average life expectancy following diagnosis is usually only a few months.

On **CT**, primary CNS lymphoma usually appears as well-circumscribed, slightly hyperdense lesions that enhance uniformly with contrast medium. The lesions are periventricular and are seldom associated with edema (Palacios et al. 1982; Spillane et al. 1982). These tumors appear markedly different, however, in AIDS patients (Whelan et al. 1983; Gill et al. 1985). Noncontrast CT scans in AIDS patients generally show hypodense regions with mass effects. These areas enhance irregularly with contrast medium, often presenting a nodular or ringlike pattern. Surrounding edema may be prominent. Multifocality occurs in approximately 30%–43% of primary CNS lymphomas by CT criteria (Kazner et al. 1978; Enzmann et al. 1979; Spillane et al. 1982; Cellerier et al. 1984) and is typical in AIDS-associated cases. Thus lymphoma cannot be excluded in a patient presenting with multiple masses, although toxoplasmosis or other infections may be more likely causes. The corresponding **MR** appearance consists of ill-defined regions of decreased signal intensity on T1-weighted images which, along with the surrounding edema, give a high signal on T2-weighted images. In AIDS patients the appearance of CNS lymphoma on both CT and MR scans is identical to that of other focal masses in AIDS.

Because of the severely immunocompromised status of AIDS patients, multiple diffuse diseases may be present simultaneously. We have seen six AIDS patients who presented with contrast-enhancing lesions typical of toxoplasmosis in whom, despite application of antitoxoplasmosis therapy, some lesions continued to grow. In these patients biopsy specimens from several lesions demonstrated the concomitant occurrence of lymphoma and toxoplasmosis (Fig. F29).

Systemic Lymphoma

Primary CNS lymphomas more frequently involve the brain parenchyma than do systemic lymphomas, which usually invade the meninges (Levitt et al. 1980; Pagani et al. 1981). Because the meninges are involved, symptoms often include radiculopathy and cranial nerve neuropathies as well as headache and altered mental status (Mackintosh et al. 1982). The pathology is consistent with leptomeningeal spread and, less commonly, with frank parenchymal metastases. Histologically these tumors are most often high-grade lymphomas (Mackintosh et al. 1982). Extension of systemic lymphoma to the CNS has been reported in 19%–22% of AIDS patients with lymphoma (Ziegler et al. 1984; Ioachim et al. 1985). **CT** and **MR** usually do not demonstrate leptomeningeal spread. This negative finding correlates well with reports that meningeal enhancement is rare (Pagani et al. 1981; Palacios et al. 1982). We have seen several patients who had hydrocephalus associated with leptomeningeal spread of systemic lymphoma. Parenchymal metastases in secondary lymphoma resemble the foci of primary CNS lymphoma. Secondary lymphoma can also affect the spinal canal in the form of lymphomatous masses compressing the spinal cord (Snider et al. 1983; Ziegler et al. 1984; Case Records of the Massachusetts General Hospital 1986). In this instance, as in other CNS involvement, high-grade lymphomas are seen histologically.

Kaposi's Sarcoma

Kaposi's sarcoma involving the CNS is unusual in AIDS patients, although several histologically proved cases have been reported (Gorin et al. 1985; Kelly et al. 1984; Levy RM et al. 1984). When it does occur, **CT** demonstrates contrast-enhancing parenchymal masses typical of brain metastases. These lesions are often hemorrhagic. Although the **MR** features of Kaposi's sarcoma metastatic to the brain have not been reported, the lesions would presumably appear similar to brain metastases of other lesions. Because MR imaging is more sensitive to subacute bleeding than CT, any hemorrhagic component would most likely show up as regions of high signal intensity on T1-weighted images. This appearance might help suggest the diagnosis.

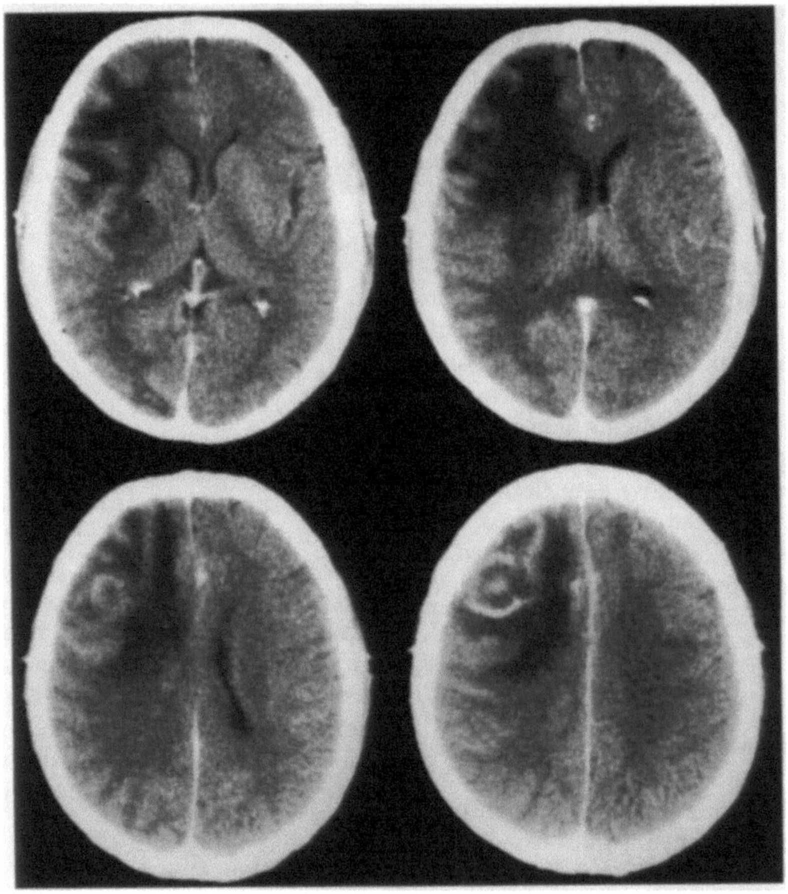

Fig. F27. Cerebral toxoplasmosis in a 37-year-old AIDS patient with a 4-week history of cerebral seizures. Neurologic exam disclosed right-sided weakness. Post-contrast CT demonstrates a mass lesion of the left frontal region with conspicuous edema involving the entire left hemisphere. An irregular enhancement pattern is observed. There is minimal displacement of midline structures

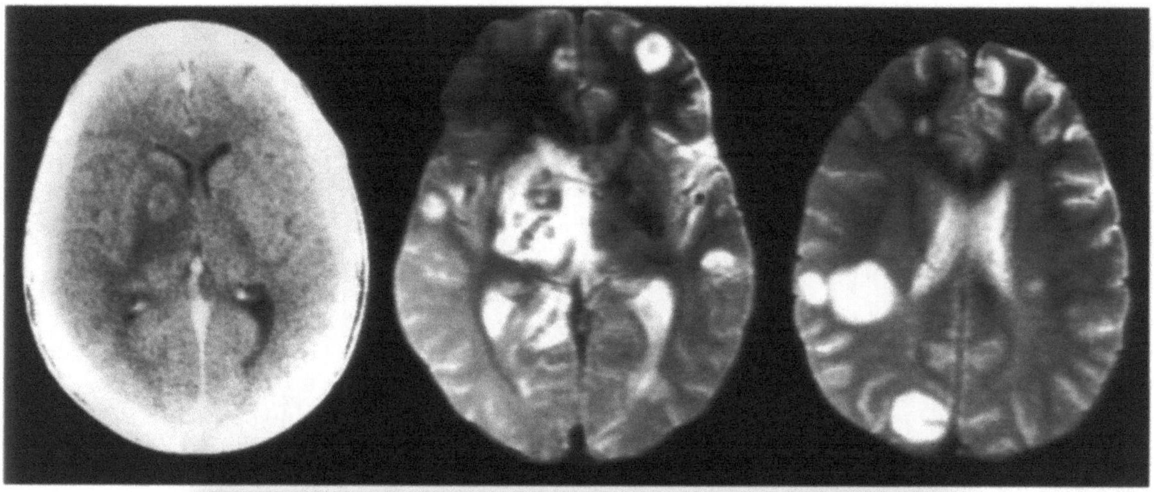

a–c

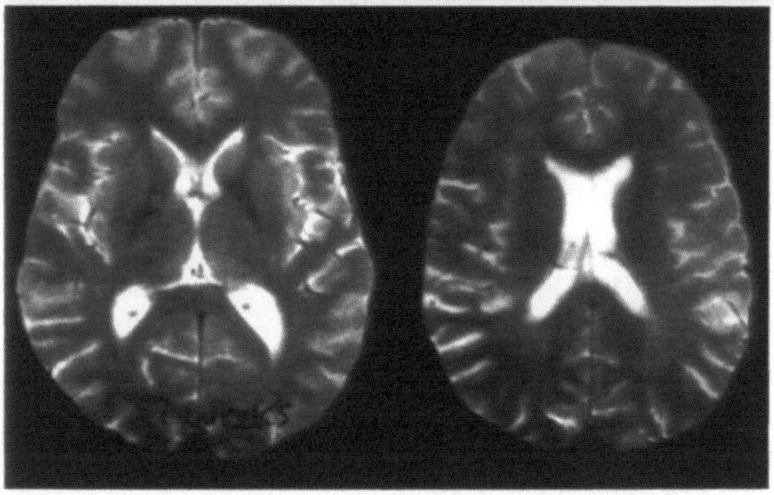

d e

Fig. F 28 a–e. Toxoplasmosis in a 31-year-old man with AIDS. **a** Postcontrast CT shows a mildly enhancing focus in the left basal ganglia with surrounding edema. **b, c** T2-weighted MR images (SE 2000/70) confirm the abnormality in the left basal ganglia, again with surrounding edema. However, several other foci of high signal are also noted. The presence of multiple, widely scattered foci of high signal intensity in a patient with this history is most consistent with toxoplasmosis. Other etiologies, such as other opportunistic infections or lymphoma, are less likely. **d, e** Remarkable resolution of the lesions is noted on this repeat MR scan following 7 weeks' treatment with pyrimethamine and sulfadiazine. Only a few traces of abnormal high signal remain (imaging parameters same as in **b, c**)

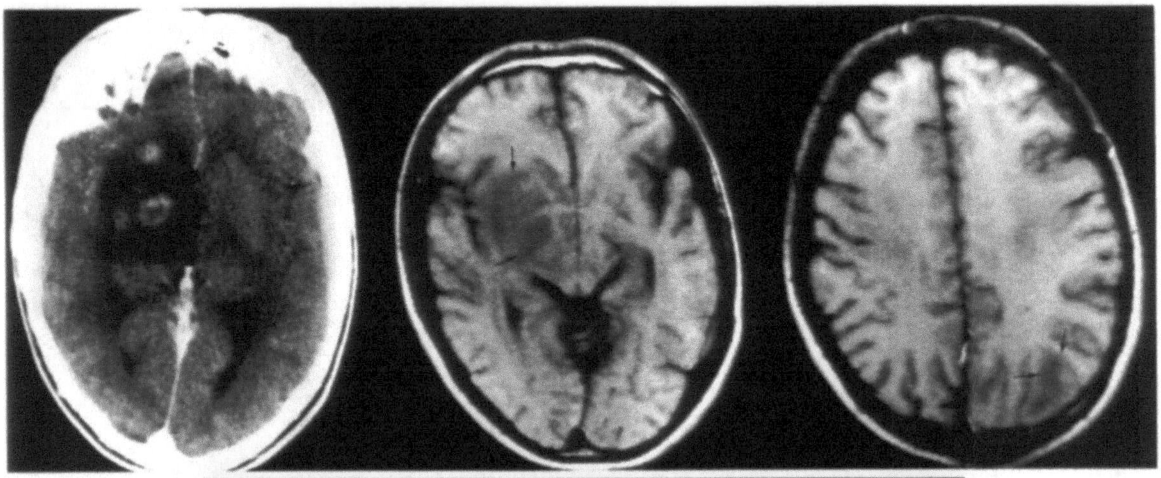

a–c

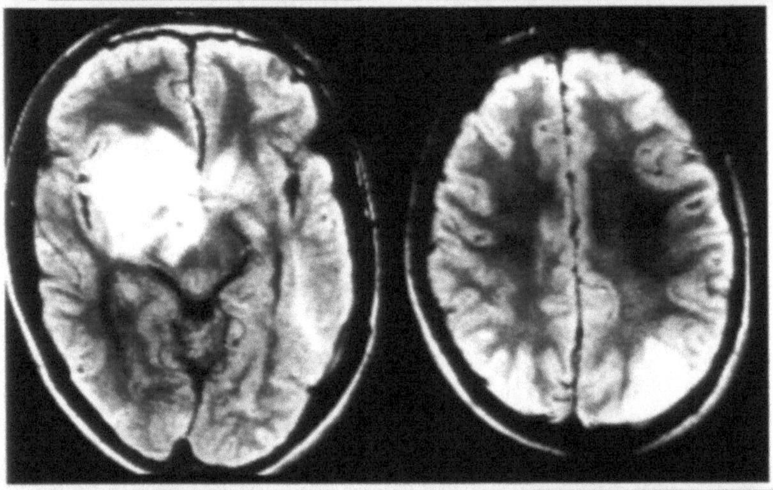

d, e

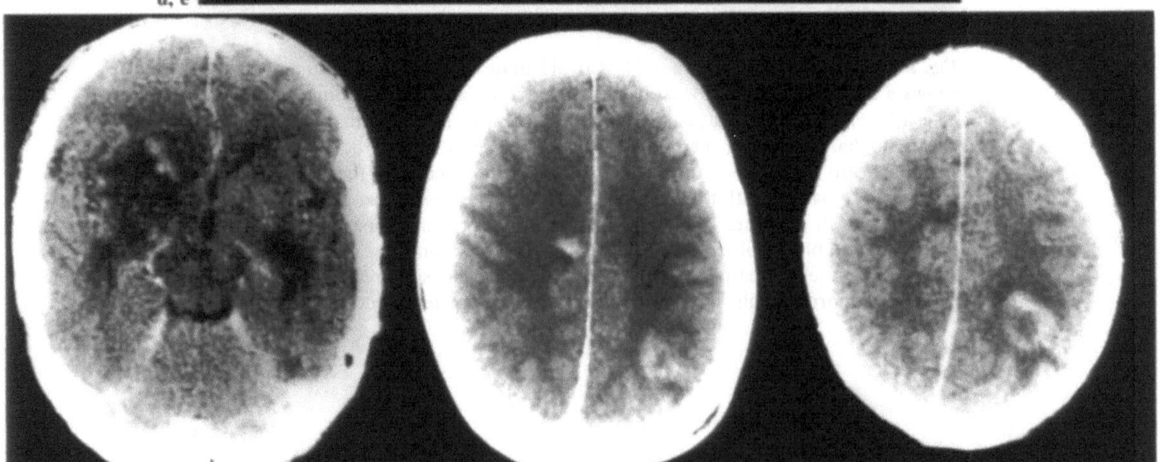

f–h

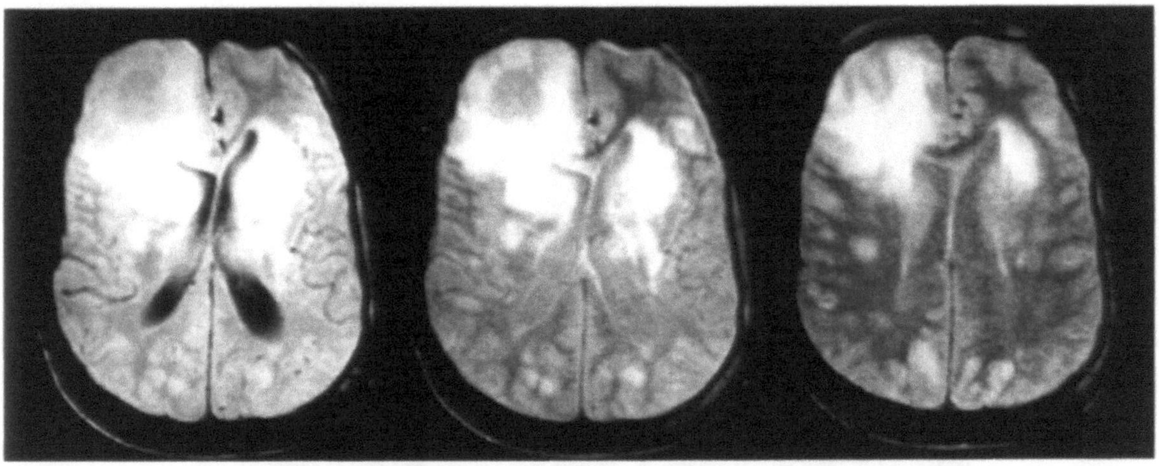

Fig. F 30. Toxoplasmosis (histologically proved) in a 30-year-old man with AIDS, headache, and right-sided weakness. MR: *left* SE 1600/35, *center* SE 1600/70, *right* SE 1600/90. Marked hyperintensity is apparent in the left frontal and right paraventricular regions. The left frontal hyperintensity contains a low-signal area representing a circumscribed focus with surrounding edema. In addition, multiple hyperintensities of varying size are seen over both hemispheres, predominantly in the white matter. These foci are displayed most clearly on the T2-weighted images

◄

Fig. F 29 a–h. Lymphoma and toxoplasmosis in a 40-year-old man with AIDS and right-sided weakness. **a** Contrast-enhanced CT demonstrates several ring or nodular lesions in the inferior portions of the left basal ganglia. Considerable mass effect and surrounding edema are visible. Additional lesions were seen superiorly, in the left centrum semiovale and right parieto-occipital region, in higher sections. **b, c** T1-weighted MR scans (SE 500/30) show ill-defined areas of low signal (*arrows*) corresponding to the CT abnormalities. **d, e** T2-weighted images (SE 2000/30) show high signal in the inferior portions of the left basal ganglia and in the right parieto-occipital region. In addition, a small focus near the left centrum semiovale may also be somewhat increased in signal intensity. The overall appearance is nonspecific. When the patient did not improve clinically with antitoxoplasmosis therapy, biopsy of the left basal ganglia lesion was performed. It revealed a malignant lymphoma, and the patient was started on radiation therapy. **f–h** After 1 month of radiotherapy the lesions in the left basal ganglia largely resolved. Some ill-defined hypodensity is still present in this region, but most of the mass effect and enhancement have disappeared. However, the right parieto-occipital lesion has grown in the interval. Repeat biopsy identified this lesion as toxoplasmosis

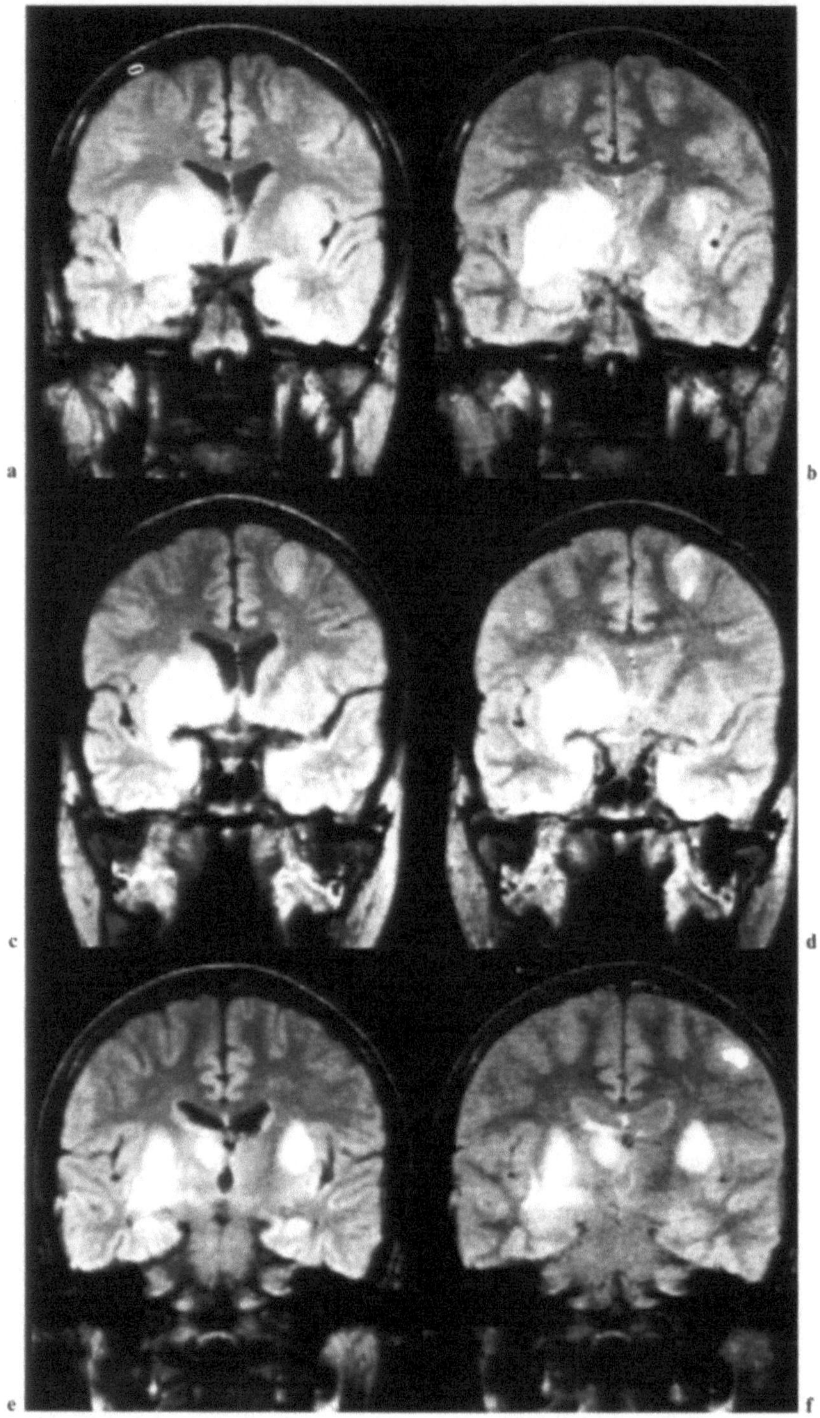

Fig. F31a–f. Cerebral toxoplasmosis in a 37-year-old man with AIDS, headache, fever, and visual disturbances. MR: **a** SE 1600/35, **b** SE 1600/70, **c** SE 1600/35, **d** SE 1600/70, **e** SE 1600/35, **f** SE 1600/70, all coronal. The scans demonstrate multiple circumscribed foci in the region of the left basal ganglia with compression of the left lateral ventricle, high in the right parietal region, and medial to the sylvian cistern on the right side

Fig. F33a–d. CMV encephalitis (histologically proved) in a 31-year-old man with fever, impaired consciousness, and cerebral seizures. MR: **a** SE 1600/35, **b** SE 1600/70, **c** SE 1600/35, **d** SE 1600/70. Multiple foci of low signal intensity and variable size occur bilaterally in the region of the basal ganglia and in the white matter of both hemispheres

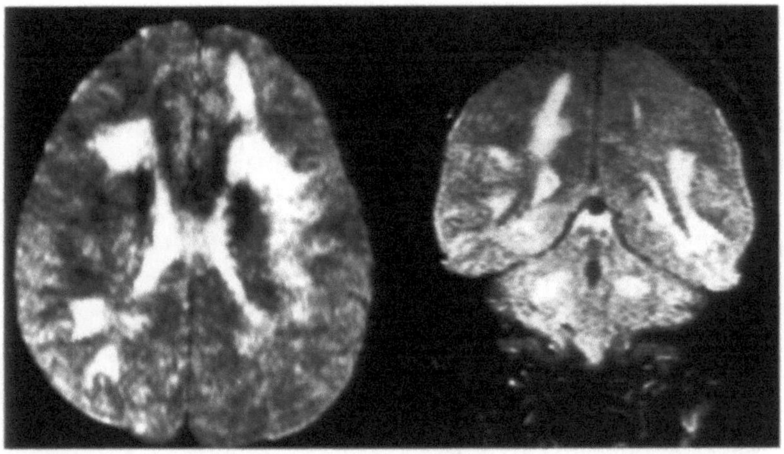

Fig. F 32. Progressive multifocal leukoencephalopathy in a 34-year-old man with AIDS and altered mental status. T2-weighted axial and coronal MR images (SE 2020/120) reveal multiple foci of high signal intensity in the white matter. There may also be minor extension into the gray matter. The patchy nature of the lesions and their essential confinement to the white matter are very typical of progressive multifocal leukoencephalopathy

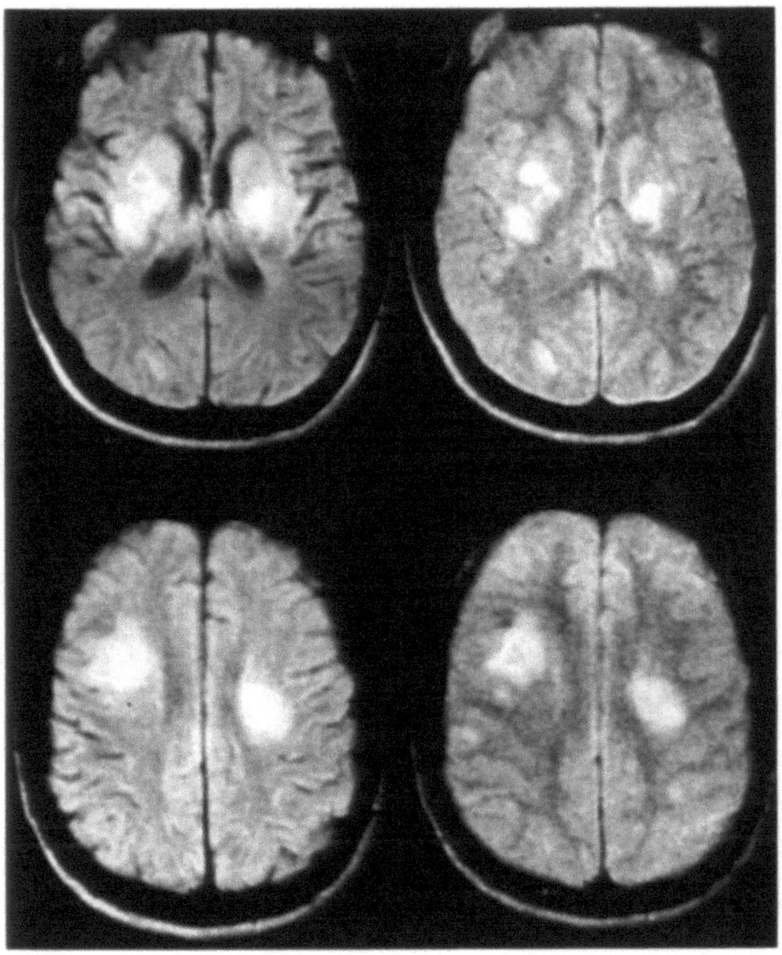

a b c d F 33

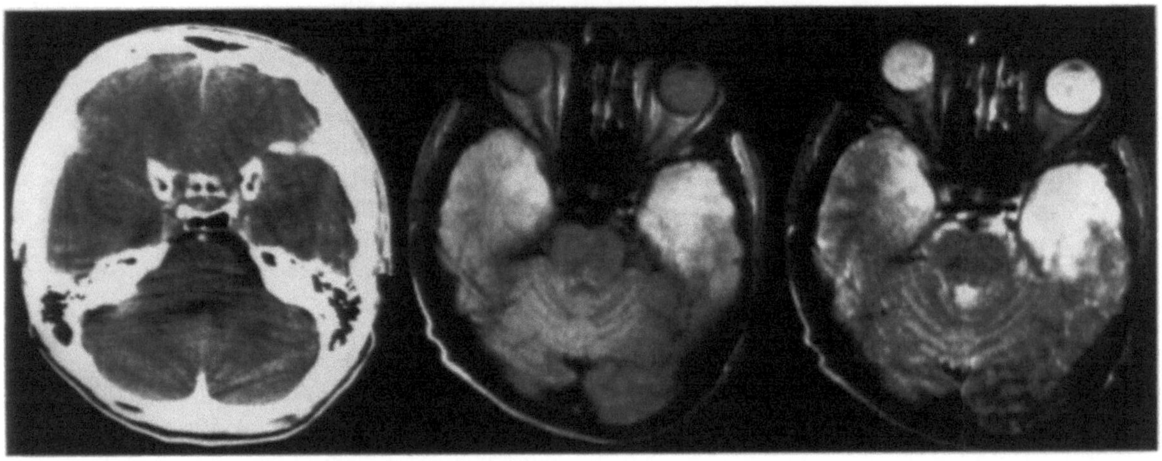

Fig. F34. Herpes simplex viral encephalitis in a 35-year-old woman with positive HIV antibody test in the blood, whose husband died of AIDS 1 month earlier, presenting with 3 days of confusion, headache, and high fevers. *Left:* Postcontrast CT reveals mild mass effect and subtle hypodensity in the right temporal lobe. *Center* and *right* T2-weighted images (SE 2000/60 and 2000/120) show massive changes in the right temporal lobe with diffuse high signal due to edema and inflammatory exudate. The left temporal lobe is also abnormal, a finding which was missed on the CT scan. The involvement of both temporal lobes is strongly suggestive, if not pathognomonic, of herpes simplex encephalitis. (Case courtesy of Dr. Charles M. Elkin, New York City)

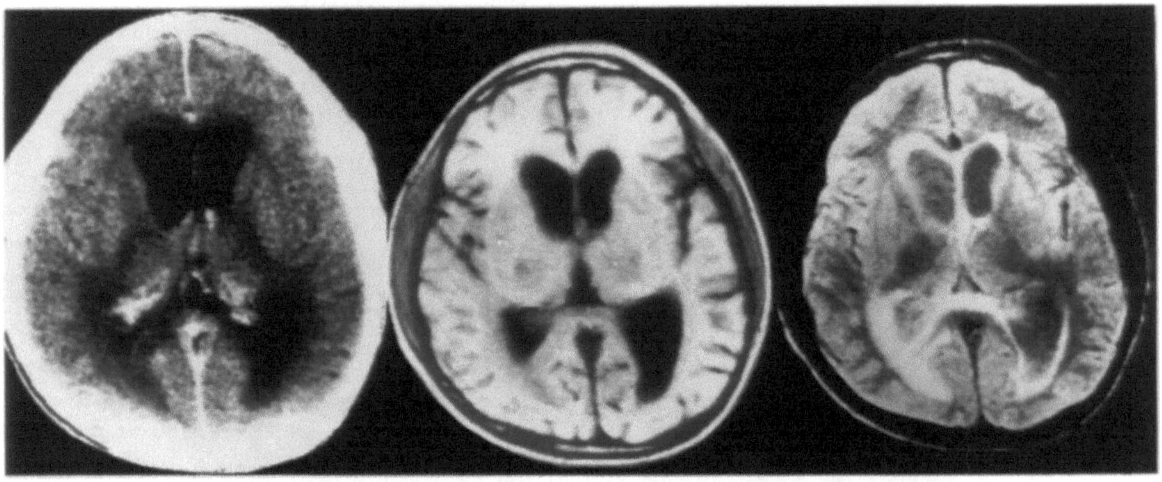

Fig. F35. Cytomegalovirus ependymitis in a 28-year-old man with AIDS, somnolence. *Left* Postcontrast CT shows a thin rim of faint enhancement surrounding prominent lateral ventricles. Slight hypodensity in the periventricular white matter is also apparent. *Center* T1-weighted MR (SE 500/30) confirms the prominent ventricles. The T2-weighted image (SE 2000/30) additionally shows a thick rim of high signal encircling the ventricles. This rim is more prominent that one would expect in pure hydrocephalus. The overall appearance in a patient with this clinical history is consistent with cytomegalovirus ependymitis, which was demonstrated at autopsy

5. Cysts

a) Arachnoid Cysts

Arachnoid cysts are the most commonly encountered cystic lesions in the cranial cavity. They may be congenital or acquired in early childhood, and their site of predilection is the *sylvian fissure* (Figs. F 36, 37). Their extra-axial location on the brain surface causes a bulging of the cranial bone overlying the cyst. There may be concomitant displacement of the brain parenchyma and ventricles. The mass effect is variable, but most commonly there is a marked separation of the temporal lobe from the cranial vault with compression of the ipsilateral ventricles.

The **CT** diagnosis of arachnoid cyst is based on the isodensity of the cystic fluid to CSF. Frequently the patient has an antecedent history of minor head trauma causing the cyst wall to rupture and discharge its contents into the subdural space (Fig. F 37). This is especially common in children. In terms of treatment planning, it is important to determine whether an arachnoid cyst communicates freely with the subarachnoid space or forms a closed mass. This can be established by CT following the intrathecal administration of contrast medium.

On **MR** the cyst fluid has long T1 and T2 relaxation times and is isointense to CSF. Because of its very long T2 times, the cyst gives an increasingly intense signal on the even echoes of a multi-echo sequence in relation to the uniform loss of signal in the brain parenchyma (Kjos et al 1985) (Figs. F 39, 40).

Less common sites of occurrence of arachnoid cysts are the *chiasmatic cistern* and the *quadrigeminal region.* Large saccular cysts may form in these regions, especially in children, and hydrocephalus may develop due to cyst obstruction of the CSF flow (Figs. F 42, 43).

Arachnoid cysts are occasionally found in the cerebellopontine angle or adjacent to the cisterna magna. A large cisterna magna may simulate an arachnoid cyst on CT and MR scans (Figs. F 45, 50–52). Arachnoid cysts *in the posterior fossa* of infants can pose special problems of differential diagnosis (Figs. F 44, 46–49). This is because the adjacent, compressed cerebellar tissues may show some degree of contrast enhancement, simulating the appearance of a ring-enhancing tumor (Fig. F 48). Indeed, differentiation from any cystic posterior fossa tumor, such as angioblastoma, can be a difficult task. The intense contrast enhancement of the angiomatous nodule and the higher attenuation values of the tumor cyst should, however, serve to differentiate the lesions. An epidermoid cyst may be mistaken for an arachnoid cyst if it lacks peripheral calcifications or if artifacts from sharp density gradients in the posterior fossa distort the CT analysis of absorption coefficients (Figs. F 45, 46).

MR provides additional information helpful in classifying the cyst contents. Specifically, the protein content of the cyst has known effects on the relaxation times and proton signals, and this yields additional criteria for differentiating an arachnoid cyst from a tumor cyst.

b) Dandy-Walker Cysts

The diagnosis of a Dandy-Walker cyst rarely presents difficulties owing to the typical changes that are associated with this anomaly. The malformation of the fourth ventricle is accompanied by absence or hypoplasia of the cerebellar vermis with obstruction of the foramina of Magendie and Luschka, resulting in hydrocephalus. CSF occupies most of the enlarged posterior fossa, communicating with the dilated fourth ventricle. The contour of the ventricle is indented by the remnants of the cerebellum. The elevated confluence of the sinuses and the abnormally upright position of the tentorium complete the CT presentation. An enlarged cisterna magna or cysts of the posterior fossa (Fig. F 49) can resemble a Dandy-Walker cyst, but they are not associated with elevation of the sinus confluence (Archer et al. 1978) (Figs. F 50–52).

c) Other Cysts

"Simple cysts" of the posterior fossa cannot always be identified as CSF-filled cavities by density measurements and so are apt to be mistaken for angioblastoma (Figs. F53, 54).

Non-neoplastic cysts are occasionally found in the cerebral hemispheres (see Fig. D6.24). Their etiology is highly variable and cannot always be ascertained (Fig. F55). The cyst wall may even contain calcifications, mimicking the appearance of a tumor.

d) Primary Aqueduct Stenoses and Obstructions of the Foramina of Luschka and Magendie

In *primary aqueduct stenosis* caused by inflammatory disease, compromise of CSF flow leads to dilatation of the first three ventricles while the fourth ventricle retains a normal shape, size, and position. Contrast enhancement of the vermis, however, can mimic a mass lesion in this region ("pseudotumor vermis"). Doubts are resolved by **MR** imaging. The midsagittal scan affords proof of aqueduct stenosis and confirms the normal anatomy of the cerebellar vermis (Fig. F56). In the future, it is expected that MR measurements of CSF flow dynamics or an absence of pulsatile flow will provide a means of establishing the diagnosis of aqueduct stenosis.

Obstruction of the foramina of Luschka and Magendie results in extreme dilatation of the fourth ventricle, which may resemble a cystic cerebellar tumor or other intra-axial cyst (Fig. F57). Again, MR images are helpful in the sagittal plane and in demonstrating flow-related phase changes in the CSF.

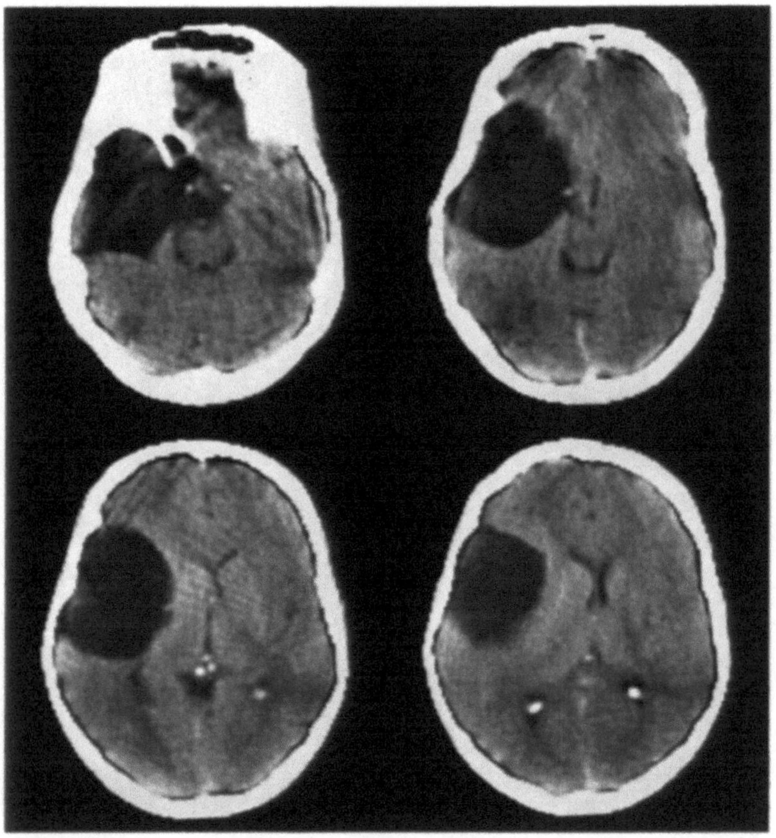

Fig. F36. Large arachnoid cyst in the left temporal region. Bulging and thinning of the cranium over the fluid-filled cavity are noted on the higher sections. Conspicuous mass effect is present. The attenuation of the cyst is 9–11 HU

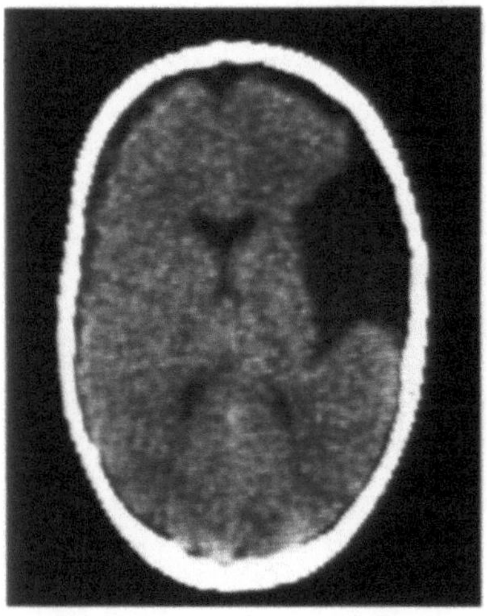

Fig. F37. Arachnoid cyst of the right temporal region in a 6-year-old child. Subdural effusions developed after minor trauma causing rupture of the cyst wall. Noncontrast CT

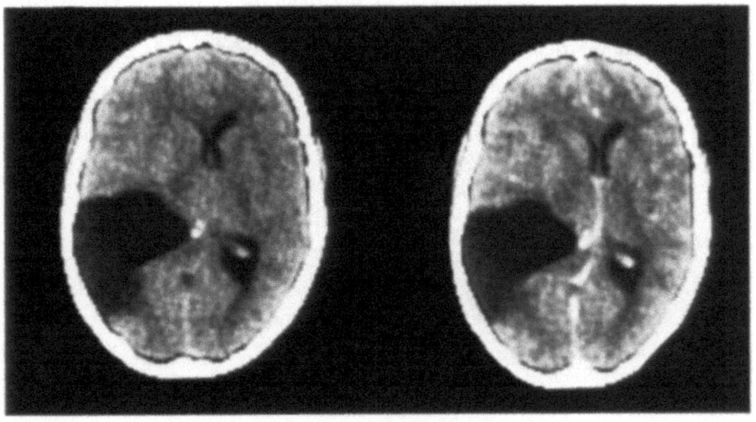

Fig. F38. Large arachnoid cyst at the junction of the left temporal and occipital lobes in a 58-year-old woman. There is significant mass effect with displacement of midline structures. The lesion is isodense to CSF and does not enhance with contrast medium. *Left* precontrast CT scan, *right* postcontrast scan

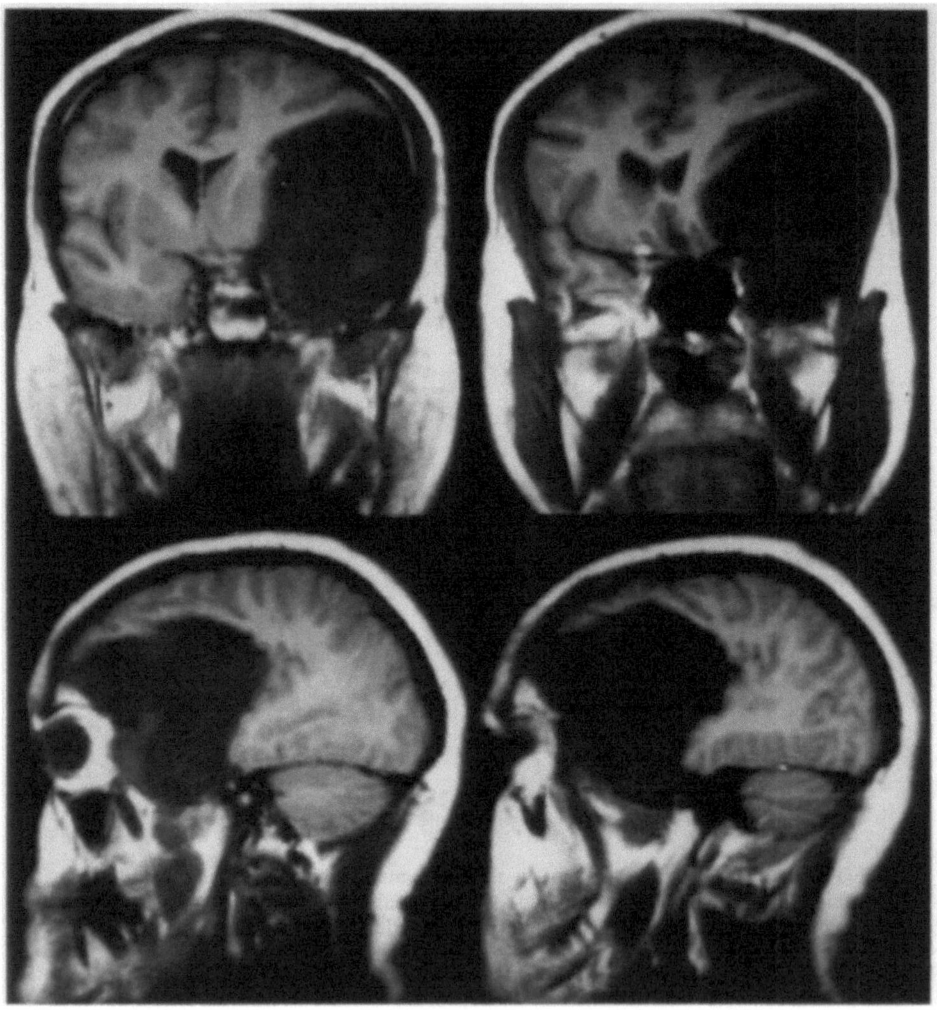

Fig. F39. Arachnoid cyst in the right frontotemporoparietal region of a 37-year-old man. SE 400/30 MR images show a smoothly delineated cyst causing significant mass effect and displacing the ventricular system toward the opposite side

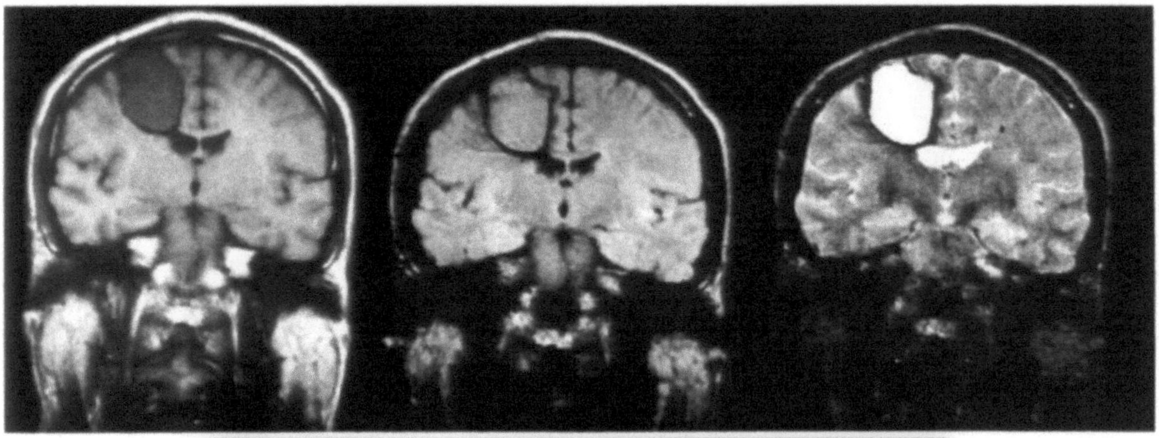

a–c

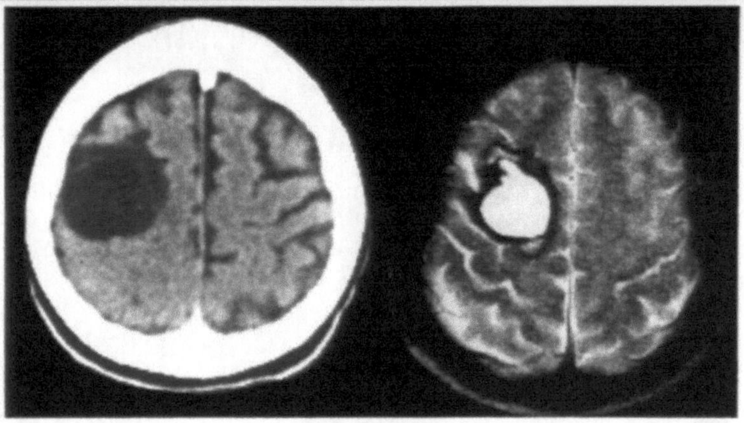

d e

Fig. F 40 a–e. Arachnoid cyst in the left centroparietal region of a 45-year-old man with a 6-month history of right-sided jacksonian seizures. A smoothly delineated, circumscribed hypodense lesion is visible on CT (**d**). MR: **a** SE 500/30, **b** SE 2000/35, **c** SE 2000/120, **e** SE 2000/120. The cyst, hypodense on the CT scan, gives an intense signal on the T2-weighted MR images (**c, e**). Again, the margins of the lesion are smooth

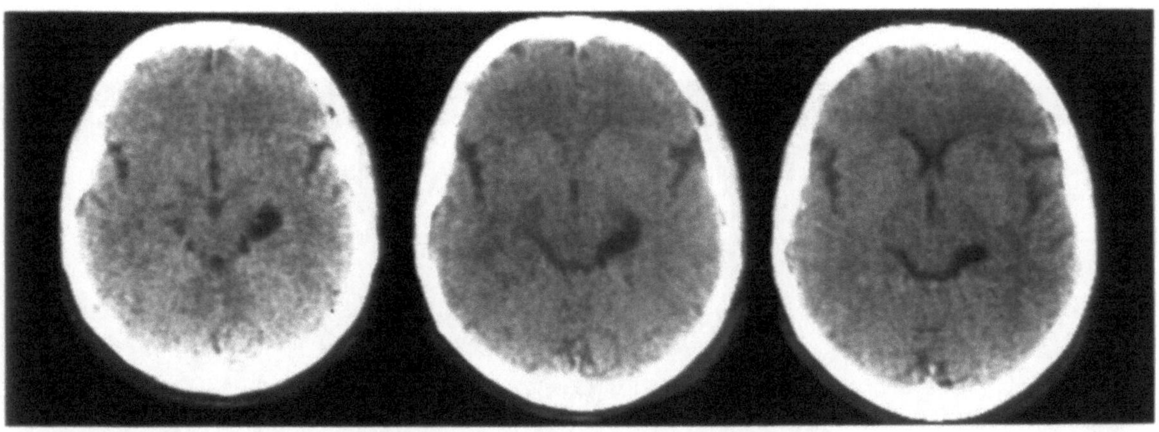

Fig. F 41. Circumscribed arachnoid cyst of the right ambient cistern in a 38-year-old woman with diffuse headache and diplopia. Noncontrast CT scans reveal a circumscribed area of low density in the region of the right ambient cistern

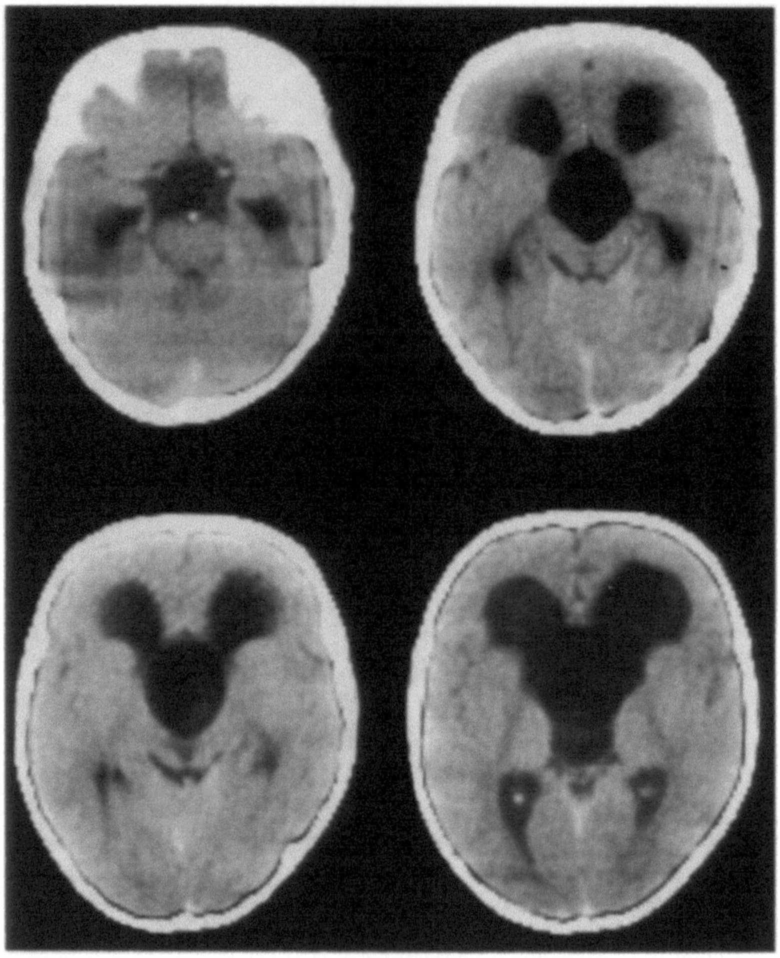

Fig. F42. Arachnoid cyst in the region of the chiasmatic cistern in a 6-year-old child with severe hydrocephalus due to bilateral obstruction of the foramina of Monro. The cyst contents are isodense to the intraventricular CSF. Postcontrast CT

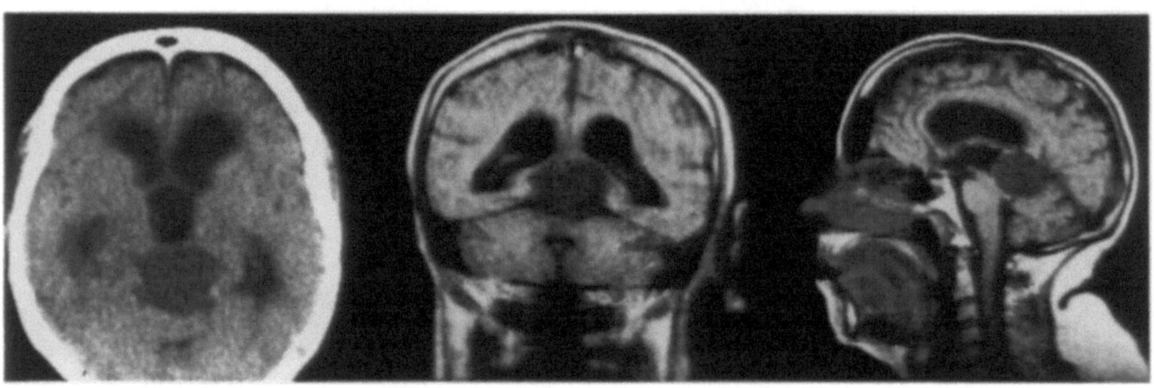

Fig. F43. Arachnoid cyst of the quadrigeminal plate in a patient with a 1-year history of headaches and a 2-week history of gait disturbance and a tendency to fall backward. CT (*left*) clearly delineates the cyst in the quadrigeminal plate region and shows the dilated third and lateral ventricles. MR: *center* coronal, *right* midsagittal, SE 400/35. The cyst gives a uniform MR signal that is slightly hyperintense to CSF. A similar difference in densities is seen on the CT scan

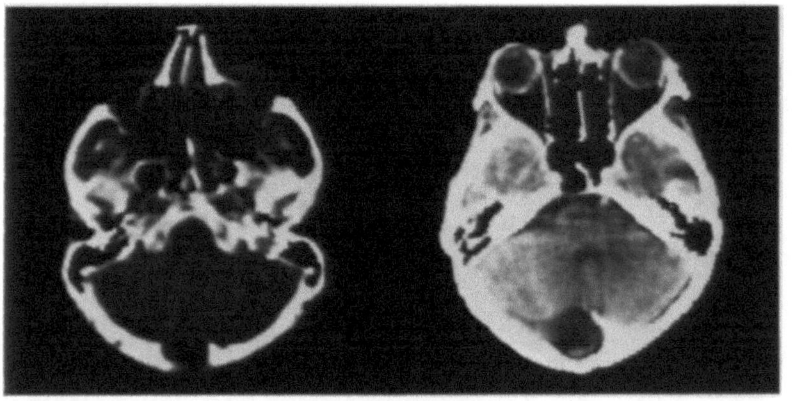

Fig. F44. Arachnoid cyst in the posterior fossa, contiguous to bone, in a 51-year-old woman. Characteristic bony changes help in forming a diagnosis

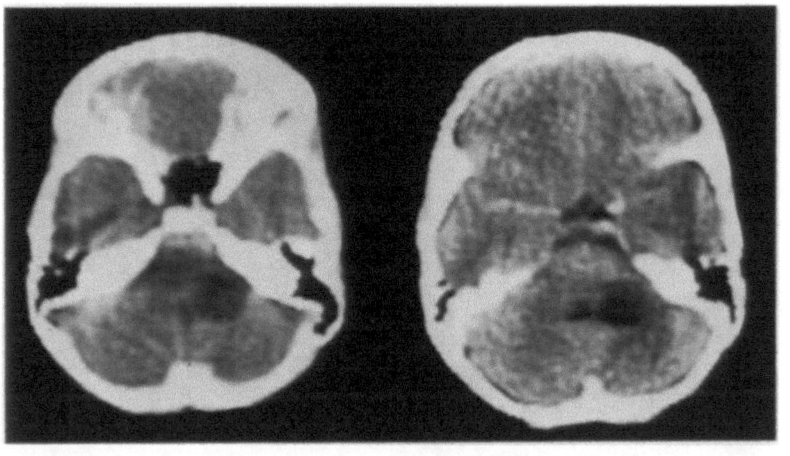

Fig. F45. Arachnoid cyst in the right cerebellopontine angle region of an 8-year-old girl with clinical symptoms of a cerebellopontine angle mass. Postcontrast CT

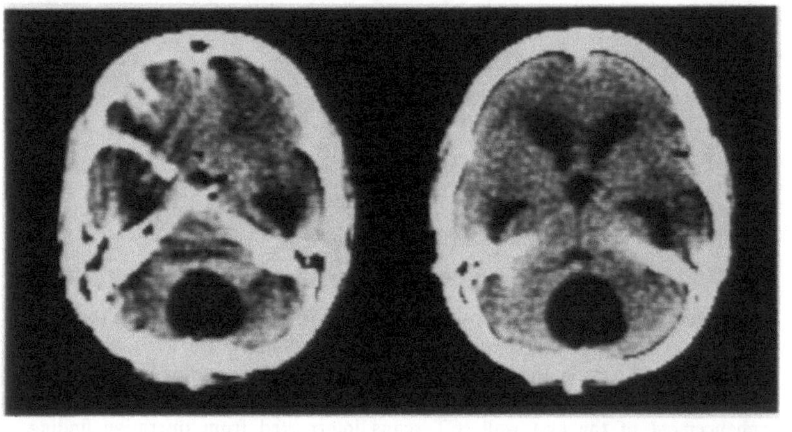

Fig. F46. Arachnoid cyst in the posterior fossa, arising from the cisterna magna, in a 50-year-old man. The lesion compresses the vermis and obstructs the fourth ventricle, causing hydrocephalus. Differentiation is required from an epidermoid cyst. Angioblastoma is less likely due to the CSF isodensity of the cyst contents

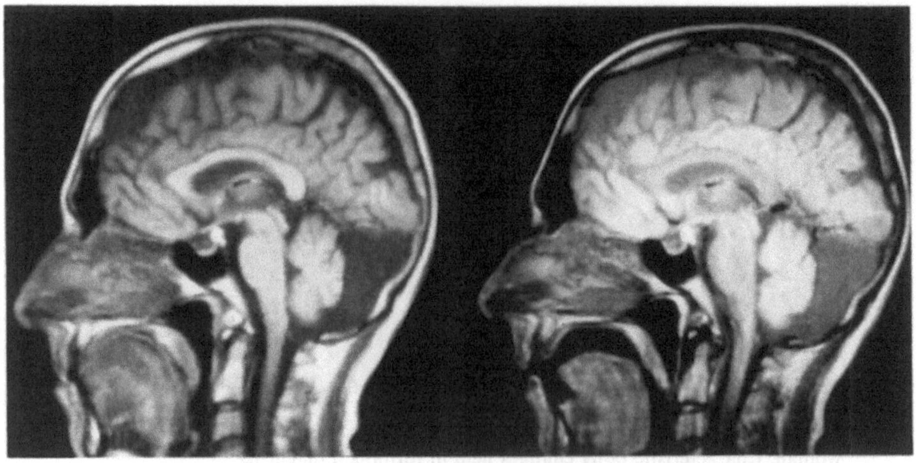

Fig. F47. Arachnoid cyst in the posterior fossa of a 43-year-old man with progressive tetraparesis and alcohol-related cachexia and polyneuropathy. MR: *left* SE 400/30, *right* SE 1600/35

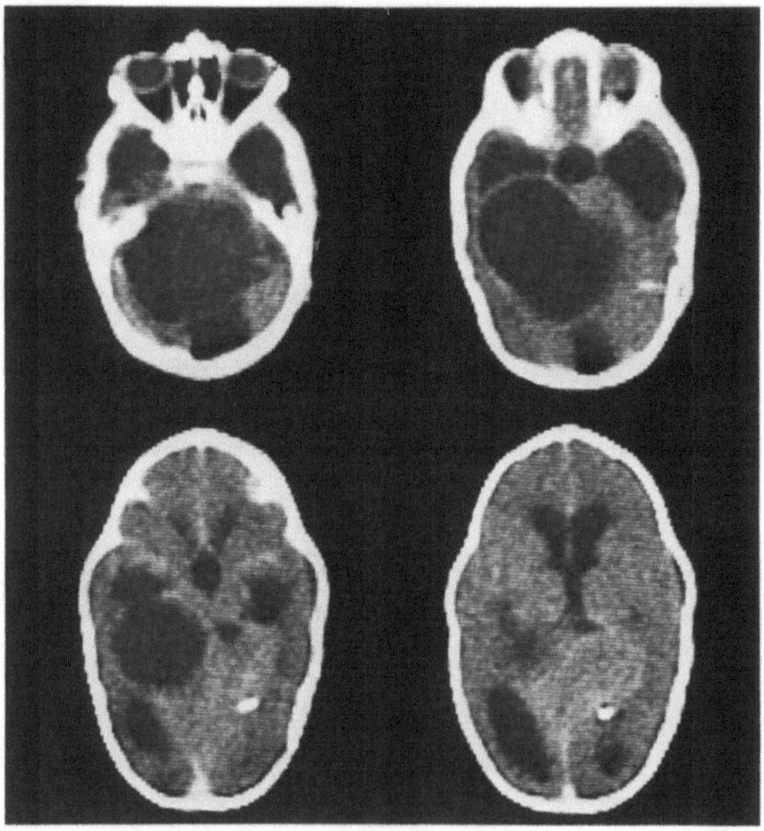

Fig. F48. Large arachnoid cyst in the posterior fossa of an 8-month-old infant. The cyst extends through the tentorium to a point below the left temporal lobe and has caused torsion and elevation of the cerebellum (lighter area to the *right* of the cyst in the *lower* scans). The vertical position of the tentorium mimics contrast enhancement of the cyst wall (CT scans interpreted from operative findings). Postcontrast CT

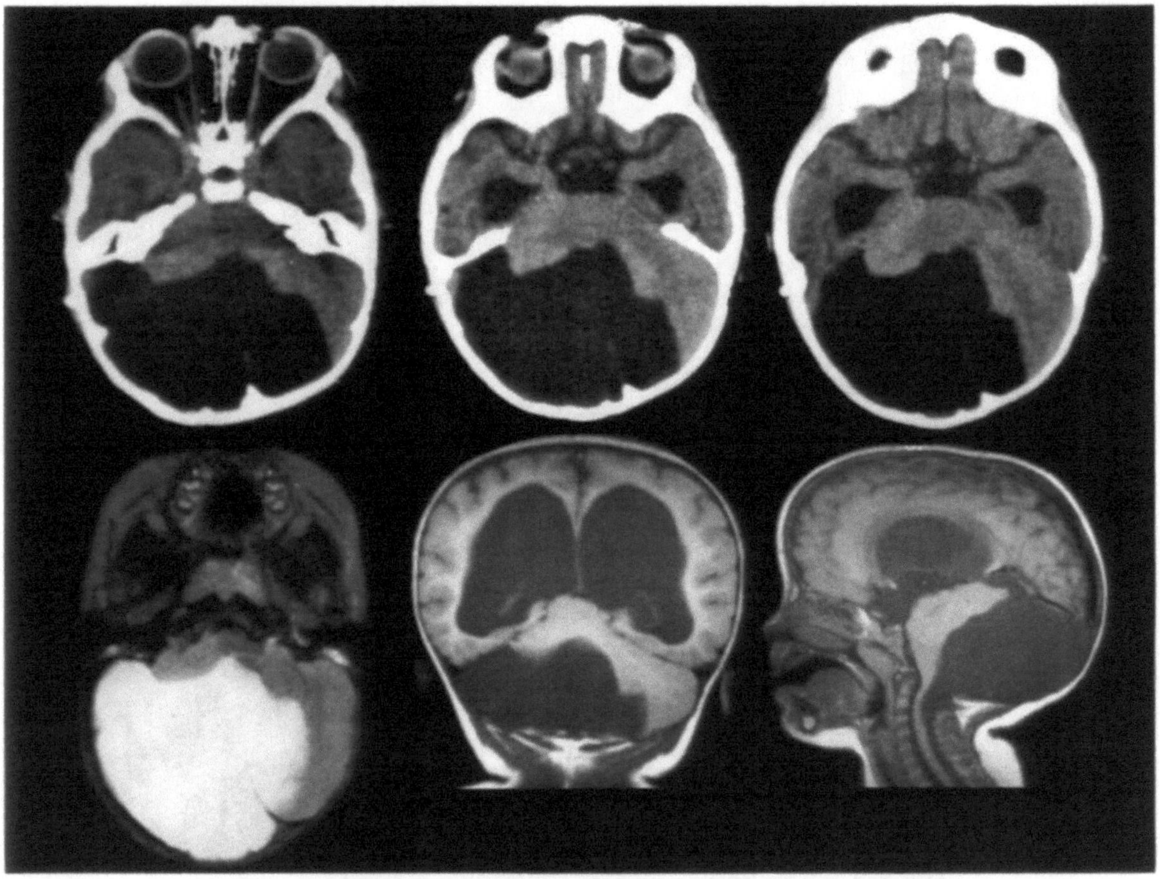

a–c

d–f

Fig. F 49 a–f. Arachnoid cyst in an 18-month-old girl with marked cranial enlargement. CT: **a–c.** MR: **d** SE 3000/90; **e, f** SE 700/30. The very large, circumscribed arachnoid cyst to the left of the cerebellum is well demonstrated even on the CT scans

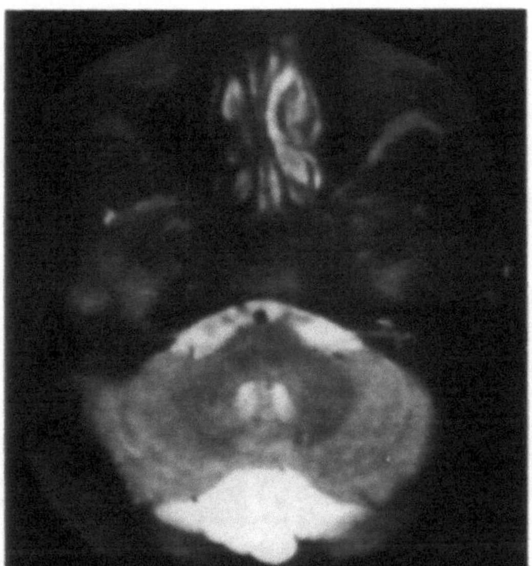

Fig. F 50. Large cisterna magna in a 17-year-old male with headache and normal neurologic findings. MR: SE 3000/90

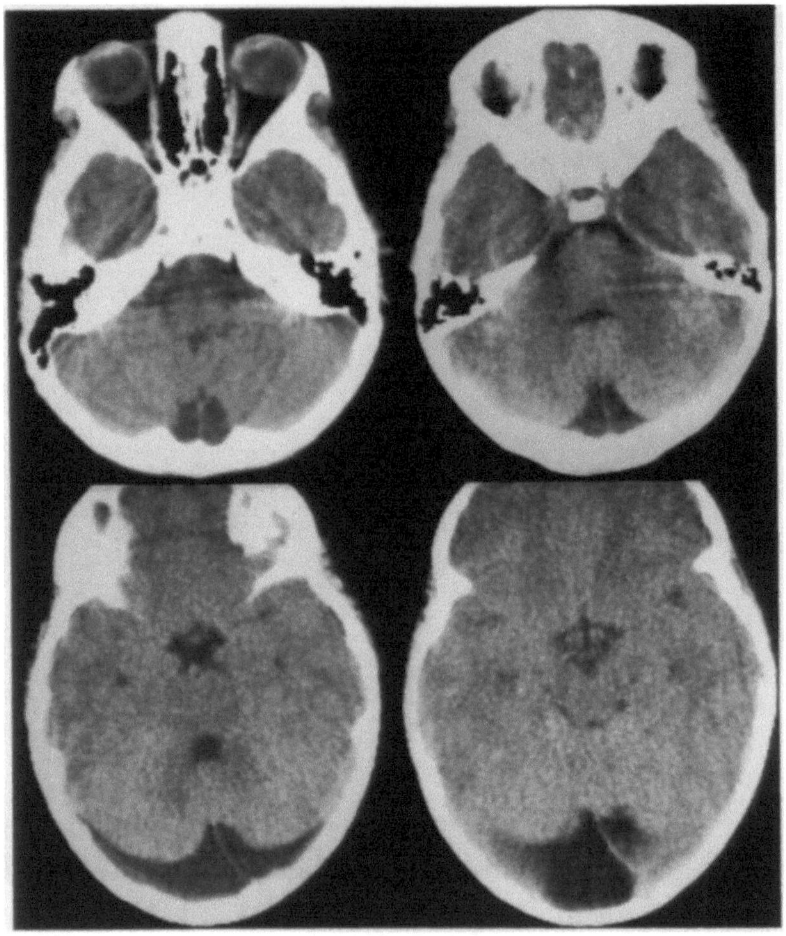

Fig. F 51. Large cisterna magna in an 8-year-old boy. Noncontrast CT demonstrates a large cisterna magna over both cerebellar hemispheres, more prominent on the left side

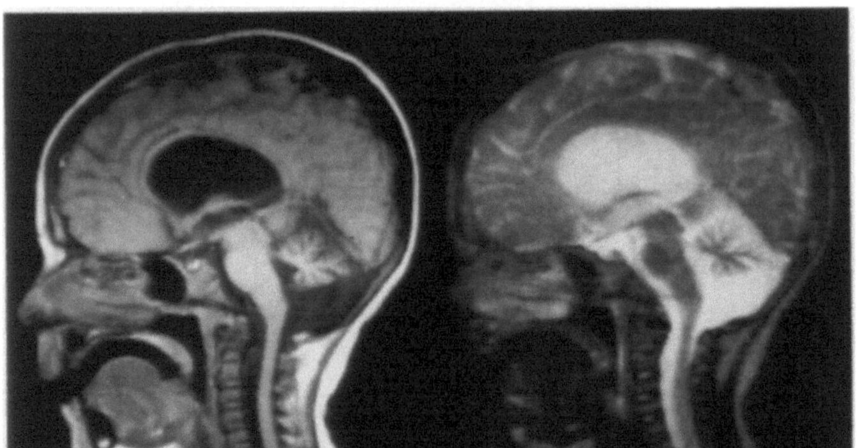

Fig. F 52. Large cisterna magna associated with cerebellar hypoplasia and narrowing of the corpus callosum in a 6-year-old boy with mental retardation, growth retardation, growth hormone deficiency, and secondary hypothyroidism. MR: *left* SE 400/30, *right* SE 1600/150. There is hydrocephalic expansion of the ventricles, and the cerebellum and corpus callosum are hypoplastic. The enlarged cisterná magna appears hyperintense on the T2-weighted image

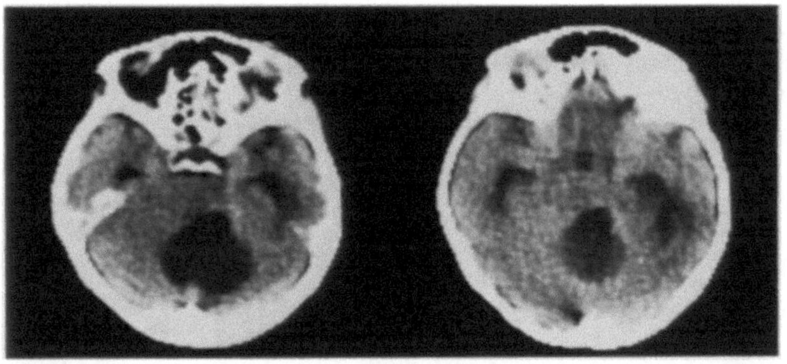

Fig. F53. "Simple" cerebellar cyst in the vermis region of a 69-year-old woman with cerebellar symptomatology. The attenuation values in the cyst are greater than those of CSF (18 HU). The lesion is indistinguishable from an angioblastomatous cyst

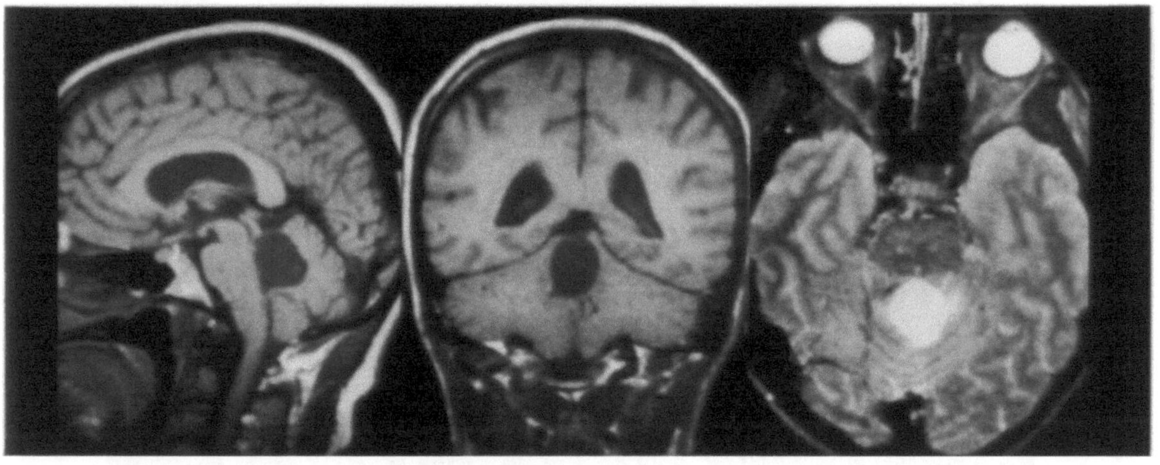

Fig. F54. Primary cerebellar cyst in the superior vermis of a 57-year-old woman with 6 weeks of severe ataxia. MR: *left* and *center* SE 500/30, *right* SE 3000/90. The primary cerebellar cyst cannot be differentiated from the fourth ventricle on the images presented

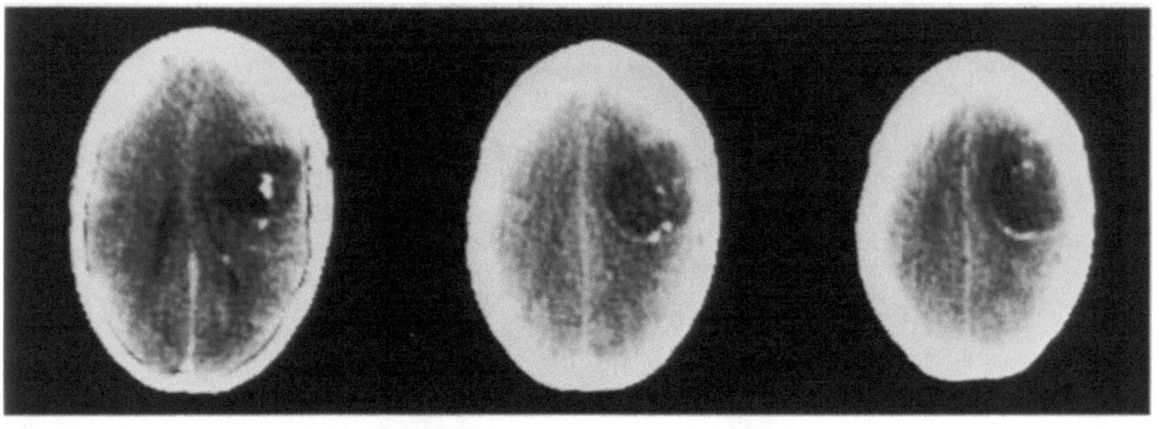

Fig. F55. Large cyst with specks of calcification in the right frontoprecentral region of a 36-year-old woman. CT findings were misinterpreted as oligodendroglioma. Operation disclosed a smooth-walled cyst with peripheral calcifications. Fibrin threads with calcifications were found in the cyst, possibly indicating an old hemorrhage. Postcontrast CT

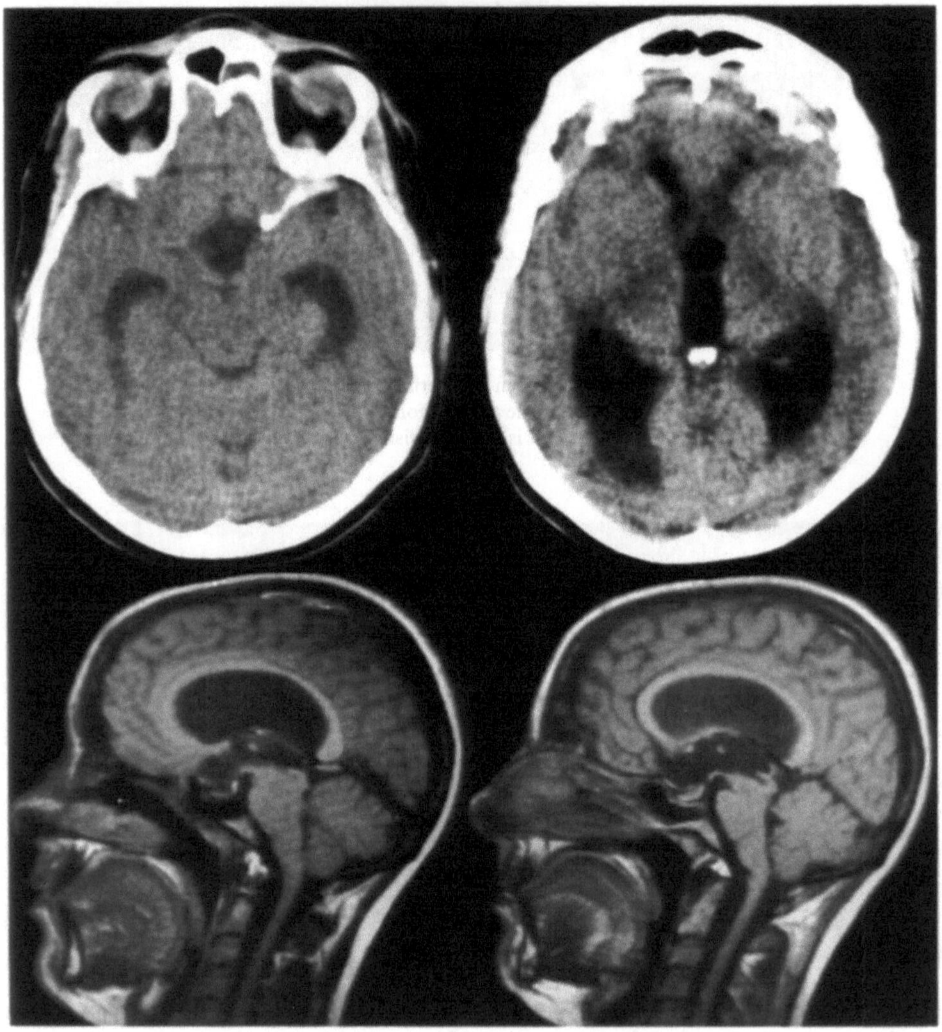

Fig. F 56. Aqueduct stenosis in a 23-year-old woman with headache. CT: *top* noncontrast. MR: *bottom* SE 500/30. Both examinations show dilatation of the lateral ventricles and third ventricle, but the aqueduct stenosis is appreciated only on the MR images

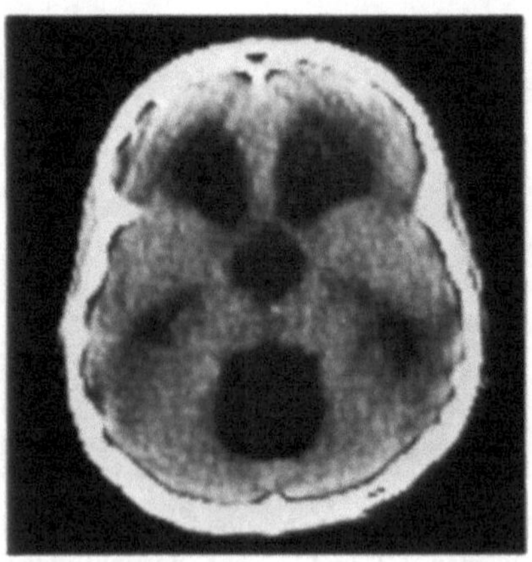

Fig. F 57. Severe postinflammatory expansion of the fourth ventricle secondary to obstruction of the foramina of Luschka and Magendie in a 34-year-old woman with severe truncal ataxia. There is also marked dilatation of the remaining ventricles

6. Postoperative Lesions and Radionecrosis

The effects of oncologic therapies on the brain parenchyma can complicate the differential diagnosis of intracranial masses. *Postoperative lesions* may include a transient blood-brain barrier lesion lasting about 3 weeks and the long-term formation of granulation tissue at the periphery of the surgical cavity, producing ring enhancement on imaging studies. This ring pattern can mimic a brain abscess, residual tumor, or recurrent growth on CT and MR, and no quantitative criteria are available for differentiating them (see p. 7). In some cases the patient's clinical condition will deteriorate as secretions are retained in the operative cavity. Reoperation usually discloses only old blood and a strongly xanthochromic fluid within the affected area. The perifocal edema often present in cases of this kind tends to direct suspicion toward a brain abscess rather than some other disorder. However, the edema does not contribute to differential diagnosis (Fig. F58). Similar problems are posed by *radionecrosis*. Animal studies demonstrate a garland pattern of contrast enhancement 17 weeks after the conclusion of radiotherapy due to incipient blood-brain barrier lesion in the irradiated area. By week 22, CT shows decreased density of the brain parenchyma as a result of edema and incipient necrosis of glial cells and neurons (O'Neil et al. 1977).

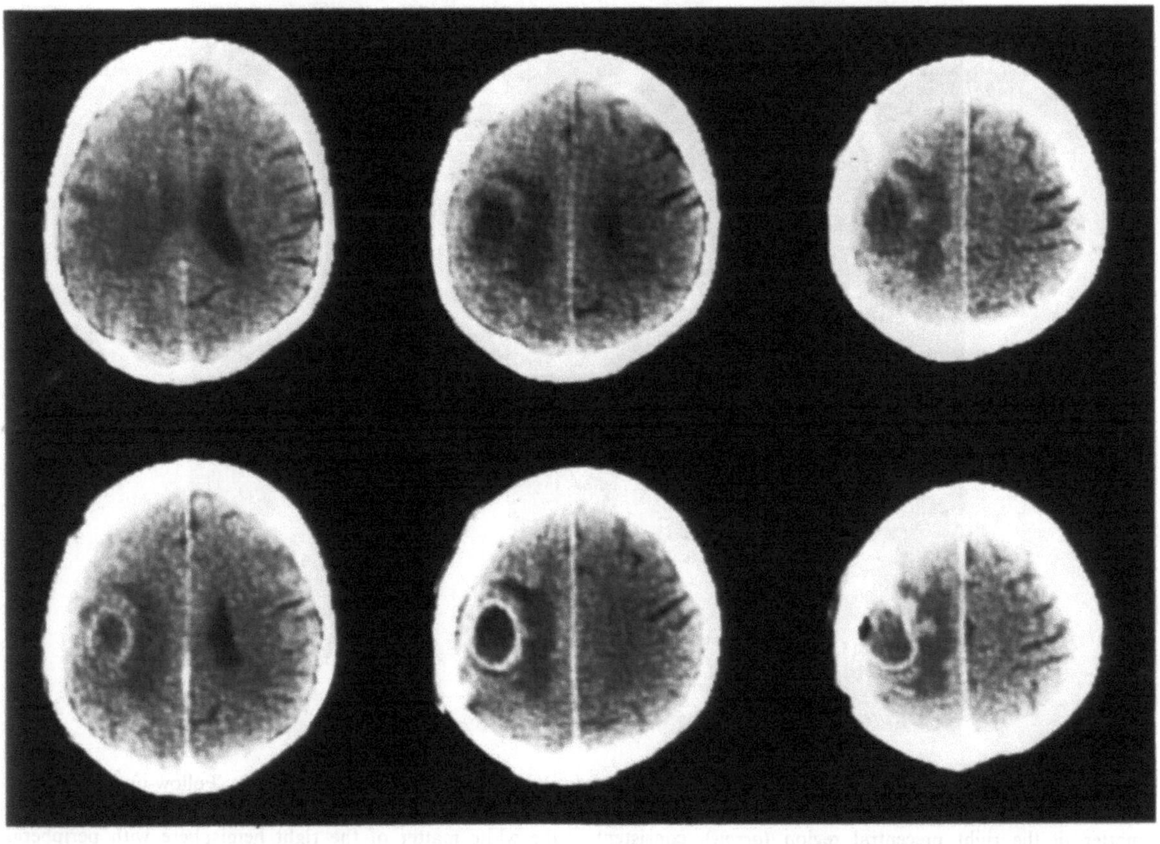

Fig. F58. Status following removal of a meningioma of the left parietal convexity. Initial improvement was followed by increasing weakness in the right arm. CT at 1 month after tumor removal shows a ringlike lesion resembling an abscess in the former operative area with marked perifocal edema. Residual air is also visible. Reoperation disclosed a noninflammatory collection of brownish-green hematomatous fluid in the surgical cavity

Clinical manifestations of radionecrosis generally appear after a latent period of 9–19 months. The lesion appears on **CT** as a circumscribed mixed density consisting of a necrotic center; a dense, strongly enhancing rim; and surrounding edema (Fig. F 59). **MR** also demonstrates a tripartite lesion with the central necrosis and surrounding edema appearing slightly hypointense on T1-weighted images and giving a high signal on T2-weighted images. Interposed between these zones is a ring that enhances brightly with Gd-DTPA. MR is more sensitive than CT in detecting intracranial radionecrosis, and the morphologic substrate of the radiation response can be visualized at an earlier stage. However, the prolongations of T1 and T2 are nonspecific, so neither modality is able to distinguish the lesion from a recurrent tumor.

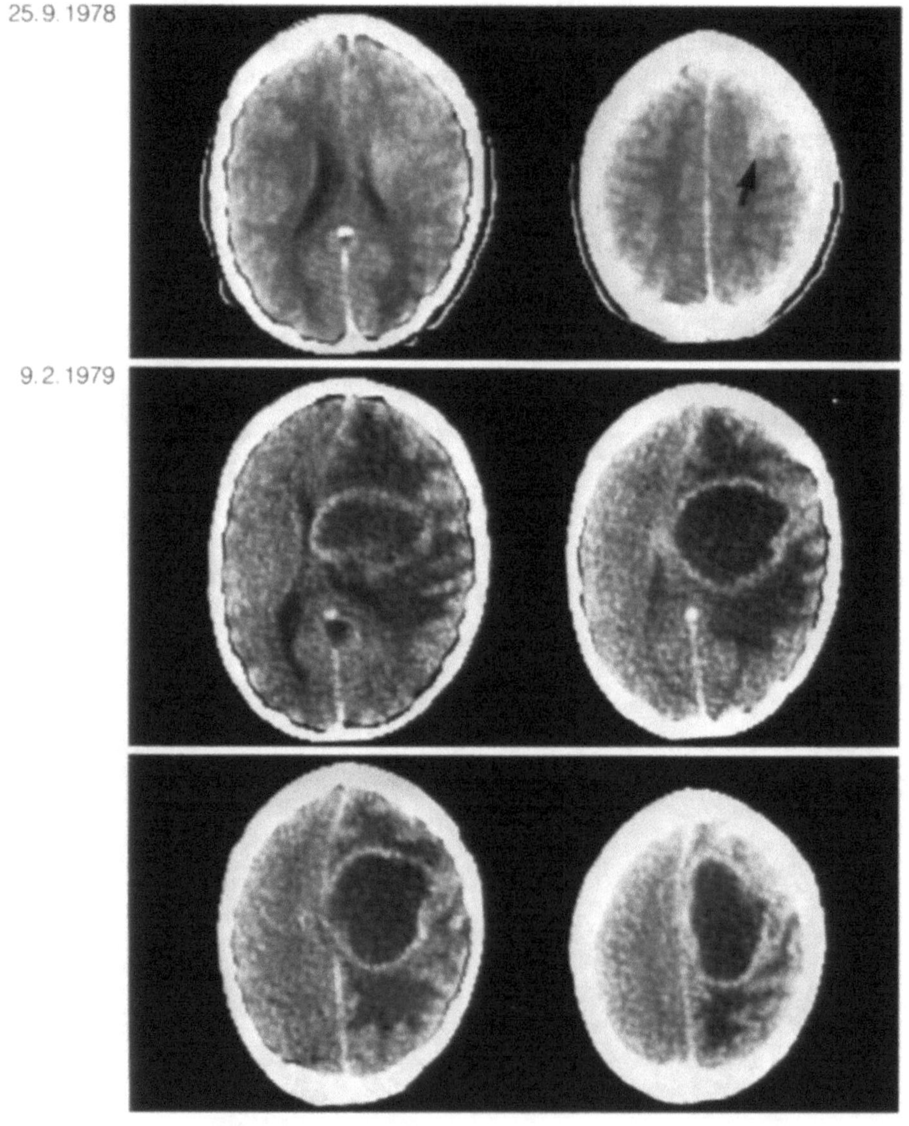

Fig. F 59. Radionecrosis in a 15-year-old male. Preoperative CT (*top*) shows a slightly hyperdense tumor in the white matter of the right precentral region (*arrow*), consistent with anaplastic oligodendroglioma (confirmed at operation). The patient received 50 Gy of radiation to the tumor. Two months after the conclusion of radiotherapy, the patient began to take a downhill course marked by profound mental changes and left-sided hemiparesis. Follow-up scans taken 4 months after operation show a large hypodense lesion in the white matter of the right hemisphere with peripheral rim enhancement and extensive perifocal edema. Conspicuous mass effect is present. Acute radiation necrosis was diagnosed and confirmed at operation

7. Acute Demyelinating Diseases

a) Disseminated Encephalomyelitis

The acute phase or exacerbation of *disseminated encephalomyelitis* is characterized by the appearance of multiple plaques up to several centimeters in diameter occurring chiefly in the paraventricular, parietal, and subcortical white matter. **CT** displays them as foci of decreased density. Their contours may be ill-defined or sharp and cystlike. Contrast enhancement is caused by breakdown of the blood-brain barrier and is proportional to the acuteness and activity of the disease. The enhancement may be ringlike or homogeneous.

During remission the lesions develop into low-density defects that do not enhance. In chronic cases, however, CT may show an absence of demyelination residues, or enhancing parenchymal lesions may be detected in patients who are clinically asymptomatic.

MR is particularly sensitive in detecting acute foci of demyelination in the brainstem and posterior fossa, and it is generally sensitive in detecting the chronic form of the lesions. On the negative side, the plaques of disseminated encephalomyelitis are difficult to distinguish from CSF on T2-weighted images, and they may contrast very poorly with the white matter on T1-weighted images. The variability of the relaxation times depends on the development and prominence of lesion formation and is eliminated by administering Gd-DTPA. Gadolinium enhancement is not helpful in establishing the stage of the disease, however, since fresh plaques and chronic lesions have similar appearances on the MR scan (Edwards et al. 1986; Grossman et al. 1986) (Figs. F60, 61).

The differential diagnosis of disseminated encephalomyelitis is aided by the clinical presentation, CSF findings, and the typical peri- and paraventricular location of the lesions. With imaging, serial examinations may be necessary to differentiate the various stages of the disease from cerebral metastases and from multiple infarcts. The finding of periventricular areas of high signal intensity or individual foci in the cerebral white matter becomes less specific in older patients and more difficult to correlate with clinical findings.

b) Diffuse Sclerosis

The acute form of diffuse sclerosis likewise is associated with contrast enhancement of affected areas on the **CT** scan. The area has irregular borders, very low central density, and a narrow enhancing rim (Fig. F62).

The foci of high signal on T2-weighted **MR** images correlate with the patient's neurologic deficits, but the parenchymal changes do not provide criteria useful for making a specific diagnosis.

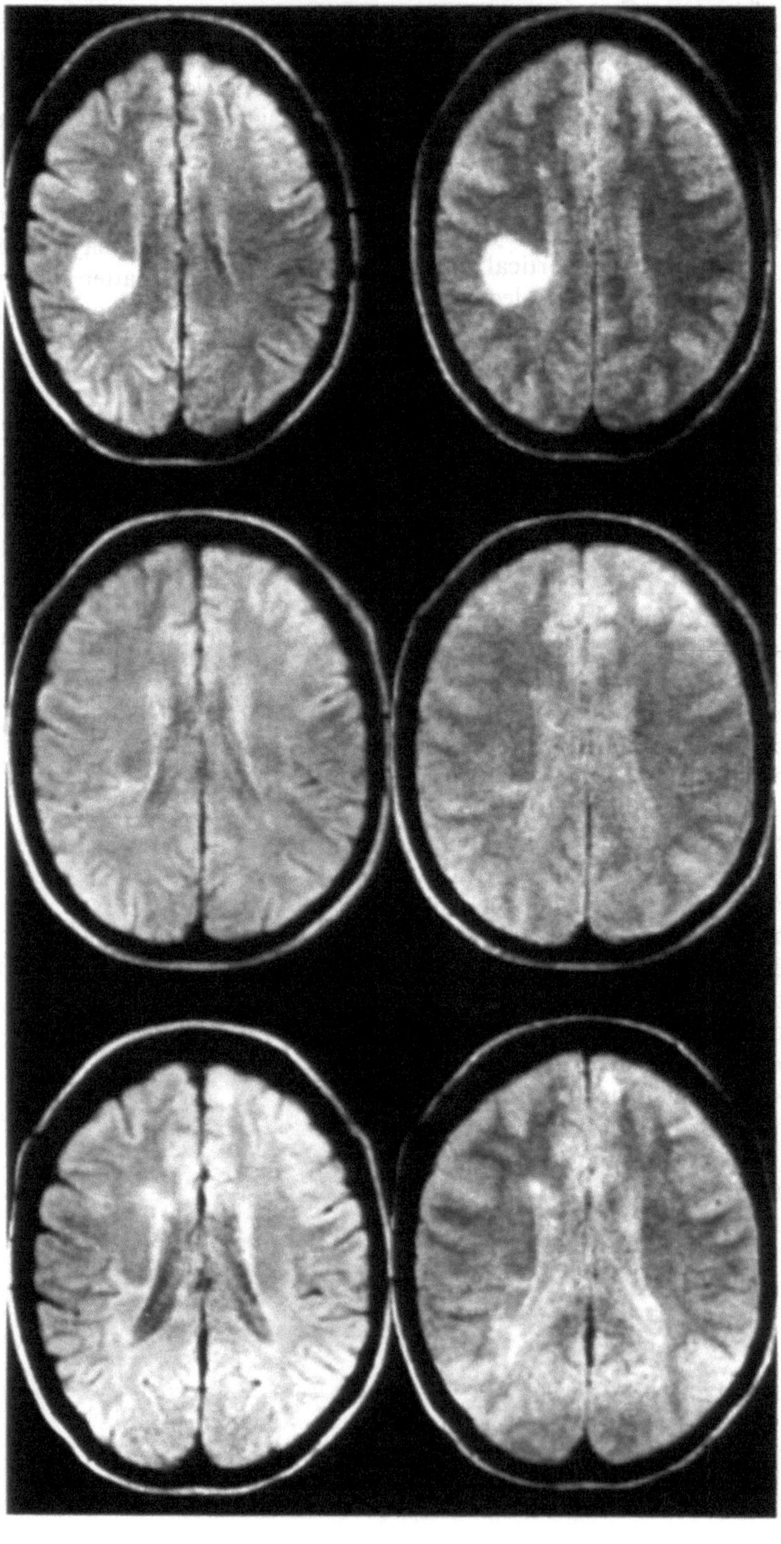

a b c d e f

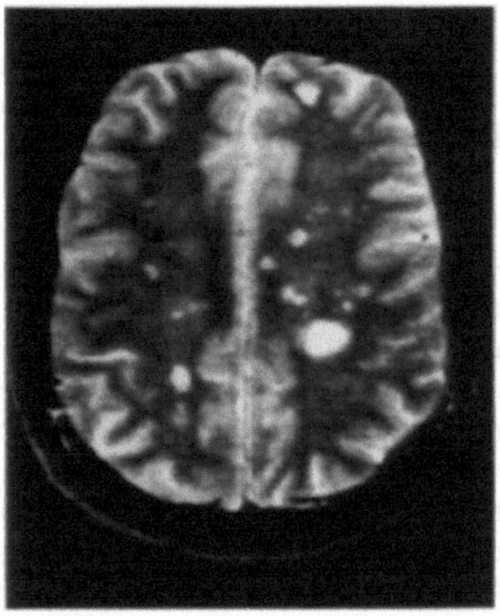

Fig. F61. Disseminated encephalomyelitis in a 48-year-old man with changing neurologic symptoms. MR (SE 3200/90) demonstrates multiple hyperintense lesions of varying size over both hemispheres. Small areas of circumscribed enhancement were also visible on postcontrast CT

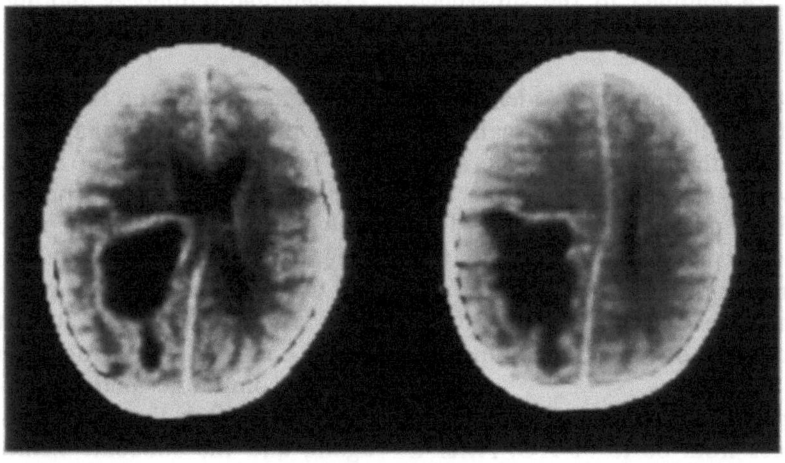

Fig. F62. Postcontrast CT shows, in a 12-year-old boy, an irregular ("maplike") low-density area in the middle and posterior portions of the left cerebral hemisphere with peripheral enhancement, initially interpreted as a tumor. Histologic examination revealed an acute form of diffuse sclerosis

Fig. F60a–f. Multiple sclerosis in a 45-year-old woman with a 3-month history of dizziness, right hemiparesis, atactic gait disturbance, and bilateral decrease of vision. Serial MR examinations were performed: **a** SE 1600/35, **b** SE 1600/70 (July 1984); **c** SE 1600/35, **d** SE 1600/70 (December 1984); **e** SE 1600/35, **f** SE 1600/70 (September 1986). Multiple hyperintense lesions are seen over both hemispheres and are most prominent in the left paraventricular and right frontal regions. As neurologic symptoms regressed, the MR abnormalities disappeared. Image **f** shows only small hyperintensities in the right frontal and left paraventricular areas

8. Intracranial Hemorrhages

a) Spontaneous Intracranial Hemorrhages

Over 60% of *spontaneous hemorrhages* are believed to be caused by hypertension and arteriosclerotic disease. Less frequent causes are microangiomas, inflammations of the cerebral vessels, and coagulation disturbances (Figs. F63, 64). Hypertensive hemorrhages typically occur in the basal ganglia, and in half of the cases the hemorrhage spreads into the ventricles (Grumme et al. 1979). Less frequently there may be extension of bleeding into the pons, the cerebellum, or the cerebral white matter (Fig. F66). In older hypertensive patients, amyloid angiopathy should be considered as a potential cause of the hemorrhage in cases where multiple hematomas occur spontaneously and are confined to the superficial cortex (Patel et al. 1984; Sobel et al. 1986) (Fig. F65).

Generally it is not difficult to identify an intracranial hemorrhage on the **CT** scan. The density of the hematoma represents the average of the absorption coefficients of the erythrocytes (80 HU) and blood plasma (22 HU). Thus, extravascular coagulated blood that is devoid of plasma appears hyperdense on CT, the attenuation values relating directly to the level of the hematocrit or the hemoglobin fraction (Wende et al. 1980).

The absorption coefficient of an acute hematoma ranges from 60 to 90 HU. After a minimum of 3 days, the hematoma acquires a low-density border (20–28 HU) caused by liquefaction of the blood, centripetal resorption, and perifocal edema. This hypodense rim enlarges and causes mass effect over a 3-week period. Meanwhile the density of the clotted blood diminishes until it is isodense to the brain parenchyma. At this stage postcontrast CT may show ring enhancement of the hematoma with a mixed-density center. This ring pattern is seen a minimum of 7 days after the acute event and disappears within 2 months as the hematoma is reabsorbed and a cavity is formed (Weisberg 1980).

In rare cases, spontaneous intracranial hemorrhage may be caused by a brain tumor (apoplectic glioblastoma, metastases). The hemorrhage may be masked by the tumor on initial CT scans and escape detection. Serious consideration should be given to this cause in younger patients who have an intracranial hemorrhage at an atypical site.

Lateral pontine hemorrhages present as a "pontine angle mass" on CT scans. The high density of the mass on the plain scan, the absence of contrast enhancement, and the sudden onset of neurologic abnormalities, usually involving the trigeminal and statoacoustic nerves, serve to identify the lesion as a hemorrhage. Rupture of a microangioma is the most frequent cause (Fig. F67).

As on CT, hemoglobin determines the appearance of intracranial hemorrhages on the **MR** image. Acute hematomas less than 1 week old appear isointense to the gray matter on T1-weighted sequences and give a hypointense signal on T2-weighted sequences (Gomori et al. 1985).

Animal studies on the progression of relaxation times in hemorrhages have shown that the T1 and T2 values of the lesion are longer than those of the brain parenchyma immediately after the hemorrhage occurs. Within 48 h they become equal to the parenchymal values and remain so for a period of 3–5 days. This shortening of relaxation times is caused by the conversion of hemoglobin to the paramagnetic compound methemoglobin. At the end of the first week the relaxation times lengthen again, and the subacute hemorrhage appears as an area of increased signal on T1- and T2-weighted images (Di Chiro et al. 1986). Chronic hematomas (more than 1 month old) likewise appear hyperintense on MR.

We can appreciate, then, the complementary roles of CT and MR in the diagnosis of intracranial hemorrhage. While CT is more sensitive in detecting the fresh hemorrhage that appears isointense to parenchyma on the MR image, MR is better able to demonstrate the subacute hematoma, which appears isodense on CT.

b) Old Hemorrhages, Chocolate Cysts

The *chronic stage of intracranial hemorrhages* presents a variety of imaging appearances. Within 6 weeks the hematoma loses its isodense character and becomes a well-defined area of low density. Clotted residues can produce a sedimentation effect in the dependent part of the lesion (Fig. F 68). If it does not show peripheral enhancement, the hemorrhagic cavity will resemble a cystic astrocytoma on the **CT** scan (Fig. F 69). Usually, however, narrow peripheral enhancement will be observed around the lesion, whose contents are isodense to CSF. This serves to distinguish the hematoma from an abscess or mixed-density tumor. Recurrent bleeding in an organized hematoma creates the picture of a hyperdense, well-circumscribed mass showing little contrast enhancement and minimal perifocal edema. This differs from the appearance of recurrent bleeding outside the original hematoma boundaries, which presents the features of a tumoral hemorrhage (Lee et al. 1986).

Chocolate cysts are most likely to develop in association with microangiomas. This lesion consists of poorly absorbed blood constituents, usually in the form of a brownish fluid, contained within a membranous sac (see Fig. C 4).

Chocolate cysts appear on **CT** as high-density areas that do not enhance further with intravenous contrast (Figs. F 70, 71). The lesion may persist for a long period, in some cases for years, and it may retain its high density. The absence of enhancement, growth tendency, and perifocal edema serve to distinguish chocolate cysts from solid, hyperdense tumors.

MR imaging offers additional criteria for differentiating *old hemorrhages* from tumors. As the hematoma enters the chronic stage, its relaxation times undergo a further change which differs in degree for T1 and T2. The result is an increase in the signal intensity of the hemorrhage, which typically is surrounded by a narrow, dark band on T2-weighted images. This low-signal ring represents paramagnetic hemosiderin deposits and smaller amounts of calcium deposits in the wall of the hemorrhagic cavity.

c) Chronic Subdural Hematomas

Chronic subdural hematomas are *isodense* on CT scans, so detection must rely on indirect signs such as unilateral ventricular distortion, white matter compression, lateral disparity in the width of the sylvian fissure, and nonvisualization of cortical markings. Evidence of cortical separation from the inner table is an additional indirect sign (Grumme et al. 1976).

A *diffuse glioma* of the cerebral hemisphere that expands the brain volume without altering its density has a similar appearance (see Fig. D 1.55). The growth can be differentiated from chronic hematoma by the infusion of contrast medium, which will delineate the hematoma through enhancement of the cerebral cortex or possibly of the hematoma capsule.

Bilateral isodense chronic subdural hematomas are manifested by a decrease in the distance between the tips of the frontal horns with a reduction in the angle between them ("rabbit ear" sign, Marcu and Becker 1977) (Figs. F 72, 73). In addition, the lateral ventricles appear abnormally narrow in the region of the pars centralis. Again, the contrast-enhanced **CT** scan is helpful for delineating the hematomas through cortical enhancement. **MR** imaging also allows for definitive diagnosis.

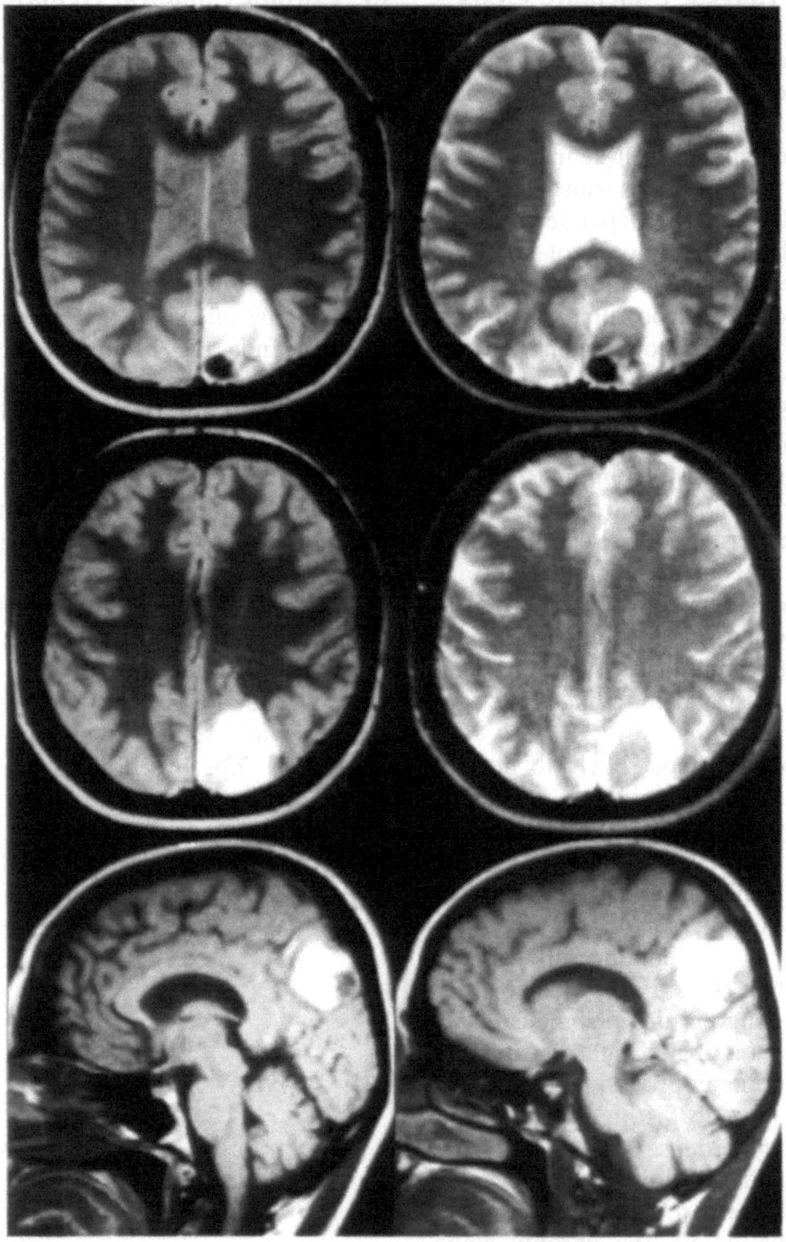

a b c d e f

Fig. F 63 a–f. Intracerebral hemorrhage in the right occipital region of a 39-year-old woman with microangioma. Ten days before admission the patient experienced abrupt headache and mild weakness on the left side. MR: **a, c** SE 3000/30, **b, d** SE 3000/90, **e, f** SE 700/30. Both the T1- and T2-weighted images show a circumscribed area of high signal intensity (blood) bordered posteriorly by a hypointense or signal-free area representing the angioma (blood flowing in large vessels creates a signal void)

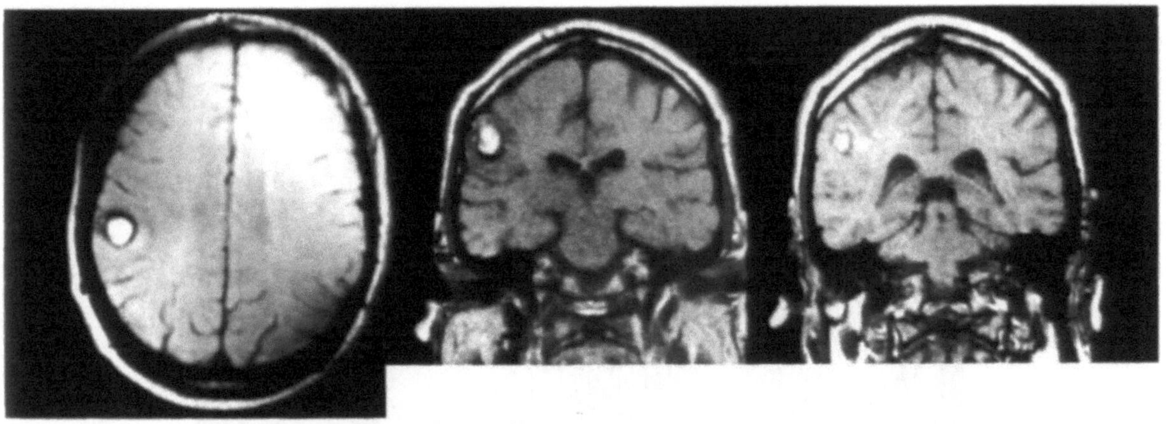

Fig. F 64. Intracerebral hemorrhage in the left parietal region of a 41-year-old man with a 1-week history of hemiparesis. MR: *left* SE 2000/30, *center* and *right* SE 500/30 coronal. A hyperintense area with a dark border is seen in the left parietal region. A microangioma with hemorrhage was confirmed at operation

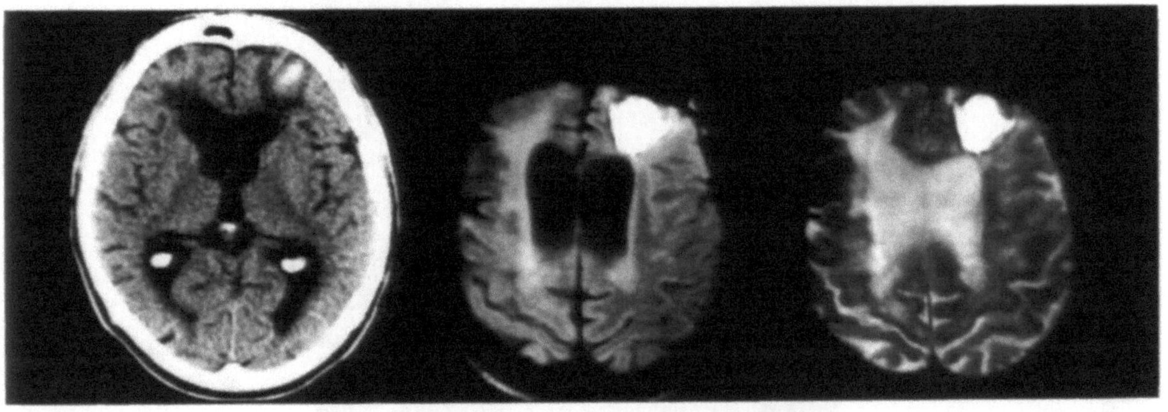

Fig. F 65. Intracerebral hemorrhage in the right frontal region of a 66-year-old man with a 2-week history of severe headache. CT: *left* noncontrast. MR: *center* SE 800/35, *right* SE 2500/120. Plain CT shows a hypodense area in the right frontal region with central increased density (blood). There is associated internal hydrocephalus and periventricular lucency. Both MR sequences show an area of very high signal intensity in the right frontal region consistent with a circumscribed hemorrhage. There is internal hydrocephalus with periventricular hyperintensity

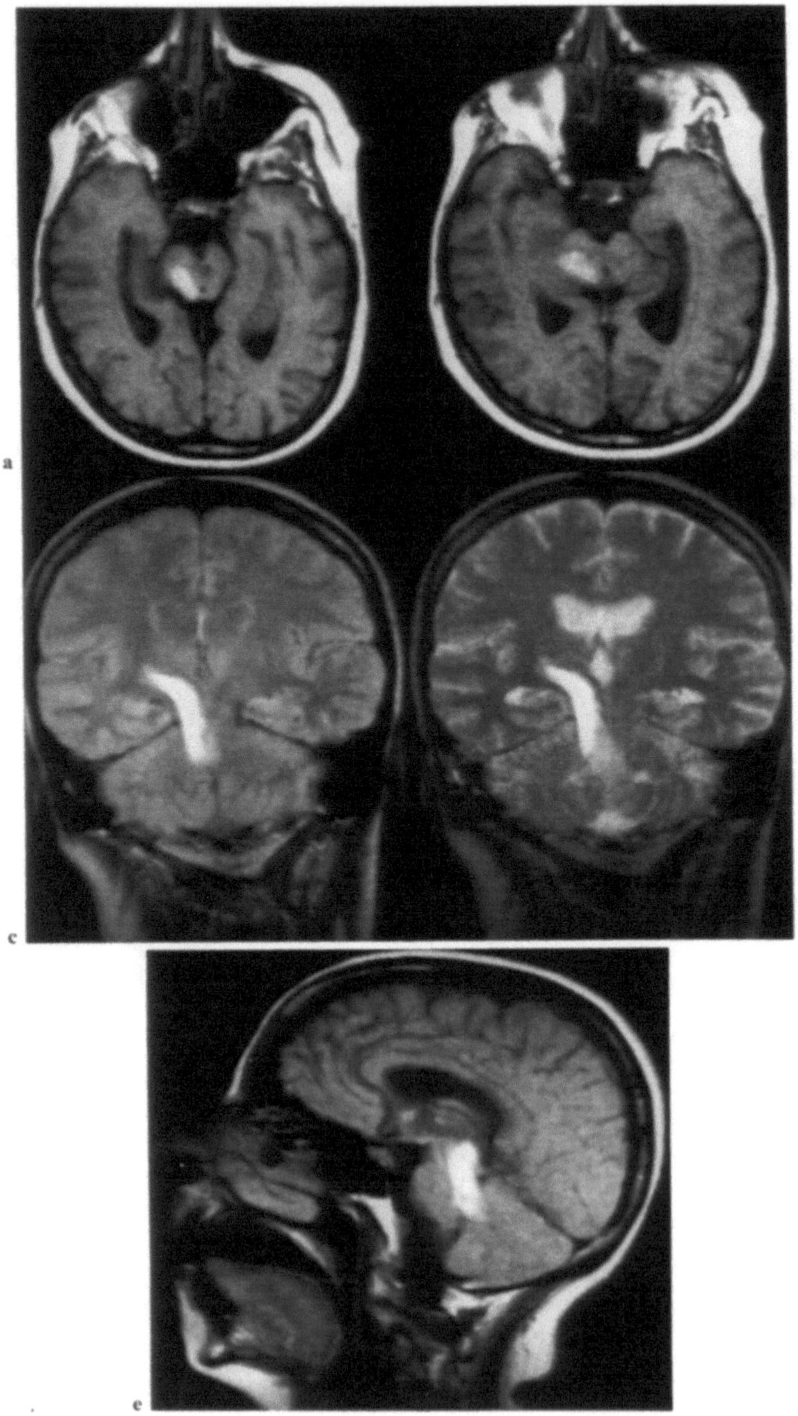

a b c d e

Fig. F66a–e. Intracerebral hemorrhage in a 48-year-old woman with sudden loss of consciousness and right hemiparesis. MR: **a, b** SE 700/30 axial; **c** SE 1800/60, **d** SE 1800/120, coronal; **e** SE 1800/35 parasagittal. The hemorrhage appears as a circumscribed area of high intensity on all sequences

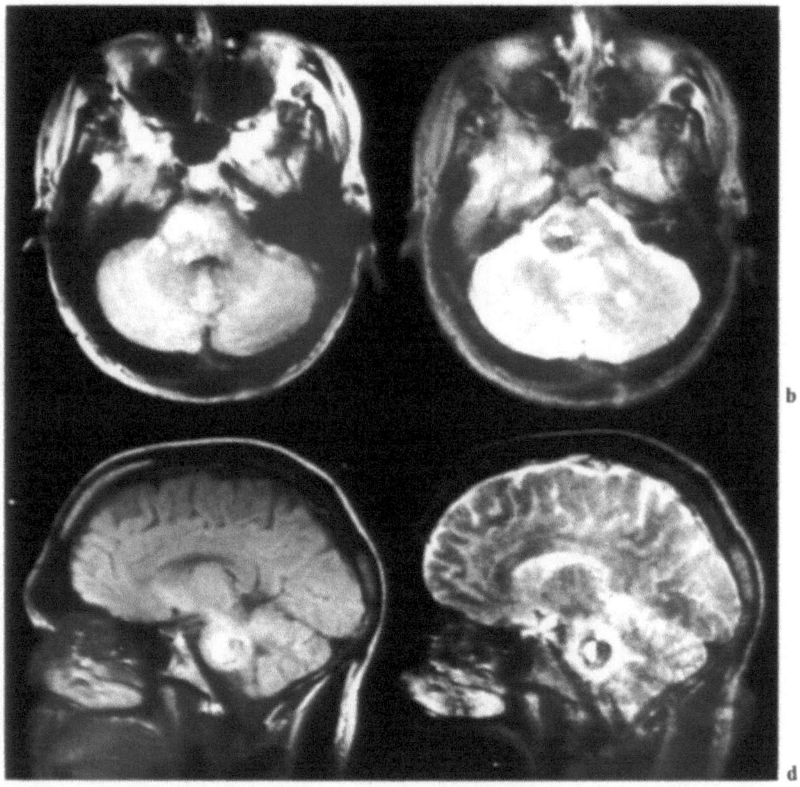

Fig. F 67 a–d. Pontine hemorrhage from microangioma in a 33-year-old man with a 3-week history of changing left-sided hemiataxia. MR: **a, c** SE 2500/30, **b, d** SE 2500/120. There is obvious expansion of the pons by the hemorrhage. The thrombosed microangioma with high-signal hemorrhage is visible within the hyperintense edematous zone (**d**)

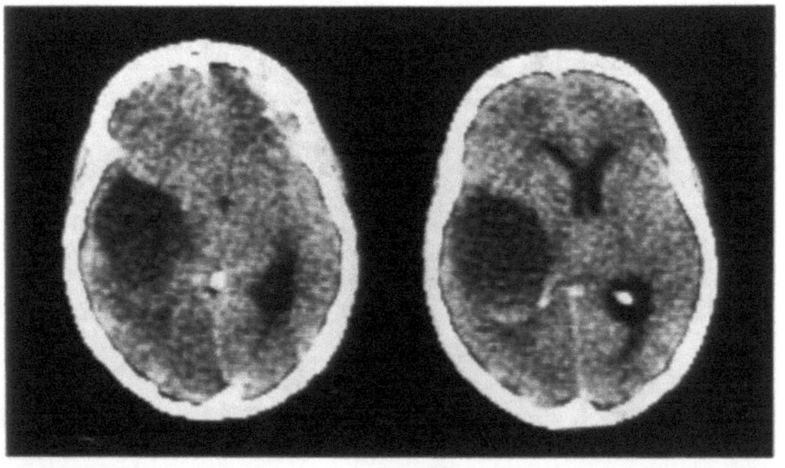

Fig. F 68. Old, liquefied intracerebral hematoma in the left temporal lobe of a 29-year-old man with no history of an acute event. A slight sedimentation effect is apparent (foci of increased density in the dependent portions of the hematoma cavity in the *right* scan). The lesion was originally thought to be a low-grade astrocytoma. Postcontrast CT

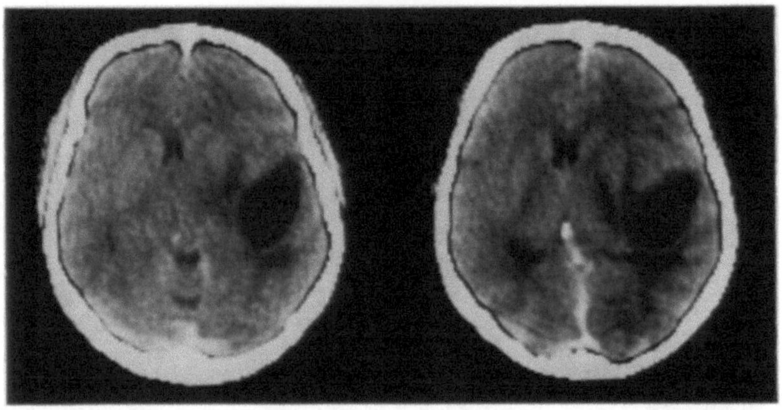

Fig. F69. Old hemorrhage in the right temporal lobe with mass effect and finger-shaped perifocal edema in a 37-year-old male. The lesion does not enhance with contrast. CT findings resemble those of cystic astrocytoma. Postcontrast study

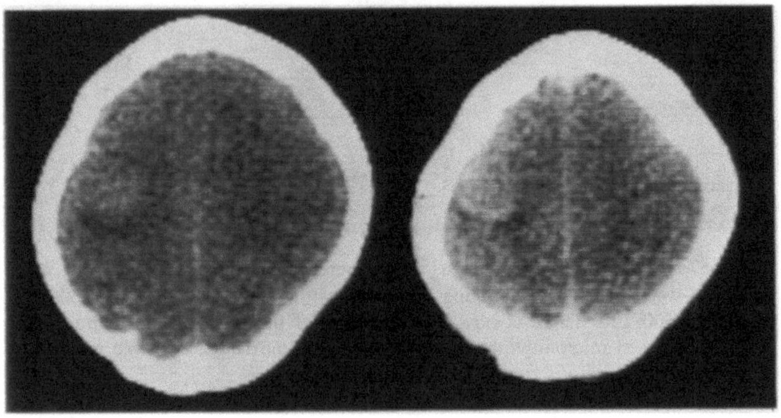

Fig. F70. Chocolate cyst in the left parietal region of a 30-year-old man, initially diagnosed as a tumor. Histologic diagnosis: microangioma with old hemorrhage. The patient had a 3-week history of sensory abnormalities in the right hand and jacksonian seizures. Postcontrast CT scans show no enhancement

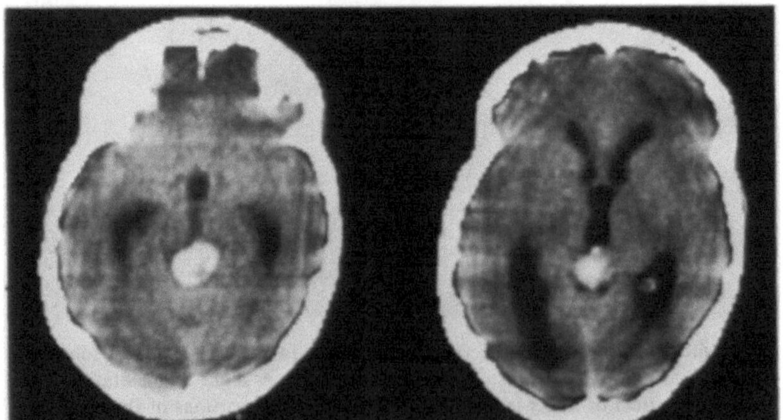

Fig. F71. Chocolate cyst with microangioma in the midbrain of a 23-year-old woman with subarachnoid hemorrhage. The lesion is indistinguishable from a calcified pinealoma on CT

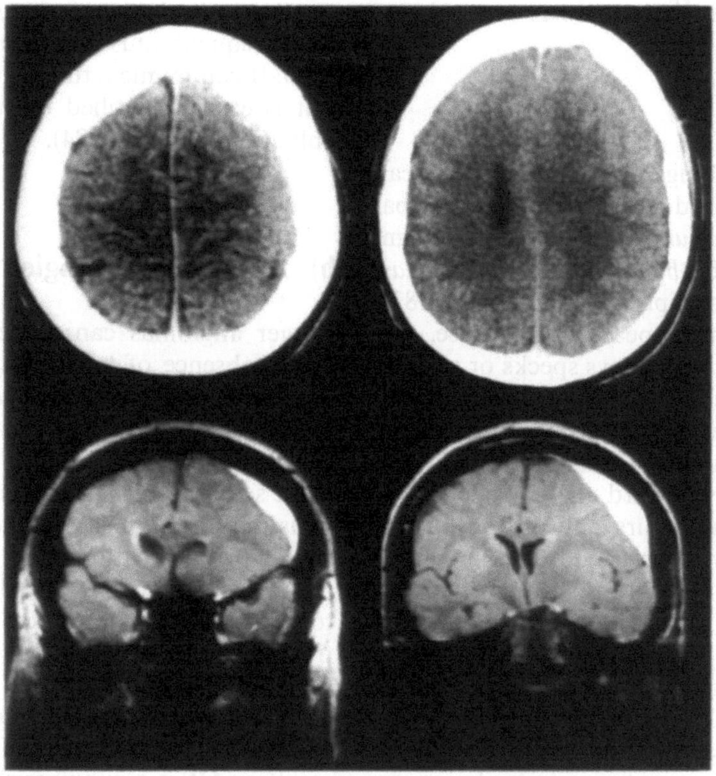

Fig. F72a–d. Chronic subdural hematoma in the right parietal region of a 63-year-old man with a history of mental deterioration. CT: **a, b**. MR: **c, d** SE 2500/30 coronal. The hematoma is isodense on the CT scans and gives a bright signal on the MR sequences. The only CT evidence of the lesion is a mass effect on the right side

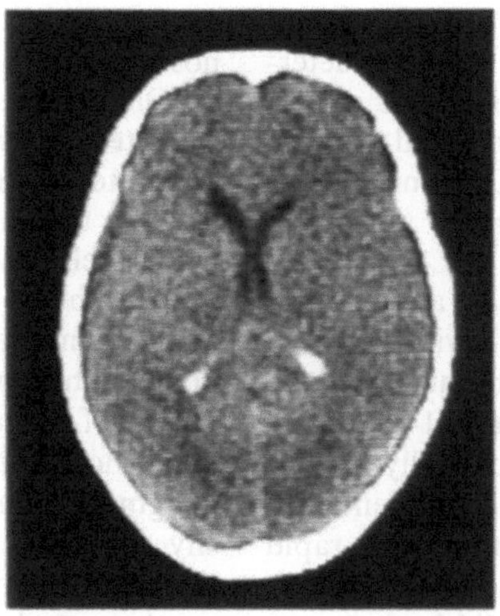

Fig. F73. Bilateral, isodense chronic subdural hematoma in a 67-year-old man. Bilateral pressure from the lesion is responsible for the acute angle between the frontal horns ("rabbit ear" sign)

9. Vascular Malformations

a) Aneurysms

Vascular outpouchings up to 3 mm in size can be directly visualized in 97% of aneurysm patients by *high-resolution CT scans* taken immediately after the *bolus injection of contrast medium* (CT angiography; Schmid et al. 1987).

The aneurysm appears hyperdense, enhances uniformly, and shows specks or plaques of calcification in its wall. Any thrombosis of the aneurysmal sac will produce a ring pattern, typically with an increase of density toward the periphery (i.e., toward the capsule). Contrast enhancement occurs only in the part of the aneurysm that is traversed by flowing blood (Figs. F74–83).

In terms of **differential diagnosis**, large aneurysms in the supra- and parasellar region can mimic pituitary adenomas or meningiomas (Kazner and Lanksch 1979) (Fig. F77).

Intense contrast enhancement should always arouse suspicion of a vascular lesion, especially if wall calcifications are also present. Thrombosed aneurysms are most likely to be mistaken for a neoplasm (Figs. F74, 76, 81, 82). Subarachnoid hemorrhage can prevent the direct visualization of the aneurysm on **CT** scans. In 70% of cases subarachnoid hemorrhage, chiefly in the basal cisterns, is the only CT manifestation of the hemorrhagic event, and the site of the aneurysm must be determined by noting the distribution and spread of the hemorrhage. It should be noted that the absorption coefficients of the CSF, initially altered by the hemorrhage, return to normal in just 3–10 days.

MR is helpful in these cases, as it clearly differentiates the low signal of flowing blood in arteries and aneurysms from the higher signal of clotted blood with its short T1 and long T2 relaxation times. Even in partially thrombosed aneurysms, characteristic differences in the signal characteristics of areas with rapid blood flow versus compact material serve to distinguish the lesion from a solid brain tumor (Figs. F80, 83).

Aneurysmal dilatation of the vein of Galen is an infrequent cause of hydrocephalus in children. It can mimic a tumor of the pineal region but is easily identified by its intense contrast enhancement (Fig. F84).

b) Arteriovenous Angiomas

Larger angiomas can cause mass effect even in the absence of hemorrhage (Figs. F87, 88). The *intense contrast enhancement of the angioma*, which often appears as a slightly hyperdense, homogeneous, vermiform structure on plain scans, is considered typical of arteriovenous malformations. It is not unusual to find specks of calcification in the angioma, and this feature, together with the demonstration of a tortuous vascular mass, should allow a definitive diagnosis to be made. The prevalence of the malformation can result in underperfusion of the adjacent brain parenchyma, leading to an atrophic reduction in the brain volume. The result on **CT** is a circumscribed hypodensity at the periphery of the angioma with no evidence of mass effect or the typical finger-like pattern of peritumoral white matter edema.

Angiomas located in the midbrain or caudal brainstem can mimic the appearance of a pontine tumor after the administration of contrast medium (Fig. F89). As in all other cases, angiography is necessary to establish the diagnosis.

On **MR**, scrutiny of the T1- and T2-weighted images reveals a tangled mass of hypointense structures conforming topographically to the angiomatous nodule and its draining vessels. Evaluation of the multi-echo sequence shows an increasing nonhomogeneity of the veins traversing the image volume, with poor definition of contours and increasing intensity of the malformation noted in every second echo. Despite the capability for varying the imaging parameters, we are not yet able to classify accurately the vessels feeding or draining the malformation with MR, and angiography continues to be a necessary examination in the workup of these cases (see Figs. C6, F90–92).

c) Sturge-Weber Syndrome

Sturge-Weber syndrome is characterized by the appearance of extensive garlandlike calcifications along the cortical gyri as early as 2 months after birth. They occur mostly in the temporo-parieto-occipital region and occasionally in the frontal region and are always ipsilateral to the facial nevus. **CT** shows evidence of local cerebral atrophy with enlargement of the external CSF spaces and thickening or abnormal smallness of the cranium overlying the affected portion of the brain (Fig. F93).

The CT appearance of the disease is completed on postcontrast scans by the detection of leptomeningeal angiomas and of widened deep cerebral veins with an absence of superficial drainage.

MR is of comparable diagnostic value, although the gyriform calcifications are not visualized.

d) Basilar Artery Ectasia

Hyperdense on plain CT scans, the *ectatic basilar artery* appears on postcontrast scans as a wide, intensely enhancing band with a tortuous course that may extend into the cerebellopontine angle. If the ectasia is pronounced, the vessel may resemble a tumor on some CT projections (Figs. F85, 86). However, differentiation is accomplished even without angiography by noting the enhancement kinetics on CT scans and also by *demonstrating flow-related phenomena on the MR image.*

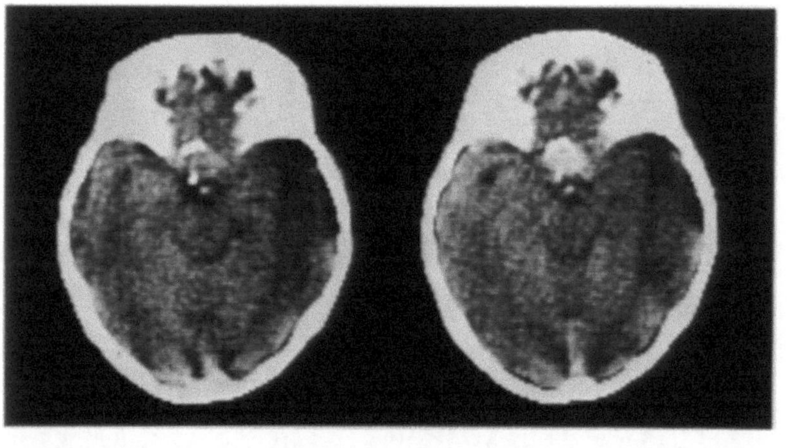

Fig. F74. Ophthalmic carotid aneurysm in a 65-year-old woman. Plain CT shows peripheral calcification in the aneurysm wall (*left*). Postcontrast scan shows intense enhancement of the aneurysmal sac (*right*)

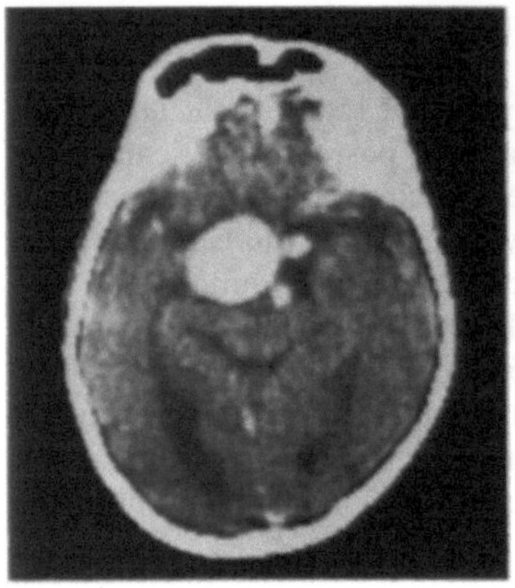

a

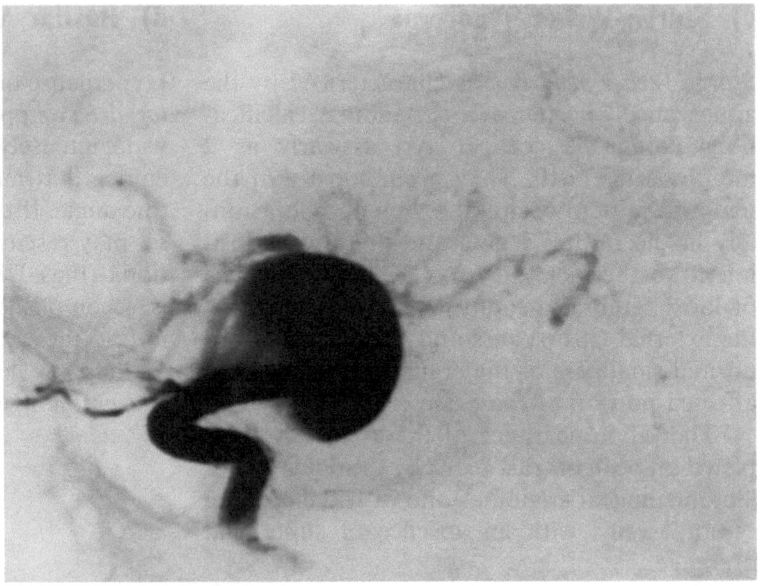

b

Fig. F75a, b. Giant aneurysm of the supraclinoidal portion of the left internal carotid artery in a 64-year-old man. **a** Postcontrast CT shows very intense, homogeneous enhancement of the aneurysmal sac and of the right internal carotid and basilar arteries, which appear to the right of the aneurysm. **b** Angiogram of the same patient

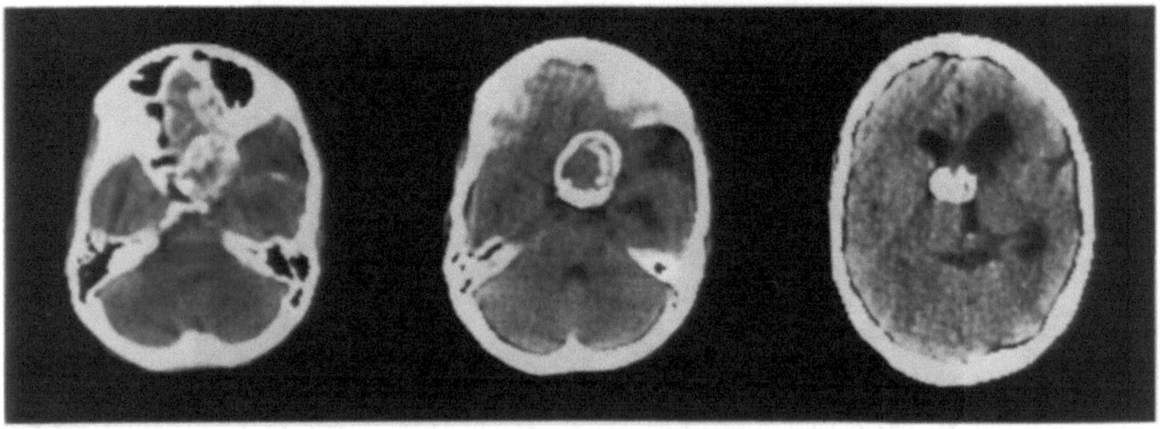

Fig. F76. Large aneurysm of the right internal carotid artery in a 29-year-old man. Scans show the heavily calcified aneurysmal sac on various planes of section. The plaque-like calcifications in the capsule of the aneurysm are typical

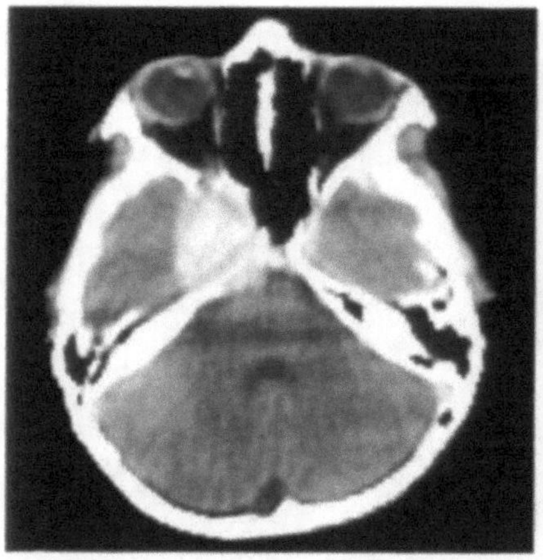

Fig. F77. Left infraclinoidal carotid aneurysm in a 10-year-old boy. Note the densely enhancing aneurysmal sac and the erosive changes in the left sphenoid wing and left petrous apex. This finding does not support a diagnosis of meningioma. Postcontrast CT

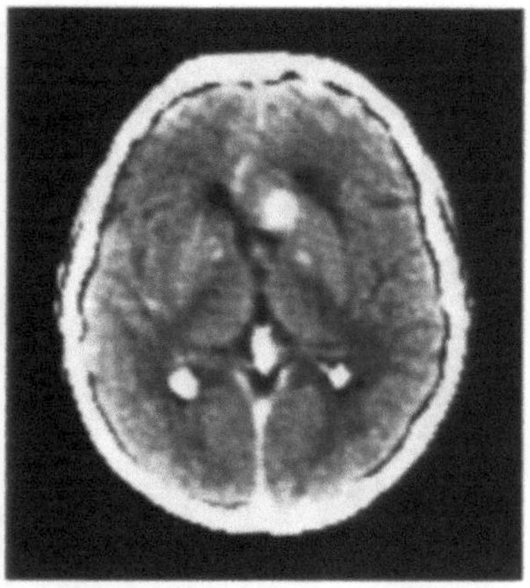

Fig. F78. Cherry-size aneurysm at the intracranial carotid bifurcation on the right side with upward extension and compression of the right frontal horn in a 52-year-old man. A funnel-shaped zone of edema extends from the tip of the right frontal horn to the external capsule. Bilateral calcifications in the basal ganglia are present as an incidental finding. Postcontrast CT

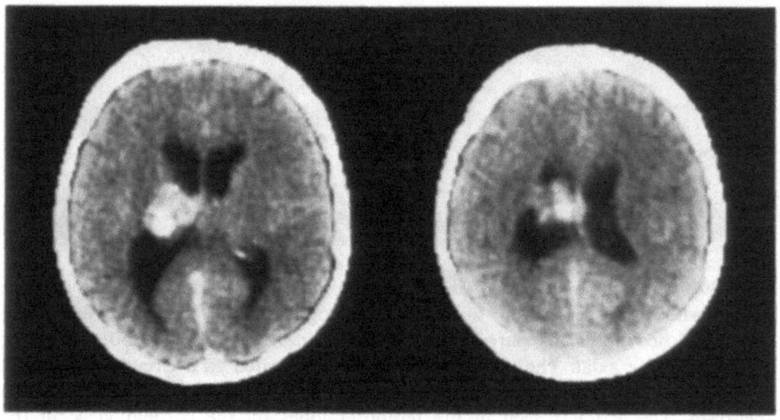

Fig. F79. Partially calcified aneurysm of the left posterior choroidal artery in a 47-year-old man. The intraventricular site of the aneurysm may cause confusion with a ventricular tumor such as choroid plexus papilloma or meningioma. Postcontrast CT

a–c

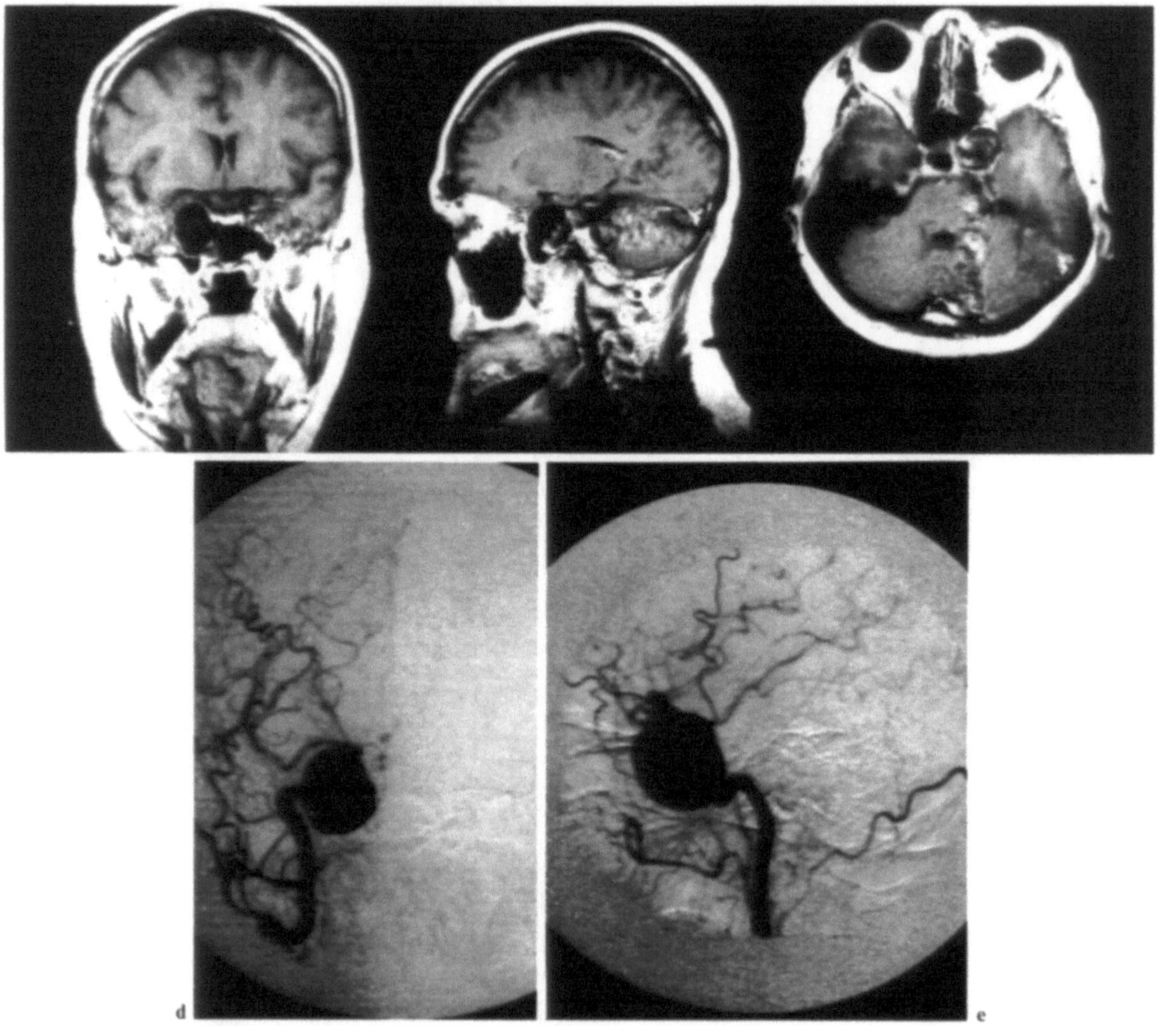

d e

Fig. F 80 a–e. Giant aneurysm of the right internal carotid artery in a 57-year-old woman with an 8-week history of diplopia and right parietal headache. Neurologic exam disclosed abducens paresis on the right side. MR: SE 400/30 **a** coronal, **b** parasagittal, **c** axial. The aneurysm is clearly delineated as a circumscribed area of signal void. The slightly hyperintense areas signify partial thrombosis of the aneurysm. The artifacts seen in the temporal lobes on the coronal view, in the cerebellar region on the parasagittal view, and on the axial image are caused by the pulsation of the vascular malformation. **d, e** Right carotid arteriograms in the sagittal and lateral projections

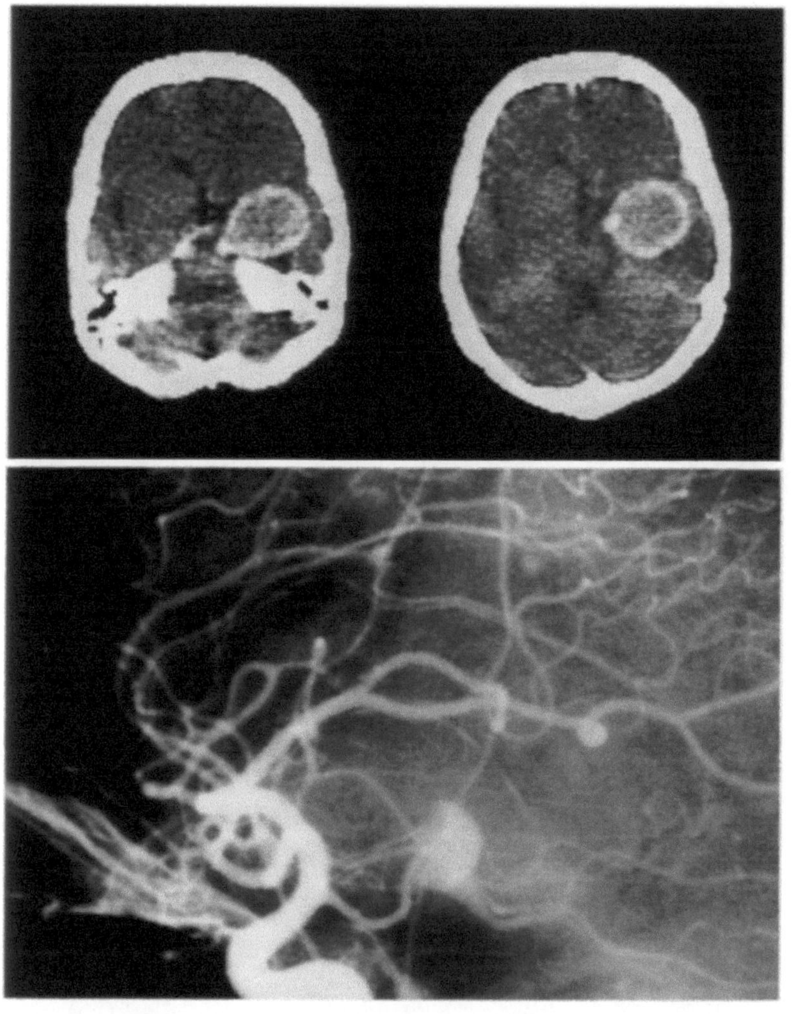

Fig. F81. Heavily thrombosed aneurysm of the right posterior cerebral artery in a 59-year-old woman. The calcified aneurysmal sac presents a bull's-eye pattern that is appreciated even on the noncontrast scan. Enhancement is confined to the medial wall of the sac (*above*). The diagnosis was confirmed by angiography (*below*) and at operation

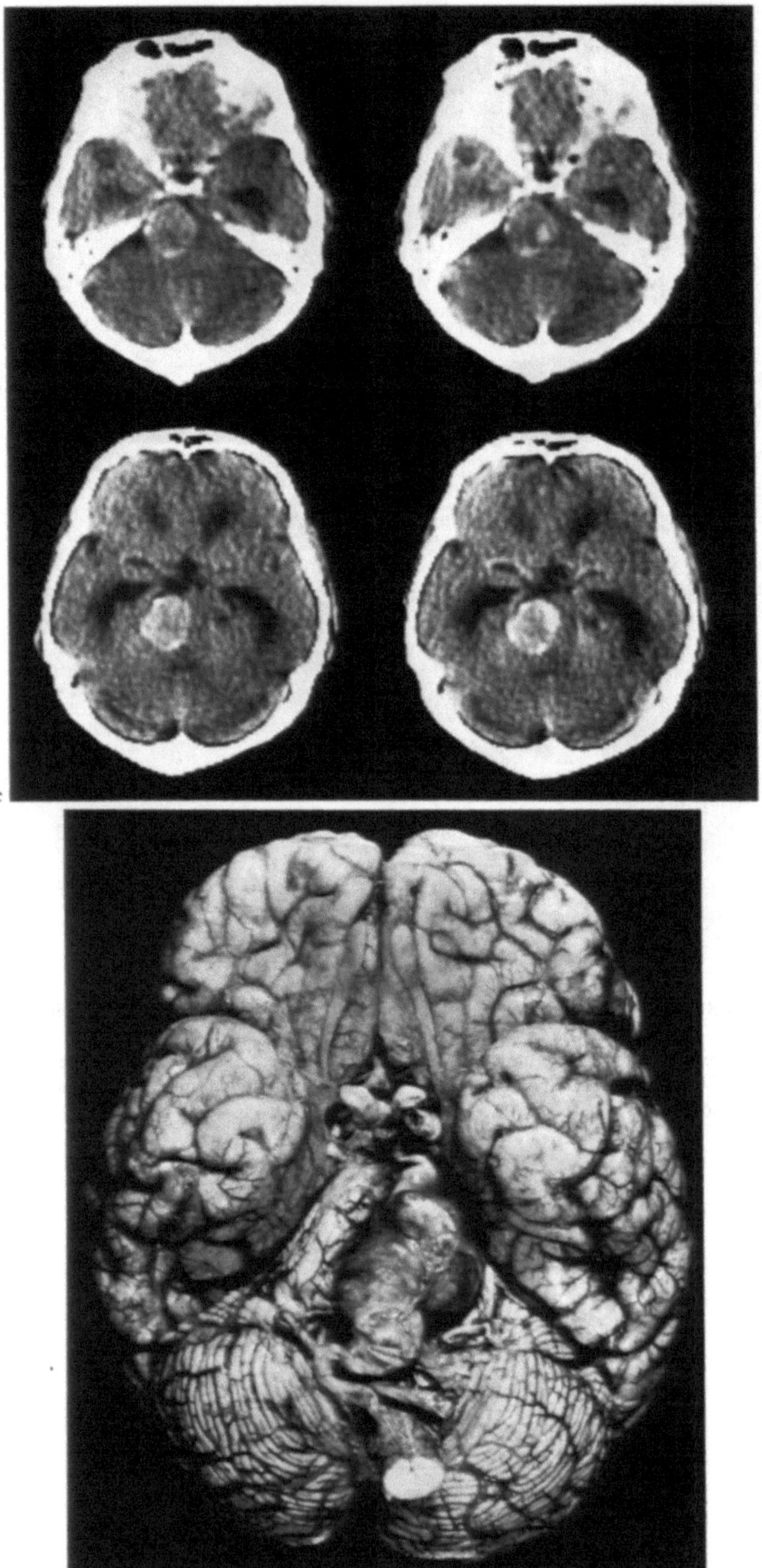

a b c d e

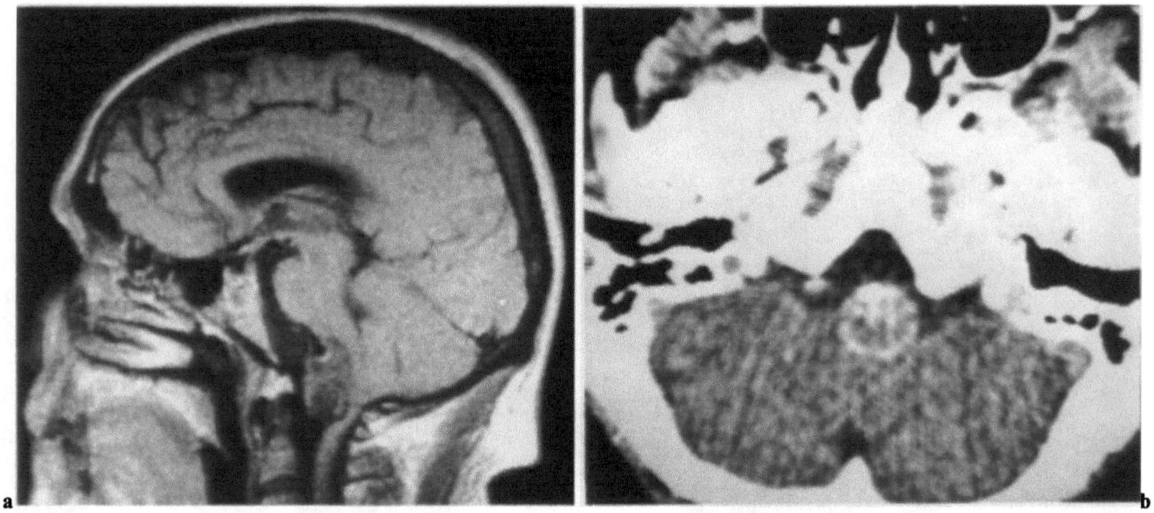

Fig. F83a, b. Vertebral artery aneurysm in a 57-year-old man with headache and vertigo. **a** MR: SE 400/35. **b** Postcontrast CT shows a circular area of irregular enhancement corresponding to the vertebral artery aneurysm demonstrated by angiography. A specific diagnosis cannot be made from the MR findings. The mass effect of the vascular malformation is conspicuous

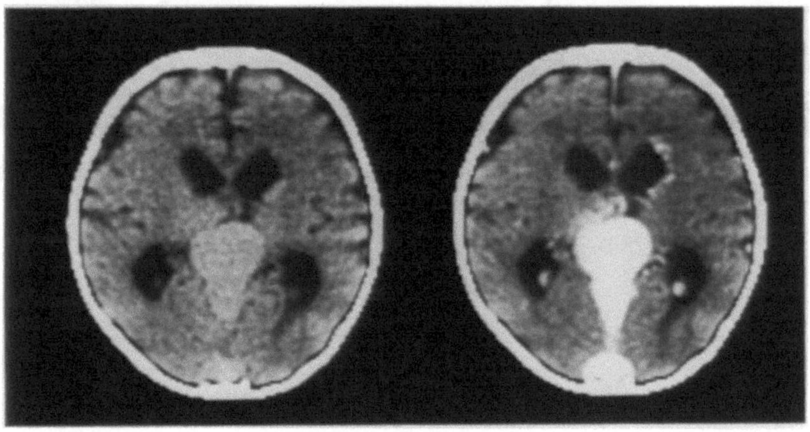

Fig. F84. Intensely enhancing vein of Galen aneurysm in a 2-year-old child. The aneurysmal sac appears slightly hyperdense on the noncontrast CT scan (*left*). Numerous ectatic veins are seen in the ventricle wall after administration of contrast medium (*right*). The lesion is drained chiefly by the expanded sinus rectus

Fig. F82a–e. Very large arteriosclerotic aneurysm of the basilar artery in a 68-year-old woman with signs of increased intracranial pressure. **a–d** The CT scans demonstrate a large mass lesion at the left pyramidal apex with peripheral calcifications and patchy enhancement (**a, c** plain scans; **b, d** postcontrast scans). The presumptive diagnosis of a partially thrombosed basilar aneurysm was confirmed at autopsy 2 years after the insertion of a CSF shunt (**e**). The cause of death was carotid artery occlusion

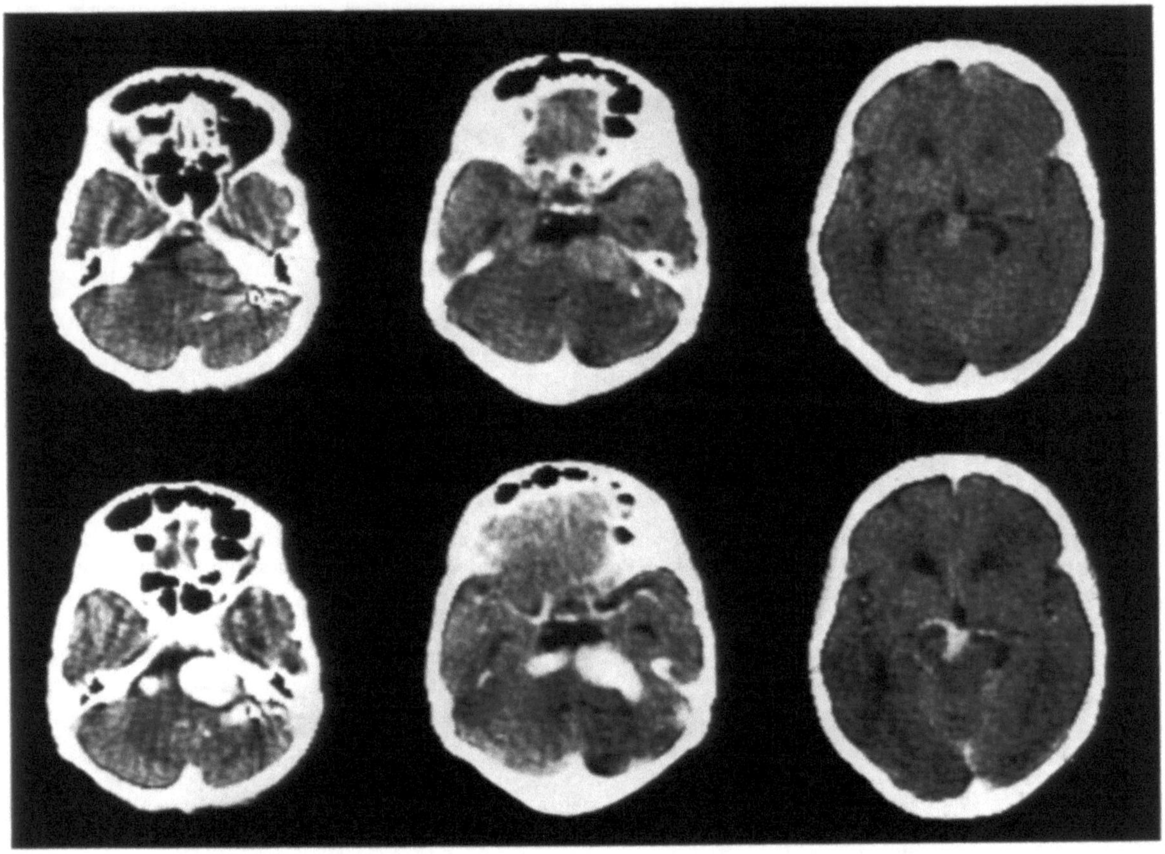

Fig. F 85. Basilar artery ectasia with fusiform expansion and marked tortuosity of the vessel. The CT sections simulate the presence of two separate lesions (*top row* precontrast, *bottom row* postcontrast)

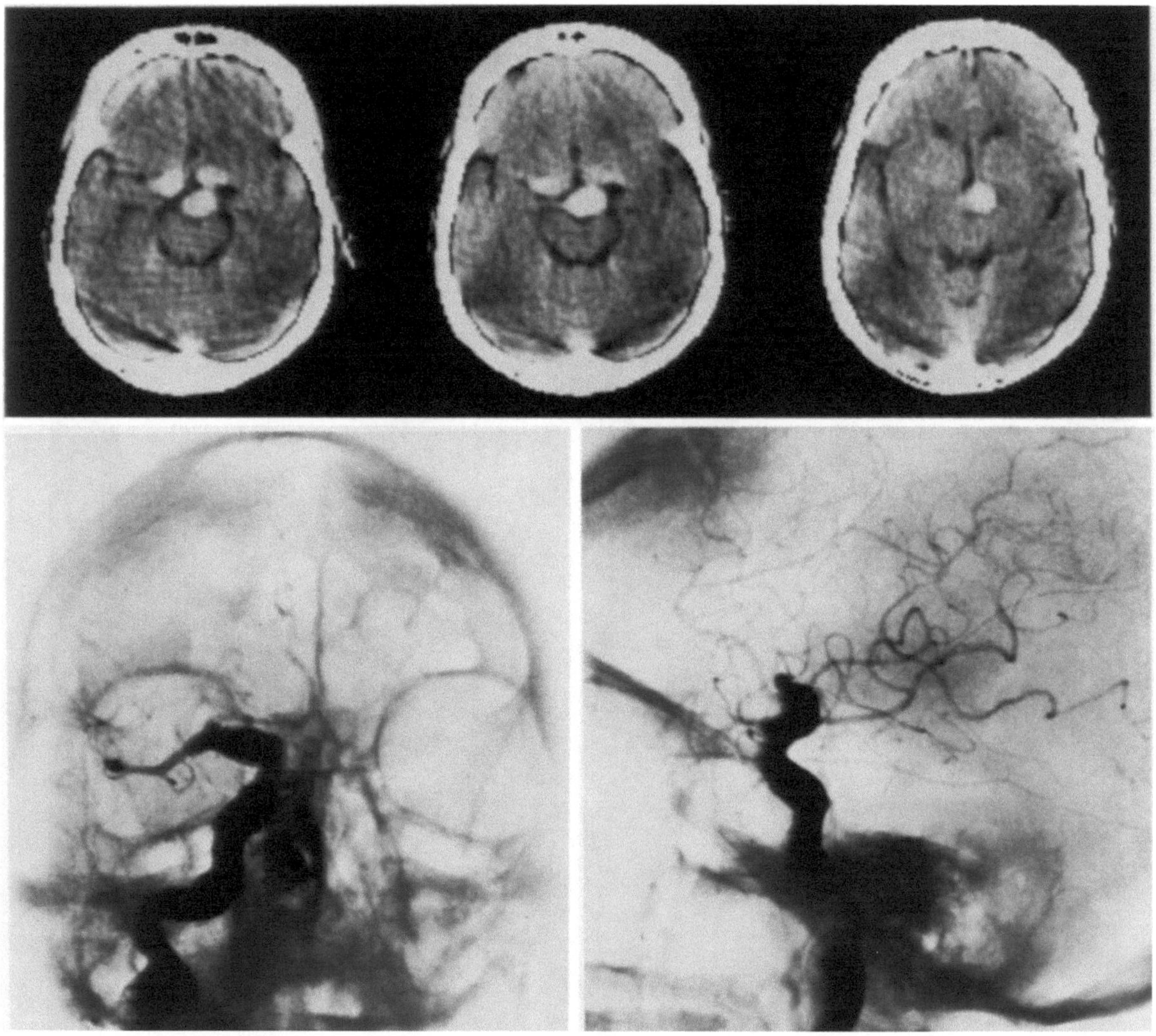

Fig. F 86. Massive fusiform dilatation of both internal carotid arteries and the basilar artery in a 67-year-old woman. Contrast-enhanced CT scans clearly demonstrate the dilated vessels in cross-section (*top*). The right carotid angiograms are pictured below

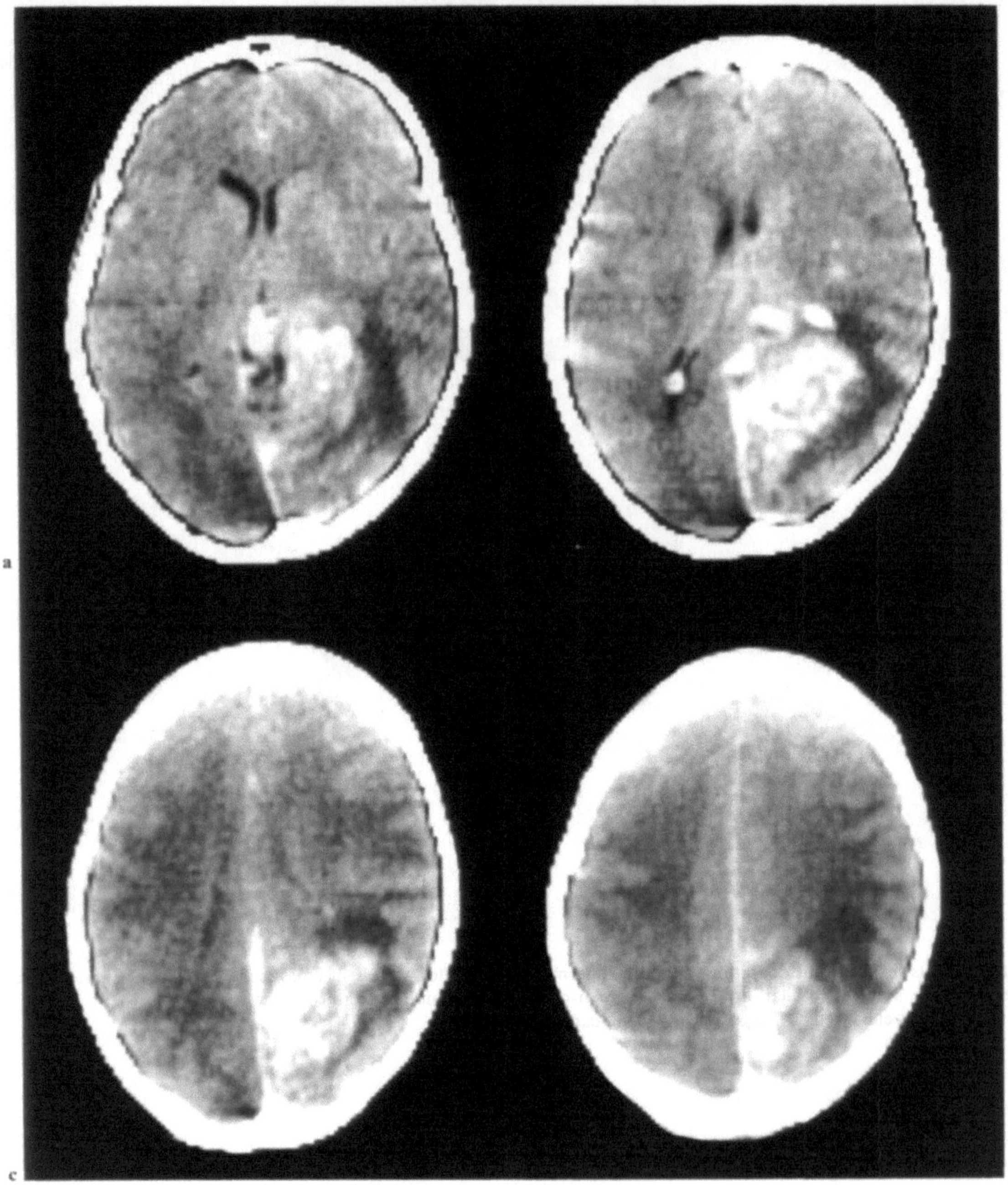

a b c d

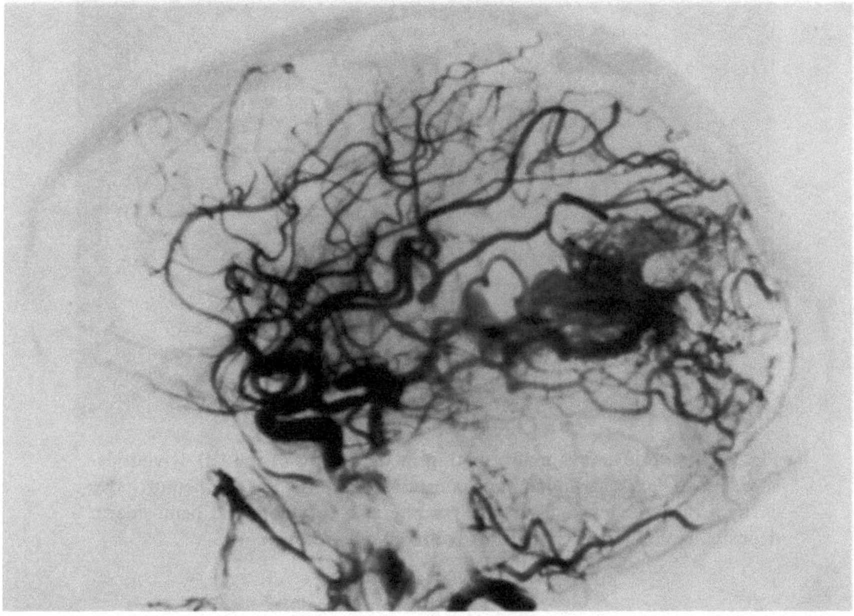

e

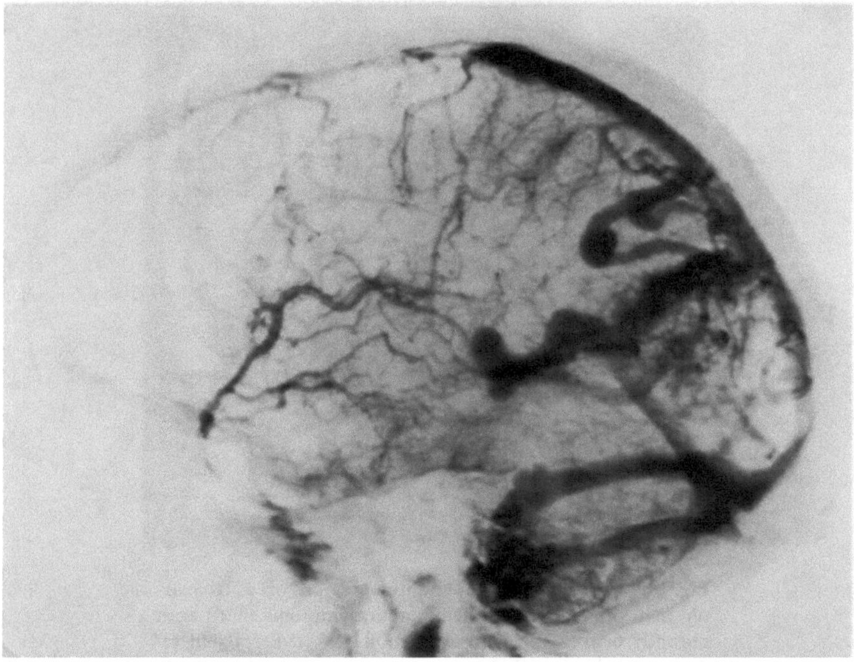

f

Fig. F87a–f. Very large angioma in the right occipital lobe, supplied mainly by the right posterior cerebral artery, in a 48-year-old woman (**e, f**). Note the unusually strong mass effect with anterior displacement of the choroid plexus, compression of the right occipital horn, and perifocal edema (**a–d**). The lesion could easily be mistaken for a tumor. Postcontrast CT

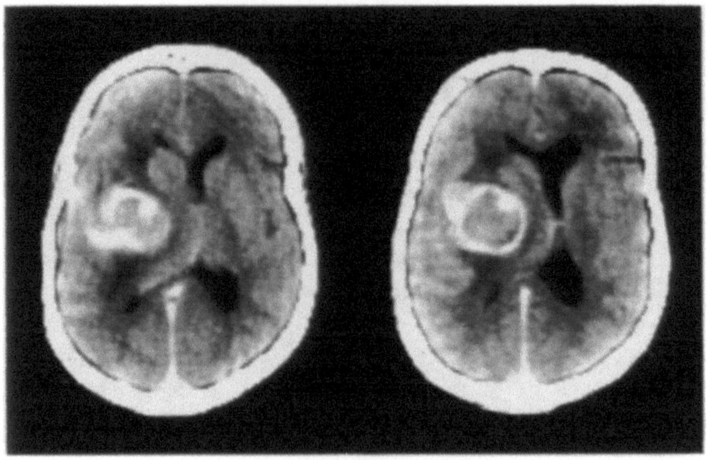

Fig. F88. Arteriovenous malformation in the region of the left sylvian fissure in a 40-year-old woman. Postcontrast CT scans show the hemorrhagic cavity as a hyperdense mass with peripheral blood clots and hemosiderin deposits. Note the ring pattern of contrast enhancement

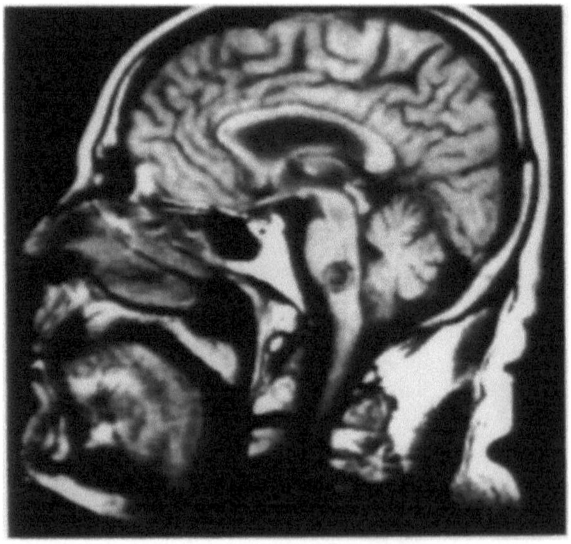

Fig. F89. Angioma in the pontine region of a 64-year-old man presenting with hemiparetic symptoms that began abruptly 6 weeks prior to evaluation. MR (SE 500/30) reveals a predominantly hypointense, "punched out" area in the region of the pons

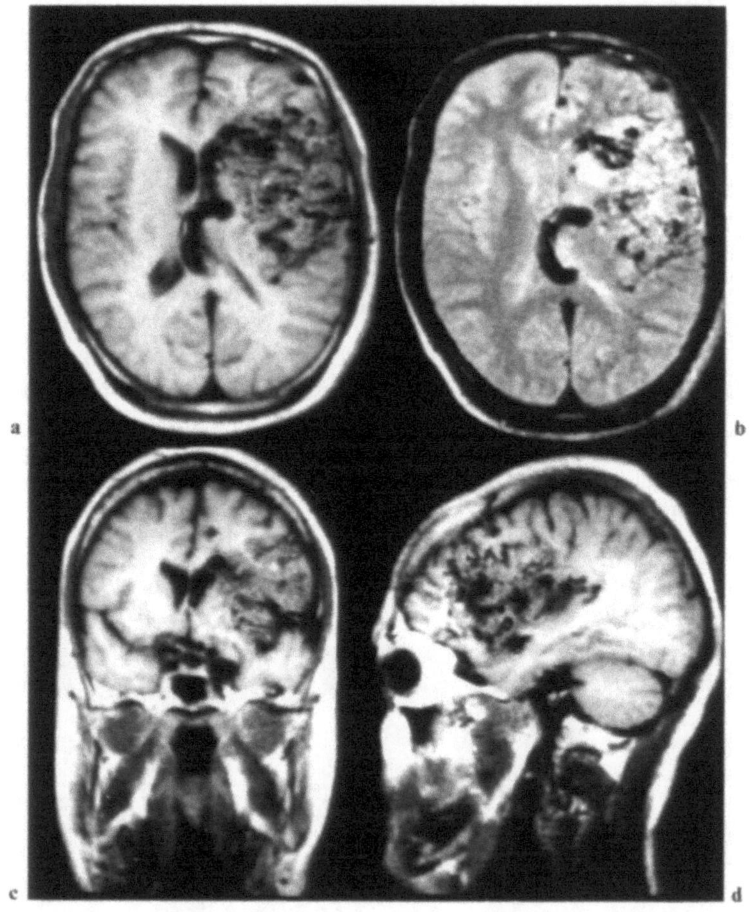

Fig. F90a–d. Arteriovenous angioma in the right parietal region of a 46-year-old man with headache, mild left-sided weakness chiefly affecting the arm and face, and disturbances of memory. MR: **a** SE 400/30, **b** SE 1600/70, axial; **c** SE 400/30 coronal; **d** SE 400/30 parasagittal. Images show a large, irregular area with patchy foci of signal void. The venous drainage of the angioma is clearly displayed

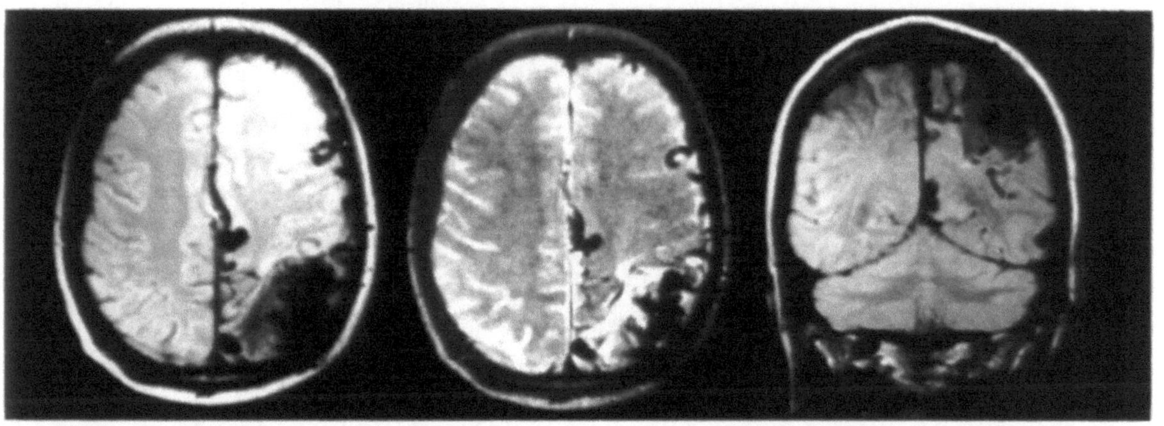

Fig. F91. Right parieto-occipital angioma in a 51-year-old man with a 10-year history of seizures. Neurologic findings were normal. MR: *left* SE 2500/30, *center* SE 2500/120, *right* SE 2500/30. The irregular signal voids are clearly delineated in both the axial and coronal views

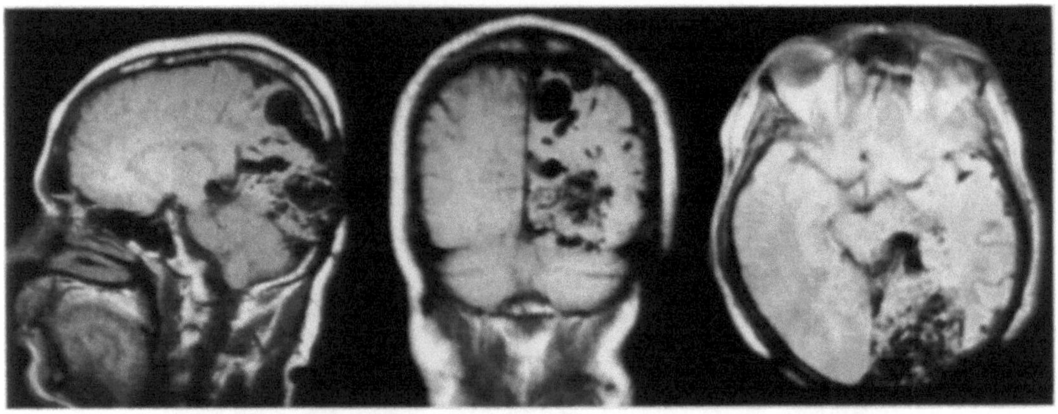

Fig. F92. Intra- and extracranial angioma in a 50-year-old man with a history of seizures. The extracranial components of the angioma were removed elsewhere 8 years previously. MR: *left* and *center* SE 400/30, *right* SE 1600/35. Scans show irregular areas of signal void in the right occipital region. The extensive venous drainage is clearly visible in all projections

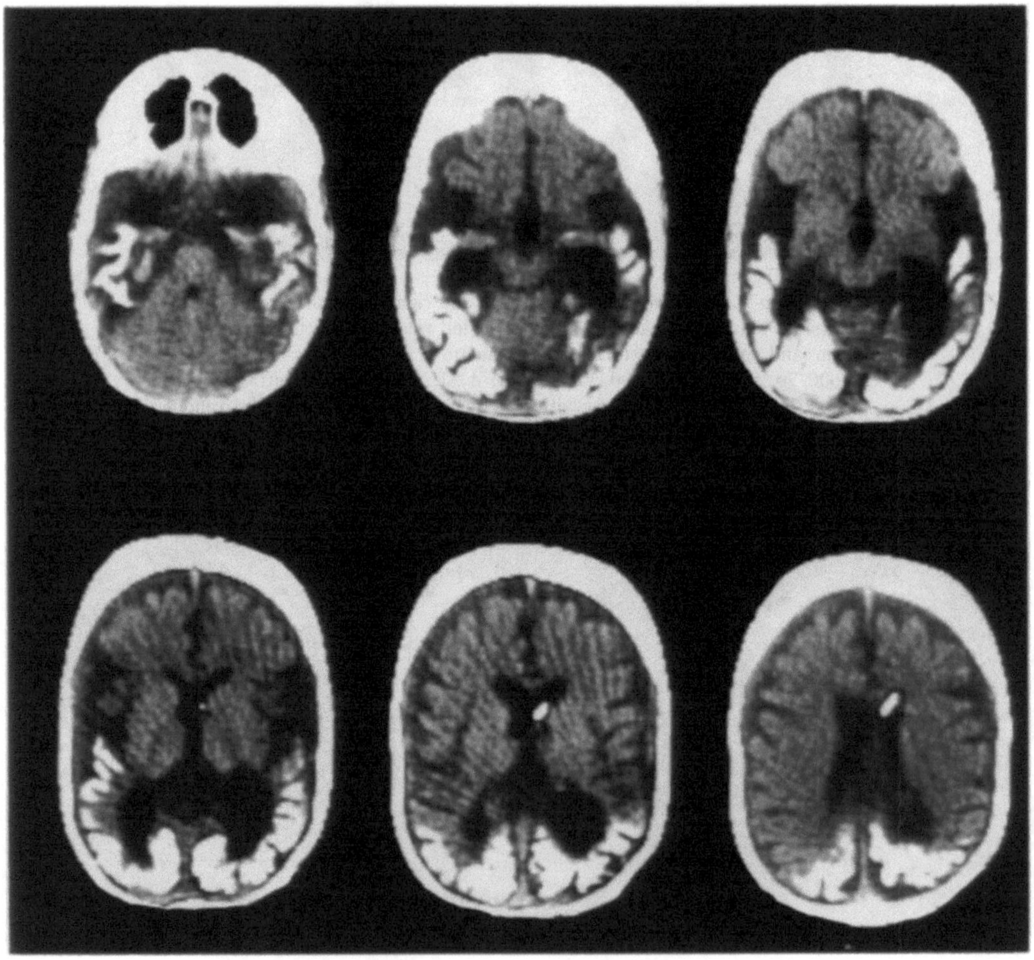

Fig. F93. Sturge-Weber syndrome in a 10-year-old boy. CT scans show bilateral calcifications in the temporo-occipital cortex with general atrophic involutionary change. A ventricular shunt was previously implanted

10. Cerebral Infarction (Arterial and Venous)

a) Postinfarction Edema with Mass Effect

Cerebral infarction can cause mass effect as a result of edema as well as hemorrhage into the infarcted area. Since the location of the infarction corresponds to a particular vascular territory, there should be no difficulty in establishing a diagnosis when proper consideration is given to the antecedent history, the acute event, and other clinical data (see diagram in Fig. F94). The development of *postinfarction edema* is characterized on **CT** by an initially subtle decrease in the density of the brain parenchyma. This may be detected as early as 3 h after the onset of symptoms, although only 20% of patients manifest CT changes within 8 h of their stroke (Aulich and Fenske 1977). As early as 24 h post infarction, the edema may attain a degree sufficient to cause up to 5 mm of midline displacement, and this may exceed 10 mm in exceptional cases. Edema tends to be most pronounced when there is carotid artery occlusion or total occlusion of the middle cerebral artery (Fig. F95). The mass effect is greatest between the 3rd and 5th days and then declines steadily over a 14-day period. Mass effect and edema resolve completely by 4 weeks at the latest, and this serves to distinguish the infarction from inflammatory disease and malignant glioma (Wende et al. 1979).

Special attention should be given to postinfarction edema associated with occlusion of the cerebellar arteries (Wilson and Moseley 1977). Severe cerebellar swelling develops in only 1–2 days, obstructing the flow of CSF and precipitating hydrocephalus. Immediate external CSF drainage is indicated in these cases (Figs. F96, 97).

MR demonstrates a linear prolongation of the T1 and T2 relaxation times which parallels the development of edema in the infarcted area. A 3% increase in brain water occurs within 4 h of the infarction, and animal experiments have shown that cerebral ischemia is demonstrable only 30 min to 2 h after the vascular occlusion (Levy et al. 1983; Brant-Zawadzki et al. 1986) (Fig. F97). The superiority of MR rests not only on the earlier and more accurate detection of the hyperintense postinfarction edema but also on its ability to resolve infarcts only 1–2 cm in size in the area supplied by the vertebrobasilar system, an area extremely difficult to evaluate with CT. What is more, the occluded vessel loses the signal characteristics of flowing blood on the MR image and instead displays the high signal intensity of thrombosis, making it possible to visualize the site of the occlusion directly.

b) Cerebral Infarction in the Stage of Blood-Brain Barrier Disruption

Most of these lesions show contrast enhancement on **CT** from about the end of the 1st week to the 4th week after the acute event. Enhancement is maximal between days 12 and 21. Various patterns and intensities of enhancement may be seen depending on the degree of BBB breakdown or of reactive hyperemia:

a) Intense peripheral enhancement, imparting a ring- or garlandlike border to the lesion (Fig. F100).
b) Faint reticular enhancement of the cortical area affected by the infarction (Fig. F98).
c) Homogeneous enhancement of an initially hypodense infarcted area, which then becomes isodense. If CT is performed immediately after the contrast medium is administered, a false-negative study may be obtained.
d) Circumscribed nodular, ring- or garland-enhancing foci within an initially hypodense infarcted area, which may be mistaken for a tumor (Fig. F103).
e) Intense enhancement of an initially isodense infarct. Conformity to a vascular territory should preclude a misdiagnosis of tumor (Fig. F99).
f) Intense enhancement at the periphery of the infarcted area, which may arouse suspicion of angioma. Persistence or delayed clearing of the enhancement helps in forming a diagnosis (Fig. F100).

In the phase of BBB disruption, **MR** offers comparable diagnostic efficacy to CT only when Gd-DTPA enhancement is used. Noncontrast MR is of limited value at this stage due to the isointensity of the infarct to brain parenchyma on T1-weighted images (Figs. F101, 102).

c) Postinfarction Hemorrhage with Mass Effect

We have found that bleeding in an infarct is a relatively uncommon event that occurs mostly in posterior cerebral artery occlusions and less frequently in middle cerebral artery occlusions (Fig. F105). The "flea-bitten" pattern of hemorrhages in the infarcted area commonly seen in postmortem examinations is not appreciated on the **CT** scan, and the blood collections must be fairly large before they can be discerned (Figs. F103, 104). The finding of hyperdense blood clots within the edematous vascular territory mainly requires differentiation from tumoral hemorrhage (Fig. F105). The previously mentioned changes in relaxation times during the course of a hemorrhage give **MR** imaging comparable diagnostic accuracy. As in CT, however, petechial hemorrhages are below the threshold of detectability by MR.

d) Cerebral Venous or Sinus Thrombosis with Edema and/or Hemorrhage

Cerebral venous and sinus thromboses are accompanied by circumscribed edema, which usually is indistinguishable from brain edema due to other causes. The superior sagittal sinus is most commonly thrombosed and appears hyperdense on plain **CT** scans, consistent with clotted blood. The ventricular system appears narrowed or obliterated, and the density of adjacent parenchyma is decreased in patchy areas or more generally, especially in the white matter. The presence of small or occasionally larger, confluent parenchymal hemorrhages along the interhemispheric fissure is also characteristic (Fig. F106). Postcontrast scans demonstrate multiple punctate foci of enhancement representing congested venous collaterals. These indirect signs of venous occlusion supplement efforts to demonstrate the thrombus directly on CT images. The thrombus itself may appear on nonenhanced scans as a dense, bandlike structure within the sinus. After 1–2 weeks the thrombus becomes isodense and appears on the enhanced scan as a filling defect most commonly located at the confluence of the sinuses.

On **MR**, the failure of venous drainage is evidenced by a *hyperintense zone* replacing the normally low signal of flowing blood. In the acute phase the thrombus gives a low intensity signal on T2-weighted images like that of a fresh blood clot, but within a short time the thrombus is demonstrated in very high contrast, first on T1-weighted sequences and then on T2-weighted sequences, and a definitive diagnosis is easily made.

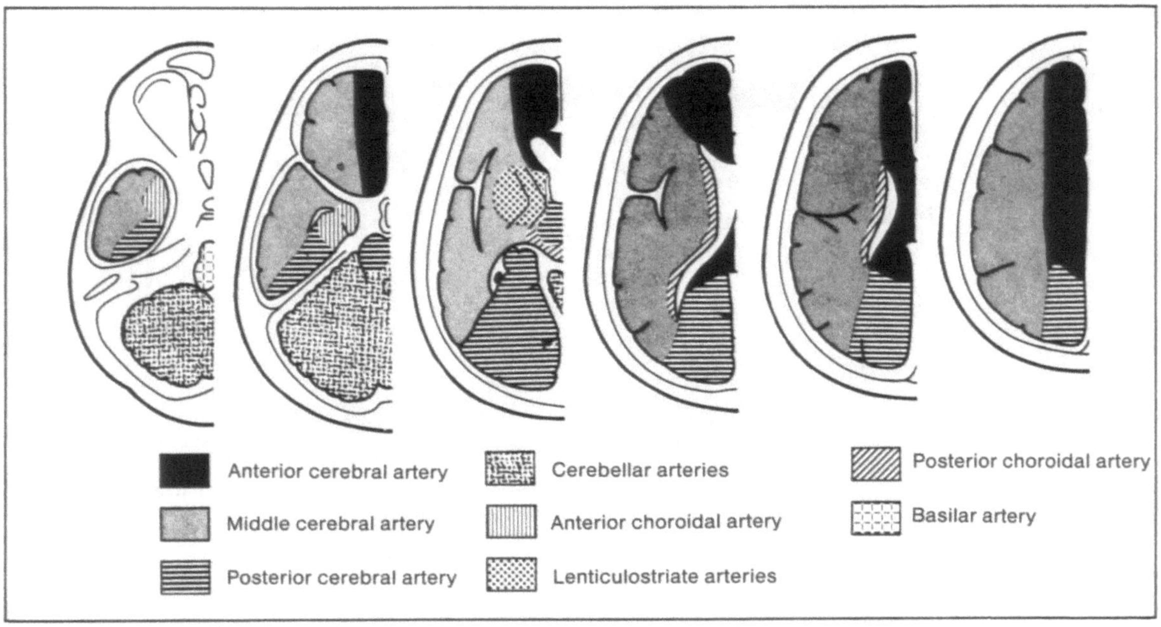

Fig. F94. Schematic representation of the areas of the brain supplied by the cerebral arteries [from S. Lange et al. (1977) Computed tomography of the brain, by kind permission of Schering AG]

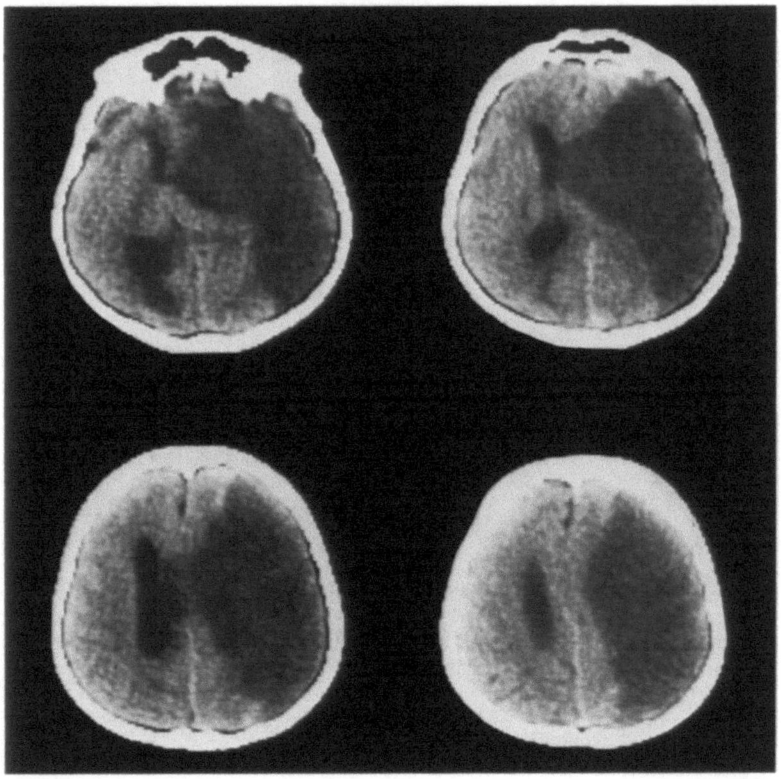

Fig. F95. CT findings 11 days after right middle cerebral artery occlusion in a 36-year-old man. The infarction involves the whole of the right middle cerebral artery territory. There is significant mass effect with compression of the ventricular system on the right side and marked displacement of midline structures (displacement is 15 mm in the region of the septum pellucidum). Postcontrast CT

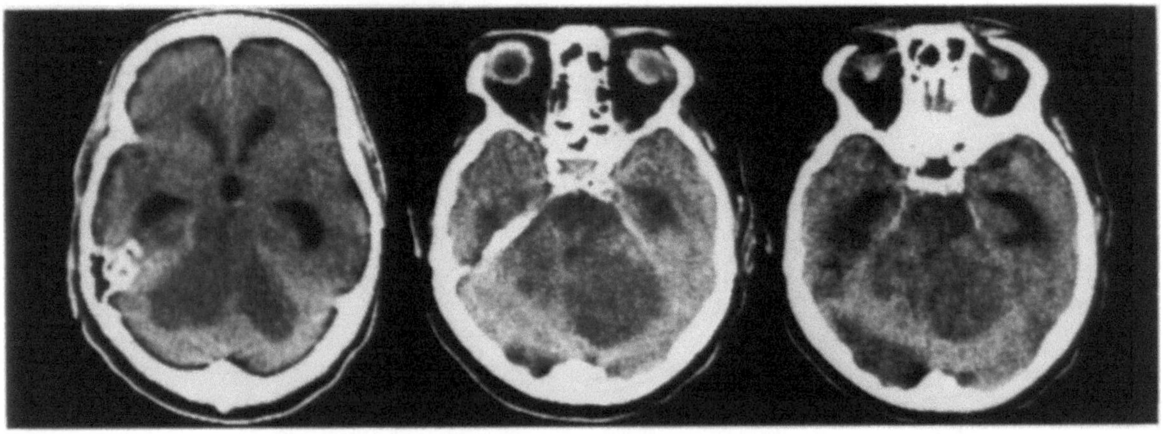

Fig. F96. Basilar artery occlusion in a 68-year-old woman with acute loss of consciousness and tetraparesis. CT demonstrates cerebellar and brainstem infarction and tension hydrocephalus with displacement and partial obstruction of the fourth ventricle

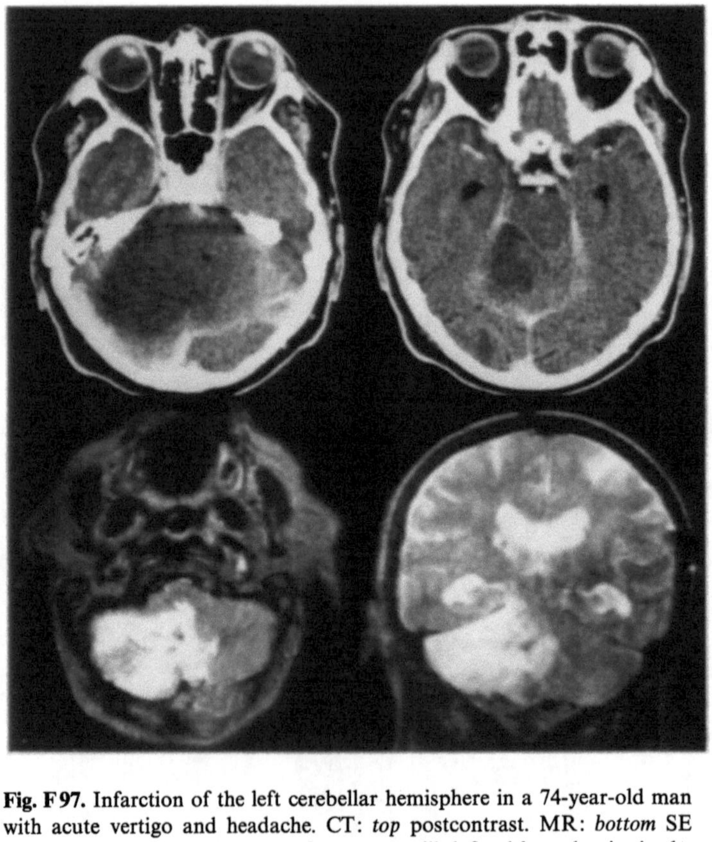

Fig. F97. Infarction of the left cerebellar hemisphere in a 74-year-old man with acute vertigo and headache. CT: *top* postcontrast. MR: *bottom* SE 2500/120. CT shows the infarcted area as an ill-defined hypodensity in the left portion of the cerebellum. MR displays the lesion more clearly as an area of high signal intensity

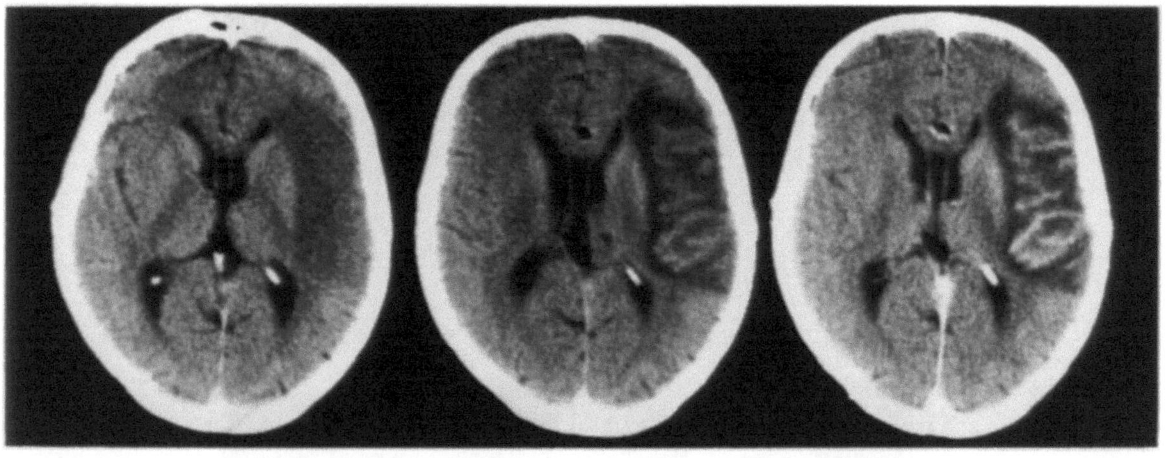

Fig. F98. Infarction due to right middle cerebral artery occlusion in a 59-year-old man with left hemiplegia of apoplectiform onset. Plain CT scan (*left*) shows decreased density in the area supplied by the right middle cerebral artery, consistent with infarction. Follow-up scans taken 1 week later (*center* plain, *right* postcontrast) clearly delineate the infarcted area. The postcontrast scan shows garlandlike enhancement of the cerebral cortex. Incidental findings are a septum pellucidum cyst and midline lipomas rostral and dorsal to the corpus callosum

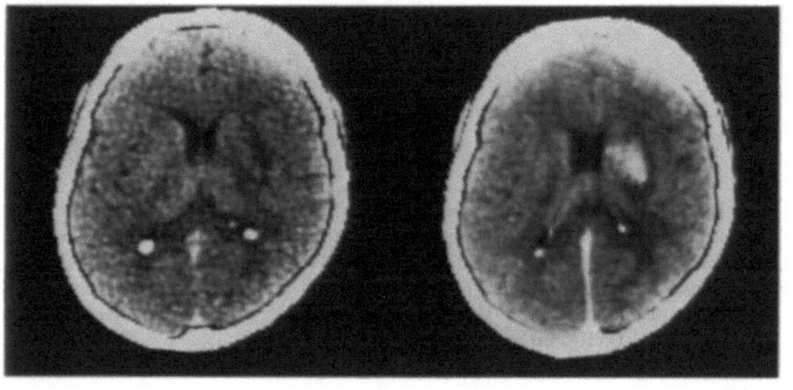

Fig. F99. Infarction of the right basal ganglia in a 49-year-old man. Plain CT (*left*) shows a finger-shaped zone of edema with mild compression of the right frontal horn. Postcontrast CT (*right*) shows marked enhancement of the infarcted area (14 days after the acute event)

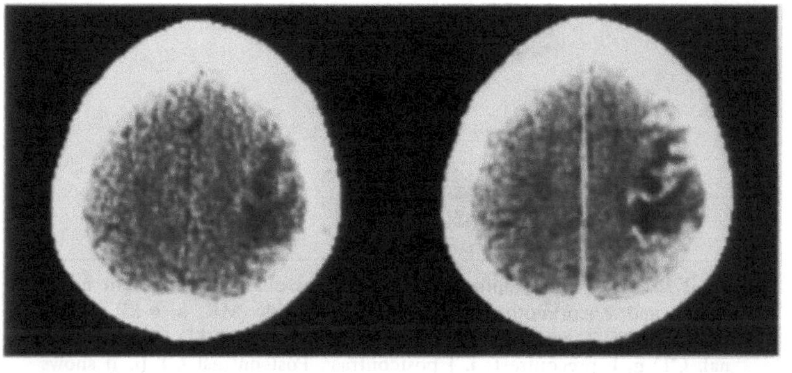

Fig. F100. Right middle cerebral artery occlusion in the stage of disturbance of the blood-brain barrier. The garland pattern of enhancement in the cortex can simulate arteriovenous angioma

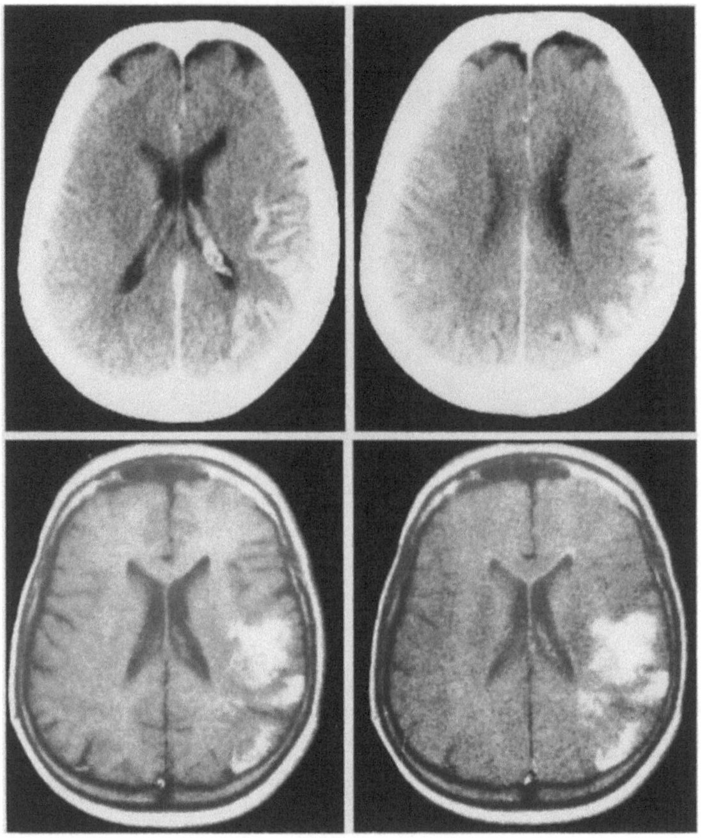

a b c d

Fig. F 101 a–d. Infarction involving part of the right middle cerebral artery territory in a 54-year-old woman with left hemiparesis. CT: **a, b** postcontrast. MR: **c** SE 500/35, **d** SE 500/70. CT 4 weeks after the stroke shows a partial infarction of the right middle cerebral artery territory with disturbance of the blood-brain barrier. The infarcted area gives an intense signal on the Gd-DTPA-enhanced MR images

Fig. F 102 a–j. Cerebral infarction in a 56-year-old man with right hemianopia and sensorimotor deficits on the right side. MR: **a, b** SE 700/35 before Gd-DTPA; **d, e** SE 700/35 post Gd-DTPA; **c, f** SE 1800/60 coronal. CT: **g, h** precontrast; **i, j** postcontrast. Postcontrast CT (**i, j**) shows marked enhancement in the thalamus and hypothalamus consistent with a posterior cerebral artery occlusion. These same areas show enhancement on the post-Gd-DTPA MR images

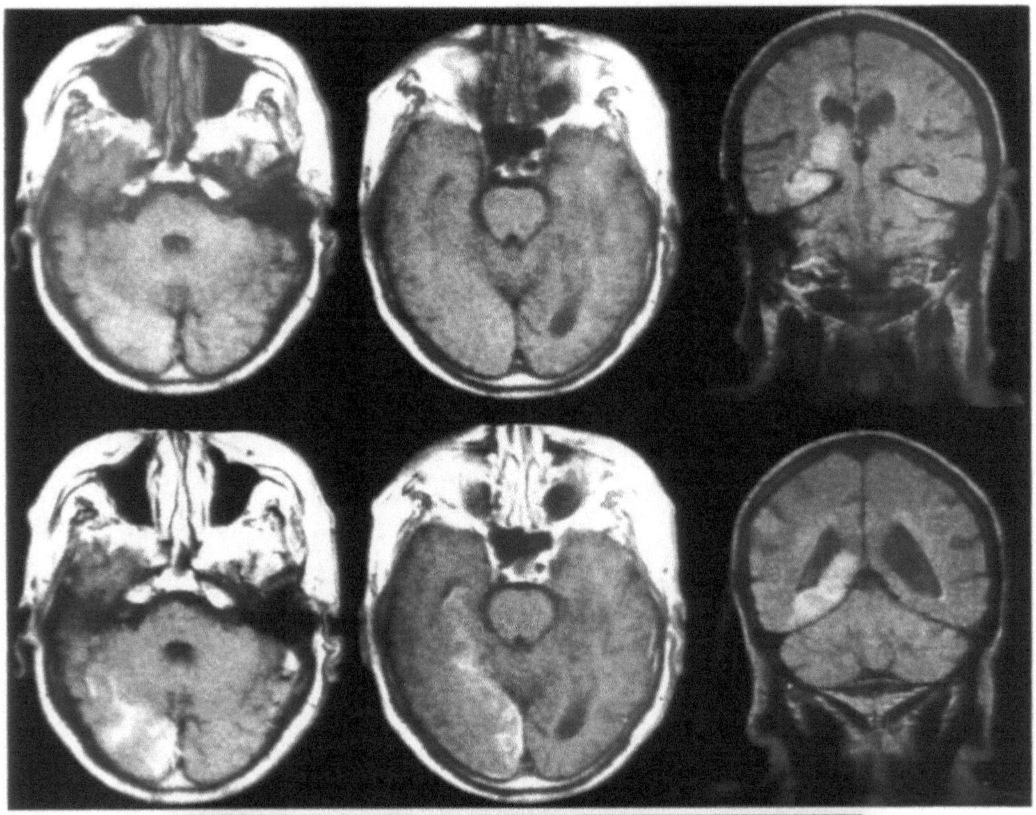

a–c

d–f

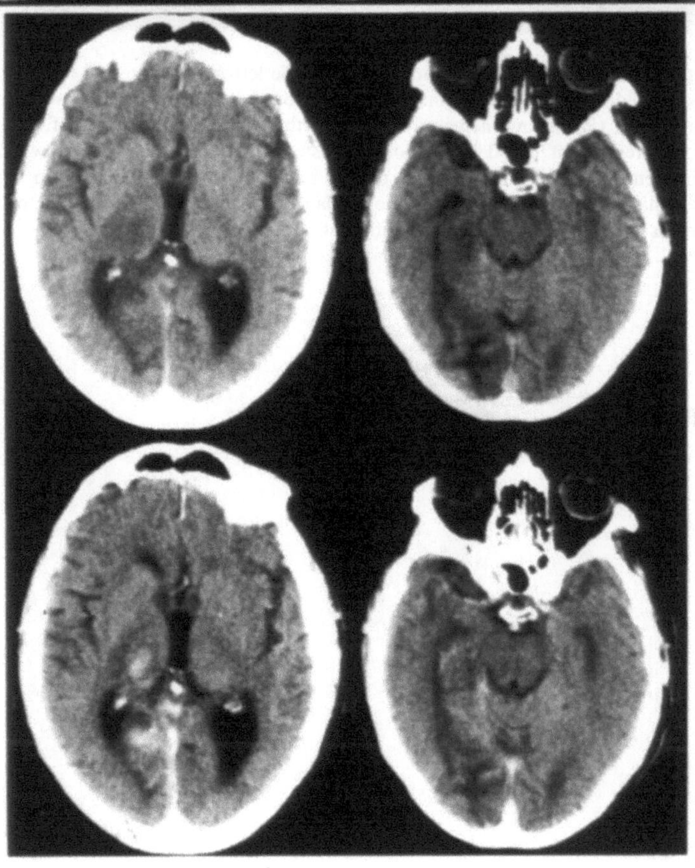

g h

i j

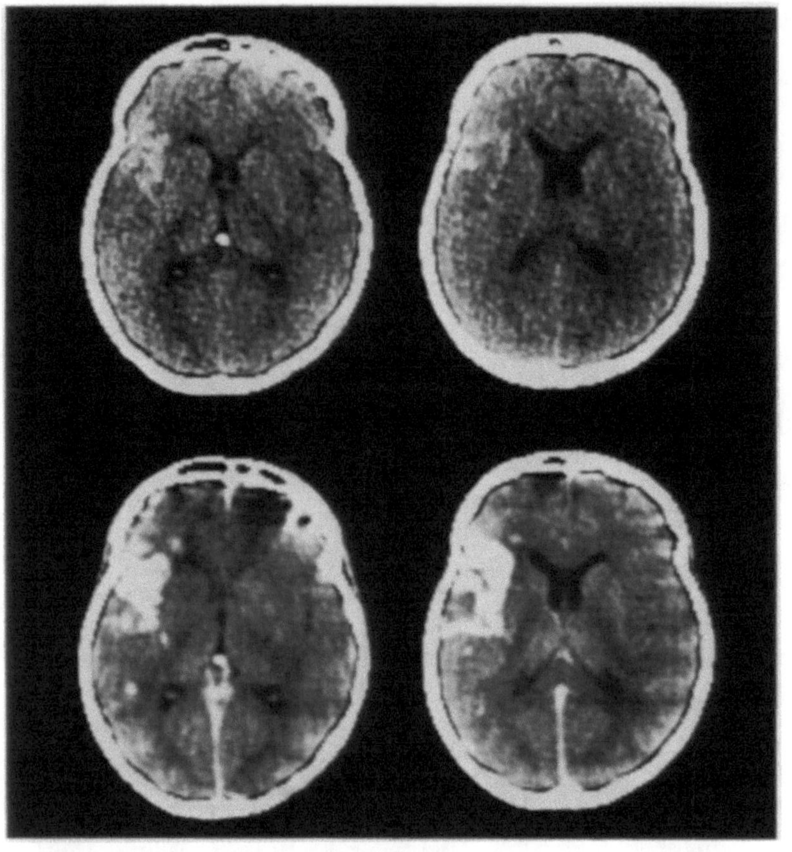

Fig. F 103. Hemorrhagic infarction involving the left middle cerebral territory in a 36-year-old woman. CT examination was performed 18 days after the acute event. Plain scans (*top*) show increased density in the region of the sylvian fissure due to the presence of blood in the cortex. Postcontrast scans (*bottom*) show intense enhancement of the infarcted area due to breakdown of the blood-brain barrier, resembling the appearance of a tumor or large AV angioma. The absence of mass effect is the principal criterion for differential diagnosis

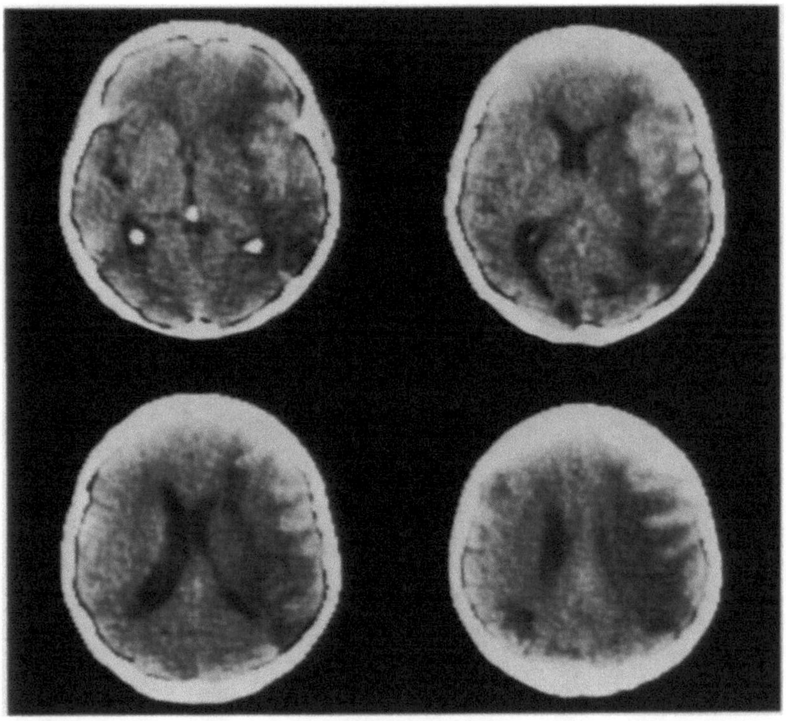

Fig. F104. Hemorrhagic infarction secondary to right middle cerebral artery occlusion in a 59-year-old woman. Marked hyperdensity of the cortex is caused by extravasated blood in the brain tissue. Noncontrast CT

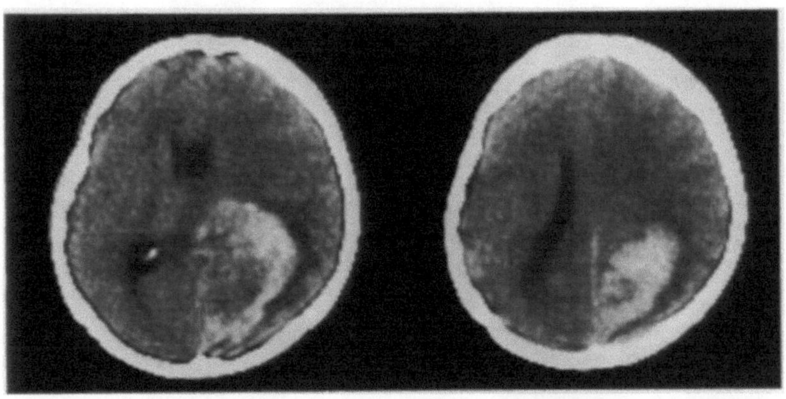

Fig. F105. Right posterior cerebral artery occlusion in a 62-year-old man. CT 10 days after the acute event shows hemorrhage into the infarcted area with significant mass effect. The findings were initially interpreted as an intratumoral hemorrhage

28.11.1986

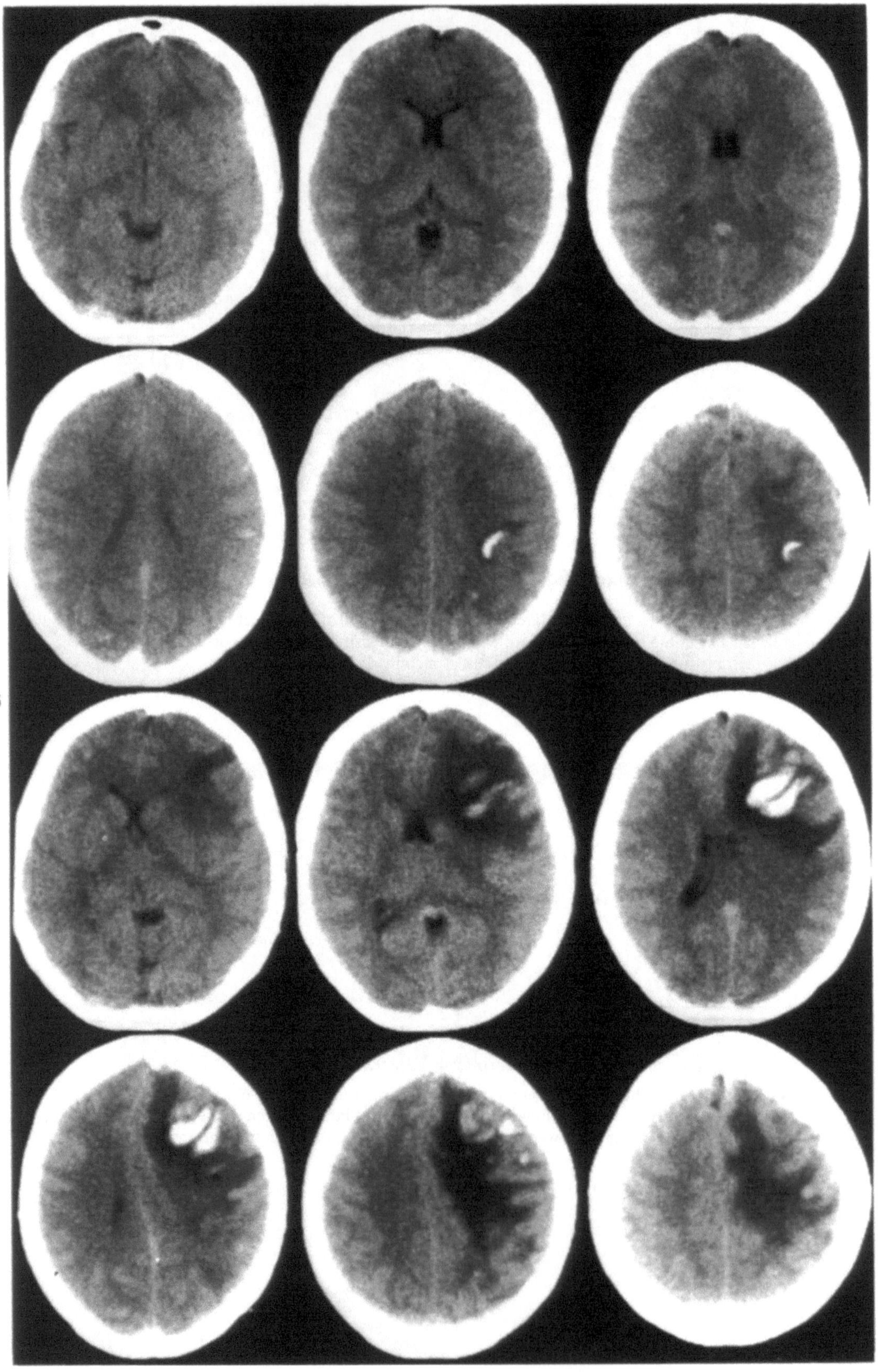

5.12.1986

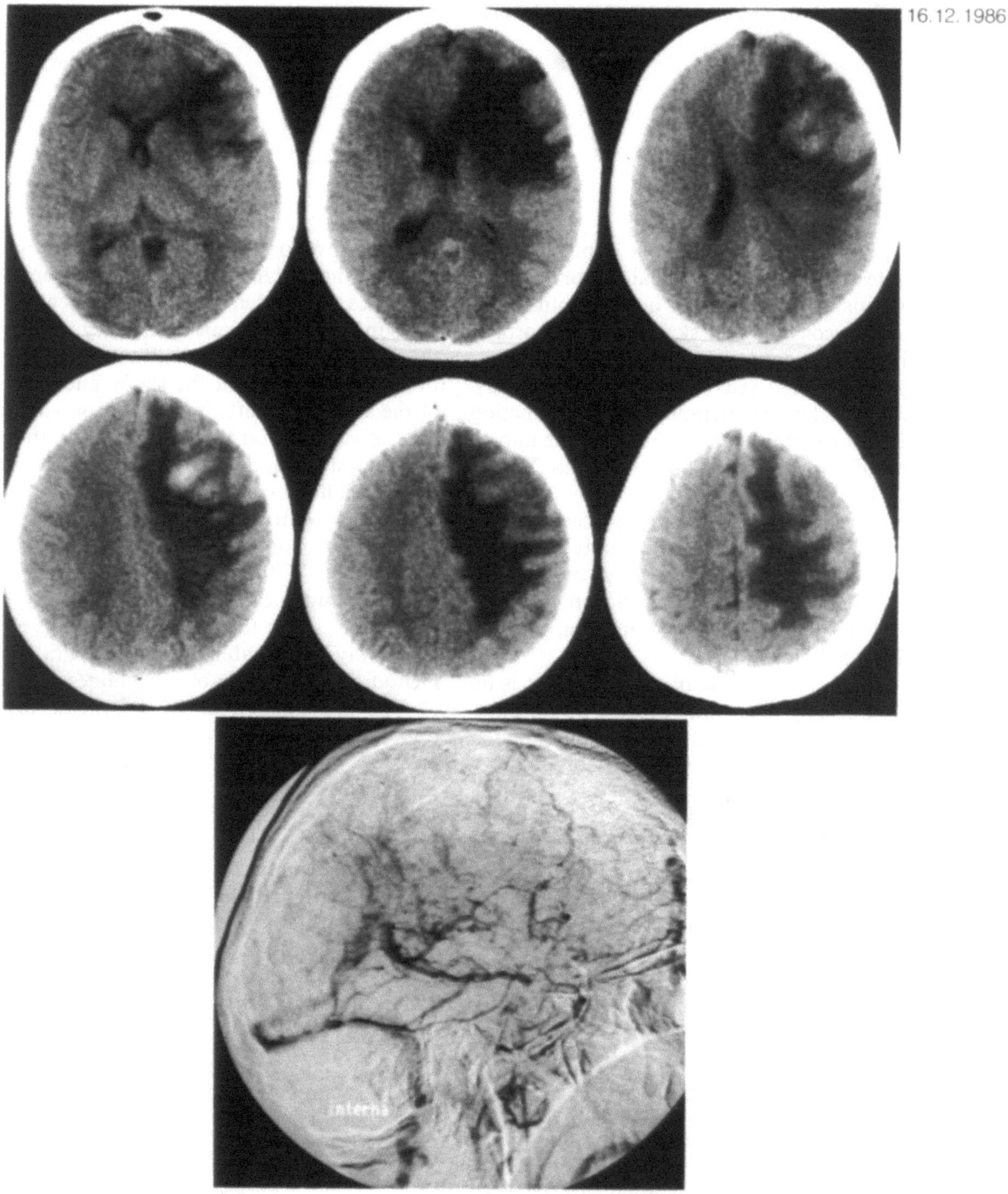

Fig. F 106. Sinus thrombosis developing 12 days post partum in a 28-year-old woman. The patient presented with left hemiparesis, grand mal seizures, and increasing somnolence. CT scans taken on November 28, 1986 show decreased density over the right hemisphere with a comma-shaped bleed in the parietal region. Follow-up scans 1 week later show increased edema in the right hemisphere with displacement of midline structures. There is marked enlargement of the intracerebral hemorrhage. Scans taken a further 11 days later show a further increase in edema with reabsorption of the hemorrhage. Angiography reveals complete obstruction of the superior and inferior sagittal sinus with opacification of collateral veins

G. CT and MR Imaging of Orbital Lesions

In the past, the diagnosis of orbital lesions manifested clinically by unilateral or bilateral proptosis and/or impaired ocular motility has relied on conventional skull films and orbital radiographs, sonography, fluorescein angiography, internal and external carotid angiography, and ophthalmic venography. The introduction of CT, however, has greatly reduced the importance of invasive diagnostic procedures (Wende et al. 1977).

Conventional radiography and tomography can demonstrate changes in the bony orbit such as thickening, increased density, destruction, malformation, and fracture. But these studies are incapable of demonstrating intraorbital soft-tissue lesions.

Sonographic examination of the orbit is indicated in all patients who present with proptosis, ocular displacement, or limitation of ocular motility, as well as in optic atrophy of unknown cause. The procedure is risk-free and can confirm or exclude a mass lesion with high confidence when performed by an experienced examiner (Ossoinig 1978; Dallow 1986; Rochels 1986). Sonography can also establish the nature of an orbital tumor in a high percentage of cases.

Internal carotid angiography demonstrates the ophthalmic artery, which lies on the medial side of the bony orbit and may be displaced by large tumors. It should be noted, however, that the range of anatomic variation is considerable, and a definitive diagnosis cannot always be made. Moreover, definite tumor staining is rarely seen on these angiograms. Selective opacification of the external carotid artery and its terminal branches is always a necessary adjunct, because many orbital tumors are supplied by branches of the external carotid, and selective contrast injection is necessary to demonstrate a tumor stain.

Orbital venography is a powerful technique for detecting orbital tumors and inflammatory processes. It can demonstrate displacements of the superior ophthalmic vein, irregularities in the caliber of the vein, and sites of stenosis. Frequently changes in the shape and position of the superior ophthalmic artery provide specific information on the location and nature of orbital lesions and can differentiate a tumor from an inflammatory process.

On the negative side, all contrast examinations used to diagnose orbital lesions before the advent of CT required hospitalization and involved a significant degree of patient risk and discomfort. Also, the cause of proptosis could not always be established despite the implementation of all available techniques.

The introduction of CT has made neuro-ophthalmologic evaluations simpler, more comfortable, and less hazardous (Ambrose et al. 1974; Baker et al. 1974; Gawler et al. 1974; Lloyd 1975; Momose et al. 1975; New and Scott 1975; Nover et al. 1976; Ostertag et al. 1976; Wende and Aulich 1976; Wackenheim et al. 1977; Hilal 1979; Jacobs et al. 1980; Wende et al. 1980; Piepgras 1981; Lloyd 1982; Forbes et al. 1982; Mancuso and Hanafee 1985; Peyster and Hoover 1984; Voigt et al. 1984; Bourjat and Wackenheim 1986; Ruchman et al. 1986).

Examination Technique

CT scans of the orbit are obtained with a different head position than is used for scanning of the brain. The gantry angulation for orbital CT should be approximately +10° to +20°, with scans performed parallel to Reid's baseline. Anatomic variations will require minor adjustments of the head position, and the quality of the scan is the only criterion for an optimum technique (Salvolini et al. 1978). It should be stressed that thinner slices are required for orbital CT than for examinations of the brain (1.5 mm to a maximum of 5 mm).

Axial scans with a 1.5-mm slice thickness eliminate errors due to partial volume effects (Swenson et al. 1982). Approximately 20–25 slices are necessary to demonstrate the orbit completely on the axial plane. This series may then be supplemented by direct coronal scans (Daniels et al. 1982). Coronal scans are made at an angle of about 70°–80° to Reid's baseline and afford an optimum view of the roof and floor of the orbit. Pathology in these areas may be missed on axial scans.

Some authors recommend extending the head 65° for direct coronal scans to eliminate molar artifacts (Tadmor et al. 1978; Forbes et al. 1982). Contiguous 1.5-mm axial sections can be computer-reformatted to obtain a coronal display. This can be done in all planes to generate special region-of-interest views. While reformatted images in other planes generally do not add to the diagnostic content of the study, they can aid the clinician in appreciating anatomic details (Unsöld et al. 1980, 1982).

Unsöld et al. (1980) note that the entire course of the optic nerve is optimally defined on the axial CT scan when the patient looks upward during the examination. The course of the nerve then becomes straight rather than sinusoidal.

The orbit can be visualized in its entirety on the different CT sections, which demonstrate not only the bony structures of the orbital wall, optic canal, and paranasal sinuses but also the globe of the eye, the optic nerve, and the extraocular muscles. The position of the optic nerve can be assessed with the globe oriented in various directions of gaze (Di Chiro et al. 1976). The sclera and lens are easily identified as separate structures. Intraorbital fat appears as a low-density zone behind the globe. The detection of intraorbital masses is rarely difficult since all tumors of this region except for lipomas and dermoid cysts have a significantly higher CT density than the surrounding fatty tissue.

Indications

CT is indicated for the diagnostic evaluation of primary and secondary tumors of the orbital region, ocular motility disturbances, proptosis, traumatic lesions, vascular malformations, and all other types of malformation.

Radiation Dose to the Patient

CT does not pose a significant radiation hazard to patients. The maximum radiation dose to the eye in standard CT examinations of the brain (from scattered radiation) is approximately 4.4 mGy. Reports vary on the dose delivered to the eye in orbital examinations. This depends on the number of slices, the overlapping of slices, and the effect of gantry angulation. Another factor to be considered is the doubling of the exposure that occurs when orbital scans are taken before and after the infusion of contrast medium.

Nemec and Roth (1976) and Tadmor and New (1978) report that the dose to the eye may be as high as 105 mGy depending on the number of slices obtained. However, these figures date from a time when thin-section CT scanning was not possible. Today it is reasonable to assume a dose of 31 mGy to the lens of the eye based on the use of up-to-date CT equipment and a total of 25 contiguous 1.5-mm axial sections. Increasing the slice thickness to 5 mm and obtaining both axial and direct coronal scans would result in a lenticular dose of 45 mGy (Forbes et al. 1982). Lund and Halaburt (1982) measured doses of 4 mGy to 273 mGy in 16 patients. These authors state that the individual dose is influenced by the gantry angulation, the head position, the thickness and number of CT slices, and finally by the KV and mA ratings of the scanner. Wilms et al. (1983) claim that the radiation dose from an orbital CT examination does not exceed 90 mGy.

In 1977 the International Commission for Radiation Protection established 264 mGy as the upper limit for the yearly lenticular dose in persons who work with radiation. However, Charles and Lindop (1977) argued that this dose limit was too high and recommended that it be lowered to 132 mGy.

In summary, it may be said that the combined use of conventional radiographic techniques (standard skull films and special views, tomography, carotid angiography and ophthalmic venography) exposes the patient to significantly higher dose levels of radiation than does CT.

Complications

CT is intrinsically harmless. Complications arise solely as a result of hypersensitivity to contrast media in certain patients. The frequency of these reactions can be minimized by careful history taking (see also p. 16).

CT and MR Appearance of Orbital Masses

Our findings in 1043 patients with orbital mass lesions are summarized in Table 12. The main diagnostic categories of the lesions are described below.

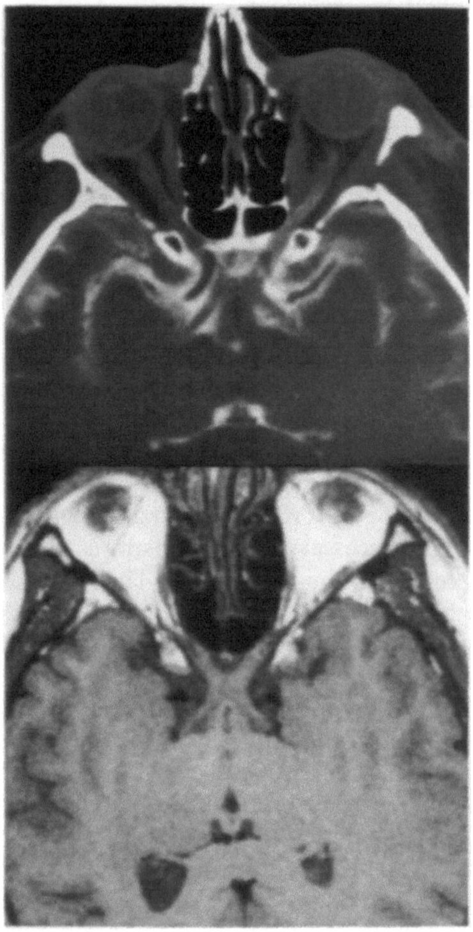

a

b

Fig. G1a, b. Normal appearance of the optic chiasm **a** on CT after the intrathecal infusion of Amipaque and **b** on MR (SE 400/26)

Table 12. Patients with orbital lesions examined by CT

Type of orbital lesion	Number of patients	
Benign tumors		310
Cavernous hemangioma	63	
Meningioma involving the orbit (sphenoid wing, olfactory groove)	72	
Optic sheath meningioma	30	
Pilocytic astrocytoma of the optic nerve	37	
Neurinoma	15	
Lipoma	14	
Epidermoid or dermoid cyst	25	
Fibroma	23	
Angioleiomyoma	2	
Adenoma of lacrimal gland	29	
Malignant tumors		239
Primary carcinoma of the orbit and metastases	102	
Lymphoma	46	
Melanoma	36	
Sarcoma (fibrosarcoma, rhabdomyosarcoma)	28	
Hemangioendothelioma	7	
Basalioma	13	
Neuroblastoma	4	
Plasmocytoma	1	
Myoblastoma	1	
Histiocytoma	1	
Inflammatory processes		152
Pseudotumor	55	
Myositis	48	
Mucocele or pyocele	29	
Abscess	8	
Orbital cellulitis	9	
Giant cell granuloma	3	
Malformations		46
Buphthalmos	6	
Sphenoid aplasia	12	
Arteriovenous angioma	18	
Fibrous dysplasia	6	
Cyst	3	
Orbital encephalocele	1	
Trauma		42
Hematoma or foreign body	35	
Carotid-cavernous fistula	7	
Endocrine ophthalmopathy		254
Total number of patients		1043

1. Benign Tumors

Cavernous Hemangioma (Fig. G2–6)

Cavernous hemangioma is the most common primary benign orbital tumor (8%–16%, Jacobs et al. 1980). This malformation can occur at any age but is most prevalent in the second to fourth decades. Females are affected twice as often as males. The tumor typically develops in the lateral part of the muscle cone or at the medial orbital border, and it can impinge upon and seriously compromise the function of the optic nerve. Histologically, cavernous hemangioma is an encapsulated mass composed of separate chambers of varying size with an endothelial lining. Some of the chambers contain blood, some are obliterated by fibrosis, and some are calcified. Local expansion of bone may occur (Davis et al. 1980).

CT shows cavernous hemangioma as a well-defined soft-tissue mass whose density differs markedly from that of normal orbital fat (Baker et al. 1974; Momose et al. 1975; Lester and Gyldensted 1976; Savoiardo et al. 1983). Contrast enhancement is dense but not always homogeneous, thus serving to distinguish cavernous hemangioma from neurinoma. In most cases the optic nerve is clearly demarcated from the cavernous hemangioma on CT sections.

MR demonstrates a smooth-bordered mass that is isointense to brain on T1-weighted images and so is easily distinguished from surrounding orbital fat. On T2-weighted images the lesion gives an intense signal compared with orbital fat (slow blood flow through the tumor) (Fries et al. 1987).

Meningioma (Figs. G7, 8, 10)
(see also Chap. D2a and Meningiomas p. 232ff)

Meningiomas constitute 3%–7% of all orbital tumors (Jacobs et al. 1980) and are more common in females than males. Histologic examination shows an encapsulated, solid lesion that is frequently calcified and rarely cystic.

Most orbital meningiomas invade the orbit and paranasal sinuses secondarily from a primary site on the tuberculum sellae, sphenoid wing, or olfactory groove. Osteoplastic sphenoid wing meningiomas initially form a carpetlike growth in the periorbita. With passage of time the soft tumor components thicken and, in conjunction with the bony changes, exert significant pressure on the orbital contents leading to conspicuous proptosis.

CT scans and X-rays of orbital meningioma show thickening and increased density of the bone as well as the intracranial, extracranial, and intraorbital extension of soft tumor components. The lesion enhances densely on postinfusion scans.

MR generally does not yield significant additional information (see Fig. D2.43).

Optic Sheath Meningioma
(Figs. G9, 11–13)

These tumors arise from the meninges of the optic nerve. Histologic examination often reveals cells of the meningoendothelial type (Swenson et al. 1982). All ages are affected, but the peak incidence is from adolescence to middle age, with females predominating. Optic sheath meningiomas are less common than pilocytic astrocytomas of the optic nerve. They tend to recur and to invade the cranial cavity through the optic canal.

CT may show enlargement and increased density in all or part of the optic nerve. The tumor has smooth margins and presents a fusiform or tubular configuration (Lloyd 1982), although its appearance is highly variable.

The meningiomatous sheath enhances densely after contrast injection and is easily distinguished from the nerve itself (Daniels et al. 1982). Slice thicknesses of 1.5 mm are required (Peyster and Hoover 1984). Intratumoral calcifications are frequent.

Differential Diagnosis

Optic glioma: Here the nerve and tumor are indistinguishable from each other following contrast enhancement.

Non-neoplastic enlargement of the optic nerve is seen in papilledema (choked disc), optic neuritis (Gawler et al. 1974), endocrine ophthalmopathy, pseudotumor, toxoplasmosis, tuberculosis, sarcoidosis, optic sheath hematoma, and occlusion of the central retinal vein (Peyster et al. 1983).

Density measurements of the optic nerve are especially helpful in differentiating papilledema from drusen of the optic disc, since the high calcium content of the drusen gives them a significantly higher density than in the normal or choked disc (Frisen et al. 1978).

An additional study, though one made largely obsolete by thin-section CT, is densitometry of the optic sheath following the intrathecal injection of a nonionic contrast medium. Because the optic nerve sheath includes an intraorbital prolongation of the subarachnoid space, enhancement of the optic nerve may be seen following the lumbar injection of contrast medium (Manelfe et al. 1978; Fox et al. 1979).

On **MR**, long T2 times result in high signal intensities. Low signal intensities indicate the presence of calcium (Mancuso and Hanafee 1985).

Extension of the tumor into the optic canal is demonstrated better with MR than with CT. In most cases the tumor is clearly demarcated from the optic nerve on the MR image.

Optic Glioma (Figs. G14–16)

Pilocytic astrocytomas (formerly called spongioblastomas) originate from glial cells, usually astrocytes and rarely oligodendrocytes (Swenson et al. 1982). They are most prevalent in childhood, with 80% occurring in the first year of life. A second peak occurs between 20 and 60 years of age (malignant astrocytoma) (Mancuso and Hanafee 1985). Optic gliomas in the latter age range tend to show a higher grade of malignancy than in juveniles (Spoor et al. 1980). The tumor grows slowly and does not metastasize. It is relatively rare and coexists with von Recklinghausen's disease in 10%–

50% of cases (Cogan 1974). Histologically the tumor is covered by intact dura, and tumor cells infiltrate the optic nerve. As tumor growth progresses there is increasing proliferation in the meninges, and the nerve becomes expanded (Swenson et al. 1982). Small calcifications are occasionally found in the tumor (Peyster and Hoover 1984).

The **CT** appearance of optic glioma resembles that of optic sheath meningioma in that a variable length of the optic nerve shows thickening and increased density. Unlike optic sheath meningiomas, however, optic gliomas do not enhance significantly with intravenous contrast medium.

Differential diagnosis should include sarcoidosis of the optic nerve (Som et al. 1982). Besides cranial nerve dysfunctions, expansion of the optic nerve may be the only evidence of the sarcoidosis. The expanded nerve enhances markedly with intravenous contrast.

MR is superior for demonstrating tumor extension into the chiasmatic region. Differentiation from optic sheath meningioma is frequently possible. Meningiomas enhance more intensely with Gd-DTPA than gliomas, providing yet another criterion for differential diagnosis.

Neurinoma (Figs. G17, 18)

Neurinomas are commonly found in association with von Recklinghausen's disease (neurofibromas). The tumor has smooth margins and is not adherent to the optic nerve. Histologic examination shows a diffuse proliferation of Schwann cells and fibroid elements. Neurinomas most commonly occur in the lateral portion of the orbit. Multiplicity is seen in von Recklinghausen's disease.

CT demonstrates a smooth-bordered, homogeneous mass. The CT density is similar to that of meningiomas, and contrast enhancement is pronounced. The tumor does not infiltrate the bony orbital walls.

Fibroma

Fibromas are rare, congenital, well-defined, solid tumors that most commonly occur on the roof of the orbit. They are encapsulated, and histologic examination reveals a simple fibrillary structure.

CT shows a smooth-bordered tumor that is usually well demarcated from other orbital structures (globe, optic nerve). The tumor enhances markedly with intravenous contrast.

MR displays both fibromas and neurinomas as smooth-bordered masses that are indistinguishable from other types of tumor.

Lipoma

Lipomas have a soft consistency and are very mobile. Histologically they present a regular structure with fatty tissue, a fibrillary network, and a thin fibrous capsule.

The **CT** and **MR** appearance is similar to that of dermoids having the density of fatty tissue. Thus diagnosis must rely on indirect evidence of a mass lesion with displacement of normal structures. Lipomas appear hyperintense on all MR sequences.

Epidermoid Cyst

Epidermoid cysts are congenital malformations composed of epidermal plaques delimited by a capsule.

CT density values are similar to CSF, providing good contrast with orbital fatty tissue (see also Chap. D6g).

Dermoid Cyst (Figs. G19, 20)

This lesion forms 1%–2% of orbital tumors but is the most common congenital tumor of the orbital region. Its rate of growth is very slow. It typically occurs in proximity to the lacrimal gland or bony sutures. Bone changes are frequent (80% in the series of Kingsley et al. 1986). The cyst contains an oily material in which hairs and cholesterol crystals are embedded (see p. 392).

CT and **MR** demonstrate a circumscribed area of very low density consistent with fatty tissue. The densities in the tumor may vary because of its nonhomogeneous composition. Dermoid cysts do not show contrast enhancement on postinfusion scans.

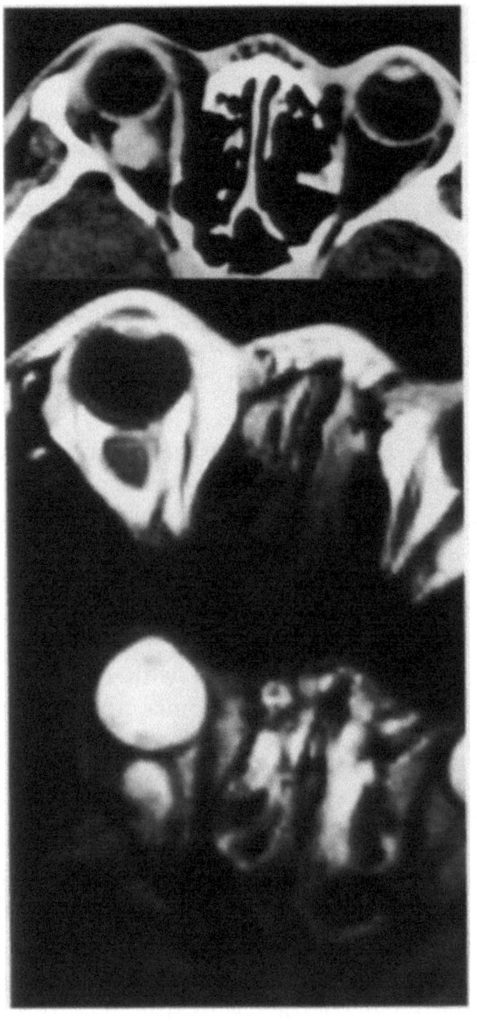

Fig. G2. Retrobulbar hemangioma on the left side detected incidentally in a 27-year-old man. CT: *top* contrast-enhanced. MR: *center* SE 400/30, *bottom* SE 1600/180. CT shows a hyperdense, well-defined retrobulbar mass displacing the optic nerve mediad. The tumor gives a low signal on the T1-weighted sequence (*center*) and a high signal on the heavily T2-weighted sequence (*bottom*)

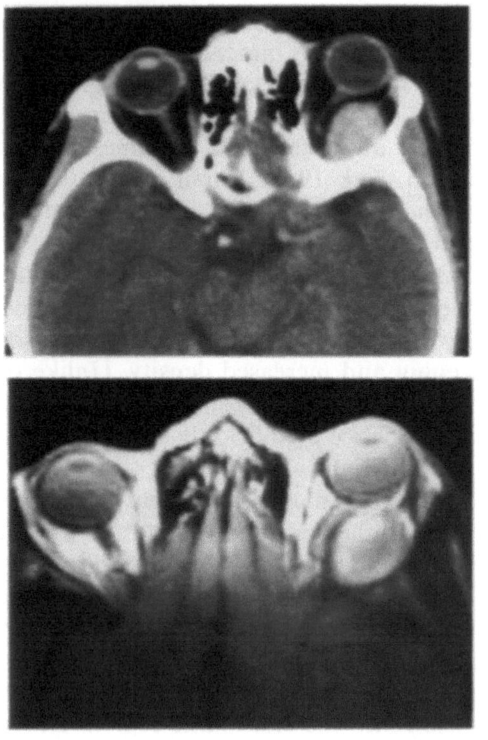

Fig. G3. Cavernous hemangioma in the right orbit of a 48-year-old man with 9 months of increasing right-sided proptosis. CT: *top* contrast-enhanced. MR: *bottom* SE 2000/30. Both examinations show a well-defined tumor with smooth margins. The optic nerve is displaced mediad

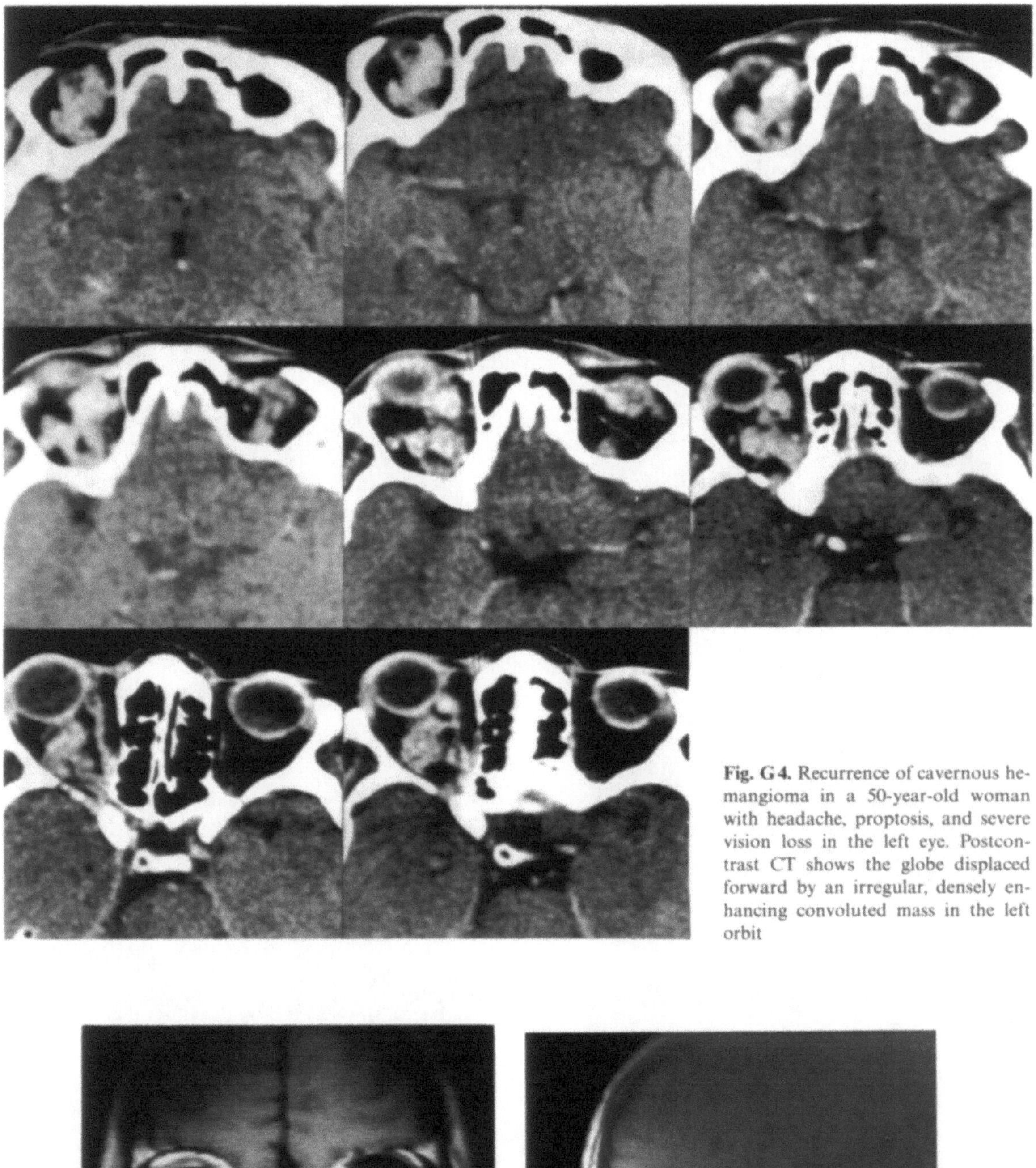

Fig. G4. Recurrence of cavernous hemangioma in a 50-year-old woman with headache, proptosis, and severe vision loss in the left eye. Postcontrast CT shows the globe displaced forward by an irregular, densely enhancing convoluted mass in the left orbit

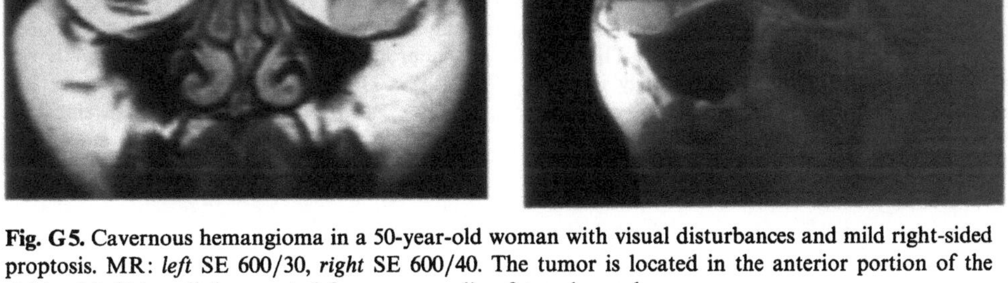

Fig. G5. Cavernous hemangioma in a 50-year-old woman with visual disturbances and mild right-sided proptosis. MR: *left* SE 600/30, *right* SE 600/40. The tumor is located in the anterior portion of the right orbit. It is well demarcated from surrounding fat and muscle

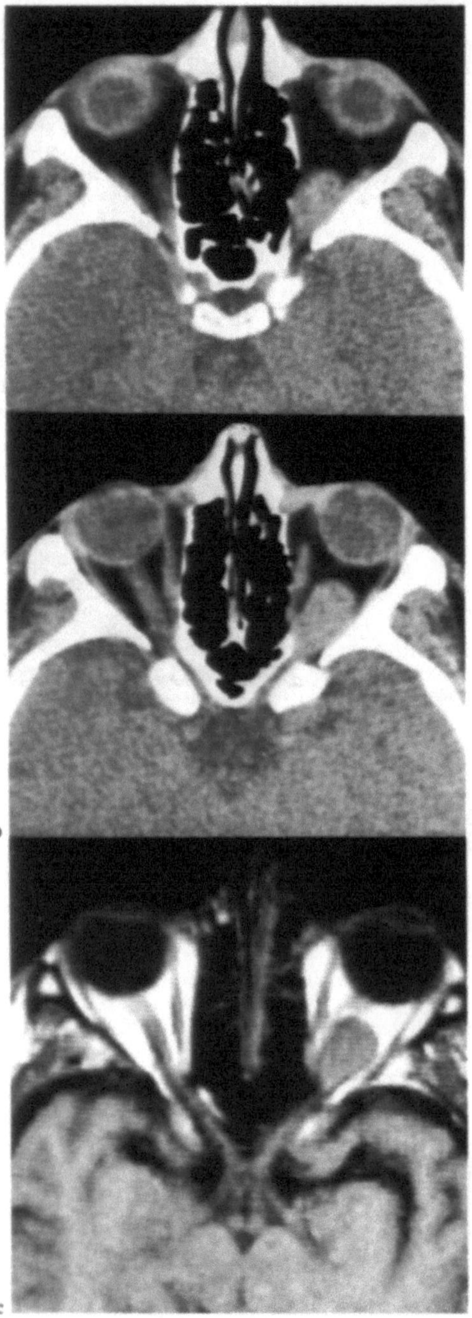

a

b

c

Fig. G6a–c. Cavernous hemangioma in a 39-year-old man with a 1-year history of visual disturbances. CT (**a, b**) shows a large, hyperdense tumor in the right orbital cone. MR: **c** SE 400/30. The smoothly delineated tumor stands out clearly in the orbital fat, and optic nerve displacement is apparent. The optic chiasm is optimally defined on the MR image

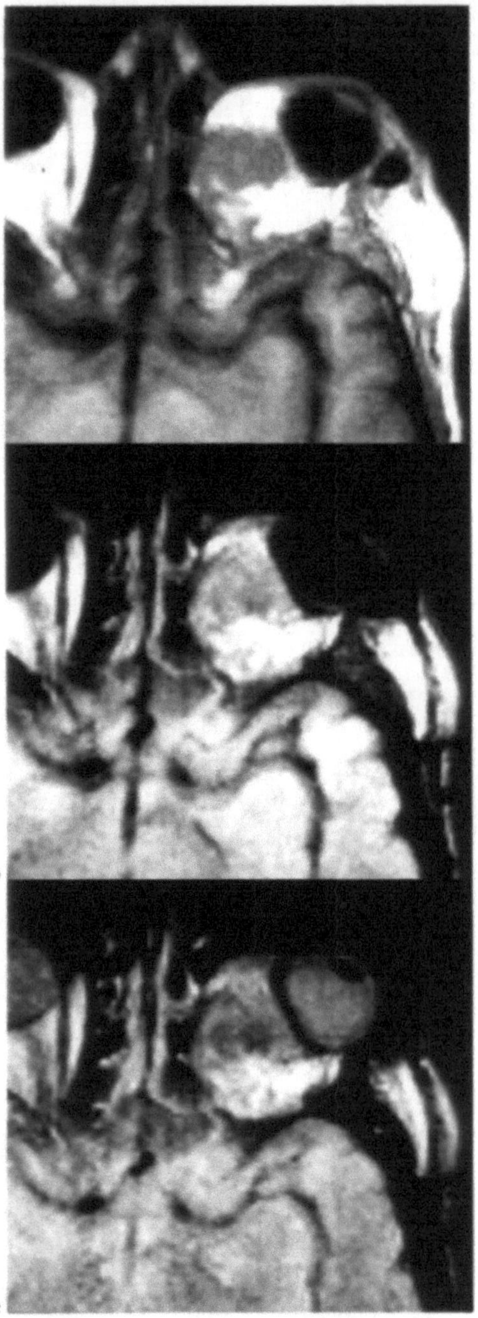

a

b

c

Fig. G7a–c. Endotheliomatous meningioma in a 59-year-old man with a 10-year history of increasing proptosis, amaurosis, and severe limitation of ocular motility on the right side. MR: **a** SE 400/30, **b** SE 1600/35, **c** SE 1600/70. Images reveal a large tumor causing extreme lateral displacement of the right globe with destruction of the orbital wall. The tumor extends into the temporal muscle

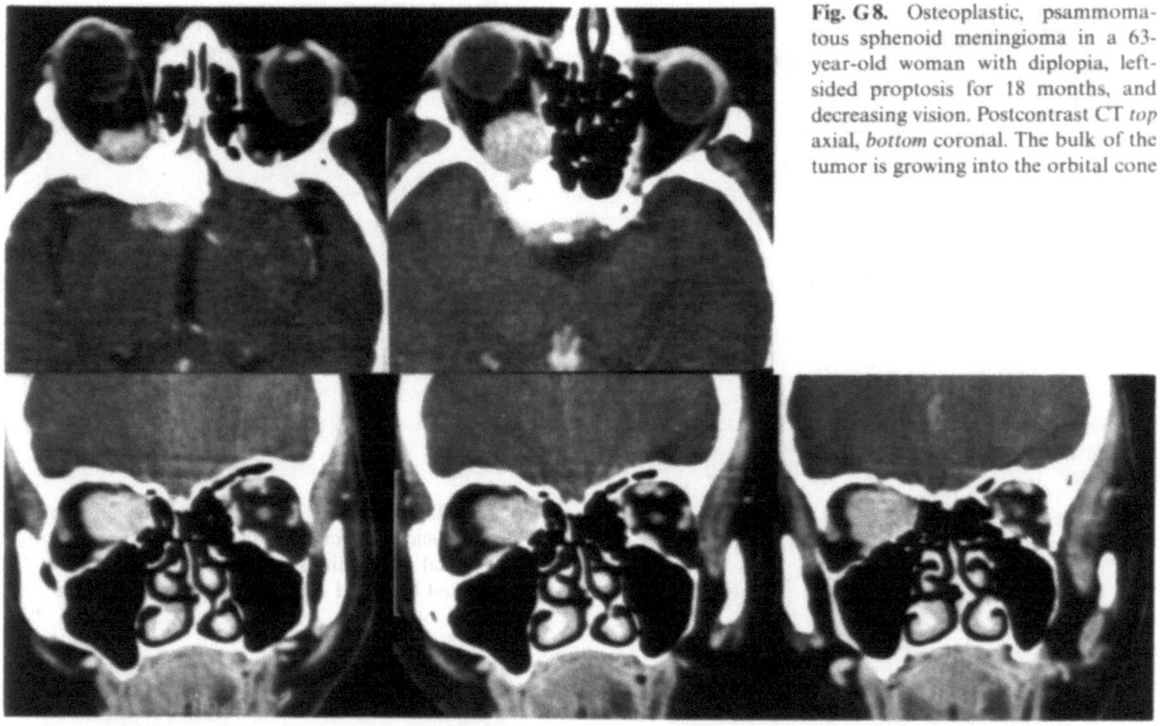

Fig. G8. Osteoplastic, psammomatous sphenoid meningioma in a 63-year-old woman with diplopia, left-sided proptosis for 18 months, and decreasing vision. Postcontrast CT *top* axial, *bottom* coronal. The bulk of the tumor is growing into the orbital cone

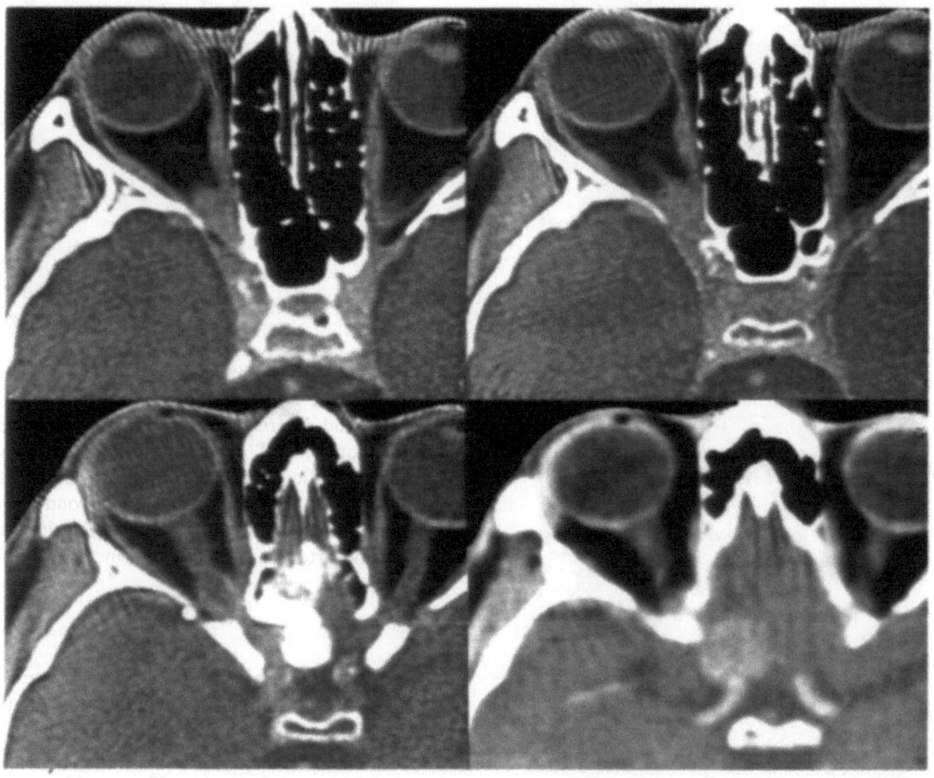

Fig. G9. Optic sheath meningioma of the left side in a 47-year-old woman with 6 months of blurred vision in the left eye and progressive visual acuity loss. Postcontrast CT shows distention of the left optic nerve by tumor, especially at the optic foramen. The tumor extends to the optic chiasm, showing marked enhancement in that region

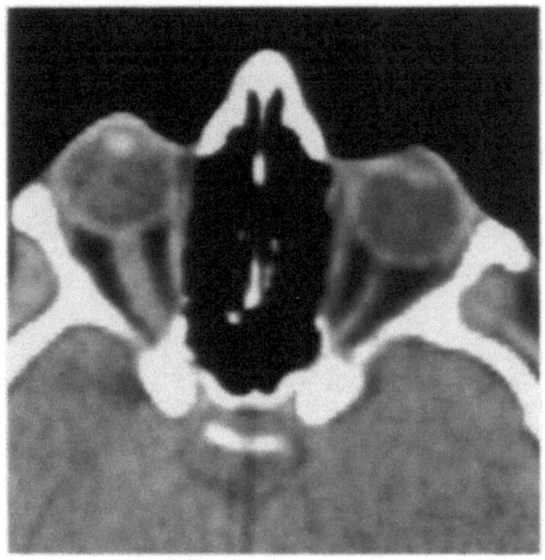

Fig. G11. Optic sheath meningioma of the left side in a 48-year-old woman with left-sided proptosis and visual disturbances. CT shows marked thickening and increased density of the left optic nerve

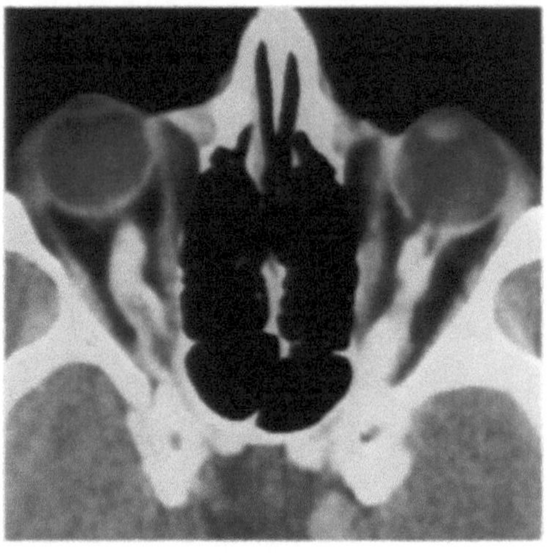

Fig. G12. Bilateral, calcified optic sheath meningioma in a 44-year-old man with right-sided amaurosis and severely decreased vision in the left eye. Postcontrast CT demonstrates bilateral expansion of the optic nerves, which show calcific attenuation values. The tumor extends beyond the orbital cone. Aneurysmatic dilatation of the right internal carotid artery is present as an incidental finding

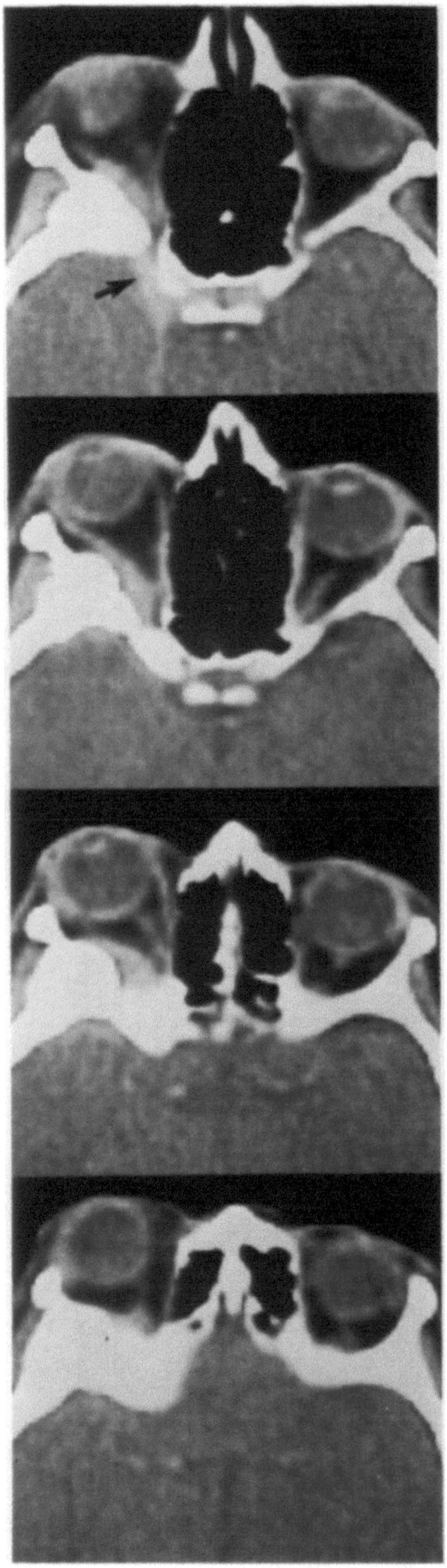

Fig. G10. Osteoplastic meningioma of the left sphenoid wing with soft-tissue components on the lateral orbital wall extending into the orbital cone and temporal fossa in a 48-year-old woman with left-sided proptosis. The tumor has invaded the cavernous sinus through the optic foramen (*arrow*). The bone is greatly expanded. Postcontrast CT

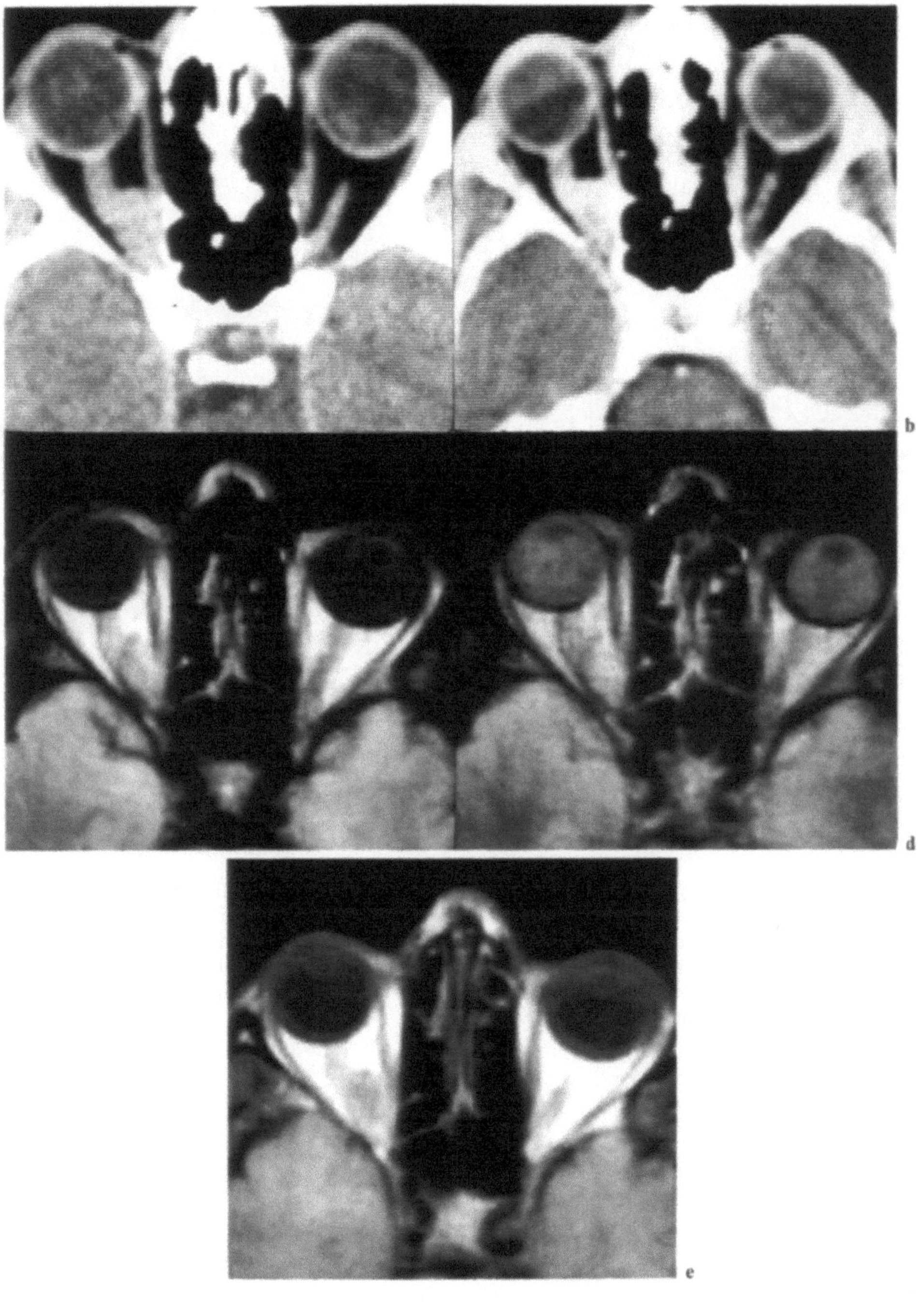

a b c d e

Fig. G13a–e. Optic sheath meningioma in a 48-year-old woman with a 4-year history of deteriorating vision in the left eye and temporal headache. Postcontrast CT (**a, b**) shows expansion of the left optic nerve with tumor filling the orbital cone. MR: **c** SE 1600/35, **d** SE 1600/70, **e** SE 400/30. The tumor margins are poorly defined in the orbital cone. The left globe is displaced anteriorly

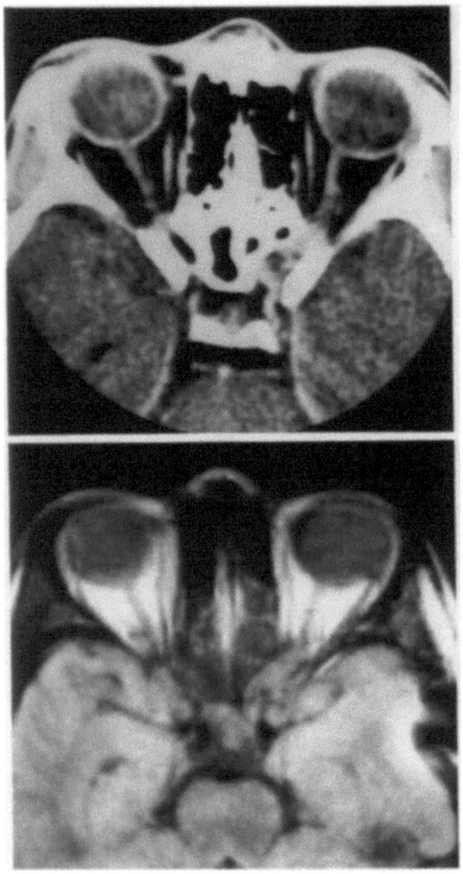

Fig. G14. Optic glioma in a 26-year-old woman with 6 years of slowly progressive visual deterioration in the right eye. CT: *top* postcontrast. MR: *bottom* SE 1600/35. CT and MR demonstrate expansion of the right optic nerve. There is intracranial extension of tumor through the foramen

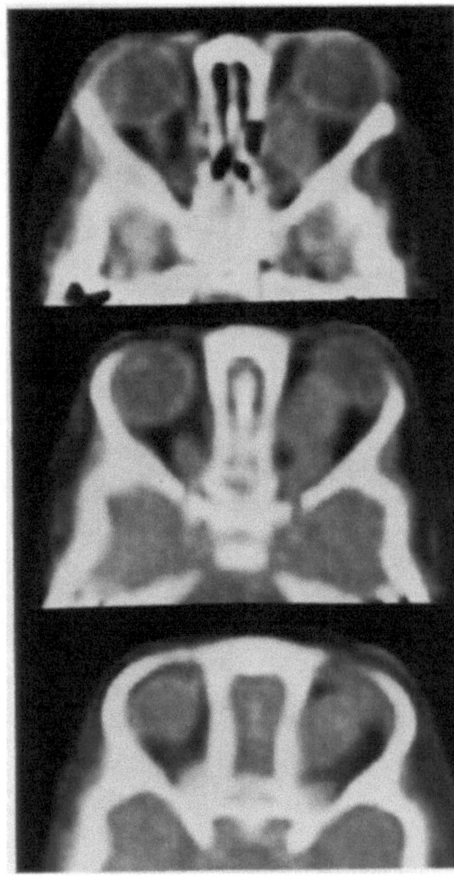

Fig. G15. Bilateral optic glioma in an 11-month-old child with neurofibromatosis. Scans show a markedly distended and tortuous right optic nerve. The tumor on the left side affects only the posterior portions of the optic nerve

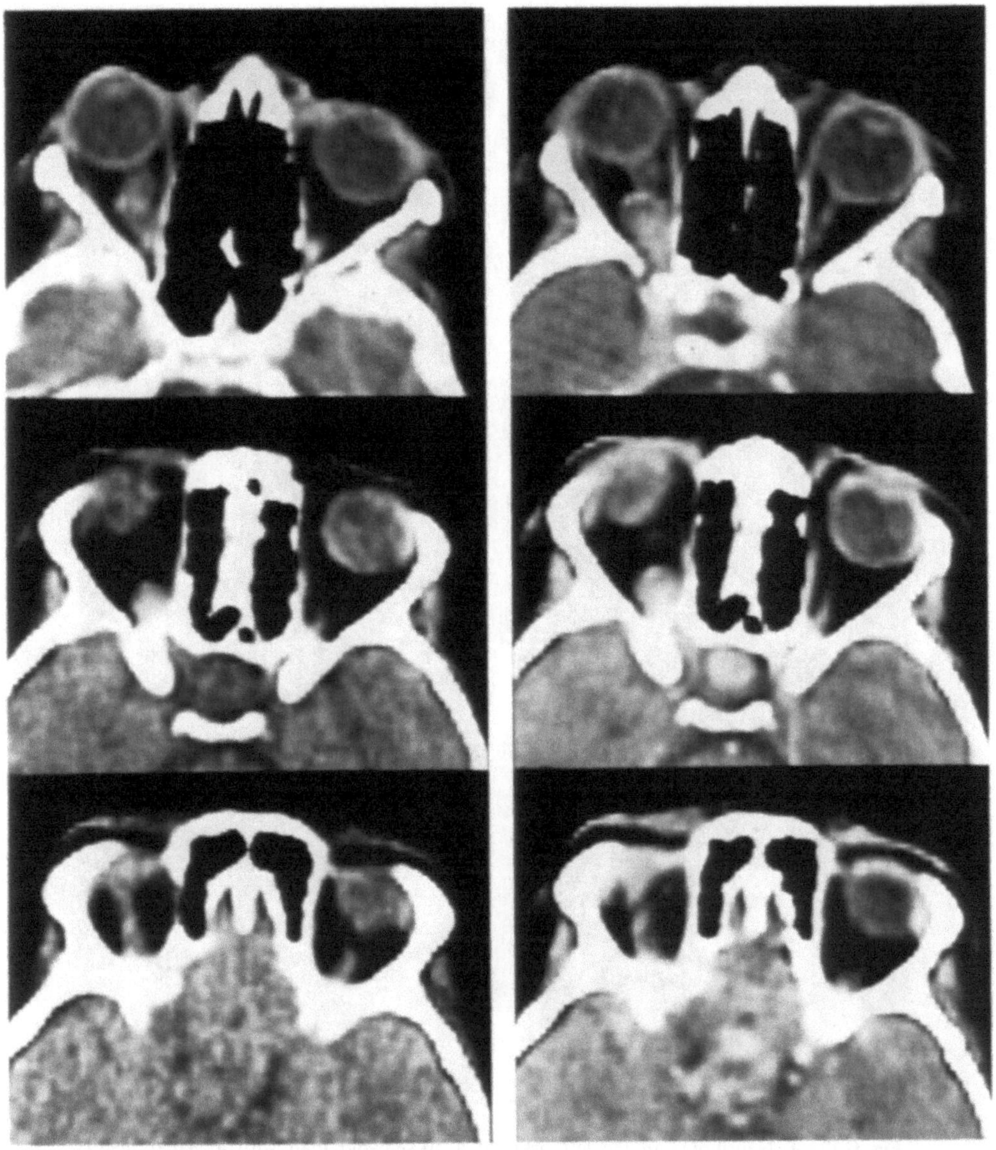

Fig. G16. Optic glioma with extension into the hypothalamus in an 18-year-old female. *Left* plain CT scans, *right* postcontrast scans. The left optic nerve is markedly expanded posteriorly. The intracranial extensions involving the optic chiasm and hypothalamus enhance markedly on the postinfusion scans

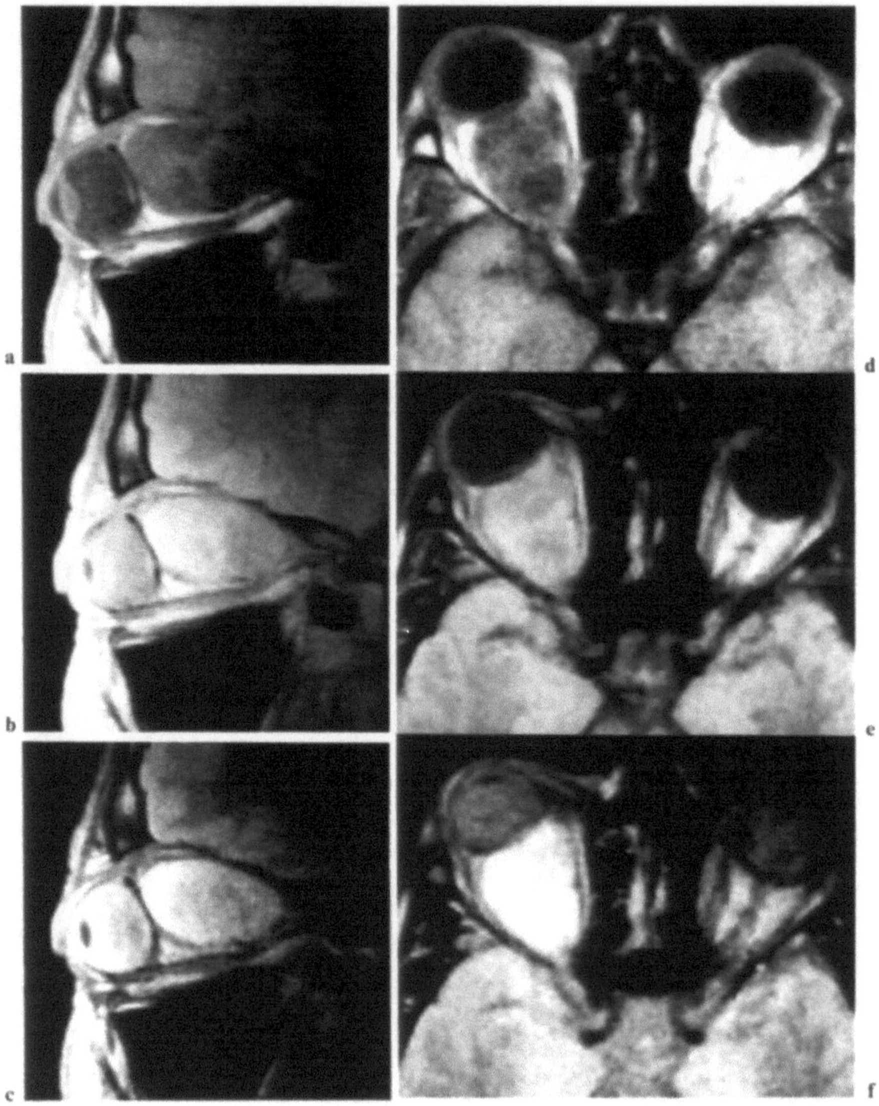

Fig. G17a–f. Neurinoma in the left orbit of a 50-year-old man with a 3-year history of left-sided proptosis and decreased ocular motility in all directions. He presented with significant visual acuity loss, chemosis, and papilledema; no visual field loss. MR: **a** SE 400/35, **b** SE 1600/35, **c** SE 1600/70 parasagittal, **d** SE 400/35, **e** SE 1600/35, **f** SE 1600/70 axial. Images reveal a large, smoothly delineated intraorbital tumor that fills almost the entire left orbit and is indenting the globe

Fig. G18a, b. Multiple neurofibromas in both orbits, more prominent on the left side, in a 34-year-old woman with von Recklinghausen's disease. There is severe bilateral proptosis, and the right orbit is almost completely filled with tumor masses. The right globe is displaced laterally downward (coronal scan, **b**). There is partial aplasia of the left sphenoid wing with disruption of the bony contour

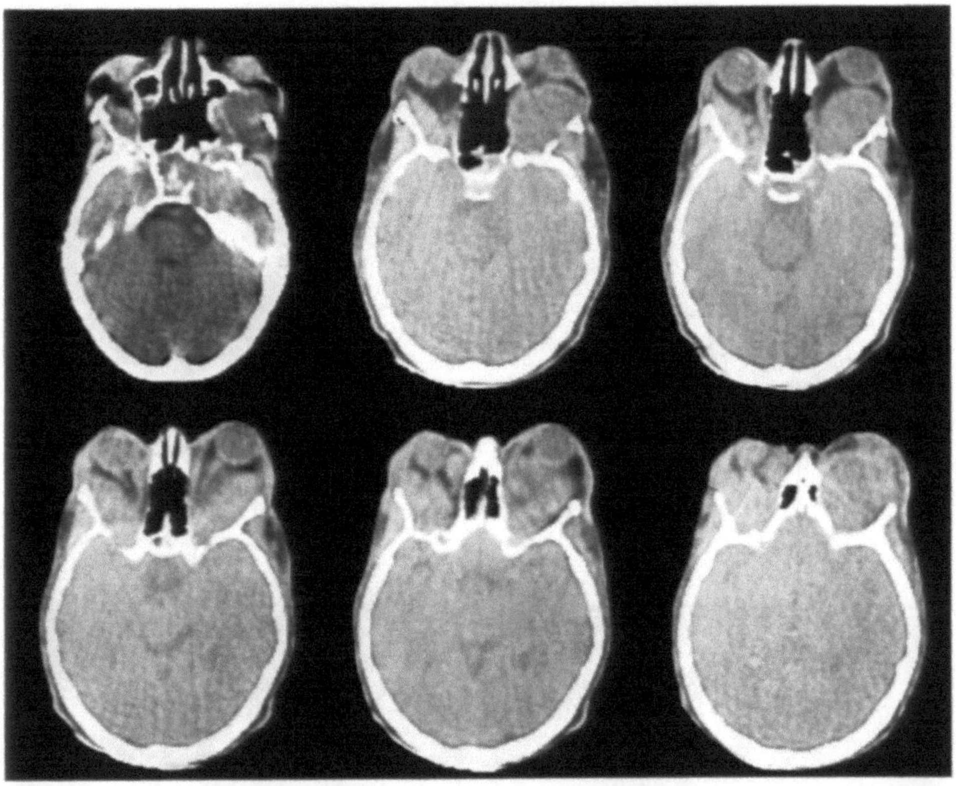

a

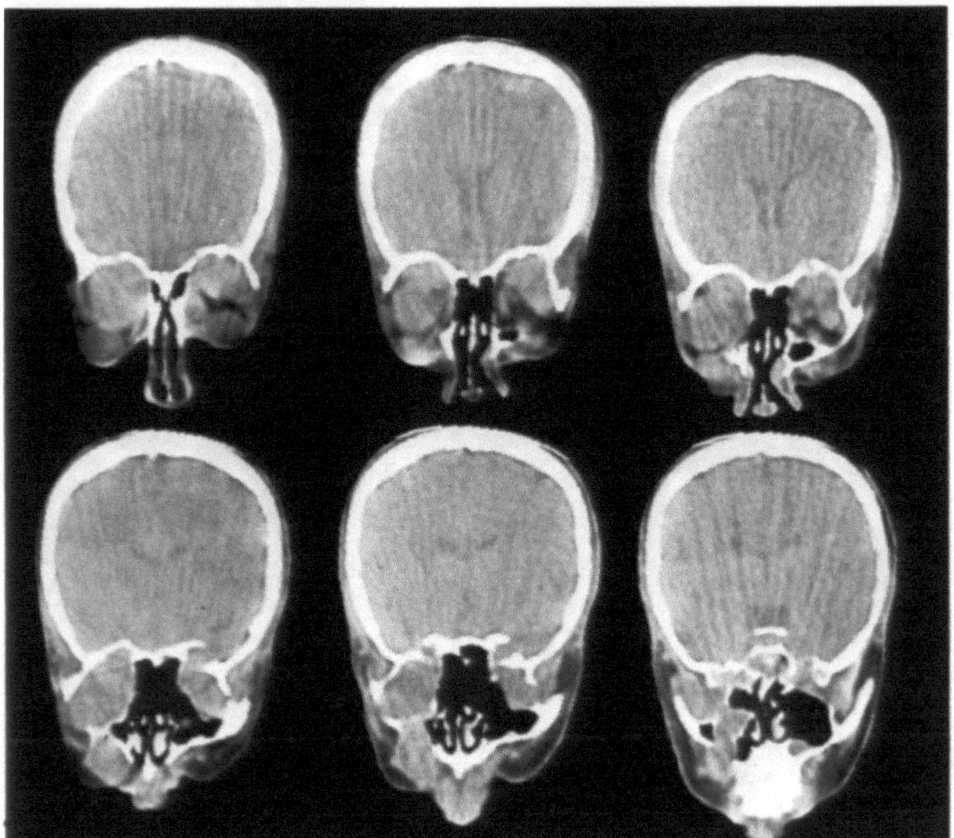

b

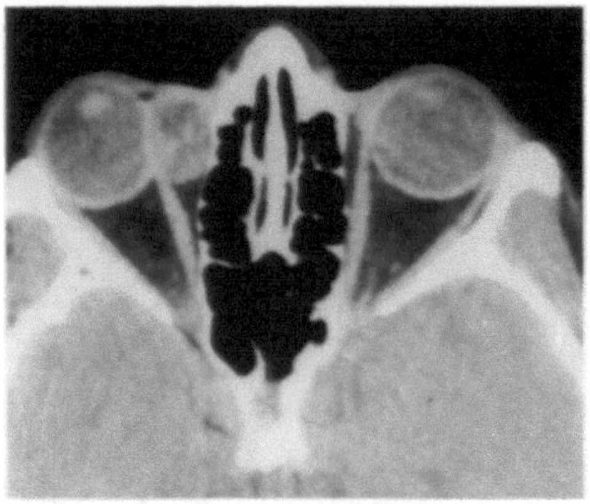

Fig. G19. Dermoid cyst in a 53-year-old woman with a "swelling" at the inner canthus of the left eye. CT demonstrates a smooth-bordered mass medial to the left globe

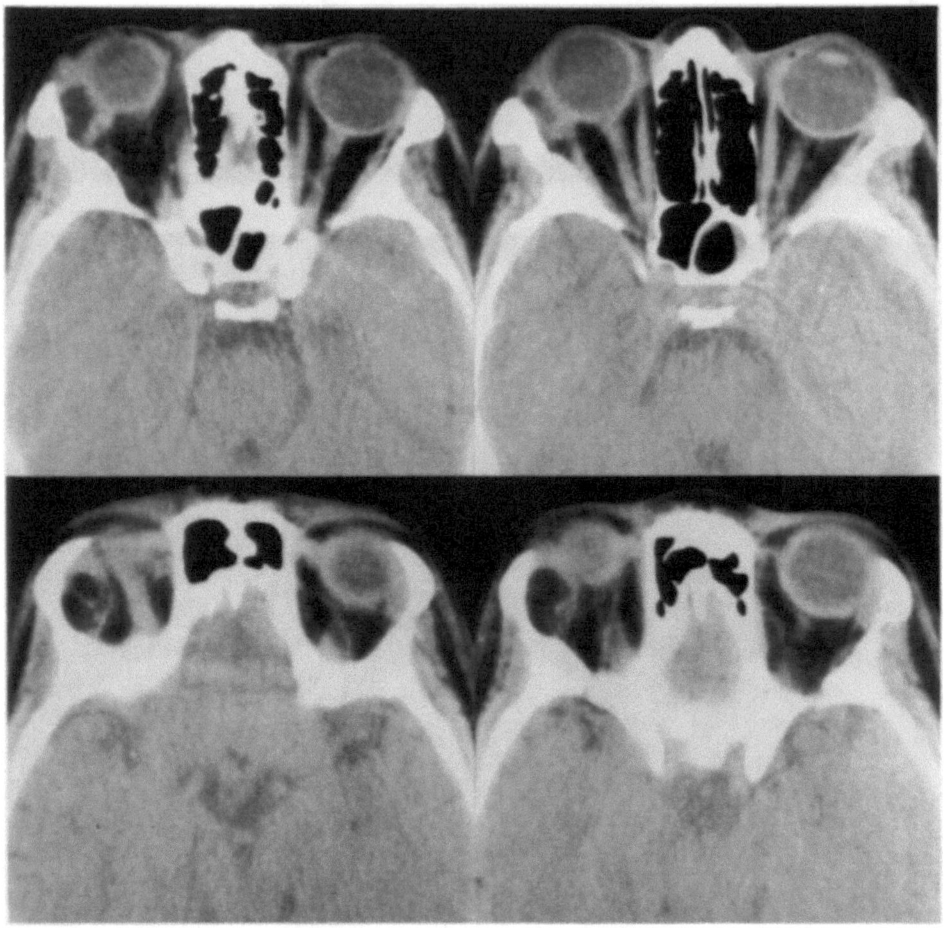

Fig. G20. Dermoid cyst in a 32-year-old woman with moderate proptosis of the left eye. CT reveals a smoothly delineated, mixed-density mass lateral to the left globe

2. Malignant Tumors

Malignant tumors such as carcinomas, sarcomas, malignant lymphomas, and tumors metastatic to primary malignancies can occur in the orbits and may cause destruction of orbital bone. A malignant growth presenting as a well-defined soft-tissue mass in the orbital region with no associated bone destruction is indistinguishable from a benign tumor (Gawler et al. 1974; Lampert et al. 1974; Momose et al. 1975).

Tumors of the Lacrimal Glands
(Figs. G21, 23, 24)

These tumors may be benign or malignant. Between 50% and 60% are pleomorphic adenomas, 5%–10% are carcinomas in pleomorphic adenomas, and 20%–30% are adenoid cystic carcinomas. Other carcinomas account for 5%–10%. Pleomorphic adenomas have cystic components and so are difficult to distinguish from the benign epithelial cysts that can occur in the lacrimal gland.

The benign forms are slow-growing, and most have smooth margins. Both benign and malignant tumors may contain calcifications. Ultimately the differential diagnosis must rely on histologic examination.

CT demonstrates a mass in the upper temporal portion of the orbit, adjacent to or behind the globe, resembling the appearance of a carcinoma or metastasis. The tumor enhances with intravenous contrast medium. Benign tumors are often well-defined, whereas malignancies tend to have ill-defined margins (Peyster and Hoover 1984; Mancuso and Hanafee 1985).

MR shows a lesion of relatively low signal intensity, like muscle, that is readily distinguishable from fat. Pleomorphic adenomas display a nonhomogeneous signal pattern on T2-weighted sequences.

Carcinomas and Metastases
(Figs. G21–23, 25, 27–29, 31, 40)

Primary orbital carcinomas originate from the lacrimal gland or eyelid. Secondary carcinomas invade the orbit from neighboring tissues.

Adenoid Cystic Carcinomas
Histologically these tumors (formerly called cylindromas) are composed of cylindrical cavities lined with columnar epithelium and filled with mucus. Growth is rapid, and extension to the intra- and extracranial space is very common. Primary orbital growths may arise from the lacrimal gland, but more commonly the orbit is involved secondarily by extension from the paranasal sinuses.

Metastases
Comprising 2%–9% of orbital tumors (Jacobs et al. 1980), metastases can arise from carcinoma of the lung, uterus, gastrointestinal tract (common), kidney (rare), thyroid, prostate, pancreas, or breast.

The major sources of orbital metastases are breast carcinoma in women and lung carcinoma in men. In children, metastases are most commonly from neuroblastoma, Ewing's sarcoma, and Wilms' tumor.

The **CT** features of carcinoma and metastases are variable. The lesions show considerable variation in density and extent. Some have well-defined margins, while others are poorly demarcated from their surroundings. Evidence of bone destruction helps in forming a diagnosis. Most of the tumors enhance with contrast medium, and this serves to delineate them more sharply. Enophthalmos may occur with tumors metastatic to scirrhous breast carcinoma. This is associated with atrophy of the ocular muscles and shrinkage of the orbital fat with retraction of the globe (Peyster and Hoover 1984).

The **MR** signal of these tumors has a relatively low intensity that is easily distinguished from orbital fat. Sites of tumor-related bone destruction are not visualized with MR.

Malignant Lymphomas (Figs. G33–37)

Malignant lymphomas constitute 7%–14% of all orbital tumors. Most are autochthonous, and a few are metastatic. They occur in all portions of the orbit, but the majority are extraconal. The growth may envelop the optic nerve or lie behind the globe. Concomitant ocular and orbital involvement has been described (Grimson et al. 1982).

Malignant lymphomas may be a manifestation of systemic disease, or they may arise in the orbit primarily with no lymphomatous disease elsewhere (Robertson et al. 1986).

The tumors grow by infiltration. Immunocytic lymphoma is the most common histologic type.

CT demonstrates a more or less clearly circumscribed soft-tissue mass of relatively high density (35–40 HU) that shows marked contrast enhancement. The tumor is often contiguous to the globe. The extraocular muscles and optic nerve may be enveloped by tumor to the extent that their boundaries are poorly defined. Pseudotumor and metastases can present a similar CT appearance. Bone destruction is unusual (Peyster and Hoover 1984). Circumscribed forms tend to affect the lacrimal gland, while diffuse forms affect the muscle cone (Mancuso and Hanafee 1985).

On **MR** the hypointense lymphoma is readily distinguishable from orbital fat.

Ocular Melanomas with Orbital Invasion (Figs. G38, 39)

From 1% to 4% of all orbital tumors are malignant melanomas of the choroid. They occur in all age groups but are most common in the sixth and seventh decades. These heavily vascularized growths arise from the melanoblasts of the choroid and invade the orbit along scleral neurovascular channels.

CT should be performed whenever it is suspected that a melanoma has invaded the posterior orbit from the globe. The tumor appears hyperdense on plain scans and enhances after contrast injection. The enhancement is most intense 20–30 s post injection and then declines (serial CT, 6 scans/min) (Heller et al. 1982).

On **MR**, T2-weighted sequences demonstrate the melanoma as an area of low signal in the hyperintense vitreous. The reverse is true on T1-weighted images, which clearly differentiate the high signal of the melanoma from the hypointense vitreous. This pattern is characteristic of melanotic melanomas but not of amelanotic forms.

Sarcomas (Figs. G30, 32)

These tumors consist of fibrosarcomas and rhabdomyosarcomas, the latter being the most common tumor of childhood. Sarcomas grow rapidly and invade surrounding structures. Clinical signs include proptosis and palpebral edema.

The **CT** and **MR** features are similar to those of carcinomas and metastases. There may be bone destruction, or the tumor may be nodular and well demarcated. The tumor appears solid on CT and enhances homogeneously with contrast medium (Peyster and Hoover 1984).

Retinoblastomas

These congenital, possibly hereditary malignant tumors of the retina have a prevalence of 1:17000 to 1:34000. They may infiltrate the brain along the optic nerve, and may metastasize to liver and bone by the hematogenous route. Calcifications are present in some 95% of cases. CT reveals a mass lesion of high density (Peyster and Hoover 1984; Lindahl 1986).

Neuroblastomas (Fig. G26)

These tumors occur in early childhood and are uncommon thereafter. Their natural history is one of rapid growth and metastasis.

CT and **MR** display retinoblastomas and neuroblastomas as large tumors that are indistinguishable from other malignancies. Both modalities demonstrate the tumor well, but calcifications in the tumor are not visualized with MR.

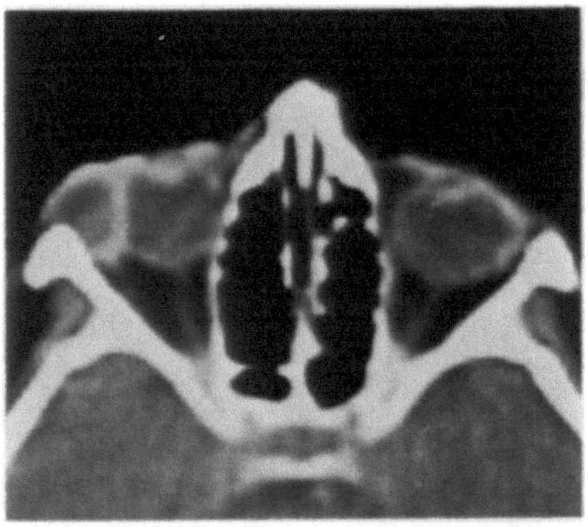

Fig. G21. Carcinoma of the left lacrimal gland in a 76-year-old man. Postcontrast CT reveals a smoothly delineated tumor in the anterolateral portion of the left orbit with peripheral enhancement

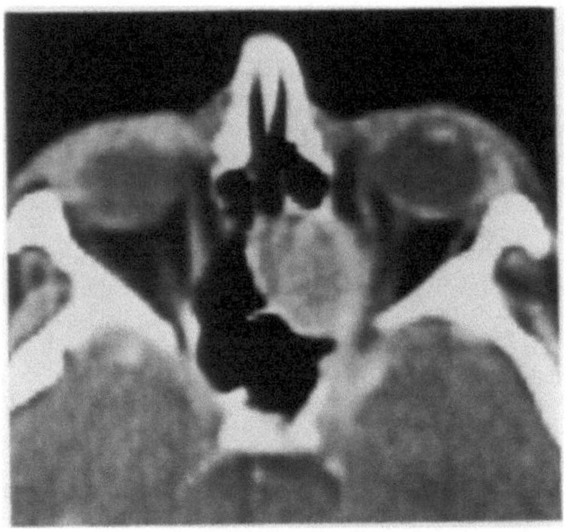

Fig. G22. Ethmoid carcinoma with invasion of the right orbit in a 38-year-old man. The tumor appears smoothly delineated and enhances with contrast medium. It is not clearly distinguishable from a mucocele or pyocele on the CT scan

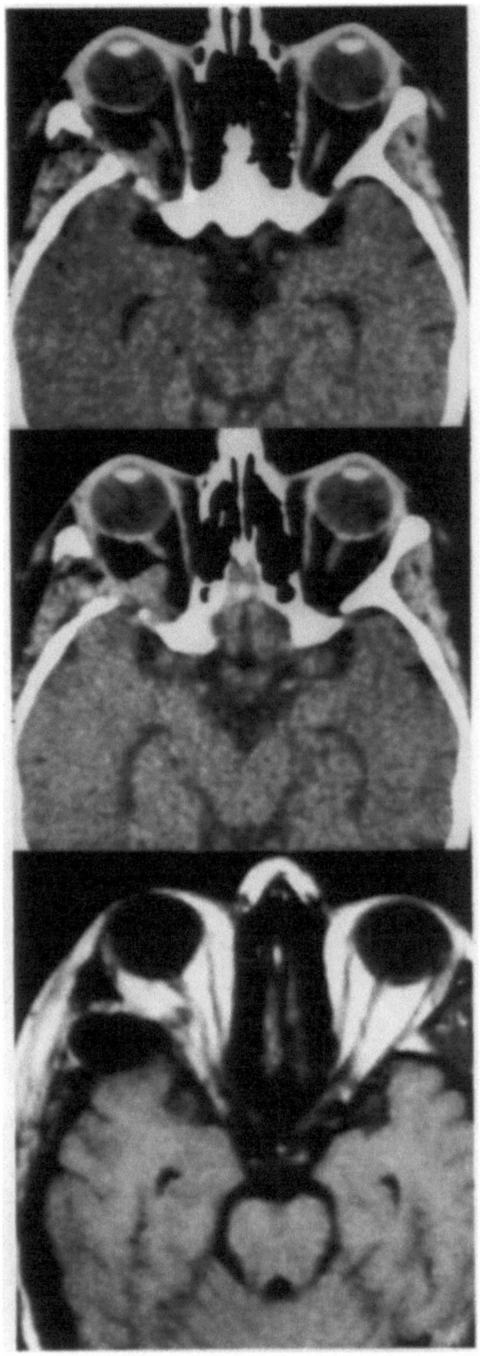

Fig. G23. Adenoid cystic carcinoma of the left lacrimal gland in a 44-year-old woman with twinging pains at the lateral canthus of the left eye for 2 years and left-sided proptosis. CT: *top* precontrast, *center* postcontrast. MR: *bottom* SE 400/30. CT shows destructive bone change in the left sphenoid. Contrast shows a moderately enhancing tumor in the posterior part of the left orbit displacing the optic nerve and infiltrating the lateral rectus muscle. T1-weighted MR demonstrates the solid tumor component, whose low signal contrasts sharply with the hyperintense fat

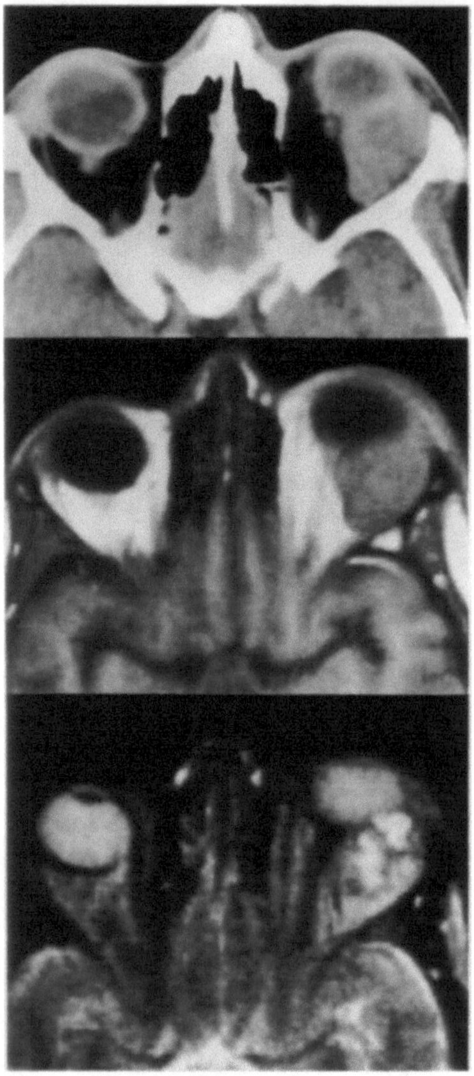

a

b

c

Fig. G24. Pleomorphic adenoma in the right orbit of a 28-year-old man with slowly progressive right-sided proptosis. CT: *top* noncontrast. MR: *center* SE 400/30, *bottom* SE 1600/180. CT shows a mass of soft-tissue attenuation in the right orbit (**a**), which has a similar appearance on the T1-weighted image (**b**). The T2-weighted image shows a mixed signal pattern with hyperintense cystic components and less intense solid components (**c**)

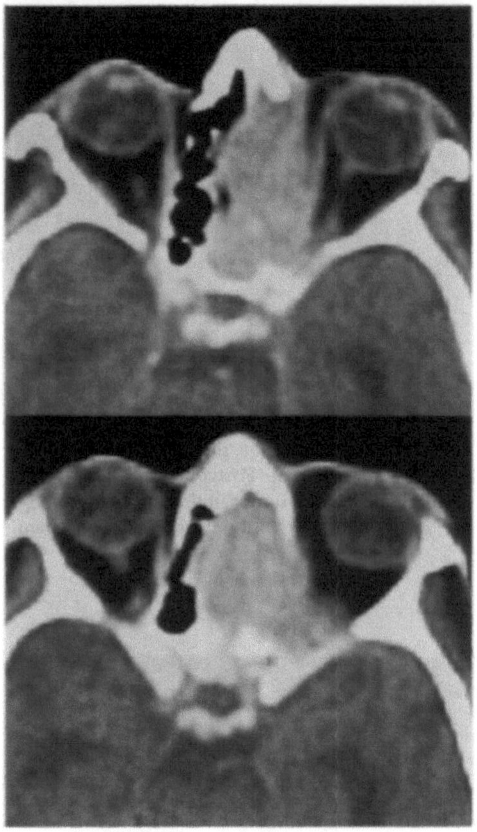

Fig. G25. Inverted papilloma with carcinoid elements involving the right ethmoid cells, the nasal cavity, and the right maxillary sinus with invasion of the right orbit, whose medial bony wall is destroyed. Postcontrast CT

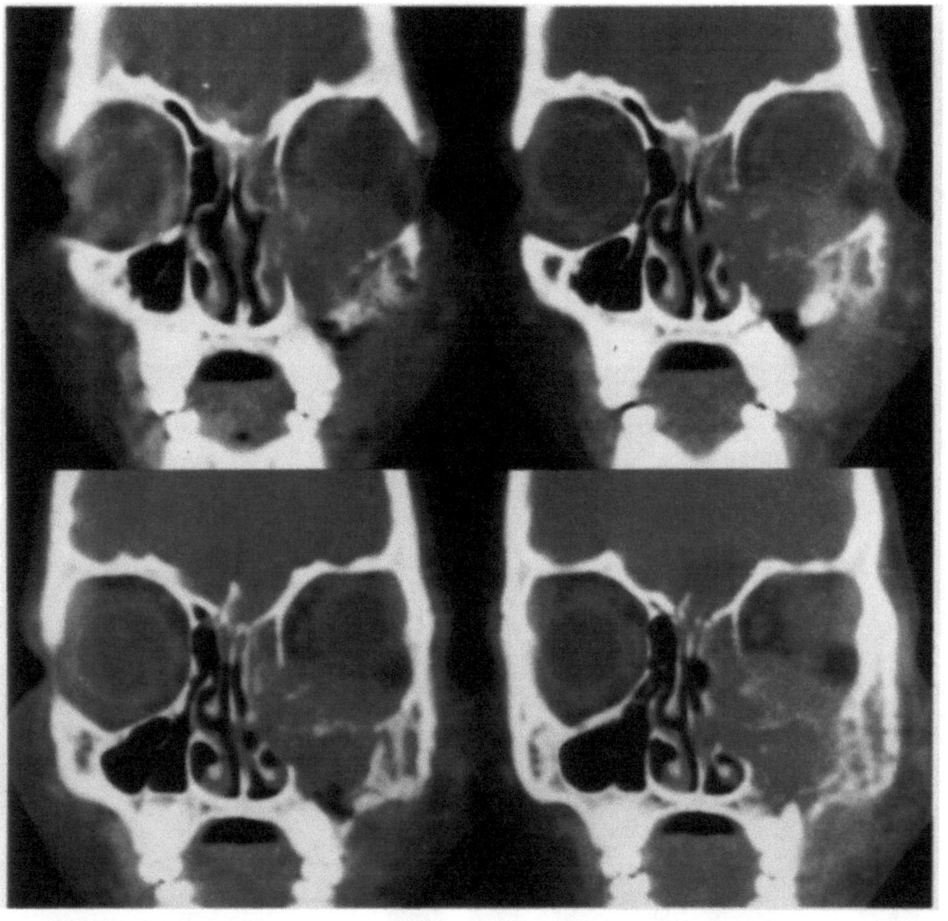

Fig. G26. Neuroblastoma in an 8-year-old girl with decreased vision in the right eye for 3 months and marked swelling in the right half of the face. Coronal CT scans reveal an osteolytic lesion widely infiltrating the right maxillary bone. There is orbital invasion with involvement of the inferior rectus muscle, anterior sclera, and right ethmoid cells. Structures of calcific density are present in the affected area

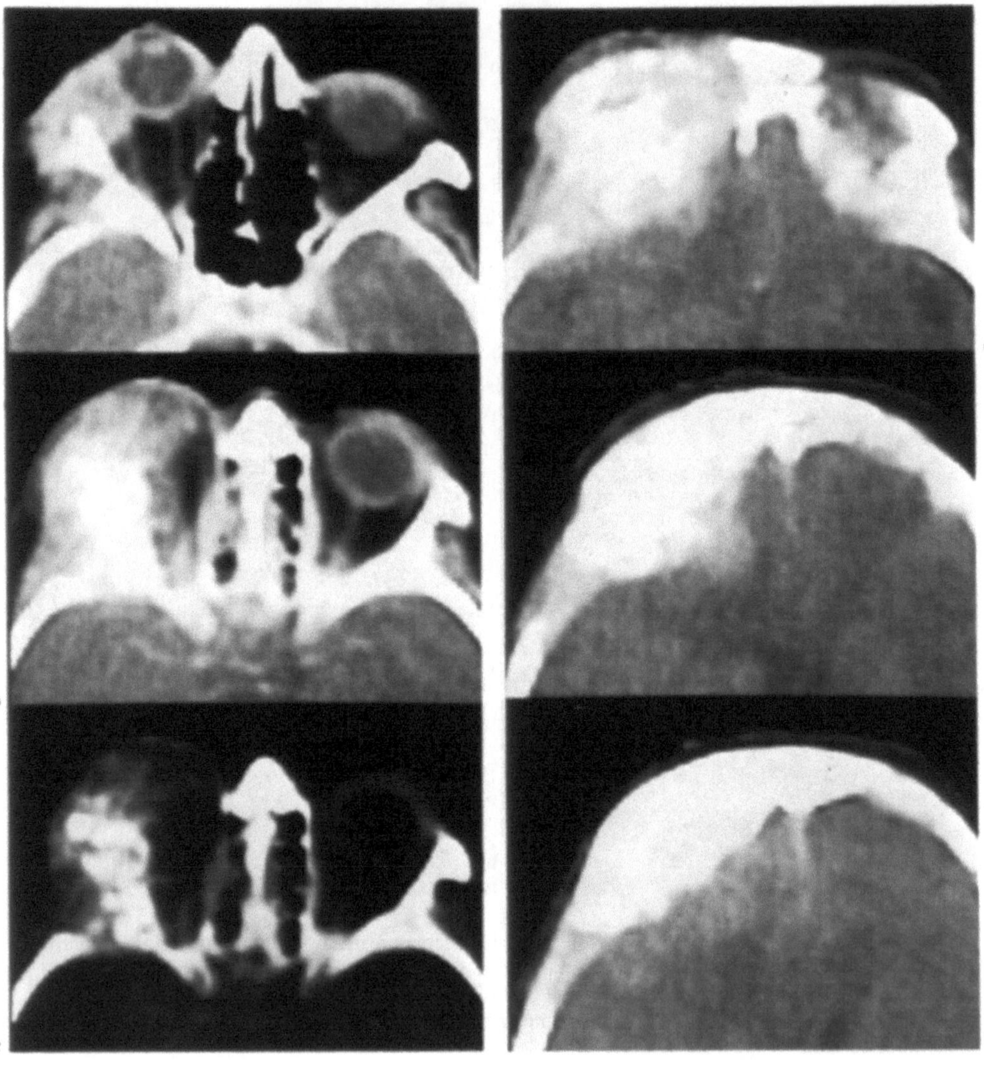

a b c d e f

Fig. G 27 a–f. Tumor of the left orbit and adjacent cranium, metastatic from breast carcinoma, in a 60-year-old woman. Scans indicate osteoplastic and osteoclastic bone changes with soft-tissue masses in the anterior part of the left orbit. The osteoplastic changes are seen most clearly on sections **c** to **f**. There is intracranial extension with midline displacement and compression of the left frontal horn (**e**)

Fig. G 28 a–h. Metastasis of an unknown primary carcinoma in the right orbit of a 50-year-old man. The tumor has displaced the intact lamina papyracea mediad. The lesion is well delineated and shows faint peripheral contrast enhancement. The globe is displaced downward and laterally. The coronal scan (**h**) shows marked destruction of the orbital roof

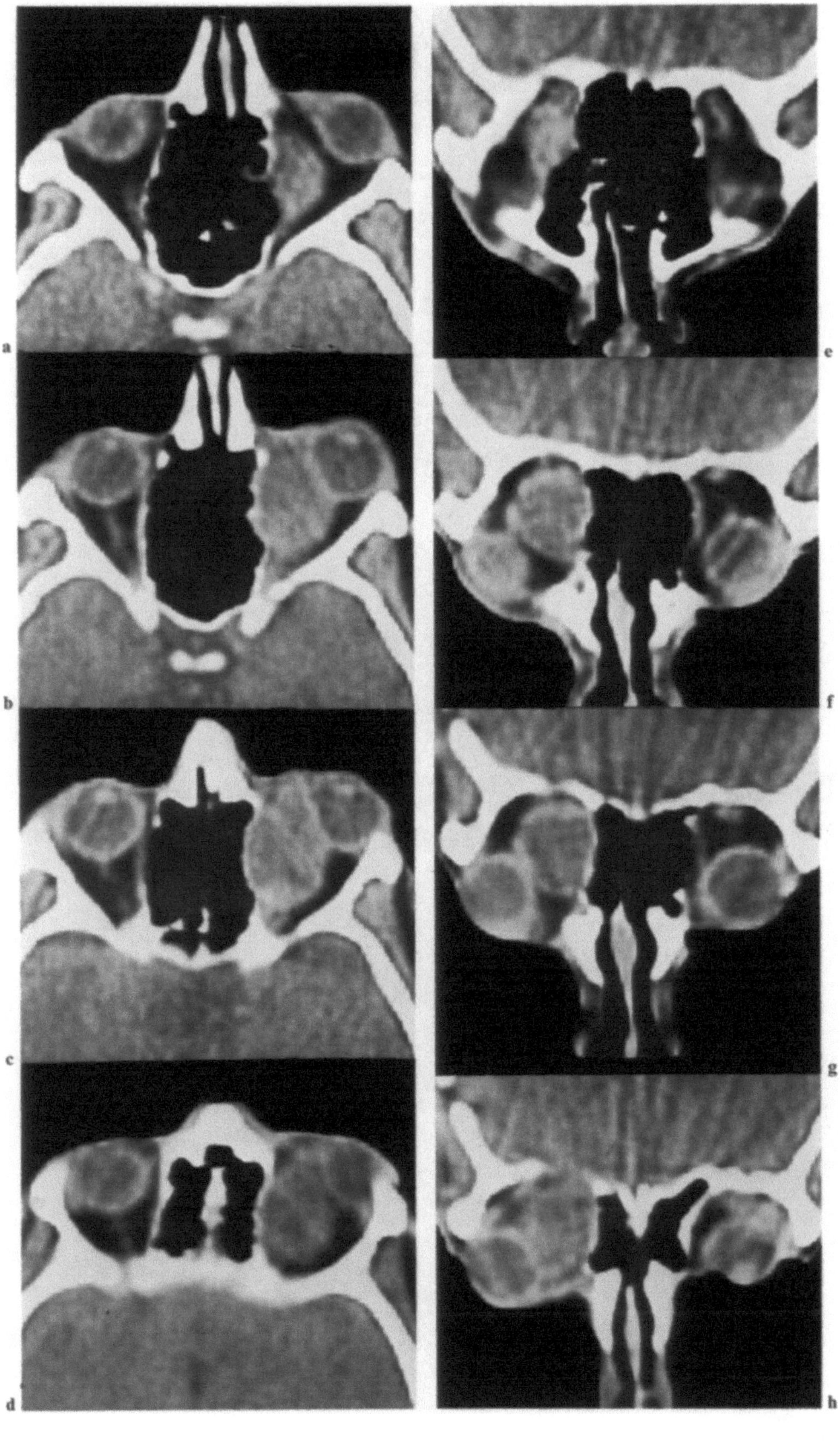
a
b
c
d
e
f
g
h

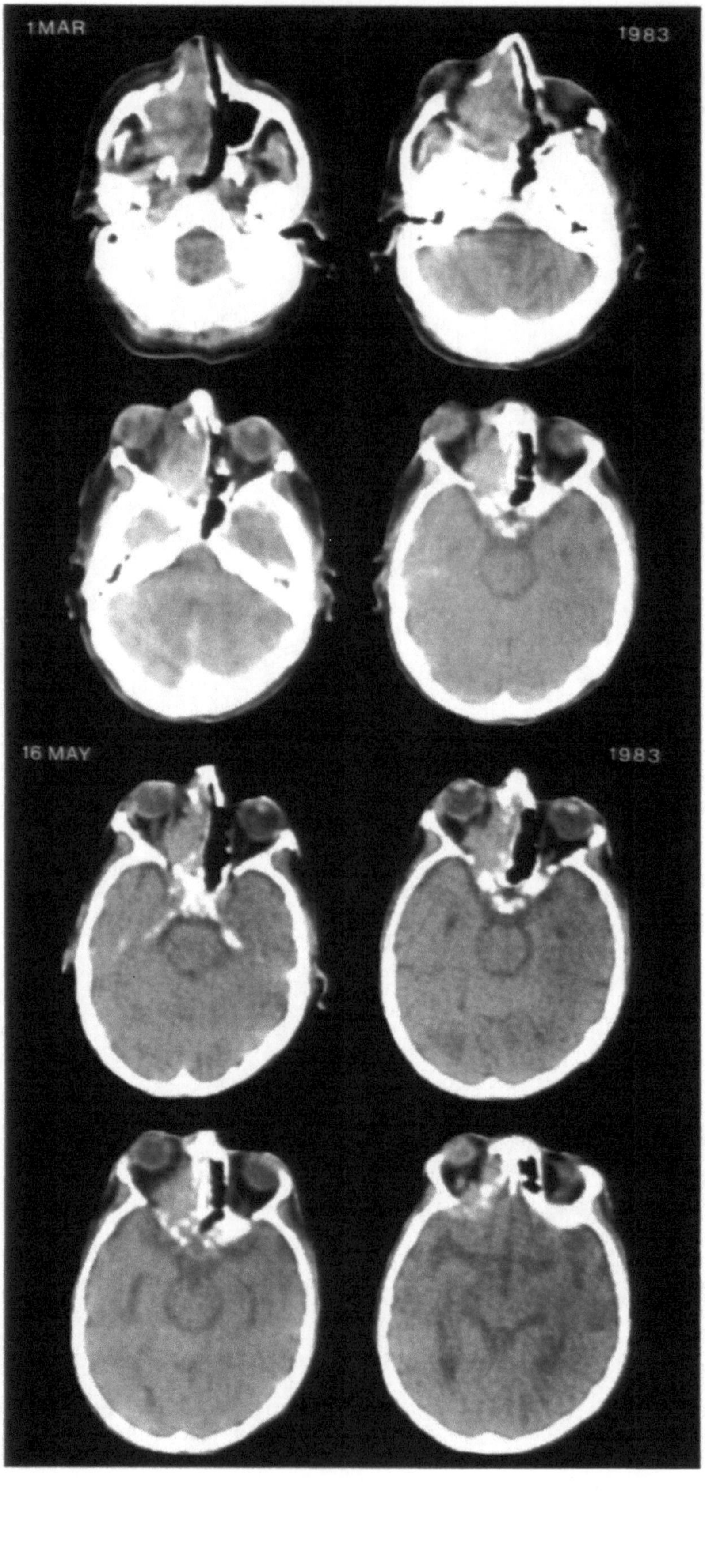

G 29

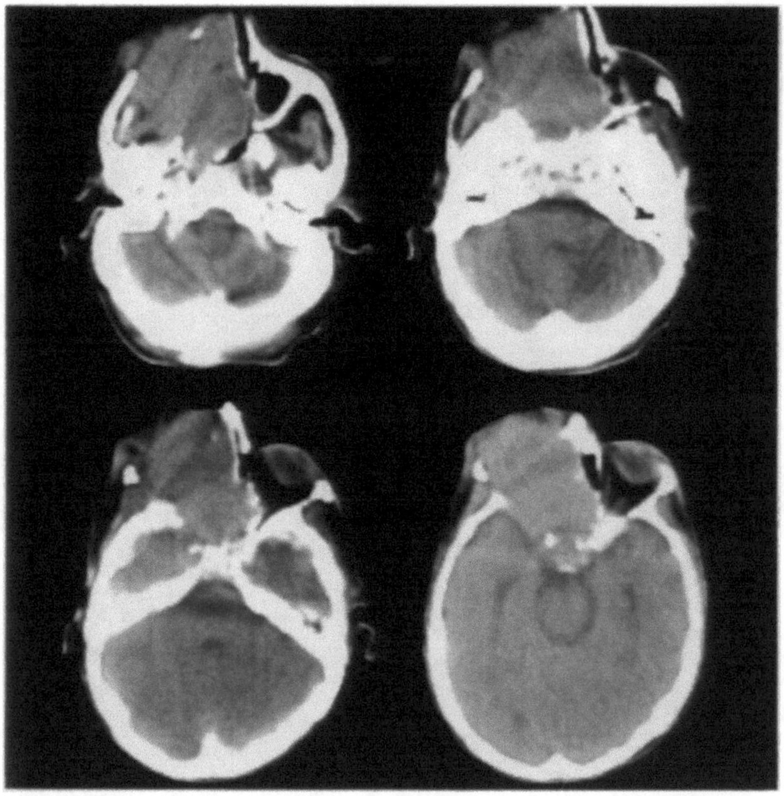

Fig. G29. Paranasal sinus carcinoma in a 75-year-old man with swelling and pain in the left half of the face. Patient underwent initial CT examination in March 1983, a second examination $2^1/_2$ months later, and a third after a further 8 months. The original examination disclosed a large mass lesion with bone destruction in the left maxillary sinus and left ethmoid cells, and extension into the retromaxillary space. Reexamination after chemotherapy showed regression of disease. The third examination disclosed extensive new tumor growth despite resumption of cytostatic therapy. The tumor now extends into the cranial cavity, and there is extensive bone destruction

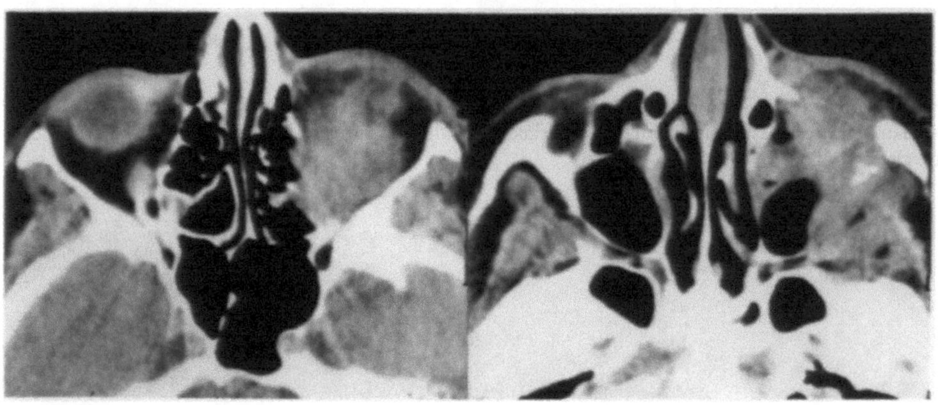

Fig. G30. Fibrosarcoma in a 48-year-old woman with pain and swelling in the right half of the face. CT reveals a large tumor in the right maxillary sinus with destructive changes in all bony walls. There is invasion of the right orbit and ethmoid cells with incipient breakthrough into the retromaxillary space

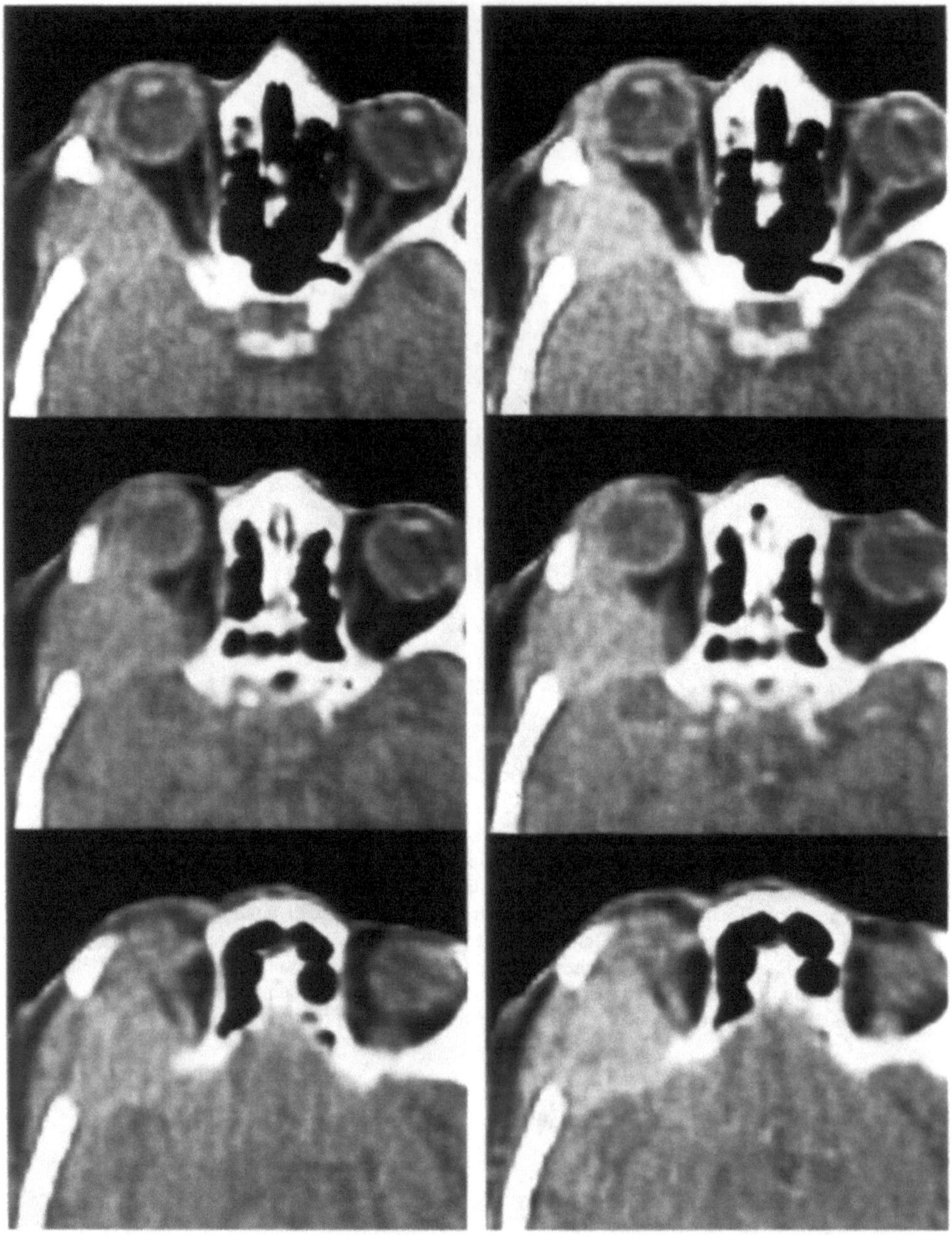

Fig. G31. Metastasis with extensive destruction of the left greater sphenoid wing in a 71-year-old woman. The soft-tissue mass enhances markedly on the postinfusion scans (*right*), and its borders are clearly defined

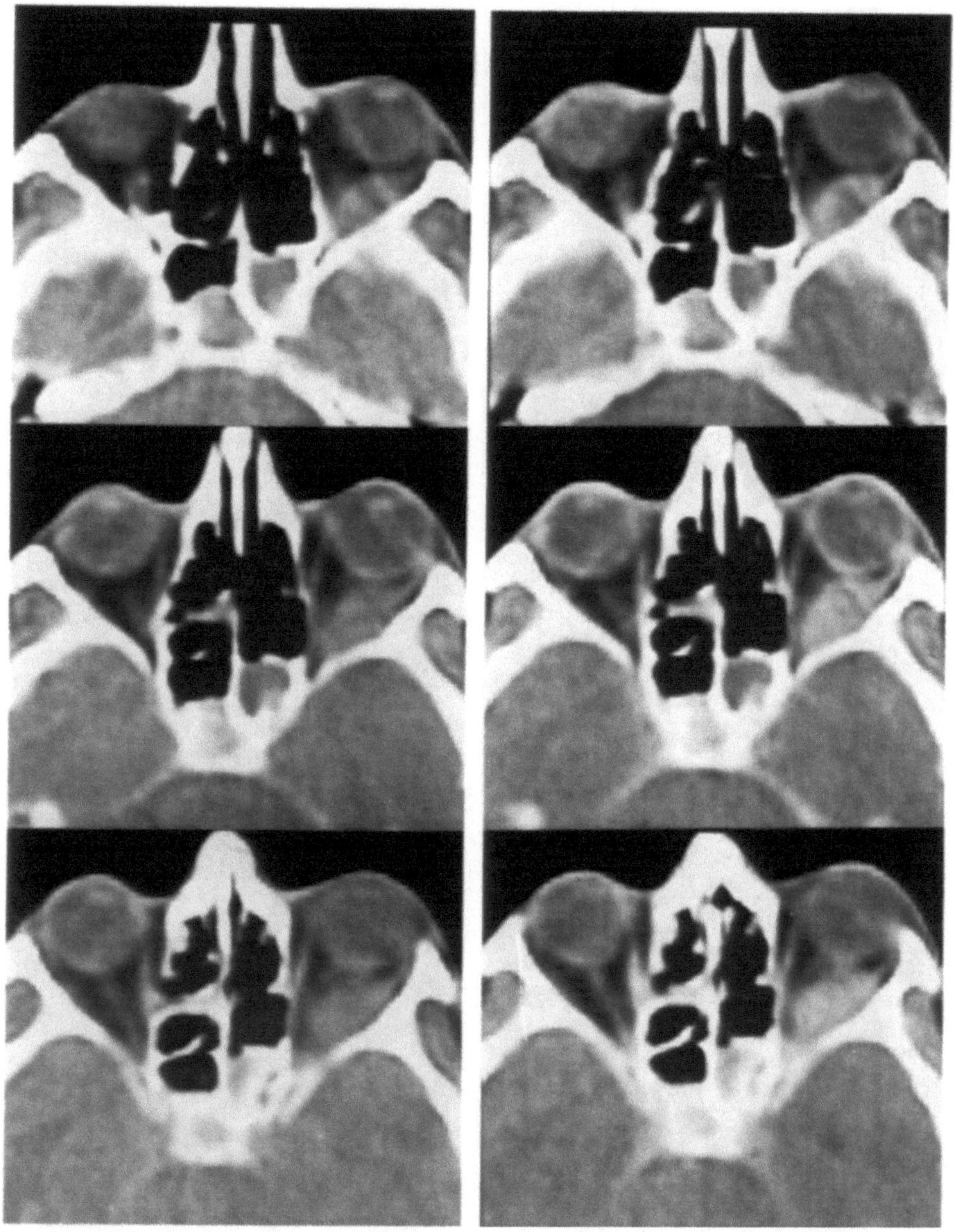

Fig. G32. Rhabdomyosarcoma in the right orbit of a 60-year-old man with right-sided proptosis. The lateral rectus muscle cannot be delineated from the tumor. CT findings aroused suspicion that the tumor was attached to the lateral rectus. The tumor tissue enhances intensely with contrast medium (*left* precontrast, *right* postcontrast)

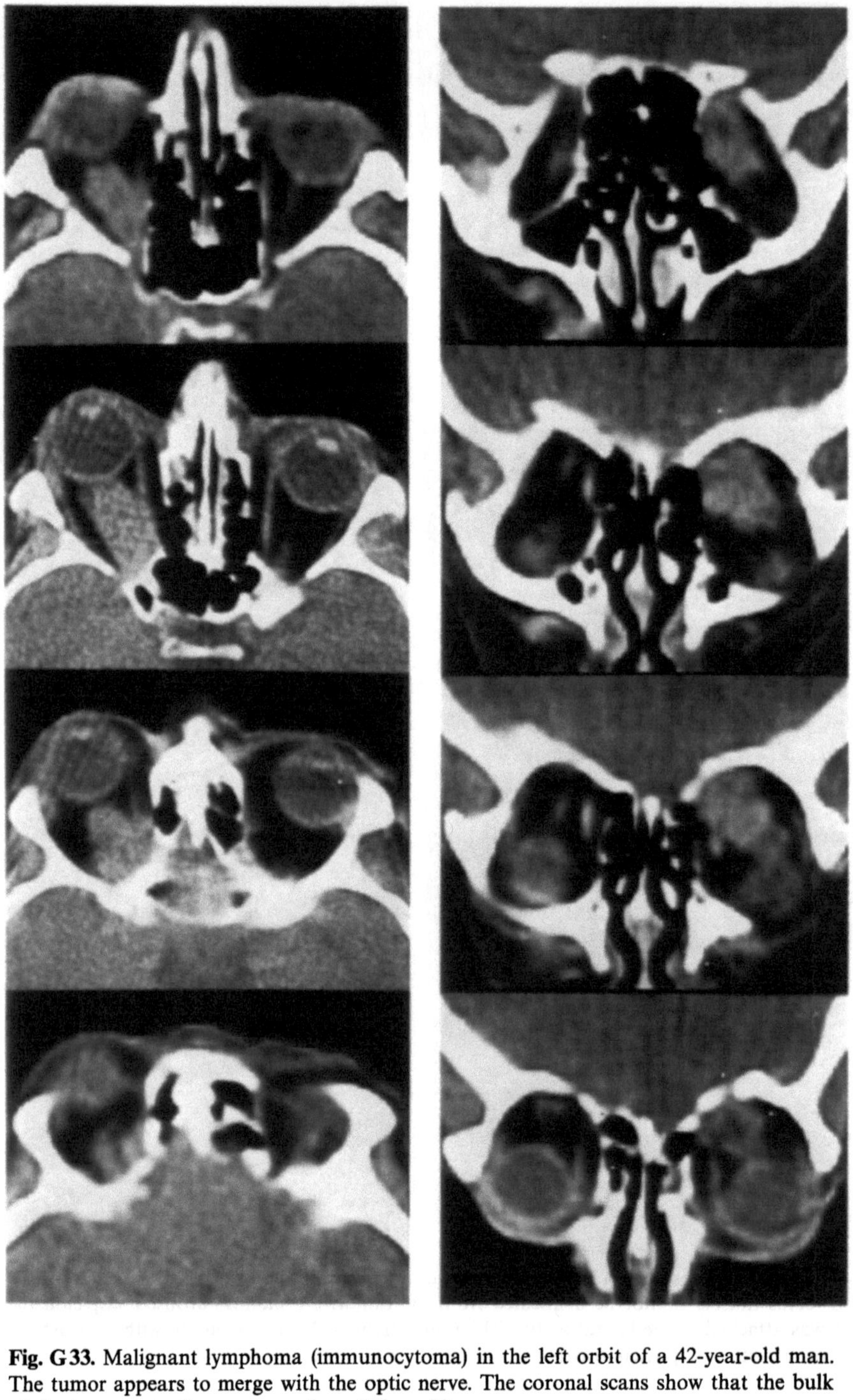

Fig. G33. Malignant lymphoma (immunocytoma) in the left orbit of a 42-year-old man. The tumor appears to merge with the optic nerve. The coronal scans show that the bulk of the tumor is in the upper portion of the orbit

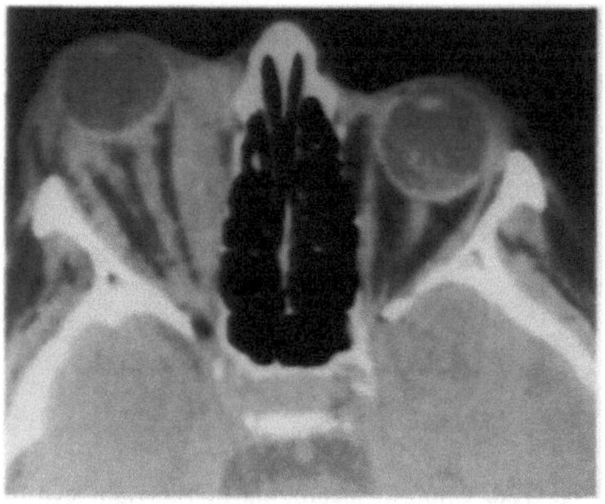

Fig. G34. Lymphoma in a 58-year-old woman with a painful swelling in the left orbital region. Proptosis is very conspicuous on the left side. CT demonstrates a soft-tissue mass in the medial part of the left orbit displacing the globe laterally and anteriorly. The tumor extends into the orbital cone and also involves the lateral rectus muscle

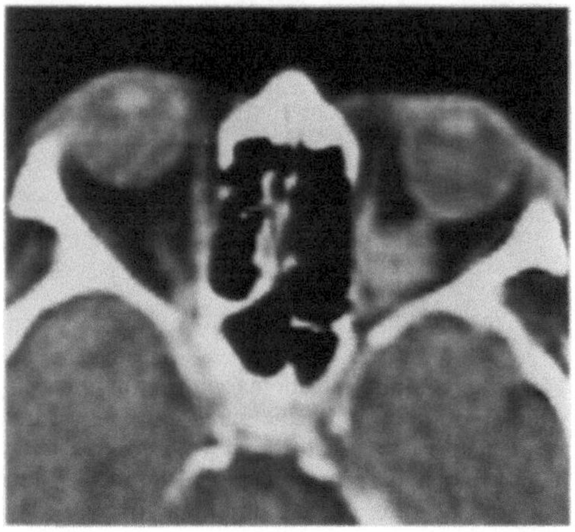

Fig. G35. Malignant lymphoma in the right orbit of a 68-year-old man. CT shows a smoothly contoured soft-tissue mass of relatively high density that cannot be separated from the optic nerve. The right orbital cone is filled by tumor

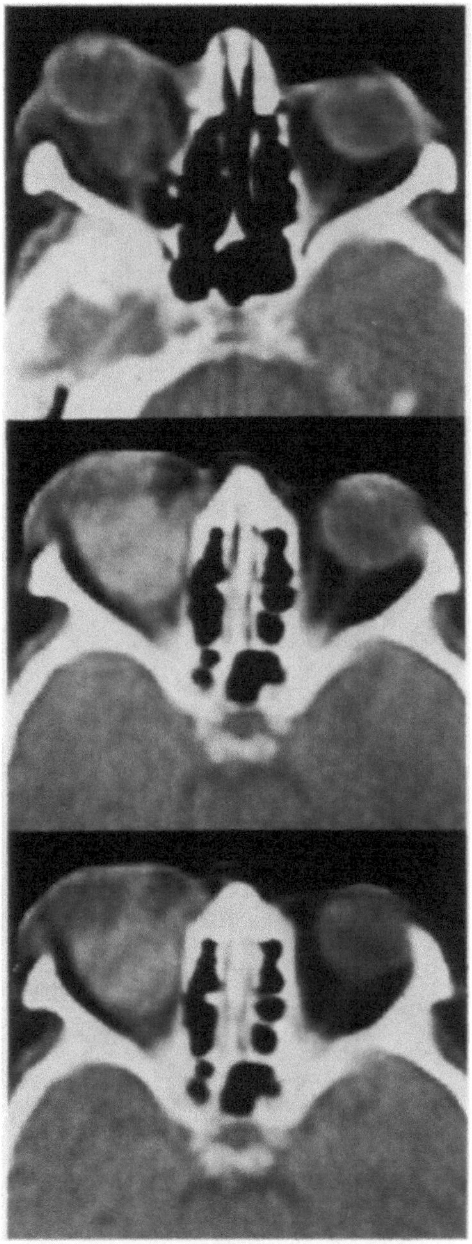

Fig. G36. Malignant lymphoma (immunocytoma) of the left orbit in an 82-year-old woman. Scans show a nonhomogeneous mass filling the upper portions of the left orbit and extending into the left upper eyelid

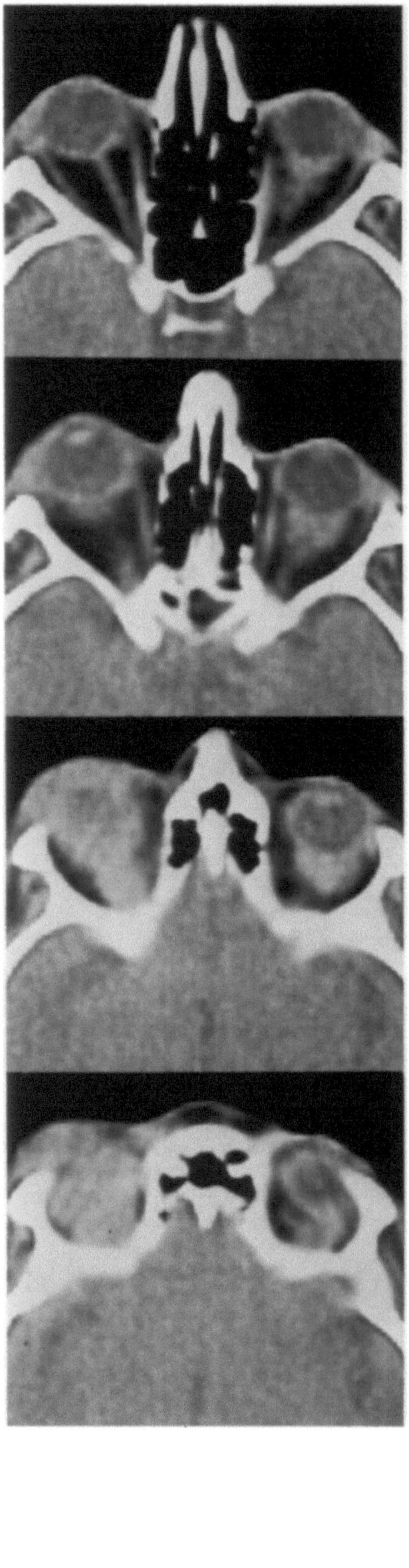

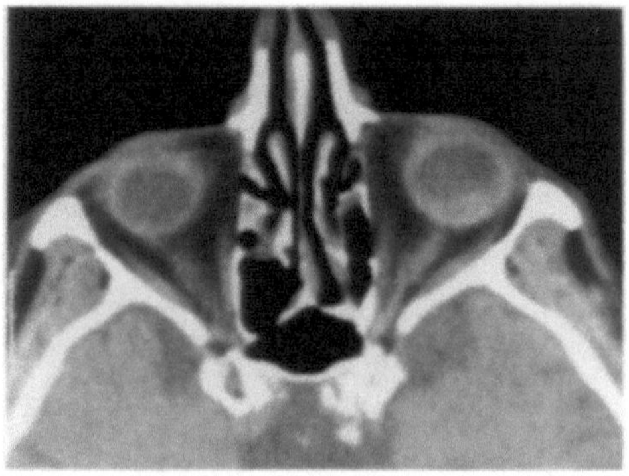

Fig. G 38. Choroid melanoma in the right eye of an 86-year-old man with visual disturbances. CT shows a conspicuous, circumscribed area of increased density with relatively smooth contours in the posterior part of the right globe

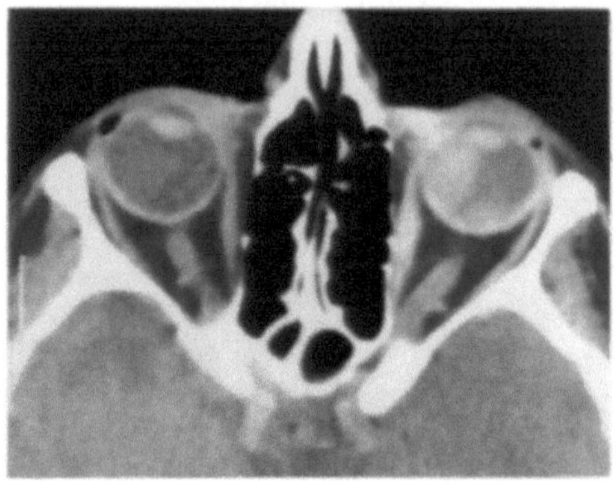

Fig. G 39. Choroid melanoma with retinal detachment and infiltration of the sclera in a 70-year-old woman with visual disturbances. CT reveals a circumscribed hyperdense process in the medial and posterior portions of the right globe

Fig. G 37. Brill-Symmers disease (lymphoreticulosis) involving both orbits in a 39-year-old woman. The soft-tissue masses abut upon the globe and infiltrate surrounding structures

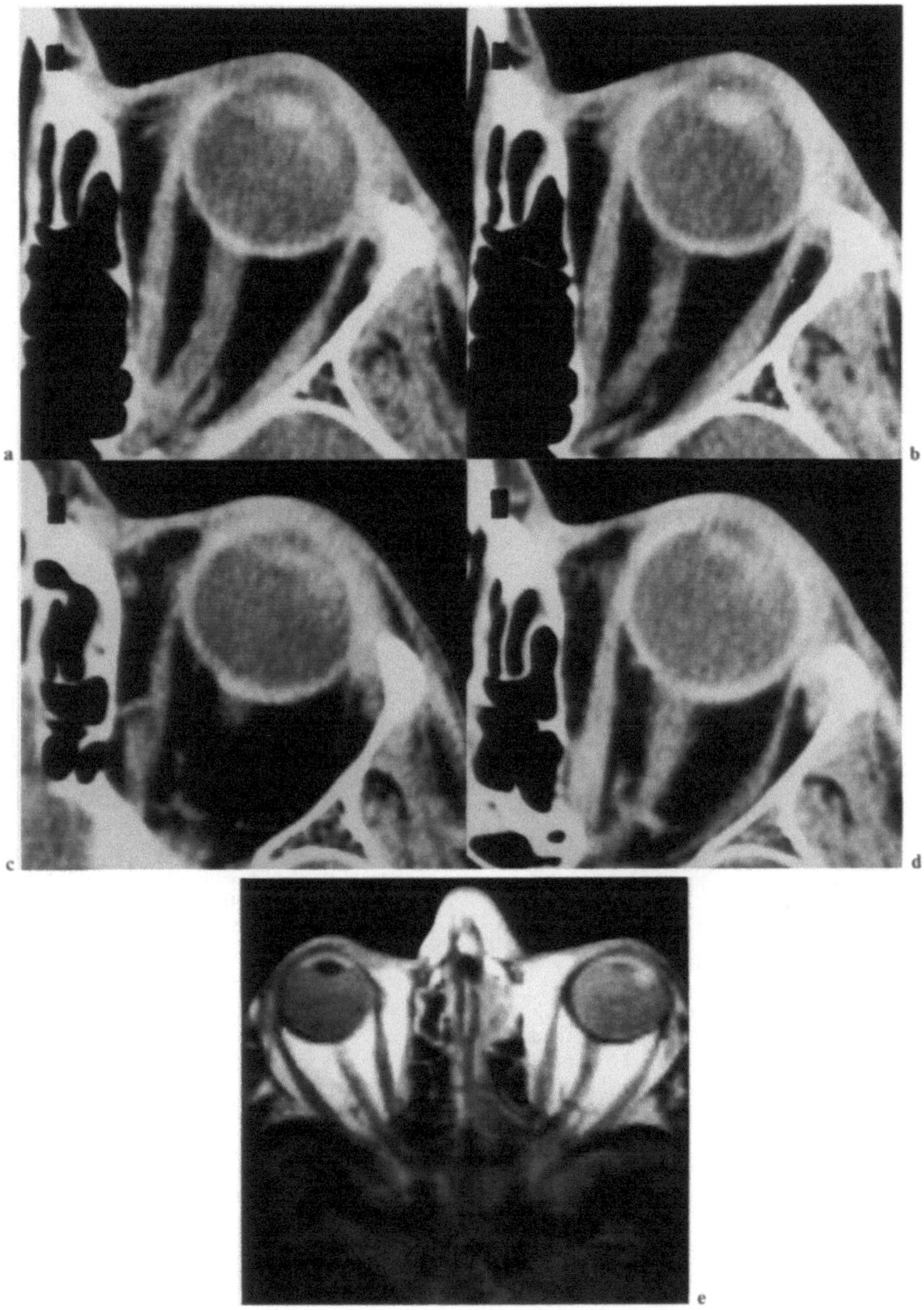

Fig. G40a–e. Metastatic adenocarcinoma without scleral penetration in a 57-year-old man with visual disturbances. CT (**a–d**) shows a circumscribed hyperdensity in the anterior and lateral portion of the right globe. MR (**e**, SE 400/30) displays the lesion as a circumscribed area of increased signal intensity in the right globe

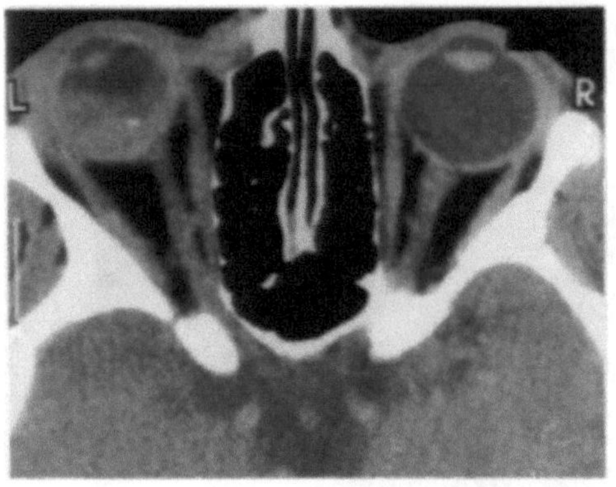

Fig. G41. Choroid hemangioma with hemorrhage in an 18-year-old female with visual disturbances in the left eye. CT shows increased density in the central and posterior portions of the left globe

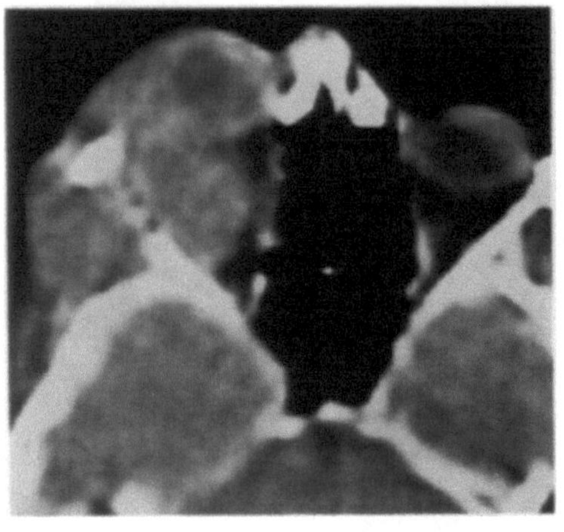

Fig. G42. Hemangioendothelioma in the left orbit with destruction of the lateral orbital wall and extension into the temporal fossa in a 37-year-old man. CT findings are consistent with the diagnosis of an orbital malignancy

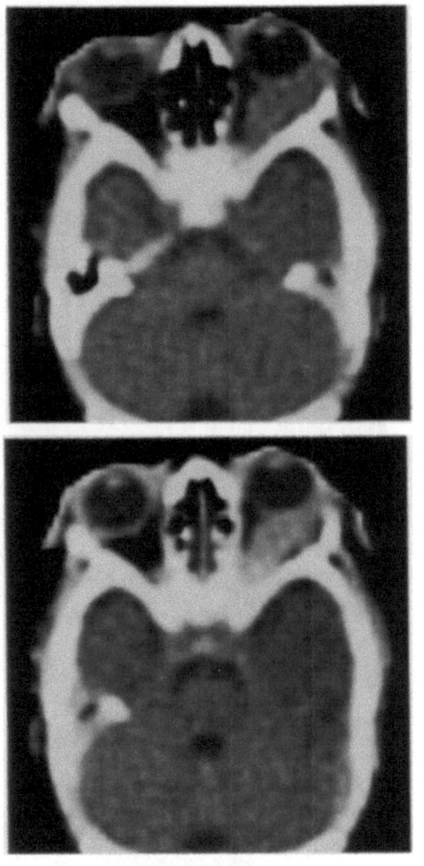

Fig. G43. Hemangioendothelioma in the right orbit of a 2-month-old infant. Scans demonstrate a soft-tissue mass almost completely filling the right orbit. The very intense contrast enhancement signifies a richly vascular tumor

3. Inflammatory Processes

Pseudotumors (Figs. G44, 45)

Pseudotumors account for 8% of all orbital tumors. While they have many of the characteristics of true neoplasms, they actually represent a chronic inflammation or reactive hyperplasia. Most common after 45 years of age, pseudotumors are a product of a nonspecific, chronic inflammation in and around the blood vessels supplying the extraocular muscles. The mass grows rapidly and is associated with the presence of lipophages, necrosis, and foreign body reaction. Orbital involvement is generally unilateral, and there may be thickening of one or more of the extraocular muscles. Diffuse infiltration of the entire orbit can occur (Peyster and Hoover 1984; Mancuso and Hanafee 1985).

An important point to consider in differential diagnosis is that pseudotumor may be the initial manifestation of a lymphoma. Pseudotumor is virtually indistinguishable from infiltrating metastases in older patients (Harr et al. 1982), especially in cases where there is associated erosion of bone (Edwards et al. 1982). Differentiation from myxoma can be accomplished only by histologic examination (Voigt et al. 1984). Bilateral pseudotumors can be difficult to distinguish from endocrine exophthalmopathy.

CT usually shows a soft-tissue mass of regular shape causing significant mass effect and proptosis. The mass may completely fill the orbit. Frequently, normal muscular and optic nerve contours are obliterated. The lesion has smooth margins (Momose et al. 1975; Enzmann et al. 1976; Lester and Gyldensted 1976) and is roughly isodense to muscle. It does not enhance after contrast injection (Mancuso and Hanafee 1985).

MR demonstrates nonspecific changes (Mancuso and Hanafee 1985) and a nonhomogeneous signal pattern.

Mucoceles and Pyoceles (Figs. G47, 48, 50–52)

These lesions are characterized by an accumulation of secretions or cyst formation leading to expansion of the paranasal sinuses. Histologic examination shows epithelial cysts containing a mucous or purulent material. The wall of the sac may protrude into the orbit and displace the globe outward, causing proptosis. These changes in the paranasal sinus region are very clearly demonstrated on conventional tomograms. The diagnosis relies on demonstrating a bulge in the bony wall of the ethmoid or frontal sinus.

CT shows a soft-tissue mass arising from the paranasal sinuses and causing expansion or erosion of bone. A specific diagnosis can be made only if CT demonstrates characteristic associated changes in the paranasal sinuses (Leo et al. 1980; Perugini et al. 1982; Mafee et al. 1986). In some cases the mucocele or pyocele may be indistinguishable from a malignant tumor. The lesions do not enhance with intravenous contrast medium.

MR allows for differentiation among tumor, hemorrhage, and inflammation owing to their different signal intensities (see Chap. E).

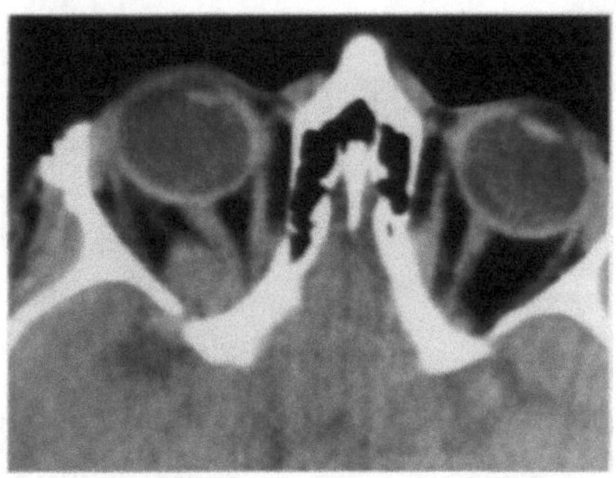

Fig. G44. Pseudotumor in a 26-year-old woman with left pupillary mydriasis and mild left-sided proptosis. Her vision was normal. CT shows marked displacement of the left optic nerve by a rounded, well-defined mass in the posterior portion of the orbit. There is proptosis of the affected side

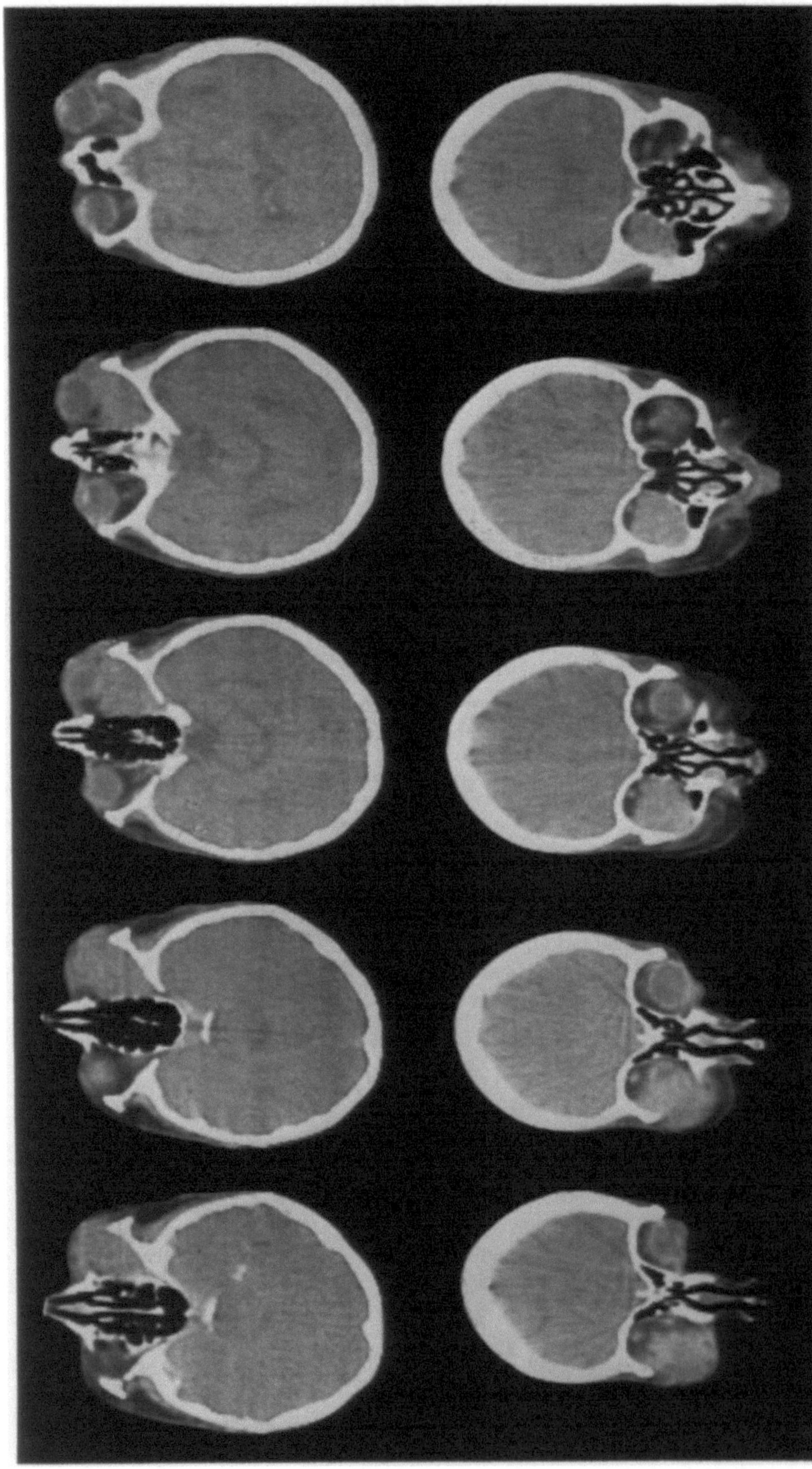

Fig. G45. Pseudotumor in the right orbit of a 79-year-old woman. The right orbit is almost completely filled by "tumor." Only the superior and medial ocular muscles are demarcated from the tumor on the coronal views. There is no evidence of bone destruction

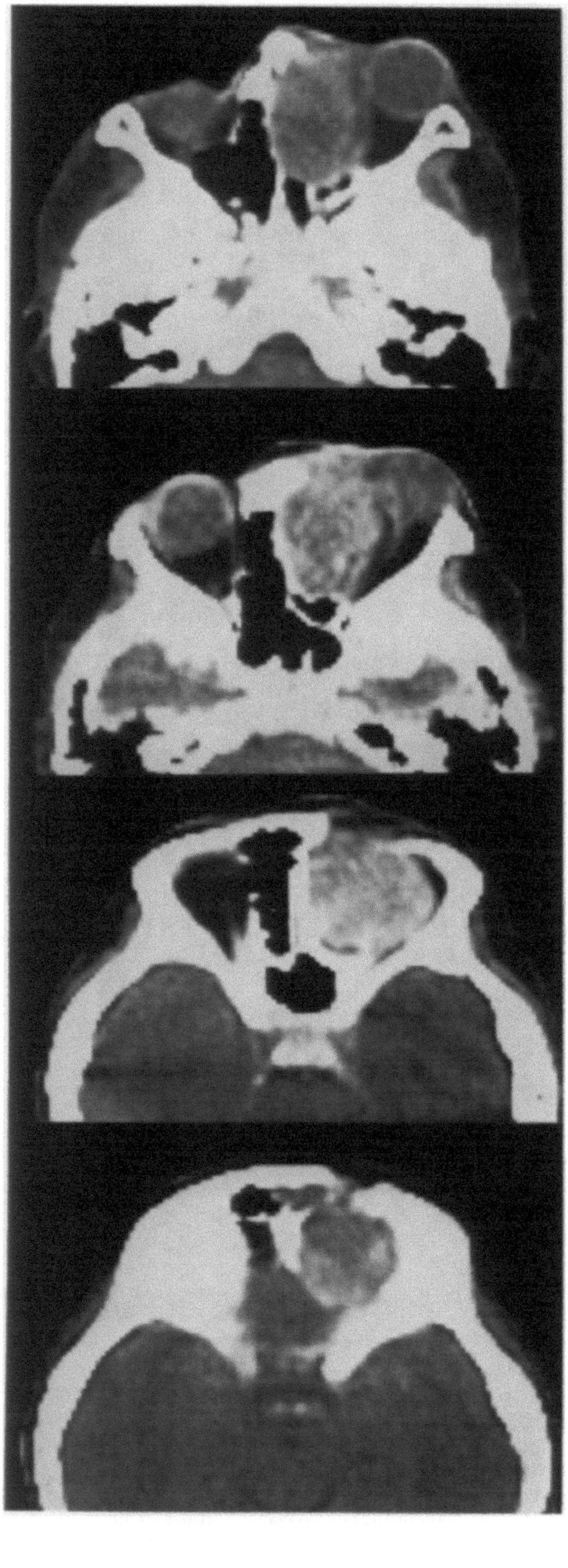

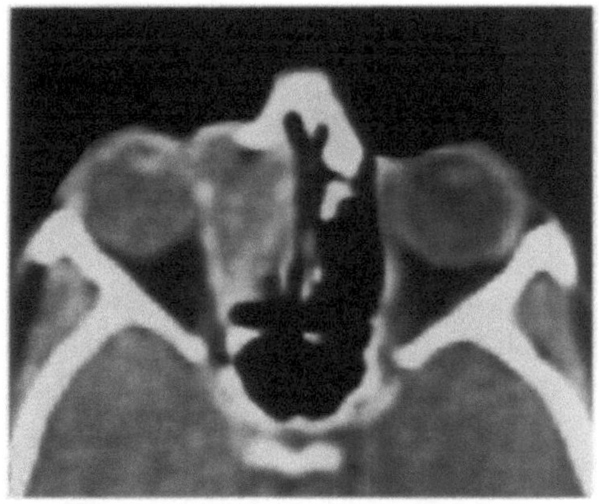

Fig. G47. Mucocele arising from the left ethmoid cells in a 14-year-old boy. The intact lamina papyracea bulges into the orbit, and the left globe is displaced laterally

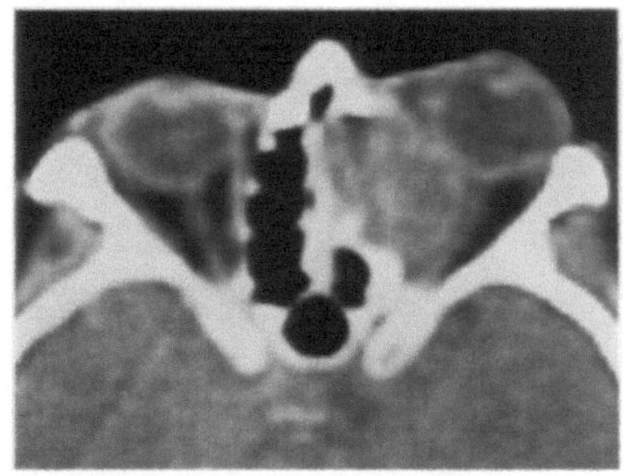

Fig. G48. Pyocele of the right ethmoid cells penetrating the right orbit in a 69-year-old woman. The lesion has eroded through the bone separating the ethmoid cells from the orbit and resembles a malignant tumor

Fig. G46. Giant cell granuloma of the ethmoid bone and right orbit in a 28-year-old woman. CT reveals a soft-tissue mass with associated bone destruction, resembling ethmoid carcinoma. Differentiation is also required from mucocele and pyocele

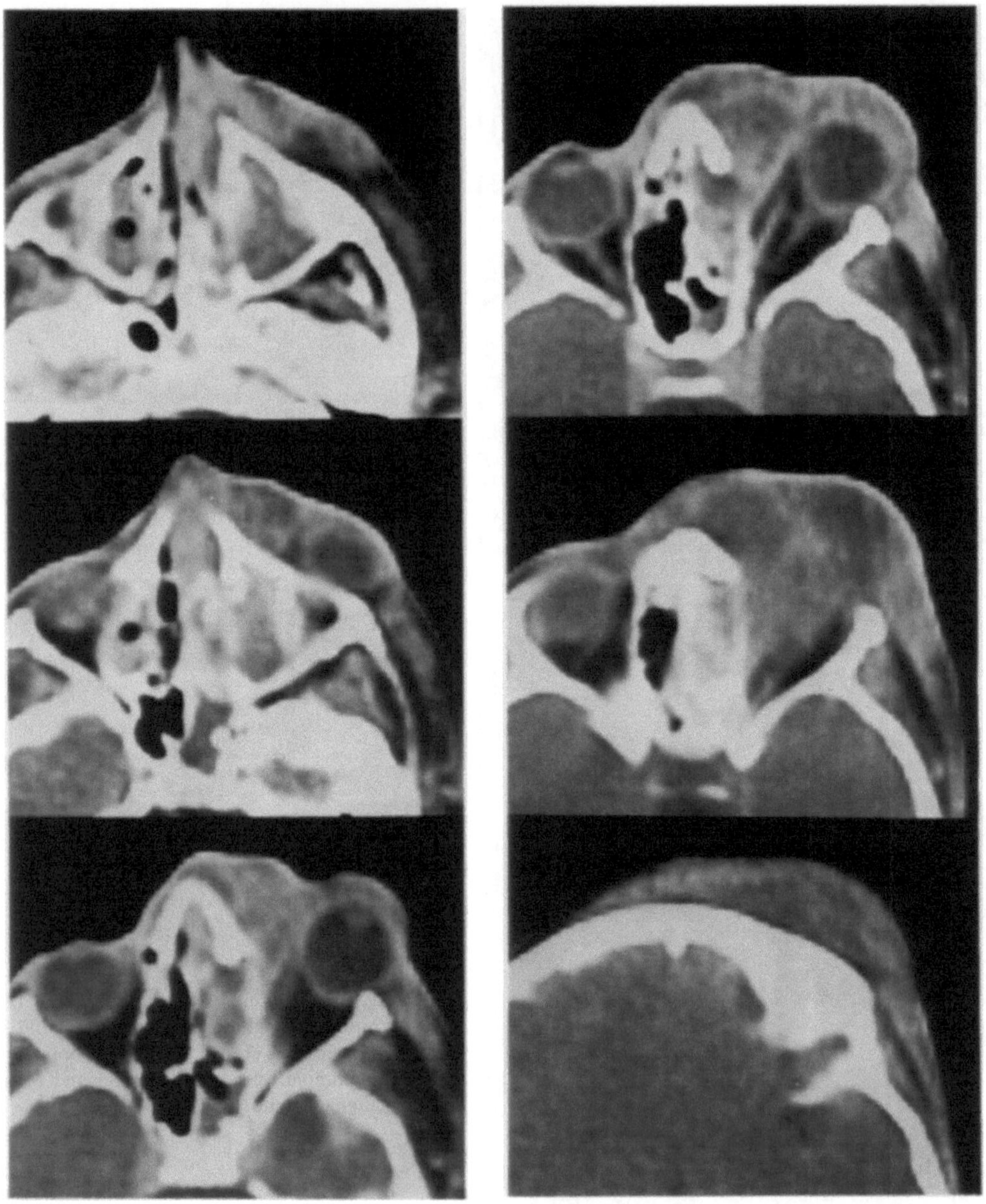

Fig. G49. Orbital cellulitis arising from the right ethmoid bone in an 11-year-old girl. CT reveals massive soft-tissue swelling with anterolateral displacement of the right globe. There is swelling of both lids and of the right frontal scalp. There is opacification of both maxillary sinuses and the right ethmoid

Fig. G50a–h. Bilateral mucoceles in a 50-year-old man. Axial CT scans show bilateral soft-tissue opacity of the ethmoid cells with bony destruction of the laminae papyracea. A soft-tissue mass in the left orbit is contiguous to the globe. A smaller soft-tissue mass appears in the upper medial portion of the right orbit (section **c**). The coronal scans show bilateral opacification of the ethmoid cells with bilateral destruction of the medial orbital walls. There is a large soft-tissue mass above the left globe, which is displaced downward and forward. Section **h** reveals another soft-tissue mass in the superomedial portions of the right orbit (*arrow*)

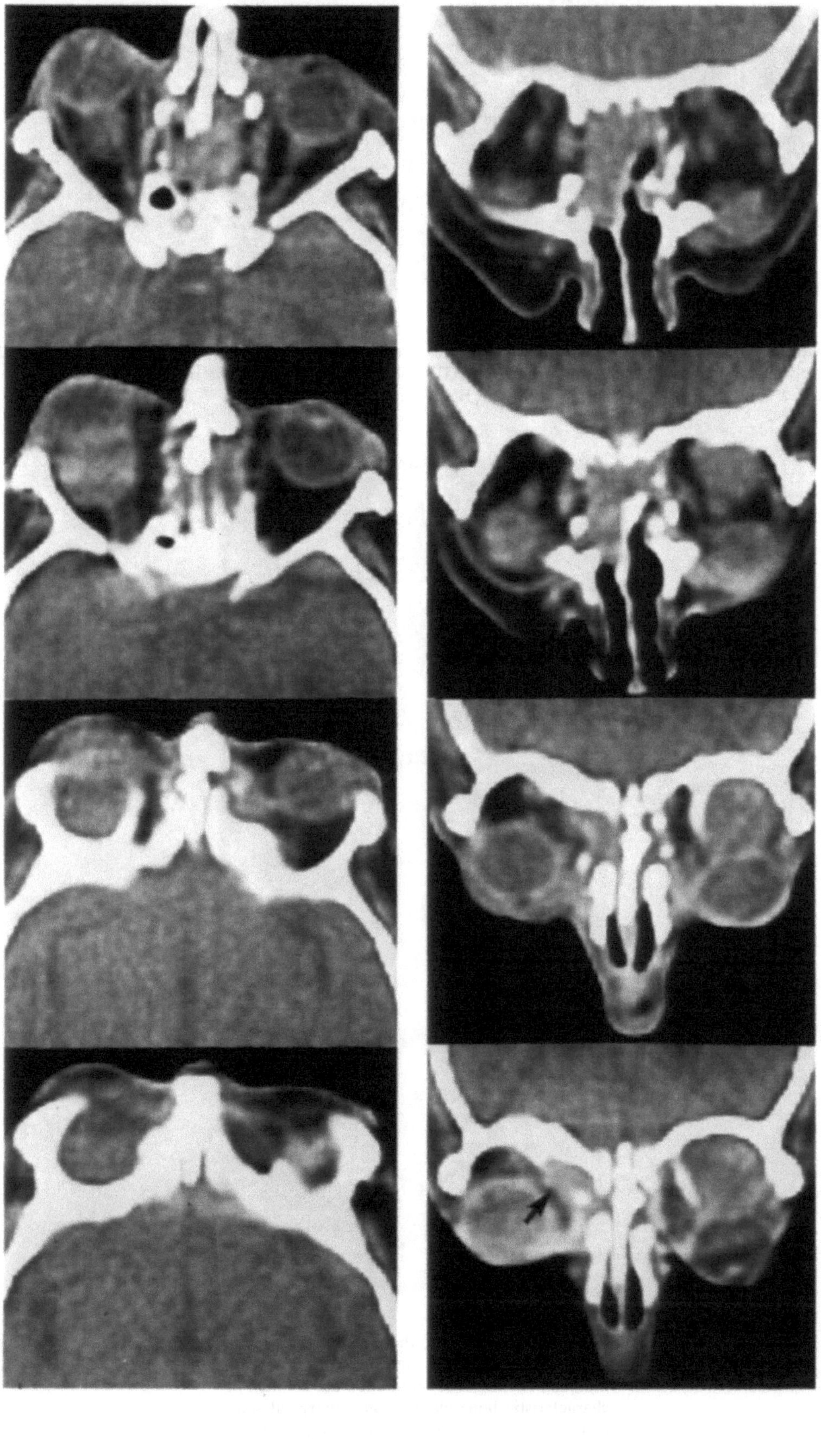

a b c d e f g h

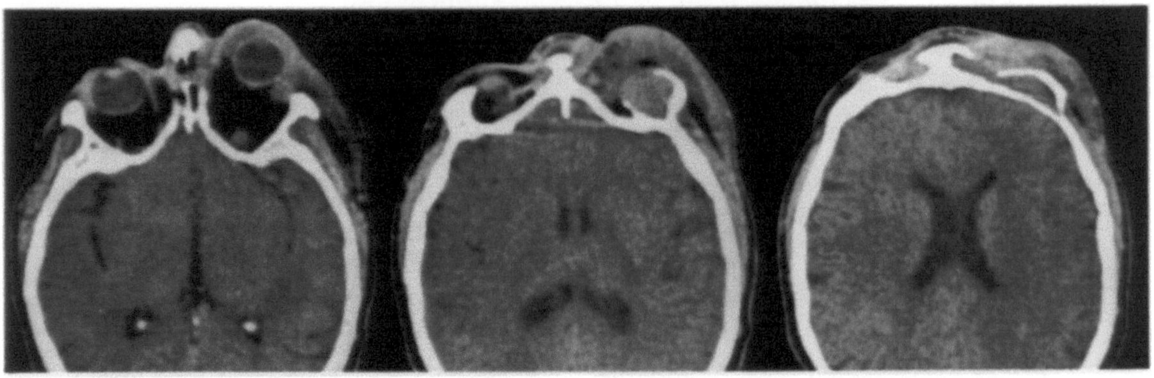

Fig. G51. Pyocele in the right frontal sinus of a 46-year-old man with recurring bouts of sinusitis following an old fracture involving the right frontal sinus and orbital roof. CT demonstrates a soft-tissue mass in the region of the right frontal sinus with extension into the right orbit. There is significant soft-tissue swelling about the forehead and upper lid with proptosis on the right side

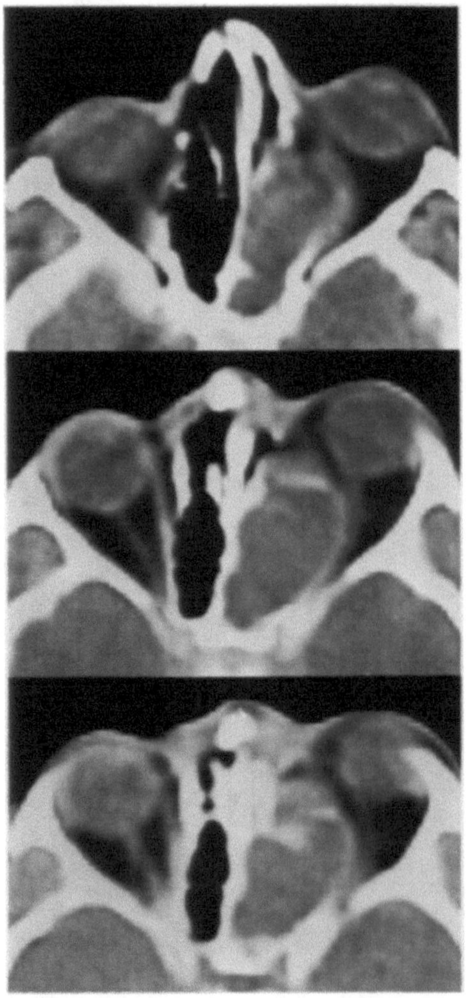

Fig. G52. Mucocele of the right ethmoid cells with penetration of the right orbit in a 44-year-old man. Prolonged inflammation has resulted in characteristic bone changes with marginal sclerosis. The lamina papyracea is bowed outward into the right orbit

4. Malformations and Posttraumatic States

Buphthalmos (Fig. G 53)

Buphthalmos is a marked enlargement of the globe and corneal diameter (macrocornea, diameter >12 mm) secondary to the increased intraocular pressure of congenital glaucoma.

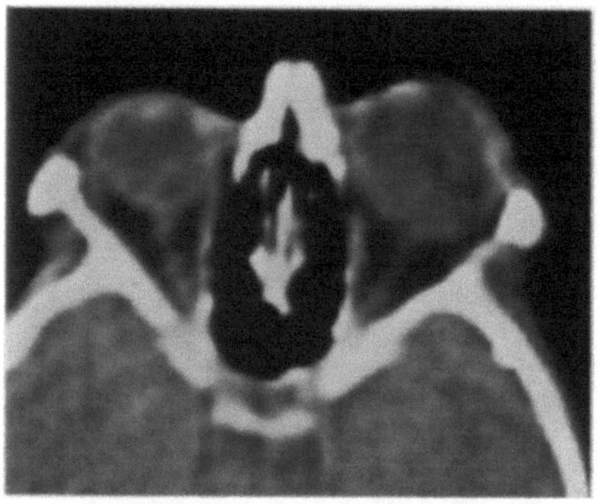

Fig. G 53. Buphthalmos of the right eye secondary to glaucoma in a 70-year-old woman

Sphenoid Aplasia (Fig. G 54)

This anomaly is seen with some frequency in patients with neurofibromatosis. It may coexist with buphthalmos or microphthalmos.

Carotid Cavernous Fistula (Figs. G 56, 57)

This abnormal communication between the internal carotid artery and cavernous sinus may occur spontaneously or as a sequel to trauma. It is characterized by a marked, often pulsating exophthalmos with significant dilatation of the superior ophthalmic vein. The lesion is easily detected by CT, especially on contrast-enhanced scans (Sanders 1976).

Besides carotid cavernous fistula, a sinus thrombosis or arteriovenous ångioma can lead to exophthalmos with secondary muscle swelling. The diagnosis is established by angiography (Voigt et al. 1984).

Arteriovenous Angiomas and Other Vascular Malformations (Figs. G 59, 60)

These malformations are distinguished from cavernous hemangioma on CT by their irregular structure and borders and by the ill-defined zones of mixed density within the lesion. They enhance with intravenous contrast. Irregular calcifications may be present in some cases.

Differentiation from the well-defined cavernous hemangioma is not difficult owing to the irregular borders of the angioma and its heterogeneous density (Momose et al. 1975). On the other hand, CT findings may be completely normal despite the clinical finding of significant exophthalmos. It is imperative that these cases be evaluated by ophthalmic venography or angiography (Lloyd 1982).

Very extensive arteriovenous hemangiomas of the scalp and face can develop in children and may involve the orbit.

AV malformations are conspicuous on MR images owing to the "flow defect" seen in the enlarged retrobulbar vessels.

Trauma

Even small orbital fractures are displayed with great clarity on thin-section CT scans. Circumscribed blood collections in the orbital region are also visualized. MR can demonstrate these hemorrhages with equal clarity but does not permit evaluation of the bony orbit.

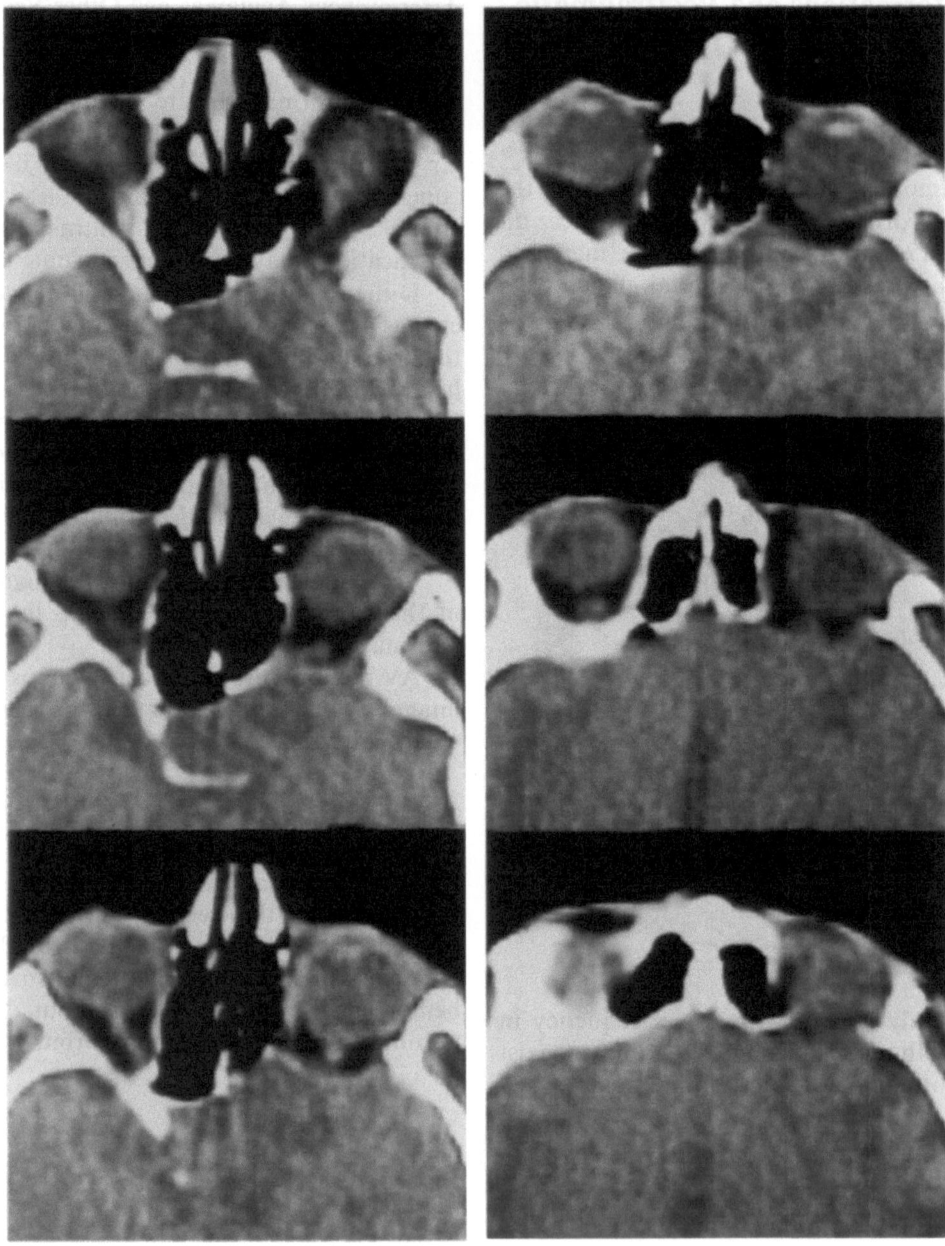

a b c d e f

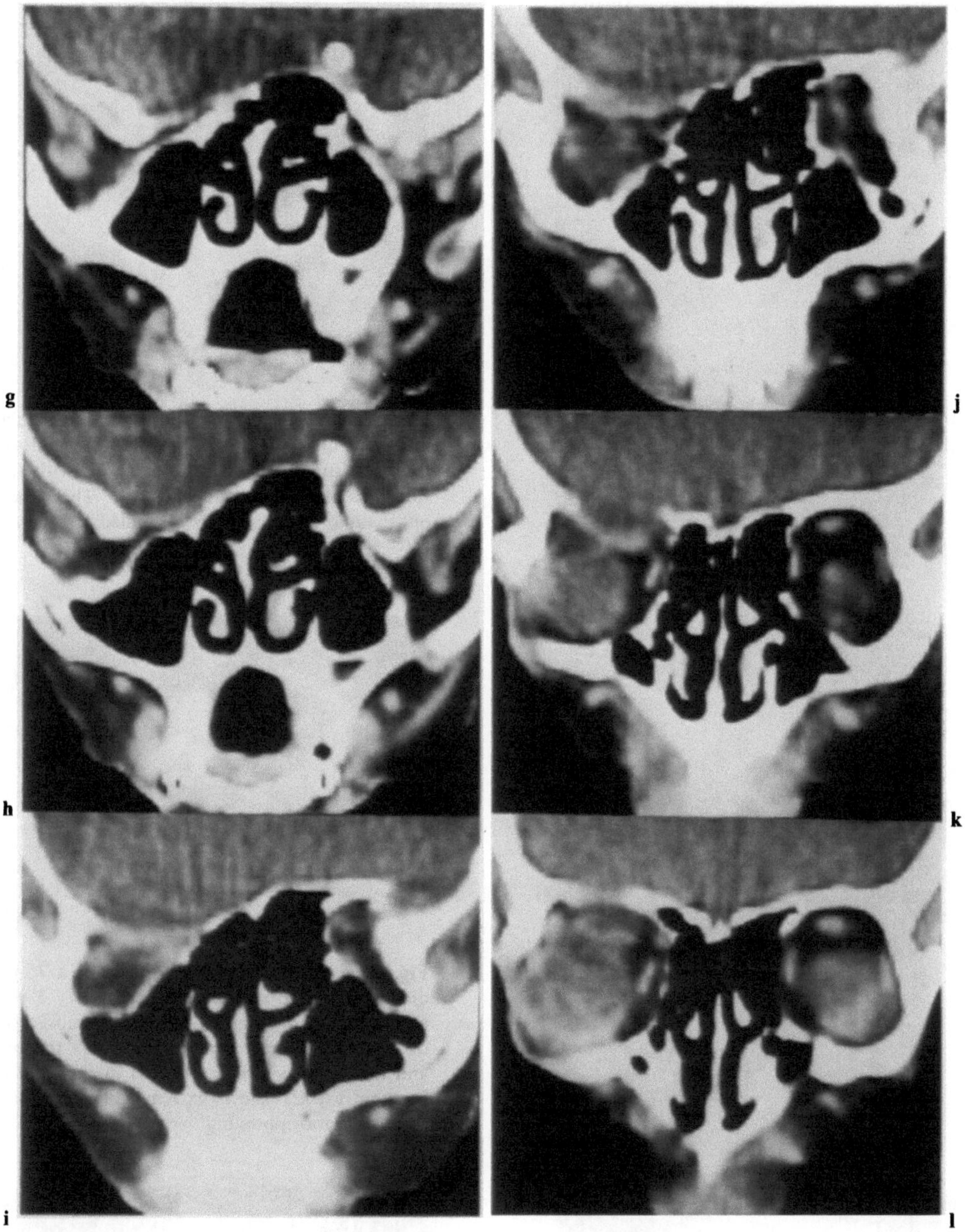

Fig. G54a–l. Partial aplasia of the right sphenoid in a 37-year-old man with neurofibromatosis. Axial and coronal projections are shown. There is buphthalmos of the right eye (**c**, **d**)

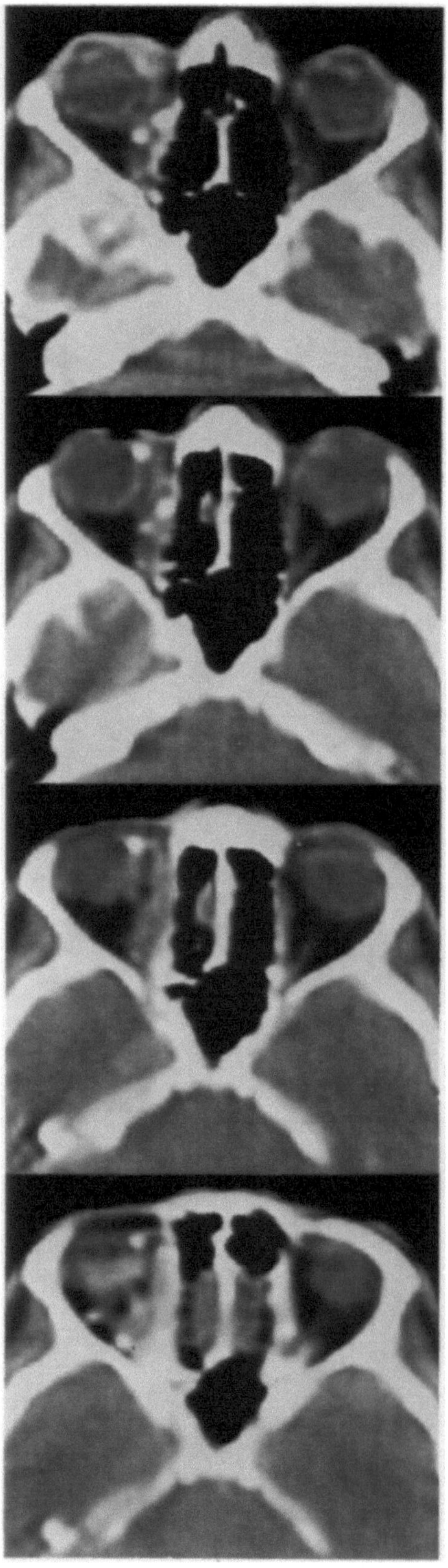

Fig. G55. (Legend see p. 619)

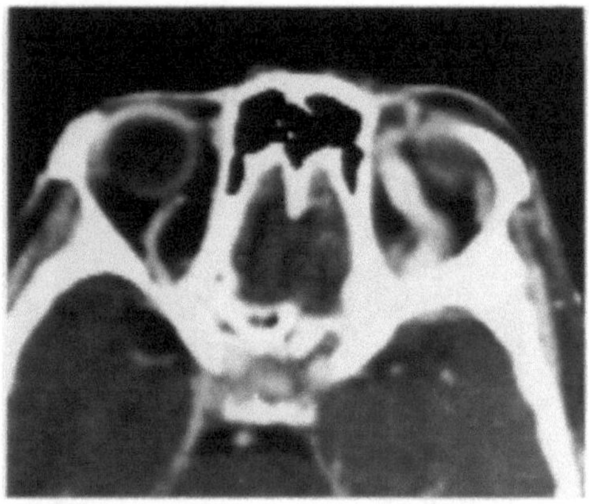

Fig. G56. *Spontaneous* carotid-cavernous fistula in a 65-year-old woman with a dural AV malformation. She presented with diplopia and with right-sided exophthalmos and chemosis. The superior ophthalmic vein is greatly distended. Postcontrast CT

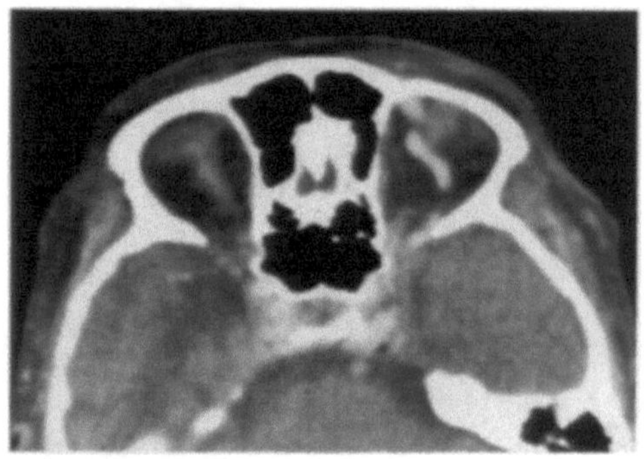

Fig. G57. Carotid-cavernous fistula in a 76-year-old woman who sustained a *head injury* 3 weeks earlier. She had progressive exophthalmos, a bruit over the right orbit synchronous with the pulse, and increasing visual acuity loss in the right eye. Postcontrast CT shows extreme dilatation of the right superior ophthalmic vein

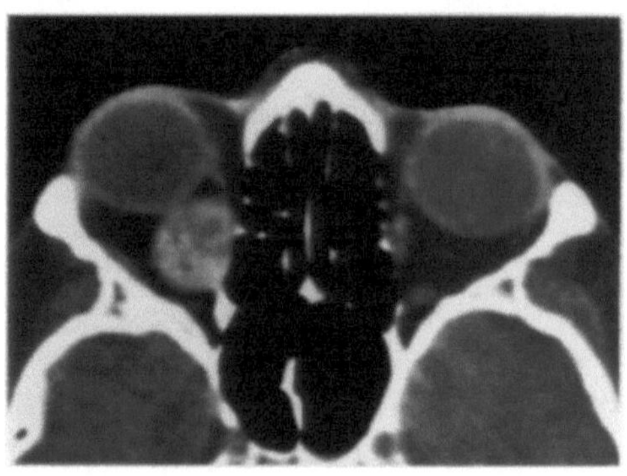

Fig. G58. Spontaneous retrobulbar hemorrhage in a 73-year-old woman with diplopia and left-sided exophthalmos. Follow-up CT examination showed normal orbital findings

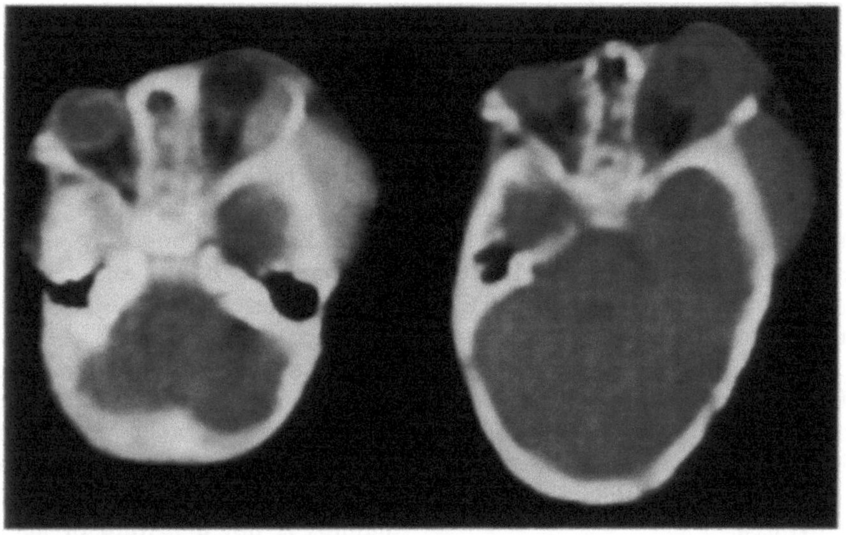

Fig. G59. Arteriovenous hemangioma of the right scalp, right upper lid, and right orbit in a 7-month-old infant. Scans show an intensely enhancing soft-tissue mass (*left*) in the right temporal fossa, the lateral portion of the right orbit, and in the right upper eyelid

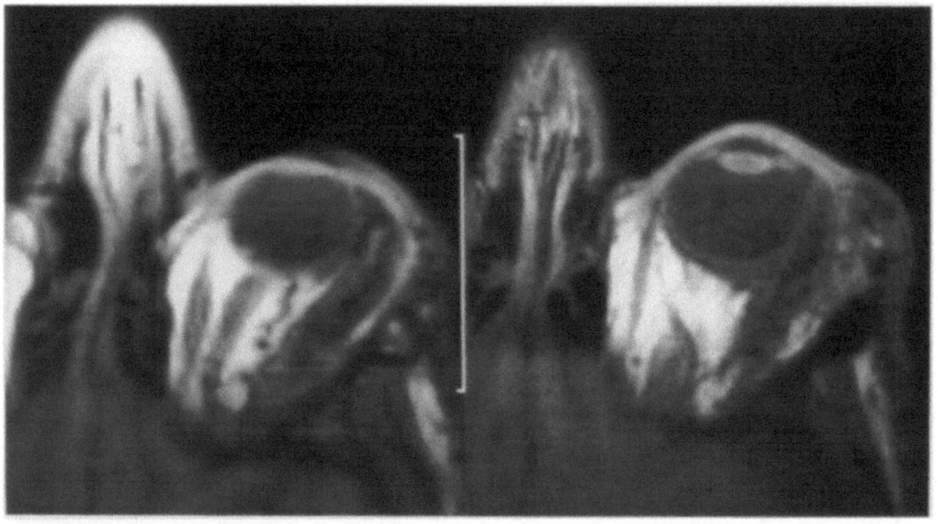

Fig. G60. Arteriovenous malformation in the right orbit of a 22-year-old male with pulsating exophthalmos. MR (SE 400/30) reveals garlandlike areas of signal void in the region of the thickened right lateral rectus muscle

Fig. G55. Varicocele with phleboliths in an 18-year-old male. Scans reveal an elongated soft-tissue mass in the medial portions of the left orbit. Multiple calcifications are seen in the course of the lesion

5. Endocrine Ophthalmopathy
(Figs. G61–64)

Exophthalmos is unilateral in 10%–20% of cases. There is local infiltration of the orbital tissue by lymphocytes, leukocytes, and mast cells. Other features are destruction of muscle fibers, increased mucopolysaccharides in the orbital tissue, lipomatosis, and increased water content in the muscles. Later the muscles undergo fibrosis and degeneration. There is progressive exophthalmos, and the globe may protrude past the eyelids. The muscular pressure causes expansion of the orbital cone, which is most pronounced at the level of the muscle bellies and particularly affects the nasal wall of the lamina papyracea.

CT shows fusiform expansion of one or more extraocular muscles, resulting in a variety of presentations. Almost always there is bilateral involvement of the extraocular muscles, even if the patient is clinically asymptomatic. The inferior rectus muscle is affected with the greatest frequency and severity, followed by the medial rectus (Inoue and Inoue 1978; Enzmann et al. 1979; Hilal 1979; Wing et al. 1979; Voigt et al. 1984).

The thickening of the muscles is fusiform and nonhomogeneous, sparing their tendinous origins and insertions. It is possible for only one muscle to appear abnormal on the CT scan while the other muscles appear normal, but most cases present with uniform, symmetrical thickening and increased density of the muscles (Bergström 1975; Brismar et al. 1976; Enzmann et al. 1976; Nowinski and Flanagan 1986). The muscle changes are proportional to the severity of the disease, and CT readily documents the positive response of these changes to therapy.

MR shows a marked increase in the volume of retrobulbar fat. As on CT, muscular thickening spares the sites of origin and insertion.

Differentiation is required from pseudotumor, metastatic carcinoma infiltrating the extraocular muscles, vascular congestion secondary to cavernous sinus fistulas or AV malformations, and tumors or aneurysms in the anterior part of the floor of the middle fossa (Trokel and Jakobiec 1981; Walsh and Hoyt 1985). Exophthalmos may also be seen with prolonged steroid use and general obesity, but in these cases the ocular muscles are not thickened, and both sides are affected equally (Peyster and Hoover 1984). Acromegaly is usually associated with marked bilateral thickening of the extraocular muscles. This phenomenon is not hormone-dependent but depends on the duration of the disease. Exophthalmos is not a feature of acromegaly (Dal Pozzo and Boschi 1982).

The major condition to be differentiated from endocrine ophthalmopathy is *myositis*, in which case the swelling involves the whole muscle including its tendinous attachments (Figs. G65, 66).

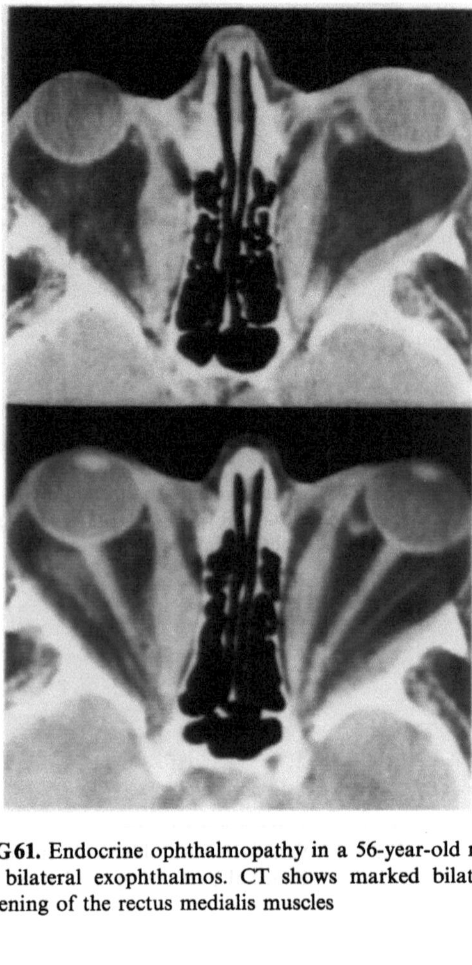

Fig. G61. Endocrine ophthalmopathy in a 56-year-old man with bilateral exophthalmos. CT shows marked bilateral thickening of the rectus medialis muscles

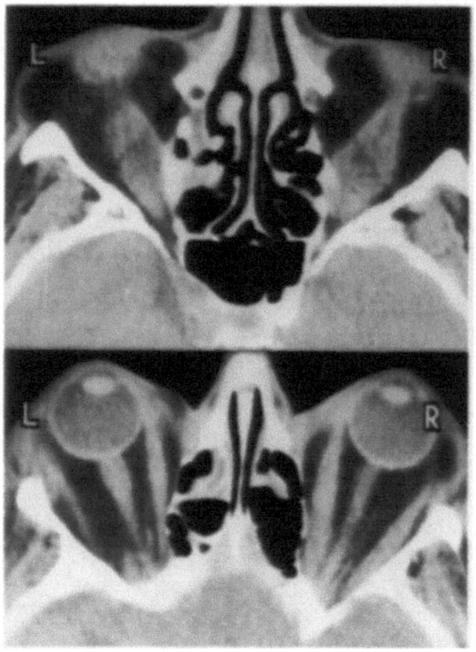

a

b

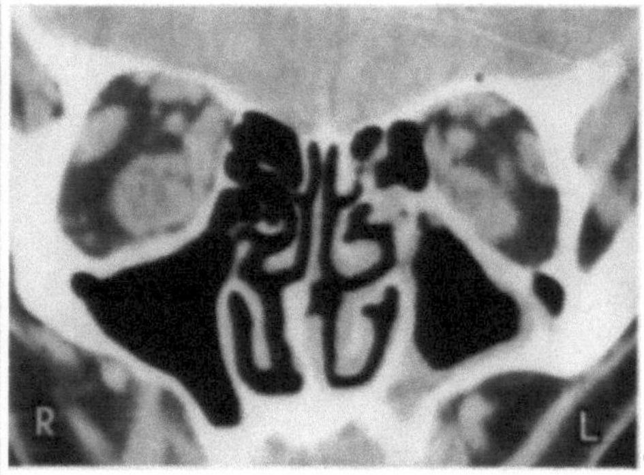

c

Fig. G62a–c. Endocrine ophthalmopathy in a 45-year-old man with bilateral exophthalmos. CT (**a**, **b** axial, **c** coronal) shows bilateral thickening of the extraocular muscles, especially of the rectus inferior

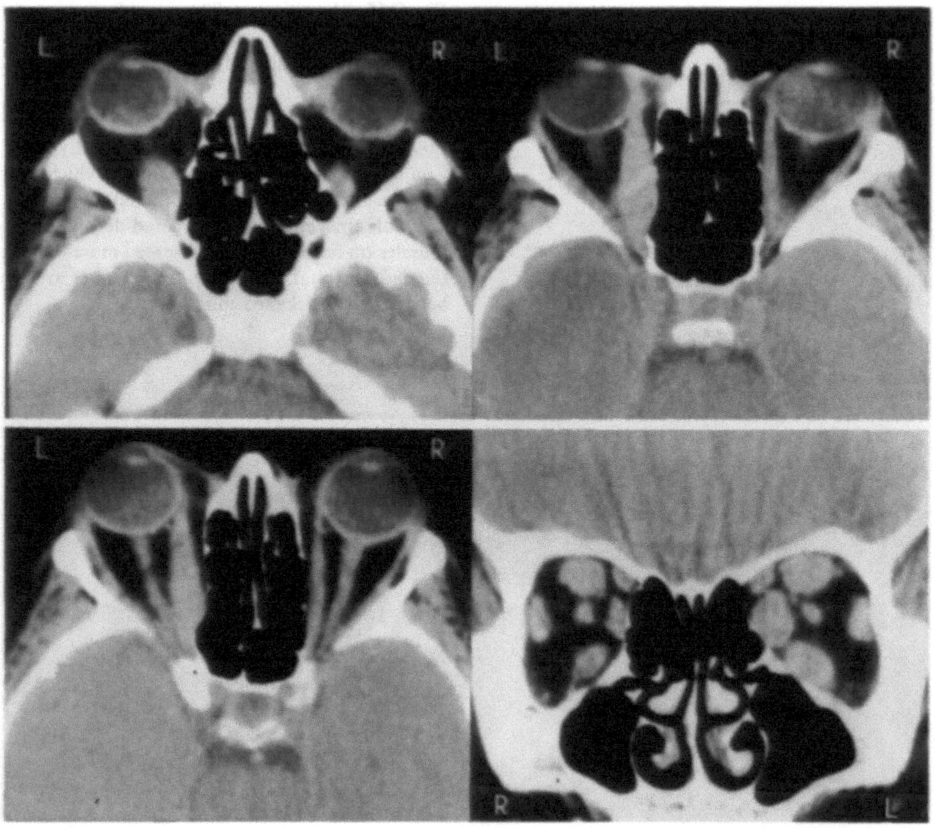

a b c d

Fig. G63a–d. Endocrine ophthalmopathy in a 48-year-old woman with bilateral exophthalmos. CT **a**, **b**, **c** axial, **d** coronal. Involvement of the individual ocular muscles is best appreciated on the coronal scan

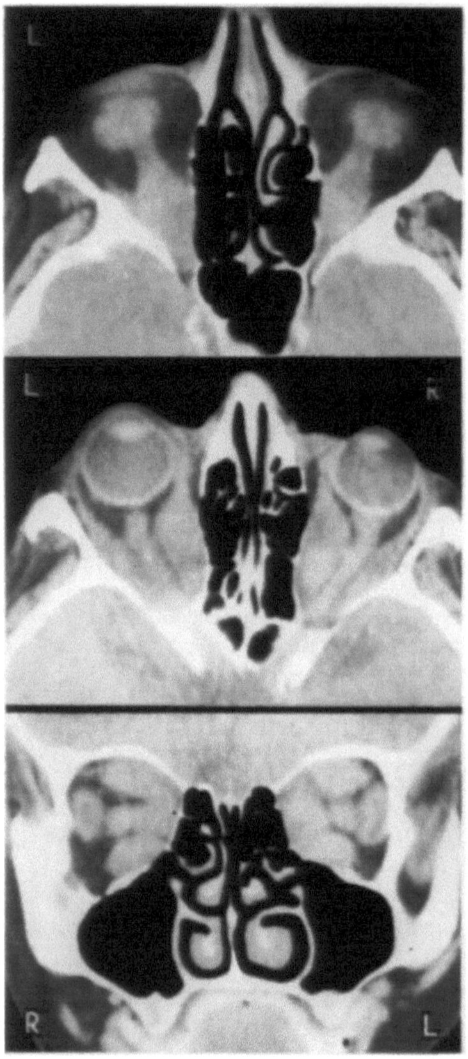

a

b

c

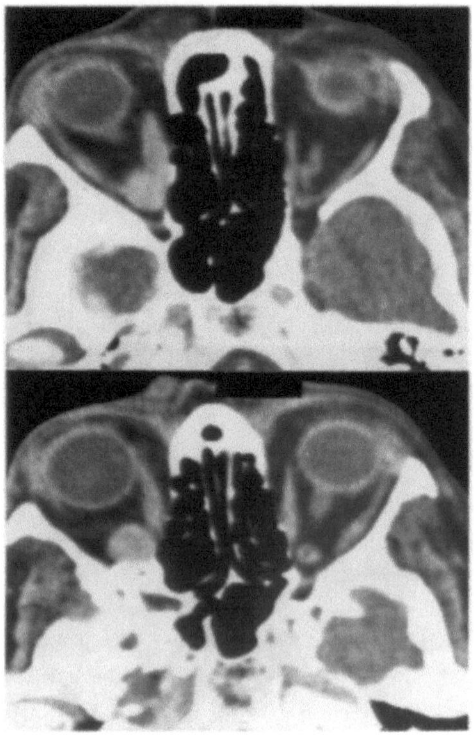

Fig. G65. Myositis in a 70-year-old woman with visual impairment in the left eye and diplopia. CT shows swelling of the inferior, medial, and lateral rectus muscles

Fig. G64a–c. Endocrine ophthalmopathy in a 45-year-old woman with marked exophthalmos, which is more prominent on the left side. CT (**a**, **b** axial, **c** coronal) shows considerable thickening and increased density of all extraocular muscles on both sides. The diseased muscle tissue fills almost the entire orbital cone. Both optic nerves are clearly defined between the thickened muscles

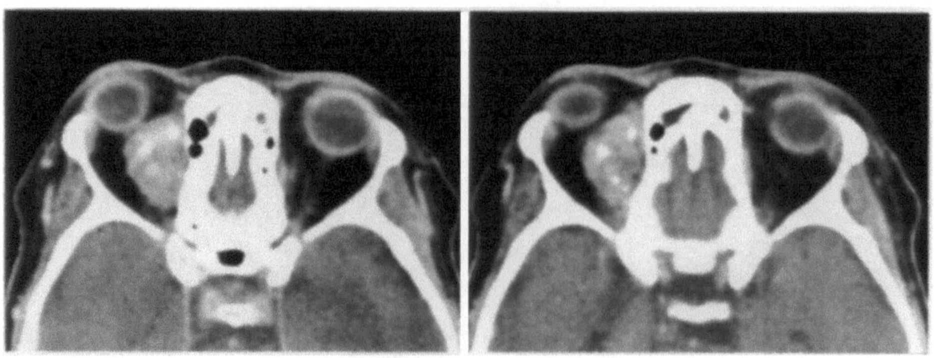

Fig. G66. Chronic myositis in a 59-year-old man with a 1-year history of increasing left-sided exophthalmos. CT reveals a soft-tissue "mass" in the medial portion of the left orbit displacing the left globe laterally and anteriorly. Stippled calcifications are seen within the mass

Summary

Orbital tumors are easy to detect with CT because all (except for dermoids and lipomas) display higher densities than the surrounding fatty tissue. Thus, the normal orbit presents an ideal background for the CT detection of a space-occupying lesion.

Comparing the efficacy of CT, ultrasound, ophthalmic venography, carotid angiography, and conventional tomography in the diagnosis of orbital pathology, Ambrose (1975) and Ambrose et al. (1974) found that CT had an accuracy rate of 84% compared with 89% for ophthalmic venography, 82% for sonography, and 71% for tomography. Moseley and Bull (1975) confirmed the high diagnostic accuracy of CT in a similar comparison. Lloyd and Ambrose (1977) compared the diagnostic accuracy of CT with that of other modalities (sonography, ophthalmic venography, conventional tomography) in the evaluation of 75 primary orbital tumors. They found a 91% accuracy rate for CT and orbital venography, approximately 86% for ultrasound, and 73% for tomography. Gyldensted et al. (1977) reported a diagnostic accuracy of 98% for CT in their patients (histologically confirmed tumors) as opposed to 82% for sonography. Forbes et al. (1982) reported on 133 orbital tumors, for which CT yielded a positive diagnosis in 96%. It should be emphasized that the latest generation of CT scanners employing 1.5-mm sections yield better diagnostic results than earlier instruments. These scanners provide better information on the location and extent of tumors, and images can be quickly reformatted in multiple planes.

As early as 1976, Maier-Hauff and Wilske noted the superiority of diagnostic ultrasound over CT in establishing the nature of orbital tumors. Bigar et al. (1982) and Li et al. (1984) also emphasized the value of sonography for tissue discrimination.

Bigar et al. cite the following advantages of CT: optimum tomographic imaging, and simple conduct of the examination in a cooperative patient. They point out that sonography offers the advantages of low equipment costs, cost-effective technique, and convenience for short-term follow-ups. They claim that the primary role of sonography is in screening for orbital disease, with equivocal or clearly pathologic findings in that study providing a basis for further special examinations. A significant disadvantage of sonography is the relative inaccessibility of the posterior portions of the orbit to ultrasound imaging.

It has been our experience (Nover et al. 1982) that both CT and sonography should be performed in patients with a suspected orbital tumor. This combination can provide the highest possible accuracy in establishing the location and nature of the disease. It is rarely possible to make a specific diagnosis on the basis of CT findings alone (Wackenheim et al. 1977; Mortelmans et al. 1978). Of course, lesions such as cavernous hemangioma are easily distinguished from optic glioma by their characteristic imaging features. Differentiation between meningioma and cavernous hemangioma also can be accomplished by noting the confinement of cavernous hemangioma to the extraconal space. Generally, however, it is not possible even to distinguish benign from malignant tumors in the absence of destructive bone changes (Wende et al. 1977; Unsöld et al. 1979). We have found that contrast-enhanced CT scans rarely provide additional information, since benign and malignant tumors show similar levels of enhancement (Wende et al. 1977). Forbes et al. (1982) note that contrast enhancement may be helpful in forming a diagnosis but is not essential. Peyster et al. (1983), on the other hand, state that contrast injection is indicated for most CT examinations of the orbit. Clearly, contrast medium should be used to differentiate an optic sheath meningioma from an optic glioma, for that is the only way to distinguish the optic sheath meningioma from the optic nerve itself (Daniels et al. 1982).

The major criteria for the differential diagnosis of the most common orbital lesions are summarized in Table 13.

If differentiation between a tumor and an inflammatory process cannot be accomplished, ophthalmic venography is recommended as an adjunctive study. This procedure can demonstrate compression of the superior ophthalmic vein associated with inflammatory disease of the muscle cone. Venous displacement is not observed, however (Lloyd et al. 1975; Brismar et al. 1976; Peeters 1977; Peeters et al. 1977; Wende et al. 1977).

No definitive statement can be made regarding the **MR imaging of orbital disease.**

The examination time is relatively long, and the bright signals from fatty tissue and from volume averaging in the thick sections make it difficult to resolve small structures of low signal intensity (Han et al. 1984). Because orbital tumors have approximately the same signal characteristics as the optic nerve, they are not easily differentiated from the nerve (Daniels et al. 1984). Li et al. (1984) note that MR provides excellent discrimination between cysts and tumors, but they also stress the disadvantage of a long examination time. Nonvisualization of bony structures is cited as another disadvantage (Edwards et al. 1985; Grossniklaus et al. 1985; Mödder 1986).

Recent studies indicate that MR examinations using surface coils and 1.5-tesla magnets yield results that are comparable if not superior to those obtained with high-resolution CT (Bilaniuk et al. 1985; Schenck et al. 1985; Zimmerman et al. 1985; Atlas et al. 1986; Sobel et al. 1986; Sullivan and Harms 1986; Krahe et al. 1987), and that MR is especially well suited for follow-up examinations (Sobel et al. 1984). However, the T1 and T2 relaxation times of benign and malignant orbital tumors show significant overlap, so it is not possible to differentiate them on MR images (Char et al. 1985).

Given the advantages and disadvantages cited above, it is fair to state that MR imaging does not yet offer an effective alternative to CT in diagnosing many types of orbital disease.

Table 13. CT criteria for the differential diagnosis of the most common lesions occurring in the orbital muscle cone (modified from Unsöld et al. 1979)

Type of lesion	Shape	Demarcation from optic nerve, extraocular muscles, and orbital fat	Bony changes	Orbital apex
Cavernous hemangioma	Round or oval soft-tissue mass	Clear demarcation from orbital fat, ocular muscles, and optic nerve	Large hemangiomas may expand the orbit; no bone defects or hyperostosis	Even large tumors spare a small triangular area at the apex
Optic sheath meningioma	Apparent thickening of the optic nerve and/or irregular soft-tissue mass	Good demarcation from orbital fat; contiguous to optic nerve	Hyperostosis may occur in adjacent bone	Usually filled
Optic glioma	Soft-tissue mass, usually club-shaped, in the course of the optic nerve	Good demarcation from orbital fat, enlargement of optic nerve	Optic canal is usually expanded	Extends to the apex
Neurinoma	Conical soft-tissue mass whose tip fills the orbital apex	Good demarcation from orbital fat; soft-tissue mass envelops the optic nerve	Usually none	Filled
Metastasis	Irregular or occasionally rounded soft-tissue mass	Usually extends diffusely into the orbital fat, tends to involve extraocular muscles and optic nerve; smooth delineation is rare	Erosive changes are common; osteoplastic metastases produce hyperostosis	Often filled
Lymphoma	Irregularly shaped soft-tissue mass	Often is contiguous to the globe and sharply demarcated from orbital fat; soft-tissue mass often envelops the ocular muscles and optic nerve	Usually none	Orbital apex may be filled
Pseudotumor	Irregularly shaped soft-tissue mass	Poor demarcation from orbital fat; ocular muscles and optic nerve are frequently enveloped by tumor; thickening of extraocular muscles is common	Hyperostosis of adjacent bone may occur in chronic cases	Orbital apex may be filled
Endocrine ophthalmopathy	Fusiform expansion of the extraocular muscles	Usually good demarcation from orbital fat	None	Usually obliterated by soft-tissue masses

H. Impact of CT and MR on the Diagnostic Evaluation of Neurologic and Neurosurgical Diseases

Today CT and MR are considered to be the most important and most reliable methods for the diagnosis of brain tumors. The sensitivity of these modalities in the detection of intracranial tumors approaches 100%. The extraordinary value of both methods is based not only on this high detection rate but also on their ability to localize tumors in relation to vital centers, assess their mass effect, and establish the tissue type of the lesion (= specificity).

The capabilities of CT and MR have been demonstrated in the preceding chapters, and the adjunctive role of other neuroradiologic procedures has been discussed. Here we shall briefly review these techniques and attempt to define their place in the diagnostic workup of neurologic and neurosurgical diseases.

Pneumoencephalography fell into disfavor after the introduction of CT and was used only occasionally for, say, the delineation of small suprasellar masses. This procedure has become obsolete since the introduction of MR imaging, which can detect even the smallest intrasellar tumors. The same is true of ventriculography, which has been completely superseded by less invasive techniques (Wende et al. 1982).

Radionuclide scanning for the detection of brain tumors, once widely practiced, was relegated to a secondary position by the advent of CT. Today, with the availability of CT and MR, isotope scans are rarely if ever performed.

New imaging techniques such as PET (positron emission tomography) and SPECT (single photon emission computed tomography) have not yet gained wide clinical application. They are very costly and are available at only a few centers.

The real domain of nuclear medicine is in function studies such as blood flow measurements in cerebrovascular disease, although this type of disease can be evaluated more effectively by serial cerebral angiograms, especially in patients with asymptomatic stenoses, transient ischemic attacks (TIA), and prolonged intermittent neurologic deficits (PRIND). *Doppler sonography* is an appropriate adjunct in these conditions owing to its high accuracy in detecting vascular stenoses in the extracranial portion of the carotid artery. Recent technical advances in this technique include two-dimensional real-time imaging of the cervical vessels and transcranial Doppler sonography, which is gaining in importance.

Regarding the role of *cerebral angiography*, it is still standard practice at most neurosurgical centers to perform angiography prior to neurosurgical intervention in patients with positive CT or MR scans, except in a few situations such as posttraumatic hematoma, classic hypertensive mass hemorrhage, and cerebellar neoplasms. Angiography is the only means of gaining a clear impression of the tumor blood supply prior to surgery and establishing the location and configuration of the vessels that feed and drain heavily vascularized tumors. Angiography may be omitted in cases where CT and MR can define the large vessels supplying a tumor. This particularly applies to tumors of the sellar region as well as poorly vascularized low-grade gliomas and isolated meningiomas of the cerebral convexity.

Angiography continues to have an absolute indication, however: the detection of vascular lesions. While CT and MR can demonstrate the end result of a vascular occlusion, the brain infarct, they are unable to visualize smaller arteriosclerotic lesions in vessel walls. Small vascular occlusions also escape detection by CT and MR when there is an adequate collateral supply. Angiography is also the procedure of choice for diagnosing aneurysms, arteriovenous malformations, and inflammatory vascular lesions, even though most AV angiomas are clearly depicted on the MR image.

In patients evaluated for a *fresh subarachnoid hemorrhage*, CT should be performed first in order to establish the location and extent of the hemorrhage. The examination is simple, fast, and not very cost-intensive. MR, on the other hand, cannot demonstrate blood in the initial hours after the acute event, and it is unable to furnish a diagnosis even in the initial three to four days following the hemorrhage.

If the patient's condition permits, angiography should be the next study performed after CT, as it is the only way to demonstrate the aneurysm clearly and elucidate its vascular supply. The angiographic evaluation of an aneurysm should include not only the vessels in proximity to the hemorrhage but also the other large cerebral vessels. We know that some 8%–20% of aneurysm patients have multiple vascular malformations involving the cerebral vessels. The decisive question in selecting patients for panarteriography is whether or not operative treatment is proposed for asymptomatic aneurysms that have not previously bled. There is still diversity of opinion on this issue.

Sequelae to head injuries, malformations, and atrophic processes can be detected easily and cost-effectively with CT, and additional neuroradiologic studies are rarely necessary. MR imaging has little if any role in the evaluation of these disorders.

CT and MR can demonstrate any tumor or inflammatory process in the *orbital region*, and *sonography* is indicated as an adjunct. Only this combination can establish both the *site* and the *nature* of an orbital mass lesion.

What then is **the role of MR imaging in the evaluation of neurologic and neurosurgical diseases**? Our experience in this area is based on comparative studies of CT and MR conducted at participating centers in Berlin, Mainz, and Augsburg (Kazner et al. 1985; Kretzschmar et al. 1985) and on the *Recommendations on the optimum diagnostic utilization of MR imaging* proposed in 1986 by the MR study group of the German Society of Radiology (Felix, Berlin; Friedmann, Cologne; Frommhold, Tübingen; Lissner, Munich). These recommendations are summarized in Tables 14 and 15, which have been modified in the light of further experience acquired since early 1986.

In assessing the role of MR, it is convenient to divide intracranial tumors into tumors of the skull base, tumors of the cerebrum and midline, and tumors of the posterior fossa.

There is no question but that MR is more sensitive than CT in detecting soft-tissue masses of the *skull base*. There are no troublesome artifacts from bone, and the MR study provides a natural, primary subtraction image. This can also be a disadvantage, however, since bone defects and other bony changes are not visualized. In a patient with suspected olfactory groove meningioma, for example, CT would be the preferred modality for demonstrating the neoplasm.

Thus, while MR is better able to define the extent of a soft-tissue tumor, CT is superior for demonstrating subtle bone changes. There are cases, therefore, in which CT and MR provide complementary information, and each modality should be employed to overcome the limitations of the other.

Larger *pituitary neoplasms* are readily demonstrated by CT. High-resolution thin-section CT is required for the detection of microadenomas, and even the smallest of these lesions are displayed with clarity following the bolus injection of contrast material. In patients with larger pituitary tumors, MR offers the advantage of demonstrating not only the tumor but also its relation to the carotid arteries and cavernous sinus. It is anticipated that *thinner MR sections* will prove superior to thin-section CT studies in the detection of microadenomas.

MR is decidedly superior to CT in detecting *tumors of the clivus and pons*. The clivus is well delineated on MR images owing to its content of fatty bone marrow, and bone changes involving the clivus are readily demonstrated. A distinct advantage of MR is its ability to determine whether a tumor is intra- or extra-axial in location. CT lacks this capability, and often it is impossible to determine whether a "brainstem tumor" on the CT scan actually arises from the brainstem or whether it is a clivus tumor infiltrating or displacing the brainstem. MR images in the coronal or midsagittal projection can resolve this question.

MR is also superior to CT in demonstrating the extension of pontine tumors such as pilocytic or fibrillary astrocytomas into the medulla oblongata or spinal cord. An accurate assessment of this extension is important in planning effective radiotherapy.

CT is very sensitive (> 90%) in detecting *malignant tumors of the cerebrum* such as glioblastomas, high-grade astrocytomas, anaplastic oligodendrogliomas, and metastases. CT findings also are very specific in terms of suggesting a histologic diagnosis. This speci-

Table 14. Comparison of CT and MR in the diagnosis of intracranial tumors (from *Recommendations on the optimum diagnostic utilization of MR imaging*, German Society of Radiology, January 1986; supplemented, modified, and expanded)

Tumor type/location	Value of MR relative to CT	Remarks
Astrocytoma (II)	MR≫CT	Advantages of MR: high sensitivity owing to good contrast resolution, superior definition of extent
Astrocytoma, anaplastic (III)[a]	MR=CT	Often neither modality can clearly distinguish tumor from edema
Oligodendroglioma, mixed glioma	MR≥CT	Only larger tumor calcifications are seen with MR, so specificity is higher with CT; but MR is superior for defining extent
Glioblastoma[a]	MR=CT	
Pilocytic astrocytoma	MR>CT	Advantages of MR: demonstration of tumor at all major sites without artifacts, free plane selection, usually good demarcation from brainstem
Pontine glioma	MR> CT	Advantages of MR: demonstration of tumor without artifacts, superior definition of tumor boundaries and extent
Ependymoma	MR≥CT	Advantages of MR: allows better evaluation of adjacent brain structures, especially the region of the foramen of Monro, the pineal region, and the fourth ventricle Advantage of CT: demonstration of calcifications
Medulloblastoma	MR>CT	Advantages of MR: demonstration of tumor without artifacts, arbitrary plane selection
Malignant lymphoma	MR>CT	Advantage of MR: superior demonstration of diffuse tumor growth
Pineal tumors	MR≥CT	Advantages of MR: high sensitivity, excellent definition of surrounding anatomic structures on midsagittal view Advantage of CT: better demonstration of calcifications
Meningioma[a]	MR≤CT	Advantages of CT: high sensitivity and *specificity*, demonstration of calcifications. MR is comparable only with Gd-DTPA enhancement, is superior only for lesions at the skull base and craniospinal junction
Acoustic neurinoma	MR>CT	Advantages of MR: demonstration of intrameatal tumor without cisternal gas insufflation, concurrent visualization of intra- and extrameatal tumor components; more sensitive than CT, free of artifacts. Neither modality is superior for larger tumors, although MR, with its multiplanar capacity, can better define the relation of the tumor to the brainstem. Gd-DTPA enhancement is necessary for MR
Pituitary adenoma	MR≥CT	Advantages of MR: demonstration of tumor without artifacts on any desired plane, assessment of its relations to the major arteries, cavernous sinus, and midline structures. CT and MR are about equal in detecting microadenomas
Hemangioblastoma	MR≥CT	CT can demonstrate practically all hemangioblastomas, but MR defines anatomic relations better and without artifacts (posterior fossa!). Gd-DTPA enhancement gives excellent definition of the tumor nodule
Hamartoma (of temporal lobe)	MR>CT	MR demonstrates the tumor without artifacts, is more sensitive than CT
Craniopharyngioma	MR≥CT	Advantages of MR: confident differentiation from pituitary adenoma owing to signal intensity of cyst contents, arbitrary plane selection, no artifacts Advantage of CT: demonstration of typical calcifications
Colloid cyst, third ventricle	MR=CT	CT is satisfactory except for cases with isodense cyst contents
Lipoma	MR=CT	CT is almost always satisfactory

Table 14 (continued)

Epidermoid, dermoid, teratoma	MR≥CT	Advantages of MR: artifact-free demonstration of the tumor, which usually lies near the skull base or in the posterior fossa; detailed visualization of tumor contents CT: generally satisfactory; can demonstrate calcifications, supporting the diagnosis
Skull base tumors	MR=CT	Advantage of MR: demonstration of soft tumor components in the bony skull base Advantage of CT: visualization of bony changes The two modalities are complementary
Metastases[a]	MR=CT	MR and CT have roughly equal value except in the posterior fossa. MR is usually unnecessary if an optimum CT scan is obtained

[a] CT and MR are of equal value after Gd-DTPA enhancement.

ficity applies not just to cerebral malignancies but also to benign *meningiomas*. MR imaging may be omitted in the workup of many these tumors, as there are only a few cases in which it will yield significant additional information.

The situation is somewhat different with *low-grade astrocytomas* and uncalcified *oligodendrogliomas*, which may produce a negative CT scan in their early stages. In some cases CT may show only an effacement of cortical gyri directing suspicion toward the presence of a tumor. These low-grade astrocytomas are considered to be an absolute indication for MR, because they can always be detected with that modality.

MR is the examination of choice for tumors of the midline, i.e., tumors located in the region of the third ventricle and of the pineal body, which occasionally are difficult to detect with CT. The midsagittal MR examination is particularly valuable and can provide information not obtainable with any other diagnostic method.

Most *posterior fossa tumors* such as medulloblastomas, pilocytic astrocytomas, ependymomas, and hemangioblastomas can be successfully evaluated with CT on the basis of their shape and location, their pattern of contrast enhancement, and their mass effect on surrounding brain. In many cases these features are sufficient to provide a precise histologic diagnosis. Again, however, MR is superior in defining the tumor extent, especially when Gd-DTPA is used, owing to the absence of bone artifacts and the capacity for variable plane selection. MR is far superior to CT in defining the relations of a tumor to the floor of the fourth ventricle and to the brainstem.

Tumors in the cerebellopontine angle (acoustic neurinomas) once were inaccessible to CT diagnosis if they were very small and did not extend beyond the internal auditory canal. Later the combination of CT and pneumocisternography became the examination of choice for these lesions (Sortland 1978). It was unnecessary to use positive contrast media, and angiography often was not required. Today MR is considered the optimum modality for detecting these tumors, and even the smallest intracanalicular neoplasms can be diagnosed owing to the marked rise of signal that occurs after the infusion of Gd-DTPA.

We may summarize the advantages and disadvantages of MR relative to CT in the detection of intracranial mass lesions as follows:

Advantages of MR

1. No artifacts from bone; no motion artifacts in cooperative patients.
2. Ability to image on multiple planes. Direct images on the sagittal and coronal planes are far superior to reformatted CT scans.
3. Excellent visualization of the craniocervical junction on multiple planes. CT cannot accomplish this with the same accuracy.
4. Differentiation between intra- and extra-axial tumors.
5. No exposure to ionizing radiation; no known side effects.

Table 15. Comparison of CT and MR in the diagnosis of non-neoplastic intracranial masses

Type of lesion	Value of MR relative to CT	Remarks
1. Inflammatory processes		
a) Brain abscess	MR=CT	Post Gd-DTPA MR is equivalent to postcontrast CT
b) Subdural empyema/epidural abscess	MR≥CT	Advantages of MR: high sensitivity, superior definition of extent, free plane selection
c) Meningoencephalitis	MR>CT	Advantages of MR: as above
2. Granulomas	MR=CT	Granulomas require contrast enhancement for clear definition on MR and CT
3. Parasites	MR=CT	Advantage of MR: more detailed depiction of lesions near the midline. Poor specificity Advantage of CT: better visualization of calcifications
4. AIDS-associated brain diseases	MR>CT	Advantage of MR: higher sensitivity
5. Cysts	MR=CT	
6. Postoperative lesions and radionecrosis	MR>CT	Advantage of MR: earlier and clearer depiction of changes in irradiated brain tissue
7. Acute demyelinating diseases Disseminated encephalomyelitis, diffuse sclerosis	MR>CT	Advantage of MR: high sensitivity (90% vs 50% in CT). MR specificity also higher than that of CT by detection of multiple peri- and paraventricular white matter lesions
8. Intracranial hemorrhages		
a) Spontaneous hemorrhages	MR<CT	Advantage of CT: high density values are specific for hemorrhage
b) Old hemorrhages, chocolate cysts	MR>CT	Advantage of MR: highly specific detection of blood even in isodense hematomas
9. Vascular malformations		
a) Aneurysms	MR>CT	Advantage of MR: signal void in perfused portions of a giant aneurysm is pathognomonic and distinguishes the lesion from a brain tumor
b) AV angiomas	MR>CT	Advantage of MR: signal void of flowing blood is pathognomonic even without contrast medium
10. Cerebral infarction	MR>CT	Advantages of MR: earlier detection than with CT, high sensitivity, visualization of pons and medulla oblongata without artifacts
11. Sinus thrombosis	MR>CT	Advantage of MR: direct visualization of the thrombosed vascular segment

Disadvantages of MR

1. High costs.
2. Problems in the examination of uncooperative or unconscious patients and of children. May be contraindicated in claustrophobic patients. Psychological preparation is essential.
3. Small calcifications in tumors (e.g., in oligodendrogliomas or craniopharyngiomas) usually are not visualized at conventional field strengths.
4. Nonvisualization of bony structures. Erosive bone changes are not demonstrated.
5. Poor specificity in identifying tumor types except when contrast media are used, lengthening the examination time.
6. Patients with cardiac pacemakers are not candidates for MR examination. Nor are patients who have undergone surgery for a brain tumor or aneurysm within the past 6 months that involved the insertion of ferromagnetic material (the field may dislodge metallic clips).

In summary, we would recommend the following approach to **selecting the most appropriate imaging modality or modalities for the diagnosis of brain tumors:**

Given the current availability of MR units, CT should be the initial examination for the diagnosis of brain tumors. If the initial CT scan is positive and gives adequate information on the site and nature of the tumor, it generally will be unnecessary to proceed with MR. However, if the surgeon requires additional information for planning an operative procedure and may reasonably expect to obtain that information from the MR image, then an MR examination should be performed.

If the initial CT study is negative or inconclusive *and* the patient manifests progressive neurologic deficits, MR should definitely be performed, as it is more sensitive than CT, particularly in detecting lesions of the midbrain or craniospinal junction as well as low-grade astrocytomas.

Thus, the optimum sequence of examinations must be determined on a case-by-case basis. The routine utilization of all modalities, especially CT and MR, would lead to exorbitant expense and would place an unnecessary burden on the patient.

Technical advances in MR imaging (shorter scan times, lower costs, thinner sections, increased use of contrast media) will undoubtedly broaden the role of this modality in the diagnosis of intracranial disease. The extent to which MR may supersede or replace other modalities, especially CT, remains unclear. At present MR is not available everywhere, and its costs remain extremely high. These high costs are a compelling reason to regard MR as something more than an adjunctive study. Given the capabilities of MR, and indeed its necessity in many cases, we can and must find ways to reduce the need for other diagnostic procedures.

Table 14 can easily give the impression that MR is superior to CT. However, when we consider the relative frequencies of the specific tumor types, a different picture emerges. In approximately 55% of all tumors (anaplastic astrocytomas, glioblastomas, cerebral metastases, meningiomas), the CT examination is entirely adequate or even superior to MR. In another 30% of patients the advantages of MR are relatively minor, and in only 15% is MR clearly and consistently superior to CT.

In the case of tumors which enhance intensely on contrast CT, such as meningiomas, glioblastomas, metastases, most anaplastic astrocytomas, and oligodendrogliomas, MR can equal the diagnostic value of CT only after contrast enhancement with Gd-DTPA.

It is noteworthy that the few authors to date who have critically compared the results of CT and MR in patients with brain tumors (Kazner et al. 1985; Kretzschmar et al. 1985; Bradley 1986; Haughton et al. 1986) were unable to demonstrate a general superiority of one modality over the other.

Given the current state of technology and especially the different numbers of CT and MR units currently available, CT and MR should be regarded as complementary examinations. In certain cases, however, both modalities should be available to the neuroradiologist and neurosurgeon in order to provide an optimum basis for decisions on how to proceed.

References

A. Introduction

Ambrose J (1974) Computerized x-ray scanning of the brain. J Neurosurg 40:679–695

Berger H (1929) Über das Elektrenkephalogramm des Menschen. Arch Psychiatr Nervenkr 87:527–570

Bloch F, Hansen WW, Packard M (1946) Nuclear induction. Phys Rev 70:474–485

Dandy WE (1918) Ventriculography following the injection of air into the cerebral ventricles. Ann Surg 68:5–11

Dandy WE (1919) Roentgenography of brain after injection of air into spinal canal. Ann Surg 70:397–403

Di Chiro G, Brooks RA (1979) The 1979 nobel prize in physiology or medicine. Science 206:1060–1062

Hounsfield GN (1973) Computerized transverse axial scanning (tomography): Part I. Description of system. Br J Radiol 46:1016–1022

Hounsfield GN (1976) Historical notes on computerized axial tomography. J Can Assoc Radiol 27:135–142

Lauterbur PC (1973) Image formation by induced local interactions: examples employing nuclear magnetic resonance. Letter to the editor. Nature 242:190–191

Leksell L (1955/1956) Echo-encephalography. I. Detection of intracranial complications following head injury. Acta Chir Scand 110:301–315

Moniz E (1927) L'encephalographie artérielle, son importance dans la localisation des tumeurs cérébrales. Rev Neurol (Paris) 32:72

Moore GE (1948) Radioactive localization of brain tumors. J Am Med Wom Assoc 137:1228–1229

Purcell EM, Torrey HC, Pound RV (1946) Resonance absorption by nuclear magnetic moments in a solid. Phys Rev 69:37–38

Selverstone B, Solomon AK (1948) Radioactive isotopes in the study of intracranial tumors. Trans Am Neurol Assoc 73:115–119

B. Classification of Brain Tumors

Ackerman LV, Rosai J (1974) Surgical pathology, 5th edn. Mosby, St Louis, pp 1248–1249

Andres KH (1967) Über die Feinstruktur der Arachnoidea und Dura mater von Mammalia. Z Zellforsch 79:272–295

Bailey P (1932) Cellular types in primary tumors of the brain. In: Penfield W (ed) Cytology and cellular pathology of the nervous system, vol III. Hafner, New York, pp 905–951

Bailey P, Bucy PC (1929) Oligodendrogliomas of the brain. J Path Bact 32:735–751

Bailey P, Cushing H (1926) A classification of the tumors of the glioma group on a histogenetic base with a correlated study of prognosis. Lippincott, Philadelphia

Bailey P, Cushing H (1930) Gewebsverschiedenheit der Hirngliome. Fischer, Jena

Bailey P, Hiller G (1924) The interstitial tissues of the central nervous system. J Nerv Ment Dis 59:337–361

Bergstrand H (1932) Über das sogenannte Astrocytom des Kleinhirns. Virchows Arch 287:538–548

Broders AC (1926) Carcinoma: grading and practical application. Arch Path 2:376–380

Bruns L (1914) Klinik der Hirngeschwülste. In: Krause F (Hrsg) Die allgemeine Chirurgie der Gehirnkrankheiten, Bd II (neue deutsche Chirurgie, Bd 12). Enke, Stuttgart, S 19–104

Bunge RP, Bunge MB, Ris H (1962) Electron microscopic observations on normal, demyelinating, and remyelinating white matter. proc IV. Internat Congr Neuropath, Bd 11. Thieme, Stuttgart, S 136–142

Cooper ERA (1935) The relation of oligocytes and astrocytes in cerebral tumours. J Path Bact 41:259–266

Earle K (1980) Persönl Mitteilung

Eder M (1977) Pathologie des Wachstums und der Differenzierung. In: Eder M, Gedigk P (Hrsg) Lehrbuch der allgemeinen Pathologie und der pathologischen Anatomie, 30. Aufl. Springer, Berlin Heidelberg New York, S 240

Fleischhauer K (1972) Ependyma und subependymal layer. In: Bourne GH (ed) The structure and function of nervous tissue, vol VI. Academic Press, New York London, pp 1–46

Friede RL (1978) Gliofibroma: a peculiar neoplasia of collagen forming glia-like cells. J Neuropathol Exp Neurol 37:300–313

Friede RL, Pollak A (1978) The cytogenic basis for classifying ependymomas. J Neuropathol Exp Neurol 37:103–118

Golgi C (1894) Untersuchungen über den feineren Bau des centralen und peripheren Nervensystem. Fischer, Jena

Gullotta F, Schindler F, Schmutzler R, Weeks-Seifert (1985) GFAP in brain tumor diagnosis: possibilities and limitations. Pathol Res Pract 180:54–60

Henschen F (1934) Referat über Gliome. Verh Dtsch Pathol Ges 27. Tagg. Fischer, Jena, S 8–39

Henschen F (1955) Tumoren des Zentralnervensystems und seiner Hüllen. In: Scholz W (Hrsg) Handb spez path Anat, Bd XIII/3. Springer, Berlin Göttingen Heidelberg, S 413–1040

Hofer H (1965) Die circumventrikulären Organe des Zwischenhirns. In: Hofer H, Schultz AH, Starck D (Hrsg) Handb Primat, Bd II. Lief 13. Karger, Basel New York

Hortega P del Río (1921) La glia de escasas radiaciónes (oligodendroglia). Arch Neurobiol (Madr) 2:Nr 1

Jellinger K (1977) Geschwülste des Nervensystems und seiner Anhänge. In: Holzner JH (Hrsg) Spezielle Pathologie II, 2. Aufl. Urban & Schwarzenberg, Berlin Wien Baltimore, S 217

Jellinger K, Radaszkiewicz Th (1976) Involvement of the central nervous system in malignant lymphomas. Virchows Arch A 370:345–362

Kaufmann E (1922) Lehrbuch der speziellen pathologischen Anatomie, 7. und 8. Aufl, Bd II. de Gruyter, Berlin Leipzig, S 1488 ff

Kepes JJ (1979) "Xanthomatous" lesions of the central nervous system: definition, classification and some recent observations. In: Zimmerman HM (ed) Progress in Neuropathology, vol 4. Raven, New York, pp 197–213

Kepes JJ, Rubinstein LJ, Eng LF (1979) Pleomorphic xanthoastrocytoma: a distinctive meningocerebral glioma of young subjects with relatively favorable prognosis. Cancer 44:1839–1852

Kernohan JW, Mabon RF, Svien HJ, Adson AW (1949) A simplified classification of the gliomas. Proc Staff Meet Mayo Clin 24:71–75

Kleihues P, Schultze B (1968) Zellproliferation und Proteinsynthese der Neuroglia beim experimentellen Hirnödem. Acta Neuropathol (Berlin) [Suppl] IV:121–124

Koelliker A (1896) Handbuch der Gewebelehre des Menschen. 6. Aufl. Bd II. Engelmann, Leipzig

Kuhlendahl H, Stochdorph O (1968) Über das Vorkommen des sog Kleinhirnastrocytoms (Bergstrand-Tumor) im Großhirn. Beitr Neurochir, H 15. Barth, Leipzig

Lenhossék Mv (1895) Der feinere Bau des Nervensystems im Lichte neuester Forschungen. Fischer, Berlin

Leonhardt H (1980) Ependym und circumventriculäre Organe. In: Oksche A (Hrsg) Handb, mikr Anat, Bd 4/10. Springer, Berlin Heidelberg New York, S 177–666

Lhermitte J, Duclos P (1920) Sur un ganglioneurome diffus du cortex du cervelet. Bull Assoc Franc Etude Cancer 9:99–106

Merrem G (1962) Die klinisch-biologische Wertigkeit der Hirngeschwülste. Sitzber Sächs Akad Wissensch Leipzig, Math-Nat Wiss Kl 105:H 2. Akademie-Verl Berlin

Niessing K (1980) Materialquelle, Entwicklung und Differenzierung der Neuroglia. In: Oksche A (Hrsg) Handb mikr Anat, Bd 4/10. Springer, Berlin Heidelberg New York, S 54–113

Penfield W (1932) Neuroglia: normal and pathological. In: Penfield W (ed) Cytoloy and cellular pathology of the nervous system, vol II. Hafner, New York, pp 423–479

Priesel A (1922) Über Gewebsmißbildungen in der Neurohypophyse und dem Infundibulum des Menschen. Virchows Arch 238:423–440

Ramón y Cajal S (1913) Contribución al conocimiento de la neuroglia del cerebro humano. Trab Lab Invest Biol Madrid 11:255–315

Ribbert H (1904) Geschwulstlehre für Ärzte und Studierende. Cohen, Berlin

Rindfleisch E (1878) Lehrbuch der pathologischen Gewebelehre, 5. Aufl. Engelmann, Leipzig

Ringertz N (1950) Grading of gliomas. Acta Path Scand 27:51–64

Ringertz N, Nordenstam H (1951) Cerebellar astrocytomas. J Neuropathol Exp Neurol 10:343–367

Rorke LB (1983) The cerebellar medulloblastoma and its relationship to primitive neuroectodermal tumors. J Neuropathol Exp Neurol 42:1–15

Rubinstein LJ (1972) Tumors of the central nervous system. Atlas of tumor pathology, 2nd ser, fasc 6. Armed Forces Institute of Pathology. Washington DC

Rubinstein LJ (1982) Tumors of the central nervous system. Atlas of tumor pathology, 2nd ser, fasc 6, Suppl. Armed Forces Institute of Pathology, Washington DC

Russell DS, Rubinstein LJ (1977) Pathology of tumours of the nervous system, 4th edn. Arnold, London

Scheithauer BW, Rubinstein LJ (1978) Meningeal mesenchymal chondrosarcoma. Cancer 42:2744–2752

Scherer HJ (1936) Etude sur les gliomes. Comportement des différents gliomes vis-à-vis des cellules ganglionnaires. Bull Assoc Franc Cancer 25:470–493

Schmincke A (1930) Zur Kenntnis der Zirbelgeschwülste. Ein Ganglioglioneurom der Zirbel. Beitr Pathol Anat 83:279–288

Sternberg C (1921) Ein Choristom der Neurohypophyse bei ausgebreiteten Ödemen. Zentralbl Pathol 31:585–591

Stochdorph O (1955) Die Gewebsbilder der Hirngewächse und ihre Ordnung. Veröff morph Path, H 60. Fischer, Stuttgart

Stochdorph O (1981) Klassifikation der Hirngeschwülste. In: Kazner E, Wende S, Grumme Th, Lanksch W, Stochdorph O (Hrsg) Computertomographie intrakranieller Tumoren. Springer, Berlin Heidelberg New York, S 2–16

Stroebe H (1895) Über Entstehung und Bau der Gehirngliome. Beitr Pathol Anat 18:405–486

Tumor-Histologie-Schlüssel (ICD-o-DA) (1978) Jacob W, Scheida D, Wingert F (Hrsg) Springer, Berlin Heidelberg New York

Virchow R (1862) Die Cellularpathologie in ihrer Begründung auf physiologische und pathologische Gewebelehre. Hirschwald, Berlin

Virchow R (1864–65) Die krankhaften Geschwülste, Bd I–III. Hirschwald, Berlin

Weindl A, Fahlbusch R, Stochdorph O (1975) Ultrastruktur eines Tumors der Lamina terminalis. Zentralbl Pathol 119:227

Weiser G, Aichner F, Mayr, U (1985) Elektronenmikroskopische Befunde bei einem Astroblastom. Verh Dtsch Ges Pathol 69. Tagg. Fischer, Stuttgart New York, S 470

Willis RA (1948) Pathology of tumours. Butterworth, London

Wolff JR (1980) Zit n Oksche A. Anmerkungen zum histologischen Überblick. In: Oksche A (Hrsg) Handb mikr Anat, Bd 4/10. Springer, Berlin Heidelberg New York, S 141–144

Zülch KJ (1956) Biologie und Pathologie der Hirngeschwülste. In: Olivecrona H, Tönnis W (Hrsg) Handb Neurochir, Bd III. Springer, Berlin Göttingen Heidelberg, S 1–702

Zülch KJ (1979) Histological typing of tumours of the central nervous system (Internat Histol Classific of Tumours, No 21). World Health Organisation. Geneva

Zülch KJ (1986) Brain tumors. Their biology and pathology. 3rd, completely rev. ed. Springer, Berlin Heidelberg New York Tokyo

C. Technique of CT and MR Examinations

General, Atlases, Monographs

Baert A, Jeanmart L, Wackenheim A (ed) (1978) Clinical computer tomography. Springer, Berlin Heidelberg New York

Caillé JM, Salamon G (1980) Computerized tomography. Springer, Berlin Heidelberg New York

Diebler C, Dulac O (eds) (1987) Pediatric neurology and neuroradiology. Cerebral and cranial diseases. Springer, Berlin Heidelberg New York London Paris Tokyo

Du Boulay GH, Moseley IF (eds) (1977) Computerised axial tomography in clinical practice. Springer, Berlin Heidelberg New York

Gonzalez CF, Grossman ChB, Palacios E (1976) Computed brain and orbital tomography. Techniques and interpretation. Wiley, New York London Sidney Toronto

Jabbour JT, Ramey DR, Roach St (1977) Atlas of computerized tomography scans in pediatric neurology. Med Examination Publ. Huber, Bern Stuttgart Wien

Kazner E, Lanksch W, Steinhoff H, Wilske J (1975) Die axiale Computer-Tomographie des Gehirnschädels: Anwendungsmöglichkeiten und klinische Ergebnisse. Fortschr Neurol Psychiatr 43:487–574

Krayenbühl H, Yasargil MG, Huber P (1979) Zerebrale Angiographie für Klinik und Praxis, 3. Aufl. Thieme Stuttgart

Kretschmann HJ, Weinrich W (1984) Neuroanatomie der kraniellen Computertomographie. Thieme, Stuttgart New York

Lange S, Grumme Th, Meese W (1977) Zerebrale Computer-Tomographie. Schering, Berlin

Lanksch W, Kazner E (eds) (1976) Cranial computerized tomography. Springer, Berlin Heidelberg New York

Latchaw RE (ed) (1985) Computed tomography of the head, neck and spine. Year Book Medical Publ, Chicago

Ledley RS, Huang HK, Mazziotta JC (1977) Cross-sectional anatomy – An atlas for computerized tomography. Williams & Wilkins, Baltimore

Lee SH, Rao KCVG (eds) (1983) Cranial computed tomography. McGraw-Hill, New York St Louis San Francisco Auckland Bogotá Guatemala Hamburg Johannesburg Lisbon London Madrid Mexico Montreal New Delhi Panama Paris San Juan Sao Paulo Singapore Sydney Tokyo Toronto

Lee SH, Rao KCVG (1987) Cranial computed tomography and MRI, 2nd edn. McGraw-Hill, New York St Louis San Francisco Auckland Bogotá Hamburg Johannesburg Lisbon London Madrid Mexico Milan Montreal New Delhi Panama Paris San Juan Sao Paulo Singapore Sydney Tokyo Toronto

Lindgren E (ed) (1975) Computer tomography of brain lesions. Acta Radiol [Suppl] (Stockh) 346

Mori K (1985) Anomalies of the central nervous system. In: Nadjmi M, Piepgras U, Vogelsang H (eds) Neuroradiology and neurosurgery. Thieme, Stuttgart New York

New PFJ, Scott WR (1975) Computed tomography of the brain and orbit (EMI-Scanning). Williams & Wilkins, Baltimore

Newton TH, Potts DG (eds) (1983) Advanced imaging techniques. In modern neuroradiology, vol 2. Clavadel, San Anselmo

Norman D, Korobkin M, Newton Th (eds) (1977) Computed tomography 1977. Mosby, St Louis

Oldendorf WH (1980) The quest for an image of brain computerized tomography in the perspective of past and future imaging methods. Raven, New York

Oliva L (ed) (1976) The new image in tomography. Excerpta Medica, Amsterdam Oxford

Piepgras U (1984) Neurokutane Systemerkrankungen. Thieme, Stuttgart New York

Quisling RG (1980) Correlative neuroradiology. A topographic approach to cerebral angiographic and CT interpretation. Wiley, New York Chichester Brisbane

Radü EW, Kendall BE, Moseley IF (1987) Computertomographie des Kopfes. Technische Grundlagen – Interpretation – Klinik, 2. Aufl. Thieme, Stuttgart New York

Ramsey RG (1977) Advances exercises in diagnostic radiology. Saunders, Philadelphia

Ramsey RG (1978) Computertomographie des Gehirns. In: Squire LF (Hrsg) Übungen in radiologischer Diagnostik, Bd VII. Thieme, Stuttgart

Rosenberg RN, Heinz ER (eds) (1984) Neuroradiology. In: The clinical neurosciences. Churchill Livingstone, New York Edinburgh London Melbourne

Ruggiero G, Sabattini L, Scialfa G (1979) Tomografia computerizzata del cervello. Il Pensiero Scientifico, Roma

Sager W-D, Ladurner G (Hrsg) (1979) Computertomographie. Derzeitige Stellung in Radiologie und Klinik. Thieme, Stuttgart

Salamon G, Huang YP (1980) Computed tomography of the brain. Springer, Berlin Heidelberg New York

Samii M (ed) (1986) Surgery in and around the brain stem and the third ventricle. Springer, Berlin Heidelberg New York

Sarwar M (ed) (1985) Computed tomography of congenital brain malformations. Nijhoff, Boston The Hague Dordrecht Lancester

Schinz (1986) Radiologische Diagnostik, Bd V, Teil 1: Schädel – Gehirn. Frommhold W, Dihlmann W, Stender H-St, Thurn P (Hrsg). Thieme, Stuttgart New York

Unsöld R, Ostertag CB, Degroot J, Newton TH (eds) (1982) Computer reformations of the brain and skull base. Anatomy and clinical application. Springer, Berlin Heidelberg New York

Vignaud J, Boulin A, Aubin ML, Berges O, Jardin C, Korach G, Le Roux B (1987) Tomodensitométrie cranio-encéphalique. Vigot, Paris

Wackenheim A, Babin E (1978) Tomodensitométrie cranio-cérébrale. Masson, Paris

Wackenheim A, du Boulay GH (eds) (1980) Choices and characteristics in computerized tomography. Kugler, Amsterdam

Weisberg LA, Nice C, Katz M (eds) (1978) Cerebral computed tomography. A text atlas. Saunders, Philadelphia London Toronto

Yamada H (ed) (1983) Pediatric cranial computed tomography. Igaku-Shoin, Tokyo New York

Yock DH jr (1985) Computed tomography of CNS disease. Year Book Medical Publ, Chicago

C.1. Technique of CT Examination

Ahmed M, Doe RP, Nuttall FQ (1974) Triiodothyronine thyrotoxicosis following iodide ingestion. A case report. J Clin Endocrinol Metab 38:574

Alexander RD, Berkes StL, Abuelo JG (1978) Contrast mediainduced oliguric renal failure. Arch Intern Med 138:381
Alta JF (1977) Computerized tomography of the head-part III. Nebr Med J 62:415–422
Ambrose J (1973) Computerized transverse axial scanning (tomography): Part 2. Clinical application. Br J Radiol 46:1023–1047
Ambrose J (1974) Computerized X ray scanning of the brain. J Neurosurg 40:679–695
Ambrose J (1974) The EMI scanner: clinical use. Br J Hosp Med 11:14–21
Ansari Z, Baldwin DS (1976) Acute renal failure due to radiocontrast agents. Nephron 17:28–40
Ansell G, Tweedie MCK, West CR, Price Evans DA, Couch L (1980) The current status of reactions due to intravenous contrast media. Invest Radiol 15:32–39
Balsys R, Janousek JE, Batnitzky S, Templeton AW (1979) Peripheral enhancement in computerized cranial tomography: a non-specific finding. Surg Neurol 11:207–216
Baltzer G (1978) Akutes Nierenversagen nach intravenöser Urographie bei Diabetikern – ein erhöhtes Risiko? Internist (Berlin) 19:649–651
Barshay ME, Kaye JH, Goldman R, Coburn JW (1973) Acute renal failure in diabetic patients after intravenous infusion pyelography. Clin Nephrol 1:35
Berdon WE, Schwartz RH, Becker J, Baker DH (1969) Tamm-Horsfall proteinuria. Radiology 92:714–722
Berezin AF (1977) Acute renal failure, diabetes mellitus, and scanning. Ann Intern Med 86:829–830
Bergman LA, Wilson MR, Dunea G (1968) Acute renal failure after drip-infusion pyelography. N Engl J Med 279:1277
Bergvall U (1975) Temporal course of contrast medium enhancement in differential diagnosis of intracranial lesions with computer tomography. In: Salamon G (ed) Advances in cerebral angiography. Springer, Berlin Heidelberg New York, pp 348–388
Blum M, Weinberg U, Shenkman L, Hollander CS (1974) Hyperthyroidism after iodinated contrast medium. N Engl J Med 291/1:24–25
Bockenheimer S (1980) Vorteile und Risiken der Meatozisternographie mit wässrigem Kontrastmittel. Laryngol Rhinol Otol (Stuttg) 59:786–789
Boroff RD, Pribram HFW (1978) Coronal and sagittal reconstruction in computerized tomography. Surg Neurol 9:85–93
Brown RC (1985) Re: Obtaining informed consent for intravenous contrast-enhanced radiography: Pros and Cons. (Letter to the editor). Radiology 155:256–257
Carvallo A, Rakowski TA, Argy WP Jr, Schreiner GE (1978) Acute renal failure following drip infusion pyelography. Am J Med 65:38
Cramer BC, Parfrey PS, Hutchinson AT, Baran D, Melanson DM, Ethier RE, Seely JF (1985) Renal function following infusion of radiologic contrast material. A prospective controlled study. Arch Intern Med 145/1: 87–89
Dahlstrom K, Andrew E, Sveen K (1982) The clinical evaluation of iohexol (Omnipaque). Farmakoterapi 3:58–65
Davis JM, Davis KR, Newhouse J, Pfister RC (1979) Expanded high iodine dose in computed cranial tomography: a preliminary report. Radiology 131:373–380
Dean RE, Andrew JH, Read RC (1964) The red cell factor in renal damage from angiographic media. J Am Med Wom Assoc 187:27–31
Diaz-Buxo JA, Wagoner RD, Hattery RR, Palumbo PJ (1975) Acute renal failure after excretory urography in diabetic patients. Ann Intern Med 83:155–158
Diebler C, Dulac O (eds) (1987) Pediatric neurology and neuroradiology. Cerebral and cranial diseases. Springer, Berlin Heidelberg New York London Paris Tokyo
Doust BD, Redman HC (1972) The myth of 1 ml/kg in angiography. Radiology 104:557–560
Drayer BP, Rosenbaum AE, Higman HB (1977) Cerebrospinal fluid imaging using serial metrizamide. CT cisternography. Neuroradiology 13:7–17
Du Boulay GH, Moseley IF (eds) (1977) Computerised axial tomography in clinical practice. Springer, Berlin Heidelberg New York
Du Boulay GH, Radu EW (1978) How should one investigate the posterior fossa? Neuroradiology 15:253–261
Dudzinski PJ, Petrone AF, Persoff M, Callaghan EE (1971) Acute renal failure following high-dose excretory urography in dehydrated patients. J Urol 106:619–621
Elke M, Ferstl A (1974) Notfallsituationen in der Röntgendiagnostik. Thieme, Stuttgart
Ethier R, Sherwin A, Taylor S (1975) Computerized angiotomography. The use of 100 cc Hypaque M 60%. Clinical and experimental results. Presented at the first International Symposium on Computerized Axial Tomography, Montreal 1974
Fiegler W, Langer M, Hedde JP, Scheer M, Felix R, Kazner E (1986) Vergleich von computertomographischen Veränderungen und klinischen Verläufen nach Bestrahlung von intrakraniellen Tumoren und Metastasen. Strahlenther Onkol 162:145–151
Fiegler W, Langer M, Scheer M, Kazner E (1986) Reversible computertomographische Veränderungen nach Hirntumorbestrahlung durch Strahlenfrühreaktion ("early-delayed-reaction"). Radiologe 26:206–209
Gado MH, Phelps ME, Coleman RE (1975) An extravascular component of contrast enhancement in cranial computed tomography. Part I: The tissue blood ratio of contrast enhancement. Radiology 117:589–593
Gado MH, Phelps ME, Coleman RE (1975) An extravascular component of contrast enhancement in cranial computed tomography. Part II: Contrast enhancement and the blood tissue barrier. Radiology 117:595–597
Gado MH, Eichling J, Currie M (1977) Quantitative aspects of CT images. In: Norman D, Korobkin M, Newton ThH (eds) Computed tomography 1977. Mosby, St Louis
Glanz S, Geehr RB, Duncan ChC, Piepmeier JM (1980) Metrizamide-enhanced CT for evaluation of brainstem tumors. AJNR 1:31–34
Gleysteen JJ, Aldrete JS, Rutsky EA (1976) Cholegraphy-induced acute renal failure: Its relation to subsequent surgical therapy. South Med J 69:173–176
Grainger RG (1979) Formulation and clinical introduction of low osmolality contrast media. 3. Asian-Oceanian Congress of Radiology, Singapore, 28. Oct–3. Nov 1979
Greitz T, Hindmarsh T (1974) Computer assisted tomography of intracranial CSF circulation using a watersoluble contrast medium. Acta Radiol 15:497–507
Hammer B (1980) Experiences with intrathecally enhanced computed tomography. Neuroradiology 19:221–228
Hammer B (1984) Soll bei der CT-Untersuchung des Hirnin-

farktes Kontrastmittel gegeben werden? Radiology 24/5:235–239
Hammer B, Deisenhammer E (1985) Iotrol, a new water-soluble non-ionic dimeric contrast medium for intrathecal use. Neuroradiology 27:337–341
Hanaway J, Black J (1977) Renal failure following contrast injection for computerized tomography. J Am Med Wom Assoc 238:2056
Hayman LA, Evans RA, Hinck VC (1979) Rapid high dose (RHD) contrast computed tomography of perisellar vessels. Radiology 131:121–123
Hayman LA, Evans RA, Fahr LM, Hinck VC (1980) Renal consequences of rapid high dose contrast CT. AJNR 1:9–11
Hayman LA, Evans RA, Hinck VC (1980) Delayed high iodine dose contrast computed tomography. Cranial neoplasms. Radiology 136:677–684
Herrmann J, Krüskemper HL (1978) Gefährdung von Patienten mit latenter und manifester Hyperthyreose durch jodhaltige Röntgenkontrastmittel und Medikamente. Dtsch Med Wochenschr 103:1434–1443
Hindmarsh T (1975) Elimination of water-soluble contrast media from the subarachnoid space. Investigation with computer tomography. Acta Radiol 346:45–49
Hindmarsh T (1977) Computer cisternography for evaluation of CSF flow dynamics. Acta Radiol 355:269–279
Hobbs BB (1981) Adverse reactions to intravenous contrast agents in Ontario, 1975–1979. J Assoc Canadienne Radiol 31:8–10
Holtas S (1984) Iohexol in patients with previous adverse reactions to contrast media. Invest Radiol 19/6:563–565
Hounsfield GN (1980) Computed medical imaging. Nobel Lecture, Dec 8, 1979. J Comput Assist Tomogr 4:655–674
Huck W (1978) The combined use of horizontal and frontal CT-scanning in intracranial lesions. Surg Rev 1:133–138
Huckman MS (1975) Clinical experience with the intravenous infusion of iodinated contrast material as an adjunct to computed tomography. Surg Neurol 4:297–318
Isherwood I, Pullan BR, Ritchings RT (1978) Radiation dose in neuroradiological procedures. Neuroradiology 16:477–481
Jacobs L, Kinkel W (1976) Computerized axial transverse tomography in normal pressure hydrocephalus. Neurology (Minneap) 26:501–507
Just HW, Goldenberg M (1979) Computed tomography of the enlarged cisterna magna. Radiology 131:385–391
Kamdar A, Weidmann P, Makoff DL, Massry SG (1977) Acute renal failure following intravenous use of radiographic contrast dyes in patients with diabetes mellitus. Diabetes 26:643–649
Kazner E, Lanksch W (1977) Computertomographische Strukturanalyse pathologischer Prozesse im Schädelinnenraum. Festschr Klinikum Großhadern. II. Teilinbetriebnahme 1977. Demeter, Gräfelfing
Kirkpatrick JB (1978) The blood-brain barrier: Its role in contrast studies. Comput Tomogr 2:189–196
Kleinknecht D, Deloux J, Homberg JC (1974) Acute renal failure after intravenous urography: Detection of antibodies against contrast media. Clin Nephrol 2:116–119
Kramer RA, Janetos GP, Perlstein G (1975) An approach to contrast enhancement in computed tomography of the brain. Radiology 116:641–647
Krumlovsky FA, Simon N, Subramanyam S, Greco F del, Roxe D, Pomaranc MM (1978) Acute renal failure. Association with administration of radiographic contrast material. J Am Med Wom Assoc 239:125–127
Lalli AF (1980) Contrast media reactions: Data analysis and hypothesis. Radiology 139:1–12
Lanksch W, Oettinger W, Baethmann A (1977) Diagnosis of brain edema using CT. Excerpta Medica. CT-Symposium, 10. Sept, 1976 Amsterdam, pp 13–25
Lasser EC, Berry C, Talner L, Santini L, Lang E, Study Participants (1984) National study of contrast media reactions (NSCMR) preliminary communication Association of University Radiologists 32nd Annual Meeting, Newport Beach, California 1984
Latchaw RE, Payne JR, Gold LHA (1978) Effective atomic number and electron density as measured with a computed tomography scanner: computation and correlation with brain tumor histology. J Comput Assist Tomogr 2:199–208
Latchaw RE, Payne JTh, Loewenson RB (1980) Predicting brain tumor histology: Change of effective atomic number with contrast enhancement. AJNR 1:289–294
Lewander R, Bergström M, Bergvall U (1978) Contrast enhancement of cranial lesions in computed tomography. Acta Radiol [Diagn] (Stockh) 19:529–552
Manelfe C, Guiraud B, Espagno J, Rascol A (1978) Cisternographie computérisée au metrizamide. Rev Neurol (Paris) 134:471–484
Maurer HJ (1980) Risiken bei Kontrastmitteluntersuchungen. Dtsch Ärztebl 77:1555–1564
McCullough EC, Payne Th (1978) Patient dosage in computed tomography. Radiology 129:457–463
Meeker TC (1978) Computerized axial tomography and acute renal failure. J Am Med Wom Assoc 240:2247–2248
Morgan C, Hammack WJ (1966) Intravenous urography in multiple myeloma. N Engl J Med 275:77–79
Myers GH jr, Witten DM (1971) Acute renal failure after excretory urography in multiple myeloma. Am J Roentgenol 113:583–588
Naidich TP, Kricheff II, Leeds NE (1977) Computerized tomography of the tentorium cerebelli. In: du Boulay GH, Moseley IF (eds) Computerised axial tomography in clinical practice. Springer, Berlin Heidelberg New York, pp 29–35
Norman D, Korobkin M, Newton ThH (eds) (1977) Computed tomography 1977. Mosby, St Louis
Norman D, Enzmann DR, Newton ThH (1978) Comparative efficacy of contrast agents in computed tomography scanning of the brain. J Comput Assist Tomogr 2:319–321
Palin MR (1979) Contrast dose for enhancement of computed tomograms of the brain. Br J Radiol 52:620–623
Peeters FLM (1977) Einige Beispiele falsch negativer Diagnosen bei der Computer-Tomographie. Radiologe 17:171–176
Perry BJ, Bridges C (1973) Computerized transverse axial scanning (tomography): Part 3. Radiation dose considerations. Br J Radiol 46:1048–1051
Pierach CA (1979) Transitorische Urämie durch Kontrastmittel – ein Risikofaktor bei niereninsuffizienten Diabetikern. Dtsch Med Wochenschr 104:148–149
Pillay VKG, Robbins PC, Schwartz FD, Kark RM (1970) Acute renal failure following intravenous urography in

patients with longstanding diabetes mellitus and azotemia. Radiology 95:633–636
Pinto RS, Handel StF, Sadhu VK (1979) CT metrizamide cisternography in the recognition of intrasellar cistern. Am J Roentgenol 133:320–321
Port FK, Wagoner RD, Fulton RE (1974) Acute renal failure after angiography. Am J Roentgenol 121:544–550
Pullicino P, Kendall BE (1980) Contrast enhancement in ischaemic lesions. I. Relationship to prognosis. Neuroradiology 19:235–239
Rapoport S, Bookstein JJ, Higgins CB, Carey PH, Sovak M, Lasser EC (1982) Experience with metrizamide in patients with previous severe anaphylactoid reactions to ionic contrast agents. Radiology 143:321–325
Reimann H-J, Tauber R, Kramann B, Gmeinwieser J, Schmidt U, Reiser M (1986) Prämedikation mit H_1- und H_2-Rezeptorantagonisten vor intravenöser Kontrastmitteldarstellung der ableitenden Harnwege. Fortschr Röntgenstr 144/2:169–173
Robinson JS, Arzola DD, Moody RA (1980) Acute renal failure following cerebral angiography and infusion computerized tomography. Case report. J Neurosurg 52:111–112
Rosenbaum AE, Drayer BP (1977) CT cisternography with metrizamide. Acta Radiol [Suppl] (Stockh) 355:323–337
Sachs Ch, Ericson K, Erasmie U, Bergström M (1979) Incidence of basal ganglia calcifications on computed tomography. J Comput Assist Tomogr 3:339–344
Sackett JF, Strother CM, (1977) Computer tomography and subarachnoid metrizamide for evaluation of cerebrospinal fluid flow. Acta Radiol [Suppl] (Stockh) 355:338–344
Savoie JC, Massin JP, Thomopoulos P, Leger F (1975) Iodine-induced thyrotoxicosis in apparently normal thyroid glands. J Clin Endocrinol Metab 41:685
Schmidt RC (1980) Mental disorders after myelography with metrizamide and other water-soluble contrast media. Neuroradiology 19:153–157
Schöter I, Wappenschmidt J (1978) Difficulties in the interpretation of computerized tomography. Adv Neurosurg 6:131–136
Schrott KM, Behrends B, Clauss W, Kaufmann J, Lehnert J (1986) Iohexol in der Ausscheidungsurographie. Fortschr Med 7:153/51–156/54
Schwartz WB, Hurwitt A, Ettinger A (1963) Intravenous urography in the patient with renal insufficiency. N Engl J Med 269:277–283
Scott WR (1980) Seizures: A reaction to contrast media for computed tomography of the brain. Radiology 137:359–361
Shafi T, Chou SY, Porush JG, Shapiro WB (1978) Infusion intravenous pyelography and renal function. Effects in patients with chronic renal insufficiency. Arch Intern Med 138:1218–1221
Shehadi WH, Toniolo G (1980) Adverse reactions to contrast media. Radiology 137:299–302
Shrivastava PN, Lynn SL, Ting JY (1977) Exposures to patient and personel in computed axial tomography. Radiology 125:411–415
Slasky B, Lenkey JL (1981) Acute renal failure, contrast media, and computer tomography. Urology XVIII:309–313
Spring DB, Akin JR, Margulis AR (1984) Informed consent for intravenous contrast-enhanced radiography: A national survey of practice and opinion. Radiology 152:609–613
Sprung C, Grumme T (1979) Use of CT cisternography, RISA cisternography and the infusion test for predicting shunting results in normal pressure hydrocephalus (NPH). Adv Neurosurg 7:350–360
Steinhoff H, Lange S (1976) Principles of contrast enhancement in computerized tomography. In: Lanksch W, Kazner E (eds) Cranial computerized tomography. Springer, Berlin Heidelberg New York, pp 60–68
Swartz RD, Rubin JE, Leeming BW, Silva P (1978) Renal failure following major angiography. Am J Med 65:31
Talner LB (1972) Urographic contrast media in uremia. Radiol Clin North Am 10/3:421–432
Talner LB, Davidson AJ (1968) Renal hemodynamic effect of contrast media. Invest Radiol 3:310–317
Tschakert H (1983) Contrast medium tolerance in computed tomography. Fortschr Röntgenstr [Suppl] 118:156–161
Van Zee B, Hoy WE, Talley TE, Jaenike JR (1978) Renal injury associated with intravenous pyelography in nondiabetic and diabetic patients. Ann Intern Med 89:51–54
Wagoner RD (1978) Acute renal failure associated with contrast agents. Arch Intern Med 138:353
Wall BF, Green DAS (1979) The radiation dose to patients from EMI brain and body scanners. Br J Radiol 52:189–196
Warren SE, Bott JC, Thornfeldt C, Swerdlin AH, Steinberg SM (1978) Hazards of computerized tomography: Renal failure following contrast injection. Surg Neurol 10:335–336
Weinrauch LA, Healy RW, Leland OS jr, Goldstein HH, Kassissieh SD, Libertino JA, Takacs FJ, Elia JA de (1977) Coronary angiography and acute renal failure in diabetic azotemic nephropathy. Ann Intern Med 86:56–59
Weinrauch LA, Healy RW, Leland OSt jr, Goldstein HH, Libertino JA, Rakacs FJ, Bradley RF, Gleason RE, Elia JA de (1978) Decreased insulin requirement in acute renal failure in diabetic nephropathy. Arch Intern Med 138:399–402
Wende S, Speck U (1981) Das Kontrastmittel-Risiko bei der Computer-Tomographie. Radiologe 21:268–273
Wende S, Ludwig B, Simon RS, Kretzschmar K (1980) Hyperdensity factors. In: Caille JM, Salamon G (eds) Computerized tomography. Springer, Berlin Heidelberg New York, pp 146–151
Wende S, Voigt K, Hammer B, du Boulay G, Scheithauer R (1986) Zur Problematik tödlicher Kontrastmittelzwischenfälle nach einer Computertomographie. Digitale Bilddiagn 6:15–17
Wing SD, Osborn AG (1977) Normal and pathologic anatomy of the corpus callosum by computed tomography. J Comput Assist Tomogr 1:183–192
Wing SD, Osborn AG, Wing RW (1978) The vertex scan: an important component of cranial computed tomography. Am J Roentgenol 130:765–767
Zimmerman RA, Bilaniuk LT, Gallo E (1978) Computed tomography of the trapped fourth ventricle. Am J Roentgenol 130:503–506
Zito JL, Davis KR, Hesselink JR (1980) Low-dose metrizamide cisternography with pluridirectional tomography: A useful adjunct to computed tomographic cisternography. Surg Neurol 14:169–174
Zülch KJ, Wende S (1977) The actual state of computerized tomography (CT) – computer assisted tomography (CAT). J Neurol 215:233–240

C.2. Technique of MR Examination

Berry I, Brant-Zawadzki M, Osaki L, Brasch R, Murovic J, Newton TH (1986) Gd-DTPA in clinical MR of the brain: 2. Extraaxial lesions and normal structures. Am J Neuroradiology 7:789–793

Bradley WG, Waluch V, Yadley RA, Wycoff RR (1984) Comparison of CT and MR in 400 patients with suspected disease of the brain and cervical spinal cord. Radiology 152:695–702

Brant-Zawadzki M, Davis PL, Crooks LE, Mills CM, Norman D, Newton TH, Sheldon P, Kaufman L (1983) NMR demonstration of cerebral abnormalities: Comparison with CT. Am J Roentgenol 140:847–854

Brant-Zawadzki M, Norman D, Newton TH, Kelly WM, Kjos B, Mills CM, Dillon W, Sobel D, Crooks LE (1984) Magnetic resonance of the brain: The optimal screening technique. Radiology 152:71–77

Brant-Zawadzki M, Berry I, Osaki L, Brasch R, Murovic J, Norman D (1986) Gd-DTPA in clinical MR of the brain: 1. Intraaxial lesions. Am J Neuroradiology 7:781–788

Brant-Zawadzki M, Norman D (eds) (1987) Magnetic resonance imaging of the central nervous system. Raven, New York

Brasch RC (1983) Work in Progress: Methods of contrast enhancement for NMR imaging and potential applications. Radiology 147:781–788

Bydder GM, Young IR (1985) MR imaging: Clinical use of the inversion recovery sequence. J Comput Assist Tomogr 9:659–675

Bydder GM, Kingsley DPE, Brown J, Niendorf HP, Young IR (1985) MR imaging of meningiomas including studies with and without Gadolinium-DTPA. J Comput Assist Tomogr 9:690–697

Carr DH, Brown J, Bydder GM, Weinmann HJ, Speck U, Thomas DJ, Young IR (1984) Intravenous chelated Gadolinium as a contrast agent in NMR imaging of cerebral tumours. Lancet 1:484–486

Carr DH, Brown J, Bydder GM, Steiner RE, Weinmann HJ, Speck U, Hall AS, Young IR (1984) Gadolinium-DTPA as a contrast agent in MRI: Initial clinical experience in 20 patients. Am J Roentgenol 143:215–224

Claussen C, Laniado M, Kazner E, Schörner W, Felix R (1985) Application of contrast agents in CT and NMR: Their potential in imaging of brain tumors. Neuroradiology 27:164–171

Claussen C, Laniado M, Schörner W, Niendorf HP, Weinmann HJ, Fiegler W, Felix R (1985) The use of Gadolinium-DTPA in magnetic resonance imaging of glioblastomas and intracranial metastases. Am J Neuroradiology 6:669–674

Claussen C, Laniado M, Weinmann HJ, Schörner W (1987) Paramagnetic contrast media in magnetic resonance. In: Taveras JM, Ferrucci JT (eds) Radiology, vol 3. Lippincott, Philadelphia, pp 1–11

Felix R, Semmler W, Schörner W, Laniado M (1985) Kontrastmittel in der magnetischen Resonanztomographie. Eine Übersicht. Teil 1: Physiko-chemische und pharmakologische Grundlagen von MR-Kontrastmitteln am Beispiel von Gadolinium-DTPA. Fortschr Röntgenstr 142:641–646

Felix R, Schörner W, Laniado M, Semmler W (1985) Kontrastmittel in der magnetischen Resonanztomographie. Eine Übersicht. Teil 2: Biologische Grundlagen, Untersuchungstechnik und klinische Anwendung von Gadolinium-DTPA in der Diagnostik intracranieller Tumoren. Fortschr Röntgenstr 143:9–14

Felix R, Schörner W, Laniado M, Niendorf HP, Claussen C, Fiegler W, Speck U (1985) Brain tumors: MR imaging with Gadolinium-DTPA. Radiology 156:681–688

Gademann G (1984) NMR-tomography of the normal brain. Springer, Berlin Heidelberg New York

Graif M, Bydder GM, Steiner RE, Niendorf HP, Thomas DGT, Young IR (1985) Contrast-enhanced MR imaging of malignant brain tumors. Am J Neuroradiology 6:855–862

Grodd W, Brasch RC (1986) Magnetopharmazeutische Kontrastveränderungen in der Kernspintomographie. Fortschr Röntgenstr 145:130–139

Haase A, Frahm J, Matthaei D, Hänicke W, Merboldt KD (1986) FLASH imaging. Rapid NMR imaging using low flip-angle pulses. J Magn Reson 67:217–225

Heindel W, Steinbrich W, Friedmann G (1986) Magnetische Resonanztomographie (MR) bei Hirntumoren: Gegenüberstellung der Ergebnisse Multiechotechnik und Gadolinium-DTPA. Fortschr Röntgenstr 145:158–162

Henning J, Nauerth A, Friedburg H, Ratzel D (1984) Ein neues Schnellbildverfahren für die Kernspintomographie. Radiologe 24:579–580

Higer HP, Bielke G (1986) Gewebecharakterisierung mit T_1, T_2 und Protonendichte: Traum und Wirklichkeit. Fortschr Röntgenstr 144:597–605

Kilgore DP, Breger RK, Daniels DL, Pojunas KW, Williams AL, Haughton VM (1986) Cranial tissues: Normal MR appearance after intravenous injection of Gd-DTPA. Radiology 160:757–761

Kressel HY (ed) (1986) Magnetic resonance annual. Raven, New York

Kressel HY (ed) (1987) Magnetic resonance annual. Raven, New York

Laniado M, Weinmann HJ, Schörner W, Felix R, Speck U (1984) First use of Gd-DTPA/dimeglumine in man. Physiol Chem Phys Med NMR 16:157–165

Laniado M, Niendorf HP, Schörner W, Felix R (1986) Spin-echo and inversion-recovery sequences for Gadolinium-DTPA-enhanced MRI of intracranial tumors. Acta Radiol [Suppl] 369:469–471

Lissner J, Seiderer M (Hrsg) (1987) Klinische Kernspintomographie. Enke, Stuttgart

Loeffler W, Oppelt A (1981) Physical principles of the NMR tomography. Eur J Radiol 1:338–344

Maravilla KR, Mickey B, Peshock RM, Weinreb JC, Riley HK, Diehl J (1986) Tumor characterization by Gd-DTPA-enhanced magnetic resonance imaging. In: Runge VM, Claussen C, Felix R, James AE (eds) Contrast agents in magnetic resonance imaging. Excerpta Medica, Princeton, pp 106–110

Margulis AR, Higgins CB, Kaufman L, Crooks LE (eds) (1983) Clinical magnetic resonance imaging. Radiology Research and Education Foundation, San Francisco

Niendorf HP, Semmler W, Laniado M, Felix R (1986) Some aspects of the use of contrast agents in magnetic resonance imaging. Diagn Imag Clin Med 55:25–36

Niendorf HP, Laniado M, Semmler W, Schörner W, Felix R (1987) Dose administration of Gadolinium-DTPA in MR of intracranial tumors. An intraindividual study. Am J Neuroradiology 8:803–815

Oppelt A, Graumann R, Barfuß H, Fischer H, Hartl W, Schajor W (1986) FISP: Eine neue schnelle Pulssequenz für die Kernspintomographie. Electromedica 54:15–18
Partain L, James AE, Rollo RD, Price RD (eds) (1983) Nuclear magnetic resonance. Saunders, Philadelphia London
Price AC, Runge VM (1986) Optimization of pulse sequence in Gd-DTPA enhanced magnetic resonance imaging. In: Runge VM, Claussen C, Felix R, James AE (eds) Contrast agents in magnetic resonance imaging. Excerpta Medica, Princeton, pp 99–102
Pykett IL, Newhouse H, Buonanno FS, Brady TJ, Goldman MR, Kistler JP, Pohost GM (1982) Principles of nuclear magnetic resonance imaging. Radiology 143:157–168
Ramm B, Semmler W, Laniado M (1986) Einführung in die MR-Tomographie. Enke, Stuttgart
Rinck PA, Meindl S, Higer HP (1985) Brain tumors: Detection and typing by use of CPMG sequences and in vivo measurements. Radiology 157:103–106
Roth K (1984) NMR-Tomographie und -Spektroskopie in der Medizin. Springer, Berlin Heidelberg New York Tokyo
Runge VM, Schörner W, Niendorf HP, Laniado M, Köhler D, Claussen C, Felix R, James AE (1985) Initial evaluation of Gadolinium-DTPA for contrast-enhanced magnetic resonance imaging. Magn Reson Imaging 3:27–35
Runge VM, Clanton JA, Price AC, Herzer WA, Allen JH, Partain CL, James AE (1985) Evaluation of contrast-enhanced MR imaging in a brain-abscess model. Am J Neuroradiol 6:139–147
Runge VM, Claussen C, Felix B, James AE Jr (eds) (1986) Contrast agents in magnetic resonance imaging. Proceedings of an international workshop, January 1986, San Diego, California. Excerpta Medica, Amsterdam Hong Kong Princeton Sydney Tokyo
Sander B (1987) Improved clinical application of FLASH imaging using multi slice technique. Topical conference on fast magnetic resonance imaging techniques, 15.–17.5.1987, Cleveland
Schörner W, Felix R, Laniado M, Lange L, Weinmann HJ, Claussen C, Fiegler W, Speck U, Kazner E (1984) Prüfung des kernspintomographischen Kontrastmittels Gadolinium-DTPA am Menschen: Verträglichkeit, Kontrastbeeinflussung und erste klinische Ergebnisse. Fortschr Röntgenstr 140:493–500
Schörner W, Laniado M, Claussen C, Kazner E, Niendorf HP, Felix R (1986) Magnetische Resonanztomographie (MR) intracranieller Tumoren: Kontrastmittelanwendung versus T_2-gewichtete Tomogramme. Fortschr Röntgenstr 144:315–322
Schörner W, Laniado M, Niendorf HP, Schubert C, Felix R (1986) Time dependent changes in image contrast in brain tumors after Gadolinium-DTPA. Am J Neuroradiology 7:1013–1020
Semmler W, Felix R (1984) Kontraste in der Kernspintomographie. Fortschr Röntgenstr 141:259–267
Semmler W, Laniado M, Felix R (1985) Der Einfluß von Kontrastmitteln auf die Grauabstufung in der magnetischen Resonanztomographie. Fortschr Röntgenstr 142:123–130
Weinmann HJ, Brasch RC, Press WR, Wesbey GE (1984) Characteristics of Gadolinium-DTPA complex: A potential NMR contrast agent. Am J Roentgenol 142:619–624
Weinmann HJ, Laniado M, Mützel W (1984) Pharmacokinetics of Gadolinium-DTPA/dimeglumine after intravenous injection into healthy volunteers. Physiol Chem Phys Med NMR 16:167–171
Weiss T, Mitsch E, Laniado M, Sander B, Kornmesser W, Deimling M, Felix R (1987) Schnelle Kernspintomographie: Erste Untersuchungsresultate mit der neuen Gradienten-Echo-Sequenz. Fortschr Röntgenstr 146:214–222
Wende S, Thelen M (Hrsg) (1983) Kernspin-Tomographie in der Medizin. Theorie – Praxis – Klinische Ergebnisse. Springer, Berlin Heidelberg New York Tokyo

C.3. MR Spectroscopy

Aue WP, Müller S, Cross TA, Seelig J (1984) Volume-selective-excitation: A novel approach to topical NMR. J Mag Res 56:350–354
Baleriaux D, Arnold DA, Segebarth C, Luyten PR, den Hollander JA (1986) 31P MR-evaluation of human brain tumour response to therapy. Abstr Mag Res Med 1:41–42
Bruhn H, Frahm J, Gyngell ML, Merboldt KD, Hänicke W, Sauter R (1988) Localized proton spectroscopy of tumours in vivo. Abstr Soc Magn Reson Med 1:253
Heindel W, Bunke J, Steinbrich W, Friedmann G (1987) Human brain tumours: evaluation by image-guided localized P31 MR-spectroscopy. Abstr Mag Res Med 1:153
den Hollander J, Luyten PR (1987) Image guided localized ^{1}H and ^{31}P NMR spectroscopy of humans. NMR Ann NY Acad Sci 508:386–398
Luyten PR, den Hollander JA (1985) Target imaging using volume-selective-excitation. Abstr Soc Mag Res Med 2:1021
Luyten PR, den Hollander JA (1986) Observation of metabolites in the human brain by MR spectroscopy. Radiology 161:795–798
Luyten PR, Marien AJH, Sijtma B, den Hollander JA (1986) Solvent-suppressed spatially resolved spectroscopy. An approach to high-resolution NMR on a whole-body MR-system. J Mag Res 67:148–155
Luyten PR, Berkelbach vd Sprenkel JW, van Rijen PC, Tulleken CAF, den Hollander JA (1987) Cerebral lactate detected by localized ^{1}H NMR spectroscopy in patients with local infarction. Abstr Soc Mag Res Med 2:533
Marien AJH, Segebarth C, Baleriaux D, Luyten PR, den Hollander JA (1987) Quantitative analysis of localized ^{31}P NMR spectra of human brain tumors. Abstr Soc Mag Res Med 1:494
Ordidge RJ (1985) Localized chemical shift measurements in phosphorus and protons. Abstr Soc Mag Res Med 1:131–132
Roth K (1984) NMR Tomographie und Spektroskopie in der Medizin. Springer, Berlin Heidelberg New York Tokyo, S 31
Segebarth C, Baleriaux D, Arnold DL, Luyten PR, den Hollander J (1987) Image guided ^{31}P MR spectroscopy of human brain tumours in situ, effects of treatment. Radiology 165:215–219

D. Brain Tumors

General, Overviews

Allen JH (1977) Computerized tomography for diagnosis of brain neoplasms. J Tenn Med Assoc 70:18–20

Ambrose J (1973) Computerized transverse axial scanning of the brain. Proc R Soc Med 66:833–834

Ambrose J (1974) Computerized x-ray scanning of the brain. J Neurosurg 40:679–695

Amundsen P, Dugstad G, Syvertsen AH (1978) The reliability of computer tomography for the diagnosis and differential diagnosis of meningiomas, gliomas, and brain metastases. Acta Neurochir (Wien) 41:177–190

Araki T, Inouye T, Suzuki H, Machida T, Iio M (1984) Magnetic resonance imaging of brain tumors: Measurements of T_1. Radiology 150:95–98

Assmann II, Schäfer W, Schumann E, Stahl M, Schneider A (1977) The complex radiological diagnosis of brain tumours. Arch Geschwulstforsch 47:369–373

Aulich A, Wende S, Meese W, Meinig G, Reulen HJ (1976) Follow-up studies in cerebral tumors using CT. In: Lanksch W, Kazner E (eds) Cranial computerized tomography. Springer, Berlin Heidelberg New York, pp 135–142

Baker HL Jr, Houser OW (1976) Computed tomography in the diagnosis of posterior fossa lesions. Radiol Clin North Am 14:129–147

Baker HL Jr, Thomas JE (1975) Computierte transaxiale Tomographie des Kopfes (EMI-Scan). Klinische Erfahrung mit einer neuen diagnostischen Methode zur Hirnuntersuchung. Fortschr Röntgenstr 123:293–299

Baker HL Jr, Houser OW, Campbell JK (1980) National cancer institute study: Evaluation of computed tomography in the diagnosis of intracranial neoplasms. Radiology 136:91–96

Banna M, Molot MJ, Kapur PL, Groves J (1975) Computer tomography of the brain in Hamilton. Can Med Assoc J 113:303–307

Becker H, Bittenbring G (1977) Computer-Tomographie und klassische Neuroradiologie bei Problemfällen. Nervenarzt 48:663–669

Becker H, Schäfer M, Klös G (1976) Localization of recurrent brain tumors by means of computerized tomography. In: Lanksch W, Kazner E (eds) Cranial computerized tomography. Springer, Berlin Heidelberg New York, pp 143–150

Berger PE, Kirks DR, Gilday DL, Fitz ChR, Harwood-Nash DC (1976) Computed tomography in infants and children: intracranial neoplasms. Am J Roentgenol 127:129–137

Besenski N, Gvozdanovic V, Nutrizio V, Simunic S, Jelicic J, Lupret V (1978) Comparative study of computed tomography and ventriculography with water soluble contrast media. Neuroradiology 16:540–542

Bilaniuk LT, Zimmerman RA, Littman P, Gallo E, Rorke LB, Bruce DA, Schut L (1980) Computed tomography of brain stem gliomas in children. Radiology 134:89–95

Brant-Zawadzki M, Badami JP, Mills CM et al (1984) Primary intracranial tumor imaging: A comparison of magnetic resonance and CT. Radiology 150:435–440

Brismar J, Stromblad L-G, Salford LG (1978) Impact of CT in the neurosurgical management of intracranial tumors. Neuroradiology 16:506–509

Brooks RA, Di Chiro G (1976) Principles of computer assisted tomography (C.A.T.) in radiographic and radioisotopic imaging. Phys Med Biol 21:689–732

Buncher CR (1980) National cancer institute study: Evaluation of computed tomography in the diagnosis of intracranial neoplasms. II. Was randomization necessary? Radiology 136:651–655

Bydder GM, Pennock JM, Steiner RE et al. (1984) The NMR diagnosis of cerebral tumors. Magn Reson Med 1:5–29

Clar H-E, Bock WJ, Grote W, Nau HE, Weichert HC (1979) Klassifikation der Tumoren der Sellaregion mit Hilfe der Computertomographie (CT) und der Enzephalographie. Neurochirurgia (Stuttg) 22:153–159

Clar H-E, Bock WJ, Weichert HC (1979) Comparison of encephalotomograms and computerized tomograms in midline tumours in infants. Acta Neurochir (Wien) 50:91–101

Collard M, Dupont H (1975) Tomographie axiale transverse computérisée par Emi-Scanner. Résultat de 1000 observations. J Belge Radiol 58:289–328

Collard M, Dupont H (1977) L'apport clinique de la tomodensitometrie cérébrale (EMI-Scanner). Etude critique de 3000 dossiers. Acta Neurol Belg 77:230–242

Cushing H (1932) Intracranial tumors. Thomas, Springfield/IL

Davis DO (1977) CT in the diagnosis of supratentorial tumors. Semin Roentgenol 12:97–108

Davis DO, Pressman BD (1974) Computerized tomography of the brain. Radiol Clin North Am XII:297–313

Delavelle J, Megret M (1980) CT sagittal reconstruction of posterior fossa tumors. Neuroradiology 19:81–88

Dohrmann GJ, Geehr RB, Robinson F, Allen WE III, Orphanoudakis SC (1978) Small hemorrhages vs calcifications in brain tumors: difficulty in differentiation by computed tomography. Surg Neurol 10:309–312

Dosch JC, Wackenheim A (1978) Density of intracranial masses in computer tomography. J Belge Radiol 61:291–296

Du Boulay GH, Marshall J (1975) Comparison of EMI and radioisotope imaging in neurological disease. Lancet 2:1294–1297

Du Boulay GH, Teather D, Harling D, Clarke G (1977) Improvement in the computer-assisted diagnosis of cerebral tumors. Br J Radiol 50:849–854

El Gammal T, McDaniel FE (1979) The target sign: a CT finding in tumors of the corpus callosum. J Comput Assist Tomogr 3:533–535

Elke M, Wiggli U, Huenig R (1977) Praktische Gesichtspunkte zur Diagnose intracranieller Tumoren durch die Computer-Tomographie (CT). Radiologe 17:157–170

Englund E, Brun A, Larsson EM, Gyorffy-Wagner Z, Persson B (1986) Tumours of the central nervous system. Proton magnetic resonance relaxation times T_1 and T_2 and histopathologic correlates. Acta Radiol [Diagn] (Stockh) 27:653–659

Enzmann DR, Krikorian J, Yorke C, Hayward R (1978) Computed tomography in leptomeningeal spread of tumor. J Comput Assist Tomogr 2:448–455

Fahlbusch R, Grumme Th, Aulich A, Wende S, Steinhoff H, Lanksch W, Kazner E (1976) Suprasellar tumors in the CT scan. In: Lanksch W, Kazner E (eds) Cranial computerized tomography. Springer, Berlin Heidelberg New York, pp 114–127

Fischgold H (1977) La tomographie axiale transverse (CT) de la tête en Allemagne Fédérale. J Radiol Électrol 58:620, 640, 646

Fitz CR, Harwood-Nash DC, Resjo IM (1978) Metrizamide ventriculography and computed tomography in infants and children. Neuroradiology 16:6–9

Foerster O, Gagel O (1939) Das umschriebene Arachnoidalsarkom des Kleinhirns. Z Ges Neurol Psychiat 164:565–580

Gado M, Huete I, Mikhael M (1977) Computerized tomography of infratentorial tumors. Semin Roentgenol 12:109–120

Gardeur D, Metzger J (1978) Tomodensitométrie (CT Scanner) en pathologie tumorale intra-cranienne. Doin Editeurs, Paris

Gawler J (1976) Computerized tomography and conventional radiology in the investigation of intracranial and orbital disease. J Belge Radiol 59:225–238

Gawler J, du Boulay GH, Bull JWD, Marshall J (1974) Computer assisted tomography (EMI scanner). Its place in investigation of suspected intracranial tumours. Lancet II:419–423

Gawler J, du Boulay GH, Bull JWD, Marschall J (1976) A comparison of computer assisted tomography (EMI scanner) with conventional neuroradiologic methods in the investigation of patients clinically suspected of intracranial tumor. J Can Assoc Radiol 27:157–169

Gawler J, du Boulay GH, Bull JWD, Marshall J (1976) Computerized tomography (the EMI scanner): a comparison with pneumoencephalography and ventriculography. J Neurol Neurosurg Psychiatry 39:203–211

Gonzalez CF, Grossman ChB, Placios E (1976) Computed brain and orbital tomography. Wiley, New York London Sidney Toronto

Graif M, Steiner RE (1986) Contrast enhanced magnetic resonance imaging of tumours of the central nervous system: A clinical review. Br J Radiol 59:865–873

Greitz T (1975) Computer tomography for diagnosis of intracranial tumours compared with other neuroradiologic procedures. Acta Radiol [Diagn] (Stockh) 346: 14–20

Grumme Th, Meese W, Lange S (1976) Die axiale Computer-Tomographie des Schädels (CT Scan) in der Neuropädiatrie. Monatsschr Kinderheilkd 124:751–762

Grumme Th, Meese W, Lange S (1976) Kraniale Computertomographie (EMI-Scan). Wert und Einsatzmöglichkeit. Dtsch Med Wochenschr 20:765–769

Grumme Th, Steinhoff H, Wende S (1976) Diagnosis of supratentorial tumors with computerized tomography. In: Lanksch W, Kazner E (eds) Cranial computerized tomography. Springer, Berlin Heidelberg New York, pp 80–89

Grumme Th, Aulich A, Kazner E, Kretzschmar K, Lanksch W, Meese W (1978) Typical findings with computerized tomography in tumors of the posterior fossa. Adv Neurosurg 5:159–165

Grumme Th, Kretzschmer K, Ebhardt G, Lanksch W, Lange S (1978) Intracerebral space-occupying lesions with brain density (isodense lesions). Adv Neurosurg 6:75–79

Hacker H, Steudel W, Becker H (1976) Control studies in brain tumors and early detection of tumors using CT. In: Lanksch W, Kazner E (eds) Cranial computerized tomography. Springer, Berlin Heidelberg New York, pp 133–134

Hanigan WC, Wright SM, Wright RM (1986) Clinical utility of magnetic resonance imaging in pediatric neurosurgical patients. J Pediatr 108:522–529

Harwood-Nash DC (1975) Computed cranial tomography in children with intracranial neoplasms. In: Salamon G (ed) Advances in cerebral angiography. Springer, Berlin Heidelberg New York, pp 349–352

Harwood-Nash DC, Fitz Cr, Reilly BJ (1975) Cranial computed tomography in infants and children. Can Med Assoc J 118:546–549

Hayman LA, Evans RA, Hinck VC (1980) Delayed high iodine dose contrast computed tomography. Cranial neoplasms. Radiology 136:677–684

Henderson SD (1979) Pathology in computed tomography of the brain. Thomas, Springfield/IL

Hilal SK, Chang DH (1978) Specificity of computed tomography in the diagnosis of supratentorial neoplasms. Consideration of metastases and meningiomas. Neuroradiology 16:537–539

Houser OW, Baker HL Jr, Campbell JK (1975) Recent advances in neuroradiology. Some aspects of computerized transaxial tomography of the head. Minn Med 58:122–128

Huckman MS, Fox JS, Ramsey RG, Penn RD (1976) Computed tomography in the diagnosis of pseudotumor cerebri. Radiology 119:593–597

Huk W, Heindel W, Deimling M, Stetter E (1983) Nuclear magnetic resonance (NMR) tomography of the central nervous system: Comparison of two imaging sequences. J Comput Assist Tomogr 7/3:468–475

Hyman RA, Loring MF, Liebeskind AL, Naidich JB, Stein HL (1978) Computed tomographic evaluation of therapeutically induced changes in primary and secondary brain tumors. Neuroradiology 14:213–218

Jänisch W, Güthert H, Schreiber D (1976) Pathologie der Tumoren des Zentralnervensystems. Fischer, Jena

Jooma R, Kendall BE (1982) Intracranial tumors in the first year of life. Neuroradiology 23:267–274

Jooma R, Hayward RD, Grant DN (1984) Intracranial neoplasms during the first year of life: Analysis of one hundred consecutive cases. Neurosurgery 14:31–41

Kazner E, Steinhoff H (1979) Aspect of rare intracranial tumors in the CT scan. In: Gerhardt P, Kaick G van (eds) Total body computerized tomography. Thieme, Stuttgart, pp 301–312

Kazner E, Aulich A, Grumme Th (1975) Results of computerized axial tomography with infratentorial tumors. In: Lanksch W, Kazner E (eds) Cranial computerized tomography. Springer, Berlin Heidelberg New York, pp 90–103

Kazner E, Lanksch W, Steinhoff H, Wilske J (1975) Die axiale Computer-Tomographie des Gehirnschädels – Anwendungsmöglichkeiten und klinische Ergebnisse. Fortschr Neurol Psychiatr 43:487–574

Kazner E, Lanksch W, Steinhoff H (1976) Cranial computerized tomography in the diagnosis of brain disorders in infants and children. Neuropaediatrie 7:136–174

Kazner E, Grumme Th, Lanksch W, Wende S (1977) Computed tomography (CT) and the operative indications for brain tumors. A cooperative study of 3 university hospitals. Int Congress Series 433 "Neurological Surgery". Excerpta Medica. Amsterdam Oxford, pp 28–36

Kazner E, Grumme Th, Steinhoff H, Aulich A (1977) Diagnosis of posterior fossa tumors in infants and children by means of axial computerized tomography (CT). J Neurosurg Sci 21:205–210

Kazner E, Grumme Th, Lanksch W, Wilske J (1978) Limitations of computed tomography in the detection of posterior fossa lesions. Adv Neurosurg 5:166–170

Kazner E, Meese W, Kretzschmar K (1978) The role of computed tomography in the diagnosis of brain tumors in infants and children. Neuroradiology 16:10–12

Kazner E, Steinhoff H, Wende S, Mauersberger W (1978) Ring-shaped lesions in the CT scan – differential diagnostic considerations. Adv Neurosurg 6:80–85

Kazner E, Grumme Th, Wende S (1979) Hirntumoren im Computertomogramm. Dtsch Ärztebl 76:1299–1312

Kendall BE, Jakubowski J, Pullicino F, Symon L (1979) Difficulties in diagnosis of supratentorial gliomas by CAT scan. J Neurol Neurosurg Psychiatry 42:485–492

Kernohan J, Sayre GP (1952) Tumors of the central nervous system. Atlas of tumor pathology. Sect X, fasc 35 and 37. Armed Forces Inst Pathol, Washington

Kernohan J, Sayre GP (1956) Tumors of the pituitary gland and infundibulum. Atlas of tumor pathology, Sect X, fasc 36. Armed Forces Inst Pathol, Washington

Ketonen L (1978) Computerized tomography for diagnosis of supratentorial tumors. Acta Neurol Scand 57:153–164

Kingsley DP, Kendall BE (1979) The CT scanner in posterior fossa tumours of childhood. Br J Radiol 52:769–776

Kobayashi N (1976) Brain tumor and EMI scan. Jpn J Clin Radiol 21:745–746

Komiyama M, Yagura H, Baba M, Yasui T, Hakuba A, Nishimura S, Inoue Y (1987) MR imaging: Possibility of tissue characterization of brain tumors using T_1 and T_2 values. AJNR 8:65–70

Krayenbühl H, Yasargil MG, Huber P (1979) Zerebrale Angiographie für Klinik und Praxis, 3. Aufl. Thieme, Stuttgart

Kretzschmar K, Aulich A, Schindler E, Lange S, Grumme Th, Meese W (1978) The diagnostic value of CT for radiotherapy of brain tumors. Neuroradiology 14:245–250

Kretzschmar K, Grumme Th, Steinhoff H (1978) Der Wert der Computer-Tomographie und Angiographie für die Diagnose supratentorieller Hirntumoren. Neuroradiology 16:487–490

Krishna Rao CVG, Kishore PRS, Bartlett J, Brennan TG (1980) Computed tomography in the postoperative patient. Neuroradiology 19:257–263

Kucharczyk W, Brant-Zawadzki M, Sobel D, Edwards MB, Kelly WM, Norman D, Newton TH (1985) Central nervous system tumors in children: Detection by magnetic resonance imaging. Radiology 155:131–136

Lange S, Aulich A, Lanksch W (1976) Image artefacts in computerized tomography. In: Lanksch W, Kazner E (eds) Cranial computerized tomography. Springer, Heidelberg Berlin New York, pp 69–72

Lange S, Grumme Th, Meese W, Wüllenweber R, zum Winkel K (1976) Die axiale Computertomographie des Gehirns. Roentgenblätter 29:211–221

Lange S, Grumme Th, Meese W (1977) Zerebrale Computertomographie. Schering, Berlin

Lange S, Steinhoff H, Aviles Ch, Kazner E, Grumme Th (1979) Kontrastmittelkinetik in zerebralen Tumoren. Fortschr Röntgenstr 130:666–669

Lanksch W, Kazner E (1976) CT findings in brain edema. In: Lanksch W, Kazner E (eds) Cranial computerized tomography. Springer, Berlin Heidelberg New York, pp 344–355

Lanksch W, Grumme Th, Kazner E (1978) Die Schädelhirnverletzungen im Computertomogramm. Springer, Berlin Heidelberg New York

Lee BC, Kneeland JB, Cahill PT, Deck MD (1985) MR recognition of supratentorial tumors. AJNR 6: 871–878

Lee KF, Lin SR (1979) Neuroradiology of sellar and juxtasellar lesions. Thomas, Springfield/IL

Leonardi M, Fabris G, Pencot T (1979) Localization of brain tumors by means of CT scan. J Neurosurg Sci 23:231–233

Lin SR, Crane MD, Lin ZS, Bilaniuk L, Plaschke WM Jr, Marshall L, Spataro RF (1978) Characteristics of calcification in tumors of the pineal gland. Radiology 126:721–726

Logue V (1977) Tumors above and below the tentorium. The radiological management of cerebral tumors. In: du Boulay GH, Moseley IF (eds) Computerized axial tomography in clinical practice. Springer, Berlin Heidelberg New York, pp 76–84

MacDonald AF, Carrill JM, Dendy PP, Keyes WI, Mallard JR (1978) Evaluation of X ray CT (EMI scan) and isotope brain studies, including radioisotope axial tomography. Neuroradiology 16:575

Manes P, Babin E, Wackenheim A (1978) Contribution of histograms to the computer tomographic study of brain tumours. J Belge Radiol 6:297–312

Marks JE, Gado M (1977) Serial computed tomography of primary brain tumors following surgery, irradiation and chemotherapy. Radiology 125:119–125

Maroon JC, Bank WO, Drayer BP, Rosenbaum AE (1977) Intracranial biopsy by computerized tomography. J Neurosurg 46:740–744

Mass S, Norman D, Newton TH (1978) Coronal computed tomography: Indications and accuracy. Am J Roentgenol 131:875–879

McAllister VL, Appleby A, Hall K (1978) Contribution of computed tomography to the diagnosis and management of posterior fossa masses. Xtract 3:2–14

McAllister VL, Hankinson J, Sengupta RP (1978) Problems in diagnosis with computerized tomography. Adv Neurosurg 6:61–74

McGeachie RE, Gold LHA, Latchaw RE (1977) Periventricular spread of tumor demonstrated by computed tomography. Radiology 125:407–410

Meese W, Grumme Th, Lange S (1977) Die zerebrale axiale Computertomographie. Therapiewoche 27:2008–2019

Messina AV (1977) Cranial computerized tomography. A radiologic pathologic correlation. Arch Neurol 34:602–607

Messina AV, Potts DG, Rottenberg D, Patterson RH (1976) Computed tomography: demonstration of contrast medium within cystic tumors. Radiology 120:345–347

Metzger J, Gardeur D, Nachanakian A, Millard JC (1978) Comparaison des tomodensitométrie. Cinégammagraphie et angiographie dans diagnostics. Topographique et histologique pré-opératoires de 300 tumeurs intracraniennes sus-tentorielles. Neuroradiology 16:495–498

Michotey P, Moseley IF, Lecaque G, Palmieri P (1977) Tumours and other lesions of the visual pathways. The comparative values of various neuroradiological investigations in the diagnosis of intracranial optic pathway lesions. In: du Boulay GH, Moseley IF (eds) Computerised axial tomography in clinical practice. Springer, Berlin Heidelberg New York, pp 147–153

Mundinger F, Ostertag Ch (1976) Computerized tomography in stereotactic interstitial curie therapy of cerebral midline tumors. In: Lanksch W, Kazner E (eds) Cranial computerized tomography. Springer, Berlin Heidelberg New York, pp 110–113

Nadjmi M (1978) Vergleichende computertomographische und angiographische Befunde der Tumoren der hinteren Schädelgrube. Roentgenblätter 31:210–220

Naidich TP, Lin JP, Leeds NE, Kricheff II, George AE, Chase NE, Pudlowski RM, Passalaqua A (1976) Computed tomography in the diagnosis of extraaxial posterior fossa masses. Radiology 120:333–339

Naidich TP, Lin JP, Leeds NE, Pudlowski RM, Naidich JB (1977) Primary tumors and other masses of the cerebellum and fourth ventricle: Differential diagnosis by computed tomography. Neuroradiology 14:153–174

New PFJ, Scott WR (1975) Computed tomography of the brain and orbit. EMI scanning. Williams & Wilkins, Baltimore/MD

New PFJ, Scott WR, Schnur JA, Davis KR, Taveras JM (1974) Computerized axial tomography with the EMI scanner. Radiology 110:109–123

New PFJ, Scott WR, Schnur JA, Davis KR, Taveras JM, Hochberg FH (1975) Computed tomography with the EMI scanner in the diagnosis of primary and metastatic intracranial neoplasms. Radiology 75–87

Norman D, Enzmann DR, Levin VA, Wilson ChB, Newton TH (1976) Computed tomography in the evaluation of malignant glioma before and after therapy. Radiology 121:85–88

Obrador S (1977) Study of 100 patients with intracranial tumors using computed axial tomography. Zh Vorpr Neirokhir 4:3–12

Oi S (1977) Computerized axial tomography in the diagnosis of multiple brain tumors-correlation with angiography and nuclear scanning. Neurol Surg (Tokyo) 5:833–840

Olivecrona H (1967) The surgical treatment of intracranial tumors. In: Handbuch der Neurochirurgie, Bd IV, Teil 4. Springer, Berlin Heidelberg New York, S 1–301

Osborn AG, Heaston DK, Wing SD (1978) Diagnosis of ascending transtentorial herniation by cranial computed tomography. Am J Roentgenol 130:755–760

Osborn AG, Williams RG, Wing SD (1978) Low attenuation lesions in the midline posterior fossa: Differential diagnosis. J Comput Assist Tomogr 2:319–329

Papo I, Caruselli G, Menichelli F, Pasquini U, Salvolini U (1978) The reliability of computerized axial tomography in the diagnosis of infratentorial mass lesions; a neurosurgical appraisal. Acta Neurochir (Wien) 41:311–326

Paxton R, Ambrose J (1974) The EMI scanner: A brief review of the first 650 patients. Br J Radiol 47:530–565

Pertuiset B, Nachanakian A, Gardeur D, Yacoubi A, Ancri D, Metzger J, Kujas M (1979) Protocole d'exploration des tumeurs cérébrales sustentorielles. Neurochirurgie 25:11–18

Petermann SB, Steiner RE, Bydder GM (1984) Magnetic resonance imaging of intracranial tumors in children and adolescents. Am J Neuroradiol 5:703–709

Philippo J, Gardeur D, Nachanakian A, Metzger J (1979) Approche diagnostique pré-opératoire des tumeurs de la fosse postérieure de l'adulte. Neurochirurgie 25:139–146

Piepgras U, Huber G, Emde H, Fuchs U (1978) Vergleich der Ergebnisse von Computertomographie und Isotopendiagnostik bei pathologischen Prozessen des infratentoriellen Bereiches. Roentgenpraxis 31:221–238

Probst FP, Liliequist B (1979) Assessment of posterior fossa tumors in infants and children by means of computed tomography. Neuroradiology 18:9–18

Pullicino P, Thomson EJ, Moseley IF, Zilkha E, Shortman RC (1979) Cystic intracranial tumours. Cyst fluid, biochemical changes and computerised tomographic findings. J Neurol Sci 44:77–85

Randell CP, Collins AG, Young IR et al. (1983) Nuclear magnetic resonance imaging of posterior fossa tumors. Am J Roentgenol 141:489–496

Rappaport ZH, Epstein F (1978) Computerized axial tomography in the preoperative evaluation of posterior fossa tumors in children. Childs Brain 4:170–179

Roberson GH, Taveras JM, Tadmor R, Kleefield J, Ellis G (1977) Computed tomography in metrizamide cisternography – importance of coronal and axial views. J Comput Assist Tomogr 1:241–245

Rothe R, Fischer K (1976) Comparison between computerized tomography and conventional contrast-medium methods in the diagnosis of brain tumors. In: Lanksch M, Kazner E (eds) Cranial computerized tomography. Springer, Berlin Heidelberg New York, pp 183–187

Rubinstein LJ (1972) Tumors of the central nervous system. Atlas of tumor pathology. 2. ser fasc 6, Suppl. Armed Forces Inst Pathol, Washington

Ruggiero G, Sabattini L, Nuzzo G (1977) Computerized tomography and encephalography. Neuroradiology 13:45–49

Russel DS, Rubinstein LJ (1971) Pathology of tumours of the nervous system. Arnold, London

Sartor K, Richert S (1979) Konventionell-radiographische und computerassistierte Zisternographie der hinteren Schädelgrube mit Metrizamid. Roentgenforschung 130:472–478

Sartor K, Karnaze MG, Winthrop JD, Gado M, Hodges FJ (1987) MR imaging in infra-, para- and retrosellar mass lesions. Neuroradiology 29:19–29

Schellinger D, Axelbaum StP, Di Chiro G (1976) An analysis of the first one thousand cerebral ACTA scans. Fortschr Röntgenstr 125:211–213

Schörner W, Treisch J, Felix R, Kazner E (1986) Indikationen der magnetischen Resonanztomographie in der Diagnostik cerebraler Erkrankungen. Erfahrungsbericht über 1200 Untersuchungen. Fortschr Geb Röntgenstr Nuklearmed Ergänzungsband 144:210–220

Sheldon JJ, Maulsby G, Leborgne JM (1979) The differential diagnosis of supratentorial enhancing lesions on computed tomography. Rev Interam Radiol 4:109–113

Sorel L, Rucquoy Ponsar M, Harmant J (1978) Electroencephalogramme et tomographie assistée par calculateur dans 393 cas d'epilepsie. Etude des correspondances des localisations EEG et des localisations decouvertes par la tomographie assistée par calculateur. Acta Neurol Belg 78:242–252

Spiess H (1979) CT-Ergebnisse bei Affektionen des Chiasmas und der Sehbahn. Klin Monatsbl Augenheilkd 174:816–823

Sprung C, Grumme T (1980) CT images of periventricular lucency (PVL) in various forms of hydrocephalus. Adv Neurosurg 8:172–182

Steinhoff H, Aviles Ch (1976) Contrast enhancement response of intracranial neoplasms – its validity for the differential diagnosis of tumors in CT. In: Lanksch W, Kazner E (eds) Cranial computerized tomography. Springer, Berlin Heidelberg New York, pp 151–161

Steinhoff H, Kazner E, Lanksch W, Grumme Th, Meese W, Lange S, Aulich A, Wende S (1978) The limitations of computerized axial tomography in the detection and differential diagnosis of intracranial tumors. A study based on 1304 neoplasms. In: Bories J (ed) The diagnostic limitation of computerized axial tomography. Springer, Berlin Heidelberg New York, pp 40–49

Steudel WI, Beck U, Becker H, Hacker H (1976) Perifocal edema in computerized tomography and EEG changes in patients with tumors of cerebral hemispheres. In: Lanksch W, Kazner E (eds) Cranial computerized tomography. Springer, Berlin Heidelberg New York, pp 188–200

Strand RD, Baker RA, Ordia IJ, Arkins TJ (1978) Metrizamide ventriculography and computed tomography in lesions about the third ventricle. Radiology 128: 405–410

Syvertsen AH, Dugstad G, Amundsen P (1976) Computerized tomography in brain tumors correlated to histology, angiography, gas encephalography, and isotope encephalography. In: Lanksch W, Kazner E (eds) Cranial computerized tomography. Springer, Berlin Heidelberg New York, pp 167–170

Thomalske G, Grau H, Schäfer M, Hacker H (1976) The significance of cranial computerized tomography for the diagnosis of certain expansive lesions of the midline. In: Lanksch W, Kazner E (eds) Cranial computerized tomography. Springer, Berlin Heidelberg New York, pp 104–109

Thomson JLG (1976) Computerised axial tomography and the diagnosis of glioma: A study of 100 consecutive histologically proven cases. Clin Radiol 27:431–444

Thron A, Bockenheimer S (1979) Giant aneurysms of the posterior fossa suspected as neoplasms on computed tomography. Neuroradiology 18:93–97

Van Kirk OC, Cornell SH, Jacoby CG (1979) Posterior fossa intra-axial tumors: A comparison of computed tomography with other imaging methods. J Comput Assist Tomogr 3:31–50

Vouge M, Pasquini U, Salvolini U (1980) CT findings of atypical forms of phakomatosis. Neuroradiology 20:99–101

Wende S, Aulich A, Kretzschmar K, Grumme Th, Meese W, Lange S, Steinhoff H, Lanksch W, Kazner E (1977) Die Computertomographie der Hirngeschwülste. Eine Sammelstudie über 1658 Tumoren. Radiologe 17:149–156

Wende S, Aulich A, Kretzschmar K, Lange S, Grumme Th, Meese W, Lanksch W, Kazner E, Steinhoff H (1977) CAT investigations of the development of cerebral edema and the effects of its treatment in patients with brain tumours. In: du Boulay GH, Moseley IF (eds) Computerised axial tomography in clinical practice. Springer, Berlin Heidelberg New York, pp 118–122

Wende S, Aulich A, Schindler E, Grumme Th, Meese W, Lange S, Kazner E, Steinhoff H, Lanksch W (1977) A German multicentre study of intracranial tumours. In: du Boulay GH, Moseley IF (eds) Computerised axial tomography in clinical practice. Springer, Berlin Heidelberg New York, pp 111–117

Von Wild K, Grau H, Neubauer M, Althoff P-H (1976) The importance of cranial computerized tomography in diagnosis and continous follow-up of space-occupying lesions of the sellar region. In: Lanksch W, Kazner E (eds) Cranial computerized tomography. Springer, Berlin Heidelberg New York, pp 128–132

Wilson JL, Moseley IF (1977) A diagnostic approach to cerebellar lesions. In: du Boulay GH, Moseley IF (eds) Computerised axial tomography in clinical practice. Springer, Berlin Heidelberg New York, pp 123–133

Wing SD, Anderson RE, Osborn AG (1980) Dynamic cranial computed tomography: Preliminary results. AJNR 1:135–139

Yates AJ, Becker LE, Sachs LA (1979) Brain tumors in childhood. Childs Brain 5:31–39

Zimmerman RA, Bilaniuk LT (1980) Computed tomography of acute intratumoral hemorrhage. Radiology 135:355–359

Zimmerman RD, Leeds NE, Naidich TP (1977) Ring blush associated with intracerebral hematoma. Radiology 122:707–711

Zülch KJ (1956) Die Hirngeschwülste in biologischer und morphologischer Darstellung. Barth, Leipzig

Zülch KJ (1975) Atlas of gross neurosurgical pathology. Springer, Berlin Heidelberg New York

Zülch KJ (1980) Principles of the new health organization (WHO) classification of brain tumors. Neuroradiology 19:59–66

Zülch KJ (1986) Brain tumors, 3rd, completely revised edn. Springer, Berlin Heidelberg New York Tokyo

D. 1. Autochthonous Tumors

Aarabi B, Long DM, Miller NR (1978) Enlarging optic chiasmal glioma with stable visual acuity. Surg Neurol 10:175–177

Afra D, Norman D, Levin VA (1980) Cysts in malignant gliomas. Identification by computerized tomography. J Neurosurg 53:821–825

Araki C, Matsumotos S (1969) Statistical reevaluation of pinealoma and related tumors in Japan. J Neurosurg 30:146–149

Artigas J, Cervos-Navarro J, Iglesias-Rozas JR, Ebhardt G (1985) Review article. Gliomatosis cerebri: clinical and histological findings. Clin Neupathol 4:135–148

Auff E, Reisner Th, Toifl K, Perneczky A (1981) Primäre diffuse Melanoblastose der Leptomeningen und CT-Veränderungen. Neurochirurgia (Stuttg) 24:35–37

Barrer SJ, Simeone FA, Han SS (1980) An unusual presentation of an oligodendroglioma. J Neurosurg 53:560–561

Beers GJ, Manson J, Carter AP, Bell R (1986) Intracranial histiocytosis X; a case report. J Comput Tomogr 10:237–241

Berge JH van den, Blaauw G (1980) Subdural cysts and diencephalic tumor. Surg Neurol 13:267–272

Bhimani S, Virapongse C, Spencer D, Kim J (1983) CT-

appearance of cerebellar glioblastoma multiforme. J Comput Assist Tomogr 7:889–891
Bilaniuk LT, Zimmerman RA, Littmann PH, Gallo E, Rorke LB, Bruce DA, Schut L (1980) Computed tomography of the brain stem gliomas in children. Radiology 134:89–95
Boethius J, Collins VP, Edner G, Lewander R, Zyajicek J (1978) Stereotactic biopsies and computer tomography in gliomas. Acta Neurochir (Wien) 40:223–232
Bohm P, Meusers P, Lehmann HJ et al. (1984) Zur Diagnostik primärer Non-Hodgkin-Lymphome des Zentralnervensystems. Fortschr Neurol Psychiatr 52:284–291
Bolender NF, Cromwell LD, Graves V et al. (1983) Interval appearance of glioblastomas not evident in previous CT examinations. J Comput Assist Tomogr 7:599–603
Bradac GB, Schörner W, Bender A, Felix R (1985) MRI (NMR) in the diagnosis of brain-stem tumors. Neuroradiology 27:208–213
Brant-Zawadzki M, Enzmann DR (1978) Computed tomographic brain scanning in patients with lymphoma. Radiology 129:67–71
Bruce DA, Allen JC (1985) Tumor staging for pineal region tumors of childhood. Cancer 56:1792–1794
Budka H, Podreka I, Reisner Th, Zeiler K (1980) Diagnostic and pathomorphological aspects of glioma multiplicity. Neurosurg Rev 3:233–241
Burke DP, Gabrielsen TO, Knake JE, Seeger JF, Oberman HA (1980) Radiology of olfactory neuroblastoma. Radiology 137:367–372
Butler AR, Horii StC, Kricheff II, Shannon MB, Budzilovich GN (1978) Computed Tomography in Astrocytomas. Radiology 129:433–439
Butler AR, Passalaqua AM, Berenstein A, Kricheff II (1978) The contrast-enhanced CT scan and the radionuclide brain scan: Parallel mechanismus of action in the detection of supratentorial astrocytomas. Neuroradiology 16:491–494
Chan RC, Thompson GB, Durity FA (1983) Primary choroid plexus papilloma of the cerebellopontine angle. Neurosurgery 12:334–336
Chang CG, Kageyama N, Kobayashi T et al. (1981) Pineal tumors: Clinical diagnosis, with special emphasis on the significance of pineal calcification. Neurosurgery 8:656–668
Cho SoS, HO J (1980) Multiple primary germinomas (ectopic pinealoma) of the brain. Neurochirurgia (Stuttg) 23:147–150
Clarenbach P, Kleihues P, Metzel E, Dichganz J (1979) Simultaneous clinical manifestation of subependymoma of the fourth ventricle in identical twins. J Neurosurg 50:655–659
Claussen C, Laniado M, Schörner W, Niendorf H-P, Weinmann H-J, Fiegler W, Felix R (1985) Gadolinium-DTPA in MR Imaging of glioblastomas and intracranial metastases. AJNR 6:669–674
Claveria LE, Kendall BE, du Boulay GH (1977) Computerised axial tomography in supratentorial gliomas. In: du Boulay GH, Moseley IF (eds) Computerised axial tomography in clinical practice. Springer, Berlin Heidelberg New York, pp 85–93
Demierre B, Stichnoth FA, Hori A, Spoerri O (1986) Intracerebral ganglioglioma. J Neurosurg 65:177–182
Dewes W, Braunke H, Gormanns R (1986) Malignes fibröses Histiozytom des ZNS. Fortschr Röntgenstr 145:231–233
Diba J, Frowein RA, Stammler A (1979) Gangliocytoma: operability and follow-up. Neurosurg Rev 2:46–53
Diwan RV, Diwan VG, Bellon EM (1982) Brain involvement in chronic lymphocytic leukemia. J Comput Assist Tomogr 6:812–814
Dorne HL, O'Gorman AM, Melanson D (1986) Computed tomography of intracranial gangliogliomas. AJNR 7:281–285
Ebhardt G, Meese W (1979) Malignant lymphomas of the brain. Adv Neurosurg 4:303–308
Enzmann DR, Norman D, Levin V, Wilson Ch, Newton ThH (1978) Computed tomography in the follow-up of medulloblastomas and ependymomas. Radiology 128:57–63
Enzmann DR, Krikorian J, Norman D, Kramer R, Pollock J, Faer M (1979) Computed tomography in primary reticulum cell sarcoma of the brain. Radiology 130:165–170
Fortuna A, Celli P, Ferrante L, Turano C (1979) A review of papillomas of the third ventricle. J Neurosurg Sci 61–76
Frank G, Ferracini R, Spagnolli F et al. (1985) Primary intracranial lymphomas. Surg Neurol 23:3–8
Friedman WA, Fries JK, Quisling RG (1979) Ganglioglioma of the medulla oblongata. Surg Neurol 12:105–108
Furtrell NN, Osborn AG, Cheson BD (1981) Pineal region tumors: Computed tomographic-pathologic spectrum. AJNR 2:415–420
Ganti SR, Hilal SK, Stein BM, Silvera AJ, Mavad M, Sane P (1986) CT of pineal region tumors. Am J Roentgenol 146:451–458; AJNR 7:97–104
Gastaldo JA, Buchheit WA (1977) Bilateral subfrontal glioma simulating a meningioma. Surg Neurol 7:105–106
Geehr RB, Dohrmann GJ, Rothman SLG et al. (1979) Subarachnoid spread of ependymoma: Diagnosis and evaluation of therapy by computerized tomography. Ann Neurol 6:538–539
Gittens WO, Huetis WS, Sangalang VE (1980) Oligodendroglioma of the cerebellum. Surg Neurol 13:237–240
Glanz S, Geehr RB, Duncan ChC, Piepmeier JM (1980) Metrizamide-enhanced CT for evaluation of brainstem tumors. AJNR 1:31–34
Graif M, Pennock JM (1986) MR Imaging of Histiocytosis X in the central Nervous System. AJNR 7:21–23
Gregorius FK, Crandall PH, Baloh RW (1976) Positional vertigo with cerebellar astrocytoma. Surg Neurol 6:283–286
Gudeman SK, Sullivan HG, Rosner MJ, Becker DP (1979) Surgical removal of bilateral papillomas of the choroid plexus of the lateral ventricels with resolution of hydrocephalus. J Neurosurg 50:677–681
Halmagyi GM, Bignold LP, Allsop JL (1979) Recurrent subependymal giant-cell astrocytoma in the absence of tuberous sclerosis. J Neurosurg 50:106–109
Handa J, Nakano Y, Handa H (1978) Computed tomography in the differential diagnosis of low-density intracranial lesions. Surg Neurol 10:179–185
Hase U, Hock H, Schindler E (1979) Tumoren der Pinealisregion Teil I. Neurochirurgia (Stuttg) 22:107–117
Hase U, Hock H, Schindler E, Schürmann K (1979) Tumoren der Pinealisregion Teil II. Neurochirurgia (Stuttg) 22:118–129
Hayek J, Valavanis A (1982) Computed tomography of gliomatosis cerebri. Comput Radiol 6:93–98

Heiss E (1981) Ein Medulloblastom im hohen Lebensalter (Fallbericht). Neurochirurgia (Stuttg) 24:142–143
Holtas S, Nyman U, Cronquist S (1984) Computed tomography of malignant lymphoma of the brain. Neuroradiology 26:33–38
Huber A, Isler W, Spiess H (1979) Optikus- und Chiasmagliome (mit spezieller Berücksichtigung des Computertomogramms). Klin Monatsbl Augenheilkd 174:833–842
Hueftle MG, Han JS, Kaufman B, Benson JE (1985) MR imaging of brain stem gliomas. J Comput Assist Tomogr 9:263–267
Iglesias-Rozas JR (1987) Die computergestützte Charakterisierung der Mischgliome anhand histologischer, immuno-histologischer, elektronenmikroskopischer und klinischer Merkmale. Habilitationsschrift FU Berlin
Izquierdo JM, Rougerie J, Lapras C, Sanz F (1979) The so-called ectopic pinealomas. A cooperative study of 15 cases. Childs Brain 5:505–512
Jack CR jr, Reese DF, Scheithauer BW (1986) Radiographic findings in 32 cases of primary CNS lymphoma. Am J Roentgenol 146:271–276
Jazy FK, Shehata WM, Tew JM et al. (1980) Primary intracranial lymphoma of the dura. Arch Neurol 37:528–529
Jellinger K, Radaskiewicz T, Slowik F (1975) Primary malignant lymphomas of the central nervous system in man. Acta Neuropathol [Suppl] (Berl) VI:95–102
Joyce P, Bentson J, Takahashi M, Winter J, Wilson G, Byrd S (1978) The accucary of predicting histologic grades of supratentorial astrocytomas on the basis of computerized tomography and cerebral angiography. Neuroradioly 16:346–348
Kawakami Y, Tabuchi K, Ohnishi R et al. (1985) Primary central nervous system lymphoma. J Neurosurg 62:522–527
Kazner E, Steinhoff H, Wende S, Mauersberger W (1978) Ringshaped lesions in the CT scan-Differential diagnostic considerations. Adv Neurosurg 6:80–85
Kazner E, Wilske J, Steinhoff H, Stochdorph O (1978) Computer assisted tomography in primary malignant lymphomas of the brain. J Comput Assist Tomogr 2:125–134
Kelly PJ, Daumas-Duport C, Kisbert DB, Kall BA, Scheithauer BW (1987) Imaging-based stereotaxic serial biopsies in untreated intracranial glial neoplasms. J Neurosurg 66:865–874
Kendall BE, Jakobowski J, Pullicino P, Symon L (1979) Difficulties in diagnosis of supratentorial gliomas by CAT scan. J Neurol Neurosurg Psychiatry 42:485–492
Khan A, Fulco JD, Shende A, Rosenthal A, Marc JA (1980) Focal histiocytosis X of the parietal lobe. J Neurosurg 52:431–433
Kieffer SA, Salibi NA, Kim RC et al. (1982) Multifocal glioblastoma: Diagnostic implications. Radiology 143: 709–710
Kilgore DP, Strother CM, Starshak RJ, Haughton VM (1986) Pineal germinoma: MR imaging. Radiology 158:435–438
Kingsley D, Kendall BE (1977) Dependent layering of contrast medium in cystic astrocytomas. Neuroradiology 14:107–110
Kingsley DPE, Kendall BE (1979) The CT scanner in posterior fossa tumours of childhood. Br J Radiol 52:769–776
Kishikawa T, Mumaguchi Y, Fukui M et al. (1981) Primary intracranial sarcomas: Radiological diagnosis with emphasis on arteriography. Neuroradiology 21:25–31
Kramer RA (1977) Vermian pseudotumor: a potential pitfall of CT brain scanning with contrast enhancement. Neuroradiology 13:229–230
Kretzschmar K, Grumme Th, Steinhoff H (1978) Der Wert der Computer-Tomographie und Angiographie für die Diagnose supratentorieller Hirntumoren. Neuroradiology 16:487–490
Krol G, Farmer P, Stein S, Tenner M, Rothmann L (1979) Carcinoma of choroid plexus in a premature infant. J Comput Assist Tomogr 3:530–532
Lanzieri CF, Sabato U, Sacher M (1984): Third ventricular lymphoma: CT findings. J Comput Assist Tomogr 8:645–647
Laster DW, Ball MR, Moody DM et al. (1984) Results of nuclear magnetic resonance with cerebral glioma. Comparison with computed tomography. Surg Neurol 22:113–122
Lee DH, Norman D, Newton TH (1987) MR Imaging of pineal cysts. J Comput Assist Tomogr 11:586–590
Lee YY, Castillo M, Nauert C, Moser RP (1985) Computed tomography of gliosarcoma. AJNR 6:527–531
Lee YY, Glass JP, Van Eys J, Wallace S (1985) Medulloblastoma in infants and children: Computed tomographic follow-up after treatment. Radiology 154:677–682
Lewander R (1979) Contrast enhancement with time in gliomas. Stereotactic computer tomography following contrast medium infusion. Acta Radiol 30:689–702
Longo M, Fiumara F, Pandolfo I et al. (1982) Metastases dans l'espace sous-arachnoidien dues a un medulloblastome; etude tomodensitométrique. J Radiol 63:279–281
Mamourian AC, Towfighi J (1986) Pineal cysts: MR Imaging. AJNR 7:1081–1086
Markwalder T-M, Huber P, Markwalder RV, Seiler RW (1979) Primary intraventricular oligodendrogliomas. Surg Neurol 11:25–28
Mauersberger W (1981) The determination of absorption values as an aid in computer tomographic differentiation between cerebral abscess and glioblastoma. Adv Neurosurg 9:36–40
McCullough DC, Huang HK, de Michelle D, Manz HJ, Sinks LF (1979) Correlation between volumetric CT imaging and autopsy measurements of glioblastoma size. Comput Tomogr 3:133–141
McDonnell P, Miller NR (1983) Chiasmatic and hypothalamic extension of optic nerve glioma. Arch Ophthalmol 101:1412–1415
Mikhael MA (1977) Case report: diminished density surrounding a meningioma, verified to be an overlying cystic astrocytoma. J Comput Assist Tomogr 1:349–351
Miller EM, Mani RL, Townsend JJ (1976) Cerebellar glioblastoma multiforme in an adult. Surg Neurol 5:341–343
Nass R, Whelan MA (1981) Gangliogliomas. Neuroradiology 22:67–71
Neuwelt EA, Glasberg M, Frenkel E, Clark WK (1979) Malignant pineal region tumors. J Neurosurg 51:597–607
North C, Segall HD, Stanley P, Zee C-S, Ahmadi J, McComb JG (1985) Early CT detection of intracranial seeding from medulloblastoma. AJNR 6:11–13
Packer RJ, Sutton LN, Rorke LB et al. (1984) Intracranial embryonal cell carcinoma. Cancer 54:520–524
Packer RJ, Zimmerman RA, Luerssen TG et al. (1985) Brainstem gliomas of childhood: Magnetic resonance imaging. Neurology 35:397–401
Pagani JJ, Libshitz HI, Wallace S, Hayman LA (1981) Cen-

tral nervous system leukemia and lymphoma. Am J Roentgenol 137:1195–1201
Palacios E, Gorelick PB, Gonzalez CF, Fine M (1982) Malignant lymphoma of the nervous system. J Comput Assist Tomogr 6:689–701
Pedersen H, Gjerris F, Klinken L (1981) Computed tomography of benign supratentorial astrocytomas of infancy and childhood. Neuroradiology 21:87–91
Peterman SR, Steiner RE, Bydder GM, Thomas DJ, Tobias JS, Young IR (1985) Nuclear magnetic resonance imaging (NMR), (MRI), of brain stem tumors. Neuroradiology 27:202–207
Picard C, Copty M, Lavoie G et al. (1979) A primary choroid plexus papilloma of the cerebellopontine angle. Surg Neurol 12:123–127
Price AC, Runge VM, Allen HA, Partain CL, James AE jr (1986) Primary glioma: diagnosis with magnetic resonance imaging. J Comput Assist Tomogr 10:325–334
Rao KCVG, Itani A, Levine H et al. (1980) CT findings in multicentric glioblastoma: diagnostic-pathologic correlation. J Comput Assist Tomogr 4:187–192
Richardson RR, Siqueira EB, Cerullo LJ (1979) Malignant glioma: its initial presentation as intracranial hemorrhage. Acta Neurochir (Wien) 46:77–84
Ringertz N (1950) "Grading" of gliomas. Acta Pathol Microbiol Scand 27:51–64
Ringertz N, Tola JH (1950) Medulloblastoma. J Neuropathol Exp Neurol 9:354–372
Rommel T, Hamer J (1983) Development of ganglioglioma in computed tomography. Neuroradiology 24:237–239
Rosenbaum TJ, McCarty CS, Büttner H (1979) Uveitis and cerebral reticulum cell sarcoma. J Neurosurg 50:660–664
Rubinstein LJ (1964) Morhological problems of brain tumors with mixed cell population. Acta Neurochir [Suppl] (Wien) X:141–165
Sabattini L, Piazza GC, Finizia FS (1980) Programmed serial CT scans in the surgical and radio-chemotherapeutic management of cerebral gliomas. J Neurosurg Sci 24: 33–36
Sahart A, Feinsod M, Beller AJ (1980) Choroid plexus papilloma: hydrocephalus and cerebrospinal fluid dynamics. Surg Neurol 13:476–478
Sarmiento J, Ferrer L, Pons L, Ferrer E (1979) Cerebral mixed tumor: Osteo-chondrosarcoma-glioblastoma multiforme. Acta Neurochir (Wien) 50:335–341
Savoiardo M, Harwood Nash DC, Tadmor R et al. (1981) Gliomas of the intracranial anterior optic pathways in children. The role of computed tomography, angiography, pneumoencephalography, and radionuclide brain scanning. Radiology 138:601–610
Sawhny BS, Dohn DF (1980) Neuroendocrinological aspects of histiocytosis X of the central nervous system. Surg Neurol 14:237–239
Schindler E, Kretzschmar K, Aulich A, Wende S, Kutzner J (1977) Serial CT studies of a metastatic pinealoma with reference to the radiotherapeutic problems. Neuroradiology 14:127–132
Schlarb H, Schirmer M (1978) Pinealoma with initial spinal manifestation. Adv Neurosurg 6:221–224
Schneider GH, Sager WD, Lepuschütz H et al. (1981) Intrakranielles Germinom: Typisches Computertomographisches Bild und Strahlentherapie. Fortschr Röntgenstr 135:422–425
Silverman C, Marks JE (1981) Prognostic significance of contrast enhancement in low-grade astrocytomas of the adult cerebrum. Radiology 139:211–213
Sogg RL, Donaldson SS, Yorke CH (1978) Malignant astrocytoma following radiotherapy of a craniopharyngioma. J Neurosurg 48:622–627
Spillane JA, Kendall BE, Moseley IF (1982) Cerebral lymphoma: Clinical radiological correlation. J Neurol Neurosurg Psychiatry 45:199–208
Stefanko SZ, Talerman A, Mackay WM, Vuzevski VD (1979) Infundibular germinoma. Acta Neurochir (Wien) 50:71–78
Steinhoff H, Lanksch W, Kazner E, Grumme Th, Meese W, Lange S, Aulich A, Schindler E, Wende S (1977) Computed tomography in the diagnosis and differential diagnosis of glioblastomas. Neuroradiology 14:193–199
Steinhoff H, Grumme Th, Kazner E, Lange S, Lanksch W, Meese W, Wüllenweber R (1978) Axial transverse computerized tomography in 73 glioblastomas. Acta Neurochir (Wien) 42:45–56
Stephenson WM, Merlis AL (1985) Computed tomography of primary melanoma of the leptomeninges Case reports. J Comput Assist Tomogr 9:337–342
Stevens JM, Kendall BE, Love S (1984) Radiological features of subependymoma with emphasis on computed tomography. Neuroradiology 26:223–228
Sutton LN, Packer RJ, Rorke LB et al. (1983) Cerebral gangliogliomas during childhood. Neurosurgery 13:124–128
Swartz JD, Zimmerman RA, Bilaniuk LT (1982) Computed tomography of intracranial ependymomas. Radiology 143:97–101
Tadmor R, Davis KR, Roberson GH, Kleinman GM (1978) Computed tomography in primay malignant lymphoma of the brain. J Comput Assist Tomogr 2:135–140
Takeuchi J, Handa H, Nagata I (1978) Suprasellar germinoma. J Neurosurg 49:41–48
Takeuchi J, Handa H, Otsuka S, Takebe Y (1979) Neuroradiological aspects of suprasellar germinoma. Neuroradiology 17:153–159
Tanghetti B, Gatta G, Giunta F, Marini G (1980) Multiple gliomas of the brain. Report of three cases. J Neurosurg Sci 24:155–159
Tans JThJ, de Jongh IE (1977) Computed tomography of supratentorial astrocytoma. Clin Neurol Neurosurg 80: 156–168
Tchang S, Scotti G, Terbrugge K, Melancon D, Belanger G, Milner C, Ethier R (1977) Computerized tomography as a possible aid to histological grading of supratentorial gliomas. J Neurosurg 46:735–739
Thompson JL (1976) Computerised axial tomography and the diagnosis of glioma: a study of 100 consecutive histologically proven cases. Clin Radiol 27:431–441
Tibbs PA, Challa V, Mortara RH (1978) Isolated histiocytosis X of the hypothalamus. J Neurosurg 49:929–934
Tibbs PA, Mortara RH (1980) Primary glioblastoma multiforme of the cerebellum. A case report. Acta Neurochir 52:13–18
Tomasello F, Albanese V, Bernini FP, Picozzi P (1981) Choroid plexus papilloma of the third ventricle. Surg Neurol 16:69–71
Turcotte JF, Copty M, Bédard F, Michaud J, Verret S (1980) Lateral ventricle choroid plexus papilloma and communicating hydrocephalus. Surg Neurol 13:143–146
Vaghi M-A, Visciani A, Passerini A, Longone V, Broggi G (1986) Magnetic resonance in the study of cerebral gliomas. Radiol Med (Torino) 72:431–438

Valavanis A, Imhof HG, Klaiber R, Dabir K (1981) The diagnosis of solitary primary reticulum cell sarcoma of the posterior fossa with computed tomography. Neuroradiology 21:213–217

Veiga-Pires JA, Dossetor RS, van Nieuwenhuizen O (1978) CT scanning for papilloma of choroid plexus. Neuroradiology 17:13–16

Vonofakos D, Marcu H, Hacker H (1979) Oligodendrogliomas: CT patterns with emphasis on features indicating malignancy. J Comput Assist Tomogr 3:783–788

Wagle V, Melanson D, Ethier R, Betrand G, Villemure J-G (1987) Choroid plexus papilloma: magnetic resonance, computed tomography, and angiographic observations. Surg Neurol 27:466–468

Weinstein ZR, Downey EF Jr (1983) Spontaneous hemorrhage in medulloblastomas. AJNR 4:986–988

Weisberg LA (1979) Computed tomography in the diagnosis of brain stem gliomas. J Comput Assist Tomogr 3:145–153

Weisberg LA (1980) Cerebral computed tomography in the diagnosis of supratentorial astrocytoma. J Comput Assist Tomogr 4:87–105

Weisberg L (1981) Computed tomographic findings of intracranial gliosis. Neuroradiology 21:253–257

Weisberg LA (1982) Computerized tomographic findings in medulloblastomas. Comput Radiol 6:83–91

Weisberg LA (1982) Computed tomographic findings in cerebellar astrocytoma. Comput Radiol 6:137–144

Weisberg LA (1983) Thalamic gliomas: Clinical and computed tomographic correlations. Comput Radiol 7:229–235

Weisberg LA (1984) Clinical and computed tomographic correlations of pineal neoplasms. Comput Radiol 8:285–292

West CGH (1982) Misleading enhancement characteristics of meningeal malignant lymphoma on serial scanning. Comput Radiol 6:205–208

Woodman R, Shin K, Pineo G (1985) Primary non-Hodgkin lymphoma of the brain. Can Medicine 64:425–430

Woodrow PK, Gajarawala J, Pinck RL (1981) Computed tomographic documentation of a non-enhancing posterior fossa medulloblastoma: An uncommon presentation. J Comput Assist Tomogr 5:41–43

Yamashita J, Handa H, Yumitori K, Abe M (1980) Reversible delayed radiation effect on the brain after radiotherapy of malignant astrocytoma. Surg Neurol 13:413–417

Yang PJ, Knake JE, Gabrielsen TO et al. (1985) Primary and secondary histiocytic lymphoma of the brain: CT features. Radiology 154:683–686

Zee CS, Segall HD, Miller C et al. (1982) Less common CT features of medulloblastoma. Radiology 144:97–102

Zimmerman HM (1975) Malignant lymphomas of the nervous system. Acta Neuropathol [Suppl] (Berl) VI:69–74

Zimmerman RA, Bilaniuk LT (1979) Computed tomography of intracerebral gangliogliomas. J Comput Assist Tomogr 3:24–30

Zimmerman RA, Bilaniuk LT (1980) CT of primary and secondary craniocerebral neuroblastoma. AJNR 1:431–434

Zimmerman RA, Bilaniuk LT, Bruno L, Rosenstock J (1978) Computed tomography of cerebellar astrocytoma. Am J Roentgenol 130:929–933

Zimmerman RA, Bilaniuk LT, Pahlajani H (1978) Spectrum of medulloblastomas demonstrated by computed tomography. Radiology 126:137–141

Zimmerman RA, Bilaniuk LT, Wood JH et al. (1980) Computed tomography of pineal, parapineal, and histologically related tumors. Radiology 137:669–677

Zimmerman RA, Bilaniuk LT, Packer R et al. (1985) Resistive NMR of brain stem gliomas. Neuroradiology 27:21–25

Zimmerman RD, Leeds NE, Naidich TP (1977) Ring blush associated with intracerebral hematoma. Radiology 122:707–712

D.2. Meningeal Tumors

Amano K, Miura N, Tajika Y et al. (1980) Cystic meningioma in a month-old infant. Case report. J Neurosurg 52:829–833

Andrioli GC, Rigobello L, Iob I, Casentini L (1981) Multiple Meningiomas. Neurochirurgia (Stuttg) 24:67–69

Aydin Y, Yolas C, Konte H, Aydin IH (1985) Cystic meningiomas: Report of two cases. Neurosurgery 16:87–89

Becker D, Norman D, Wilson CB (1979) Computerized tomography and pathological correlation in cystic meningiomas. Neurosurgery 50:103–105

Bilaniuk LT, Zimmerman RA, Spagnoli M, Goldberg HI MRI of meningiomas. 4th Annual Meeting, Society of Magnetic Resonance in Medicine, 19.–23.8.85, London; Book of Abstracts, S 312

Bonnal J, Born JD, Tremoulet M (1979) Meningiomes multiples intracraniens. Neurochirurgie 25:78–83

Bradac GB, Ferszt R, Bender A, Schoerner W (1986) Peritumoral edema in meningeomas: A radiological and histological study. Neuroradiology 28:304–312

Bradley WG, Kortman KE, Zung TTM (1985) MRI of intracranial meningiomas. 4th Annual Meeting, Society of Magnetic Resonance in Medicine, 19.–23.8.85, London; Book of Abstracts, S 317–318

Bydder GM, Kingsley DPE, Brown J, Niendorf HP, Young IR (1985) MR Imaging of Meningiomas Including Studies with and without Gadolinium-DTPA. J Comput Assist Tomogr 9:690–697

Cabezudo JM, Vaquero J, Garcia-De-Sola R et al. (1981) Meningioma of the anterior part of the third ventricle. Acta Neurochir 56:219–231

Claveria LE, Sutton D, Tress BM (1977) The radiological diagnosis of meningiomas, the impact of EMI scanning. Br J Radiol 50:15–22

Cushing H, Eisenhardt J (1938) Meningeomas. Thomas, Springfield/IL

Dell S, Ganti SR, Steinberger A, McMurtry J (1982) Cystic meningiomas: a clinicoradiological study. J Neurosurg 57:8–13

Dietemann JL, Heldt N, Burguet JL et al. (1982) CT findings in malignant meningiomas. Neuroradiology 23: 207–209

Dosch JCI, Wackenheim A (1978) Hypodense meningioma: Computer tomographic examination of a meningioma. J Belge Radiol 61:325–334

Fine M, Brazis P, Palacios E, Neri G (1980) Computed tomography of sphenoid wing meningiomas: Tumor location related to distal edema. Surg Neurol 13:385–390

Fleury P, Bocquet L, Carou J-P, Poiver J, Marsault C, Basset J-M, Coupez D, Sterkers O, Compère J-F, Pansier P (1979) Meningioma of the ear simulating a glomus tumor. Apropos of 2 cases. Ann Otolaryngol Chir Cervicofac 96:469–491

Fornari M, Savoiardo M, Morello G, Solero CL (1981) Meningiomas of the lateral ventricles. Neuroradiological and surgical considerations in 18 cases. J Neurosurg 54:64–74

Genua E, Pappada G, Regalia F, Arrigoni M (1983) Multiple Meningiomas. Report of nine cases. Acta Neurochir (Wien) 68:33–43

Giromini D, Pfeiffer J, Tzonos T (1981) Über zwei Fälle von Ventrikelmeningeomen im Kindesalter. Neurochirurgia 24:144–146

Ito J, Kadekaru T, Hayano M et al. (1981) Meningioma in the tela choroidea of the third ventricle: CT and angiographic correlations. Neuroradiology 21:207–211

Just M, Higer HP, Grigat M, Voth D, Bockenheimer S, Pfannenstiel P (1986) Nativdarstellung von Meningiomen im NMR-Tomogramm – Retrospektive Kontrastoptimierung durch Bildsynthese. Digitale Bilddiagn 6:156–160

Kadis GN, Mount LA, Ganti SR (1979) The importance of early diagnosis and treatment of the meningiomas of the planum sphenoidale and tuberculum sellae: a retrospective study of 105 cases. Surg Neurol 12:367–371

Kendall B, Pullicino P (1979) Comparsion of consistency of meningiomas and CT appearances. Neuroradiology 18:173–176

Kim KS, Rogers LF, Lee C (1983) The dural lucent line: Characteristic sign of hyperostosing meningioma en plaque. Am J Roentgenol 141:1217–1221

Kolluri VRS, Reddy DR, Reddy PK, Naidu MRC, Devi S (1987) CT-findings in cystic meningiomas. Acta Neurochir 87:31–33

Lusins JO, Nakagawa H (1981) Multiple meningiomas evaluated by computed tomography. Neurosurgery 9:137–141

Mani RL, Hedgcock MW, Mass SI, Gilmor RL, Enzmann DR, Eisenberg RL (1978) Radiographic diagnosis of meningioma of the lateral ventricle. J Neurosurg 49:249–255

Markwalder T-M, Seiler RW, Markwalder RV, Huber P, Markwalder HM (1979) Meningioma of the anterior part of the third ventricle in a child. Surg Neurol 12:29–32

Mawhinney RR, Buckley JH, Holland IM, Worthington BS (1986) The value of magnetic resonance imaging in the diagnosis of intracranial meningiomas. Clin Radiol 37:429–439

Mikhael MA (1977) Diminished density surrounding a meningioma, verified to be an overlying cystic astrocytoma. J Comput Assist Tomogr 1:349–351

Mikhael MA, Ciric IS, Wolff AP (1885) Differentiation of cerebellopontine angle neuromas and meningiomas with MR imaging. J Comput Assist Tomogr 9:852–856

Miwa Y, Sakai N, Yamada H et al. (1985) Meningioma of the third ventricle in a child. Nerv Syst Child 10:37–42

Möller A, Hatam A, Olivecrona H (1978) The differential diagnosis of pontine angle meningioma and acoustic neuroma with computed tomography. Neuroradiology 17:21–33

Nagahiro S, Matsukado Y, Uemura S (1982) Posterior fossa meningioma with special reference to false localizing sign. Neurol Med Chir (Tokyo) 22:421–428

Nahser HC, Grote W, Loehr E, Gerhard L (1981) Multiple meningiomas. Clinical and computed tomographic observations. Neuroradiology 21:259–263

Nakagawa H, Lusins JO (1980) Biplane computed tomography of intracranial meningiomas with extracranial extension. J Comput Assist Tomogr 4:478–483

Nauta HJW, Rucker WS, Horsey WJ, Bilbao JM, Gonsalves C (1979) Xanthochromic cysts associated with meningioma. J Neurol Neurosurg Psychiatry 42:529–535

New PFJ, Aronow S, Hesselink JR (1980) National cancer institute study: Evaluation of computed tomography in the diagnosis of intracranial neoplasms. IV. Meningiomas. Radiology 136:665–675

New PFJ, Hesselink JR, O'Carroll CP, Kleinman GM (1982) Malignant Meningiomas. CT and histologic criteria, including a new CT-Sign. AJNR 3:267–276

Price HI, Danziger A, Richter I, Batnitzky S (1980) Computed tomographic findings in intracranial meningioma. Isr J Med Sci 16:743–747

Pullicino P, Kendall BE, Jakubowski J (1980) Difficulties in diagnosis of intracranial meningiomas by computed tomography. J Neurol Neurosurg Psychiatry 43:1022–1029

Rausing A, Ybo W, Stenflo J (1970) Intracranial Meningioma – A population study of ten years. Acta Neurol Scand 46:102–110

Russel DS, Rubinstein LJ (1977) Pathology of tumors of the nervous system, 4th edn. Williams & Wilkins, Baltimore

Russell EJ, George AE, Kricheff II, Budzilovich G (1980) Atypical computed tomographic features of intracranial meningioma. Radiology 135:673–682

Sartor K, Kühne D (1978) Meningeome mit Beziehung zum Tentorium cerebelli: Computertomographische und angiographische Aspekte. Fortschr Röntgenstr 128:651–661

Savoiardo M, Lodrini S (1980) Hypodense area within a meningeoma: Metastasis from breast cancer. Neuroradiology 20:107–110

Schröder BA, Samanaweera RN, Starshak RJ, Oechler HW (1987) Intraparenchymal meningioma in a child: CT und MR findings. J Comput Assist Tomogr 11:192–193

Servo A, Laskelainen J, Wahlstrom T, Haltia M (1985) Diagnosis of intracranial haemangiopericytomas with angiography and CT scanning. Neuroradiology 27:38–43

Shapir J, Coblentz C, Malanson D, Ethier R, Robitaille Y (1985) New CT finding in aggressive meningioma. AJNR 6:101–102

Spagnoli MV, Goldberg HI, Grossman RI, Bilaniuk LT, Gomori JM, Hackney DB, Zimmerman RA (1986) Intracranial meningiomas: High-field MR imaging. Radiology 161:369–375

Stevens JM, Ruiz JS, Kendall BE (1983) Observation on peritumoral oedema in meningioma. Part I: Distribution, spread, and resolution of vasogenic oedema seen on computed tomography. Neuroradiology 25:71–80

Stevens JM, Ruiz JS, Kendall BE (1983) Observation on peritumoral oedema in meningioma. Part II. Mechanisms of oedema production. Neuroradiology 25:125–131

Sutton C, Claveria LE (1977) Meningiomas diagnosed by scanning: a review of 100 intracranial cases. In: du Boulay GH, Moseley IF (eds) Computerised axial tomography in clinical practice. Springer, Berlin Heidelberg New York, pp 102–110

Tans JThJ, de Jongh IE (1977) Computed tomography of supratentorial meningioma. Clin Neurol Neurosurg 80:10–21

Treisch J, Schörner W, Laniado M, Felix R (1987) Charakteristika intrakranieller Meningeome in der magnetischen Resonanztomographie. Fortschr Röntgenstr 146:207–214

Vassilouthis J, Ambrose J (1978) Intraventricular meningioma in a child. Surg Neurol 10:105–107

Vassilouthis J, Ambrose J (1979) Computerized tomography scanning appearances of intracranial meningiomas. An attempt to predict the histological features. J Neurosurg 50:320–327

Weisberg LA (1979) Computed tomography in the diagnosis of intracranial meningioma. J Comput Assist Tomogr 3:115–124

Wiggli U, Elke M, Müller HR, Hünig R, Wüthrich R (1976) The CT pattern of meningioma – is it specific? In: Lanksch W, Kazner E (eds) Cranial computerized tomography. Springer, Berlin Heidelberg New York, pp 162–166

Wills K, Teather D, du Boulay GH (1982) An improvement in computer-aided diagnosis of meningiomas after CT. Neuroradiology 22:255–257

Zimmerman RA (1984) MRI in intracranial meningiomas. 3rd Annual Meeting, Society of Magnetic Resonance in Medicine, 13.–17.09.1984, New York. Abstracts, pp 779–780

Zimmerman RD, Fleming CA, Saint-Louis LA, Lee BCP, Manning JJ, Deck MDF (1985) Magnetic resonance imaging of meningiomas. AJNR 6:149–157

D.3. Neurinomas

Bocquet M, Vignaud J, Cosnard G, Iba-Zizen MT (1984) IRM du neurinome de l'acoustique. J Neuroradiol 11:263–273

Boggan JE, Rosenblum ML, Wilson CB (1979) Neurilemmoma of the fourth cranial nerve. J Neurosurg 50:519–521

Canale DJ, Bebin J (1972) Von Recklinghausen disease of the nervous system. Handbook of Clinical Neurology XIV. North Holland, Amsterdam

Canigiani G (1978) Nativdiagnostik mit Tomographie der Kleinhirnbrückenwinkel-Tumoren. In: Plester D, Wende S, Nakayama N (Hrsg) Kleinhirnbrückenwinkel-Tumoren. Springer, Berlin Heidelberg New York, S 92–120

Daniels DL, Haughton VM (1987) Magnetic resonance imaging of the sella and temporal bone. In: Kressel HY (ed) Magnetic resonance annual 1987. Raven, New York

Daniels DL, Millen StJ, Meyer GA, Pozunas KW, Kilgore DP, Shaffer KA, Williams AL, Haughton VM (1987) MR detection of tumor in the internal auditory canal. AJNR 8:249–252

Davis KR, Parker SW, New PFJ, Roberson GH, Taveras JM, Ojemann RJ, Weiss AD (1977) Computed tomography of acoustic neuroma. Radiology 124:81–86

Deutsch EC (1984) Von Recklinghausen's neurofibromatosis with mutliple intracranial tumors. Ear Nose Throat J 63:18–30

Dossetor RS, de Winter J, Nurick S (1979) Diagnosis of a small acoustic neuroma by metrizamide computerassisted cisternography. Br J Radiol 52:667–668

Dubois PJ, Drayer BP, Bank WO, Deeb ZL, Rosenbaum AR (1978) An evaluation of current diagnostic radiologic modalities in the investigation of acoustic neurilemmomas. Radiology 126:173–179

Fink LH, Early CB, Bryan RN (1978) Glossopharyngeal schwannomas. Surg Neurol 9:239–245

Gardeur D, Palmieri A, Mashaly R (1983) Cranial computed tomography in the phakomatoses. Neuroradiology 25:293–304

Glowacki J (1963) Multiple cerebral tumors accompanying Recklinghausen's disease. Folia Med Cracov 5:99–130

Goebel HH, Shimokawa K, Schaake Th, Kremp A (1979) Schwannoma of the sellar region. Acta Neurochir (Wien) 48:191–197

Goldberg R, Byrd S, Winter J, Takahashi M, Joyce P (1980) Varied appearance of trigeminal neuroma on CT. Am J Roentgenol 134:57–60

Gyldensted C, Lester J, Thomsen J (1976) Computer tomography in the diagnosis of cerebellopontine angle tumors. Neuroradiology 11:191–197

Hatam A, Möller A, Olivecrona H (1979) Evaluation of the internal auditory meatus with acoustic neuromas using computed tomography. Neuroradiology 17:197–200

Heller M, Wohrle M, Jend HH et al. (1983) Aussagekraft der CT in der Diagnostik von Tumoren der Kleinhirnbrückenwinkelregion. Vergleich der verschiedenen radiologischen, klinischen und otologischen Untersuchungsverfahren. Fortschr Geb Roentgenstr Nuklearmed Ergänzungsband 139:48–55

Higer HP, Just M, Vahldiek G, Gutjahr P, Pfannenstiel P (1987) MRT bei Neurofibromatose und tuberöser Sklerose. Fortschr Röntgenstr 147:64–68

Huete I, Corrales M (1979) Cisternographie computérisée dans le diagnostic des petits neurinomes de l'acoustique. J Neuroradiol 6:335–340

Jacoby ChG, Go RT, Beren RA (1980) Cranial CT of neurofibromatosis. AJNR 1:311–315

Jacoby ChG, Go RT, Beren RA (1980) Cranial CT of neurofibromatosis. Am J Roentgenol 135:553–557

Kanter WR, Eldridge R, Fabricant R, Allen JC, Koerber T (1980) Central neurofibromatosis with bilateral acustic neuroma: genetic, clinical and biochemical distinctions from peripheral neurofibromatosis. Neurol 30:851–859

King TT, Ambrose J (1977) CAT scanning in tumours of the cerebellopontine angle. In: du Boulay GH, Moseley IF (eds) Computerised axial tomography in clinical practice. Springer, Berlin Heidelberg New York, pp 134–138

Kingsley DPE, Brooks GB, Leung AWL, Johnson MA (1985) Acoustic neuromas: Evaluation by magnetic resonance imaging. Am J Neuroradiol 6:1–5

Kricheff II, Pinto RS, Bergeron RT, Cohen N (1980) CT-air-cisternography and canalography in the diagnosis of small acoustic neuromas. AJNR 1:57–63

Latack JT, Kartush JM, Kemink JL et al. (1985) Epidermoidomas of the cerebellopontine angle and temporal bone. Radiology 157:361–366

Lichtenstein BW (1949) Neurofibromatosis (Von Recklinghausen's disease of the nervous system). Arch Neurol Psychiat 62:822–839

Martuza RL, Ojemann RG (1982) Bilateral acoustic neuromas: clinical aspects, pathogenesis and treatment. Neurosurgery 10:1–12

Mikhael MA, Ciric JS, Wolff AP (1987) MR diagnosis of acoustic neuromas. J Comput Assist Tomogr 11:232–235

Mironov A (1984) Gegenwärtiger Stand der neuroradiologischen Diagnostik von Kleinhirnbrückenwinkel-Tumoren. Radiologe 24:493–501

Osborn JD (1975) A comparative study of special petrous views and tomography in the diagnosis of acoustic neuromas. Br J Radiol 48:996–999

Öztürk S, Sprung C, Maier-Hauff K (1987) Multiple primäre intrakranielle Tumoren. 2. Arbeitstagung Neuroonkologie der Deutschen Gesellschaft für Neurochirurgie. 1987, Tübingen

Pearce J (1967) The central nervous system pathology in multiple neurofibromatosis. Neurology 17:691–697

Piepgras U (1984) Neurokutane Systemerkrankungen. Eine synoptische Darstellung aus radiologischer Sicht. Thieme, Stuttgart New York

Pinto RS, Kricheff II, Bergeron RT, Cohen N (1982) Small acoustic neuromas: Detection by high resolution gas CT cisternography. Am J Roentgenol 139:129–132

Robbins B, Marschall WH Jr (1978) Computed tomography of acoustic neurinoma. Radiology 128:367–370

Robinson JS, Lopes J, Moody R (1979) Intracranial hypoglossal neurilemmoma. Surg Neurol 12:496–498

Rodriguez HA, Berthrong M (1966) Multiple primary intracranial tumours in Von Recklinghausen's neurofibromatosis. Arch Neurol 14:467–475

Rosenbaum AE, Drayer BP, Dubois PJ, Black FO (1978) Visualization of small extracanalicular neurilemmomas by metrizamide cisternographic enhancement. Arch Otolaryngol 104:239–243

Rosenbloom SB, Carson BS, Wand H et al. (1985) Cerebellopontine angle lipoma. Surg Neurol 23:134–138

Salvoloni U, Pasquini U, Babin E, Gasquez P (1978) Von Recklinghausen's disease and computer tomography. J Belge Radiol 61:313–318

Schepps S, Reiser M, Ingianni G, Hölscher M (1986) Diagnostik der Neurofibromatose durch Kernspintomographie. Fortschr Röntgenstr 144:473–476

Schnegg JF, de Tribolet N (1984) Neurinoma of the facial nerve associated with parietal meningeoma. Surg Neurol 21:19–22

Schubiger O, Valavanis A, Menges H (1978) Computed tomography for small acoustic neuromas. Neuroradiology 15:287–290

Schubiger O, Valavanis A, Hayek J, Dabir K (1980) Neuroma of the cavernous sinus. Surg Neurol 13:313–316

Sortland O (1978) X-ray diagnosis of expanding lesions in the cerebellopontine angle. Meeting Nord Soc Radiol, Oslo, June 1978

Sortland O (1979) Computed tomography combined with gas cisternography for the diagnosis of expanding lesions in the cerebellopontine angle. Neuroradiology 18:19–22

Swartz JD (ed) (1986) Imaging of the temporal bone. A text atlas. Thieme, Stuttgart New York

Thomsen J, Gyldensted C, Lester J (1977) Computer tomography of cerebellopontine angle lesions. Arch Otolaryngol 103:65–69

Tritthart H, Lepuschütz H (1979) Wertigkeit der axialen Computertomographie in der Diagnostik intrakanalikulärer Gewächse des Nervus statoacusticus. In: Sager WD, Ladurner G (eds) Computertomographie. Thieme, Stuttgart, S 21–23

Van der Hoeve J (1933) Les phacomatoses de Bourneville, de Recklinghausen et de von Hippel-Lindau. Acta Neurol Psychiatr Belg 33:752–762

Valavanis A, Schubiger O, Wellauer J (1978) Computed tomography of acoustic neuromas with emphasis on small tumour detectability. Neuroradiology 16:598–600

Valavanis A, Schubiger O, Naidich TP (eds) (1987) Clinical imaging of the cerebello-pontine angle. Springer, Berlin Heidelberg New York London Paris Tokyo

Vassilouthis J, Richardson AE (1979) Acoustic neurinoma in a child. Surg Neurol 12:37–39

Vignaud J, Jardin C, Rosen L (eds) (1986) The ear. Diagnostic imaging. Masson, New York Paris Barcelona Mexico City Milan Sao Paulo

Wende S (1980) Die kombinierte Anwendung von Computertomographie und Luftzisternographie bei Kleinhirnbrückenwinkeltumoren. Fortschr Röntgenstr 132:666–667

Wende S, Nakayama N (1978) Zisternographie mit negativen und positiven Kontrastmitteln. In: Plester D, Wende S, Nakayama N (Hrsg) Kleinhirnbrückenwinkel-Tumoren. Springer, Berlin Heidelberg New York, S 121–143

Zimmerman RA, Bilaniuk LT, Metzger RA, Grossman RI, Schut L, Bruce DA (1983) Computed tomography of orbital-facial neurofibromatosis. Radiology 146:113–116

D.4. Pituitary Adenomas

Ahmadi J, North CM, Segall HD, Zee CS, Weiss MH (1985) Cavernous Sinus Invasion by Pituitary Adenomas. AJNR 6:893–898

Bajraktari X, Bergström M, Brismar K, Goulatie R, Greitz T, Grepe A (1977) Diagnosis of intrasellar cisternal herniation (empty sella) by computer assisted tomography. J Comput Assist Tomogr 1:105–116

Banna M, Baker HL Jr, Houser OW (1980) Pituitary and parapituitary tumours on computed tomography. A review article based on 230 cases. Br J Radiol 53:1123–1143

Bilaniuk LT, Zimmerman RA, Wehrli FW, Snyder PJ, Goldberg HI, McFall RI, Redington RW (1984) MRI of pituitary lesions using 1.0 to 1.5 T field strength. Radiology 153:415–418

Bonneville JF, Cattin F, Dietemann JL (1986) Computed tomography of the pituitary gland. Springer, Berlin Heidelberg New York Tokyo

Brennan ThG jr, Krishna Rao CVG, Robinson W, Itani A (1977) Tandem lesions: chromophobe adenoma and meningioma. J Comput Assist Tomogr 1:517–520

Citrin CM, Davis DO (1977) Computerized tomography in the evaluation of pituitary adenomas. Invest Radiol 12:27–35

Daniels D, Pojunas KW, Kilgore DP, Pech P, Meyer GA, Williams AL, Haughton VM (1986) MR of the Diaphragma sellae. AJNR 7:765–769

Daniels DL, Haughton VM (1987) Magnetic resonance imaging of the sella and temporal bone. In: Kressel HY (ed) Magnetic resonance annual 1987. Raven, New York

Davis PC, Hoffman JC, Tindall GT, Braun IF (1985) CT-surgical correlation in pituitary adenomas: evaluation in 113 patients. AJNR 6:464

Donovan Post MJ, David NJ, Glaser JS, Safran A (1980) Pituitary apoplexy: Diagnosis by computed tomography. Radiology 134:665–670

Gardeur D, Nachanakian A, Kulesza E, Metzger J (1979) La tomodensitométrie dans les adenomes hypophysaires. Ann Radiol 22:489–499

Gross CE, Binet EF, Esguerra JV (1979) Metrizamide cisternography in the evaluation of pituitary adenomas and the empty sella syndrome. J Neurosurg 50:472–476

Gyldensted C, Karle A (1977) Computed tomography of intra- and juxtasellar lesions. A radiological study of 108 cases. Neuroradiology 14:5–13

Hall K, McAllister VL (1980) Metrizamide cisternography in pituitary and juxtapituitary lesions. Radiology 134:101–108

Hankins CA, Zamani AA, Rumbaugh CL (1985) Prolactinomas. Clinical presentation, radiologic assessment, and therapeutic options. Invest Radiol 20:345–354

Hatam A, Bergström M, Greitz T (1979) Diagnosis of sellar and parasellar lesions by computed tomography. Neuroradiology 18:249–258

Haughton VM, Prost R (1986) Pituitary fossa: Chemical shift effect in MR imaging. Radiology 158:461–462

Haughton VM, Rosenbaum AE, Williams AL, Drayer B (1980) Recognizing the empty sella by CT: The infundibulum sign. AJNR 1:527–529

Hemminghytt S, Kalkhoff KR, Daniels LD, Williams LA, Grogan PJ, Haughton MV (1983) Computed tomographic study of hormon-secreting microadenomas. Radiology 146:65–69

Hoffmann JC jr, Tindall GT (1980) Diagnosis of empty-sella syndrome using Amipaque cisternography combined with computerized tomography. J Neurosurg 52:99–102

Huk JW, Fahlbusch R (1985) NMR imaging of the region of the sella turcica. Neurosurg Rev 141–150

Kaplan CH (1985) CT of the sella turcica after transsphenoidal resection of pituitary adenomas. AJNR 6:723–732

Kazner E, Fahlbusch R, Lanksch W, Rothe R, Scherer U, Steinhoff H, Grumme Th, Lange S, Meese W, Aulich A, Wende S (1978) Computerized tomography in diagnosis and follow-up examination of pituitary adenomas. In: Fahlbusch R, v Werder K (eds) Treatment of pituitary adenomas. Thieme, Stuttgart, pp 101–114

Kucharczyk W (1987) The pituitary gland and sella turcica. In: Brandt-Zawadzki M, Norman D (eds) Magnetic resonance imagings of the central nervous system. Raven, New York

Lee BCP, Deck MDF (1985) Sellar and juxtasellar lesion detection with MR. Radiology 157:143–147

MacPherson P, Anderson DE (1981) Radiological differentiation of intrasellar aneurysms from pituitary tumours. Neuroradiology 21:177–183

Maravilla KR, Kirks DR, Maravilla AM, Diehl JT (1978) Computed tomography in the evaluation of sella and parasellar lesions: The value of sagittal and coronal reconstructions. Comput Tomogr 2:237–249

Muhr C, Bergstrom K, Enoksson P, Hugosson R, Lundberg PO (1980) Follow-up study with computerized tomography and clinical evaluation 5 to 10 years after surgery for pituitary adenoma. J Neurosurg 52:144–148

Nakagawa Y, Matsumoto K, Fukami T, Takese K (1984) Exploration of the pituitary stalk and gland by high-resolution CT. Comparative study of normal subjects and cases with microadenoma. Neuroradiology 26:473–478

Numaguchi Y, Kishikawa T, Ikeda J et al. (1981) Neuroradiological manifestations of suprasellar pituitary adenomas, meningiomas and craniopharyngiomas. Neuroradiology 21:67–74

Okony T, Sudo M, Momoi T, Takao T, Ito M, Konishi Y, Yoshioka M, Suzuki J, Nakano Y (1980) Pituitary hyperplasia due to hypothyroidism. J Comput Assist Tomogr 4:600–602

Patel DV, Shields MC (1979) Intraventricular hemorrhage in pituitary apoplexy. J Comput Assist Tomogr 3:829–831

Pojunas KW, Daniels DL, Williams AL, Haughton VM (1985) Comparison of MR and CT imaging of pituitary microadenomas. AJNR 6:464

Pojunas KW, Daniels DL, Williams AL, Haughton VM (1986) MR imaging of prolactin-secreting microadenomas. AJNR 7:217–222

Quencer RM (1980) Lymphocytic adenohypophysitis: Autoimmune disorder of the pituitary gland. AJNR 1:343–345

Reich NE, Zelch JV, Alfidi RJ, Meaney TF, Duchesneau PM, Weinstein MA (1976) Computed tomography in the detection of juxtasellar lesions. Radiology 118:333– 334

Rilliet B, Mohr G, Robert F, Hardy J (1981) Calcifications in pituitary adenomas. Surg Neurol 15:249–255

Robertson WD, Newton TH (1978) Radiological assessment of pituitary microadenomas. Am J Roentgenol 13:489–492

Sakoda K, Mukada K, Yonezawa M et al. (1980) CT scan of pituitary adenomas. Neuroradiology 20:249–253

Sheldon P, Molyneux A (1979) Metrizamide cisternography and computed tomography for the investigation of pituitary lesions. Neuroradiology 17:83–87

Smaltino F, Bernini FP, Muras I (1980) Computed tomography for diagnosis of empty sella associated with enhancing pituitary microadenoma. J Comput Assist Tomogr 4:592–599

Snow BR, Lavyne HM, Lee CPB, Morgello S, Patterson HR (1986) Craniotomy versus transsphenoidal excision of large pituitary tumors: The usefulness of MRI in guiding the operative approach. Neurosurgery 19 (1) 59–64

Syvertsen A, Haughton VM, Williams AL, Cusick JF (1979) The computed tomographic appearance of the normal pituitary gland and pituitary microadenomas. Radiology 133:385–391

Taylor HC, Wilson DJ, Schumacher OP (1979) Pituitary stones and associated hypopituitarism. J Am Med Wom Assoc 242:751–752

Teasdale E, Teasdale G, Mohsen F, Macpherson P (1986) High-resolution computed tomography in pituitary microadenoma: Is seeing believing? Clin Radiol 37:227–232

Teng MMH, Gado M, Sartor K (1985) MRI of pituitary adenoma and the normal pituitary gland: A quantitative study. AJNR 6:463

Tenner MS, Weitzner Jr I (1980) Pitfalls in the diagnosis of erosive changes in expanding lesions of the pituitary fossa. Radiology 137:393–396

Turski PA, Watanabe TJ, Chambers EF, Newton ThH (1981) Contrast enhancement of the normal and abnormal pituitary gland. In: Felix R, Kazner E, Wegener OH (eds) Contrast media in computed tomography. Excerpta Medica, S 157–164

Vignaud J, Aubin ML, Bories J (1979) Value of computer assisted tomography in the exploration of the sellar and suprasellar structures. Rev Neurol 135:41–50

Weisberg LA (1977) Pituitary apoplexy. Association of degenerative change in pituitary adenoma with radiotherapy and detection by cerebral computed tomography. Am J Med 63:109–115

Wolpert SM, Post KD, Biller BJ, Molitch ME (1979) The value of computed tomography in evaluating patients with prolactinomas. Radiology 131:117–119

D.5. Hemangioblastomas

Cornell SH, Hibri NS, Menezes AH, Fraf CJ (1979) The complementary nature of computed tomography and angiography in the diagnosis of cerebellar hemangioblastoma. Neuroradiology 17:201–205

Ganti SR, Silver AJ, Hilal SK, Mawad ME, Sane P (1982) Computed tomography of cerebellar hemangioblastomas. J Comput Assist Tomogr 6:912–919

Heiss E, Albert F (1982) Computertomographische Befunde bei Kleinhirnangioblastomen. Fortschr Geb Röntgenstr Nuklearmed Ergänzungsband 136:151–156

McDonnell DE, Pollock P (1978) Cerebral cystic hemangioblastoma. Surg Neurol 10:195–199

Nishimoto A, Kawakami Y (1980) Surgical removal of hemangioblastoma in the fourth ventricle. Surg Neurol 13:423–427

Obrador S, Martin-Rodriguez JG (1977) Biological factors involved in the clinical features and surgical management of cerebellar hemangioblastomas. Surg Neurol 7:79–85

Seeger JF, Burke DP, Knake JE, Gabrielsen TO (1981) Computed tomographic and angiographic evaluation of hemangioblastomas. Radiology 138:65–73

Tomasello F, Albanese V, Iannotti F, Dilorio G (1980) Supratentorial hemangioblastoma in a child. J Neurosurg 52:578–583

D.6. Dysontogenetic Tumors

Ahmadi J, Miller CA, Segall HD, Park SH, Zee CS, Becker RL (1985) CT patterns in histopathologically complex carvernous hemangioms. AJNR 6:389–393

Ambrose J (1974) Computerized x-ray scanning of the brain. J Neurosurg 40:679

Amendola MA, Garfinkle WB, Ostrum BJ, Katz MR, Katz RI (1978) Preoperative diagnosis of a ruptured intracranial dermoid cyst by computerized tomography. J Neurosurg 48:1035–1037

Antunes JL, Louis KM, Ganti SR (1980) Colloid cysts of the third ventricle. Neurosurgery 7:450–455

Arita N, Bitoh S, Ushio Y, Hayakawa T, Hasegawa H, Fujiwara M, Ozaki K, Parkhen L, Mori T (1980) Primary pineal endodermal sinus tumor with elevated serum and CSF alphafetoprotein levels. J Neurosurg 53:244–248

Auque J, Marchal JC, Bracard S, Berchet T, Fauve M, Hepner H, Lepoire J (1985) Current diagnostic criteria for intracranial epidermoid and dermoid cysts. Neurochirurgie 31/1:47–50

Baudrillard JC, Scherpereel B, Rousseaux P, Lerais JH, Toubas O, Auqier F, Guyot JF, Lacour PY (1986) Rupture of a cerebral dermoid cyst. Apropos of a case: x-ray computed tomography aspects. J Radiol 67:111–113

Boesel CP, Suhan JP, Bradel EJ (1983) Ultrastructure of primitive neuroectodermal neoplasms of the central nervous system. Cancer 42:194–201

Boissonnot L, Drouineau J, Roualdes G, Morin H, Neau JP, Bataille B (1986) Spontaneous rupture of intracranial dermoid cyst. Clinical and radiological study. J Radiol 67:917–919

Bosch DA, Rähn T, Backlund EO (1978) Treatment of colloid cysts of the third ventricle by stereotactic aspiration. Surg Neurol 9:15–18

Braun IF, Naidich ThP, Leeds NE (1977) Dense intracranial epidermoid tumors: Computed tomographic observations. Radiology 122:717–719

Bruhlmann Y, de Tribolet N, Berney J (1985) Intracerebral cavernous angiomas. Neurochirurgie 31 (4):271–279

Budku H (1974) Intracranial lipomatous hamartomas (intracranial "lipomas"). Acta Neuropathol (Berl) 28:205–222

Bullard DE, Osborne D, Cook WA Jr (1982) Colloid cyst of the third ventricle presenting as a ring-enhancing lesion on computed tomography. Neurosurgery 11:790–791

Cabezudo JM, Vaquero J, Garcia-De-Sola R et al. (1981) Computed tomography with craniopharyngiomas: A review. Surg Neurol 15:422–427

Claussen C, Lohkamp F, Rebien W, Kuttig H (1977) Computertomographische Diagnostik, Therapieplanung und Verlaufskontrolle beim Kraniopharyngeom. Strahlentherapie 153/11:744–753

Clavici G, Heppner F (1979) The operative approach to lipomas of the corpus callosum. Neurochirurgia (Stuttg) 22:77–81

Davidson HD, Ouchi T, Steiner RE (1985) NMR imaging of congenital intracranial germinal layer neoplasms. Neuroradiology 27:301–303

Dee RH, Kishore PRS, Young HF (1980) Radiological evaluation of cerebello-pontine angle epidermoid tumor. Surg Neurol 13:293–296

Diebler C, Ponsot G (1983) Hamartomas of the tuber cinereum. Neuroradiology 25:93–101

Eberts TJ, Ransburg RC (1979) Primary intracranial endodermal sinus tumor. J Neurosurg 50:246–252

Evans DC, Netsky MG, Allen VE, Kasantikul V (1979) Empty sella secondary to suprasellar colloid cyst of foregut (respiratory) origin. J Neurosurg 51:114–117

Faerber EN, Wolpert SM (1978) The value of computed tomography in the diagnosis of intracranial lipomata. J Comput Assist Tomogr 2:297–299

Fawcitt RA, Isherwood I (1977) Intracranial epidermoid and dermoid tumors. In: du Boulay GH, Moseley IF (eds) Computerised axial tomography in clinical practice. Springer, Berlin Heidelberg New York, pp 94–101

Fitz CR, Wortzmann G, Harwood-Nash DC, Holgate RC, Barry JF, Boldt DW (1978) Computed tomography in craniopharyngiomas. Radiology 127:687–691

Frank G, Cacciari E, Cristi G et al. (1982) Hamartomas of the tuber cinereum and precocious puberty. Childs Brain 9:222–231

Friedman RB, Segal R, Latchaw RE (1986) Computerized tomographic and magnetic resonance imaging of intracranial lipoma. J Neurosurg 65:407–410

Ganti SR, Antunes JL, Louis KM, Hilal SK (1981) Computed tomography in the diagnosis of colloid cysts of the third ventricle. Radiology 138:385–391

Gendell H, Maroon I, Wisotzkey H (1976) Epidermoid of the fourth ventricle: discovery by computerized tomography. Surg Neurol 5:37–39

Godt P, Stöppler L (1979) Infratentorielle Epidermoide und Dermoide im kranialen Computertomogramm. Fortschr Röntgenstr 131:368–371

Gomez MR, Mellinger JF, Reese DF (1975) The use of computerized transaxial tomography in the diagnosis of tuberous sclerosis. Mayo Clin Proc 50:553–556

Guner M, Shaw MDM, Turner JW, Steven JL (1976) Computed tomography in the diagnosis of colloid cyst. Surg Neurol 6:345–348

Gyldensted C, Karle A (1977) Computed tomography of intra- and juxtasellar lesions. A radiological study of 103 cases. Neuroradiology 14:5–13

Handa J, Handa H, Nakano Y, Mukai T (1979) Radiolucent intracranial dermoid cyst. Report of an unusual case. Neuroradiology 17:211–214

Hart MN, Earle KM (1973) Primitive neuroectodermal tumors of the brain in children. Cancer 32:890–897

Healy JF, Brahme FJ, Rosenkrantz H (1980) Dermoid cysts and their complications as manifested by computed cranial tomography. Comput Tomography 4:111–115

Herpers MJHM, Budka H (1985) Primitive neuroectodermal tumors including the medulloblastoma: glial differentiation signaled by immunoreactivity for GFAP is restricted to the pure desmoplastic medulloblastoma ("arachnoidal sarcoma of the cerebellum"). Neuropathology 4/1:12–18

Hinshaw DB jr, Ashwal S, Thompson JR, Hasso AN (1983) Neuroradiology of primitive neuroectodermal tumors. Neuroradiology 25:87–92

Hoffmann HJ (1985) Craniopharyngeomas. Can J Neurol Sci 12:348–352

Hubschmann O, Kasoff S, Doniger D, Llena J, Leeds N (1976) Cavernous hemangioma in the pineal region. Surg Neurol 6:349–351

Hughes DS, Osborn RE (1986) Corpus callosal lipoma: report of 2 cases and review of the literature. J Am Osteopath Assoc 86:564–567

Isherwood I, Pullan BR, Rutherford RA, Strang FA (1977) Electron density and atomic number determination by computed tomography. Part I: Methods and limitations. Part II: A study of colloid cysts. Br J Radiol 50:613–619

Ishikawa M, Handa H, Moritake K, Mori K, Nakano Y, Aii H (1980) Computed tomography of cerebral cavernous hemangiomas. J Comput Assist Tomogr 4:587–591

Kazner E, Stochdorph O, Wende S, Grumme Th (1980) Intracranial lipoma. Diagnostic and therapeutic considerations. J Neurosurg 52:234–245

Kobayashi T, Yoshida J, Kageyama N, Mori O, Ogawa H (1985) Successful treatment of dwarfism and hypogonadism after total removal of craniopharyngeoma. Neurol Med Chir (Tokyo) 25/19:61–65

Kosnick EJ, Boesel CP, Bay J, Sayers MP (1978) Primitive neuroectodermal tumors od the central nervous system in children. J Neurosurg 48:741–746

Krainer L (1935) Die Hirn- und Rückenmarkslipome. Virchows Arch 295:107–142

Laster DW, Moody DM, Ball MR (1978) Computerized cranial tomography of free intracranial fat in congenital tumors. Comput Tomogr 2:257–265

Lee BC, Deck HD (1985) Sellar and juxtasellar lesion detection with MR. Radiology 157:143–147

Lee BCP, Gawler J (1978) Tuberous sclerosis. Comparison of computed tomography and conventional neuroradiology. Radiology 127:403–407

Lipper MH, Kishore PRS, Ward JD (1981) Craniopharyngioma: Unusual computed tomographic presentation. Neurosurgery 9:76–78

Malik GM, Horoupian DS, Boulos RS (1980) Hemorrhagic (colloid) cyst of the third ventricle and episodic neurologic deficits. Surg Neurol 13:73–77

McDonnell DE (1977) Pineal epidermoid cyst: its surgical therapy. Surg Neurol 7:387–391

Michels LG, Rutz D (1982) Colloid cysts of the third ventricle. A radiologic-pathologic correlation. Arch Neurol 39:640–643

Mikhael MA, Mattar AG (1978) Intracranial pearly tumors: the roles of computed tomography, angiography, and pneumoencephalography. J Comput Assist Tomogr 2:421–429

Mori K, Handa H, Gi H, Mori K (1980) Cavernomas in the middle fossa. Surg Neurol 14:21–31

Murphy MJ, Risk WS, Van Gilder JC (1980) Intracranial dermoid cyst in Goldenhar's syndrome. J Neurosurg 53:408–410

New PFJ, Scott WR (1975) Computed tomography of the brain and orbit. EMI scanning. Williams & Wilkins, Baltimore/MD

Numaguchi Y, Kishikawa T, Fukui M, Sawada K, Kitamura K, Matsuura K, Russell WJ (1979) Prolonged injection angiography for diagnosing intracranial cavernous hemangiomas. Radiology 131:137–138

Papo I, Scarpelli M, Caruselli G (1980) Intrinsic third ventricle craniopharyngiomas with normal pressure hydrocephalus. Neurochirurgia (Stuttg) 23:80–88

Powell MP, Torrens MJ, Thomson JLG, Horgan JG (1983) Isodense colloid cysts of the third ventricle: A diagnostic and therapeutic problem resolved by ventriculoscopy. Neurosurgery 13:234–237

Probst FP, Erasmie U, Nergardh A, Brun A (1979) CT-appearances of brain lesions in tuberous sclerosis and their morphological basis. Ann Radiol 22:171–183

Ramina R, Ingunza W, Vonofakis D (1980) Cystic cerebral cavernous angioma with dense calcification. J Neurosurg 52:259–262

Rodiek S (1983) Die computertomographische Manifestation intrakranieller Lipome und Fettkörper. Fortschr Geb Röntgenstr Nuklearmed Ergänzungsband 138:50–53

Rosario M, Becker DH, Conlay FK (1981) Epidermoid tumors involving the fourth ventricle. Neurosurgery 9:9–13

Sackett JF, Messina AV, Petito CK (1975) Computed tomography and magnification vertebral angiotomography in the diagnosis of colloid cysts of the third ventricle. Radiology 116:95–100

Savoiardo M, Passerini A (1978) CT, angiography and RN scans in intracranial cavernous hemangiomas. Neuroradiology 16:256–260

Savoiardo M, Strada L, Passerini A (1983) Intracranial cavernous hemangiomas: Neuroradiologic review of 36 operated cases. Am J Neuroradiol 4:945–950

Schijman E, Monges J, Cragnaz R (1986) Congenital dermal sinuses, dermoid and epidermoid cysts of the posterior fossa. Childs Nerv Syst 2:83–89

Simard JM, Garcia-Bengochea F, Ballinger WE jr, Mickle JP, Quisling RG (1986) Cavernous angioma: a review of 126 collected and 12 new clinical cases. Neurosurgery 18/3:162–172

Sperling MR, Wilson G, Engel J jr, Babb TL, Phelps M, Bradley W (1986) Magnetic resonance imaging in intractable partial epilepsy: correlative studies. Ann Neurol 20/1:57–62

Suemitsu T, Nakajima SI, Kuwajima K, Nihei K, Kamostuta S (1979) Lipoma of the corpus callosum: report of a case and review of the literature. Childs Brain 5:476–483

Tadmor R, Davis KR, Roberson GH, New PFJ, Taveras JM (1977) Computed tomography in extra-dural epidermoid and xanthoma. Surg Neurol 7:371–375
Tahmouresie A, Kroll G, Shoeart W (1979) Lipoma of the corpus callosum. Surg Neurol 11:31–34
Takakura K (1985) Intracranial germ cell tumors. Clin Neurosurg 32:429–444
Uken P, Sato Y, Smith W (1986) MR findings of malignant intracranial teratoma in a neonate. Pediatr Radiol 16:504–505
Vaquero J, Cabezudo JM, Leunda G, Carrillo R, Bravo G (1980) Intraorbital and intracranial glial hamartoma. J Neurosurg 53:117–120
Vaquero J, Manrique M, Oya S, Cabezudo JM, Bravo G (1980) Calcified telangiectatic hamartomas of the brain. Surg Neurol 13:453–457
Vighetto A, Davenas C, Bret P, Aimard G (1985) Pseudo-optic neuritis as a manifestation of craniopharyngeoma. Rev Neurol 141:490–492
Vonderrahe AR, Niemer WT (1944) Intracranial lipoma. J Neuropathol Exp Neurol 3:344–354
Wakai S, Segawa H, Kitahara S, Asano T, Sano K, Ogihara R, Tomita S (1980) Teratoma in the pineal region in two brothers. J Neurosurg 53:239–243
Wallace D (1976) Lipoma of the corpus callosum. J Neurol Neurosurg Psychiatry 39:1178–1185
Weaver EN Jr, Coulon RA (1979) Excision of a brain-stem epidermoid cyst. J Neurosurg 51:254–257
Weisberg LA (1984) Clinical-computed tomographic correlations in colloid cysts of the third ventricle. Comput Radiol 8:157–163
Weiss Th, Mitsch E, Kazner E (1986) Zystische Veränderungen der hinteren Schädelgrube im Kernspintomogramm. Fortschr Röntgenstr 145/5:590–597
Willis RA (1953) Pathology of tumours. Butterworth, London
Yamasaki T, Handa H, Moritake K (1985) Cavernous angioma in the fourth ventricle. Surg Neurol 23/3:249–254
Yamasaki T, Handa H, Yamashita J, Paine J, Tashiro Y, Uno A, Ishikawa H, Asato R (1986) Intracranial and orbital cavernous angiomas. J Neurosurg 64:197–208
Yock DH jr (1980) Choroid plexus lipomas associated with lipoma of the corpus callosum. J Comp Assist Tomogr 4:678–682
Zilkha A (1981) Computed tomography of colloid cysts of the third ventricle. Clin Radiol 32:397–401
Zimmerman RA, Bilaniuk LT, Dolinskas C (1979) Cranial computed tomography of epidermoid and congenital fatty tumors of maldevelopmental origin. CT J Comput Tomogr 3:40–50

D.7. Intracranial Tumors of Skeletal Origin

(see references Chap. E)

D.8. Locally Invasive Tumors

(see references Chap. E)

D.9. Intracranial Metastases

Anand AK, Potts DG (1982) Calcified brain metastases: Demonstration by computed tomography. Am J Neuroradiol 3:527–529
Bushe KA (1972) Intrakranielle Metastasen. Bedeutung und therapeutisches Konzept. Langenbecks Arch Chir 332:369–375
Butler AR, Kricheff II (1978) Non contrast CT scanning: Limited value in suspected brain tumor. Radiology 126:689–693
Butler AR, Leo JS, Lin JP, Boyd AD, Kricheff II (1979) The value of routine cranial computed tomography in neurologically intact patients with primary carcinoma of the lung. Radiology 131:399–401
Cairncross JG, Chernik NL, Kim JH, Posner JB (1979) Sterilization of cerebral metastases by radiation therapy. Neurology Minneap 29:1195–1202
Cushing H (1935) Intrakranielle Tumoren. Springer, Berlin
Davis PC, Friedman NC, Fry SM, Malko JA, Hoffmann CJ jr, Braun IF (1987) Leptomeningeal metastasis: MR imaging. Radiology 163:449–454
Deck MDF, Messina AV, Sackett JF (1976) Computed tomography in metastatic disease of the brain. Radiology 119:115–120
Dublin AB, Norman D (1979) Fluid-fluid level in cystic cerebral metastatic melanoma. J Comput Assist Tomogr 3:650–652
Dyment PG, Rothner AD, Duchesneau PM, Weinstein MA (1976) Computerized tomography in the detection of intracranial metastases in children. Pediatrics 58:72–77
Elke M, Hünig R, Wiggli U, Friedrich R, Müller HR, Wüthrich R (1976) The diagnosis of intracranial metastases: the efficiency of CT and scintigraphy in patients investigated by both methods. In: Lanksch W, Kazner E (eds) Cranial computerized tomography. Springer, Berlin Heidelberg New York, pp 171–176
Enzmann DR, Kramer R, Norman D, Pollock J (1978) Malignant melanoma metastatic to the central nervous system. Radiology 127:177–180
Fink LH (1979) Metastasis of prostatic adenocarcinoma simulating a falx meningioma. Surg Neurol 12:253–258
Ginaldi S, Wallace S, Shalen P, Luna M, Handel S (1981) Cranial computed tomography of malignant melanoma. Am J Roentgenol 136:145–149
Handa J, Nakasu Y, Kamijyo Y (1980) Calcified metastatic carcinoma of the brain. Surg Neurol 14:67–70
Healy JF, Marshall WH, Brahme FJ, White F (1981) CT of intracranial metastases with skull and scalp involvement. Am J Neuroradiol 2:335–338
Henschen F (1955) Tumoren des ZNS und seiner Hüllen. In: Scholz W (Hrsg) Nervensystem. (Handbuch der speziellen pathologischen Anatomie und Histologie, Bd XIII/3). Springer, Berlin Göttingen Heidelberg, S 413–1040
Hooper RG, Tenholder MF, Underwood GH, Beechler CR, Spratling L (1984) Computed tomographic scanning of the brain in initial staging of bronchogenic carcinoma. Chest 85/6:774–776
Jaeckle KA, Krol G, Posner JB (1985) Evolution of computed tomographic abnormalities in leptomeningeal metastases. Ann Neurol 17:85–89
Jänisch W, Güthert H, Schreiber D (1976) Pathologie der Tumoren des Zentralnervensystems. Fischer, Jena
Jones JN (1977) Unique presentation of a metastatic adenocarcinoma diagnosed pre-operatively by C.T. Scan J Neurol 214:229–234
Kawakami Y, Yamada O, Tabuchi K et al. (1980) Primary intracranial choriocarcinoma. J Neurosurg 53:369–374
Kazner E, Schulz B, Kern A, Trempenau B, Laniado M,

Treisch J, Schörner W, Felix R (1985) Vergleich zwischen Computertomographie und Magnetresonanztomographie unter Einschluß paramagnetischer Kontrastmittel bei 165 Patienten mit Hirntumoren. Digitale bildgebende Verfahren, integrierte digitale Radiologie. 4. Grazer Radiol Sympos 03–05 Okt 1985

Kretzschmar K, Kühnert A, Wende S, Müller W (1985) Diagnostik der Hirntumoren mit CT und/oder MR? Digitale bildgebende Verfahren, integrierte digitale Radiologie. 4. Grazer Radiol Sympos. 03–05 Okt 1985

Krishna Rao CVG, Govindan S (1979) Intracranial choriocarcinoma. J Comput Assist Tomogr 3:400–404

Lopez-Pousa S, Ojeda B, Lopez-Lopez JJ et al. (1981) The correlation between clinical symptomatology and computerized tomography in brain metastasis secondary to breast and lung neoplasias. Comput Tomography 5:17–23

MacDonald J, Parker JC, Brown S, Page LK, Wolfe DE (1978) Cerebral metastasis from a malignant thymoma. Surg Neurol 9:58–60

Mintz BJ, Tuhrim S, Alexander S, Yang WC, Shanzer S (1984) Intracranial metastases in the initial staging of bronchogenic carcinoma. Chest 86/6:850–853

New PFJ, Scott WR, Schnur JA, Davis KR, Taveras JM, Hochberg FH (1975) Computed tomography with the EMI scanner in the diagnosis of primary and metastatic intracranial neoplasms. Radiology 114:75–87

Nosaka Y, Nagao S, Tabuchi K, Nishimoto A (1979) Primary intracranial epidermoid carcinoma. J Neurosurg 50:830–833

Percy AK, Elveback LR, Okazaki H, Kurland LT (1972) Neoplasms of the CNS: epidemiological considerations. Neurology (Minneap) 22:40–48

Posner JB (1977) Management of central nervous system metastases. Semin Oncol 4:81–91

Potts DG, Abbott GF, von Sneidern JV (1980) National cancer institute study: Evaluation of computed tomography in the diagnosis of intracranial neoplasms. III. Metastatic tumors. Radiology 136:657–664

Ringelstein EB, Zeumer H, Hacke W, Keulers P (1981) Indikation zur kranialen Computertomographie bei metastasierenden Tumoren. Eine klinisch-computertomographische Vergleichsuntersuchung. Dtsch Med Wochenschr 106:1566–1571

Rubinstein LJ (1972) Tumors of the central nervous system. Atlas of tumor pathology, second series, fasc 6. Armed Forces Institute of Pathology, Washington

Smith VC, Kasdon DL, Hardy RC (1980) Metastatic brain tumor from the prostate. Surg Neurol 14:189–191

Störtebecker TP (1954) Metastatic tumors of the brain from a neurosurgical point of view. A follow-up study of 158 cases. J Neurosurg 11:84–111

Tarver RD, Richmond BD, Klatte VC (1984) Cerebral metastases from lung carcinoma: Neurological and CT correlation. Work in Progress. Radiology 153:689–692

Weaver DD, Cross DL, Winn R, Jane JA (1984) Computed tomographic findings in metastatic dural carcinomatosis. Surg Neurol 21:190–194

Weisberg LA (1979) Computerized tomography in intracranial metastases. Arch Neurol 36:630–634

Weisberg LA (1985) Computerized tomographic findings in intracranial metastatic malignant melanoma. Computerized Radiol 9/6:365–372

Weisberg LA (1985) Solitary cerebral metastases. Clinical and computed tomographic correlations. Arch Neurol 42:336–341

Ya-Yen Lee, Glass JP, Geoffray A, Wallace S (1984) Cranial computed tomographic abnormalities in leptomeningeal metastasis. Am J Roentgenol 143:1035–1039

Zülch KJ (1986) Brain tumors. Their biology and pathology, 3rd completely revised edn. Springer, Berlin Heidelberg New York Tokyo

E. Skull Base and Cranial Vault

Alvarez-Berdecia A, Schut I, Bruce DA (1979) Localized primary intracranial Ewing's sarcoma of the orbital roof. J Neurosurg 50:811–813

Bass IS, Haller JO, Berdon WE, Barlow B, Carsen G, Khakoo Y (1985) Nasopharyngeal carcinoma: clinical and radiographic findings in children. Radiology 156:651–654

Becker H, Grau H, Hacker H, Ploder KW (1978) The base of the skull: a comparison of computed and conventional tomography. J Comp Assist Tomogr 2:113–118

Biller J, Heredia S, Palacios E, Fine M (1980) Malignant nasopharyngeal tumors. Surg Neurol 14:197–201

Bradac GB, Simon RS, Grumme T, Schramm J (1977a) Limitations of computed tomography for diagnostic neuroradiology. Neuroradiology 13:243–247

Bradac GB, Simon RS, Grumme T (1977b) Routine neuroradiological diagnosis with the EMI 5005 body scanner. Neuroradiology 14:133–137

Bradac GB, Schramm J, Grumme T, Simon RS (1978a) Wert und Grenzen der Computertomographie in der Studie von Prozessen der Schädelbasis. Neuroradiology 16:438–439

Bradac GB, Schramm J, Grumme T, Simon RS (1978b) CT of the base of the skull. Neuroradiology 17:1–5

Brusis T, Mödder U (1984) HNO Röntgen-Aufnahmetechnik und Normalbefunde. Springer, Berlin Heidelberg New York Tokyo

Brusis T, Mödder U (1986) HNO Röntgen-Atlas. Pathologische Befunde. Springer, Berlin Heidelberg New York Tokyo

Bydder GM, Kingsley DPE, Brown J, Niendorf HP, Young IR (1985) MR imaging of meningiomas including studies with and without gadolinium-DTPA. J Comp Assist Tomogr 9:690–697

Caillé JM, Dop A, Constant P, Renaud-Salis JL (1977) CAT studies of tumors of the skull base and face. In: du Boulay GH, Moseley IF (eds) Computerised axial tomography in clinical practice. Springer, Berlin Heidelberg New York, pp 139–146

Carter BL, Carmody CS (1978) Computed tomography of the face and neck. Semin Röntgenol 13:257–266

Caughran M, White TJ III, Gerald B, Gardner G (1980) Computed tomography of jugulotympanic paragangliomas. J Comp Assist Tomogr 4:194–198

Chandler JR, Goulding R, Moskowitz L, Quencer R (1984) Nasopharyngeal angiofibromas: staging and management. Ann Otol Rhinol Laryngol 93:322–329

Claussen C, Lochner B (1983) Dynamische Computertomographie. Grundlagen und klinische Anwendung. Springer, Berlin Heidelberg New York Tokyo

Claussen C, Singer R (1979) Progress in the diagnosis of cranio-facial injuries and tumors by computer tomography. J Maxillofac Surg 7:210–217

Claussen C, Lohkamp F, Spenneberg H, Krastel A, Singer

R (1978) Computertomographie des Gesichtsschädels. 2. Kongreß der internat. Ges für Kiefer- und Gesichtschir, 1.–3. Sept 1976, Basel, und In: Pape H, Bethman E (eds) Acta Chir Max, Fac. Barth, Leipzig

Claussen C, Lochner B, Köhler D, Banzer D (1982) Dynamische Computertomographie bei Gesichtsschädeltumoren. Fortschr Röntgenstr 136:144–150

Daniels DL, Williams AL, Haughton VM (1984) Jugular foramen: anatomic and computed tomography study. AJR 142:153–158

De la Cruz A (1984) Polytomographic evaluation of the clivus and petrous apices: a new view. Laryngoscope 94:153–164

Dickson RI, Flores AD (1985) Nasopharyngeal carcinoma: evaluation of 134 patients treated between 1971–1980. Laryngoscope 95:276–286

Dillon WP, Mills CM, Kjos BO, DeGroot H, Brant-Zawadzki M (1984) Magnetic resonance imaging of the nasopharynx. Radiology 152:731–738

Dop A, Constant P, Renaud-Salis JL, Caillé JM (1976) Interès de la tomodensitométrie en pathologie tumorale de la base du crane du massif facial. J Neuroradiol 3:193–214

Duncavage JA, Campbell BH, Hanson GA, Kun LE, Hanson RM, Toohill RJ, Malin TC (1983) Diagnosis of malignant lymphomas of the nasal cavity, paranasal sinuses and nasopharynx. Laryngoscope 93:1276–1280

Dutton J (1978) Intracranial solitary chondrome. J Neurosurg 49:460–463

Freyschmidt J (1980) Knochenerkrankungen im Erwachsenenalter. Röntgenologische Diagnose und Differentialdiagnose. Springer, Berlin Heidelberg New York

Galanski M, Dickob M, Wittkowski W (1986) CT-Zisternographie der basalen Zisternen. Fortschr Röntgenstr 145:149–157

Graber HR, Zaunbauer W, Haertel M (1986) Zur computertomographischen Diagnose und Differentialdiagnose maligner Nasennebenhöhlentumoren. Fortschr Röntgenstr 144:405–412

Grodd W, Lenz M, Baumann R, Schroth G (1984) Kernspintomographische Untersuchungen des Gesichtsschädels. Fortschr Röntgenstr 141:517–524

Hammerschlag SB, Wolpert SM, Carter BL (1977) Computed tomography of the skull base. J Comput Assist Tomogr 1:75–80

Hanafee WN, Hoover HA (1983) Differential diagnosis of nasopharyngeal tumors by computed tomography scanning. Arch Otolaryngol 109:43–47

Harrison DFN (1984) Osseous and fibro-osseous conditions affecting the craniofacial bones. Ann Otol Rhinol Laryngol 93:199–203

Helpap B (1978) Extraadrenale Paraganglien und Paragangliome. Normale und pathologische Anatomie, Bd 37. Thieme, Stuttgart, S 1–89

Hesselink JR, New PF, Davis KR, Weber AL, Robertson GH, Taveras JM (1978) Computed tomography of the paranasal sinuses and face. Part I: normal anatomy. J Comput Assist Tomogr 2:559–567

Howell CG, van Tessel P, Gammal TE (1984) High resolution computed tomography in neonatal nasopharyngeal teratoma. J Comput Assist Tomogr 8:1179–1181

Huk W, Schiefer W (1978) Computertomographie bei Prozessen der Schädelbasis und der Orbitae: Kombinierte Anwendung von Horizontal- und Frontalschnitten. Fortschr Röntgenstr 128:8–11

Irnberger T (1985) Die fibröse Knochendysplasie und das ossifizierende Knochenfibrom im orbitalen und periorbitalen Bereich unter besonderer Berücksichtigung der CT. Fortschr Röntgenstr 143:569–574

Ischebeck W, Thal HU, Nabakowski R (1978) Computerized tomography of the posterior fossa and the upper cervical spine. Adv Neurosurg 5:171–175

Jend-Rossmann I, Crone-Münzebrock W, Grabbe E (1984) Die Computertomographie der Schädelbasisfrakturen. Fortschr Röntgenstr 140:147–151

Kido DK, Gould R, Taati F, Duncan A, Schnur J (1978) Comparative sensitivity of CT scans, radiographs and radionuclide bone scans in detecting metastatic calvarial lesions. Radiology 128:371–375

König H, Kurtz B (1984) Computertomographie der Felsenbeine. Fortschr Röntgenstr 141:129–135

König H, Kurtz B, Strohm M (1984) Hochauflösende und dynamische Computertomographie in der Diagnostik von Glomus-tympanicum- und Glomus-jugulare-Tumoren. Fortschr Röntgenstr 141:642–646

König H, Lenz M, Sauter R (1986) Temporal bone region: high-resolution MR imaging using surface coils. Radiology 159:191–194

Köster O, Strähler-Pohl HJ (1985) Stellenwert der hochauflösenden CT in der Diagnostik der erworbenen Mittelohrcholesteatome. Fortschr Röntgenstr 143:322–326

Krayenbühl H, Yasargil MG (1975) Cranial chordomas. Progr Neurol Surg 6:435–463

Krayenbühl H, Yasargil MG (1979) Zerebrale Angiographie für Klinik und Praxis, 3. Aufl. Thieme, Stuttgart

Latack JT, Kartush JM, Kemink JL, Graham MD, Knake JE (1985) Epidermoidomas of the cerebellopontine angle and temporal bone: CT and MR aspects. Radiology 157:361–366

Latack JT, Hutchinson RJ, Heyn RM (1987) Imaging of rhabdomyosarcomas of the head and neck. AJR 8:353–359

Lenz M, König H, Sauter R, Schrader M (1985) Kernspintomographie bei Erkrankungen im Bereich des Felsenbeins. Fortschr Röntgenstr 143:623–634

Lenz M, König H, Sauter R, Schrader M (1985) Kernspintomographie des Felsenbeins und Kleinhirnbrückenwinkels. Fortschr Röntgenstr 143:1–8

Liliequist B, Forsell A (1976) Computertomography of the neurocranium. Acta Radiol [Diagn] (Stockh) 17:399–404

Lloyd GAS, Du Boulay GH, Phelps PD, Pullicino P (1979) The demonstration of the auditory ossicles by high resolution CT. Neuroradiology 18:243–248

Lohkamp F, Claussen C (1977) Computertomographie des Gesichtsschädels (Teil I). Darstellbarkeit bestimmter Strukturen und tiefliegender Regionen. Fortschr Röntgenstr 126:292–299

Lohkamp F, Claussen C (1977) Die Bedeutung der Computertomographie für die TNM-Klassifikation der Gesichtsschädelmalignome im Bereich der Nasennebenhöhle, des Nasopharynx und der Parotis. Laryngol Rhinol Otol (Stuttg) 56:739–748

Lohkamp F, Claussen C, Spenneberg H (1977) Computertomographie des Gesichtsschädels (Teil II). Pathologische Veränderungen. Fortschr Röntgenstr 126:513–520

Lucarelli G, Fornari M, Savoiardo M (1980) Angiography and computerized tomography in the diagnosis of aneurysmal bone cyst of the skull. J Neurosurg 53:113–116

Mafee MF, Valvassori GE, Shugar MA, Yannias DA, Dob-

ben GD (1983) High resolution and dynamic sequential computed tomography. Use in the evaluation of glomus complex tumors. Arch Otolaryngol 109:691–696
Manelfe C, Rochiccioli P (1979) CT of septo-optic dysplasia. Am J Roentgenol 133:1157–1160
Maravilla KR, Mickey B, Peshock RM, Weinreb JC, Riley HK, Diehl J (1986) Tumor characterization by Gd-DTPA-enhanced magnetic resonance imaging. In: Runge VM, Claussen C, Felix R, James AE (eds) Contrast agents in magnetic resonance imaging. Excerpta Medica, Princeton Amsterdam
Marsman JWP (1979) Tumors of the glomus jugulare complex (chemodectomas) demonstrated by cranial computed tomography. J Comput Assist Tomogr 3:795–799
Meyer JE, Oot RF, Lindfors KK (1986) CT appearance of clival chordomas. J Comput Assist Tomogr 10:34–38
Michael AS, Mafee MF, Valvassori GE, Tan WS (1985) Dynamic computed tomography of the head and neck: differential diagnostic value. Radiology 154:413–419
Mitnick JS, Pinto RS (1980) Computed tomography in the diagnosis of eosinophilic granuloma. J Comp Assist Tomogr 4:791–793
Mödder U, Rose KG, Friedmann G, Heuser L (1978) Zum Aussagewert von Computertomographie und Filmtomographie des Gesichtsschädels und der Schädelbasis. Laryngol Rhinol Otol (Stuttg) 57:305–313
Mödder U, Friedmann G, Gode A, Rose KG (1979) Computertomographie des Gesichtsschädels und des pharyngealen Raumes. Fortschr Röntgenstr 131:249–256
Namba K, Aschenbrenner C, Nikpour M, van Gilder JC (1979) Primary rhabdomyosarcoma of the tentorium with peculiar angiographic findings. Surg Neurol 11:39–43
Osborn AG, Anderson RW, Wing SD (1980) Sagittal CT scans in the evaluation of deep facial and nasopharyngeal lesions. J Comput Tomogr 1:19–24
Parkinson D, Hay R (1986) Neurofibromatosis. Can Surg Neurol 25:109–113
Parsons C, Hodson N (1979) Computed tomography of paranasal sinus tumors. Radiology 132:641–645
Potter GD (1970) Sclerosis of the base of the skull as a manifestation of nasopharyngeal carcinoma. Radiology 94:35–38
Raffel C, Wright DC, Gutin PH, Wilson CB (1985) Cranial chordomas: clinical presentation and results of operative and radiation therapy in twentysix patients. Neurosurg 17:703–710
Sarwar M (1979) Primary sellar-parasellar esthesioneuroblastoma. Am J Roentgenol 133:140–141
Schindler E, Aulich A, Wende S (1978) Value and limits of computerized axial tomography in ORL. Adv Otorhinolaryngol 24:9–20
Schroth G, Gawehn J, Marquardt B, Schabet M (1986) MR imaging of esthesioneuroblastoma. J Comput Assist Tomogr 10:316–319
Schwarz CW (1940) Cranial osteomas from a roentgenologic viewpoint. Am J Roentgenol 44:188–196
Scotti G, Harwood-Nash DC (1982) Computed tomography of rhabdomyosarcomas of the skull base in children. J Comput Assist Tomogr 6:33–40
Silver AJ, Sane P, Hilal SK (1984) CT of the nasopharyngeal region. Normal and pathologic anatomy. Radiol Clin North Am 22:161–176
Som PM, Shugar JMA (1980) The CT classification of ethmoid mucoceles. J Comput Assist Tomogr 4:199–203
Som PM, Biller HF, Lawson W, Sacher M, Lanzieri CF (1984) Parapharyngeal space masses: an updated protocol based upon 104 cases. Radiology 153:149–156
Som PM, Lawson W, Biller HF, Lanzieri CF (1986) Ethmoid sinus disease: CT evaluation in 400 cases. Part I. Nonsurgical patients. Radiology 159:591–597
Takahashi M, Tamakawa Y, Shindo M, Kono A (1977) Computed tomography of the paranasal sinuses and their adjacent structures. J Comput Assist Tomogr 1:295–311
Taveras JM, Ferrucci JT (1987) Neuroradiology and radiology of the head and neck. Radiology Vol 3, Diagnosis – Imaging – Intervention. Lippincott, Philadelphia
Treisch J, Schörner W (1986) Topographische Diagnostik von Chordomen mit der magnetischen Resonanztomographie (MRT). Fortschr Röntgenstr 144:232–234
Treisch J, Schörner W, Laniado M, Felix R (1987) Charakteristika intrakranieller Meningeome in der magnetischen Resonanztomographie. Fortschr Röntgenstr 146:207–214
Uhlenbrock D, Radtke J, Beyer HK, Machtens E, Pastoors H (1986) Ergebnisse der Kernspintomographie bei Tumoren des Gesichtsschädels. Fortschr Röntgenstr 144: 322–327
Unsöld R, Ostertag CB, DeGroot J, Newton TH (1982) Computer reformations of the brain and skull base. Anatomy and clinical application. Springer, Berlin Heidelberg New York
Valvassori GE, Potter GD, Hanafee WN, Carter BL, Buckingham RA (1984) Radiologie in der Hals-Nasen-Ohren-Heilkunde. Thieme, Stuttgart New York
Vibhakar SD, Eckhauser C, Bellon EM (1983) Computed tomography of the nasopharynx and neck. CT 7:259–265
Virapongse C, Sarwar M, Bhimani S, Crelin ES (1984) Skull phylogeny: an investigation using radiography and high-resolution computed tomography. Am J Neuroradiol 5:147–154
Vogelsang H, Scharek G, Stolke D, Becker H (1985) CT-Befunde bei Chordomen der Schädelbasis. Fortschr Röntgenstr 142:369–373
Weber AL, Tadmor R, Davis R, Robertson G (1978) Malignant tumors of the sinuses. Radiologic evaluation including CT scanning, with clinical and pathological correlation. Neuroradiology 16:443–448
Weinstein AM, Levine H, Duchesneau P, Tucker HM (1978) Diagnosis of juvenile angiofibroma by computed tomography. Radiology 126:703–705
Wende S, Kazner E, Grumme T (1979) Die radiologische Diagnostik von Läsionen der Schädelbasis, der hinteren Schädelgrube und der Orbita. In: Sager WD, Ladurner G (eds) Computertomographie. Derzeitige Stellung in Radiologie und Klinik. Thieme, Stuttgart, pp 13–21
Whelan MA, Reede DL, Meisler W, Bergeron RT (1984) CT of the base of the skull. Radiol Clin North Am 22:177–217
Wiggli UME, Müller HR, Hünig R, Wüthrich R (1976) Analysis of osseous structures of the skull base. In: Lanksch W, Kazner E (eds) Cranial computerized tomography. Springer, Berlin Heidelberg New York, pp 399–402
Wolfe III JT, Scheithauer BW, Dahlin DC (1983) Giant-cell tumor of the sphenoid bone. Review of 10 cases. J Neurosurg 59:322–327
Zanella FE, Mödder U, Benz-Bohm G, Thun F (1984) Die

Neurofibrose im Kindesalter. Fortschr Röntgenstr 141:498–504
Zimmerman RA, Bilaniuk LT (1977) Computed tomography of sphenoid sinus tumors. J Comput Assist Tomogr 1:22–32

F. Non-neoplastic Intracranial Masses

Overviews

Kazner E, Klein W, Stochdorph O (1978) Möglichkeiten und Aussagewert der Computertomographie bei nicht tumorbedingten raumfordernden intrakraniellen Prozessen. Roentgenpraxis 31:181–198
Ruggiero G, Sabattini L (1976) La tomographie axiale avec ordinateur dans les maladies non tumorales. J Neuroradiol 3:313–330
Williams RG, Osborn AG (1980) Low-attenuation lesions in the middle cranial fossa: differential diagnosis. J Comput Assist Tomogr 4:89–97

F.1. Inflammatory Lesions

Allo MD, Silva J, Kauffman CA, Dicks RE III (1979) Enlarging histoplasmomas following treatment of meningitis due to histoplasma capsulatum. J Neurosurg 51:242–244
Aulich A, Lange S, Steinhoff H, Schindler E, Wende S (1976) Diagnosis and follow-up studies in brain abscesses using CT. In: Lanksch W, Kazner E (eds) Cranial computerized tomography. Springer, Berlin Heidelberg New York, pp 366–371
Bannister G, Williams B, Smith S (1981) Treatment of subdural empyema. J Neurosurg 55:82–88
Benator RM, Magill HL, Gerald B, Igarashi M, Fitch SJ (1985) Herpes simplex encephalitis: CT findings in the neonate and young infant. AJNR 6:539–543
Bilaniuk LT, Zimmerman RA, Brown L, Yoo HJ, Goldberg HI (1978) Computed tomography in meningitis. Neuroradiology 16:13–14
Blaquiere RM (1983) The computed tomographic appearances of intra- and extracerebral abscesses. Br J Radiol 56:171–181
Borovich B, Braun J, Honigman S, Joachims HZ, Peyser E (1981) Supratentorial and parafalcial subdural empyema diagnosed by computerized tomography. J Neurosurg 54:105–107
Brant-Zawadzki M, Enzmann DR, Placone RC, Sheldon P, Britt RH, Brasch RC, Crooks LA (1983) NMR imaging of experimental brain abscess: comparison with CT. AJNR 4:250–253
Buge A, Metzger J, Rancurel G, Gardeur D, Eohanno F, Pertuiset BF (1979) Les aspects tomodensitométriques (C.T. Scan) des encephalites aigues necrosantes herpetiques (7 cas) premieres tentatives therapeutiques par l'isoprinosine. Rev Neurol 135:401–416
Bullock MRR, Welchman JM (1982) Diagnostik and prognostic features of tuberculous meningitis on CT scanning. J Neurol Neurosurg Psychiatry 45:1098–1101
Byrne E, Brophy BP, Perrett LV (1979) Nocardia cerebral abscess: new concepts in diagnosis, management and prognosis. J Neurol Neurosurg Psychiatry 42:1038–1045
Carter BL, Bankoff MS, Fisk JD (1983) Computed tomographic detection of sinusitis responsible for intracranial and extracranial infections. Radiology 147:739–742
Casselman ES, Hasso AN, Ashwal S, Schneider S (1980) Computed tomography of tuberculous meningitis in infants and children. J Comput Assist Tomogr 4:211–216
Chiu LC, Jensen JC, Cornell SH, Christie JH (1977) Computerized tomography of brain abscess. J Comput Assist Tomogr 1:33–38
Claveria LE, du Boulay GH, Moseley LF (1976) Intracranial infections: investigation by computerized axial tomography. Neuroradiology 12:59–71
Cockrill HH Jr, Dreisbach J, Lowe B, Yamauchi T (1978) Computed tomography in leptomeningeal infections. Am J Roentgenol 130:511–515
Damasio AR, van Hoesen GW (1985) The limbic system and the localisation of herpes simplex encephalitis. J Neurol Neurosurg Psychiatry 48:297–301
Danziger A, Price H, Schechter MM (1980) An analysis of 113 intracranial infections. Neuroradiology 19:31–34
Davidson HD, Steiner RE (1985) Magnetic resonance imaging in infections of the central nervous system. AJNR 6:499–504
Davis JM, Davis KR, Kleinman GM, Kirchner HS, Taveras JM (1978) Computed tomography of herpes simplex encephalitis, with clinicopathological correlation. Radiology 129:409–417
Dubois PJ, Heinz ER, Wessel HB, Zaias BW (1979) Multicystic encephalomalacia of infancy: computed tomographic findings in two cases with associated intracerebral calcifications. J Comput Assist Tomogr 3:97–102
Enzmann DR (1984) Imaging of infections and inflammations of the central nervous system: Computed tomography, ultrasound, and nuclear magnetic resonance. Raven Press, New York
Enzmann DR, Norman D, Mani J, Newton ThH (1976) Computed tomography of granulomatous basal arachnoiditis. Radiology 120:341–344
Enzmann DR, Ranson B, Norman D, Talberth E (1978) Computed tomography of herpes simplex encephalitis. Radiology 129:419–425
Enzmann DR, Britt RH, Yeager AS (1979) Experimental brain abscess evolution: Computer tomographic and neuropathologic correlation. Radiology 133:113–122
Enzmann DR, Britt RH, Placone RC, Obana W, Lyons B, Yeager AS (1982) The effect of short-term corticosteroid treatment on the CT appearance of experimental brain abscesses. Radiology 145:79–84
Enzmann DR, Britt RH, Placone R (1983) Staging of human brain abscess by computed tomography. Radiology 146:703–708
Enzmann DR, Placone RC, Britt RH (1984) Dynamic computed tomographic scans in experimental brain abscess. Neuroradiology 26:309–313
Enzmann DR, Britt RH, Obana WG, Stuart J, Murphy-Irwin K (1986) Experimental Staphylococcus aureus brain abscess. AJNR 7:395–402
Fink IJ, Danziger A, Dillon WP, Brant-Zawadzki M, Rechthand E (1984) Atypical CT findings in bacterial meningoencephalitis. Neuroradiology 26:51–54
Galbraith JG, Barr VW (1974) Epidural abscess and subdural empyema. Adv Neurol 6:257–267
Grossman RI, Wolf G, Biery D, McGrath J, Kundel H, Aronchick J, Zimmerman RA, Goldberg HI, Bilaniuk

LT (1984) Gadolinium enhanced nuclear magnetic resonance images of experimental brain abscess. J Comput Assist Tomogr 8:204–207
Hacke W, Zeumer H (1981) Computertomographie bei Herpes-simplex-Enzephalitis. Fortschr Röntgenstr 135: 426–431
Herman TE, Cleveland RH, Kushner DG, Taveras JM (1985) CT of neonatal herpes encephalitis. AJNR 6:773–775
Holtas S, Tornquist C, Cronqvist S (1982) Diagnostic difficulties in computed tomography of brain abscesses. J Comput Assist Tomogr 6:683–688
Joubert MJ, Stephanov S (1977) Computerized tomography and surgical treatment in intracranial suppuration. J Neurosurg 47:73–78
Kaufman DM, Leeds NE (1977) Computed tomography (CT) in the diagnosis of intracranial abscesses. Brain abscess, subdural empyema and epidural empyema. Neurology 27:1069–1073
Kaufman DM, Zimmerman RD, Leeds NE (1979) Computed tomography in herpes simplex encephalitis. Neurology 29:1392–1396
Kazner E (1976) Effects of computerized axial tomography on the treatment of cerebral abscess. Neuroradiology 12:57–58
Kirmani N, Tuazon CU, Ocuin JA, Thompson AM, Kramer NC, Geelhoed GW (1978) Extensive cerebral nocardiosis cured with antibiotic therapy alone. J Neurosurg 49:924–928
Kretzschmar K, Wallenfang T, Bohl J (1981) CT studies of brain abscess in cats. Neuroradiology 22:93–98
Leo JS, Weiner RL, Lin JP, Ransohoff J (1978) Computed tomography in herpes simplex encephalitis. Surg Neurol 10:313–317
Long Jr JA, Herdt JR, Di Chiro G, Cramer HR (1980) Cerebral mass lesions in torulosis demonstrated by computed tomography. J Comput Assist Tomogr 4:766–769
Luken MG III, Whelan MA (1980) Recent diagnostic experience with subdural empyema. J Neurosurg 52:764–771
Messina AV, Guido LJ, Liebeskind AL (1977) Preoperative diagnosis of brain-stem abscess by computerized tomography with survival. J Neurosurg 47:106–108
Mikhael MA (1978) Radiation necrosis of the brain: correlation between computed tomography, pathology and dose distribution. J Comput Assist Tomogr 2:71–80
Mineury K, Mori T (1980) Sparganosis of the brain. J Neurosurg 52:588–590
Moseley IF, Kendall BE (1984) Radiology of intracranial empyemas, with special reference to computed tomography. Neuroradiology 26:333–345
Moseley IF, Claveria LE, du Boulay GH (1977) Diseases of the brain parenchyma, atrophy and hydrocephalus. The role of CAT in the diagnosis and management of intracranial infection. In: du Boulay GH, Moseley IF (eds) Computerised axial tomography in clinical practice. Springer, Berlin Heidelberg New York, pp 182–190
Moussa AH, Dawson BH (1978) Computed tomography and the mortality rate in brain abscess. Surg Neurol 10:301–304
New PFJ, Davis KR, Ballantine HT (1976) Computed tomography in cerebral abscess. Radiology 121:641–646
Nielsen H, Gyldensted C (1977) Computed tomography in the diagnosis of cerebral abscess. Neuroradiology 12: 207–217
Price HJ, Danziger A (1978) Computed tomography in cranial tuberculosis. Am J Roentgenol 130:769–771
Probst FP (1980) Non-pyogenic focal encephalitis diagnosis and follow-up by computed tomography and nuclear brain scanning. Neuroradiology 20:155–158
Reisner Th (1979) Die Bedeutung der kranialen Computertomographie in der Differentialdiagnose entzündlicher Erkrankungen des Gehirns. In: Sager W-D, Ladurner G (eds) Computertomographie. Thieme, Stuttgart, S 74–78
Roberts FJ (1981) Problems in the diagnosis of tuberculous meningitis. Arch Neurol 38:319–320
Rodiek SO, Backmund H (1984) Die Herpes-simplex-Enzephalitis im Computertomogramm. Fortschr Röntgenstr 141:23–29
Rosenblum ML, Hoff JT, Norman D, Edwards MS, Berg BO (1980) Nonoperative treatment of brain abscesses in selected high-risk patients. J Neurosurg 52:217–225
Rosenblum ML, Hoff JT, Norman D, Weinstein PR, Pitts L (1978) Decreased mortality from brain abscesses since advent of computerized tomography. J Neurosurg 49:658–668
Rovira M, Romero F, Torrent O, Ibarra B (1980) Study of tuberculous meningitis by CT. Neuroradiology 19:137–141
Runge VM, Clanton JA, Price AC, Herzer WA, Allen JH, Partain CL, James RE (1985) Evaluation of contrast enhanced MR imaging in a brain-abscess model. AJNR 6:139–147
Sadhu VK, Handel SF, Pinto RS, Glass TF (1980) Neuroradiologic diagnosis of subdural empyema and CT limitations. AJNR 1:37–44
Sage MR, Dubois PJ, Oakes J, Rothman S, Heinz ER, Drayer B (1981) Rapid development of cerebral atrophy due to perinatal herpes simplex encephalitis. J Comput Assist Tomogr 5:763–766
Schiefer W, Huk W (1976) Computerized tomographic findings with brain abscesses. In: Lanksch W, Kazner E (eds) Cranial computerized tomography. Springer, Berlin Heidelberg New York, pp 360–365
Schiefer W, Klinger M (1978) Aspects of modern brain abscess diagnosis and treatment. Neurosurg Rev 1/2:37–45
Schochet SS, Sarwar M, Kelly PJ, Masel BE (1980) Symptomatic cerebral histoplasmoma. J Neurosurg 52:273–275
Schroth G, Thron A (1983) Neuroradiologische Verlaufsdiagnostik konservativ behandelter Hirnabszesse. Radiologe 23:463–470
Schroth G, Kretzschmar K, Gawehn J, Voigt K (1987) Advantage of magnetic resonance imaging in the diagnosis of cerebral infections. Neuroradiology 29:120–126
Smith HP, Hendrick EB (1983) Subdural empyema and epidural abscess in children. J Neurosurg 58:392–397
Stephanov S (1978) Experience with multiloculated brain abscesses. J Neurosurg 49:199–203
Stephanov S, Joubert MJ, Welchmann JM (1979) Combined convexity and parafalx subdural empyema. Surg Neurol 11:147–151
Tamaka R, Takeda N, Okada K, Ueki K (1979) Computerized tomography of coagulation necrosis of the brain and brain tumors. Surg Neurol 11:9–12
Thomson JLG (1976) The computed axial tomography in acute herpes simplex encephalitis. Br J Radiol 49:86–87
Tress B, Davis S (1979) Computed tomography of intracerebral toruloma. Neuroradiology 17:223–226

Tully RJ, Watts C (1979) Computed tomography and intracranial aspergillosis. Neuroradiology 17:111–113
Wallenfang T, Bohl J, Kretzschmar K (1980) Evolution of brain abscess in cats. Formation of capsule and resolution of brain edema. Neurosurg Rev 3:101–111
Weisberg LC (1986) Subdural empyema: clinical and computed tomographic correlations. Arch Neurol 43:497–500
Whelan MA, Hilal SK (1980) Computed tomography as a guide in the diagnosis and follow-up of brain abscesses. Radiology 135:663–671
Whitley RJ (1982) Herpes simplex virus infections of the central nervous system in children. Semin Neurol 2:87–96
Zimmerman RA, Bilaniuk LT (1980) CT of orbital infection and its cerebral complications. Am J Roentgenol 134:45–50
Zimmerman RA, Patel S, Bilaniuk LT (1976) Demonstration of purulent bacterial intracranial infections by computed tomography. Am J Roentgenol 127:155–165
Zimmerman RD, Russel EJ, Leeds NE, Kaufman D (1980) CT in the early diagnosis of herpes simplex encephalitis. Am J Roentgenol 134:61–66
Zimmerman RD, Leeds NE, Danziger A (1984) Subdural empyema: CT findings. Radiology 150:417–422

F.2. Granulomatous Lesions

Bhalla D, Kumar S, Pal DN et al. (1980) Aspergilloma of the frontal lobe. Acta Neurochir 55:135–139
Bhargava S, Tandon PN (1980) Intracranial tuberculomas: a CT study. Br J Radiol 53:935–945
Brooks BS, Gammal TE, Hungerford GD, Acker J, Trevor RP, Russel W (1982) Radiologic evaluation of neurosarcoidosis: role of computed tomography. AJNR 3:513–521
Brückner O, Kluge W (1981) Intracranial tuberculous abscess mimicking pyogenic brain abscess. Neurochirurgia (Stuttg) 24:147–149
Cornell SH, Jacoby CG (1982) The varied computed tomographic appearance of intracranial cryptococcosis. Radiology 143:703–707
Decker RE, Mardayat M, Marc J, Rasool A (1979) Neurosarcoidosis with computerized tomographic visualization and transsphenoidal excision of a supra- and intrasellar granuloma. Case report. J Neurosurg 50:814–816
Delaney P (1977) Neurologic manifestations in sarcoidosis: review of the literature with a report of 23 cases. Ann Intern Med 87:336–345
Eltomey AA, Olin MS, Roberts MP (1984) Cerebellopontine angle gumma. Neurosurgery 15:252–253
Ganti SR, Cohen M, Sane P, Hilal SK (1981) Computed tomography of cerebral syphilis. J Comput Assist Tomogr 5:345–347
Godt P, Stoeppler L, Wischer U, Schroeder HH (1979) The value of computed tomography in cerebral syphilis. Neuroradiology 18:197–200
Grossman RI, Davis KR, Taveras JM et al. (1981) Computed tomography of intracranial aspergillosis. J Comput Assist Tomogr 5:646–650
Guest SS, Sivit CJ, Meisler WJ, Stevens AC, Simon GL (1987) Intracranial tuberculosis due to mycobacterium bovis. Comput Radiol 11:151–154
Hirsh LF, Lee SH, Silberstein StD (1978) Intracranial tuberculomas and the CAT scan. Acta Neurochir (Wien) 45:155–161
Kaplan JG, Sterman AB, Horoupian D, Leeds NE, Zimmerman RD, Grade R (1981) Luetic meningitis with gumma: Clinical radiographic and neuropathologic features. Neurology 31:464–467
Kendall BE, Tatler GLV (1978) Radiological findings in neurosarcoidosis. Br J Radiol 51:81–92
Ketonen L, Oksanen V, Kuuliala I, Somer H (1986) Hypodense white matter lesions in computed tomography of neurosarcoidosis. J Comput Assist Tomogr 10:181–183
Ketonen L, Oksanen V, Kuuliala I (1987) Preliminary experience of magnetic resonance imaging in neurosarcoidosis. Neuroradiology 29:127–129
Leibrock L, Epstein MH, Rybock JD (1976) Cerebral tuberculoma localized by EMI Scan. Surg Neurol 5:305–306
Peatfield RC, Shawelon HH (1979) Five cases of intracranial tuberculoma followed by serial computerised tomography. J Neurol Neurosurg Psychiatry 42:373–379
Post MJD, Quencer RM, Tabei SZ (1982) CT demonstration of sarcoidosis of the optic nerve, frontal lobes, and falx cerebri: Case report and literature review. AJNR 3:523–526
Price HI, Danziger A (1978) Computed tomography in cranial tuberculosis. Am J Roentgenol 130:769–771
Rush JL, Kusske JA, Porter RW, Pribram HW (1979) Xanthogranulomas of the third ventricle. Neurosurgery 4:329–333
Szper J, Oi S, Leestma J, Kim KS, Wetzel NE (1979) Xanthogranuloma of the third ventricle. J Neurosurg 51:565–568
Terao H, Kobayashi S, Teraoka A, Okeda R (1978) Xanthogranulomas of the choroid plexus in a neuroepileptic child. J Neurosurg 48:649–653
Welchman JM (1979) Computerised tomography of intracranial tuberculomata. Clin Radiol 30:567–573
Whelan MA, Stern J (1979) Intracranial tuberculoma. Radiology 138:75–81

F.3. Parasitic Diseases

Abassioun K, Rahmat H, Ameli NO, Tafazuli M (1978) Computerized tomography in hydatid cyst of the brain. J Neurosurg 49:408–411
Bentson JR, Wilson GH, Helmer E, Winter J (1977) Computed tomography in intracranial cysticercosis. J Comput Assist Tomogr 1:464–471
Byrd SE, Locke GE, Biggers S, Percy AK (1982) The computed tomographic appearance of cerebral cysticercosis in adults and children. Radiology 144:819–823
Camas E, Esterez J, Soto M, Obrador S (1978) Computerized axial tomography for the diagnosis of cerebral cysticercosis. Acta Neurochir (Wien) 44:197–205
Hamza R, Touibi S, Jamoussi M, Bardi-Bellagha I, Chtioui R (1982) Intracranial and orbital hydatid cysts. Neuroradiology 22:211–214
Handler LC, Mervis B (1983) Cerebral cysticercosis with reference to the natural history of parenchymal lesions. AJNR 4:709–712
Jankowski R, Zimmerman RD, Leeds NE (1979) Cysticercosis presenting as a mass lesion at foramen of Monro. J Comput Assist Tomogr 3:694–696

Latovitzki N, Abrams G, Clark C, Mayeux R, Ascherl G Jr, Sciara D (1978) Cerebral cysticercosis. Neurology 28:838–842

Mazer S, Antoniuk A, Ditzel LFS, Araujo JC (1983) The computed tomographic spectrum of cerebral cysticercosis. Comput Radiol 7:373–378

McCorkell SJ, Lewall DB (1985) Computed tomography of intracerebral echinococcal cysts in children. J Comput Assist Tomogr 9:514–518

Mervis B, Lotz JW (1980) Computed tomography (CT) in parenchymatous cysticercosis. Clin Radiol 31:521–528

Ramos OM, Stiebel-Chin G, Altman N, Duchowny M (1986) Diagnosis of neurocysticercosis by magnetic resonance imaging. Pediatr Infect Dis 5:470–473

Rodriquez-Carbajal J, Salgado P, Gutierrez-Alvarado R, Escobar-Izquierdo A, Aruffo C, Palacios E (1983) The acute encephalitic phase of neurocysticercosis: Computed tomographic manifestations. AJNR 4:51–55

Suss AR, Maravilla KR, Thompson J (1986) MR imaging of intracranial cysticercosis: Comparison with CT and anatomicpathologic features. AJNR 7:235–242

Torrealba G, del Villar S, Tagle P, Arriagada P, Kase CS (1984) Cysticercosis of the central nervous system: clinical and therapeutic considerations. J Neurol Neurosurg Psychiatry 47:784–790

Vaquero J, Jimenez C, Martinez R (1982) Growth of hydatic cysts evaluated by CT scanning after presumed cerebral hydatic embolism. J Neurosurg 57:837–838

Zee C, Segall HD, Miller C, Tsai FY, Teal JS, Hieshima G, Ahmadi J, Halls J (1980) Unusual neuroradiological features of intracranial cysticercosis. Radiology 137: 397–407

Zee CS, Segall HD, Apuzzo MLJ, Ahmadi J, Dobkin WR (1984) Intraventricular cysticercal cysts: further neuroradiologic observations and neurosurgical implications. AJNR 5:727–730

F.4. Brain Diseases Associated with AIDS

Alonso R, Heiman-Patterson T, Mancall EL (1984) Cerebral toxoplasmosis in acquired immune deficiency syndrome. Arch Neurol 41:321–323

Anders K, Steinsapir KD, Iverson DJ et al. (1986) Neuropathologic findings in the acquired immunodeficiency syndrome (AIDS). Clin Neuropathol 5:1–20

Anderson KP, Atlas E, Ahern MJ et al. (1983) Central nervous system toxoplasmosis in homosexual men. Am J Med 75:877

Bagley PH, Scott DA, Smith LS et al. (1986) Cytomegalovirus infection, ascending myelitis, and pulmonary embolus (Letter). Ann Intern Med 104:587

Barre-Sinoussi F, Chermann JC, Rey F et al. (1983) Isolation of a T-lymphotropic retrovirus from a patient at risk for acquired immune deficiency syndrome (AIDS). Science 220:868

Berger JR, Moskowitz L, Fischl M et al. (1984) The neurologic complications of AIDS: frequently the initial manifestation. Neurology 34:134–135

Bredesen DE, Messing R (1983) Neurological syndromed hearlding the acquired immune deficiency syndrome. Program and Abstracts, American Neurological Association 14:141

Britton CB, Miller JR (1984) Neurologic complications in acquired immunodeficiency syndrome (AIDS). Neurol Clin 2:315–339

Britton CB, Mesa-Tejada R, Fenoglio CM et al. (1985) A new complication of AIDS: thoracic myelitis caused by herpes simplex virus. Neurology 35:1071–1074

Case records of the Massachusetts General Hospital (1986) Weekly clinicopathological exercises. Case 9-1986. A 40-month-old girl with the acquired immunodeficiency syndrome and spinal-cord compression. N Engl J Med 61:100–103

Cellerier P, Chiras J, Gray F et al. (1984) Computed tomography in primary lymphoma of the brain. Neuroradiology 26:485–492

Dix RD, Bredesen DE, Erlich KS et al. (1985) Recovery of herpes viruses from cerebrospinal fluid of immunodeficient homosexual men. Ann Neurol 18:611–614

Dix RD, Waitzman DM, Follansbee S et al. (1985) Herpes simplex virus type 2 encephalitis in two homosexual men with persistent lymphadenopathy. Ann Neurol 17:203–206

Edwards RH, Messing R, McKendall RR (1985) Cytomegalovirus meningoencephalitis in a homosexual man with Kaposi's sarcoma: isolation of CMV from CSF cells. Neurology 35:560–562

Enzmann DR, Krikorian J, Norman D et al. (1979) Computed tomography in primary reticulum cell sarcoma of the brain. Radiology 130(1):165–170

Fauci AS (1985) The acquired immunodeficiency syndrome: an update. Ann Intern Med 102:800–813

Fischl MA, Pitchenik AE, Spira TJ (1985) Tuberculous brain abscess and Toxoplasma encephalitis in a patient with the acquired immunodeficiency syndrome. JAMA 253:3428–3430

Gallo RC, Sarin PS, Gelmann EP et al. (1985) Isolation of human T cell leukemia virus in acquired immune deficiency syndrome (AIDS). Science 220:865–867

Gill PS, Levine AM, Meyer PR et al. (1985) Primary central nervous system lymphoma in homosexual men: clinical, immunologic and pathologic features. Am J Med 78:742–748

Goldstick L, Mandybur TI, Bode R, (1985) Spinal cord degeneration in AIDS. Neurology 35:103–106

Gorin FA, Bale JF, Halks-Miller M et al. (1985) Kaposi's sarcoma metastatic to the CNS. Arch Neurol 42:162–165

Greene JB, Sidhu GS, Lewin S et al. (1982) Mycobacterium avium-intracellulare: A case of disseminated life-threatening infection in homosexuals and drug abusers. Ann Intern Med 97:539–546

Helle TL, Britt RH, Colby TV (1984) Primary lymphoma of the central nervous system. Clinicopathological study of experience at Stanford. J Neurosurg 60:94–103

Ho DD, Rota TR, Schooley RT et al. (1985) Isolation of HTLV-III from cerebrospinal fluid and neural tissues of patients with neurologic syndromes related to the acquired immunodeficiency syndrome. N Engl J Med 313:1493–1497

Holtz HA, Lavery DP, Kapila R (1985) Actinomycetales infection in the acquired immunodeficiency syndrome. Ann Intern Med 102:203–205

Ioachim HL, Cooper MC, Hellman GC (1985) Lymphomas in men at high risk for acquired immune deficiency syndrome (AIDS). A study of 21 cases. Cancer 56:2831–2842

Kazner E, Wilske J, Steinhoff H et al. (1978) Computer assisted tomography in primary malignant lymphoma of the brain. J Comput Assist Tomogr 2:125–134

Kelly WM, Brant-Zawadzki M (1984) Acquired immunodeficiency syndrome: neuroradiologic findings. Radiology 149:485–491

Kleihues P, Lang W, Burger PC et al. (1985) Progressive diffuse leukoencephalopathy in patients with acquired immune deficiency syndrome (AIDS). Acta Neuropathol (Berl) 68:333–339

Kovacs JA, Kovacs AA, Polis M et al. (1985) Cryptococcosis in the acquired immunodeficiency syndrome. Ann Intern Med 102:533–538

Krupp LB, Lipton RB, Swerdlow ML et al. (1985) Progressive multifocal leukoencephalopathy: clinical and radiographic features. Ann Neurol 17:344–349

Letendre L, Banks PM, Reese DF et al. (1982) Primary lymphoma of the central nervous system. Cancer 49:939–943

Levine AM, Gill PS, Meyer PR et al. (1985) Retrovirus and malignant lymphoma in homosexual men. JAMA 254:1921–1925

Levitt LJ, Dawson DM, Rosenthal DS et al. (1980) CNS involvement in the non-Hodgkin's lymphomas. Cancer 45:545–552

Levy JA, Hoffman AD, Kramer SM et al. (1984) Isolation of lymphocytopathic retroviruses from San Francisco patients with AIDS. Science 225:840

Levy JA, Kaminsky LS, Morrow WJ et al. (1985) Infection by the retrovirus associated with the acquired immunodeficiency syndrome. Clinical, pathological, and molecular features. Ann Intern Med 103:694–699

Levy RM, Bredesen DE, Rosenblum ML (1985) Neurological manifestations of the acquired immunodeficiency syndrome (AIDS): experience at UCSF and review of the literature. J Neurosurg 62:475–495

Levy RM, Morgan WM, Rosenblum ML (1986) The neuroepidemiology of AIDS in the United States. International Conference on Acquired Immunodeficiency Syndrome (AIDS), Paris, France, June 23–25, 1986

Levy RM, Pons VG, Rosenblum ML (1984) Central nervous system mass lesions in the acquired immunodeficiency syndrome (AIDS). J Neurosurg 61:9–16

Mackintosh FR, Colby TV, Podolsky WJ et al. (1982) Central nervous system involvement in non-Hodgkin's lymphoma: an analysis of 105 cases. Cancer 49:586–595

Micozzi MS, Wetli CV (1985) Intravenous amphetamine abuse, primary cerebral mucormycosis, and acquired immunodeficiency. J Forensic Sci 30:504–510

Montagnier L (1985) Lymphadenopathy-associated virus: from molecular biology to pathogenicity. Ann Intern Med 103:689–693

Moskowitz LB, Gregorios JB, Hensley GT et al. (1984a) Cytomegalovirus. Arch Pathol Lab Med 108:873–877

Moskowitz LB, Hensley GT, Chan JC et al. (1984b) Brain biopsies in patients with acquired immune deficiency syndrome. Arch Pathol Lab Med 108:368–371

Moskowitz LB, Hensley GT, Chan JC et al. (1984c) The neuropathology of acquired immune deficiency syndrome. Arch Pathol Lab Med 108:867–872

Nielsen SL, Petito CK, Urmacher CD et al. (1984) Subacute encephalitis in acquired immune deficiency syndrome: a postmortem study. Am J Clin Pathol 82:678–682

Pagani JJ, Libshitz HI, Wallace S et al. (1981) Central nervous system leukemia and lymphoma: computed tomographic manifestations. AJR 137:1195–1201

Palacios E, Gorelick PB, Gonzalez CF et al. (1982) Malignant lymphoma of the nervous system. J Comput Assist Tomogr 6:689–701

Petito CK, Navia BA, Cho E et al. (1985) Vacuolar myelopathy pathologically resembling subacute combined degeneration in patients with acquired immunodeficiency syndrome. N Engl J Med 312:874–879

Pitchenik AE, Fischl MA, Walls KW (1983) Evaluation of cerebral-mass lesions in acquired immunodeficiency syndrome (Letter). N Engl J Med 308:1099

Pitlik SD, Fainstein V, Bolivar R et al. (1983) Spectrum of cerebral mass lesions in AIDS (Letter). N Engl J Med 308:771–772

Post MJD, Chan JC, Hensley GT et al. (1983) Toxoplasma encephalitis in Haitian adults with acquired immunodeficiency syndrome: a clinical-pathologic-CT correlation. AJNR 140:861–868

Post MJD, Kursunoglu SJ, Hensley GT et al. (1985) Cranial CT in acquired immunodeficiency syndrome: spectrum of diseases and optimal contrast enhancement technique. AJR 145:929–940

Post MJD, Hensley GT, Moskowitz LB et al. (1986) Cytomegalic inclusion virus encephalitis in patients with AIDS: CT, clinical and pathologic correlation. AJNR 7:275–280

Rosenberg SA, Berard CW, Brown BW Jr et al. (1982) National Cancer Institute sponsored study of classifications of non-Hodgkin's lymphomas, summary and description of a working formulated for clinical usage. Cancer 49:2112–2135

Price RW, Navia BA, Cho E (1986) AIDS encephalopathy. Neurol Clin 4:285–301

Shaw GM, Harper ME, Hahn BH et al. (1985) HTLV III infection in brains of children and adults with AIDS encephalopathy. Science 227:177–182

Snider WD, Simpson DM, Nielsen S et al. (1983) Neurological complications of acquired immune deficiency syndrome: analysis of 50 patients. Ann Neurol 14:403–418

So YT, Beckstead JH, Davis RL (1986) Primary central nervous system lymphoma in acquired immune deficiency syndrome: a clinical and pathologic study. Ann Neurol 20(5):566–572

Spillane JA, Kendall BE, Moseley IF (1982) Cerebral lymphoma: clinical radiological correlation. J Neurol Neurosurg Psychiatry 45:199–208

Tadmor R, David KR, Roberson GH et al. (1978) Computed tomography in primary malignant lymphoma of the brain. J Comput Assist Tomogr 2:135–140

Whelan MA, Kricheff II, Handler M et al. (1983) Acquired immunodeficiency syndrome: cerebral computed tomographic manifestations. Radiology 149:477–484

Wiley CA, Schrier RD, Denaro FJ et al. (1986) Localization of cytomegalovirus proteins and genome during fulminant central nervous system infection in an AIDS patient. J Neuropathol Exp Neurol 45:127–139

Wong B, Gold JWM, Brown AE et al. (1984) Central-nervous-system toxoplasmosis in homosexual man and parenteral drug abusers. Ann Intern Med 100:36–42

Ziegler JL, Beckstead JA, Volberding PA et al. (1984) Non-Hodgkin's lymphoma in 90 homosexual men. Relation to generalized lymphadenopathy and the acquired immunodeficiency syndrome. N Engl J Med 311:565–570

Zuger A, Louie E, Holzman RS et al. (1986) Cryptococcal disease in patient with the acquired immunodeficiency syndrome. Diagnostic features and outcome of treatment. Ann Intern Med 104:234–240

F.5. Cysts

Agnoli AL, Ellams ET (1984) Die Arachnoidalcysten. Eine klinische, neuroradiologische, computertomographische Untersuchung. Fortschr Geb Roentgenstr Nuklearmed Ergänzungsband 141:491–498

Anderson FM, Segall HD, Caton WL (1979) Use of computerized tomography scanning in supratentorial arachnoid cysts. J Neurosurg 50:333–338

Archer CR, Darwish H, Smith K jr (1978) Enlarged cisternae magnae and posterior fossa cysts simulating Dandy-Walker syndrome on computed tomography. Radiology 127:681–686

Averback P (1977) Developmental arachnoid cysts of the posterior fossa – an analysis of 13 cases. Acta Neurochir (Wien) 39:181–186

Di Rocco C, Di Trapani G, Janelli A (1979) Arachnoid cyst of the fourth ventricle and "arrested" hydrocephalus. Surg Neurol 12:467–471

Drayer BP, Rosenbaum AE, Maroon JC, Bank WO, Woodford JE (1977) Posterior fossa extraaxial cyst: Diagnosis with Metrizamide CT cisternography. Am J Roentgenol 128:431–436

Dubois PJ, Heinz ER, Wessel HB, Zaias BW (1979) Multiple cystic encephalomalacia of infancy: computed tomographic findings in two cases with associated intracerebral calcification. J Comput Assist Tomogr 3:97–102

Galassi E, Piazzi G, Gaist G, Frank F (1980) Arachnoid cysts of the middle cranial fossa: a clinical and radiological study of 25 cases treated surgically. Surg Neurol 14:211–219

Geissinger JD, Kohler WC, Robinson BW, Davis FM (1978) Arachnoid cysts of the middle cranial fossa: surgical considerations. Surg Neurol 10:27–33

Gregorius FK, Batzdorf U (1976) Diagnosis of intrathalamic cyst by computerized tomographic scan. Surg Neurol 6:191–193

Handa J, Nakano Y, Aii H (1977) CT cisternography with intracranial arachnoidal cysts. Surg Neurol 8:451–454

Hayashi T, Anegawa S, Honda E, Kuramoto S, Mori K, Murata T, Miwa S, Handa W (1979) Clinical analysis of arachnoid cysts in the middle fossa. Neurochirurgia (Stuttg) 22:201–210

Hayashi T, Kuratomi A, Kuramoto S (1980) Arachnoid cyst of the quadrigeminal cistern. Surg Neurol 14:267–273

Kasdon DL, Douglas EA, Brougham MF (1977) Suprasellar arachnoid cyst diagnosed preoperatively by computerized tomographic scanning. Surg Neurol 7:299–303

Kjos BO, Brant-Zawadzki M, Kucharczyk W, Kelly WM, Norman D, Newton TH (1985) Cystic intracranial lesions: magnetic resonance imaging. Radiology 155:363–369

MacGregor BJL, Gawler J, South JR (1976) Intracranial epithelial cysts. J Neurosurg 44:109–115

Maravilla KR, Kirks DR, Maravilla AM (1978) CT diagnosis of intracranial cystic abnormalities in children. Comput Tomogr 2:221–235

Markakis E, Heyer R, Stoeppler L, Werry H (1979) Die Aplasie der perisylviischen Region. Neurochirurgia (Stuttg) 22:211–220

Markwalder T-M, Zimmermann A (1979) Intracerebral ciliated epithelial cyst. Surg Neurol 11:195–198

Mayr U, Aichner F, Bauer G et al. (1982) Supratentorial extracerebral cysts of the middle cranial fossa. A report of 23 consecutive cases of the socalled temporal lobe agenesis syndrome. Neurochirurgia (Stuttg) 25:51–56

Mercuri S, Curatolo P, Giuffre R, di Lorenzo N (1979) Agenesis of the vermis cerebelli and malformations of the posterior fossa in childhood and adolescence. Neurochirurgia (Stuttg) 22:180–188

Murali R, Epstein F (1979) Diagnosis and treatment of suprasellar arachnoid cyst. J Neurosurg 50:515–518

Palma L, di Lorenzo N, Nicole S (1979) Developmental CSF cysts of the posterior fossa. Neurosurg Rev 2:159–169

Rao KCVG, Gunadi IK, Diaconis JN (1982) Interhemispheric intradural cyst. J Comput Assist Tomogr 6:1167–1171

Rengachary SS, Watanabe I, Brackett CE (1978) Pathogenesis of intracranial arachnoid cyst. Surg Neurol 9:139–144

Scolt LC, Deck JHN, Baim RC, Terbrugge K (1980) Interhemispheric cyst of neuroepithelial origin in association with partial agenesis of the corpus callosum. J Neurosurg 52:399–405

Servo A, Porras M, Jaaskinen J (1983) Diagnosis of ependymal intraventricular cysts of the third ventricle by computed tomography. Neuroradiology 24:155–157

Sherman JL, Citrin CM (1986) Magnetic resonance demonstration of normal CSF flow. AJNR 7:3–7

Waluch V, Bradley WG (1984) NMR even echo rephasing in slow laminar flow. J Comput Assist Tomogr 8:594–598

Yeates A, Enzmann D (1979) An intraventricular arachnoid cyst. J Comput Assist Tomogr 3:697–700

F.6. Postoperative Lesions and Radionecrosis

Brismar J, Roberson GH, Davis KR (1976) Radiation necrosis of the brain. Neuroradiological considerations with computed tomography. Neuroradiology 12:109–113

Curnes JT, Laster DW, Ball MR, Moody DM, Witcofski RL (1986) Magnetic resonance imaging of radiation injury to the brain. AJNR 7:389–394

Dooms GC, Hecht S, Brant-Zawadzki M, Berthiaume Y, Norman D, Newton TH (1986) Brain radiation lesions: MR imaging. Radiology 158:149–155

Glass JP, Hwang T-L, Leavens ME, Libshitz HJ (1984) Cerebral radiation necrosis following treatment of extracranial malignancies. Cancer 54:1966–1972

Kingsley DPE, Kendall BE (1981) CT of the adverse effects of therapeutic radiation of the central nervous system. AJNR 2:453–460

Martins AN, Johnston JS, Henry JM, Stoffel TJ, di Chiro D (1977) Delayed radiation necrosis of the brain. J Neurosurg 47:336–345

Mikhael MA (1979) Radiation necrosis of the brain: Correlation between pattern on computed tomography and dose of radiation. J Comput Assist Tomogr 3:241–249

O'Neil RR, Wakisaka S, Malamut BL (1977) Computer assisted tomography of focal cerebral radiation necrosis in the monkey. Neuropath Exp Neurol 36:950–955

Pay NT, Carella RJ, Lin JP, Kricheff II (1976) The usefulness of computed tomography during and after radiation therapy in patients with brain tumors. Radiology 121:79–83

Schmitt HP (1979) Akute und intervalläre Strahlenschäden des Zentralnervensystems. Springer, Berlin Heidelberg New York

Zülch KJ (1960) Über die Strahlensensibilität der Hirngeschwülste und die sogenannte Strahlenspätnekrose des Hirns. Dtsch Med Wochenschr 85:293–298

Zülch KJ (1963) Morphologische Veränderungen an Geschwülsten nach Bestrahlung und Schädigungsmöglichkeit am normalen Hirn. Strahlenforschung und Strahlenbehandlung IV Sonderbände Strahlentherapie 52:47–62

Zülch KJ (1969) Roentgen sensitivity of cerebral tumors and so-called late irradiation necrosis of the brain. Acta Radiol (Stockh) Ther 18:92–110

F.7. Acute Demyelinating Diseases

Atlas SW, Grossman RI, Goldberg HI, Hackney DB, Bilaniuk LT, Zimmerman RA (1986) MR diagnosis of acute disseminated encephalomyelitis. J Comput Assist Tomogr 10:798–801

Bories J, Carpena JP, Chiras J, Tamraz T, Iba-Zizen MT (1984) Imageric par résonance magnétique: Premiere résultats dans la Sclérose en plaques. J Neuroradiol 11:307–314

Bouchareine MF, Aubin ML, Vignaud J (1980) La tomodensitométrie dans la sclerose en plaques. Rev Neurol 136:481–490

Buonanno FS, Kistler JP, Lehrich JR, Noseworthy JH, New PFJ, Brady TJ (1983) ^{1}H nuclear magnetic resonance imaging in multiple sclerosis. Neurol Clin 1:757–764

Cala LA, Mastaglia FL, Black JL (1978) Computerized tomography of brain and optic nerve in multiple sclerosis. Observations in 100 patients, including serial studies in 16. J Neurol Sci 36:411, 426

Di Chiro G, Arimitsu T, Brooks RA, Morgenthaler DG, Johnston GS, Jones E, Keller MR (1979) Computed tomography profiles of periventricular hypodensity in hydrocephalus and leukoencephalopathy. Radiology 130: 661–666

Ebers GC, Vinuela FV, Feasby T, Bass B (1984) Multifocal CT enhancement in MS. Neurology 34:341–346

Edwards MK, Farlow MR, Stevens JC (1986) Multiple sclerosis: MRI and clinical correlation. AJNR 7:595–598

Eiben RM, Di Chiro G (1977) Computer assisted tomography in adrenoleukodystrophy. J Comput Assist Tomogr 1:308–314

Furuse M, Obayashi T, Tsuji S, Miyatake T (1978) Adrenoleukodystrophy. A correlative analysis of computed tomography and radionuclide studies. Radiology 126:707–710

Gerard G, Weisberg LA (1986) MRI periventricular lesions in adults. Neurology 36:998–1001

Grossman RI, Gonzalez-Scarano F, Atlas SW, Galette S, Silberberg DH (1986) Multiple sclerosis: Gadolinium enhancement in MR imaging. Radiology 161:721–725

Gyldensted C (1976) Computer tomography of the cerebrum in multiple sclerosis. Neuroradiology 12:33–42

Hall K, Gardner-Medwin D (1978) CT scan appearances in Leigh's disease (subacute necrotizing encephalomyelopathy). Neuroradiology 16:48–50

Harding AE, Radue EW, Whiteley AM (1978) Contrastenhanced lesions on computerised tomography in multiple sclerosis. J Neurol Neurosurg Psychiatry 41:754–758

Haughton VM, Ho KCh, Williams AL, Eldevik OP (1979) CT detection of demyelinated plaques in multiple sclerosis. Am J Roentgenol 132:213–215

Heinz ER, Drayer BP, Haenggeli CA, Painter MJ, Crumrine P (1979) Computed tomography in white-matter disease. Radiology 130:371–378

Huckman MS, Fox JH, Ramsey RG (1977) Computed tomography in the diagnosis of degenerative diseases of the brain. Semin Roentgenol 12:63–75

Jackson JA, Leake DR, Schneider NJ, Rolak LA, Kelley GR, Ford JJ, Appel SH, Bryan RN (1985) Magnetic resonance imaging in multiple sclerosis. AJNR 6:171–176

Kirshner HS, Tsai SI, Runge VM, Price AC (1985) Magnetic resonance imaging and other techniques in the diagnosis of multiple sclerosis. Arch Neurol 42:859–863

Lane B, Carroll BA, Pedley TA (1978) Computerized cranial tomography in cerebral diseases of white matter. Neurology 28:534–544

Loizok L, Rolfe EB, Hewazy H (1982) Cranial computed tomography in the diagnosis of multiple sclerosis. J Neurol Neurosurg Psychiatry 45:905–912

Radue EW, Kendall BE (1978) Iodine and xenon enhancement of computed tomography (CT) in multiple sclerosis (MS). Neuroradiology 15:153–158

Sheldon JJ, Siddharthan R, Tobias J, Sheremata WA, Soila K, Viamonte M (1985) MR imaging of multiple sclerosis: Comparison with clinical and CT examinations in 74 patients. AJNR 6:683–690

Steinhaus H (1980) Die kraniale Computertomographie bei multipler Sklerose. Wien Med Wochenschr 130:382–384

Taboada D, Alonso A, Olagüe R, Mulas F, Andrés V (1980) Radiological diagnosis of periventricular and subcortical leukomalacia. Neuroradiology 20:33–41

Tritschler JL, Delouvrier JJ, Masson M, Nahum H, Cambier J (1979) Apport de la tomodensitométrie cerebrale au diagnostic de la sclerose en plaques. Rev Neurol 135:455–466

Wang A-M, Morris JH, Hickey WF, Hammerschlag SB, O'Reilly GV, Rumbaugh CL (1983) Unusual CT pattern of multiple sclerosis. AJNR 4:47–50

Weinstein MA, Lederman RJ, Rothner AD, Duchesneau PM, Norman D (1978) Interval computed tomography in multiple sclerosis. Radiology 129:689–694

Wüthrich R, Gigli H, Wiggli U, Müller HR, Elke M, Hünig R (1976) CT scanning in demyelinating diseases. In: Lanksch W, Kazner E (eds) Cranial computerized tomography. Springer, Berlin Heidelberg New York, pp 239–243

Young IR, Hall AS, Pallis CA, Bydder GM, Legg NJ, Steiner RE (1981) Nuclear magnetic resonance imaging of the brain in multiple sclerosis. Lancet 2:1063–1066

F.8 and 9. Intracranial Hemorrhages, Vascular Malformations

Aarabi B, Chambers J (1978) Giant thrombosed aneurysm associated with an arteriovenous malformation. J Neurosurg 49:278–282

Amendola MA, Ostrum BJ (1977) Diagnosis of isodense

subdural hematomas by computed tomography. Am J Roentgenol 129:693–697
Babu VS, Eisen H (1979) Giant aneurysm of anterior communicating artery simulating 3rd ventricular tumor. Comput Tomogr 3:159–163
Bannister CM, Weller J (1980) Pre- and post-operative CT scans of an infant with an aneurysm of the vein of Galen – a case report. Neurochirurgia (Stuttg) 23:17–20
Bradley WG, Schmidt PG (1985) Effect of Methemoglobin on the MR appearance of subarachnoid hemorrhage. Radiology 156:99–103
Britt RH, Silverberg GD, Enzmann DR, Hanbery JW (1980) Third ventricular choroid plexus arteriovenous malformation simulating a colloid cyst. J Neurosurg 52:246–250
Byrd SH, Bentson JR, Winter J, Wilson GH, Joyce PW, O'Connor L (1978) Giant intracranial aneurysms simulating brain neoplasms on computed tomography. J Comput Assist Tomogr 2:303–307
Coin CG, Coin JW, Glover MB (1977) Vascular tumors of the choroid plexus: diagnosis by computed tomography. J Comput Assist Tomogr 1:146–148
Cone JD, Maravilla KR, Cooper PR, Diehl JT, Clark WK (1979) Computed tomography findings in ruptured arteriovenous malformations of the corpus callosum. J Comput Assist Tomogr 3:478–482
Cosnard G, Jeanbourquin D, Perfettini C, Blanc AM, Iba-Zizen MT, Cabanis EA (1987) Hématoms et IRM à 0,15 T. J Radiol 68:319–331
Daniels DL, Haughton VM, Williams AL, Strother ChM (1979) Arteriovenous malformation simulating a cyst on computed tomography. Radiology 133:393–394
Deeb JL, Jannetta PJ, Rosenbaum AE, Kerber CW, Drayer BP (1979) Tortuous vertebrobasilar arteries causing cranial nerve syndromes: screening by computed tomography. J Comput Assist Tomogr 3:774–778
De la Paz RL, New PFJ, Buonanno FS, Kistler JP, Oot RF, Rosen BR, Taveras JM, Brady TJ (1984) NMR imaging of intracranial hemorrhage. J Comput Assist Tomogr 8:599–607
Dhopesh VP, Greenberg JO, Cohen MM (1980) Computed tomography in brainstem hemorrhage. J Comput Assist Tomogr 4:603–607
Di Chiro G, Brooks RA, Girton ME, Caporale T, Wright DC, Dwyer AJ, Horne MK (1986) Sequential MR studies of intracerebral hematomas in monkeys. AJNR 7:193–199
Di Tullio MV, Stern WE (1979) Hemangioma calcificans. J Neurosurg 50:110–114
Edelman RR, Johnson K, Buxton R, Shoukimas G, Rosen BR, Davis KR, Brady TJ (1986) MR of hemorrhage: A new approach. AJNR 7:751–756
Enzmann DR, Hayward RW, Norman D, Dunn RP (1977) Cranial computed tomographic scan appearance of Sturge-Weber disease: unusual presentation. Radiology 122:721–724
Enzmann DR, Britt RH, Lyons BE, Buxton JL, Wilson DA (1981) Natural history of experimental intracerebral hemorrhage: sonography, computed tomography, and neuropathology. AJNR 2:517–526
Fierstien SB, Pribram HW, Hieshima G (1979) Angiography and computed tomography in the evaluation of cerebral venous malformations. Neuroradiology 17:137–148
Golden JB, Kramer RA (1978) The angiographically occult cerebrovascular malformation. J Neurosurg 48:292–296
Gomori JM, Grossman RI, Bilaniuk LT, Zimmerman RA, Goldberg HI (1985) High-field MR imaging of superficial siderosis of the central nervous system. J Comput Assist Tomogr 9:972–973
Gomori JM, Grossman RI, Goldberg HI, Hackney DB, Zimmerman RA, Bilaniuk LT (1986) Occult cerebral vascular malformations: high-field MR imaging. Radiology 158:707–713
Gomori JM, Grossman RI, Goldberg HI, Zimmerman RA, Bilaniuk LT (1985) Intracranial hematomas: Imaging by high-field MR. Radiology 157:87–93
Greenhouse AH, Barr JW (1979) The bilateral isodense subdural hematoma on computerized tomographic scan. Arch Neurol 36:305–307
Grumme Th, Lanksch W, Aulich A (1976) The diagnosis of chronic subdural hematoma by computerized axial tomography. In: Lanksch W, Kazner E (eds) Cranial computerized tomography. Springer, Berlin Heidelberg New York, pp 337–341
Grumme Th, Lanksch W, Kazner E, Aulich A, Meese W, Lange S, Steinhoff H, Wende S (1976) Zur Diagnose des chronischen subduralen Hämatoms im Computertomogramm. Neurochirurgia (Stuttg) 19:95–103
Grumme Th, Lanksch W, Wende S (1976) Diagnosis of spontaneous intracerebral hemorrhage by computerized tomography. In: Lanksch W, Kazner E (eds) Cranial computerized tomography. Springer, Berlin Heidelberg New York, pp 284–290
Grumme Th, Lanksch W, Kretzschmar K (1979) Intrakranielle Blutungen im Computertomogramm. Dtsch Ärztebl 24:1627–1634
Hammer B (1979) Computertomographische Diagnose der Megadolichobasilaris. Fortschr Röntgenstr 131:255–261
Handa J, Nakano Y, Okuno T, Komuro H, Handa H (1977) Computerized tomography in Moyamoya syndrome. Surg Neurol 7:315–319
Handa J, Nakano Y, Aii H, Handa H (1978) Computed tomography with giant intracranial aneurysms. Surg Neurol 9:257–263
Harwood-Nash DC, Breckbill DL (1976) Computed tomography in children: a new diagnostic technique. J Pediatr 89:343–357
Hayward RD (1976) Intracranial arteriovenous malformations. Observations after experience with computerised tomography. J Neurol Neurosurg Psychiatry 39:1027–1033
Humphreys RP (1978) Computerized tomographic definition of mesencephalic hematoma with evacuation through pedunculotomy. J Neurosurg 49:749–752
Kazner E, Lanksch W (1979) CAT findings in cerebral aneurysms and subarachnoid haemorrhage. In: Pia HW, Langmaid C, Zierski J (eds) Cerebral aneurysms. Springer, Berlin Heidelberg New York, pp 184–190
Kazner E, Lanksch W, Grumme Th, Kretzschmar K (1980) Diagnosis and differential diagnosis of spontaneous ICH with CT scan. In: Pia HW, Langmaid C, Zierski J (eds) Spontaneous intracerebral haematomas. Advances in diagnosis and therapy. Springer, Berlin Heidelberg New York, pp 178–190
Kendall BE, Claveria LE (1976) The use of computed axial tomography (CAT) for the diagnosis and management of intracranial angiomas. Neuroradiology 12:141–160
Kendall BE, Claveria LE (1977) The use of computerised axial tomography (CAT) for the diagnosis and management of intracranial angiomas. In: du Boulay GH, Mo-

seley IF (eds) Computerised axial tomography in clinical practice. Springer, Berlin Heidelberg New York, pp 261–271
Lanksch W, Grumme Th, Kazner E (1978) Schädelhirnverletzungen im Computertomogramm. Springer, Berlin Heidelberg New York
Leblanc R, Ethier R, Little JR (1979) Computerized tomography findings in arteriovenous malformations of the brain. J Neurosurg 51:765–772
Lee YY, Moser R, Bruner JM, van Tassel P (1986) Organized intracerebral hematoma with acute hemorrhage: CT pattern and pathologic correlations. AJNR 7:403–416
Lemme-Plaghos L, Kucharczyk W, Brant-Zawadzki M, Uske A, Edwards M, Norman D, Newton TH (1986) MRI of angiographically occult vascular malformations. Am J Roentgenol 146:1223–1228
Macpherson P, Teasdale GM, Lindsay KW (1979) Computed tomography in diagnosis and management of aneurysm of the vein of Galen. J Neurol Neurosurg Psychiatry 42:786–789
Maehara T, Tasaka A (1978) Cerebral venous angioma: computerized tomography and angiographic diagnosis. Neuroradiology 16:296–298
Maki Y, Semba A (1979) Computed tomography of Sturge-Weber-disease. Childs Brain 5:51–61
Marcu H, Becker H (1977) Computed tomography of bilateral isodense chronic subdural hematomas. Neuroradiology 14:81–83
Marshall WH, Easter W, Zatz LM (1977) Analysis of the dense lesion at computed tomography with dual kVp scans. Radiology 124:87–89
Martelli A, Scotti G, Harwood-Nash DC, Fitz CR, Chuang SH (1980) Aneurysms of the vein of Galen in children: CT and angiographic correlations. Neuroradiology 20:123–133
Mauersberger W (1978) Vascular deformity of the basilar artery which gave the clinical and computerized impression of a tumor. Adv Neurosurg 5:176–178
McDavid WD, Waggener RG, Sank VJ, Dennis MJ, Payne WH (1977) Correlating computed tomographic numbers with physical properties and operating kilovoltage. Radiology 123:761–762
Meese W, Aulich A, Kazner E, Wüllenweber R (1976) CT findings in angiomas and aneurysms. In: Lanksch W, Kazner E (eds) Cranial computerized tomography. Springer, Berlin Heidelberg New York, pp 291–297
Messina AV (1976) Computed tomography: contrast media within subdural hematomas. A preliminary report. Radiology 119:725–726
Michels LG, Bentson JR, Winter J (1977) Computed tomography of cerebral venous angiomas. J Comput Assist Tomogr 1:149–154
Moon KL, Brant-Zawadzki M, Pitts LH, Mills CM (1984) Nuclear magnetic resonance imaging of CT-isodense subdural hematomas. AJNR 5:319–322
Moseley IF, Holland IM (1979) Ectasia of the basilar artery: the breadth of the clinical spectrum and the diagnostic value of computed tomography. Neuroradiology 18:83–91
Müke R, Kühne D (1978) Diagnostic errors in computerized tomography in the differential diagnosis of cerebrovascular lesions. Adv Neurosurg 6:115–124
Müller HR, Wiggli U (1977) Cerebral, cerebellar and pontine haemorrhages. In: du Boulay GH, Moseley IF (eds) Computerised axial tomography in clinical practice. Springer, Berlin Heidelberg New York, pp 249–254
Nadjmi M, Ratzka M, Wodarz M (1978) Giant aneurysms in CT and angiography. Neuroradiology 16:284–286
Norman D (1977) Computed tomography in intracranial hemorrhage. In: Norman D, Korobkin M, Newton ThH (eds) Computed tomography 1977. Mosby, St Louis
Olsen WL, Brant-Zawadzki M, Hodes J, Norman D, Newton TH (1987) Giant intracranial aneurysms: MR imaging. Radiology 163:431–435
Patel DV, Hier DB, Thomas CM, Hemmat M (1984) Intracerebral hemorrhage secondary to cerebral amyloid angiopathy. Radiology 151:397–400
Peterson NT, Duchesneau PM, Westbrook EL, Weinstein MA (1977) Basilar artery ectasia demonstrated by computed tomography. Radiology 122:713–715
Petit-Perrin D, Aubin ML, Vignaud J (1979) Apport de la scanographie au diagnostic des anéurysmes géants intra-crâniens. J Neuroradiol 6:317–326
Phelps ME, Kuhl DE (1976) Pitfalls in the measurements of cerebral blood volume with computed tomography. Radiology 121:375–377
Pia HW (1980) Large and giant aneurysms. Neurosurg Rev 3:7–16
Pia HW, Langmaid C, Zierski J (1980) Spontaneous intracerebral haematomas. Advances in diagnosis and therapy. Springer, Berlin Heidelberg New York
Pinto RS, Kricheff II, Butler AR, Murali R (1979) Correlation of computed tomographic, angiographic and neuropathological changes in giant cerebral aneurysms. Radiology 132:85–92
Pressman BD, Gilbert GE, Davis DO (1975) Computerized transverse tomography of vascular lesions of the brain. Part II: Aneurysms. Am J Roentgenol 124:215–219
Pressman BD, Kirkwood JR, Davis DO (1975) Computerized transverse tomography of vascular lesions of the brain. Part I: Arteriovenous malformations. Am J Roentgenol 124:208–214
Probst FP (1980) Vascular morphology and angiographic flow patterns in Sturge-Weber angiomatosis: fact, thoughts and suggestions. Neuroradiology 20:73–78
Rao KC, Knipp HC, Wagner EJ (1981) Computed tomographic findings in cerebral sinus and venous thrombosis. Radiology 140:391–398
Sartor K (1978) Spontaneous closure of cerebral arteriovenous malformation demonstrated by angiography and computed tomography. Neuroradiology 15:95–98
Savoiardo M, Strada L, Passerini A (1983) Intracranial cavernous hemangiomas: Neuroradiologic review of 36 operated cases. AJNR 4:945–950
Schmid UD, Steiger HJ, Huber P (1987) Accuracy of high resolution computed tomography in direct diagnosis of cerebral aneurysms. Neuroradiology 29:152–159
Schubiger O, Valavanis A, Hayek J (1980) Computed tomography in cerebral aneurysms with special emphasis on giant intracranial aneurysms. J Comput Assist Tomogr 4:24–32
Schulthess GK von, Higgins CB (1985) Blood flow imaging with MR: spin phase phenomena. Radiology 157:687–695
Scotti G, Terbrugge K, Melançon D, Bélanger G (1977) Evaluation of the age of subdural hematomas by computerized tomography. J Neurosurg 47:311–315
Sobel DF, Baker E, Anderson B, Kretzschmar H (1985)

Cerebral amyloid angiopathy associated with massive intracerebral hemorrhage. Neuroradiology 27:318–321
Soeur M, Brihaye J, Moerman C (1979) Pseudo-tumoral aneurysm in the third ventricle: report of three cases. Acta Neurochir (Wien) 45:247–258
Spallone A (1979) Computed tomography in aneurysms of the vein of Galen. J Comput Assist Tomogr 3:779–782
Sundt TM jr, Piepgras DG (1979) Surgical approach to giant intracranial aneurysms. Operative experience with 80 cases. J Neurosurg 51:731–742
Tagle P, Huete I, Mendez J, Del Villar S (1986) Intracranial cavernous angioma: presentation and management. J Neurosurg 64:720–723
Terao H, Ikeda A, Kobayashi S, Teraoka A (1978) A thrombosed giant aneurysm of the internal carotid artery with brain stem displacement. Surg Neurol 10:157–168
Terbrugge K, Scotti G, Ethier R, Melancon D, Tchang S, Milner C (1977) Computed tomography in intracranial arteriovenous malformations. Radiology 122:703–705
Tsai FY, Huprich JE, Segall HD, Teal JS (1979) The contrast-enhanced CT scan in the diagnosis of isodense subdural hematoma. J Neurosurg 50:64–69
Ventureyra ECG, Ivan LP (1979) Venous malformation of the pineal region. Surg Neurol 11:225–228
Ventureyra ECG, Choo SH, Benoit B (1980) Super giant globoid intracranial aneurysm in an infant. J Neurosurg 53:411–416
Wagle WA, Smith TW, Weiner M (1984) Intracerebral hemorrhage caused by cerebral amyloid angiopathy: Radiographic-pathologic correlation. AJNR 5:171–176
Waluch V, Bradley WG (1984) NMR even echo rephasing in slow laminar flow. J Comput Assist Tomogr 8:594–598
Weisberg LA (1980) Peripheral rim enhancement in supratentorial intracerebral hematoma. Comput Tomogr 4:145–154
Welch K, Naheedy MH, Abrous IF, Strand RD (1980) Computed tomography of Sturge-Weber syndrome in infants. J Comput Assist Tomogr 4:33–36
Wende S, Ludwig B, Simon RS, Kretzschmar K (1980) Hyperdensity factors. In: Caillé M, Salamon G (eds) Computerized tomography. Springer, Berlin Heidelberg New York, pp 146–151
Zatz LM (1976) The effect of the kVp level on EMI-values. Radiology 119:683–688
Zimmerman RA, Bilaniuk LT (1978) Computed tomography of vertebrobasilar artery aneurysm. J Comput Assist Tomogr 2:39–49
Zimmerman RA, Bilaniuk LT (1979) Computed tomography of choroid plexus lesions. J Comput Assist Tomogr 3:93–103
Zimmerman RA, Bilaniuk LT, Grossman RI, Levine RS, Lynch R, Goldberg HI, Samuel L, Edelstein W, Bottomley P, Redington RW (1985) Resistive NMR of intracranial hematomas. Neuroradiology 27:16–20
Zimmerman RA, Bilaniuk LT, Hackney DB, Goldberg HI, Grossman RI (1986) Head injury: early results of comparing CT and high-field MR. Am J Roentgenol 147:1215–1222

F. 10. Cerebral Infarction

Aulich A, Fenske A (1977) Das Computertomogramm des Schlaganfalles. Akt Neurol 4:129–140
Aulich A, Wende S, Kazner E, Lanksch W, Steinhoff H, Grumme Th, Lange S, Meese W (1978) Computerized axial tomography for diagnosis and follow-up studies of cerebral infarcts and the development of brain edema. In: Bories J (ed) The diagnostic limitations of computerised axial tomography. Springer, Berlin Heidelberg New York, pp 105–109
Bech-Skriver E, Skyhøj Olsen T (1981) Transient disappearance of cerebral infarcts on CT scan, the so called fogging effect. Neuroradiology 22:61–65
Biller J, Adams HP, Dunn V, Simmons Z, Jacoby CG (1986) Dichotomy between clinical findings and MR abnormalities in pontine infarction. J Comput Assist Tomogr 10:379–385
Bonafe A, Manelfe C, Scotto B, Pradere MY, Rascol A (1985) Role of computed tomography in vertebrobasilar ischemia. Neuroradiology 27:484–493
Bories J, Derhy S, Chiras J (1985) CT in hemispheric ischaemic attacks. Neuroradiology 27:468–483
Brant-Zawadzki M, Solomon M, Newton TH, Weinstein P, Schmidley J, Norman D (1985) Basic principles of magnetic resonance imaging in cerebral ischemia and initial clinical experience. Neuroradiology 27:517–520
Brant-Zawadzki M, Pereira B, Weinstein P, Moore S, Kucharczyk W, Berry F, McNamara M, Derugin N (1986) MRS of acute experimental ischemia in rats. AJNR 7:7–11
Bryan RN, Willcott MR, Schneiders NJ, Ford JJ, Derman HS (1983) Nuclear magnetic resonance evaluation of stroke. Radiology 149:189–192
Caillé JM, Guibert F, Bidabe AM, Billerey J, Piton J (1980) Enhancement of cerebral infarcts with CT. Comput Tomogr 4:73–77
Campbell JK, Houser OW, Stevens JC, Wahner HW, Baker HL, Folger WN (1978) Computed tomography and radionuclide imaging in the evaluation of ischemic stroke. Radiology 126:695–702
Crisi G, Colombo A, de Santis M, Guerzoni MC, Calo M, Panzetti P (1984) CT and cerebral ischemic infarcts. Correlations between morphological and clinical-prognostic findings. Neuroradiology 26:101–105
Davis SM, Tress BM, Hopper JL, Kaye AH, Rossiter SC (1987) Dynamic CT brain scanning in the haemodynamic evaluation of cerebral arterial occlusion disease. Neuroradiology 29:259–265
Duyckaerts C, Hauw JJ (1985) Pathology and pathophysiology of brain ischaemia. Neuroradiology 27:460–467
Fox AJ, Bogousslavsky J, Carey LS, Barnett HJM, Vinitski S, Karlik SJ, Vinuela F, Pelz DM, Hachinski V (1986) Magnetic resonance imaging of small medullary infarctions. AJNR 7:229–233
Goldberg AL, Rosenbaum AE, Wang H, Kim WS, Lewis VL, Hanley DF (1986) Computed tomography of dural sinus thrombosis. J Comput Assist Tomogr 10:16–20
Hakim AM, Ryder-Cooke A, Melanson D (1983) Sequential computerized tomographic appearance of strokes. Stroke 14:893–897
Hecht-Leavitt C, Gomori JM, Grossman RI, Goldberg HI, Hackney DB, Zimmerman RA, Bilaniuk LT (1986) High field MRI of hemorrhagic cortical infarction. AJNR 7:581–585
Heiss WD, Herholz K, Böcher-Schwarz HG, Pawlik G, Wienhard K, Steinbrich W, Friedmann G (1986) PET,

CT, and MR imaging in cerebrovascular disease. J Comput Assist Tomogr 10:903–911
Henrikson GC, Patel DV (1985) Enhancing cerebral infarction simulating arteriovenous malformation on computed tomography. J Comput Assist Tomogr 9:502–606
Hilal SK, Maudsley AA, Simon HE, Perkman WH, Bonn J, Mawad ME, Silver AJ, Ganti SR, Sane P, Chien IC (1983) In vivo NMR imaging of tissue sodium in the intact cat before and after acute cerebral stroke. AJNR 4:245–249
Ho SU, Kim KS, Berenberg RA, Ho HT (1981) Cerebellar infarction: A clinical and CT study. Surg Neurol 16:350–352
Kashihara M, Matsumoto K (1985) Acute capsular infarction. Neuroradiology 27:248–253
Kazner E (1979) Die Bedeutung der Computertomographie für die Diagnose und Differentialdiagnose zerebraler Durchblutungsstörungen. Neurol Psychiatr (Bucur) 5:312–324
Kim KS, Walczak TS (1986) Computed tomography of deep cerebral venous thrombosis. J Comput Assist Tomogr 10:386–390
Launay M, Nidiaye M, Bories J (1985) X-ray computed tomography (CT) study of small, deep and recent infarcts (SDRJs) of the cerebral hemispheres in adults. Preliminary and critical report. Neuroradiology 27:494–508
Levy RM, Mano I, Brito A, Hosobuchi Y (1983) NMR imaging of acute experimental cerebral ischemia: time course and pharmacologic manipulations. AJNR 4:238–241
Macchi PJ, Grossman RI, Gomori JM, Goldberg HI, Zimmerman RA, Bilaniuk LT (1986) High field MR imaging of cerebral venous thrombosis. J Comput Assist Tomogr 10:10–15
Masdek JC (1983) Enhancing mass of CT: Neoplasm or recent infarction? Neurology 33:836–840
McMurdo SK, Brant-Zawadzki M, Bradley WG, Chang GY, Berg BO (1986) Dural sinus thrombosis: Study using intermediate field strength MR imaging. Radiology 161:83–86
Naeser MA, Hayward RW, Laughlin SA, Zatz LM (1981) Quantitative CT scan studies in aphasia I. Infarct size and CT numbers. Brain Lang 12:140–164
Olteanu-Nerbe V, Schmiedek P, Kazner E, Lanksch W, Marguth F (1976) Comparison of regional cerebral blood flow and computerized tomography in patients with cerebrovascular disease and brain tumors. In: Lanksch W, Kazner E (eds) Cranial computerized tomography. Springer, Berlin Heidelberg New York, pp 305–308
Ostertag ChB, Mundinger F (1978) Diagnostic errors in the interpretation of cerebral infarction. Adv Neurosurg 6:86–93
Sager WD, Ladurner G (1979) Klassifikation und Verlauf des Hirninfarktes im Computertomogramm. Fortschr Röntgenstr 131:470–475
Segall HD, Ahmadi J, McComb JG, Zee C-S, Beckert TS, Han JS (1982) Computed tomographic observations pertinent to intracranial venous thrombotic and occlusive disease in childhood. Radiology 143:441–449
Shirakuni T, Tamaki N, Matsumoto S, Fujiwara M (1985) Megadolichobasilar anomaly associated with brain stem infarction: a case report. J Comput Tomogr 9:79–81
Sipponen JT (1984) Visualization of brain infarction with nuclear magnetic resonance imaging. Neuroradiology 26:387–391
Skriver EB, Olsen TS (1982) Contrast enhancement of cerebral infarcts. Incidence and clinical value in different states of cerebral infarction. Neuroradiology 23:259–265
Somerhausen P (1980) Contrast enhancement of cerebral infarction in computer tomography. J Belge Radiol 63:561–572
Virapongse L, Mancuso A, Quisling R (1986) Human brain infarcts: Gd-DTPA-enhanced MR imaging. Radiology 161:785–794
Wall SD, Brant-Zawadzki M, Jeffrey RB, Barnes B (1981) High frequency CT findings within 24 hours after cerebral infarction. AJNR 2:553–557
Wende S, Kazner E, Grumme Th (1979) Differentialdiagnose zwischen Ödem und Erweichung im Computer-Tomogramm. Nervenarzt 50:423–425
Wilson JL, Moseley IF (1977) A diagnostic approach to cerebellar lesions. In: du Boulay GH, Moseley IF (eds) Computerised axial tomography in clinical practice. Springer, Berlin Heidelberg New York, pp 123–131
Wüllenweber R, zum Winkel K, Grumme Th, Lange S, Meese W (1976) Differentialdiagnose des Schlaganfalles im Computertomogramm. Neurochirurgia (Stuttg) 19:1–19
Yamanouchi H, Tohgi H, Tomonaga H, Jjo M (1981) Computerized tomographic evaluation of chronic ischemic lesions in cerebral white matter. Jpn J Geriat 18:297–307
Yock DH, Marshall WH (1975) Recent ischemic brain infarcts and computed tomography: Appearances pre- and post-contrast infusion. Radiology 117:599–608
Yock D, Norman D, Newton ThH (1978) Pitfalls in the diagnosis of ichaemic cerebral infarcts by computed tomography. In: Bories J (ed) The diagnostic limitations of computerised axial tomography. Springer, Berlin Heidelberg New York, pp 90–104
Zülch KJ (1985) The cerebral infarct. Springer, Berlin Heidelberg New York Tokyo

G. Orbital Lesions

Ambrose J (1973) Computerized transverse axial scanning (tomography): Part 2. Clinical application. Br J Radiol 46:1023–1047
Ambrose J (1975) New techniques in the investigations of the orbit. Trans Ophthalmol Soc UK 95:233
Ambrose J, Lloyd GAS, Wright JE (1974) A preliminary evaluation of fine matrix computerized axial tomography (EMI scan) in the diagnosis of orbital space-occupying lesions. Br J Radiol 47:747–751
Aronow S, Kadir S (1976) In vitro evaluation of the detectability of intra-orbital foreign bodies. In: Symposium on Computer Assisted Tomography in Nontumoral Diseases of the brain, spinal cord and eye. National Institute of Health, Bethesda, Maryland, October 11–15
Atlas SW, Grossman RI, Savio RP, Sergott RC, Schatz NJ, Hackney DB, Goldberg HI, Bilaniuk LT, Zimmerman RA (1986) High field surface coil MRI of orbital pseudotumor. MRI-Schering-Symposium, San Diego/USA
Baker HL, Kearns ThP, Campbell JK, Henderson JW

(1974) Computerized transaxial tomography in neuroophthalmology. Am J Ophthalmol 78:285–294

Baleriaux-Waha D, Mortelmans LL, Dupont MG, Terwinghe G, Jeanmart L (1977) The use of coronal scans for computed tomography of the orbits. Neurology 14:89–96

Bergström K (1975) Computer tomography of the orbits. Acta Radiol [Suppl] (Stockh) 346:155–160

Bergström K, Dahlin H, Gustafsson M, Nylen O (1972) Eye lens doses in carotid angiography. Acta Radiol [Diagn] (Stockh) 12:134

Bigar F, Spiess H, Artaria L (1982) Abklärung raumfordernder Orbitaprozesse: Echographie oder Computertomographie? Fortschr Ophthalmol 79:25–27

Bilaniuk LT, Schenck JF, Zimmerman RA, Hart HR, Foster TH, Edelstein WA, Goldberg HI, Grossman RI (1985) Ocular and orbital lesions: surface coil MR imaging. Radiology 156:669–674

Bourjat P, Wackenheim A (1986) Röntgendiagnostisches Vorgehen bei Orbita-Tumoren. Radiologe 26:118–122

Brant-Zawadzki M, Enzmann DR (1979) Orbital computed tomography: calcific densities of posterior globe. J Comput Assist Tomogr 3:503–508

Brismar J, Davis KR, Dallow RL, Brismar G (1976) Unilateral endocrine exophthalmos. Diagnostic problems in association with computed tomography. Neuroradiology 12:21–24

Bull JWD (1975) The changing face of neuroradiology over nearly forty years. Neuroradiology 9:111–115

Buschmann W, Linnert D (1978) Zusammenwirken von Ultraschalldiagnostik und Röntgen-Computer-Tomographie bei raumfordernden Orbitaprozessen. Klin Monatsbl Augenheilkd 173:155–170

Byrd SE, Harwood-Nash DC, Fitz CR, Barry JF, Rogovitz DM (1978) Computed tomography of intraorbital optic nerve gliomas in children. Radiology 129:73–78

Cabanis EA, Salvolini U, Rodallec A, Menighelli F, Pasquini U, Bonnin P (1978) Computed tomography of the optic nerve: Part 2: Size and shape modifications in papilledemas. J Comput Assist Tomogr 2:150–155

Char DH, Sobel D, Kelly WM, Kjos BO, Norman D (1985) Magnetic resonance scanning in orbital tumor diagnosis. Ophthalmology 92:1305–1310

Charles MW, Lindop PJ (1977) Skin and eye irradiations. Examples of some limitations of international recommendations in radiological protection. I AEA-SR-36/6:547–561

Charles MW, Lindop PJ (1977) Recommendations of the international commission on radiological protection. ICRP 26:12–23; 21

Cogan DG (1974) Tumors of the optic nerve. In: Handbook clinical neurology. North-Holland, Amsterdam

Dallow RL (1986) Ultrasonography of the eye and orbit. In: Gonzalez CG, Becker MH, Flanagan JC (eds) Diagnostic imaging in ophthalmology. Springer, New York Berlin Heidelberg Tokyo

Dal Pozzo G, Boschi MC (1982) Extraocular muscle enlargement in acromegaly. J Comput Assist Tomogr 6:706–707

Damme W van, Kosmann Ph, Wackenheim A (1977) A standardizing method for computed tomography of the orbits. Neuroradiology 13:139–140

Daniels DL, Williams AL, Syvertsen A, Eager WE, Harris GJ (1982) CT recognition of optic nerve sheath meningioma: Abnormal sheath visualization. AJNR 3:181–183

Daniels DL, Herfkins R, Gager WE, Meyer GA, Koehler PR, Williams AL, Haughton VM (1984) Magnetic resonance imaging of the optic nerves and chiasm. Radiology 152:79–83

Davis KR, Hesselink JR, Dallow RL, Grove AS jr (1980) CT and ultrasound in the diagnosis of cavernous hemangioma and lymphangioma of the orbit. J Comput Assist Tomogr 4:98–104

Diaz F, Latchow R, Duvall AJ, Quick CA, Erickson DL (1978) Mucoceles with intracranial and extracranial extensions. J Neurosurg 48:284–288

Di Chiro G, Herdt JR, Vermess M, Kollaris CR (1976) Movement of optic nerves observed by sequential CT scans with different gaze positions. Presented at the International Symposium and Course on Computerized Tomography. San Juan, Puerto Rico, April 5–9

Ducrey N (1985) Les affections orbitaires non traumatiques. Masson, Paris

Edwards JH, Hyman RA, Vacirca SJ et al. (1985) Magnetic resonance imaging of the orbit. Am J Roentgenol 144/5:1015–1020

Edwards MK, Zauel DW, Gilmor RL, Muller J (1982) Invasive orbital pseudotumor-CT demonstration of extension beyond orbit. Neuroradiology 23:215–217

Enzmann DR, Donaldson SS, Marshall WH, Kriss JP (1976) Computed tomography in orbital pseudotumor (idiopatic orbital inflammation). Radiology 120:597–601

Enzmann DR, Marshall WH, Rosenthal AR, Kriss JP (1976) Computed tomography in Graves' ophthalmopathy. Radiology 118:615–620

Enzmann DR, Donaldson SS, Kriss JP (1979) Appearance of Graves' disease on orbital computed tomography. J Comput Assist Tomogr 3:815–819

Forbes GS, Earnest F IV, Waller RR (1982) Computed tomography of orbital tumors, including late-generation scanning techniques. Radiology 142:387–394

Fox AJ, Debrun G, Vinuela F, Assis L, Coated R (1979) Intrathecal metrizamide enhancement of the optic nerve sheath. J Comput Assist Tomogr 3(5):653–656

Fries PD, Char DH, Norman D (1987) MR imaging of orbital cavernous hemangioma. J Comput Assist Tomogr 11:418–421

Frisen L, Schöldström G, Svendsen P (1978) Drusen in the optic nerve head. Arch Ophthalmol 96:1611–1614

Gagliardi FM, Nicole S, Desiato MT (1979) Orbital epidermoids and dermoids. Neurosurg Rev 2:87–91

Gawler J, Sanders MD, Bull JWD, Du Boulay G, Marshall J (1974) Computer assisted tomography in orbital disease. Br J Ophthalmol 58:571–587

Gonzalez CF, Grossman ChB, Palacios E (1976) Computed brain and orbital tomography. Wiley, New York London Sydney Toronto

Gonzalez CF, Becker MH, Flanagan JC (eds) (1986) Diagnostic imaging in ophthalmology. Springer, New York Berlin Heidelberg Tokyo

Gore RM, Weinberg PE, Kim KS, Ramsey RG (1980) Sphenoid sinus mucoceles presenting as intracranial masses on computed tomography. Surg Neurol 13:375–379

Grimson B, Cohen K, McCartney W (1982) Concomitant ocular and orbital neoplasms. J Comput Assist Tomogr 6:617–619

Grossniklaus HE, Levine M, Purnell EW (1985) Comparison of magnetic resonance imaging with computed tomography of the orbit. Orbit 4:221–230

Gyldensted C, Lester J, Fledelius H (1977) Computed tomography of orbital lesions. A radiological study of 144 cases. Neuroradiology 13:141–150

Han JS, Benson JE, Bonstelle CT, Alfidi RJ, Kaufman B, Levine M (1984) Magnetic resonance imaging of the orbit: a preliminary experience. Radiology 150:755–759

Hanaway J, Scott WR, Strother ChM (1977) Atlas of the human brain and the orbit for computed tomography. Green, St Louis/MO

Hann LE, Borden S, Weber AL (1977) Orbital teratoma in the newborn. Pediatr Radiol 5:172–174

Harr DL, Quencer RM, Abrams GW (1982) Computed tomography and ultrasound in the evaluation of orbital infection and pseudotumor. Radiology 142:395–401

Harris GJ, Jakobiec FA (1979) Cavernous hemangioma of the orbit. J Neurosurg 51:219–228

Hart WM jr, Burde RM, Klingele TG, Perlmutter JC (1980) Bilateral optic nerve sheath meningiomas. Arch Ophthalmol 98:149–151

Haughton VM, Davis JP, Eldevik OP, Gager WE (1978) Optic nerve sheath imaging with metrizamide. Invest Radiol 13:544–546

Hawkes RC, Holland GN, Moore WS et al. (1983) NMR imaging in the evaluation of orbital tumors. AJNR 4:254–256

Hedges TR III, Pozzi-Mucelli R, Char DH, Newton TH (1982) Computed tomographic demonstration of ocular calcification: Correlation with clinical and pathological findings. Neuroradiology 23:15–21

Heller M, Guthoff R, Hagemann J, Jend HH (1982) CT of malignant choroidal melanoma-morphology and perfusion characteristics. Neuroradiology 23:23–30

Hesselink JR, Davis KR, Weber AL, Davis JM, Taveras JM (1980) Radiological evaluation of orbital metastases with emphasis on computed tomography. Radiology 137:363–366

Hilal SK (1979) Computed tomography of the orbit. Ophthalmology 86:864–870

Hilal SK, Trokel SL (1977) Computerized tomography of the orbit using thin sections. Semin Roentgenol 12:137–147

Hollender L, Lysell G (1971) Radiation doses during tomography of various parts of the head. Odontol Rev 22:291–295

Hounsfield GN (1973) Computerized axial scanning (tomography): Part 1. Description of system. Br J Radiol 46:1016–1022

Huber A, Isler W, Spiess H (1979) Computertomography for diagnosis of optic nerve and chiasmal gliomas. Klin Monatsbl Augenheilkd 174:833–842

Inoue Y, Inoue T (1978) Computerized orbital tomography in dysthyroid ophthalmopathy. Jpn J Ophthalmol 22:286–296

Isherwood J, Young JM, Bowker KW, Bramall GK (1975) Radiation dose to the eyes of the patient during neuroradiological investigations. Neuroradiology 10:137–141

Jacobs L, Weisberg LA, Kinkel WR (1980) Computerized tomography of the orbit and sella turcica. Raven, New York

Kingsley DPE, Lloyd GAS, Kendall BE (1986) Radiology of orbital masses in children. Acta Radiol, Suppl 369, 654–657

Kollarits CR, Christiansen JR (1976) Computer assisted tomography for localisation of intraocular and intraorbital foreign bodies. In: Symposium on Computer assisted Tomography in nontumoral diseases of the brain, spinal cord and eye. National Institute of Health, Bethesda, Maryland, October 11–15

Kollarits CR, Moss ML, Cogan DG, Doppman JL, Di Chiro G, Cutler GB, Marx SJ, Spiegel AM (1977) Scleral calcifications in hyperparathyroidism: demonstration by computed tomography. J Comput Assist Tomogr 1:500–504

Krahe Th, Giesecke J, Herter M, Trier HG, Wolf HH, Lackner K (1987) Magnetische Resonanztomographie (MRT) der Orbita. Fortschr Röntgenstr 146:267–273

Lallemand DP, Brasch RC, Char DH, Norman D (1984) Orbital tumors in children. Characterization by computed tomography. Radiology 151:85–88

Lampert VL, Zeich JW, Cohen DN (1974) Computed tomography of the orbits. Radiology 113:351–354

Leo JS, Halpern J, Sackler JP (1980) Computed tomography in the evaluation of orbital infections. Comput Tomogr 4:133–138

Leonardi M, Barbina V, Fabris G, Penco T (1977) Sagittal computed tomography of the orbit. J Comput Assist Tomogr 1:511–512

Lester J, Gyldensted C (1976) CT of retrobulbar lesions. Int Symp Computerized Tomography, Puerto Rico, April 1976

Li KC, Poon PY, Hinton P et al. (1984) MR imaging of orbital tumors with CT and ultrasound correlations. J Comput Assist Tomogr 8:1039–1047

Lindahl S (1986) Computed tomography of retinoblastoma. Act Radiol [Diagn] (Stockh) 27:513–518

Lloyd GAS (1975) Radiology of the orbit. Saunders, London

Lloyd GAS (1982) Primary orbital meningioma: A review of 41 patients investigated radiologically. Clin Radiol 33/2:181–187

Lloyd GAS (1982) Vascular anomalies in the orbit: CT and angiographic diagnosis. Orbit 1:45–54

Lloyd GAS, Ambrose J, Wright JE (1975) New techniques in the investigation of the orbit. Trans Ophthalmol Soc UK 95:233–236

Lund E, Halaburt H (1982) Irradiation dose to the lens of the eye during CT of the head. Neuroradiology 22:181–184

Mafee MF, Dobben GD, Valvassori GE (1986) Computed tomography assessment of paraorbital pathology. In: Gonzalez CF, Becker MH, Flanagan JC (eds) Diagnostic imaging in opthalmology. Springer, New York Berlin Heidelberg Tokyo

Maier-Hauff K, Wilske J (1976) Correlation of A-scan echography and computed tomography of orbital tumors. In: Lanksch W, Kazner E (eds) Cranial computerized tomography. Springer, Berlin Heidelberg New York, pp 212–220

Mancuso AA, Hanafee WN (1985) Computed tomography and magnetic resonance imaging of the head and neck. Williams & Wilkins, Baltimore London Los Angeles Sydney

Manelfe C, Bonafe A, Fabre P, Pessey J-J (1978) Computed tomography in olfactory neuroblastoma: one case of esthesioneuroepithelioma and four cases of esthesioneuroblastoma. J Comput Assist Tomogr 2:412–420

Manelfe C, Pasquini U, Bank W (1978) Metrizamide demonstration of the subarachnoid space surrounding the optic nerves. J Comput Assist Tomogr 2:545–547

Michotey P, Moseley IF, Aubin ML, Mouly A, Farnarie Ph, Sanders MD, Aron D, Doyon D (1976) Apport de la tomographie axiale commandée par ordinateur en ophthalmologie. J Neuroradiol 3:257–276

Miller NR (1985) Walsh and Hoyt's Clinical Neuro-Ophthalmology. Williams & Wilkins, Baltimore London Los Angeles Sydney

Mödder U (1986) Orbita. In: Dihlmann W, Stender H-St (Hrsg) Radiologische Diagnostik in Klinik und Praxis, 7. Aufl, Bd V, Teil 1: Schädel – Gehirn. Thieme, Stuttgart New York

Momose KJ, Grove AS, New PFJ, Scott W (1975) The use of computed tomography in ophthalmology. Radiology 115:361–368

Mortelmans LL, Baleriaux-Waha D, Dupont MG, Jeanmart L, Potvliege R (1978) Neuroophthalmology. In: Baert A, Jeanmart L, Wackenheim A (eds) Clinical computer tomography. Springer, Berlin Heidelberg New York, pp 147–155

Moseley IF, Bull JWD (1975) Computerized axial tomography, carotid angiography and orbital phlebography in the diagnosis of space-occupying lesions of the orbit. In: Salamon G (ed) Advances in cerebral angiography. Springer, Berlin Heidelberg New York, pp 361–369

Moseley IF, Brant-Zawadzki M, Mills C (1983) Nuclear magnetic resonance imaging of the orbit. Br J Ophthalmol 67/6:333–342

Nemec HW, Roth J (1976) Über die Strahlenbelastung des Kopfes, insbesondere der Augenlinsen, bei der axialen Tomographie mit dem EMI-Scanner. Fortschr Röntgenstr 126:526–530

New PFJ, Scott WR (1975) Computed tomography of the brain and orbit (EMI-Scanning). Williams & Wilkins, Baltimore

Nover A, Schmitt J, Wende S, Aulich A (1976) Computer-Tomographie in der Ophthalmologie. Klin Monatsbl Augenheilkd 168:461–467

Nover A, Rochels R, Queckenstedt U, Wende S (1982) Vergleich echographischer, computertomographischer und histologischer Befunde bei Orbitatumoren. Fortschr Ophthalmol 79:22–24

Nowinski ThS, Flanagan JC (1986) Evaluation of exophthalmos and thyroid ophthalmopathy. In: Gonzalez CF, Becker MH, Flanagan JC (eds) Diagnostic imaging in ophthalmology. Springer, New York Berlin Heidelberg Tokyo

Ossoinig K (1977) Echography of the eye, orbit and periorbital region. In: Argen PH (ed) Orbit roentgenology. Wiley, New York

Ossoinig K (1978) Orbital disorders. In: de Vlieger M, Holmes JH, Kazner E, Kossoff G, Kratchowil A, Kraus R, Poujol J, Strandness DE (eds) Handbook of clinical ultrasound. Wiley, New York Chichester Brisbane Toronto, pp 881–904

Ossoinig K (1982) Ein neues echographisches Merkmal zur verläßlichen Differentialdiagnostik des endokrinen Exophthalmus. Klin Monatsbl Augenheilkd 180:189–197

Ostertag ChB, Unsöld R, Mundinger F (1976) Computerized tomography in neuro-ophthalmology. In: Lanksch W, Kazner E (eds) Cranial computerized tomography. Springer, Berlin Heidelberg New York, pp 202–206

Peeters F (1977) Radiological diagnosis of orbital tumors. Radiol Clin (Basel) 46:18–25

Peeters F, Kröger R, Verbeeten B jr, Versteege C (1977) The value of computer tomography, orbital venography and carotid angiography in the diagnosis of exopthalmos. Radiol Clin (Basel) 46:430–438

Perry BJ, Bridges C (1973) Computerized transverse axial scanning (tomography), Part 3: Radiation dose considerations. Br J Radiol 46:1048–1051

Perugini S, Pasquini U, Menichelli F, Salvolini U, de Micola M, Valazzi CM, Benedetti S (1982) Mucoceles in the paranasal sinuses involving the orbit: CT signs in 43 cases. Neuroradiology 23:133–139

Peyster RG, Hoover ED (1984) Computerized tomography in orbital disease and neuro-ophthalmology. Year Book Medical Publishers, Chicago London

Peyster RG, Hoover ED (1984) The orbit and neuro-ophthalmology. In: Rosenberg RN, Heinz ER (eds) The clinical neurosciences. Churchill Livingstone, New York Edinburgh London Melbourne

Peyster RG, Hoover ED, Herschey BL, Haskin ME (1983) High resolution CT of lesions of the optic nerve. AJNR 4:169–174

Piepgras U (1981) Vergleichende radiologische Diagnostik bei Orbitaprozessen. Radiologe 21:1–11

Robertson WD, Lapointe JS, Rootman J, Nugent RA, Graeb DA (1986) Orbital lymphoma: CT characteristics. Vortrag MRI-Schering-Symposium, San Diego/USA

Rochels R (1986) Ultraschalldiagnostik in der Augenheilkunde. ecomed, Landsberg

Ruchman MC, Stefanyszyn MA, Flanagan JC, Gonzalez CF, Becker MH (1986) Orbital tumors. In: Gonzalez CF, Becker MH, Flanagan JC (eds) Diagnostic imaging in ophthalmology. Springer, New York Berlin Heidelberg Tokyo

Salvolini U, Menichelli F, Pasquini U (1977) Computer assisted tomography in 90 cases of exophthalmos. J Comput Assist Tomogr 1:81–100

Salvolini U, Cabanis EA, Rodallec A, Menichelli F, Pasquini U, Iba-Zizen NT (1978) Computed tomography of the optic nerve: Part 1. Normal results. J Comput Assist Tomogr 2:141–149

Sanders M (1976) The contribution of CAT in neuroopthalmology. ESCAT Seminar, London October 1976. Trans Ophthalmol Soc UK 95:237–245

Savoiardo M, Strada L, Passerini A (1983) Cavernous hemangiomas of the orbit: Value of CT, angiography, and phlebography. AJNR 4:741–744

Schenck JF, Hart HR, Foster TH, Edelstein WA, Bottomley PA, Redington RW, Hardy CJ, Zimmerman RA, Bilaniuk LT (1985) Improved MR imaging of the orbit at 1.5 T with surface coils. AJNR 6:193–196

Schneider G, Sager WD, Spreizer H (1978) Strahlenbelastung der Orbita bei der Computertomographie mit dem EMI-Scanner CT 1010. Roentgenforschung 128: 687–690

Smith FW, Cherryman GR, Singh AK, Forrester JV (1985) Nuclear magnetic resonance tomography of the orbit at 3.4 MHz. Br J Radiol 58:947–957

Sobel DF, Mills C, Char D et al. (1984) NMR of the normal and pathologic eye and orbit. AJNR 5:345–350

Sobel DF, Moseley JF, Brant-Zawadzki M (1986) Magnetic

Resonance Imaging (MRI) of the eye and orbit. In: Gonzalez CF, Becker MH, Flanagan JC (eds) Diagnostic imaging in ophthalmology. Springer, New York Berlin Heidelberg Tokyo
Som P, Sacher M, Weitzner I et al. (1982) Sarcoidosis of the optic nerve. J Comput Assist Tomogr 6:614–616
Spoor TC, Kennerdell JS, Martinez AJ, Zorub D (1980) Malignant gliomas of the optic nerve pathways. Am J Ophthalmol 89:284–286
Sullivan JA, Harms SE (1986) Surface-coil MR imaging of orbital neoplasms. AJNR 7:29–34
Swenson SA, Forbes GS, Younge BR, Campbell RJ (1982) Radiologic evaluation of tumors of the optic nerve. Neuroradiology 3/3:310–326
Tadmor R, New PFJ (1978) Computed tomography of the orbit with special emphasis on coronal sections: Part 1. Normal anatomy. J Comput Assist Tomogr 2:24–34
Tadmor R, New PFJ (1978) Computed tomography of the orbit with special emphasis on coronal sections: Part 2: Pathological anatomy. J Comput Assist Tomogr 2:35–44
Takahashi M, Tamakawa Y (1977) Coronal computed tomography in orbital disease. J Comput Assist Tomogr 1:505–509
Trokel SL, Jakobiec FA (1981) Correlation of CT scanning and pathologic features of ophthalmic Grave's disease. Ophthalmology 88/6:553–564
Turner RM, Gutman J, Hilal SK, Behrens J, Odel J (1983) CT of drusen bodies and other calcific lesions of the optic nerve: Case report and differential diagnosis. AJNR 4:175–178
Unsöld R, Hoyt WF, Newton ThH (1979) Die computertomographischen Merkmale des kavernösen Hämangioms und ihre Bedeutung für die Differentialdiagnose im Muskeltrichter gelegener Tumoren der Orbita. Klin Monatsbl Augenheilkd 175:715–878
Unsöld R, de Groot J, Newton TH (1980) Images of the optic nerve: Anatomic CT correlation. AJNR 1:317–323
Unsöld R, Newton TH, de Groot J (1980) CT-evaluation of extraocular muscles – anatomic CT-correlations. Graefes Arch Klin Exp Ophthalmol 214/3:155–180
Unsöld R, Newton TH, Hoyt WF (1980) CT examination technique of the optic nerve. J Comput Assist Tomogr 4/4:560–563
Unsöld R, Ostertag CB, de Groot J, Newton TH (1982) Computer reformations of the brain and skull base. Springer, Berlin Heidelberg New York
Vermess M, Haynes BF, Fauci AS, Wolff SM (1978) Computer assisted tomography of orbital lesions in Wegener's granulomatosis. J Comput Assist Tomogr 2:45–48
Vignaud J, Aubin M-L (1978) Les coupes coronales (frontales) d'orbite en tomodensitométrie. J Neuroradiol 5:161–174
Voigt B, Kretzschmar K, Wende S (1984) Computertomographische Diagnostik der endokrinen Orbitopathie. Radiologe 24:468–471
Wackenheim A, van Damme W, Kosmann P, Bittighofer B (1977) Computed tomography in ophthalmology. Neuroradiology 13:135–138
Wende S, Aulich A (1976) Die Computer-Tomographie der Orbita. In: Ullerich K (Hrsg) Die gezielte Diagnostik raumfordernder Prozesse der Orbita. Enke, Stuttgart
Wende S, Aulich A, Lange S, Lanksch W, Schmitt EJ (1976) Computerized tomography in diseases of the orbital region. In: Lanksch W, Kazner E (eds) Cranial computerized tomography. Springer, Berlin Heidelberg New York, pp 201–211
Wende S, Aulich A, Nover A, Lanksch W, Kazner E, Steinhoff H, Meese W, Lânge S, Grumme Th (1977) Computed tomography of orbital lesions. A cooperative study of 210 cases. Neuroradiology 13:123–134
Wende S, Kazner E, Grumme Th (1980) The diagnostic value of computed tomography in orbital diseases. Neurosurg Rev 3:43–49
Wilms G, Smits J, Baert AL (1983) CT of the orbit: Current status with high resolution computed tomography. Neuroradiology 24:183–192
Wing WD, Hunsaker JN, Anderson RE (1979) Direct sagittal computed tomography in Graves' ophthalmopathy. J Comput Assist Tomogr 3:820–824
Wollensak J, Bleckmann H, Lange S, Grumme Th (1976) Computertomographie des Auges und der Orbita. Monatsschr Ophthalmol 168:467–475
Zimmerman LE, Sobin LH (eds) (1980) Histological typing of tumours of the eye and its adnexa. Int Histological Classification of Tumors No 24. World Health Organization, Geneva
Zimmerman RA, Bilaniuk LT, Yanoff M, Schenck JF, Hart HR, Foster TH, Edelstein WA, Bottomley PA, Redington RW, Hardy CJ (1985) Orbital magnetic resonance imaging. Am J Ophthalmol 100:312–317
Zonneveld FW (1987) Computed tomography of the temporal bone and orbit. Urban & Schwarzenberg, München Wien Baltimore

H. Impact of CT and MR on Diagnosis

Baker HL jr, Houser OW, Campbell JK (1980) National Cancer Institute Study: Evaluation of computed tomography in the diagnosis of intracranial neoplasms. I. Overall results. Radiology 136:91–96
Bradley WG jr (1986) Magnetic resonance imaging in the central nervous system: Comparison with computed tomography. In: Kressel HY (ed) Magnetic resonance annual 1986. Raven, New York
Davis KR, Taveras JM, Roberson GH, Ackerman RH (1976) Some limitations of computed tomography in the diagnosis of neurological diseases. Am J Roentgenol 127:111–123
Davis KR, Poletti CE, Roberson GH, Tadmor R, Kjellberg RN (1977) Complementary role of computed tomography and other neuroradiologic procedures. Surg Neurol 8:437–447
Gross WS, Verta MJ jr, van Bellen B, Bergan JJ, Yao JST (1977) Comparison of noninvasive diagnostic techniques in carotid artery occlusive disease. Surgery 82:271–278
Haughton VM, Rimm AA, Sobocinski KA, Papke RA, Daniels DL, Williams AL, Lynch R, Levine R (1986) A blinded clinical comparison of MR imaging and CT in neuroradiology. Radiology 160:751–755
Kazner E, Wende S, Meese W (1976) Reliability and limitations of cranial computerized tomography. In: Lanksch W, Kazner E (eds) Cranial computerized tomography. Springer, Berlin Heidelberg New York, pp 463–470
Kazner E, Schulz B, Kern A, Trempenau B, Laniado M, Treisch J, Schörner W, Felix R (1985) Vergleich zwischen Computertomographie und Magnetresonanztomogra-

phie unter Einschluß paramagnetischer Kontrastmittel bei 165 Patienten mit Hirntumoren. In: Digitale bildgebende Verfahren. Integrierte digitale Radiologie. 4. Grazer Radiologisches Symposium, 03.–05.10.1985

Kretzschmar H (1979) Die Leistungsfähigkeit der Computer-Tomographie im Vergleich zu anderen neuroradiologischen Untersuchungsverfahren. Inauguraldissertation, Johannes-Gutenberg-Universität Mainz

Kretzschmar K, Grumme Th, Steinhoff H (1978) Der Wert der Computertomographie und Angiographie für die Diagnose supratentorieller Hirntumoren. Neuroradiology 16:487–490

Kretzschmar K, Kühnert A, Wende S, Müller W (1985) Diagnostik der Hirntumoren mit CT und/oder MR? In: Digitale bildgebende Verfahren. Integrierte digitale Radiologie. 4. Grazer Radiologisches Symposium, 03.–05.10.1985

Müller A (1980) Grenzen der Computertomographie bei der Diagnose intrakranieller tumoröser Prozesse (Vergleich mit den klassischen neuroradiologischen Methoden). Inaugural-Dissertation, FU Berlin

Wende S, Kishikawa T, Hüwel N, Kazner E, Grumme Th, Lanksch W (1982) Computer-Tomographie und/oder Ventrikulographie? Radiologe 22:38–44

Subject Index

The page numbers in *italics* refer to figures

L. M. Auer, Graz/Hannover;
V. Van Velthoven, Gent

Intraoperative Ultrasound Imaging in Neurosurgery

Comparison with CT and MRI

1989. 466 figures. Approx. 180 pages. Hard cover
ISBN 3-540-50258-0

Intraoperative ultrasound is the first, and at present, only direct method available for depicting cerebral structures during neurosurgery. This atlas is a practical introduction to intraoperative ultrasound in neurosurgery and a guide to anatomy and pathomorphological diagnosis.

A short introduction to the technical basis of ultrasound is given first. It is followed by instructions for practical application of the method in the operating theater. The next, comprehensive chapter presents various intracranial pathomorphological changes in the ultrasound picture and compares them to the familiar computer tomography and MR images. A separate chapter deals with individual aspects of actual application during neurosurgical operations: ultrasound biopsy, puncture and endoscopy.

Springer-Verlag Berlin
Heidelberg New York
London Paris
Tokyo Hong Kong

Springer

MIX
Papier aus verantwortungsvollen Quellen
Paper from responsible sources
FSC® C105338

If you have any concerns about our products,
you can contact us on
ProductSafety@springernature.com

In case Publisher is established outside the EU,
the EU authorized representative is:
Springer Nature Customer Service Center GmbH
Europaplatz 3, 69115 Heidelberg, Germany

Printed by Libri Plureos GmbH
in Hamburg, Germany